D1087151

SECOND EDITION

WITH THE ASSISTANCE OF

NICHOLAS R. ANTHONISEN

B.A. (Dartmouth), M.D. (Harvard), Ph.D. (McGill).

Associate Professor of Experimental Medicine, McGill University, and Assistant Physician, Royal Victoria Hospital, Montreal.

PIERRE H. BEAUDRY, B.A., M.D. (Montreal)

Associate Professor of Pediatrics, McGill University; Assistant Physician-in-Chief and Director, Department of Respiratory Function, The Montreal Children's Hospital, Montreal.

RICHARD E. DONEVAN

M.D., C.M. (Queen's), M.Sc. (McGill), F.R.C.P.(C) F.A.C.P.

Assistant Professor, Department of Medicine, McGill University; Associate Physician, Royal Victoria Hospital; Physician, Royal Edward Chest Hospital, Montreal.

ROBERT G. FRASER, M.D.

Professor of Diagnostic Radiology, McGill University, and Diagnostic Radiologist-in-Chief, Royal Victoria Hospital, Montreal.

J. MILIC–EMILI, M.D. (Milan)

Professor of Physiology, McGill University; Assistant Professor of Experimental Medicine and Research Associate, Royal Victoria Hospital, Montreal.

J. A. PETER PARÉ, M.D.

Associate Professor of Medicine, McGill University; Joint Cardiorespiratory Service, Royal Victoria Hospital, Montreal.

W. B. Saunders Company / Philadelphia / London / Toronto

Respiratory Function in Disease

An introduction to the integrated study of the lung

DAVID V. BATES

M.D. (Cantab.), F.R.C.P. (C), F.R.C.P. (London)

Professor of Experimental Medicine and,
Chairman, Department of Physiology, McGill University;
Physician, Royal Victoria Hospital, Montreal.

PETER T. MACKLEM

B.A. (Queen's), M.D., C.M. (McGill), F.R.C.P. (C).

Associate Professor of Experimental Medicine, McGill University;
Director, Respiratory Division, Royal Victoria Hospital, Montreal.

RONALD V. CHRISTIE

M.D. (Edinburgh), M.Sc. (McGill), D.Sc. (London),
Hon. D.Sc. (Dublin & Edinburgh), F.A.C.P.,
F.R.C.P. (London, Edinburgh, & Canada),
Emeritus Professor of Medicine, McGill University,
Lately Physician-in-Chief, Royal Victoria Hospital,
and Dean of the Faculty of Medicine, McGill University.

W. B. Saunders Company: West Washington Square
Philadelphia, Pa. 19105

12 Dyott Street
London, WC1A 1DB

833 Oxford Street
Toronto, Ontario M8Z 5T9, Canada

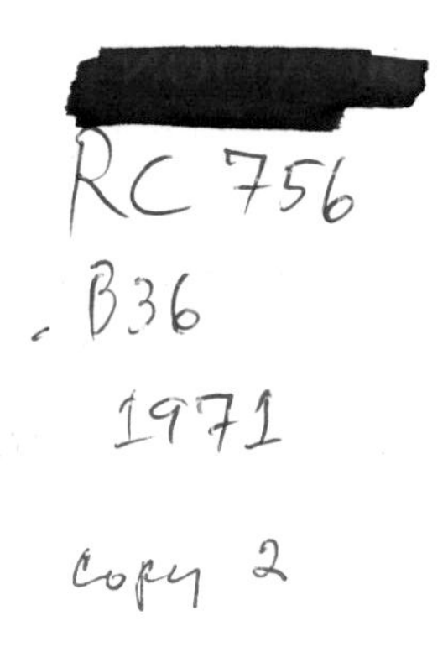

Listed here is the latest translated edition of this book together with the language of the translation and the publisher.

Italian (1st Edition)—Piccin Editore,
Padova, Italy

Respiratory Function in Disease ISBN 0-7216-1591-0

Print No.: 9 8 7 6

DEDICATION

This book is dedicated to the memory of

JONATHAN C. MEAKINS

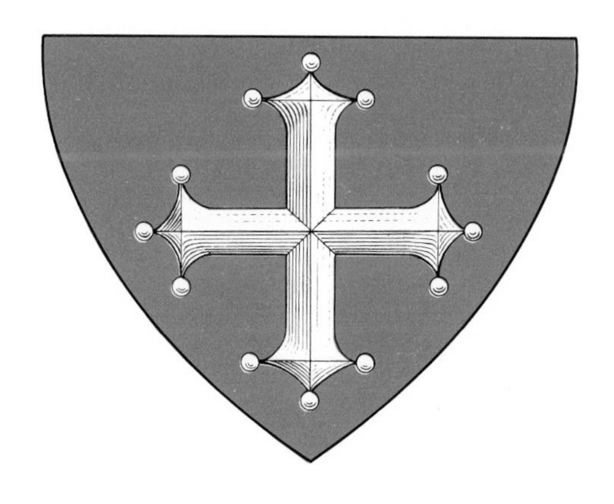

Preface to the Second Edition

The welcome given to the first edition of this book has encouraged us to bring the book up-to-date, in the hope that it will continue to prove useful in the training of physicians in the field of lung disease and as a reference source for those whose work necessitates an understanding of the lung.

Since the first edition was prepared in 1964, there have been many important advances in the understanding of pulmonary physiology and abnormalities of pulmonary function. In comparison with the state of knowledge at that time, the contribution of different-sized airways to the flow-resistance of the whole tracheobronchial tree is much better defined today, and we now understand that such measurements as the FEV_1 are insensitive indicators of changes occurring in small airways; measurements of regional lung function have clarified the effects of aging on the lung and emphasized the importance of small-airway closure in a wide variety of clinical circumstances; important new observations have been made of the hypoxemia that occurs in spasmodic asthma and in respiratory failure secondary to shock; and the treatment of respiratory failure has been greatly advanced by careful application of controlled oxygen therapy. This period has also seen the first attempts, so far unsuccessful, at human lung transplantation, and much new information has been contributed in other clinical and physiological areas.

To incorporate in a new edition these and other advances in our knowledge, extensive revision and redrafting have been necessary. Most of the first seven chapters have been entirely rewritten and the chapter on respiratory failure has been modified to a major extent. We have completely revised the sequence of presentation of pulmonary physiology and hope that we have achieved thereby a more satisfactory approach to the understanding of pulmonary function. This reorganization and updating necessitated a total rewriting of the chapters on physiology.

The additions have been accommodated in the present volume with little increase in length, since specialized books or monographs have now been published on such topics as pulmonary surfactant, pediatric chest disease, dyspnea, exercise physiology, and by our colleagues on the radiological and clinical basis of the diagnosis of lung disease. These contributions have led us to change the emphasis in some aspects of the original text and have permitted us to curtail or omit altogether detailed discussion of these areas.

Since many students and trainees should, in our opinion, be encouraged to begin their reading with early literature, we have decided not to eliminate from the present bibliography any of the references that were in the first edition, although many of these references are not now specifically referred to in the text. This bibliography, together with 1476 new references that have been added, summarizes the field of pulmonary function and respiratory physiology since 1945. We have provided an index to the now extensive bibliography that we hope will permit the physician and the trainee to make better use of the references contained within it.

Our colleagues, Dr. R.G. Fraser and Dr. J.A.P. Paré, have now published a text of their own. Their extensive involvement in the preparation of that work has limited their participation in the revision of this edition, but, nevertheless, they have both made valuable contributions. Heavy responsibilities have prevented Prof. Thurlbeck from a detailed involvement in the preparation of this new edition, but much of his original contribution has been retained and he has been good enough to edit many of the changes and supervise the drafting of the new chapter on the anatomy of the lung. His assistance in many other parts of the book is gratefully acknowledged. Dr. M.R. Becklake, who contributed much of the original section on occupational lung disease, was too heavily committed with other work to undertake the revision, but her contribution to the present volume is, nevertheless, gratefully acknowledged.

We are specially indebted to friends and colleagues who have allowed us to use illustrations for this edition, in particular, Dr. John West, Dr. Maurice McGregor, and the editors of the *Scientific American*. We are also very much indebted to all those who have made suggestions to us for the improvement of the first edition and hope that critical readers will continue to be of assistance to us in improving the present volume.

One of us (D.V.B.) wishes to record his gratitude to Dr. L. Donato and to Dr. C. Giuntini of the University of Pisa for making it possible for him to begin the task of preparation of the second edition of this volume in the comparative tranquillity of Tuscany.

Finally, we would like to acknowledge the assistance given us by the staff members of the W. B. Saunders Company, who, with their usual patience, have accepted explanations for our delay in completing this task and have dealt very expeditiously with the manuscript, once it was finally delivered into their hands.

David V. Bates

Peter T. Macklem

Ronald V. Christie

Acknowledgments

We are grateful to a number of authors for their permission to use figures and diagrams they have published: the Editors of Scientific American for Figure 1–2; the Yearbook Medical Publishers for Figure 2–27; Blackwell's Limited for Figure 2–28; Dr. K. T. Fowler for Figures 2–29 and 2–31; Dr. L. E. Farhi for Figures 2–30 and 2–34; Dr. J. B. West for Figure 2–40 and, together with the publishers of Respiration Physiology, Figures 2–35, 2–36, 2–37, and 2–38; Dr. N. C. Staub for Figure 2–43; and Dr. R. H. Shepard for Figure 2–42.

We are indebted to Dr. F. Wiglesworth for the descriptions of the pathology of Cases 11 and 22; and to Dr. Scott Dunbar for his reports on the radiographs of Cases 4, 11, 17, and 22. Dr. R. E. G. Place kindly permitted us to reproduce the bronchospirometry tracing in Case 13. We also wish to thank Dr. R. G. Fraser and other members of the staff of the Department of Radiology for the radiology reports on the new illustrative cases that have been added, and Dr. J. Hogg of the Department of Pathology for pathological reports in five of the new illustrative cases.

We are most grateful to our medical and surgical colleagues who have referred patients to us for study and who have taken a continuing interest in our research program which they have assisted in a variety of ways. Mr. J. Novaczek and his staff performed most of the routine function studies in this book and they have been responsible for the data reported on the clinical cases. Mr. L. S. Bartlett of the Cardiorespiratory Division of the Royal Victoria Hospital and Mr. K. Holeczek have been responsible for the lined diagrams in the text, and many of them have been photographed by Mr. Holeczek.

We wish to thank the medical librarians of the McGill University Medical and Osler Libraries and of the Royal Victoria Hospital who provided much assistance at varying stages of preparation of the manuscript.

We also wish to thank the Medical Research Council of Canada for its continuing support of our research program on pulmonary physiology and different aspects of chronic lung disease.

Finally, we wish to thank the various members of the staff of the W. B. Saunders Company for being unfailingly courteous and helpful to us in the preparation of this book.

DAVID V. BATES, M.D.

P. T. MACKLEM, M.D.

R. V. CHRISTIE, M.D.

Preface to the First Edition

"This book is intended mainly for those engaged in the practice and teaching of Medicine. We trust that our friends and colleagues who are concerned with the more technical and purely physiological aspects of respiration will not judge too severely our presentation of the subject. We have attempted to give physicians a working knowledge of the chemical and physiological facts concerning respiration, indicating their clinical applications and as far as possible avoiding a highly technical dissertation on the subject.

"We are fully conscious of the incompleteness in our knowledge of respiratory function. As there are many points still in dispute regarding the physiology of normal respiration, it is not surprising to find that there are even more deficiencies in our understanding of the abnormal. We have attempted to point out many of these, hoping in this way to focus attention on our ignorance. At times opposing views have been given in as impartial a manner as possible. We quite ackowledge our difficulty and perhaps weakness in not always keeping ourselves from inclining towards one or other point of view. This possible bias is in all cases quite open to correction, and we trust that the near future may settle some debatable points beyond fear of contradiction."

This was written by Jonathan C. Meakins and H. Whitridge Davies in their preface to their book "Respiratory Function in Disease," which was published in 1925. We cannot improve upon it to describe our purpose in writing this volume, which we have dedicated to the memory of Jonathan Meakins. He was a pioneer in the application of physiological methods to the problems of clinical medicine. In 1923 he developed in the McGill University Clinic of the Royal Victoria Hospital what must have been one of the first respiratory function laboratories, if not the first, to be established in any hospital. It was in this laboratory that one of us received his early training; and it has been in the same laboratory that the patients referred to in this book have been studied.

During the past forty years the contribution of physiologists and biochemists to our understanding of functional impairment in disease has been remarkable. It has led, however, to a degree of specialization tending to separate disciplines which are, by their nature, interdependent. An understanding of the clinical patterns of disease and of the morphological changes that underlie disease is still necessary if the physiological and biochemical changes that occur are to be understood in proper perspective. We are hopeful that the brief reviews of clinical patterns, radiological findings, and morphology of lung disease that we have included will be valuable to those scientists whose major interest lies outside these fields. Such sections are not aimed at the experienced chest physician, radiologist, or pathologist respectively, any more than are the sections on normal physiology written for the physiologist.

The literature on respiratory function is already so vast that we have been able to include only sufficient references to provide the essential background, and from these the reader will be able to obtain a more comprehensive bibliography.

It is our hope that our many friends and colleagues, who have not hesitated to stimulate us with their criticisms in the past, will bring to our attention any deficiencies and inaccuracies they detect in the present volume.

DVB
RVC

Montreal
1964

Contents

List of Illustrative Cases

Glossary of Terms

AIRWAY CONDUCTANCE (Gaw)—The reciprocal of airway resistance, expressed as liter/sec/cm H_2O.

AIRWAY RESISTANCE (Raw)—The pressure between the airway opening (i.e., mouth or nose) and the alveoli, in relation to simultaneous air flow; expressed as cm H_2O/liter/sec.

ALVEOLAR–ARTERIAL DIFFERENCES for O_2, CO_2, and N_2 (A-aΔ)—The difference (in mm Hg) between a measured arterial gas tension and a simultaneously measured or computed mean alveolar gas tension. The differences reflect, among other factors, abnormalities of $\dot{V}/\dot{Q}$ ratio (*see* Figure 2–34).

ALVEOLAR–ARTERIAL END-CAPILLARY GRADIENT—The pressure difference (in mm Hg) that exists between alveolar gas and pulmonary capillary blood as the latter leaves the alveolus (*see* Figure 2–43).

ALVEOLAR GAS—Expired gas that has come from alveoli. The definition of mean alveolar gas concentration is complicated by the discontinuous nature of lung ventilation and perfusion, and by the nonuniform behavior of the lung in regard to these aspects of function.

ALVEOLAR VENTILATION—If the lungs behaved as a completely uniform system, alveolar ventilation could be defined as the tidal volume minus the anatomical dead-space volume, multiplied by the respiratory frequency. In many situations, however, alveolar ventilation can be defined only in terms of the arterial P_{CO_2}, the level of which ordinarily reflects the total effective alveolar ventilation.

BLOOD-GAS TENSION—The pressure in mm Hg of a gas in the blood. Note that pressures between a liquid and a gas must always be in equilibrium, regardless of solubility, buffer systems, partition coefficients, or dissociation curves.

COMPLIANCE, DYNAMIC (C dyn)—The ratio of the tidal volume to the difference in pressure at points of zero gas flow, expressed in liters/cm H_2O.

COMPLIANCE, STATIC (C st)—The slope of a static-pressure—volume curve at a point, or the linear approximation of the nearly straight portion of such a curve, in the tidal volume range, expressed in liters/cm H_2O.

DEAD SPACE, ANATOMICAL (inert-gas dead space)—The volume of all non-gas-exchanging passages in the lung, normally comprising the upper airway and bronchial tree as far as the respiratory bronchioles.

DEAD SPACE, PHYSIOLOGICAL—A number (not a topographical volume) which by comparison with the anatomical or inert-gas dead space expresses the nonuniformity of $\dot{V}/\dot{Q}$ ratios in the lung. When expressed for a particular gas, the physiological dead space is the number that has to be used for V_D in the Bohr equation if the correct arterial tension is to be computed from inspired and mixed expired concentrations.

DIFFUSING CAPACITY (D_L)—The rate of gas transfer through a membrane in relation to a constant pressure difference across it. A simple physical concept that in biology is usually a complex measurement on account of difficulty in accurate determination of the effective pressure difference.

DIFFUSING CAPACITY COMPONENTS—Components of the total diffusing capacity ($D_{L_{CO}}$) may be summed as resistances as follows:

$$\frac{1}{D_{L_{CO}}} = \frac{1}{D_M{}^{*}} + \frac{1}{\theta V_c{}^{**}}$$

*Membrane diffusion coefficient (*q.v.*).
**Pulmonary capillary blood volume (*q.v.*).

ELASTANCE—The reciprocal of compliance, expressed in cm H_2O/liter.

ELASTIC RECOIL (Pst)—The difference between intrapleural and alveolar pressure at a given lung volume under static conditions.

FORCED EXPIRATORY VOLUME (FEV)—The volume of a maximally fast expiration starting from a full inspiration. The time in fractions of a second over which the FEV has been measured is indicated by suitable subscripts (i.e., $FEV_{0.75}$, $FEV_{1.0}$, etc.).

FUNCTIONAL RESIDUAL CAPACITY (FRC)—The volume of gas contained in the lungs at the end of a normal quiet expiration.

INERT-GAS DISTRIBUTION—The distribution of a nonexchanging gas between alveoli, theoretically perfect only when each alveolus receives from the tidal volume the same quantum of inspired gas in relation to its original volume as does every other alveolus.

INSPIRATORY CAPACITY (IC)—The volume of gas that can be taken into the lungs on a full inspiration, starting from the resting expiratory position.

KINETIC CONSTANT (θ)—The rate of combination of CO with red blood cells, expressed as ml CO/min/mm Hg/ml of blood. Affected by the oxygen tension simultaneously present.

MAXIMAL BREATHING CAPACITY (MBC)—The maximal volume of gas that can be breathed per minute by voluntary effort.

MAXIMAL MIDEXPIRATORY FLOW RATE (MMFR)—The velocity (in L/sec) of expiration over the middle third of total expired volume.

MAXIMAL STATIC NEGATIVE INTRAPLEURAL PRESSURE—The difference between intrapleural and alveolar pressure at full inspiration.

MEMBRANE DIFFUSION COEFFICIENT (D_M)—A component of total diffusing capacity that sums every factor affecting CO transfer other than pulmonary capillary blood volume (V_c) and the kinetic constant (θ). It thus includes both qualitative and quantitative aspects of the alveolar surface, together with other addition factors.

MINUTE VOLUME—The volume of gas expired per minute.

PULMONARY CAPILLARY BLOOD VOLUME (V_c)—The volume of blood in the lung in contact with alveolar gas at any instant.

RESIDUAL VOLUME (RV)—The volume of gas in the lungs that cannot be expelled by expiratory effort; hence, the total lung capacity minus the vital capacity.

RQ—The ratio of CO_2 production to oxygen uptake, as follows:

$$\frac{\dot{V}_{CO2}}{\dot{V}_{O2}}$$

TIDAL VOLUME—The volume of gas expired with each breath.

TIME CONSTANT—In pulmonary mechanics, this term is used to indicate the product of compliance and airway resistance.

TOTAL LUNG CAPACITY (TLC)—The volume of gas contained in the lungs at the end of a full inspiration.

VITAL CAPACITY (VC)—The volume of gas that can be expelled from the lungs from a position of full inspiration, with no time limit to the duration of expiration.

$\dot{V}/\dot{Q}$—The ratio between ventilation and perfusion, each being expressed in the same units.

WORK OF BREATHING—The cumulative product of instantaneous pressure developed by the respiratory muscles and volume of air moved in a breathing cycle, expressed as Kg M.

THE ANATOMY OF THE LUNG

CHAPTER 1

It is not our intention in this section to provide a comprehensive review of pulmonary anatomy, but rather to emphasize certain aspects of lung structure that play a major part in determining function or that assume particular importance when the pathological features of some pulmonary disorders are to be described. A full treatment of the anatomy of the human lung may be found in von Hayek's comprehensive volume,[23] and additional information may be found in a Ciba symposium volume[26] and in the authoritative monograph on lung morphometry by Weibel.[2224] Special monographs have been published on the mechanism of function of the chest wall and diaphragm,[4] and there is also considerable recent work on the postnatal development of the lung[819] and on the time course of appearance of pulmonary surfactant.[2359]

The upper respiratory tract has long been recognized as playing the part of an air conditioner for the lungs. Not only is it important for humidification, but it is designed to filter inspired gas and thus protect the respiratory tract. Negus[556] has written a detailed account of these functions. The ciliary system of the bronchi seems to be remarkably efficient in removing dirt by carrying it on a continuously moving blanket of mucus. Much remains to be learned about the physiology of ciliary function, but it is clear that it is easily adversely affected by a wide variety of agents.[1548, 2360]

It has been known for many years that under normal circumstances expired air is fully saturated with water vapor,[557] and Bruck[558] has investigated in detail the physiology of water loss from the lungs. The volume of water lost in this manner is extremely variable, and the generally quoted figure of 5 ml/hr/sq m of body surface area is so greatly affected by ambient conditions that it can be regarded only as a very approximate yardstick. The upper respiratory tract constitutes about half of the total anatomical dead space, and the larynx and nose together contribute about 45 per cent of the total airway resistance.

The bronchial tree exists for the purpose of conducting air to the alveolar surface. The inspired air should be evenly distributed to the alveolar capillary bed with minimum resistance to flow. In addition, the bronchi and lungs must be able to protect themselves against noxious agents, whether these be physical, chemical, or biological. The greater part of the length and the smaller part of the volume of the respiratory tract is concerned only with the conduction of air; this is made up of the bronchi and bronchioles, which are distinguished from each other by the presence of cartilage in the walls of the former. The remaining part of the tract is concerned with both conduction and gas exchange, the latter function assuming greater ascendancy as the system is followed distally. Respiratory bronchioles, alveolar ducts, atria, alveolar sacs, and the alveoli themselves make up these segments of the lung and together are often referred to as "the acinus." (*See* Figure 1–1.)

Bronchial and bronchiolar division is generally dichotomous, and usually the two branches are of approximately equal size, their total cross-sectional area being about 20 per cent greater than that of the parent branch. This is close to the predicted configuration for minimal resistance to gas flow. Where branches are equal in size, their angles of branching are equal. Where they are not the same size, the smaller branch deviates more from the line of direct continuation of the parent bronchus. The observed angles of branching are close to the ideal for the minimum volume of the conducting system. One interesting approach to understanding the system is that of Horsfield and Cumming.[2361] They have built a theoretical model of the airways that would provide maximal efficiency and then made detailed measurements of the airways of a normal human subject.[2362] The actual dimensions and angles of branching have been shown by this means to be in close conformity with the ideal, and the measurements which these authors have published are the most complete and accurate available. Where the distance from the main bronchus to the periphery of the lung is small, such as in the lung substance at the hilum, small branches come off the parent bronchus to form a spiral; these are called lateral pathways. Where the distance is large, the branches are of approximately equal size and are called axial pathways. There may be as few as six generations of bronchi and bronchioles in a lateral pathway[2343] and as many as 25 in an axial one.

The cartilages of the main-stem bronchi and the lower-lobe bronchi are horseshoe-shaped, as in the trachea, and presumably are responsible for maintaining patency of the bronchi. In the upper-lobe bronchus and in lingular and segmental bronchi of all lobes, the cartilages are less complete and consist of irregular plates. As the pathway proceeds distally, the cartilages become progressively smaller and less complete, until finally, in bronchi slightly under 1 mm in diameter, they surround only the origins of the bronchioles arising from them. The bronchial muscle lies between the open ends of the horseshoe-shaped cartilages in the major bronchi, where it is attached to the inner perichondrium about 1 mm from their ends. As the cartilages diminish in size and become irregular, the attachments extend further and further along the cartilages, until finally they encircle the bronchi. In the smaller bronchi and the bronchioles, the muscle bundles form a criss-crossed, spiral "geodesic network."

The diameters and total cross-sectional

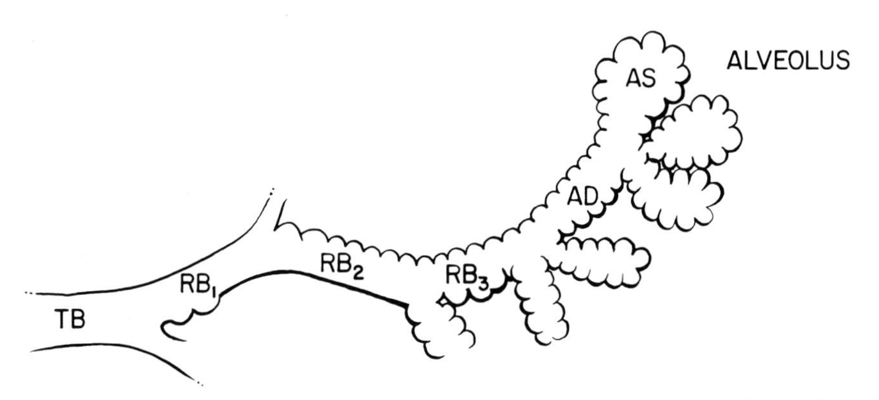

FIGURE 1–1. Diagram of the acinus or gas exchanging portion of the lung. There are three orders of respiratory bronchioles (RB) with progressively more alveoli in their walls. A third order respiratory bronchiole (RB_3) is followed by an alveolar duct (AD), whose wall is formed by alveoli. An alveolar sac (AS) succeeds the alveolar duct and represents the blind end of the respiratory passage. (Reprinted from Thurlbeck, W. M.: Pathology Annual. Chronic obstructive lung disease. Edited by Sheldon C. Sommers. New York, Appleton-Century-Crofts, Inc., Division of Meredith Corporation, 1968, with the permission of the publisher.)

TABLE 1–1 BRONCHIAL AND BRONCHIOLAR DIVISION

Structure	Generation from: Trachea	Segmental Bronchus	Terminal Bronchiole	Number	Diameter of Individual Structures	Total Cross-Sectional Area
Trachea	0			1	2.5 cm	5.0 sq cm
Main bronchi	1			2	11–19 mm	3.2 sq cm
Lobar bronchi	2–3			5	4.5–13.5 mm	2.7 sq cm
Segmental bronchi	3–6	0		19	4.5– 6.5 mm	3.2 sq cm
Subsegmental bronchi	4–7	1		38	3– 6 mm	6.6 sq cm
Bronchi		2–6		variable	variable	variable
Terminal bronchi		3–7		1000	1.0 mm	7.9 sq cm
Bronchioles		5–14		variable	variable	variable
Terminal bronchioles		6–15	0	35,000	0.65 mm	116 sq cm
Respiratory bronchioles			1–8	variable	variable	variable
Terminal respiratory bronchioles			2–9	630,000	0.45 mm	1000 sq cm
Alveolar ducts and sacs			4–12	14×10^6	0.40 mm	1.71 sq meters
Alveoli				300×10^6	0.25–0.30 mm	70 sq meters

area of the conducting system are shown in Table 1–1. There is an initial narrowing of total cross-sectional area, which then rapidly increases. It is this increase in area which is responsible for the relatively very low resistance to airflow in the small airways of the lung.

The epithelium of the bronchi is of pseudostratified ciliated type and contains numerous goblet cells. As the pathway proceeds distally, the epithelium is progressively thinner, to become single-layered in the bronchioles, and the goblet cells decrease. Although it is agreed that the function of the goblet cells and bronchial glands is the production of mucus, there is considerable uncertainty concerning other sites of mucus production.[26] In the terminal bronchioles, the goblet cells and cilia have disappeared, and the epithelium has become flattened. The origin of mucus that may be found in these bronchioles is still not known, though it has been shown that it does not originate from the mucous glands of the bronchi: von Hayek[26] believes it to be a special secretion of cells that bulge into the lumen of the terminal and preterminal bronchiole (Clara cells). There has been considerable recent interest in these cells, and it now seems unlikely that they secrete mucus. They are highly active metabolically,[2363] and Niden[2364] has suggested that these cells are the source of pulmonary surfactant. We have produced evidence[2363] that the cells contain much choline-rich phospholipid bound tightly to another substance (probably protein). It seems likely that this is the secretory product of the cell, but whether or not the material is surface active remains in question. Regardless of where it may be produced, we have found evidence that the terminal bronchioles of the cat are lined with surfactant.[2409]

Underneath the epithelium is the basement membrane; deep to this is the membrana propria, composed of loose fibrous tissue with a rich capillary network. Longitudinal bands of elastic fibers form dense bundles, causing longitudinal ridging of the bronchi, which becomes less conspicuous distally. These fibers connect with circularly arranged elastic fibers that are in relation to the muscular layer, and through them to the surrounding alveolar and septal elastic tissue, thus forming a continuum through the lungs. It is this radial tethering mechanism that is believed to play a major part in maintaining the patency of the small bronchi and bronchioles. The mucous glands belong to the membrana propria, but frequently they extend externally to the cartilage or muscle wall. The glands are mixed serous and mucous and extend out to the small bronchi. Where they lie internal to the cartilages, their maximal thickness is about one third of the total width from basement membrane to perichondrium. The peribronchial connective tissue surrounds the bronchi to the point where the bronchiolar walls become continuous with the lung parenchyma. It is continuous with the periarterial connective tissue and, near the hilum, with the perivenous connective tissue and, through it, with the interlobular septa and the pleura. The lymphatics, bronchial arteries, and nerves are present in this layer.

The last purely conducting structure, without alveoli in its walls and with a continuous bronchial epithelial lining, is the terminal bronchiole. The portion of lung distal to a terminal bronchiole is called an acinus, and it is made up of respiratory bronchioles, alveolar ducts, alveolar sacs, and alveoli. Branching is generally dichotomous until the alveolar sacs are reached. A variety of terms have been used for the structures in the acinus. The arrangement of pathways within the acinus is as complicated as in the non-alveolated conducting pathways. The divisions within the acinus follow a pattern of irregular dichotomy, and there are both lateral and axial pathways. There may be two to nine respiratory bronchioles. The last respiratory bronchiole gives rise to a complex spray of alveolar ducts and alveolar sacs in which dichotomous, trichotomous, or quadripartite divisions occur in irregular fashion. There are about 400 alveolar ducts and sacs in an acinus, and about 18 last-order terminal bronchioles arise from one terminal bronchiole. Figure 1–1 shows the classic simplified acinus in which there are three orders of respiratory bronchiole, with progressively larger numbers of alveoli in their walls as they proceed distally. A respiratory bronchiole of the second order characteristically has a branch of the pulmonary artery parallel and adjacent to one of its walls. At this point it is lined by cubical epithelium, and the opposite wall is made up of alveoli. The respiratory bronchioles are succeeded by a single order of alveolar duct, the wall of which is composed of a musculo-elastic mesh through which alveoli protrude outward. It is probably by the contraction of the few muscle fibers in this region that the closure of terminal airway units can occur.[1859] Alveolar ducts give rise to the terminal spray of alveolar sacs, which are the blind ends of the respiratory tract; their walls are lined with alveoli. Alveoli are multifaceted rather than round, with an average maximum diameter of approximately 250 μ at full inflation. The most recent estimate of the total number of alveoli in the average adult lung is 300 million.[560, 2224] Total alveolar surface area is related to body length, and varies from 40 to 100 sq m. In addition, some loss of alveolar surface area occurs with increasing age, mainly due to changes in the geometric configuration of the lung.

The alveolar capillary bed is best regarded as a pool of blood, since the network that forms it is the densest in the body, the distance between capillaries often being smaller than the capillaries themselves. Fung and Sobin[2365] have recently analyzed flow through this network on the basis of "sheet flow,"

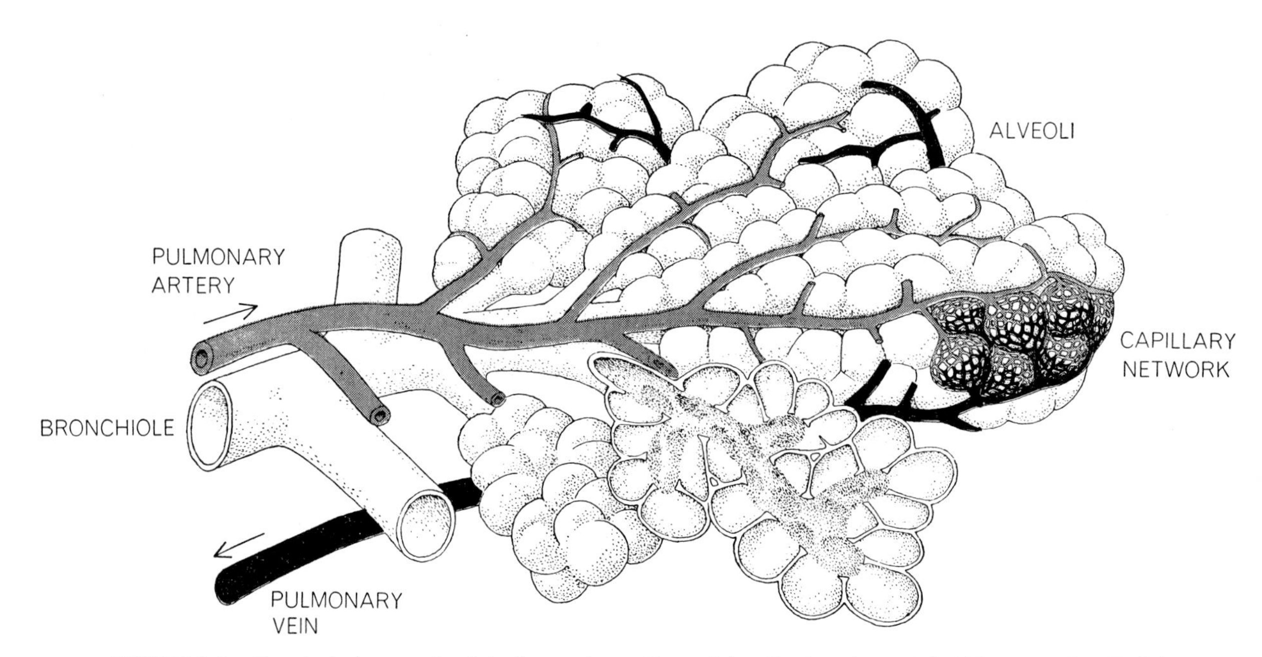

FIGURE 1–2. Terminal airway unit of the human lung. (From Scientific American, Vol. 207, No. 1, Pg. 48, July, 1962.)

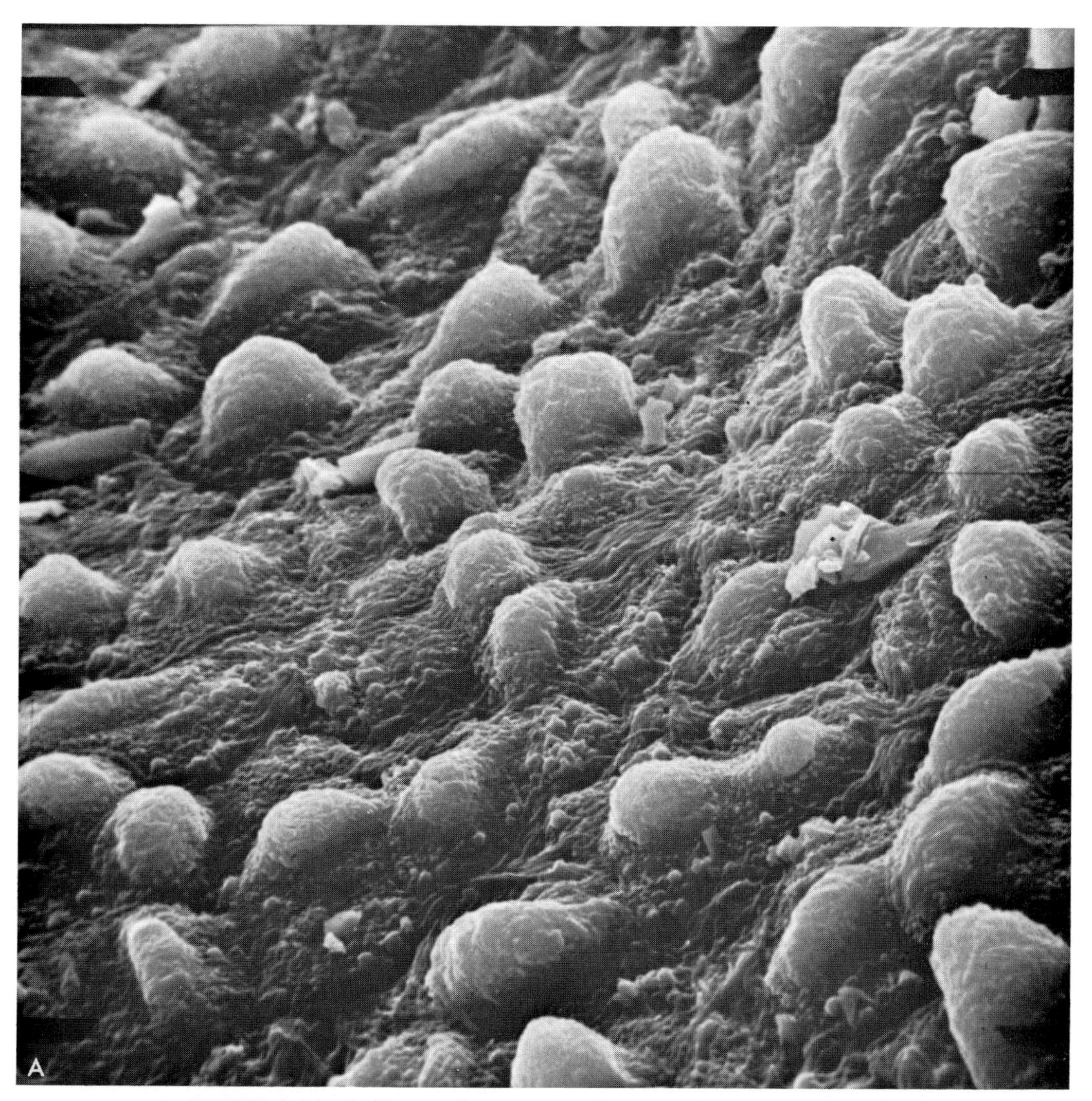

FIGURE 1–3.* *A*, Human Respiratory Terminal Bronchiole. (×2200)

The cells protruding into the lumen are Clara Cells.

*Photographed with scanning electron microscope at the Pulp and Paper Research Institute, Montreal, by Mr. Seil. Human lung preparations by Prof. W. M. Thurlbeck and Dr. N. Wang of the McGill Institute of Pathology. Enlargement by Mr. K. Holeczek, Dept. of Physiology, McGill. See reference 3832.

(*Illustration continues.*)

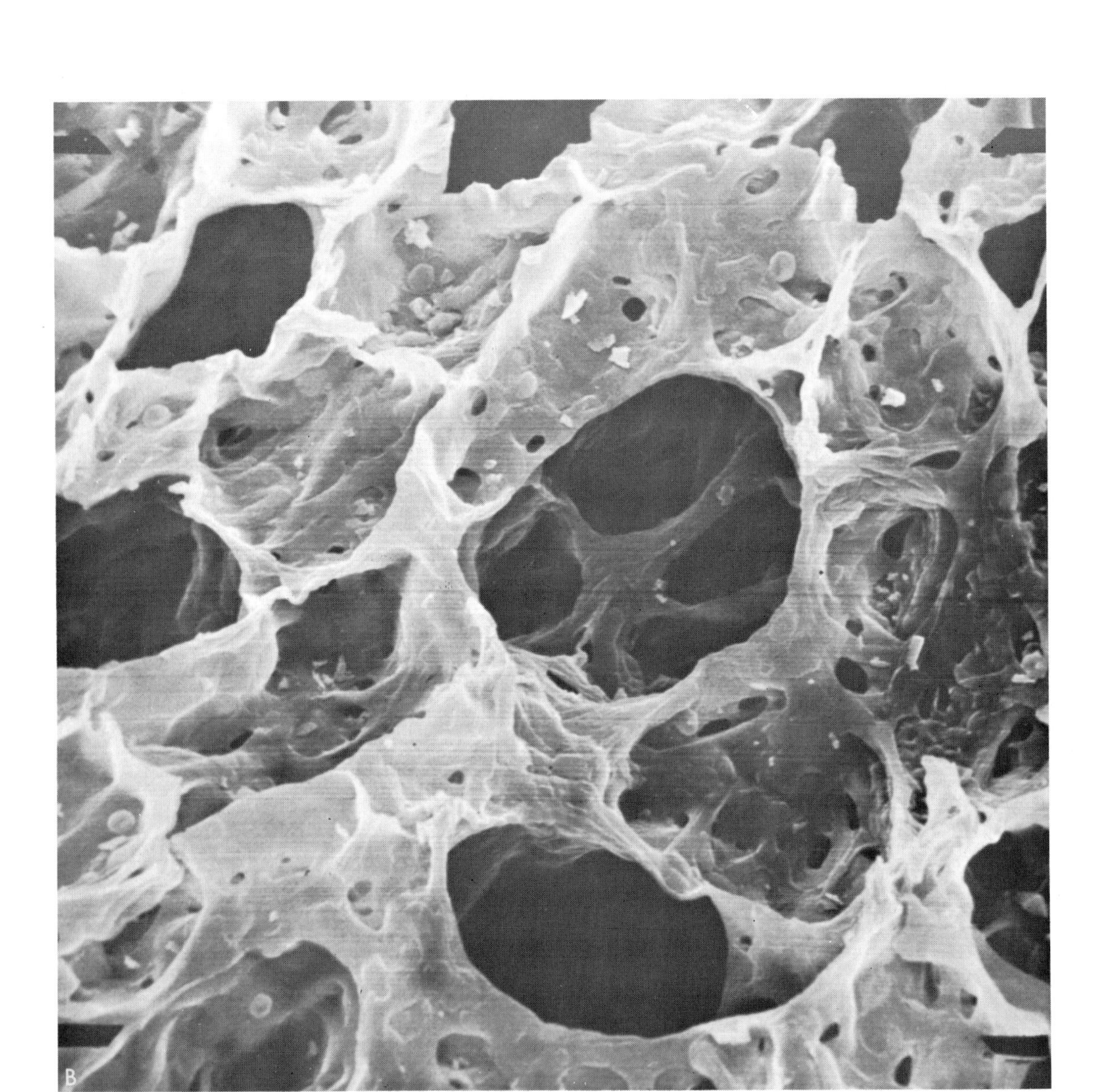

FIGURE 1–3 Continued. *B*, (ALVEOLI.)

Note the frequency of intercommunications. Mouse lung ×550.

(*Illustration continues.*)

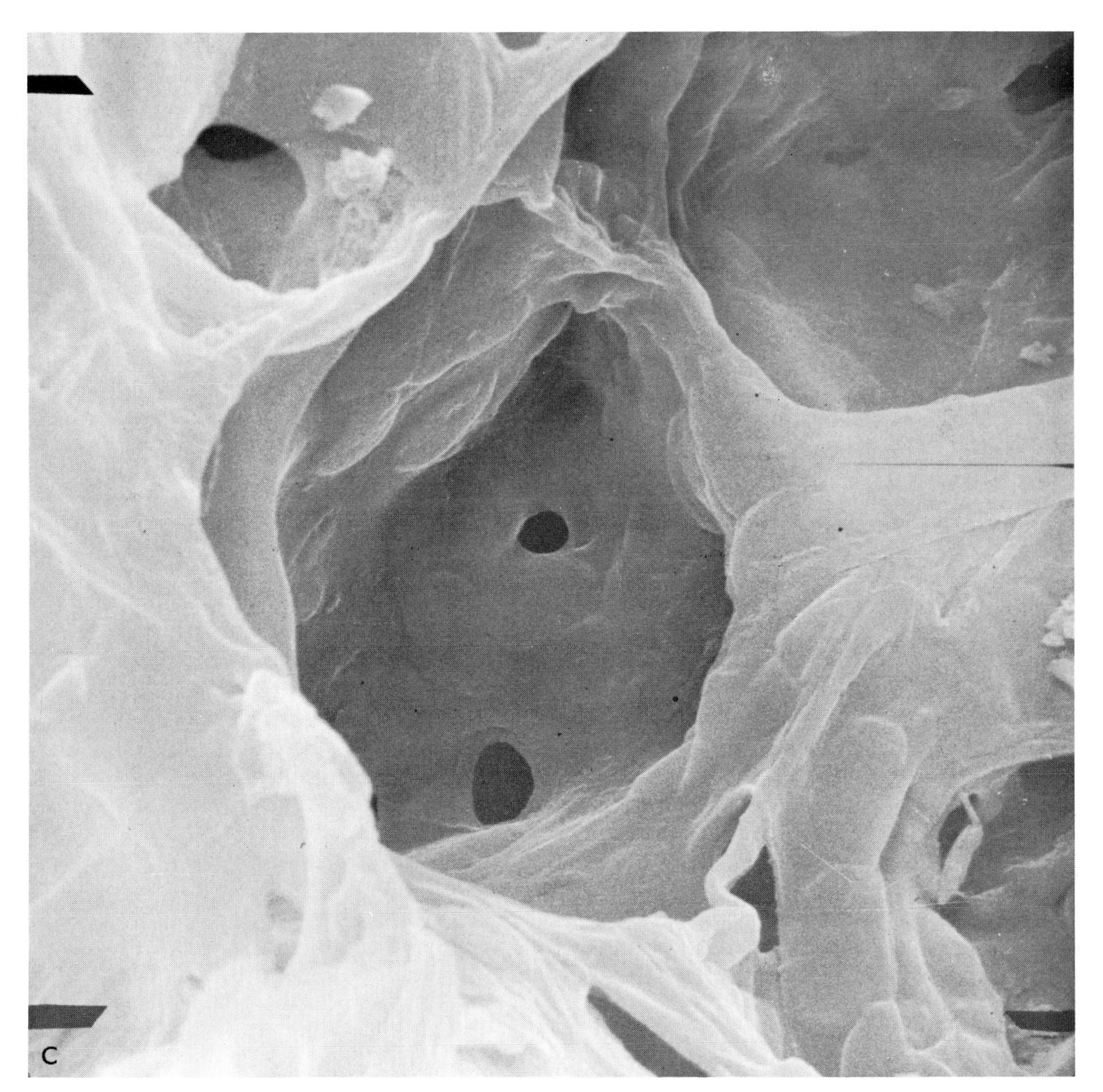

FIGURE 1-3 Continued. *C*, A SINGLE ALVEOLUS, SHOWING PORES OF KOHN.

Mouse lung ×2200.

visualizing the capillary bed as a continuous sheet space, with supporting pillars within it. Weibel and Gomez[560, 657, 1868, 2224] have pointed out that both alveolar and capillary surface areas increase with increasing lung size, and the same conclusion is supported by measurements of pulmonary capillary blood volume. When it is recalled that this rarely exceeds 300 ml even during exercise[399] and that the internal surface area is about 70 sq m, it is apparent that the structure is well adapted to permit maximal diffusion transfer of oxygen during the half-second transit of the pulmonary capillary by the red cell. Schultz[26] has computed the thickness of the pathway from alveolar gas to the plasma layer of blood in human lungs to be of the order of 0.36 to 2.50 μ, a small distance in terms of the diameter of a normal red blood cell. Tenney and Remmers[1847] have pointed out that in mammals of widely differing size, there is a close relationship between alveolar diameter and total oxygen consumption.

Although the exact nature of the gas-tissue interface in the lung was disputed for many years, recent electron microscopy has shown beyond reasonable doubt that the inner aspect of the alveoli is lined by flattened cytoplasmic extensions of alveolar lining (Type I) cells. In the sharp angles of alveoli are plumper cells with granular cytoplasm (granular pneumonocyte or Type II cells). These Type II cells are highly active metabolically and contain many cellular organelles as well as characteristic osmiophilic inclusions thought to be the origin of the surface active material which lines alveoli. The osmiophilic inclusions are believed to be derived from multivesicular bodies, although earlier work indicated a possible origin from mitochondria. The Type II cells are not phagocytic. The phagocytes and macrophages found in alveolar spaces are derived from blood cells.

THE LOBULE

This is the smallest discrete portion of the lung that is surrounded by connective tissue septa. These septa are variable in size and extent, and hence the lobule, as defined, shows considerable variation in size. However, since it forms a convenient and easily recognized unit that can be used for descriptive purposes, it should be retained as a descriptive term. This definition of the lobule corresponds to Miller's term "secondary lobule";[561] the term "primary lobule" that he used referred to an alveolar duct, its vessels, and the structures arising from them. Reid and Simon[770] have suggested a much more precise and useful definition of a lobule. They point out that an abrupt transition occurs in the distance between branches near the end of the conducting airways. The distance between branches changes from 0.5 to 1.0 cm (centimeter pattern) to 2 to 3 mm (millimeter pattern) intervals. They suggested that the cluster of terminal bronchioles which form the millimeter pattern be used as the definition of a lobule. This defines a unit of uniform size, three to five terminal bronchioles being found in these clusters.

CANALS OF LAMBERT

The distal portions of the bronchiolar tree, particularly the preterminal bronchioles, contain a number of epithelial-lined tubular communications between them and the surrounding alveoli. The physiological significance of these structures is not known, but they obviously provide an accessory route for air to pass from bronchioles directly into alveoli.

ALVEOLAR PORES

Although these are often called the pores of Kohn, von Hayek[23] attributes their original description to Henle but according to Miller, Adriani described them. They are believed to exist in all mammalian lungs, though they are relatively more common in some species than in others. In the human lung, they are openings, or discontinuities, of the alveolar wall, about 5 to 10 μ in diameter. These can be well seen in Figure 1–3. There is little doubt that they can be responsible for collateral air drift between lobules of the lung. The part these pores play in the human lung is obscure, though it is probable that, by providing alternative pathways for the passage of air, they may prevent collapse of segments of the lung when the lumen of a smaller bronchus is plugged. Enlargement of these pores has long been suggested as a mechanism of development of emphysema.

The resistance to collateral flow has only recently been quantitated. In the normal human lung this is of the order of several hundred cm H_2O/liter/sec, but in emphysema this resistance may be less than that of the conventional pathways of ventilation.[2402]

VASCULAR SYSTEM

The pulmonary arterial system accompanies the bronchial tree and divides with it and conveniently may be considered in three categories. The arteries that accompany the bronchi are elastic, and those that run with the nonrespiratory bronchioles are muscular. These muscular arteries initially are about 1000 μ in diameter but become about 100 μ at the level of the terminal bronchiole. They have a thin muscular coat enclosed between a poorly defined internal elastic lamina and a better-defined outer layer. Beyond the terminal bronchioles, the arteries lose this continuous muscle coat and become arterioles with a single elastic lamina. The arterioles continue to divide and accompany their respective branches of the respiratory tree to the level of the atria. Lateral branches are given off to supply the walls of the respiratory tree and their alveoli. Such branches, with the terminal branches around the alveolar sacs, are sometimes called the precapillary arterioles; they break up to form the capillary network of the alveoli themselves.

The bronchial arteries are inconstant in origin; they may arise from the aorta or the intercostal, subclavian, or internal mammary arteries. They supply the bronchial wall as far as the terminal bronchioles and then form one arterial plexus in the peribronchium and another in the tunica propria. In some forms of bronchiectasis, the bronchial arterial system is greatly hypertrophied and may carry significant quantities of blood into the plexus so formed.[24, 2038]

The pulmonary venous radicles arise from capillaries distal to the alveolar meshwork, from venous plexuses that correspond to the bronchial arterial plexuses, and from the capillary network of pleura. Histologically, venules are indistinguishable from arterioles other than by their position. The venous system drains into the interlobular septa, and thus does not accompany the corresponding bronchial or arterial tree. The venous drainage of the large bronchi and the tracheal bifurcation form a few small trunks (the bronchial veins) that drain into the pulmonary veins near the hilum. These veins also receive trunks from the mediastinum and anastomose with others leading to the azygos and hemiazygos veins.

ARTERIOVENOUS ANASTOMOSES

Although precapillary anastomoses between the pulmonary arteries and veins, and between bronchial and pulmonary arteries, may be found in disease, it is less clear whether these occur in the normal lung.

THE NORMAL LUNG: PHYSIOLOGY AND METHODS OF STUDY

CHAPTER 2

"Because a three-fold division of function may exist in science, between the instrument-maker, the laboratory worker, and the theorist, it has always been possible, and still is, for the strategic thinking in science to take place outside the laboratory, away from the instruments (though it may still be controlled by the accessible mathematical techniques). Thus Tycho's instruments were made by the metal-workers of Augsburg; he himself managed their use with consummate skill; and his results were interpreted by the mathematician Kepler. But the third function without the second, and the second without the first, can clearly yield only diminishing returns. The progress of science demands originality at all three levels; more than this, it may demand the existence of resources of industrial magnitude, of a glass-industry, of a gas-industry, of the great plants required to produce antibiotics and radioactive isotopes. If it seems increasingly likely that the major advances of the future will come from large institutes, freely endowed, and as the result of co-operative labours, it is no more than a fresh step in that growth of complexity, and of an increasing reliance on techniques and tools of investigation, which was typical of the scientific revolution. In a sense it is the fulfilment of Bacon's foresight."*

INTRODUCTION

The principal function of the lung is to ventilate the blood. It might seem to follow from this that measurement of the tension of respiratory gases leaving the lungs might be regarded as the only required test of function. However, the "pulmonary reserve" is so large, and mechanisms to adjust minute ventilation or to relate perfusion to ventilation within the lung may be so efficient, that these gas tensions may remain within normal limits despite the presence of extensive lung disease or marked changes in lung mechanics. In addition, it may be remarked that the symptoms of lung disease, in particular the sensation of dyspnea, bear little direct relationship to the efficiency of hemorespiratory exchange. For these reasons, measurement of the properties of the lung, such as size (or volume), expansibility (elasticity), ventilatory ability (forced expiratory volume), or efficiency of gas transfer (diffusing capacity), can often provide a much more complete picture of the state of the lung than can be gained from arterial blood gas measurements, important though these are.

It is essential for the physician to understand that no single test of lung function can ever measure all the attributes that constitute the totality. All too frequently, and often because of convenience or the appeal of simplicity, the physician or epidemiologist may extrapolate conclusions from a simple test which would not have been justifiable if more detailed laboratory techniques had been applied. Thus it may be taught that the early stages of a disease, such as pneumoconiosis, cause no impairment of lung function because the forced expiratory volume may still be

*From Hall, A. R.: *The Scientific Revolution, 1500–1800: The Formation of the Modern Scientific Attitude.* London, Longmans Green, 1954; Boston, Mass., Beacon Press (paperback ed.), 1956 ("Technical Factors," pp. 242–243).

normal; but it may later be shown that these stages are accompanied by alterations in gas exchange, particularly on exercise, that do indicate interference with normal lung function.

It is essential that anyone using pulmonary function tests for any purpose should be thoroughly familiar with his apparatus and fully conversant with calibration procedures and sources of error. This chapter is not concerned with details of methods and procedure, but is intended as a guide to the many techniques now available and as an introduction to the physiological considerations which lie behind the interpretation of derangement of function. The choice of methods of study is not an easy one, and different methods of measurement are more or less suitable when different problems confront the physician. Thus the routine methods available in a large general hospital would be expected to differ from those available in a major thoracic referral center; and these, in turn, might be quite unsuitable for field use by a department of epidemiology or for routine use to assist a pneumoconiosis panel in its work. It is generally true that the limits of interpretation of simpler tests can only be understood when very detailed and time-consuming methods of study have been used in the investigation of different diseases; but there is little place for an "evangelical" approach to particular lung function tests to cover all possible situations in which they may be of value.

SUBDIVISIONS OF LUNG VOLUME

Definitions

A long period of confusion in nomenclature of the subdivisions of lung volume ended in 1950 with the publication of a suggested standardization.[87] The terms now commonly used are indicated in Figure 2–1.

It follows from a study of these that:

$$IC = TLC - FRC,$$
$$\text{that } RV = FRC - ERV,$$

and that RV expressed as a fraction of TLC equals (FRC − ERV) divided by (FRC + IC). One of the older terms not adopted by the committee recommending these terms was "midcapacity." This designated the volume of lung being ventilated during steady-state breathing and is therefore the sum of the FRC plus half the tidal volume.

In scientific writing, it is important to provide the reader with sufficient data to enable him to calculate all of the subdivisions of lung volume if these have been measured. This can be done, for example, by giving TLC, FRC, and VC; or RV, ERV, and VC. This is a better practice than to provide only ratios, from which the basic data often cannot be computed.

The remarkable paper by Mr. John Hutchinson, a surgeon, published in 1846[89] is distinguished not only by its title, "On the

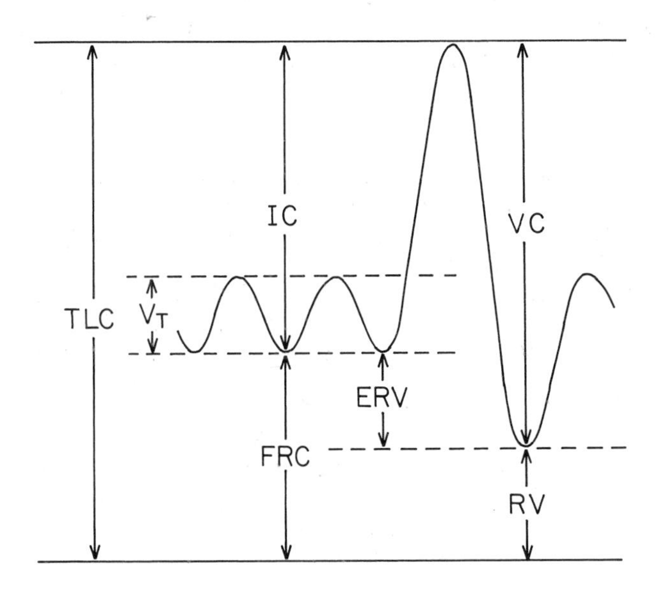

FIGURE 2–1. Subdivisions of Lung Volume:

TLC = Total lung capacity
FRC = Functional residual capacity
VC = Vital capacity
ERV = Expiratory reserve volume
RV = Residual volume
IC = Inspiratory capacity
V_T = Tidal volume.

capacity of the lungs and on the respiratory functions, with a view of establishing a precise and easy method of detecting disease by the spirometer," which might serve as a motto for respiratory physiologists, but also by the excellence of his description of apparatus and the perception with which the statistical treatment of his data was conducted.

Spirometry

A recording spirometer such as is used, or was used, for the routine measurement of basal metabolic rate provides a readily available method of measuring the vital capacity and its subdivisions. More generally useful, however, is the Wright ventilation meter (*see* page 15), if resting ventilation or a vital capacity is needed. If fast expirations are to be measured, old spirometers generally have undesirable characteristics and have generally and deservedly fallen out of use for this purpose. In order to measure absolute gas volume in the lung (TLC, FRC, and RV), one of three different methods must be employed: inert gas dilution or wash-out, whole body plethysmography, or radiological techniques.

Closed-circuit helium equilibration

In the year 1799 Davy measured the residual air, using hydrogen dilution with forced breathing.[88] From time to time this method was modified on minor points of technique, but the next real advance was made in 1923, when Van Slyke and Binger[90] described a hydrogen dilution method for the measurement of the functional residual air without forced breathing, a method suitable for clinical application. Difficulties in the analysis of hydrogen were a serious drawback, and wider use was made of an oxygen dilution method described by Christie in 1932.[91] This method, however, proved unsatisfactory in patients with uneven ventilation, because of delayed equilibrium between subject and circuit.[93] The introduction of a continuously recording thermal conductivity meter by Herrald and McMichael[104] stimulated a return to the use of hydrogen as an inert indicator gas,[106] later replaced by helium,[107, 109] which is now the gas most commonly used.

The subject is switched into a closed circuit containing a suitable percentage of helium in air, and breathes quietly until no further fall in helium takes place. Some recent publications contain useful descriptions of the method and practical details of procedure.[39, 110, 112, 113] As used originally, the circuit contained helium in oxygen, requiring a long period of oxygen breathing before the measurements were made,[98, 114] but more recently air has been used in the circuit[39] and it has been shown that this introduces no error.[110] A correction factor for the very small volume of helium taken up by the blood during the procedure has been proposed[116] but not universally adopted. It has been shown that the ideal circuit volume for use with adults is about 5 liters.[115]

Open-circuit nitrogen clearance

A new principle was introduced in 1940 by Darling,[94, 95] Cournand,[96] and their colleagues when they described the measurement of lung volume by nitrogen wash-out. This method involved the displacement of nitrogen from the lungs by oxygen breathing, and calculation of the volume of nitrogen expired by analysis of the nitrogen content of expired air. The technical details and precautions necessary to ensure accuracy with this technique have been well described,[13] and minor modifications of apparatus and method have been suggested by several authors.[97–100]

Although the nitrogen analysis of the expired gas was made initially in the Van Slyke apparatus, it may be performed more conveniently by a nitrogen meter.[102] If used for this purpose, the meter must be very carefully calibrated, since the method depends upon multiplication of a large gas volume by a value for the nitrogen concentration, and small analytical errors cause considerable changes in the FRC computed.[98]

The open-circuit technique is more simple in the sense that it requires only equipment that should be readily available in any respiratory laboratory; the expired air is collected, its volume measured, and its nitrogen content accurately measured by the Van Slyke apparatus or nitrogen meter.

The closed-circuit technique requires a specially adapted recording spirometer equipped with a katharometer. Once assembled, the apparatus seldom gives any trouble, and the measurement of lung volume is a simple matter. From the literature it is difficult to assess the relative merits of the open- and closed-circuit methods, and it is fair perhaps to say that there is no valid reason why a worker accustomed to one should change to the other. Gilson and Hugh-Jones in 1949 compared values obtained with a closed helium circuit and by the nitrogen wash-out method.[98] No systematic discrepancy was found, and they pointed out that the closed-circuit method was simpler and quicker. Goldman and Becklake[118] recently reviewed estimates of lung volume in normal subjects from different laboratories all using the closed-circuit method, and they pointed out that these show satisfactory uniformity.

There is little doubt that both the helium method and the open-circuit technique, if carefully handled, are satisfactory when normal subjects are being studied. The problem is of an entirely different order, however, in patients with pulmonary emphysema, in whom equilibration with the closed circuit or nitrogen elimination may take many minutes.[2280] In 1950 we suggested that, with the closed-circuit technique, the equilibration procedure should be continued until "mixing is complete,"[114] and showed a tracing on a patient with emphysema in which it had taken more than 10 minutes. More recently, it has been shown[102, 1786] that this period of equilibration may have to be much longer (e.g., up to 18 minutes in emphysema[1786]) if the total gas in the lung computed from a helium dilution study is to be the same as that measured by the body plethysmographic technique (*see* page 15), which measures total intrathoracic gas volume whether or not in free communication. In such patients it seems highly likely that some parts of the lung can be ventilated only through "gas drift" through small alveolar fenestrae, all normal bronchiolar connections having been destroyed. A general awareness of this problem, together with the plethysmographic evidence of very large lung volumes in some patients, has led to an increasing number of reports of patients with emphysema who have very large functional residual capacities. It is unfortunate that a circuit leak also will produce a large computed FRC, but if this is suspected the subject must be restudied. It seems probable from Emmanuel's[102] work that, if the helium closed-circuit or the nitrogen-elimination procedure is continued for long enough, values for FRC computed from these methods are not very different from those found by plethysmography.

The closed-circuit helium method has been adapted successfully for use during bronchospirometry by Fleming and West,[119] allowing the subdivisions of lung volume to be measured for each lung separately. Wright and Gilford[49] have described more recently an unusual method of measuring the subdivisions of lung volume. By placing a 6-liter bag of oxygen inside a Krogh spirometer, and using a nitrogen meter for continuous analysis at the mouth, the residual volume can be computed. These authors developed this method for survey work and show that the maximal breathing capacity can be satisfactorily measured with the same apparatus. Values determined by this method agree with those obtained with conventional techniques.

When the subdivisions of lung volume were the only laboratory measurements available, they assumed great importance in the investigation of patients with chronic lung disease. Today there are many other more useful measurements that can be made, but it should be remembered that the interpretation of more complex measurements, such as compliance and diffusing capacity, depends in part upon knowledge of lung volume.

BODY PLETHYSMOGRAPHY

The concept of plethysmography in the study of the lungs dates from 1882 when Pflüger measured his own intrathoracic gas volume by applying Boyle's Law to relate changes in alveolar pressure to simultaneous changes in lung volume.[122] He used a wooden chamber or plethysmograph which completely enclosed the subject and which was in communication with a spirometer. Technical difficulties led to abandonment of the method. Modern advances in technique have led to its revival by Comroe and Botelho as a pressure plethysmograph, an air-tight chamber in which volume changes in the intrathoracic gas can be calculated from the simultaneous rarefaction of the surrounding gas in the plethysmograph. Practical details of this method of measuring lung volume have been fully described[3, 120, 121, 1787] and elaborated in a wholly delightful manner by DuBois in the Third Bowditch Lecture.[122] A modified plethysmograph built by Schmidt and Cohn[123] is said to be more comfortable and less formidable for the patient than the original model; the authors state that they successfully studied in it a patient who had never entered a telephone booth because of claustrophobia.

The plethysmographic method of measuring the gas in the lungs yields higher values in some patients with lung cysts or emphysema than do the gas-dilution methods,[121] but such differences are reduced if the gas-dilution or gas-clearance methods are continued for a sufficiently long time.[102, 123, 1786]

Mead[124] has revived the original volume-displacement plethysmograph of Pflüger with great success. His instrument, because it is superior to the pressure plethysmograph in recording slow events, is likely to be particularly valuable to the respiratory physiologist and has the advantage of having less stringent requirements as to air leaks.

Radiological methods

Arithmetical calculation of lung volume as the product of area (determined by planimetry, from a PA chest roentgenogram) and depth (the external diameter of the chest measured with calipers) was first introduced by Hurtado and Fray in 1933.[92] Barnhard and his colleagues[1788] found good agreement between radiological methods and gas dilution or body plethysmographic determinations. Although various formulae have been published,[1788, 1796, 2369, 2370] the most accurate technique appears to be that of Loyd, String, and DuBois,[2370] who found excellent agreement between the radiological and plethysmographic determinations in normal subjects and in patients with a wide variety of lung diseases. Their overall correlation coefficient was a remarkable 0.966. They assumed that the volume of the thorax could be treated as if it were composed of five elliptical cylindroids in horizontal layers. In order to obtain the lung volume, they subtracted the volume of the heart, of both domes of the diaphragm, and of the pulmonary blood and lung tissue from the volume of the thorax. They showed that the measurements could be made just as accurately by a technician as by a physician and, with training, required only 20 minutes to complete. This is about equivalent to the man-hours required for any of the physiological measurements.

Other investigators have emphasized the importance of simultaneous spirometry,[125, 2369] which, along with a radiological determination of TLC, permits calculation of all the subdivisions of lung volume. Such a combination would be ideally suited to field studies and survey work, and it is perhaps rather surprising that it has not been more widely used.

Summary

The most commonly used methods of estimating lung volume are by nitrogen wash-out and by helium dilution. Both these techniques measure communicating gas volume, and although each has its own advocates, there is no good evidence that one is inherently better than the other. The body plethysmograph, however, measures total intrathoracic gas volume, whether or not this is in communication with the airways. It has advantages in some areas of research and has been successfully used in the field. There is much to recommend a combination of spirometric and radiographic methods, particularly in circumstances in which the maintenance and calibration of gas analysis or pressure sensing equipment may prove difficult.

The physiological factors determining lung volume are discussed in a later section (*see* pages 44–47.

VENTILATION MEASUREMENTS

Resting ventilation

Resting minute ventilation is defined as the quantity of air expired per minute ($\dot{V}_E$) and can be easily measured with a recording spirometer equipped with a soda–lime canister. It is important to correct the measured expired volume for the absorbed CO_2. In many laboratories, use of a mouthpiece with valves for the collection of expired air into a Neoprene bag is preferred to that of a spirometer. The volume of expired gas collected is then measured in a Tissot spirometer or by means of a volume meter. For bedside use, the Wright Respirometer,[1783] a pocket-sized instrument, is preferable, and this should be part of the routine equipment of a modern recovery room or intensive-care unit. From the measured resting ventilation it is possible to make an approximate estimate of alveolar ventilation if a value of dead space is assumed.

The measurement of resting ventilation plays little part in routine pulmonary assessment, since patients with advanced lung disease frequently breathe with a normal tidal volume and respiratory rate. However, the physician may observe deep sighing respirations, occurring intermittently, that may signal a psychogenic disorder, or he may wish to obtain an accurate record of resting ventilation if he suspects the presence of hypoventilation. The patterns of resting ventilation in normal subjects have been studied in detail [1782, 2371] and Bendixen, Smith, and Mead[2371] noted that men breathed at an average frequency of 16 per minute and women at 19 per minute, with much individual variation, and that sighing occurred at an average rate of 10 sighs per hour. It seems clear that intermittent deep breaths and sighing and yawning have an important physiological function.

One of the problems in the measurement of ventilation is that normal values are difficult to obtain. As soon as a subject knows that his ventilation is being measured, breathing no longer remains an unconscious process, and its pattern may well alter. In addition, the presence of a mouthpiece and noseclip even in trained normal subjects may cause the rate and depth to change. Possibly the most accurate measurements have been made by observing the frequency of breathing in a congregation during a church service.[2372] Another approach is to use magnetometers attached to the chest wall which may be monitored by telemetry to measure rate and depth of breathing when the subject is unaware that measurements are being made.[2373] Recent developments in the use and design of impedance plethysmography[2416, 2422] have demonstrated the potentiality of this technique. Tanser[3140] found a correlation coefficient of 0.97 between the tidal volume directly measured and that computed from a change in thoracic impedance, and put the method to excellent use in studying a patient with Cheyne-Stokes breathing (*see* Chapter 15).

In contrast to its insignificant role in routine pulmonary assessment, the measurement of resting ventilation plays an important but often neglected part in the management of patients who are in danger of developing respiratory failure from hypoventilation. This situation may arise in postoperative states, in barbiturate intoxication or in neuromuscular disease. In such patients the minute ventilation is a vital sign as important as the pulse rate and blood pressure and should be measured by the nursing staff at frequent intervals. There are, of course, many situations in which the minute ventilation may be normal but the alveolar ventilation may be grossly deficient. Nevertheless, the simultaneous measurement of minute ventilation (with a calculation of alveolar ventilation) whenever an arterial blood gas sample is drawn may enable the physician to avoid frequent repetition of the arterial puncture, if he follows the minute volume closely.

Bag–Box circuit

In certain types of investigation the inspired air has to be an artificial mixture of gases that differs from the atmosphere. In these circumstances the conventional spirometer circuit has many drawbacks, and it is usually preferable to use the so-called "bag–box" circuit. This consists of a Neoprene balloon suspended in an air-tight tank.[37] The tank is connected to a spirometer, and the balloon, which contains the mixture of gases to be inspired, is connected to the patient. Alternatively, if it is the expired air which is to be sampled, the subject breathes from the tank and exhales into the balloon. In either case the spirometer attached to the tank will give an accurate record of the tidal air. This device has been used both for single-breath experiments[38] and during steady-state breathing.[39] It is also useful for recording the difference between oxygen uptake and CO_2 output[37] and for studies involving gases that are very soluble in the water jacket of the conventional spirometer. In general, the total volume of the bag–box system should not exceed 50 liters; otherwise, serious error may be introduced by the inertia of the system, which also prevents accurate volume recording at high respiratory rates. Unless short periods of gas collection only are required, the method is thus unsuitable for exercise studies.

It is worth noting, however, that if recording a long period of resting breathing with the subject breathing air is required, as might be desired, for example, in the measurement of Cheyne-Stokes respiration, this may often most conveniently be performed using a bag–box circuit, since the closed spirometer circuit is not suitable for this purpose unless

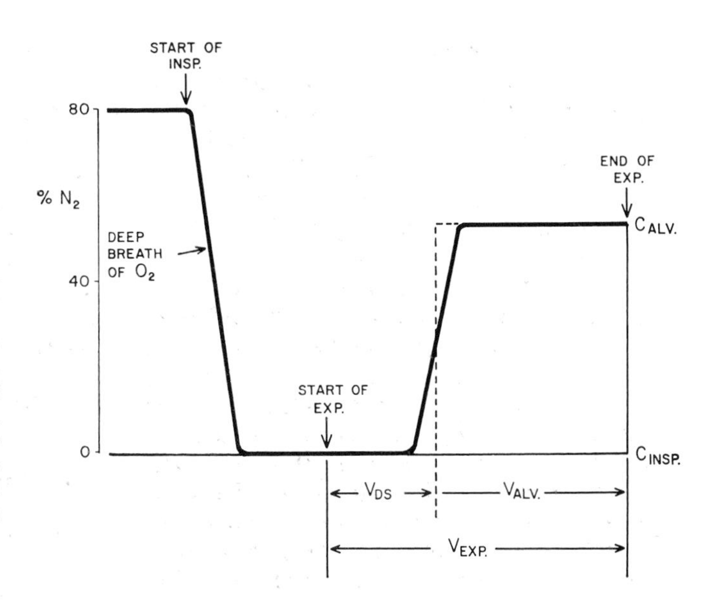

FIGURE 2–2. CALCULATION OF INERT-GAS DEAD SPACE AFTER SINGLE BREATH OF 100 PER CENT OXYGEN

This diagram illustrates the recorded nitrogen percentage at the mouth, using a fast analyzer. At the start of expiration the gas coming from the anatomical dead space contains no nitrogen. The nitrogen concentration then rises steeply until all the gas being expired is coming from alveoli. The inert-gas dead space (V_{DS}) may be calculated from the volume of expiration from the start of expiration until the point indicated on the curve of nitrogen concentration. This point is selected by determining the point at which the two triangles (made up of the dotted line and the nitrogen curve) have equal area. This method may be used even if the alveolar nitrogen concentration is not uniform (see text).

oxygen can be added continually to it. The principle has been successfully employed in an apparatus designed for field testing of pulmonary function.[40]

ANATOMICAL DEAD SPACE

A part of each breath remains within the upper airway and tracheobronchial tree and does not reach the gas-exchanging surfaces in the alveoli. Therefore it does not contribute to exchange of O_2 and CO_2. This part of the airway is referred to as the "anatomical dead space" and is commonly designated V_D. That fraction of total ventilation ($\dot{V}_E$) that enters the gas-exchanging surface is called the "alveolar ventilation" or $\dot{V}_A$. In order to measure $\dot{V}_A$ it is necessary to subtract the dead space ventilation from $\dot{V}_E$. This is given by the following expression:

$$\dot{V}_A = \dot{V}_E - fV_{D\,anat},$$

where f is the respiratory frequency. V_D may be either measured directly or estimated from body height[1801] or body weight.[267]

In 1948, Fowler described a single-breath method of measuring $V_{D\,anat}$. This method involves the simultaneous registration of expired nitrogen concentration and volume or flow, following a deep inspiration of a nitrogen-free gas. This is the same approach as that used by Comroe and Fowler[142] to measure changes in the alveolar plateau of nitrogen. The details of measurement of dead space from the tracing may be seen in Figure 2–2. From the S-shaped curve of N_2 wash-out a theoretical square wave can be derived representing the "front" between alveolar air and dead-space air, and the dead space can be calculated by computing the volume expired up to this front. The great advantage of this over other methods is that it is independent of spot alveolar sampling.

Since the original description of this technique was published, several workers have studied various factors which influence the dead space measured in this way. A very elegant series of model experiments by Birath[237] has shown that with this technique, with repeated determinations, one can estimate the volume of a 190-ml dead space at a mean of 189 ml with an SD of ±7.0 ml. It has been shown that the dead space so measured is unaffected whether oxygen, carbon dioxide, nitrogen, or helium is used as the indicator gas in resting normal subjects.[236] The value of the dead space in normal subjects decreases if the breath is held after the inspiration has been taken,[236, 238–239, 2423] and is increased by increasing the end-expiratory lung volume.[239] The change with the duration of breath-holding is rapid initially but slower thereafter, and is thought to represent diffusion occurring at the effective boundary between dead space and alveolar gas. In subjects 4 to 42 years of age it has been shown that the anatomical dead space bears a close relationship to body height.[1801]

Under normal conditions, the gas volume measured by this method is the volume of those parts of the respiratory tract which, at the beginning of expiration, contain gas whose composition is unchanged from that of inspired air. This volume approximates that of the bronchial tree down to the terminal bronchioles, and probably measures it more accurately than can be done in the cadaver. It has been shown[240] that the extrathoracic fraction of the dead space, mainly comprising the pharynx and mouth, contributes about 66 ml of dead space to the average total of about 150 ml for a normal man. This value falls from 66 ml to 35 ml with depression of the jaw and flexion of the neck, and protrusion of the jaw and neck extension increases it from 66 ml to about 105 ml. The dead space measured by this technique is smaller in the supine position than sitting,[243] and is increased with increasing age.[241, 244] The volume of the dead space is decreased after pneumonectomy,[242] and is decreased 60 per cent by tracheostomy.[245]

If the distribution of inspired gas into the alveolar spaces is uneven, as in emphysema, the alveolar N_2 plateau on expiration is steeper and may be difficult to define, but usually it is possible to do so by having the patient take a deeper breath. Thus Fowler[241] was able to show by this method that the inert-gas dead space in emphysema is minimally increased, and thereby end the uncertainty that existed in the literature as to whether the distribution defect in this disease should be characterized as an increase in dead space.

Birath has also confirmed the validity of the technique in patients with emphysema in whom no real alveolar nitrogen plateau exists.[1836] Recently a considerable body of work has been done with this technique in experiments to study the importance of gas mixing in the lung by diffusion within the gas phase. This technique is referred to later (*see* page 27).

THE BOHR EQUATION AND THE PHYSIOLOGICAL DEAD SPACE

If one complete expiration is collected in a bag, the amount (in ml) of a gas "y" it will contain must equal the fractional concentration of "y" times the volume of the expiration, or $[F_{E_y} \times V_T]$. This volume of "y" is made up of two distinct portions, (1) a volume of gas from the nonexchanging dead space, in which the concentration of "y" was the same as in the previous inspired air $[V_D \times F_{I_y}]$, plus (2) the volume of "y" derived from alveolar gas $F_{A_y} \times [V_T - V_D]$. Note that the volume of alveolar gas in the sample must equal the total volume of the sample $[V_T]$ minus the dead-space volume $[V_D]$. Hence, we may write that:

$$[F_{E_y} \times V_T] = F_{I_y} V_D + F_{A_y} [V_T - V_D]$$

or, by rearrangement:

$$F_{A_y} = \frac{V_T F_{E_y} - V_D F_{I_y}}{V_T - V_D} \quad \textit{(Equation 1)}$$

or, in terms of V_D:

$$V_D = \frac{[F_{A_y} - F_{Ey}]\, V_T}{[F_{Ay} - F_{Iy}]} \quad \textit{(Equation 2)}$$

If the inspired gas contains no "y" (as with CO_2 under normal conditions): $F_{Iy} = 0$; hence:

$$V_{D_{CO_2}} = \frac{[F_{ACO_2} - F_{ECO_2}]\, V_T}{F_{ACO_2}} \quad \textit{(Equation 3)}$$

This equation therefore provides a value for V_D valid if a single number can be used correctly to define the mean alveolar gas tension (F_{ACO_2}).

If the assumption is made that arterial P_{CO_2} is equal to alveolar P_{CO_2}, equation 3 can be rewritten in terms of gas tensions rather than fractional concentrations and appears as follows:

$$V_{D_{CO_2}} = \frac{V_T\, [P_{aCO_2} - P_{ECO_2}]}{P_{aCO_2}} \quad \textit{(Equation 4)}$$

The validity of substituting arterial for alveolar CO_2 tension is discussed later.

Since the expired tidal volume and the arterial and mixed expired CO_2 tensions can be measured easily and accurately, a value for V_{DCO_2} can be readily computed. This number is called the "physiological dead space." When arterial and mixed alveolar gas tensions are the same, the calculated anatomical and physiological dead spaces will be the same, and both are an approximate measure of the volume of the conducting airway system.

When there is a difference between arterial and alveolar CO_2 tensions (ΔA-a CO_2), the physiological dead space calculated from equation 4 will be found to be greater than the anatomical dead space, the value of the latter still remaining an approximately accurate estimate of conducting airways. The difference in these circumstances between "anatomical" and "physiological" dead space has been termed the "alveolar" dead space by Severinghaus and Stupfel.[246] It has been used by them as an index of uneven pulmonary blood flow, since this value will obviously increase when perfusion ceases to reach parts of the lung that are still ventilated. Many useful studies of the physiological dead space and the factors influencing it have been published.[273–279,1799,1840] The physiological dead space is increased in relation to anatomical dead space when there are significant volumes of lung with a high $\dot{V}/\dot{Q}$ ratio or, in other words, with a ventilation disproportionately high in relation to perfusion. The measurement of physiological dead space is therefore a measure of ventilation/perfusion discrepancy, but its magnitude cannot be interpreted rigorously as the volume of airways plus alveoli that are totally unperfused. The physiological dead space volume tells one that the lungs are behaving *as if* this volume of lung were totally unperfused, though in fact all alveoli might be perfused but the normal spread of $\dot{V}/\dot{Q}$ ratios has been extended.

The apparent change in physiological dead space that occurs in disease has been developed by Rossier and his colleagues as a test of pulmonary function.[280–282] Rossier[17] uses the term "functional dead space" for the physiological dead space and early recognized that an increase in functional dead space could be explained by the presence of uneven $\dot{V}/\dot{Q}$ ratios. He also expressed the view that inhomogeneity of gas within alveoli due to incomplete diffusion mixing might contribute to this volume. This effect is not likely to be large in normal lungs in which the alveoli are small,[260] but it might play a part in determining the very large values for physiological dead space in patients with emphysema documented by a number of authors.[283–285]

Strang[288] has reported that the ratio of physiological dead space to tidal volume is greater in newborn infants than in adults, indicating a greater unevenness of $\dot{V}/\dot{Q}$ ratios shortly after birth. Any such unevenness leads to a lowered efficiency in terms of CO_2 elimination (*see* page 73)—a consequence of considerable importance to this age group.

Alveolar Ventilation

Once the physiological dead space is known, or in a normal lung if the anatomical dead space is known, the alveolar ventilation may be calculated by subtracting the dead space ventilation from the minute ventilation.

It is of interest that, at very low tidal volumes, alveolar ventilation is greater than would be predicted from the measured anatomical dead space,[268] probably due to diffusion mixing at the interface between alveolar and dead space gas. Considerable speculation as to how the giraffe manages any alveolar ventilation at all was ended by Robin and his colleagues,[269] who found that, although the giraffe's dead space is about 1.5 liters in volume, this is not much bigger in relation to the total lung capacity of 47 liters than is the human dead space. It is believed that the giraffe has a tidal volume of about 4 liters per breath, so that at rest the ratio V_D/V_T in the giraffe is about 0.37, a value not different from the average human value of 0.3.

When the $\dot{V}/\dot{Q}$ ratios are similar throughout the lungs, as in normal subjects, an alveolar ventilation at rest of about 4 liters per minute usually is adequate. When the $\dot{V}/\dot{Q}$ ratios are unbalanced throughout the lung, or when the lung architecture is destroyed by disease, then considerably greater volumes of total ventilation may be necessary to maintain normal arterial gas tensions. A more satisfactory method of estimating alveolar ventilation in such cases may be to make the computation outlined above, using "physiological" dead space. Even though "physiological" dead space has no volume counterpart (except that it exceeds "anatomical" dead space when $\dot{V}/\dot{Q}$ ratios are not absolutely uniform throughout the lung), use of this value in place of the "anatomical" dead space does enable one to estimate what proportion of tidal volume is being used effectively in CO_2 exchange.

However, alveolar ventilation can be considered adequate only if it maintains within physiological limits the tension of the respiratory gases in the blood leaving the lung. Thus the *only* satisfactory measurement of effective alveolar ventilation in many clinical circumstances is by the measurement of arterial carbon-dioxide tension.

The arterial P_{CO_2} is inversely proportional to alveolar ventilation and, if alveolar ventilation is unchanged, is directly proportional to CO_2 production. Arterial oxygen saturation, on the other hand, is a poor reflection of the

TABLE 2–1 Change in Arterial Gas Tensions with a Falling Alveolar Ventilation, Assuming Normal Gas Distribution and Normal Diffusion, Oxygen Uptake of 300 ml/min and RQ of 0.8

Alveolar (L/Min) Ventilation	Arterial			
	Po_2 (mm Hg)	O_2 Hb (per cent)	Pco_2 (mm Hg)	pH (if no change in HCO_3)
5.0	90	95.0	40	7.40
4.0	77	93.0	50	7.32
3.0	56	86.0	67	7.24
2.0	15	22.0	100	7.15

Notice that a critical stage is reached when the alveolar ventilation has fallen to 3.0 liters/min. The patient will not be noticeably cyanosed, yet the arterial Pco_2 has reached 67 mm Hg. A further depression of ventilation—whether due to medication or a reduction in effective ventilation due, for example, to airway obstruction—causes a rapid change in arterial gas tensions.

adequacy of alveolar ventilation, because this value will fall only slightly despite a significant fall in alveolar oxygen tension. This point is illustrated in Table 2–1, in which are shown the effects of a progressive fall in alveolar ventilation upon arterial O_2 and CO_2 tensions, and upon arterial O_2 saturation.

The physician must remember that cyanosis may well not be noticeable even though arterial saturation may have dropped to 87 per cent;[1779] yet when this stage has been reached the Pco_2 will be 75 mm Hg. The continuous administration of oxygen to a patient at this stage will result in 100 per cent oxygen saturation, but the dangerous elevation of Pco_2 has not been treated until the level of alveolar ventilation has been raised. A full understanding of this important point is essential to an appreciation of the technique of management of many patients in the postoperative period or with respiratory depression from any cause. Thus it is apparent that direct measurement of arterial Pco_2 is often necessary for accurate assessment of alveolar ventilation and is the only permissible method when the lung is damaged or its architecture deranged. In subjects with normal lungs it is often useful to compute alveolar ventilation at rest, as indicated above, from measured minute ventilation and an assumed value for dead space (e.g., dead space in ml = weight in lb[267]); values so computed can be compared with standard resting requirements as calculated by Radford and conveniently presented by him in the form of a nomogram.[267] Similarly, this nomogram may be used as a guide to the correct adjustment of a ventilator (in terms of rate and depth) when the subject concerned has normal lungs (e.g., in poliomyelitis, under anesthesia, or under the effects of depressant drugs).

Maximal breathing capacity (MBC)

The maximal volume of air that a subject can breathe per minute,[41] or MBC, was proposed originally as a measure of pulmonary performance by Hermannsen in 1933.[42] It may be measured either with a spirometer,[43] or with mouthpiece, valve, and collecting bag,[13] or by using an appropriately modified gas-meter,[137] the subject being required to breathe maximally for 15 to 30 seconds. As a test of pulmonary performance the MBC has a number of limitations. Besides being dependent upon intrinsic properties of the lung such as flow resistance,[136] this measurement is influenced also by nonpulmonary factors such as motivation to ensure maximal effort, muscular force, and endurance,[56] points to be remembered in its interpretation. In addition, the MBC is a measurement greatly influenced by the tools used and procedure adopted. For instance, whatever type of circuit is used, its resistance should always be defined, since relatively minor increases in this value have been shown to cause the recording of falsely low values, particularly in patients with lung disease.[50–52]

If an open circuit is employed, low-resistance valves should be used,[53, 54] and the addition of CO_2 to the inspired gas is advisable to prevent hypocapnea and to minimize the possible bronchoconstrictor effect of low airway Pco_2.[1084] If a spirometer is used its performance characteristics should be such as to avoid errors due to resonance of the system, especially of the water column, which may occur in the older Benedict-Roth type spirometer,[43–46] but which has been overcome in the newer types of instrument.[47–49] In addition, maximal ventilatory ability, particularly in normal subjects, is dependent upon breathing frequency,[46] rates of nearly 100/min being necessary to achieve peak values. In a test in which the patient has the choice of breathing frequency, the peak may never be achieved unless he breathes at some predetermined rate. For these reasons the MBC has been replaced in many laboratories by a single-breath measurement of ventilatory ability of the type to be described next. However, some investigators have continued to prefer it to such single-breath determinations.[49]

SINGLE-EXPIRATION MEASUREMENTS

The volume of a forceful expiration starting at the full inspiratory position, measured in relation to time, was introduced as a test of respiratory performance in France and in the USA at about the same date.[57] It has been the subject of many subsequent reports.[41, 58–67] Like the MBC, this measurement can be made on a recording spirometer, provided the instrument conforms to certain technical requirements.[64] Its flow resistance must be low (usually achieved by fitting a light-weight bell, wide tubing, and removing the CO_2 absorber); the speed of response must be as high as practicable and it must be critically damped to avoid recording errors; and kymograph speed must be variable within an appropriate range (from 2 cm/sec for patients with airway obstruction, to 9 cm/sec for healthy young normal subjects). A simplified instrument capable of making this type of recording is the McKesson Vitalor.[72, 73] Analysis of tracings obtained by either technique is facilitated by the use of a calibrated scale on a plastic mask[39] which can be laid directly over the tracing.

Figure 2–3 illustrates two typical normal

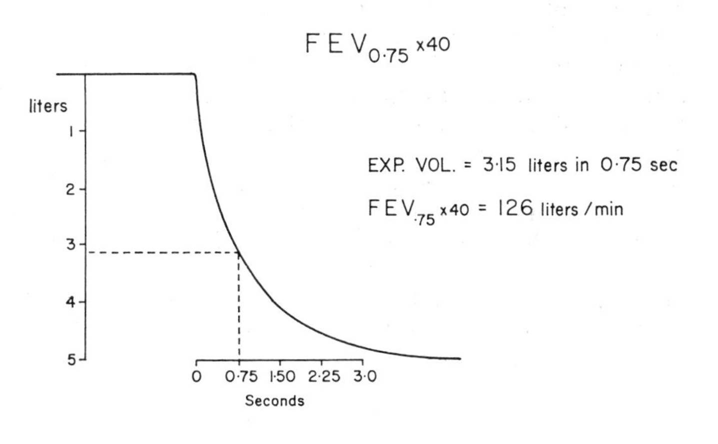

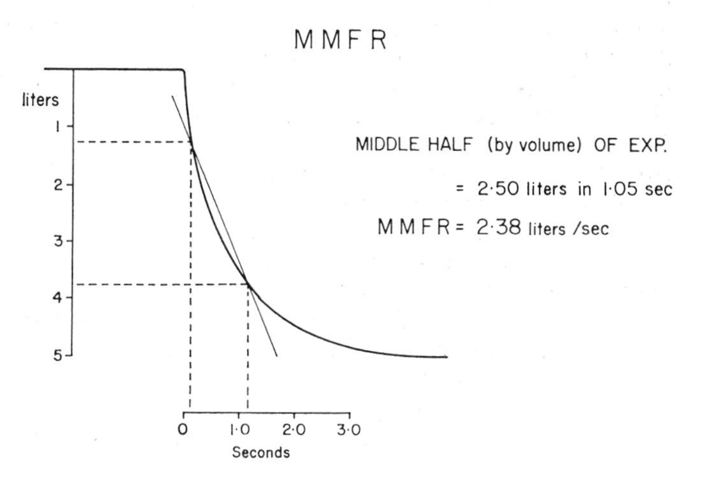

FIGURE 2–3. MEASUREMENT OF VENTILATORY FLOW RATES

A maximally fast expiration is made after a full inspiration. The $FEV_{0.75}$ is recorded by measuring the volume expired in the first three-quarters of a second after the start of expiration. The maximal midexpiratory flow rate (MMFR) is calculated by measuring the middle half by volume of the total expiration, and computing the flow rate over this volume in liters/sec. Both of these computations are facilitated by the use of transparent masks that can be placed over the tracings.

forced-expiration curves. Selection of the volume and the time period over which the tracing is to be analyzed has varied greatly, providing an example of the confusion that follows when an original test is continually modified.

The simplest analysis of the forced expiratory spirogram is to report the change in one variable (volume or time) for a fixed change in the other. Thus, if the variable of time is fixed, the curve may be described as forced expiratory volume in a fixed time, of 0.5 sec ($FEV_{0.5}$), of 0.75 sec ($FEV_{0.75}$), or of 1.0 sec ($FEV_{1.0}$).[41] Forced expiratory volumes may be expressed also as a percentage of the vital capacity $\left(\text{e.g., } \frac{FEV_{1.0}}{VC} \times 100\%\right)$.[67] In normal subjects between 20 and 30 years old. the volume expired in the first second is 87 per cent of the total; this falls to 81 per cent of the total between the ages of 50 and 60.[59] Changes during the course of the day are insignificant.[1784] $FEV_{1.0}$ has been shown to correlate closely with maximal voluntary ventilation at a frequency of 40/min.[1837]

If the $FEV_{0.75}$ is multiplied by 40, or the $FEV_{1.0}$ is multiplied by 30, it will give an approximate indication of the maximal breathing capacity in liters/min. Although this procedure has been criticized,[41, 57] it has been widely accepted in routine work. Some workers ignore the first 300 ml of air expired before the volume is measured, though this maneuver seems to make little difference to the results.[58]

Another approach is to measure the time taken to expire a given volume, as for instance the first liter from a maximal inspiration, discarding the initial 200 ml (maximal expiratory flow rate, or MEFR),[76] or the middle half of the vital capacity (maximal midexpiratory flow rate, or MMFR).[74]

It will be appreciated that any one of the measurements described above is a somewhat restricted description of the curve in Figure 2–3, in which the expiratory flow rates achieved (i.e., the slope of the curve) change throughout the expiration from high initial values to ever-decreasing values in the last part of the breath. This decline in forced expiratory flow rates parallels the decline in lung volume which occurs as the expiration proceeds, and the relationship between these two ($\dot{V}/\Delta V$) is remarkably reproducible in any one person.[68, 70, 1174] Evidence of this is the fact that any number of forced expiratory curves of an individual subject can be superimposed, provided they are matched for volume above the end expiratory level. Indeed, it appears that only in the upper portion (about 25 per cent[1174] of the vital capacity) can greater flow rates be achieved by greater effort by the subject.

Of the various simplified forms of analysis of the expiratory spirogram, there is probably little to choose between the $FEV_{1.0}$ and the $FEV_{0.75}$. There is some reason to suggest that the MMFR may be more sensitive than either of these,[2419] but all would be suitable as a laboratory procedure or field tool. The FEV and its subdivisions are dependent on the vital capacity. If this is reduced the FEV will usually also be reduced. The ratio of $FEV_{1.0}$ to vital capacity may be used to detect reductions in FEV over and above those due to the reduced vital capacity alone.

The discriminatory value of the $FEV_{0.75}$,[39] $FEV_{1.0}$,[75] and MMFR[39, 75] in detecting "bronchitis" has been documented by several groups. The MEFR, on the other hand, is theoretically a less sound measurement, being influenced by the effort made during the early part of a forced expiration, and in practice it has been shown to have a greater variance in normal subjects than have the other measurements mentioned.[76]

Another single-expiration measurement popularized recently is the peak expiratory flow rate (PFR).[79–85, 1781, 1783, 2309] Its enthusiastic adoption resulted from the development by Wright and McKerrow of an ingenious peak-flow meter,[78] a portable instrument for field use in contrast to the more accurate pneumotachograph which has been used for some years in the laboratory to measure air flow.[13, 77] The measurement of peak-flow rate during forced expiration is equivalent to a spot measurement of the slope of the expiratory spirogram at its steepest point (*see* Figure 2–3). This will obviously occur in the upper half of the vital capacity and therefore is subject to the same criticisms as the MEFR. A greater variability in results compared with those by other single-breath tests[80–83] has been found, and therefore Ritchie[82] has suggested that this test be regarded as a complement to, and not a substitute for, other single-breath tests. In addition, survey work has shown that, in practice, it is less discriminatory than $FEV_{0.75}$, $FEV_{1.0}$, and MMFR.[75, 77, 2232] Even in children—who, it is said, can perform this peak-flow test more easily than a spirogram[79, 85]—it is preferable to attempt the latter as well, and most workers agree that over the age of 3 there is no difficulty in getting the child's co-operation.[86] The Wright peak-flow meter can be adapted to measure inspiratory flow.[1780] The clinical usefulness of this measurement has not yet been clearly established.

It has been our experience that in routine work there is considerable merit in calculating both the $FEV_{1.0}$ and the MMFR from each forced expiratory tracing. This procedure makes it easier to detect errors in the calculation of either one of them during daily routine measurement. Both the FEV and the MMFR have been shown to have a smaller standard deviation on repeated testing in nonsmokers compared to smokers. Dawson,[2419] who reported this observation, also found that the difference between smokers and nonsmokers was greater in the MMFR measurements than in the measured $FEV_{1.0}$, being 0.45 liters/sec in the case of the MMFR and 0.38 liters/sec. in the case of the FEV.

The physiological factors influencing both the single forced expiration tests and the maximum breathing capacity are dependent on the overall mechanical properties of the lungs. The pioneering work of Fry and Hyatt[68–70] and Dayman[1174] has done much to elucidate these factors. Although these tests are widely assumed to be specific measurements of airway caliber, this assumption is erroneous. Events occurring when pleural pressure becomes greater than atmospheric and when intrathoracic airways are dynamically compressed are complex; but it is clear that the flow rates achieved are dependent on the elastic recoil of the lungs just as much as on the state of the airways. This is more fully discussed on pages 33–37 of this chapter.

DISTRIBUTION OF VENTILATION

SINGLE-BREATH MEASUREMENTS

The single-breath test to measure $V_{D\ anat}$ may also be used to measure how evenly inspired air is distributed to alveoli.[142] Once the dead space gas has been exhaled, the expirate consists of alveolar gas. In Figure 2–4 are shown the results of a typical test in a normal subject and in a patient with emphysema. An unchanging concentration of nitrogen would be produced if, at the end of the inspiration of oxygen, all alveoli contained the same nitrogen percentage and gas mixing within alveoli was complete. For this to be the case, assuming all alveoli had contained the same percentage of nitrogen at the start of inspiration, the inspired oxygen would have to have been distributed to each alveolus in exact proportion to its pre-existent volume. Perfect gas distribution might then be described as an unvarying ratio of V_T to V_A throughout all alveoli.

In an actual test, the change in nitrogen percentage that occurs between the 750-ml and 1250-ml volume points on the tracing is measured. In normal subjects below the age of 50 Comroe and Fowler found that this varied from 0 to 1.5 per cent N_2; in healthy men and women older than 50, Greifenstein and his co-workers,[143] from the same laboratory, found a range of 0 to 4.5 per cent. In some patients with emphysema, values as high as 12 per cent were recorded.[142] In a discussion of the possible factors that might cause an uneven gas distribution in normal subjects. Fowler[144] pointed out that gas in the bronchial tree from the previous expiration might be preferentially distributed to certain parts of the lung that filled first when an inspiration was taken. In an admirable review of the whole problem of intrapulmonary distribution of inspired gas,[145] he later pointed out for the first time that gas distribution was almost certain to be sequentially distributed in relation to time—a concept that has received support from work on lung mechanics[147] and from recent work on the effect on lung emptying of different patterns of expiratory flow.[1790]

Subsequent workers have pointed out that results of this test are much influenced by the procedure adopted, and that results are more satisfactory if there is no significant pause between the maximal inspiration and expiration;[149, 150, 2423] if the inspired volume is controlled; if the velocity of expiration is controlled;[148] if the mean of several tests on the subject is used rather than a single result;[150] and if the test is commenced from FRC, not RV.[149, 150]

Recent studies on regional gas distribution, discussed in detail later (pages 43–46), have revealed that the distribution of an inspiration is influenced in regional terms by whether the inspiration began from residual volume or from FRC.[2431]

Apart from the fact that it inevitably in-

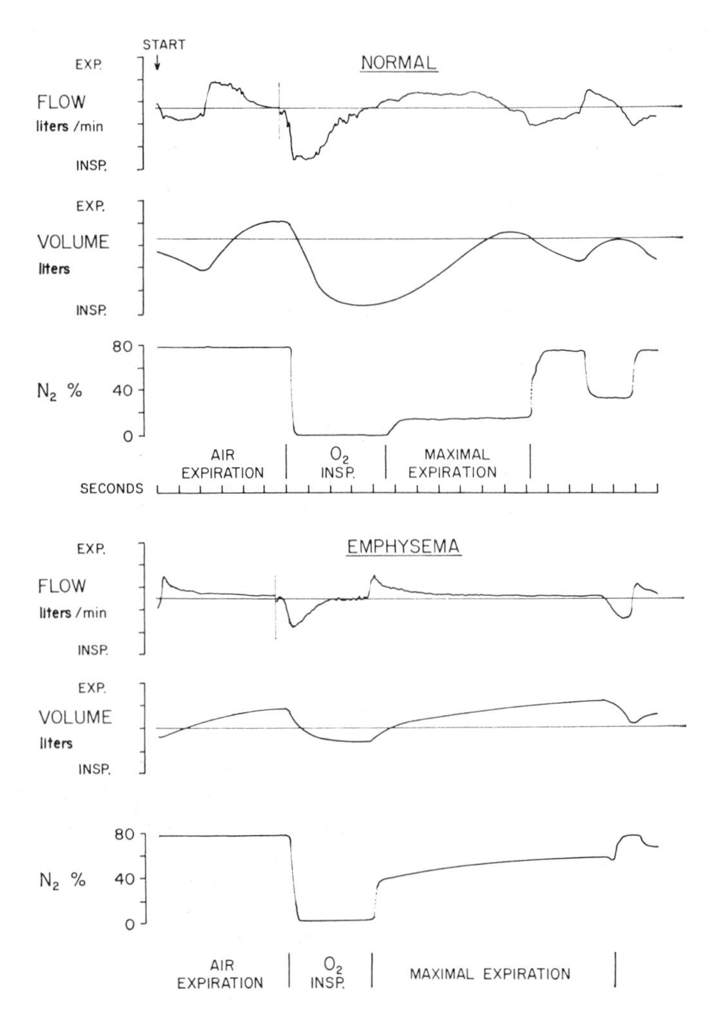

FIGURE 2–4. Change in Percentage of Expired Nitrogen after a Deep Inspiration of 100 Per Cent Oxygen

In each case the top tracing records the pneumotachographic record of flow; the middle tracing is volume change recorded from a spirometer; and the lower tracing is nitrogen percentage recorded by a fast-response nitrogen meter. The transition from inspiration to expiration is signaled by the zero flow points on the pneumotachograph record. The change in nitrogen percentage during expiration is customarily measured between the 750 and 1250 ml volumes of the expiration. Notice the steeper gradient in the case of emphysema compared to the normal.

volves the use of somewhat elaborate equipment, the single-breath measurement of gas distribution offers considerable advantages over other methods, since it is much easier to perform and calculation of the results is quick. It is obvious that it can be used only to distinguish normality from abnormality in general terms, but the same applies to all other indices of gas distribution, since they are all affected by any process that interferes with normal lung architecture or with lung expansion, or gas flow. In this sense these measurements are completely nonspecific in terms of underlying pathological condition. Comroe and Fowler[142] originally suggested that the test might be of value as a screening procedure for normality or otherwise, and it has been used successfully as a field method in population surveys.[835] It may be more sensitive than the FEV in detection of minor degrees of airway abnormality.[1789]

Stanescu and his colleagues have recently shown that this index may be significantly altered in cigarette smokers whose $FEV_{1.0}$ is not abnormal.[2772]

Open-circuit clearance

There is a very extensive bibliography of studies of gas distribution in the lung, based on analysis of sequential breaths. The first appears to be that of Gréhant[2433] in 1864, who measured lung volume using hydrogen, and observed the change with six consecutive breaths. He concluded: "Les gaz mélanges à l'air inspiré pénétrant comme lui jusqu'aux extrémités des bronches," and proposed the calculation of a coefficient of ventilation that was, in effect, a dilution index. Haldane recognized that accurate knowledge of nitrogen clearance during oxygen breathing was essential to an understanding of problems related to diving and decompression,[2] but a systematic study of nitrogen clearance began only in 1940 with the pioneer work of Darling, Cournand, and Richards.[94–96] From this endeavour came the simplest of the open-circuit gas-distribution indices. The subject breathed pure oxygen for a period of seven minutes, at the end of which time he delivered an alveolar sample for analysis. In normal people this sample was found to contain less than 2.5 per cent of nitrogen, whereas in patients with a wide variety of lung disease it was often more than double this value. It was recognized that this measurement took no account of the factors, such as minute volume and FRC, which not infrequently were abnormal in disease and which of themselves (and regardless of the uniformity of gas distribution) would play a part in determining the rate of gas clearance.

In 1950, Robertson, Siri, and Jones[153] studied serial nitrogen clearance during oxygen breathing, using a mass spectrometer for the first time in medical research. This instrument sampled expired gas continuously after the gas had passed through a 400-ml baffle box, the nitrogen in expired air then being graphed on semilogarithmic paper against time on the linear abscissa. This enabled them to divide the lung into compartments with different clearance rates. They observed that the effectiveness of ventilation was correlated with age, and characterized a few patients with different diseases in terms of the efficiency of nitrogen clearance. It has since been shown that, in the normal subject, gas distribution is little affected by alterations in rate or tidal volume,[1795] except in elderly subjects (see page 96).

In 1952, Fowler, Cornish, and Kety[154] published a detailed study of inert-gas clearance which has rightly come to be regarded as one of the major definitive studies in this field. Using a nitrogen meter sampling continuously at the mouth, together with a pneumotachygraph which produced a simultaneous record of air flow, these authors integrated the flow record with the measured nitrogen concentration, to calculate the mean expired nitrogen concentration per breath. From this information they computed the "pulmonary N_2-clearance delay per cent," by comparing the time the nitrogen molecules would have remained in the lung if all alveoli had been ventilated uniformly with the actual average time spent. It was possible also to interpret ventilation in terms of a model lung divided into several parts and to characterize the volume and clearance rates of these parts.

Following his earlier observations on gas distribution,[159] Briscoe has recently described detailed studies of uneven ventilation in normal and diseased lungs by an open-circuit technique,[160] modified to record the alveolar helium fractional concentration rather than the mean expired concentration. Results can then be expressed in terms of volume and ventilation fractions of three lung "phases"; in addition, a "clearance delay percentage" similar to that derived by Fowler was calculated. Lichtneckert and Lundgren suggested another type of analysis, in which an "alveolar-ventilation index" is computed.[1802] Although too complicated for routine use, this approach might well be valuable in investigative work. A complex statistical approach to this problem, proposed by Gómez,[1831] may represent the first successful approximation to descriptions of inert-gas distribution in terms of a continuous distribution of dilution ratios in the lung, rather than analysis by analogy with a two- or three-compartment model.[154]

A number of other workers[101, 152, 155, 157, 158, 163] approached the problem of deriving an overall index of gas distribution more simply than did Fowler, Cornish, and Kety,[154] the methods of Becklake[163] and of Luft and his colleagues[100] perhaps being best suited to clinical evaluation. Becklake derived a "clearance index" by dividing the total volume respired to clear the lung of N_2 by the measured FRC, analysis being made at the 90 per cent clearance and volume point, whereas the latter authors suggested continuing the analysis to a chosen end-expiratory nitrogen level of 0.01 per cent.

Using this technique, Edelman, Mittman, Norris, and Shock have recently reported a detailed analysis of the effect of age on ventilation uniformity.[2430] This was of particular interest, since it was shown that the uniformity of ventilation distribution in old subjects was affected by the depth of tidal volume taken—the larger the tidal volume, the more uniform the distribution. This result is explicable on the basis of airway closure and is discussed in detail in a later section. Okubo and Lenfant[2425] have recently reported an analysis of nitrogen clearance curves making use of a Laplace transform type of analysis and expressing the results as a distribution curve of lung volume and ventilation. For normal subjects these were found to be symmetrical with a relatively narrow base, whereas in patients with disease, the range of distribution was much larger.

The application of these methods of open-circuit gas-clearance analysis to problems of lung disease has been rewarding,[2341] and it is evident that neither the single-breath technique nor the closed-circuit equilibration methods can yield such apparently precise measurement of defects in gas distribution. The reason for this can be appreciated from a theoretical analysis of the limitations to the sensitivity of the two methods, excellently delineated by Visser[113] and by Nye.[161] Cumming[2859] has recently suggested that the nitrogen wash-out curve should be plotted as the amount of nitrogen remaining in the lung at the end of each breath, and he points out that, theoretically, this technique should permit differentiation between abnormalities due to diffusion and those due to other causes of non-uniform gas distribution.

Closed-circuit helium equilibration

Several variables determine the time required for equilibrium to be reached between a closed-circuit spirometer system containing an inert gas and the air in the lungs of a subject breathing into the spirometer. These are: (1) the volume of the patient's lungs; (2) the volume of the circuit; (3) the amount of air exchanged per breath; (4) the speed of gas mixing in the circuit; and (5) the speed of gas mixing in the patient.

The values for (1), (2), and (3) can be measured and, since (4) is constant in any one circuit, one may use the time course of equilibration as a measure of (5), the intrapulmonary gas distribution.

Earlier workers[1283] had appreciated that closed-circuit methods of lung-volume determination are likely to be in error in some patients with lung disease, on account of delayed equilibration. However, the first to attempt quantitation of this delay as a measure of intrapulmonary gas distribution was Birath in 1945,[106] who in a closed-circuit equilibration expressed the delay as reduction in the effective tidal volume or enlargement of dead space. This approach was taken a step further by us in 1950,[114] using a smaller circuit with a faster pump, thereby reducing the delay in equilibration within the circuit. Technical details and modification of this assembly have been described in detail recently.[39] An index of mixing efficiency was calculated by comparing the measured number of breaths taken to reach 90 per cent of the final equilibrium value with the predicted number, assuming even distribution of the entire tidal volume (including dead space) within the lung. Values for this index have been reported to vary between 45 and 80 per cent in normal subjects,[152, 163–166] deviations probably being attributable in part to differences in circuit volume and pump speed in different laboratories, both of which affect the equilibration time.

Different ways of analyzing closed-circuit equilibration data have been suggested by a number of authors,[167–169, 2276] but only that proposed by Becklake,[170] in which the prediction formula takes into account an assumed value for anatomical dead space, appears to provide an index of greater sensitivity without making the calculation procedure much more complex.

A most valuable approach to the technical problems of designing a closed circuit with minimal delay has been that developed by Nye.[161] His analysis of the theoretical limitations inherent in all closed-circuit indices of the type described here has at last enabled a clear view to be obtained of the information such measurements can and cannot be expected to give. It seems clear that there is little point in attempting to refine the closed-circuit method further, and nothing to be gained by substituting any other point for the 90 per cent equilibrium value. The technique is limited by instrumental accuracy and response time, and such indices are not sensitive to some patterns of uneven distribution that an open-circuit N_2 wash-out method may detect. In general, closed-circuit indices are at their most sensitive when the ventilation inequality is caused by a lung "compartment" of moderate volume receiving a very small fraction of each tidal volume only. This situation is encountered clinically in patients with lung cysts with pin-hole communication only to bronchi, in whom very low closed-circuit indices may be found. In a recent paper, we reported some studies on patients with bronchial asthma in whom significant abnormality of the closed-circuit helium index closely paralleled the regional ventilation defect measured by radioactive xenon.[735]

More recently, we have reported[2532] that in a group of patients with chronic bronchitis with relatively good ventilatory function the closed-circuit index of gas distribution was significantly correlated with the abnormality of gas distribution measured regionally with xenon.[133] This provides further evidence of the general usefulness of this simple index, even though it has potential limitations and sources of variability that are not easy to circumvent.

FACTORS INFLUENCING THE DISTRIBUTION OF VENTILATION

There are a considerable number of possible causes of unequal gas distribution in the lung, and among the most important are regional differences in intrapleural pressure (*see* page 43) and differing mechanical properties of various parallel pathways in the lung (*see* page 38), and airway closure (*see* page 47). Another important factor, and one on which much present attention is focused, is gaseous diffusion. By this is meant the possible limitation of gas uniformity by too slow a rate of diffusion in the gas phase. This used to be referred to as "stratified inhomogeneity" and until the last few years it was generally assumed that Rauwerda[249] had laid this ghost to rest in 1946. However, recent data and, particularly, better instrumentation have led to a re-examination of the problem.

Diffusion of gases in airspaces

As the front of inspired gas travels down the tracheobronchial tree, its velocity constantly diminishes as the total cross-sectional area of the tracheobronchial tree gets larger and larger. Reference to Table 1–1 on page 3 shows that the cross-sectional area at the level of subsegmental bronchi is about 6.6 square cm, whereas at the level of the terminal bronchioles it is 17 times this or about 116 sq cm. At about the 1-mm diameter level (terminal bronchi) the linear velocity of the gas is about equal to the velocity due to gas diffusion. Thus, although mass flow brings gas into the alveoli, oxygen must diffuse in the gas phase to reach the alveolar wall in order to be taken up. Similarly CO_2 must diffuse from the alveolar wall to a point from which it can subsequently be carried in the expired gas. Rauwerda[249] calculated that the distances involved were so short and the time available sufficiently long that there would be complete diffusion mixing in the time course of one breath. Recently, Georg and his colleagues,[2378] using a two-gas technique, have provided evidence that diffusion mixing was incomplete. Cummings and his coworkers, in a series of papers,[2374, 2375, 2859] have proposed new models for the terminal airway structure of the lung and presented additional experimental evidence that diffusion equilibrium is not complete even in normal lungs. Both groups have pointed out that the increased diffusion distances in emphysema might well lead to considerable effects, as we suggested in the first edition of this volume. Although the validity and relevance of Cummings' model has been questioned,[2376] Sikand, Cerretelli, and Farhi[2377] have reported additional experimental data that support the conclusion reached by Georg and his colleagues. This volume of work clearly raises the general problem of the probable contribution of this factor to gas non-uniformity in normal and abnormal lungs. A recent symposium[3363] on respiratory gas mass transport is most valuable in providing a discussion of interpretation of aerosol deposition and gas dead space experimental data and should be consulted by anyone interested in more detailed consideration of this problem than is possible here.

PULMONARY MECHANICS

INTRODUCTION AND SYMBOLS

Although the important conceptual ideas were available from the work of Rohrer in 1915[435] and of von Neergaard and Wirz 12 years later,[436] the extensive development of this area of knowledge had to await the introduction of fast-response electrical pressure transducers, and safe techniques for estimating pleural pressures. A valuable review of this field up to 1960 was contributed by Mead,[434] and this may be supplemented by reference to the Handbook of Physiology published in 1964.[2434]

In this section and throughout this book the following symbols relating to pulmonary mechanics will be used:

Pao	= pressure at the airway opening
Ppl	= pleural pressure
Palv	= alveolar pressure
P_L	= transpulmonary pressure
	= Pao − Ppl
Pres	= pressure difference between alveolus and mouth = Pao − Palv
Pel	= pressure difference across the alveolar wall = Palv − Ppl
Pst(l)	= static elastic recoil pressure of the lung

V_L = an arbitrary lung volume
$\dot{V}$ = flow
C = compliance
Cst = static lung compliance
Cdyn = dynamic lung compliance
R = resistance
Raw = airway resistance (cm H_2O/liter/sec)
Rtiss = viscous resistance of lung tissue
R_L = pulmonary resistance = Raw + Rtiss
Gaw = airway conductance
SGaw = specific airway conductance = Gaw/V_L
SRaw = specific airway resistance = 1/SGaw

Theoretical considerations

In order to move any structure which is at rest, or in order to change the velocity of any structure which is in motion, a force must be applied to the structure to overcome its resistance to motion or to change of motion. Resistance to motion is offered by three specific properties of the structure: its elasticity, its friction, and its inertia. Thus, according to Newton's third law, the force applied to the structure must equal the sum of (1) the force required to overcome its elasticity, (2) the force required to overcome its frictional resistance, and (3) the force required to overcome its inertia.

In the lung, inertia is negligible and can be ignored.[2413] The forces are analyzed in terms of pressures (force per unit area). The applied pressure is equal to the pressure difference across the lung.
Thus:

$$\begin{aligned} P_L &= Pao - Ppl \\ &= (Pao - Palv) + (Palv - Ppl) \\ &= Pres + Pel \qquad \textit{(Equation 1)} \end{aligned}$$

To a close approximation, Pres is the pressure required to overcome frictional resistance, and Pel is the pressure required to overcome the elasticity.

The force required to overcome the elasticity of an elastic band depends on its position, i.e., the length to which the band is stretched, but not on how fast it was stretched, i.e., its velocity. On the other hand, the force required to slide a block across a table does not depend on the position of the block on the table, but on how fast the block is moved, i.e., the friction between the block and the table surfaces. In the lungs, length is analyzed in terms of volume, and velocity in terms of flow. Thus we can write:

$$Pel \propto V_L, \text{ and}$$
$$Pres \propto \dot{V}$$

Lung compliance is defined as the change in volume per unit change in pressure, and over the tidal volume range this relationship is very nearly linear. It may be written in the following form:

$$C = \Delta V_L / \Delta Pel = V_T / \Delta Pel, \text{ and}$$

$$\Delta Pel = \frac{1}{C} \times V_T$$

At the end of a quiet expiration, (FRC), Pel has a finite value of approximately 5 cm H_2O. Therefore:

$$Pel = Pel_0 + \frac{1}{C} \times V_T \qquad \textit{(Equation 2)}$$

where Pel_0 is the elastic recoil pressure at FRC.

Resistance is defined as the pressure required to overcome frictional resistance per unit of flow. Thus:

$$R = \frac{Pres}{\dot{V}}, \qquad \textit{(Equation 3)}$$

From equations 2 and 3, and substituting for Pres and Pel in equation 1, we have:

$$P_L = Pel_0 + \frac{1}{C} \times V_T + R\dot{V} \qquad \textit{(Equation 4)}$$

Measurements of lung mechanics

The introduction of the esophageal balloon to estimate pleural pressure[440, 445, 471] represented a major step forward in overcoming the technical problems of measurement of lung mechanics. It provides a safe measurement of P_L and, when recorded simultaneously with measurements of air flow and lung volume, it gives considerable information on the mechanical properties of the lungs. The technical aspects of recording the esophageal pressure have been described and analyzed

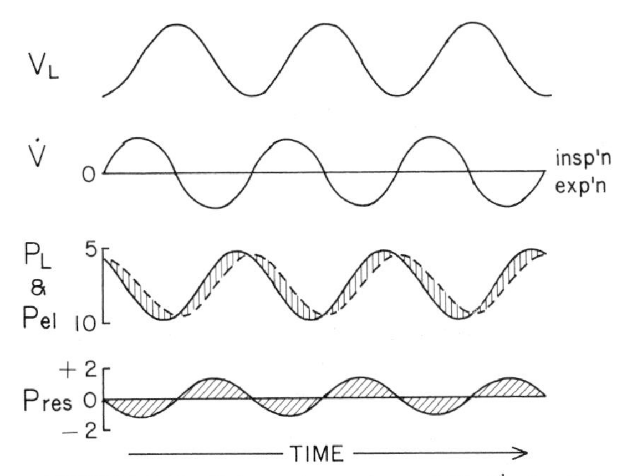

FIGURE 2–5. Schematic tracings of V_L, $\dot{V}$, P_L, Pel, and Pres during quiet breathing.

in a number of papers.[444–456, 2293, 2306] In Figure 2–5 are shown tracings of P_L, $\dot{V}$, and V_L. From such a tracing, made during spontaneous breathing, the dynamic compliance (Cdyn) and R_L can be computed. From equation 2, when flow is zero, Pres must be zero, and the only component of P_L is Pel. It follows that at points of zero flow at the extremes of tidal volume, the change in Pel may be read directly from the tracing of P_L, and compliance may be estimated as the ratio of the tidal volume to the change in P_L. Since, as noted earlier, the relationship between Pel and V_L over the tidal volume range is usually linear, Pel may be estimated from the tracing of P_L throughout the whole breath. This has been drawn graphically as the interrupted line in the third panel of Figure 2–5. Because

$$P_L = \text{Pres} + \text{Pel},$$

the shaded area must represent Pres, and this is drawn in the fourth panel of the figure. R_L may then be estimated as the ratio Pres/$\dot{V}$ at any point on the breathing cycle.

LUNG ELASTICITY

Measurements of lung compliance provide only limited information as to the elastic properties of lungs. Compliance is influenced by lung volume, by lung volume history (whether or not a deep inspiration or a full expiration has been made immediately prior to the measurement of compliance), by respiratory frequency in some normal subjects and in many diseases, and by time.

The only adequate measure of the lung's elastic properties is the static pressure–volume curve of the lung, in which absolute transpulmonary pressure is related to absolute lung volume over the whole vital capacity range, on both inflation and deflation. Such a curve is shown in Figure 2–6. The curve may be measured below FRC, but it is likely that at these lung volumes there is an artefact in the measured esophageal pressure.[2293] The curve is obtained by having the subject breathe in deeply from RV or FRC to TLC, and then breath-hold, with the glottis open for one or two seconds, at a number of different lung volumes as the inspiration proceeds. In a similar fashion, the subject breathes back out from TLC to FRC or RV. Absolute lung volume is then plotted against P_L during the breath-hold periods, and because flow is zero at these times, P_L will equal Pst. If volume is measured plethysmographically or by integration of the pneumotachygraph signal, the breath-holding maneuver may be accomplished easily by placing one's hand over the mouthpiece. If a spirometer or bag–box system is used, a manually operated three-way tap or solenoid valve may be placed in the mouthpiece assembly.

In order to correct for body size in patients with suspected lung disease, the static elastic recoil pressure may be plotted against the percentage of the predicted TLC. Figure 2–7 shows typical deflation static pressure-volume curves in normal subjects[2380] and in patients with asthma in bronchospasm,[2381] emphysema,[2381] rheumatic valvular disease,[2382, 2383] and pulmonary fibrosis.[583] In patients with emphysema the curve is shifted upward and to the left, indicating a marked loss of elastic recoil. In asthmatic subjects with bronchospasm there is also loss of recoil,[2384, 2585] but there are conflicting results from different studies of such patients in remission. We reported a slight loss of recoil in older asthmatics, but normal values in those under the age of 20 years.[583] Gold and his colleagues[2585] found that recoil returned to normal in remission, whereas Finucane and Colebatch reported that the loss of recoil persisted.[2381] Woolcock and Read[2384] found that elastic recoil returned to normal in half their patients, but apparently remained abnormal in the other half.

In patients with pulmonary fibrosis the

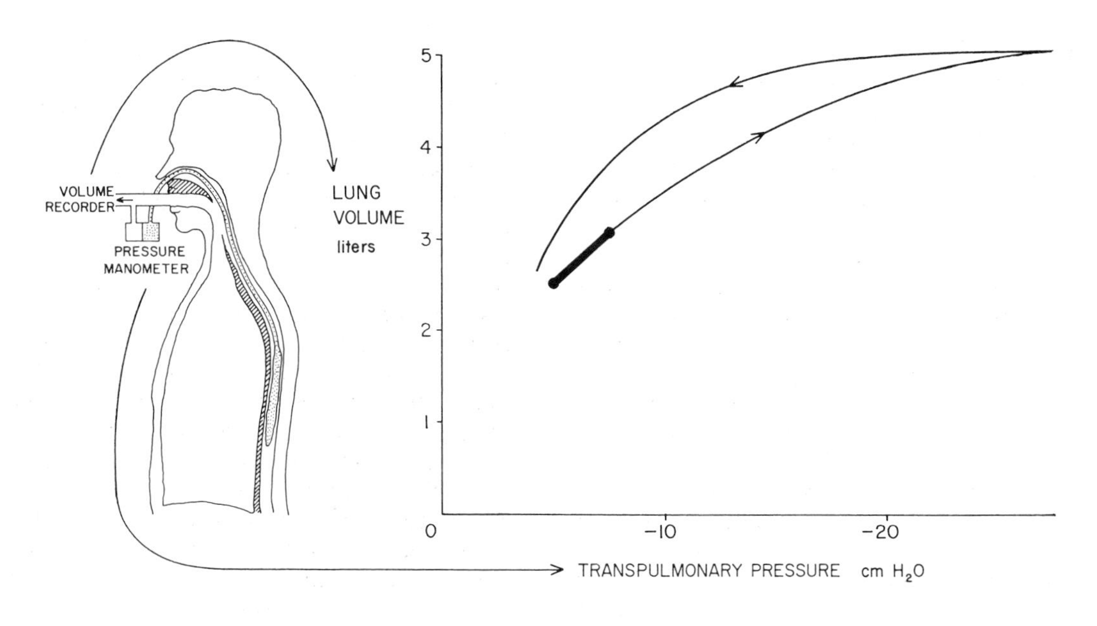

$$\text{STATIC COMPLIANCE} = \frac{\Delta V}{\Delta P} = \frac{0{\cdot}500}{2{\cdot}5} = 0{\cdot}200 \text{ liter/cm}$$

FIGURE 2–6. STATIC PRESSURE–VOLUME RELATIONSHIPS IN A NORMAL SUBJECT

The static compliance, expressed as liters per cm H_2O, is the ratio of volume change, shown on the ordinate, to pressure change, shown on the abscissa. The heavy line marks the normal range of tidal volume during a quiet inspiration, where the relationship between volume and pressure change is approximately linear. This is the value commonly used to describe the elastic properties of the lung. Note, however, that even in the normal subject, the relationship changes over the inspiratory range and that there is a difference between the inspiratory and deflation curves.

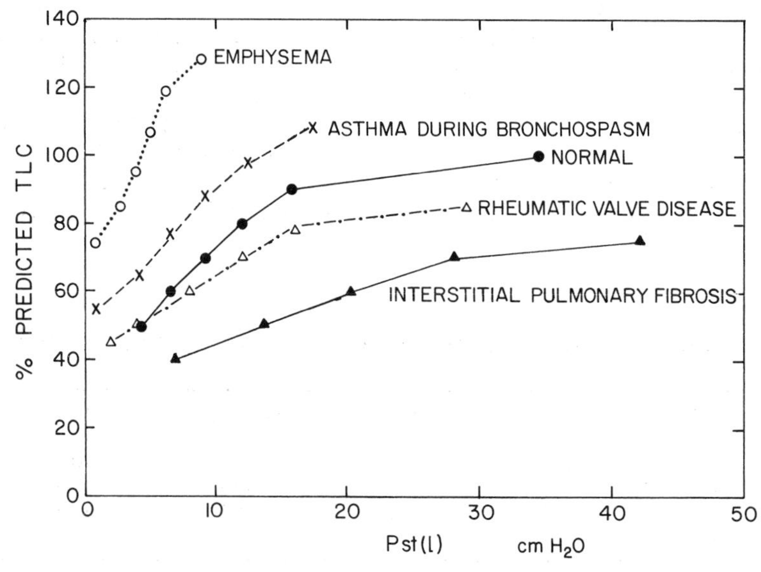

FIGURE 2–7. Static deflation pressure–volume curves in emphysema,[2414] asthma during bronchospasm,[2414] normal subjects,[2413] rheumatic valve disease.[2415, 2416] The curve for interstitial pulmonary fibrosis was obtained during inflation.[583]

curve is shifted downward and to the right, indicating a marked increase in elastic recoil at all lung volumes. In patients with rheumatic valvular disease, there is commonly an increase in recoil at high lung volumes and a decreased recoil at low lung volumes below FRC.[2383]

Many factors contribute to the shape and position of the static pressure volume curve of the lung. Lung volume history is clearly an important factor, as shown by the difference between the inflation and deflation curves in Figure 2–6. Another important factor is age, since the elastic recoil falls with age, as indicated in the data in Table 2–2. The state of the lung tissue is clearly another important determinant, as is the nature of the air–liquid interface in the lung. It is not yet clear how the recoil may change, as it apparently does in asthma, nor exactly why the aging of the lung should be associated with a loss of recoil that is disproportionate to any morphological changes.

SURFACE TENSION

Although von Neergaard in 1929 pointed out that surface tension forces were likely to be concerned with the retractive force of the lung,[521] and Macklin produced evidence that a mucoid film probably lined the surfaces of the alveoli exposed to gas,[522, 523] there was until recently no organized body of thought on the exact interrelationship between structure, mechanical forces and surface tension in the lung. Contemporary knowledge has grown at a remarkable speed from two observations made at about the same time: Radford[24, 524] observed that the pressure–volume loop of a saline-filled lung was different from that of an air-filled lung, insofar as hysteresis was much reduced when the lung was filled with fluid; and Pattle[525] showed that the fluid formed in the lung as a result of pulmonary edema had a much lower surface tension – or a much higher level of surface activity – than did plasma. The subsequent study of the physical properties of extracts of lung, pioneered by Clements and his co-workers,[526] showed that, in animals, while the surface was expanding (i.e., during inspiration), surface retractive forces were considerable, being similar to the elastic retractive forces of the lung tissue itself. However, while the surface was contracting (i.e., during expiration) these forces were very much less. Thus the pressure–volume plot of the surface extract of the lung shows considerable hysteresis and probably is responsible at least in part for the hysteresis of the pressure–volume plot of human lungs, either directly or insofar as a lining layer of such material would enable more lung units to remain open for a longer period during expiration.

Because the pressure–volume curve of the saline-filled lung shows little hysteresis (i.e., the inflation and deflation curves are almost identical), the hysteresis observed in the air-filled lung must be attributed principally to the surface tension at the air–liquid interface, and not directly to the tissues. If this is true, inspection of the curve suggests that the surface tension must be higher on inflation than on deflation because at the same lung volume, Pst(l) is greater.

A recent comprehensive monograph by Scarpelli[2429] provides an excellent review of the rapidly expanding knowledge about surfactant, based on 328 references to the literature. Earlier reviews by Pattle,[529] Clements,[527] Mead,[434] and Radford,[1856] and the proceedings of a Ciba Symposium[26] provide additional background. A discussion of contemporary evidence bearing on the site of

TABLE 2–2 NORMAL VALUES OF ELASTIC RECOIL PRESSURE [Pst(l)] AS A FUNCTION OF AGE*

AGE	50% TLC	60% TLC	70% TLC	80% TLC	90% TLC	100% TLC
13–25	5.8	9.0	12.9	16.1	20.6	45.4
25–35	4.8	6.8	9.7	12.9	17.4	35.4
34–45	3.2	5.2	7.1	10.0	13.5	39.9
45–61	3.5	5.2	7.1	9.1	12.2	26.4

*See Reference 2380.
Note: All measurements expressed in cm H_2O.

formation of the surface active material is beyond the scope of this volume.

The Frictional Resistance of Airways and Lungs

The estimation of Pres, described earlier using measurements of esophageal pressure, includes the pressure required to overcome the friction between the air and the airways and the pressure required to overcome the viscosity of lung tissues. When related to flow, it therefore measures R_L. Alveolar pressure (*see* later) may be measured indirectly, so that a measurement of airway resistance is possible. The difference between R_L and Raw is the viscous resistance of lung tissue. Although earlier estimates of this resistance had placed it as high as 20 to 40 per cent of R_L,[480, 1365] more recent measurements indicate that it is probably negligible.[2389, 2744] It is probable that a pressure difference due to static pressure–volume hysteresis, which is not flow-resistive in nature, was included in the earlier measurements.

The method of measuring R_L graphically indicated in Figure 2–5 is laborious and time-consuming. A more satisfactory technique was described by Mead and Whittenberger in which the elastic component of P_L is subtracted electrically.[471] The resultant Pres–$\dot{V}$ curve is displayed on an oscilloscope, and R_L is read directly from an overlying rotatable grid. A newer method of measuring R_L has been described[2393, 2394] in which forced oscillations are generated from a loudspeaker at or near the resonant frequency of the lung. The basis of this technique is that at the resonant frequency elastic pressures are exactly equal and opposite to inertial pressures, so that only the flow-resistive pressure is being measured. This technique may also be used to measure the resistance of the total respiratory system (i.e., lungs plus chest wall) easily and rapidly, and it does not require the passage of an esophageal balloon.

Measurement of Alveolar Pressure by Use of a Body Plethysmograph

Before the body plethysmograph was used in respiratory physiology, some estimates of alveolar pressure were obtained by measuring the mouth pressure while air flow was momentarily stopped by an electric shutter that permitted mouth pressure to equilibrate with alveolar pressure. This technique, known as the "airway interruption technique,"[472] yielded estimates of air-flow resistance similar to those obtained with an esophageal balloon.[473] Mead and Whittenberger in 1954 concluded that the form of interrupter they tested did not measure alveolar pressure correctly because the diaphragm continued to act after airway interruption had occurred.[474] Several authors doubted whether it could be used in certain patients with lung disease in whom pressure equilibrium between mouth and some alveoli at least might be slow. Clements and his colleagues in 1959[475] described a more elaborate device that interrupted air flow 10 times per second; this gave satisfactorily reproducible and accurate results in normal subjects, but the authors considered it unsuitable for patients with obstructive lung disease. Though results in such patients have been reported,[476–478, 727] its usefulness appears to be limited.

The introduction of the pressure-sealed body plethysmograph[479] represented a major step forward in the difficult problem of measuring effective alveolar pressure and, hence, distinguishing the two components of flow resistance, namely, airway resistance and tissue resistance.[480] As mentioned previously (*see* page 14), the pressure plethysmograph was reintroduced by Comroe, DuBois, and their colleagues[120, 122, 479] as an air-tight cabinet in which the subject could be seated. To measure air-flow resistance the subject is required to pant into the plethysmograph through a heated pneumotachygraph that records air flow. The alveolar pressure at any instant can be deduced from pressure changes in the plethysmograph. The change in alveolar pressure relative to mouth pressure (as must occur to cause air flow in and out of the lungs) is the result of rarefaction or compression of gas in the lungs. This leads to pressure changes within the plethysmograph which are in phase with and directly proportional to alveolar pressure. The relationship between plethysmograph and alveolar pressure can be established by a calibration study.

Mention has been made already of a volume plethysmograph described by Mead.[124] It is smaller and made of lighter materials than the pressure plethysmographs and therefore is more portable and cheaper to construct, and its requirements as to air-tightness are less exacting. Mead[124] considers that, whereas the pressure plethysmograph is obligatory to study such phenomena as pulmonary capillary flow,[122] for most respiratory purposes the simpler volume plethysmograph is quite as suitable, and measurements of air-flow resistance can easily be made with it.

A plethysmographic method has several advantages that the esophageal-balloon method lacks for the sensitive measurement of air-flow resistance, in particular the fact that measurement of esophageal pressure is unnecessary and that almost simultaneous measurements of lung volume can be made.

However, lung elastic recoil cannot be measured without use of an esophageal balloon, and many workers continue to use the latter method (i.e., stimultaneous measurement of volume, intra-esophageal pressure, and flow) for routine studies.

Factors influencing resistance

Lung volume

Resistance varies inversely with lung volume, and the relationship between the two is hyperbolic.[481] The change with lung volume is due to the increase in diameter of the airways as the lung volume increases. The elastic elements in the lung are attached not only to the pleural surface but also to the outer walls of airways and extra-alveolar blood vessels, with the result that peribronchial pressure is equal to[2395] or more negative than pleural pressure. With increasing lung volume, therefore, there is increasing traction on the outer walls of airways and their diameter increases. In dogs, the greatest changes in resistance with lung volume occur in 3- to 8-mm diameter airways.[2387] The change in resistance with volume is not simply a matter of increased elastic recoil at high lung volumes but depends upon bronchomotor tone as well.[2387] In the absence of such tone, the resistance of the tracheobronchial tree changes markedly at low lung volumes, remains relatively constant over the mid-lung volume, and then actually increases somewhat at high lung volumes, both in the dog[2387, 2744] and in man.[2396]

In assessing the significance of a measurement of resistance, it is therefore of importance to take into account the effect of lung volume.[481, 1082]

Relative resistance of central and peripheral airways

The contribution of different-sized airways to the total pulmonary resistance has been measured recently in dogs[2390, 2391, 2544, 2744] and in human lungs obtained at autopsy.[2544] In normal man and dog, the resistance of airways smaller than 2 mm in diameter has been shown to be only about 0.1 to 0.2 cm H_2O/liter/sec, and it therefore comprises only about 10 to 30 per cent of total lower pulmonary resistance. These results are in good agreement with estimates based on anatomical measurements.[2388, 2400] Since the resistance of the upper airway is about 50 per cent of the total,[1851, 2397] the resistance of the peripheral airways can account for only about 5 to 15 per cent of total pulmonary resistance. This conclusion is of major significance in relation to understanding of airway obstruction, since it follows that if the obstruction were to be selectively situated in peripheral airways, it would have little influence on R_L until it was far advanced. However, it would be likely to have a significant effect on ventilation distribution and gas exchange, since such a process would be unlikely to be uniformly distributed throughout the lung. This appears to be the case at an early stage of chronic bronchitis, when the $FEV_{1.0}$ is still almost normal.[2398, 2532] Furthermore, in advanced obstructive disease, the major site of obstruction in the absence of dynamic compression (*see* page 34) is located in airways less than 2 mm in diameter.[2544]

Airway conductance and specific conductance

Because the relationship between airway resistance and lung volume is hyperbolic, the relationship between the inverse of resistance and lung volume is linear. This inverse is called "airway conductance" and is symbolized by Gaw. This linear relationship permits the influence of lung volume to be taken into account when Gaw is expressed as the "specific airway conductance" (SGaw) or conductance per unit volume. Normal values for SGaw are given in Table 2–3.

Dynamic compression of airways

Measurement of events occurring during forced expirations is an extremely common test of lung function. It includes the FEV and its variously timed subdivisions, and

TABLE 2–3 NORMAL VALUES FOR SPECIFIC AIRWAY CONDUCTANCE AND RESISTANCE

AGE	SEX	SMOKING	SGAW (sec^{-1} cm H_2O^{-1})	SRAW (sec cm H_2O)	REF
Adult	M	NS	0.24	4.1	2379, 2767
Adult	M	S	0.23	4.3	2379, 2767
Adult	F	NS	0.22	4.5	2379
Adult	F	S	0.16	6.2	2379
20–26	F	NS & S	0.25	4.0	2385
4–18	M & F	–	0.17	5.9	481, 2386
2	M & F	–	0.17	5.9	2411
1 hr–11 days	M & F	–	0.45	2.2	668, 2412

SGAW = Specific airway conductance = airway conductance per unit lung volume
SRAW = Specific airway resistance = 1/SGAW
M = Males; F = Females
NS = Nonsmoker; S = Smoker

analyses of expiratory velocity such as the Peak Flow Rate and the Maximal Midexpiratory Flow Rate. Analysis of what occurs under these conditions is complex (*see* page 36), but it is clear that when pleural pressure becomes greater than atmospheric pressure during forced expiration and cough, it will compress and narrow those airways within which the pressure is less than pleural pressure. This phenomenon is known as "dynamic compression." Einthoven[2414] was the first to appreciate the importance of this in the pathophysiology of obstructive airway disease. Subsequently, Dayman[939] observed that in patients with emphysema, the expiratory flow reached a maximum value and then decreased, even though the pressure producing the flow continued to increase. By recording pressures in the bronchial tree, a number of workers have shown that this flow limitation can be due to collapse of large airways in human disease.[2837]

MAXIMAL EXPIRATORY FLOW-VOLUME CURVE

A major advance in understanding forced expirations came with the work of Hyatt, Schilder, and Fry.[68] They described the maximal expiratory flow volume curve (MEFV). This is illustrated in Figure 2–8, which shows a curve obtained during a forced vital capacity expiration when instantaneous expiratory airflow is plotted against lung volume instead of time (as is done for the FEV.) Flow increases rapidly, reaches a maximum at about 80 per cent of the vital capacity, and then decreases, reaching a value of zero at residual volume. The curve consists of an effort-dependent portion above about 75 per cent of VC, and an effort-independent portion below 75 per cent of VC. The effort-dependent part depends upon how rapidly the expiratory muscles can contract and is an expression of the force–velocity relationship of these muscles.[2424] The effort-independent part shows the relationship between lung volume and the maximal expiratory flow that is possible. Once sufficient effort has been used to reach this line, flow becomes limited at its maximal value, and increasing degrees of effort will not produce any further increase in flow.

On the left-hand side of Figure 2–9, flow rates during quiet breathing are shown over the tidal volume range. It is clear that there is

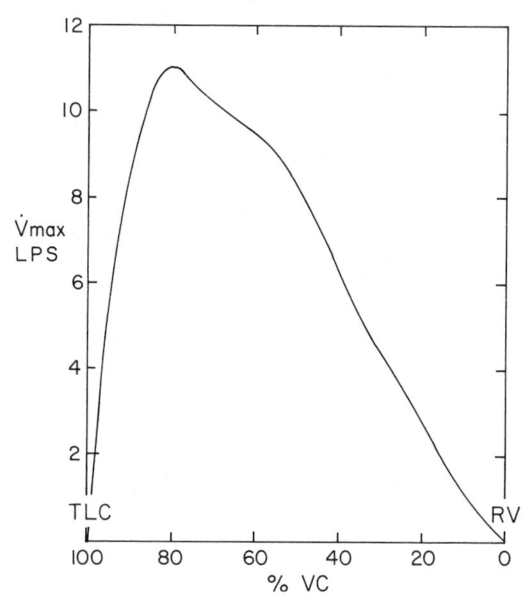

FIGURE 2–8. Normal maximal expiratory flow volume curve.

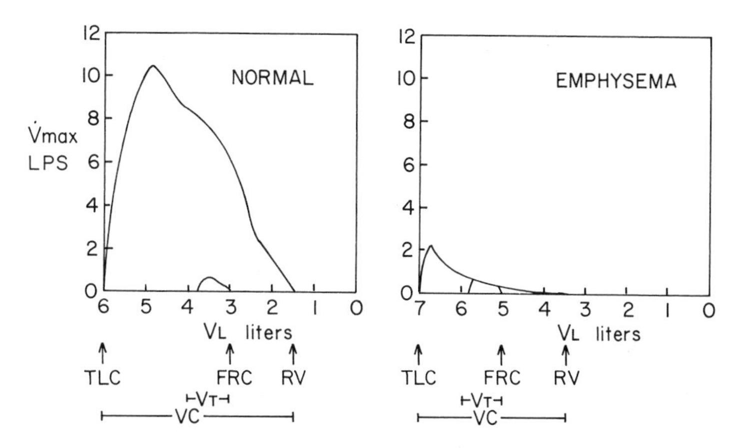

FIGURE 2–9. Left panel: Normal maximal expiratory flow volume curve together with flow rates during quiet breathing over the tidal volume range. Right panel: Maximal expiratory flow volume obtained from patient with emphysema. Flow rates during quiet breathing are the maximal ones over the tidal volume range.

a very large ventilatory reserve and that the normal person can increase both his tidal volume and flow to a considerable extent before he reaches maximal values. In fact, not even during maximal exercise do normal subjects require maximal expiratory flow.[2405] Probably the only time that maximal flow is achieved is during coughing. The MEFV curve in the patient with emphysema, shown on the right-hand side of Figure 2–9, is markedly abnormal. The slope of the curve is much reduced, and this, together with the reduction in vital capacity, severely limits the ventilatory reserve available to him. In the example shown, in order to breathe quietly at rest, the patient requires flow rates which are at his maximal possible value. This situation is typical of advanced obstructive airway disease.[485] The only way that such a patient can increase his minute ventilation is by increasing his lung volume or by decreasing the time of inspiration.

When a subject is instructed to perform a series of vital-capacity expirations of graded effort, varying from a very slow breath out to one of maximal speed and effort, a series of curves, as shown in Figure 2–10, is obtained. The intersection of these curves with the line AB shows the flows obtained as the subject passes through a specific lung volume, in this case 50 per cent of VC. Hyatt and his colleagues plotted these flows obtained at the same volume against the simultaneous values for transpulmonary pressure and obtained the isovolume pressure–flow curves similar to the example shown in Figure 2–11. At zero flow, P_L is Pst(l) at that volume, and because flow ($\dot{V}$) and P_L are measured at the same lung volume with each breath, Pst(l) remains constant. As $\dot{V}$ increases with each expiration, pleural pressure (Ppl) becomes less negative and eventually becomes positive. As it becomes more and more positive it compresses the intrathoracic airway, increasing the airway resistance until a point is reached (at a Ppl of 15 cm H_2O in Figure 2–11) beyond which further increases in pressure result in proportionate increases in resistance so that $\dot{V}$ remains constant at its maximal value for this lung volume.

Permutt and his colleagues obtained curves similar to these, using a simple mechanical analogue, the Starling resistor, illustrated in Figure 2–12. This consists of a collapsible

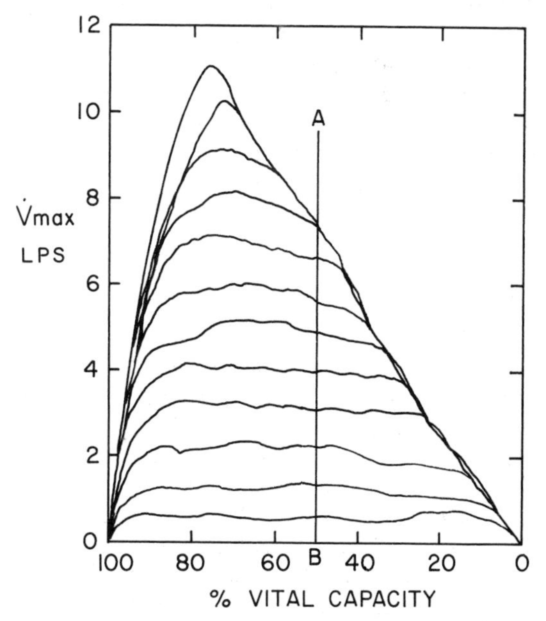

FIGURE 2–10. Flow volume curves obtained when a subject performs a series of vital capacity expirations of graded effort, varying from a very slow breath out to one of maximal speed and effort.

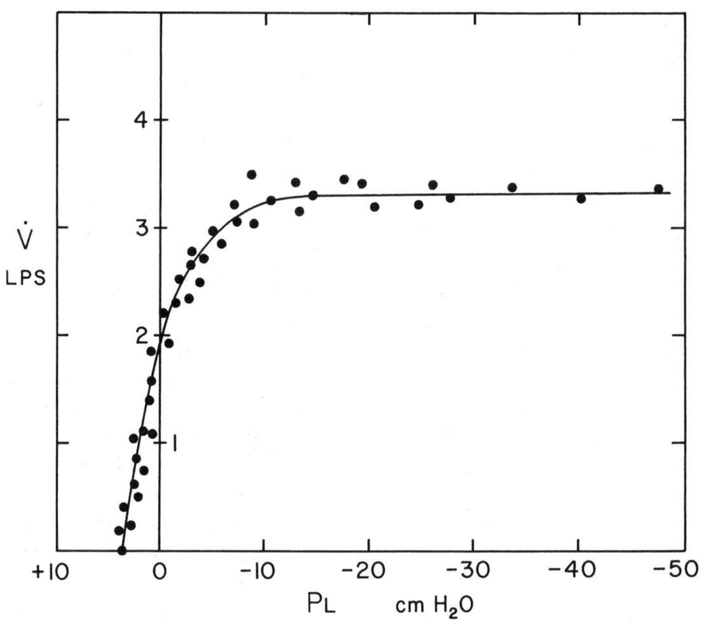

FIGURE 2–11. An example of the iso-volume pressure flow curve obtained in a normal subject at 33 per cent VC. These curves are obtained from a family of curves similar to that shown in Figure 2–10 by plotting the flows as the subject passes through a specific lung volume against the simultaneous values of transpulmonary pressure.

tube enclosed in a chamber. There is a pressure difference between the ends of the tube, $P_1 - P_3$, where P_1 is the pressure at the inlet and P_3 the pressure at the outlet. He found that when the pressure surrounding the tube, P_2, is greater than P_3, flow is dependent on the difference between P_1 and P_2 rather than that between P_1 and P_3. By keeping $P_1 - P_2$ constant and lowering P_3 from a point at which it was equal to P_1 (i.e., at which no flow was occurring) to a point at which it was less than P_2, curves could be obtained similar to isovolume pressure–flow curves. Flow increases until $P_3 = P_2$, but when P_3 is less than P_2, flow does not change but remains constant and independent of $P_1 - P_3$. Applying this concept to the lung, we see that the inlet is analogous to the alveoli and that P_1 is analogous to alveolar pressure. P_3 is the mouth pressure, and the pressure in the surrounding chamber, P_2, corresponds to Ppl.

In analyzing the similarities between the simple model and the isovolume pressure flow curve, Mead and his co-workers[2406] and Permutt and his colleagues[2407] have developed different, but complementary, concepts of how the lungs behave during a forced expiration.

Mead's concept is as follows: During forced expiration the pressure inside the airway at the alveolar end is alveolar pressure; in the trachea it is close to atmospheric pressure and may even be negative.[2408] The pressure at the outer walls of the airways is equal to pleural pressure[7] or, in the case of intrapulmonary airways, possibly slightly more

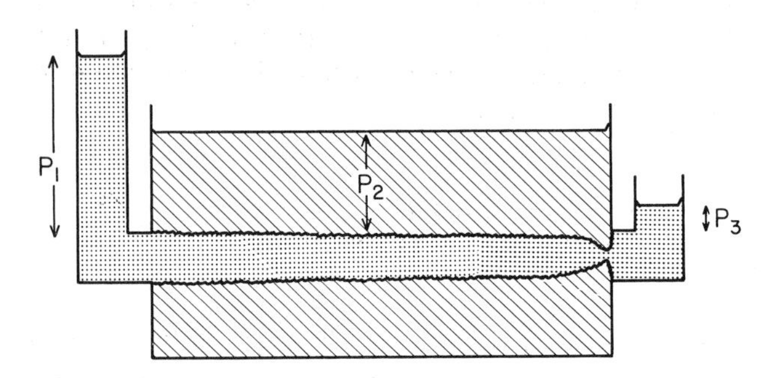

FIGURE 2–12. Diagram of a Starling resistor. This consists of a segment of collapsible tubing contained in a chamber which exerts a pressure (P_2) on the outer wall of the tube. The pressure at the inlet, producing flow through the tube, is P_1, and the pressure at the outlet is P_3. When $P_2 > P_3$ flow is independent of the total driving pressure ($P_1 - P_3$), but is proportional to $P_1 - P_2$, which is the "effective" driving pressure in this circumstance.

negative than pleural pressure. Thus, at the alveolar end the pressure inside is greater than that outside, whereas at the mouth the opposite is true. It follows that at some point or points along the airway the pressure inside is exactly equal to that outside. Such points are referred to as "equal pressure points." It is only downstream from equal pressure points that dynamic compression of airways, and therefore flow limitation, can occur. The pressure drop from alveoli to the equal pressure point (EPP) is the pressure drop from alveolar pressure to pleural pressure and therefore equals the elastic recoil pressure. At any particular lung volume (as on an isovolume pressure flow curve) the elastic recoil pressure is constant. Once peak flow is achieved (at the plateau of an isovolume pressure flow curve), flow also remains constant. Because the pressure drop from alveoli to EPP is constant, and the flow is constant, the resistance of airways between alveoli and the EPP must also be constant. This resistance is referred to as the upstream resistance. Thus, at maximum flow at any given lung volume, the lungs may be regarded as a fixed resistor (the upstream resistance) in series with a variable resistor (the airways dynamically compressed downstream from the EPP). In a series of resistors, flow may be expressed as the pressure drop down any of the segments divided by the resistance of that segment. This may be expressed as follows:

$$\dot{V}_{max} = \frac{Pst(l)}{Rus}$$

where Rus equals the resistance of airways between alveoli and the EPP. In this analysis, the elastic recoil pressure is the "effective" driving pressure producing maximum flow in the same way as the inflow pressure minus the surrounding pressure is the effective pressure-producing flow in a Starling resistor. This points up the important conclusion that maximal expiratory flow rates, whether measured as the FEV or by any of the other methods of analysis, are just as dependent on the elastic properties of the lung as they are on the state of the airways.

The analysis of Pride and Permutt[2407] takes into consideration events occurring downstream from the EPP. At some point or points downstream, the dynamic compression reaches a transmural pressure sufficiently great to narrow the airway enough to limit flow. All events downstream from this point have no influence on the flow. Upstream from this point, at any given lung volume the transmural pressures remain constant, so that the resistance of the airways between the EPP and the flow-limiting segment also remains constant. Thus, both concepts regard maximal flow from the lungs as resulting from a fixed driving pressure operating through a fixed resistor in series with a variable resistor. In the equal pressure point theory, the fixed resistor is regarded as extending from the alveoli to the equal pressure points, but in the analysis of Pride and Permutt it extends from alveoli to the flow-limiting segment. The two concepts are therefore complementary and not in conflict with each other.

There are, however, important differences between the two approaches. Mead's analysis does not take into consideration the mechanisms by which flow is limited. It does point up the major factors which determine the maximum value for flow that can be achieved, that is, the elastic properties of lungs and the resistance of smaller airways. Yet, unless properly understood, the approach can be misleading. For example, a very flaccid segment of the intrathoracic part of the trachea could act as a flow-limiting segment as soon as the pressure inside it became less than pleural pressure. The EPP would become fixed just upstream from this point and maximum flow would be less than normal. Rus would be increased because the length of the upstream segment would be longer than normal. Although it is unlikely that this would result in a marked decrease in flow,[2406] it would be wrong to conclude that flow was reduced *owing* to an increase in Rus. In fact, in this circumstance Rus is increased *owing* to the reduction in flow.

Permutt's analysis avoids the possibility of such a misinterpretation. Although somewhat more complex than Mead's approach, it takes into consideration the exact mechanism by which flow is limited and thus makes up for its additional complexity by taking into account the mechanical properties of the flow-limiting segment—a feature lacking in equal pressure point theory.

RELATIONSHIP BETWEEN AIRWAY RESISTANCE AND VENTILATION DISTRIBUTION

In a later section (*see* pages 45–47) it is shown that the variation in intrapleural pressure plays an important part in determining ventilation distribution, which is also influenced by the shape of the pressure–volume curve of the lung. In this section we discuss the interrelationship between the airways and their frictional properties, and ventilation distribution.

One of the most remarkable features of most young normal lungs is that all the millions of alveoli fill and empty synchronously during both slow and rapid breathing. In Figure 2–13 is shown a model of a two-compartment lung in which the airways are represented by the common and branched pathways and are connected to airspaces. The branch to airspace A is constricted. Let us apply a pressure change across the model of 5 cm H_2O and allow a sufficient length of time for both airspaces to fill. Assume that the volume change in each is 500 ml. The compliance of the model is the total volume change divided by the pressure change, or

$$\frac{500 + 500}{5} = 0.2 \text{ liters/cm } H_2O$$

If we had not allowed sufficient time for both airspaces to fill, the volume change in airspace A would have lagged behind that in airspace B because the airway leading to it is constricted. By adjusting the resistance to A appropriately, we could arrange that by the time B had received 500 ml at the end of inspiration, A would have received only 100 ml. Under these circumstances the measured compliance would be only

$$\frac{500 + 100}{5} \text{ or } 0.12 \text{ liters/cm } H_2O$$

Compartment A would lag behind B and asynchronous behavior would result. During slow cycle frequencies the compliance of this model would be greater than during rapid frequencies, i.e., compliance would be frequency dependent.

A detailed analysis of the mechanical principles which determine whether or not the lungs will behave synchronously was presented for the first time in the classic paper by Otis and his colleagues.[147] As they pointed out, when Cdyn falls with increasing respiratory frequency (as it does in obstructive airway disease), the lungs are behaving asynchronously and there are phase differences in filling between different parts. In most normal lungs, Cdyn is independent of respiratory frequency up to about 100 breaths per minute. Normal lungs thus behave synchronously over physiological breathing frequencies, and there is evidence that this may be true even at frequencies as high as 5 cycles per second.[2393]

Whether or not all the units within the lung behave synchronously depends upon the uniformity of the "time constants" of different units. The time constant is the product of the compliance of the unit and that part of the resistance that is not shared with other units (i.e., common pathways such as the trachea and upper airway). Otis and his colleagues[147] suggested that the fact that dynamic compliance in the normal lung was not affected by frequency meant that all the time constants must be equal or nearly so. If this were the case, it would imply that there were extraordinary structural interrelationships among pathway length, pathway diameter, and regional compliance, because the pathway

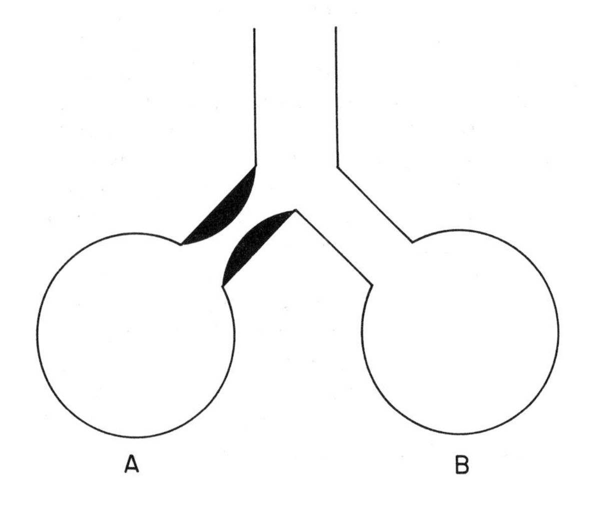

FIGURE 2–13. Two-compartment lung model illustrating the mechanical behavior of lungs when the mechanical properties of each compartment are different.

lengths are known to vary from 7 cm to 21 cm.[2362] However, the observation that the resistance of peripheral airways is low allows for less rigorous structural requirements.[2744] Units subtended by these airways have low absolute values for their individual time constants. This allows for considerable inequalities of these time constants, yet essentially synchronous behavior will still result at physiological breathing frequencies because the absolute values of the time constants are so small. The development of asynchronism depends not only on the degree of inequality of the time constants but also on the time taken to complete a breathing cycle relative to the absolute value of the time constant.

Other factors have recently been shown to be important in producing synchronous behavior. Mead and his colleagues[2401] have pointed out that because lung units are interconnected, they cannot be treated as if they were similar to a bunch of grapes hanging on a vine, from which it is possible to remove one grape without moving its neighbors. In the lung, because of common walls between alveoli, it will require more pressure to move a given unit out of phase with its neighbors than it does to move it in phase. The units are thus made interdependent, permitting a greater degree of time constant inequality before asynchrony develops.

Finally, even when small airways are considerably obstructed, producing marked time-constant discrepancies, air may enter the obstructed units through collateral channels. If this occurs sufficiently rapidly, synchronous behavior will still result.[2399, 2402] Collateral ventilation is sufficiently rapid in the dog but is slow or absent in the pig.[2399, 2403] The human lung appears to lie somewhere between the dog lung and the pig lung in this regard[2403] and asynchronous behavior in humans with airway obstruction but with a normal parenchyma is likely. Recently it has been shown that in emphysema the resistance of collateral channels is extremely low, lower, in fact, than airway resistance may be in this disease.[2402] It is to be presumed, therefore, that in some patients with emphysema, collateral channels are extremely important ventilatory pathways.

Thus, synchronous behavior is achieved in lungs in spite of time-constant inequalities of moderate degree,[2387] first, because the resistance of peripheral airways is low; second, because of interdependence of lung units; and third, because in some species, at least, ventilation of airspaces through collateral channels may occur just as rapidly as ventilation of these spaces through airways.

Work of breathing: oxygen cost of respiration

From a continuous analysis of the relationship of pressure (which is an expression of force) to volume (which is an expression of distance) during steady-state breathing conditions, it is possible to compute the work of breathing in mechanical terms. Fenn first drew attention to the various factors involved in the work of breathing, and his analysis of this aspect of pulmonary mechanics[32] provides an excellent starting point for anyone concerned with this aspect of respiration. Subsequently the work of breathing was reviewed by Otis in 1954,[443] although the reader perhaps should be advised that many contributions have been made since that date.

Normal subjects have been studied at rest and on exercise,[486–490] and during hyperventilation,[443, 2262] and the mechanical work at different respiratory rates has been measured.[491, 492] The mechanical work for a given ventilation does not appear to be influenced by athletic training;[493] it is increased in recumbency compared with the upright position largely because of an increased airway resistance when the subject is lying flat.[494] The same mechanism is mainly responsible for the increased work that accompanies orthopnea, together with some compliance change in some patients.[495, 496] It can be shown[443] that for any given system there must be a certain respiratory frequency that represents the most economical rate of breathing in terms of work that has to be done against the mechanical properties of the lung and is wasted in ventilating the dead space. It is clear that deep breaths will necessitate more work against the elastic recoil of the lung, whereas shallow breaths of high air flow at a fast rate will result in more energy loss overcoming resistance to gas flow in the airways and a wasteful ventilation of the dead space. Thus, there must be some respiratory rate for a given minute volume that represents the minimum rate of work for that particular set of circumstances. Subsequently it has been suggested that minimum "force per unit time" required from the respiratory muscles, rather than minimum work, is the predominant factor,[520] and indeed it seems a more logical mechanism than one that requires the integration of pressure and volume.

Mammals of very different size naturally breathe at rates and depths that represent their own minimal rates of respiratory work — a phenomenon clearly demonstrated by the studies of Crosfill and Widdicombe[462] and Agostoni and his colleagues.[506] The demonstration by Marshall and Christie,[507] that the observed spontaneous respiratory rate in patients with acute pneumonia also represented the most economical rate in that condition because pulmonary compliance had decreased, showed that this adaptive mechanism is capable of controlling the respiratory frequency when the mechanical characteristics of the lungs have altered. It is not known how these changes are signaled. The only physiological circumstance in which the work of breathing is reduced is reduction of atmospheric pressure (e.g., during residence at a high altitude or in decompression tanks).

Originally it seemed possible that the rate of respiratory work might be closely correlated with the sensation of dyspnea, and this proposition has been discussed by several authors.[3, 17, 495, 499–501] This complex problem is discussed in Chapter 23. It may be noted here that an excessive degree of respiratory work for a given level of ventilation does exist in emphysema,[497] mitral stenosis[498] and some other conditions, notably obesity.[502–504] Nisell has pointed out that in mitral stenosis the degree of dyspnea bears a closer relationship to respiratory pressure than to respiratory work.[505] Although the oxygen cost of breathing at rest is only about 1 per cent of the total oxygen uptake, this proportion rises considerably at very high ventilation rates, and the oxygen cost per unit ventilation increases considerably.[508, 509, 518] It may also change under different conditions of breathing,[510–515, 519] and in dogs, at least, it may be increased by breathing CO_2.[1857] If the respiratory system is mechanically abnormal, the oxygen cost of ventilation may seriously encroach on the oxygen available for external work.[510, 516, 517]

Widdicombe and Nadel explored the interrelationship that exists between anatomical dead-space volume and work of breathing at given levels of alveolar ventilation.[1858] Their calculations suggest that alterations in airway caliber might represent adjustments to ensure maintenance of a minimal work of breathing. It is of interest that the oxygen cost of breathing can be closely related to an index of respiratory force in kg/min, whereas the relationship to mechanical respiratory work in kgM/min depends upon the type of respiratory experiment performed.[520] Since the oxygen available for external work other than respiration is the difference between the total oxygen uptake and the oxygen used in breathing, in some clinical situations further exercise necessitating an increase in ventilation may reduce the oxygen supply to working muscles.

Recent studies of athletes at the extreme limit of exercise suggest that a point commonly may be reached at which any increase of ventilation would entail so great an oxygen cost for the respiratory muscles that no increased oxygen would be available for the muscles doing the external work;[2435] such an extreme situation is probably encountered only in those who have been trained to exercise to the absolute limit of their maximal oxygen uptake.

REGIONAL VENTILATION DISTRIBUTION

METHODS OF MEASUREMENT

During the past 10 years, there has been a great deal of development in the techniques that may be used to measure the regional distribution of ventilation in the lung. Until the introduction of radioactive gas techniques by Knipping and his colleagues in 1955,[330] the only method of assessing the regional distribution of ventilation was by bronchospirometry, and, as generally used, this was only of value in comparing the ventilation and oxygen uptake of one lung with that of the other. It may also be remarked that, although the physicians skilled in this technique developed great facility in it, its nature was such that studies on normal subjects were difficult to justify. As this section will indicate, the radioactive gas methods have provided new insight into the principles which underlie regional lung function. The techniques have also been employed in studying a variety of clinical conditions, and their usefulness in research and in clinical evaluation has been clearly established. In this section, only a brief summary of these techniques can be given. Many of the original papers contain useful technical data,[172, 173, 174, 175] and, more recently, we have elaborated on some of the details of instrumentation,[2456] West has reviewed the general field of radioactive gas studies,[2459] and other papers contain very useful technical details in the course of describing different kinds of research.[2457, 2460, 2461] A symposium held in Sweden in 1965[2437] provides a useful starting point and includes some debate on the relative advantages and disadvantages of different techniques.

Use of ^{133}xenon

Most methods of using ^{133}xenon make use of a comparison between the count rate recorded when the subject is equilibrated, with the gas in a closed spirometer circuit, and the count rate after a single breath or during equilibration. The technique has three variants: the detectors may be rigidly mounted and static; a pair of counters may scan the lung by being moved or by the patient being moved relative to them; or the ventilation may be studied by observing the clearance of xenon from the lung field following its delivery into the field after it has been dissolved in saline and injected into a vein. Each technique possesses advantages and disadvantages. Static counters are simpler to mount and enable wash-out and clearance studies to be undertaken; moving detectors scanning the lungs after a single breath and again after equilibration provide continuous scanning of all the lung instead of measuring in only 6 or 10 zones; and study of clearance after perfusion delivery permits an analysis of ventilation vis à vis perfusion that is not possible with tests involving inhalation alone.

Use of scintillation gamma camera and ^{135}xenon

^{135}Xenon, having a shorter half-life than ^{133}xenon, can only be used close to a production source, but it offers some advantages. The scintillation camera has been used very effectively with this gas,[2438] and also with the more easily obtained ^{133}xenon, and this technique is well suited to measurements of ventilation and perfusion distribution.[2436]

Whichever technique is used, the greater the amount of data collected, the more severe is the problem of assimilating it. Automatic data collection methods have been described,[2458] and the computer back-up of the scintillation camera[2438] may entail resources well beyond those the pulmonary function laboratory may be able to command. It seems very possible that in the next few years a general simplification of these techniques may come about, even enabling them to be used routinely or in screening studies.

Regional subdivisions of lung volume

Since most accounts of ventilatory function of the body as a whole begin with an account of the subdivisions of lung volume, it is logical to begin an account of regional ventilation distribution with a description of the *regional* subdivisions of lung volume (or the proportional inflation of different parts of the lung at different lung volumes). Measurements of the regional subdivisions of lung volume are based on the gas-dilution principle, using externally detected ^{133}xenon as the test gas.[2444] Regional volumes are expressed as a percentage of the volume of each region at TLC, i.e., TLC_r, the subscript r denoting a regional parameter. TLC_r thus denotes the volume of gas contained by a region at full inspiration (TLC). In Figure 2–14 are shown the regional subdivisions of lung volume as determined in eight normal young men, seated upright. Since, in normal subjects, at TLC the volume of the lung units ("alveoli") is probably uniform throughout the lung,[2441, 2444] regional volumes expressed as a percentage of TLC_r are also an expression of the volume of the alveoli. The upper abscissa of Figure 2–14 shows the volume "per alveolus" expressed as a percentage of the alveolar volume at TLC (i.e., TLC_{alv}).

It is apparent that at the end of a normal expiration (FRC) and of a maximal expiration (RV) the apical lung regions are more expanded than the basilar lung zones; that is to say that the regional FRC and the regional RV are both relatively greater in the upper zones of the lungs. The regional FRC (FRC_r) decreases approximately linearly with distance down the lung, whereas the regional RV (RV_r) is found to decrease progressively from the top of the lung to about its mid-level, and thereafter it remains more or less constant.

These regional differences in lung expansion can be explained by a mechanical model based on the combination of the gradient in pleural pressure in the vertical axis and the shape of the static volume–pressure curve of the lung.[2444, 2445] In upright man, there is be-

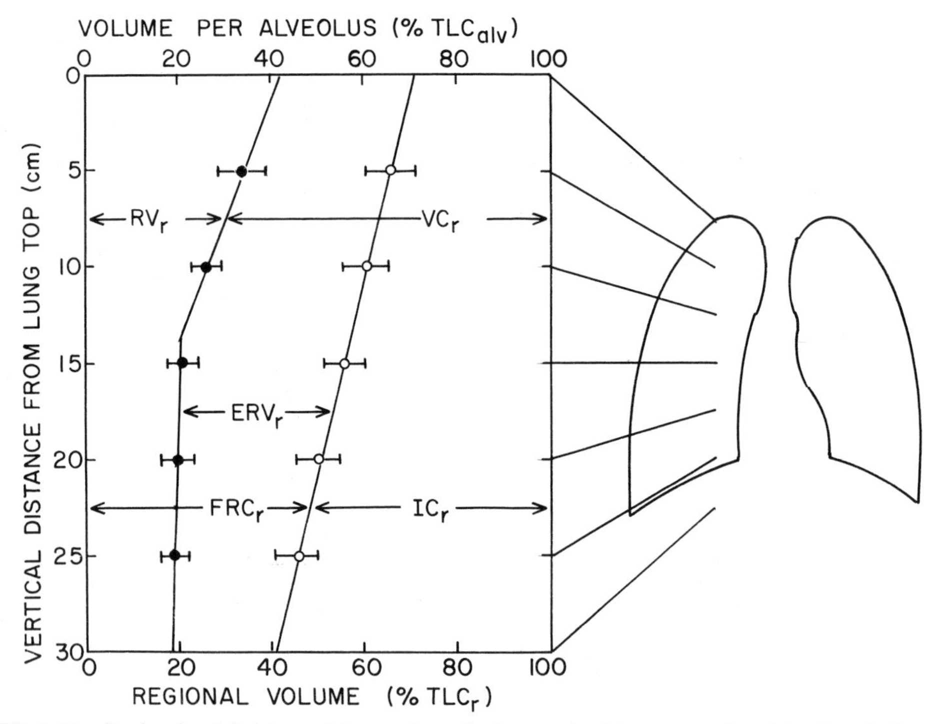

FIGURE 2–14. Regional subdivisions of lung volume in 8 normal subjects, seated upright. Bars indicate ±2 S.E. RV_r = regional residual volume; IC_r = regional inspiratory capacity; ERV_r = regional expiratory reserve volume; VC_r = regional vital capacity.

lieved to be a gradient in pleural pressure down the lung, with the more negative values toward the apex. Although its nature is not precisely understood, the gradient appears to be gravity dependent and related to the weight of the lung. For simplicity it may be assumed that pleural pressure increases at a constant rate of 0.25 cm H_2O per centimeter down the lung; thus, in a lung with a vertical length of 30 cm the total difference in pleural pressure from the top of the lung to the bottom amounts to 7.5 cm H_2O. The problem of measurement and analysis of the gradient in pleural pressure has recently been the object of study by three groups of workers.[2453, 2454, 2462] A detailed comparison of their findings is beyond the scope of this volume; however, it is clear that although much remains to be fully understood, the generalization just presented has been widely confirmed.

In Figures 2–15, 2–16, and 2–17 is shown the gradient in pleural pressure combined with the elastic properties of the lung (which are assumed to be uniform throughout the lungs). It is clear that the gradient in pleural pressure can account for the regional differences in lung expansion observed in the ^{133}xenon studies. At full inspiration (TLC) all regions are expanded nearly to a uniform degree, despite the vertical gradient in pressure, and this is because the static pressure volume curve is nearly flat near full inflation, so that the (still existent) pleural pressure difference down the lung does not cause any appreciable regional differences in expansion. As the lung volume decreases below TLC, the lung regions operate on a progressively steeper part of their pressure–volume curve, thus causing marked differences in regional expansion down the lung at these lower lung volumes.

It is important to note that at residual volume (*see* Figure 2–17) pleural pressure in dependent lung zones exceeds the airway pressure and is thus positive. This will lead to airway closure, and gas will be trapped behind the closed airways.[2392, 2450] Therefore, airway closure sets a limit to expiration from the dependent lung zones,[2444, 2450] the volume of trapped gas representing their minimal volume. The observation that the regional RV is virtually constant from about the middle of the lung to the bottom suggests that at full expiration all lung units in the lower half of the lungs have attained their minimal volume. By contrast, at least in

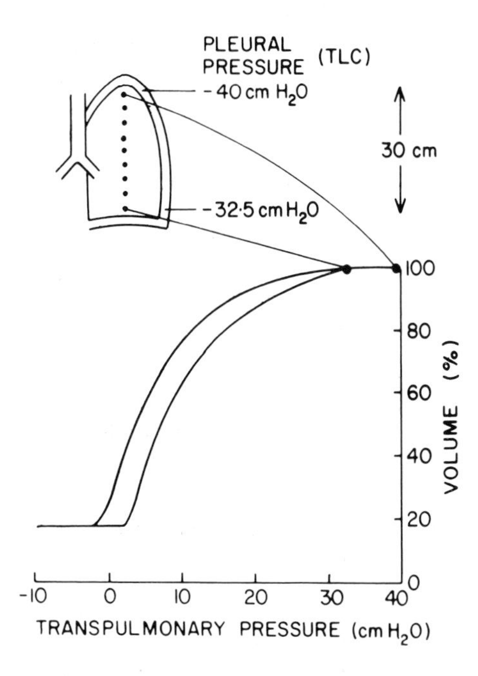

FIGURE 2–15. At maximally negative transpulmonary pressure (40 cm H_2O), the lungs are fully expanded (at TLC). Although there is a 7.5 cm H_2O difference between the top and the bottom of the lung, the volume of alveoli will be the same at the top and bottom of the lung, since the pressure-volume curve is nearly flat at this point. It is assumed that the pressure increases at a constant rate of 0.25 cm H_2O/cm vertical distance.

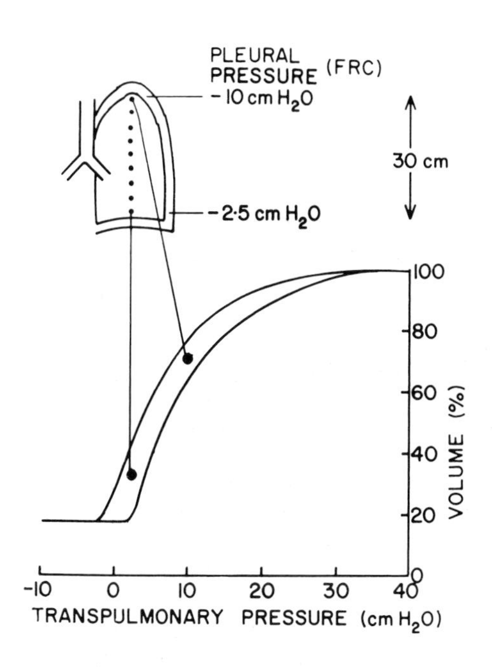

FIGURE 2–16. At FRC, because there is a 7.5 cm H_2O difference between the top and the bottom of the lung, alveoli in these regions are expanded to different degrees.

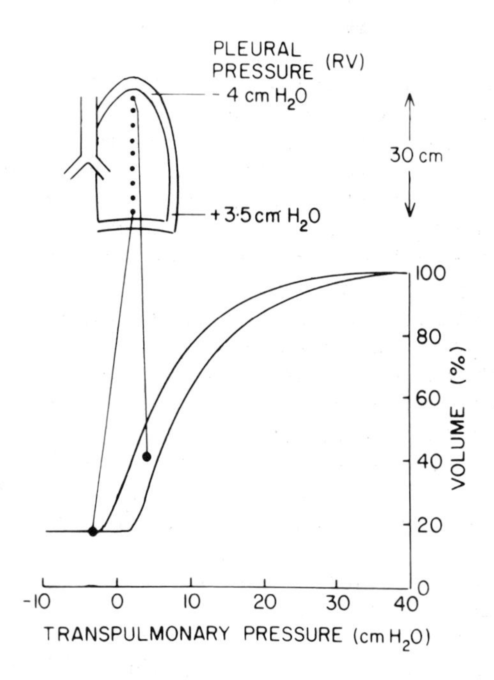

FIGURE 2–17. At residual volume (full expiration), airways at the bottom of the lung have closed, whereas airways at the top are still open because the upper lung regions are still at 40 per cent of their maximal volume.

young normal subjects, the upper lung units do not reach their minimal volume at the end of a maximal expiration.

This lung model effectively explains the changes that occur when the body position is changed and also accounts for the observed effect of aging on the lung. In the supine position, the distribution of gas between apex and base becomes more uniform,[2302] but differences in expansion will now exist between ventral and dorsal parts of the lungs (See Fig. 2–18). The pleural pressure gradient and the consequent differences in lung expansion will always occur "vertically" in the direction of gravity, while along the horizontal axis the regional distribution of gas will be almost uniform.[2442, 2444] In the lateral decubitus position, the lower lung will be better ventilated in the tidal volume range,[2442] an observation first made by Svanberg,[576] using bronchospirometry. Thus, the tidal ventilation is matched to the increased perfusion of the dependent lung by virtue of the shape of the pressure–volume curve—an interesting example of the operation of design of the system rather than of a control system. With increasing age, the shape of the pressure–volume curve changes. This will have the effect of leading to airway closure in dependent lung zones at a higher lung volume (or higher up the lung at the same lung volume) than will be the case in a young subject,[2432, 2455] and as a consequence the distribution of ventilation in the elderly subject will be critically dependent on the depth of breath taken, as Edelman and his colleagues found it to be.[2430] (See page 98).

Glazier and his colleagues[2441] have recently shown that there is a vertical gradient of alveolar size in the dog. This demonstration was made by freezing anesthetized dogs in an upright position and thus fixing the lungs in situ without alteration of the pleural pressure relationships that would be produced by opening the thorax (see Fig. 2–20).

REGIONAL DISTRIBUTION OF VENTILATION

West and Dollery[338] reported that when a normal, seated man took a breath of CO_2 labeled with radioactive oxygen ($^{15}O_2$), the ventilation per unit gas volume was greater in basal than in apical lung regions. Similar results were reported by ourselves[174] and Glaister.[2440] Using ^{133}xenon, we also observed that ventilation per unit gas volume becomes more uniform if the inspired volume is increased from resting tidal volume to a maximal inspiration.[2302] In all of these studies, inspiration was started from resting end-expiratory lung volume. A more complete analysis of the regional distribution of gas within the lung has recently been obtained by measuring the regional lung volumes at different overall lung volumes and covering the whole range of the vital capacity.[2442, 2444] Such measurements, obtained in four young,

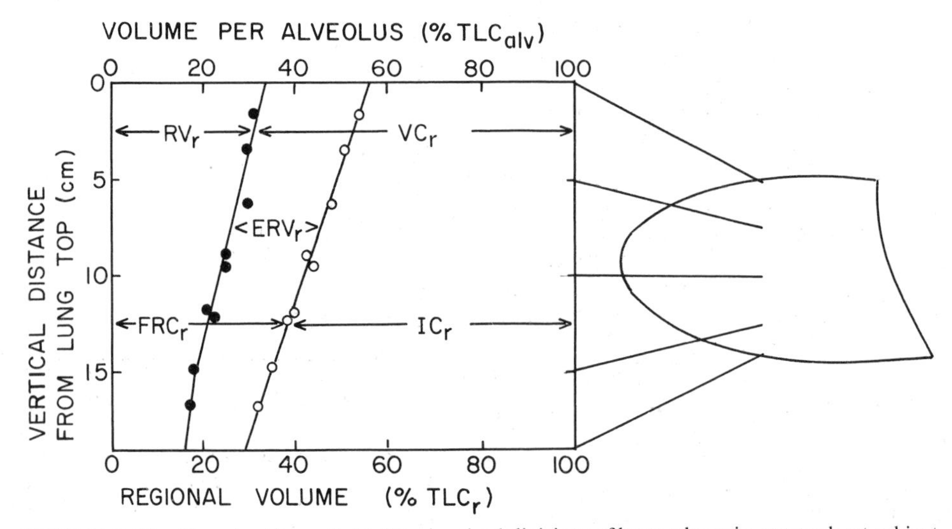

FIGURE 2–18. (See also Figure 2–14.) Regional subdivisions of lung volume in a recumbent subject.

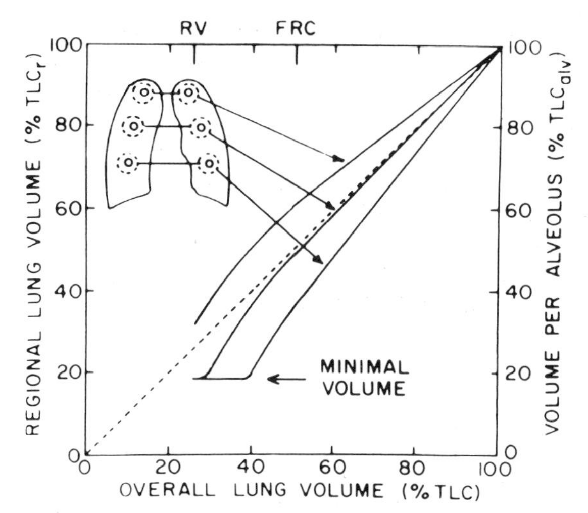

FIGURE 2–19. Proportional expansion of upper, middle, and lower zones of lungs of a normal subject, seated upright. The dotted line shows the progression expansion that would occur in all zones if there was no regional difference in intrapleural pressure. Data from studies of four healthy young men, seated upright. The lung counters were 4.5, 13.8, and 22.5 cm, respectively, from the top of the lung.

normal, and seated men, are shown in Figure 2–19. Regional volumes (V_r) existing at three vertical levels in the lung are plotted against overall lung volume. The results were obtained under quasi-static conditions, with an inspiratory airflow amounting to less than 0.5 liters/sec. This is an important experimental condition, since the distribution is considerably influenced by flow.[2446] If the alveoli of all regions had expanded uniformly, the volume of each region (expressed as a percentage of regional TLC) should always be the same as the overall lung volume (expressed as a percentage of overall TLC); that is to say that the relationship between regional and overall lung volumes should be given by the line of identity with a slope = 1. This line is shown as a broken line in the figure. It is evident that this is not the case. The upper lung regions appear to be more expanded than the units in the lower zones at all lung volumes except at full inspiration.

The slopes $\Delta V_r / \Delta V$ of the curves in Figure 2–19 indicate the rate of filling and emptying (or ventilation) of the lung units in the various lung regions in relation to the volume changes of the whole lung. It is clear that at lung volumes above FRC the *proportion* of ventilation delivered to any lung region is substantially constant, as shown by the linear relationships between regional and overall lung volumes. In this range of lung volumes, therefore, the various lung zones do not fill sequentially. The slope of the curves is greater in dependent than in upper lung zones, indicating the better ventilation of dependent lung units. When a normal subject takes a slow breath from FRC, the ventilation per alveolus is greater in dependent than in upper lung regions, but the relative distribution of ventilation is virtually independent of the volume inspired, i.e., the difference in ventilation is proportionately the same whether the subject takes a resting tidal breath or a maximal inspiration. It is to be noted that at lung volumes greater than FRC the regional distribution of gas is affected relatively little by inspiratory flow rate,[2446] and thus a plot of the slopes of the linear portion of the curves shown in Figure 2–19 against the vertical distance down the lung will describe the regional distribution of ventilation per alveolus for breaths of any magnitude and velocity, but always provided that breathing takes place over the range of lung volume in which the relationship between regional and overall lung volume is a linear one. Such a diagram is shown in Figure 2–21 in which the ventilation per alveolus is expressed as a percentage fraction of the value predicted if there were a uniform distribution of ventilation to all lung units. It is apparent that ventilation per alveolus increases approximately linearly with vertical distance down the lung. The slope of the line in this figure is an expression of the relative change in ventilation per alveolus per

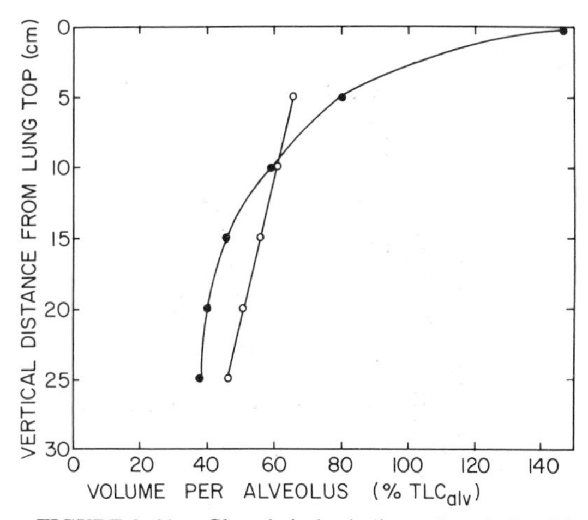

FIGURE 2–20. Closed circles indicate the relationship between vertical distance and alveolar volume in greyhound dogs, frozen, head up, at FRC (*see* reference 2441). Open circles indicate results from normal, seated man, plotted from Figure 2–14.

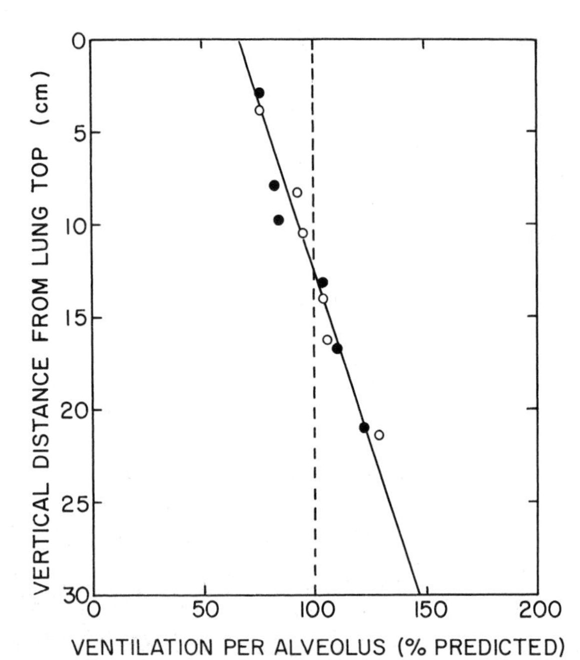

FIGURE 2–21. Relationship between vertical distance from lung top and ventilation per alveolus in a seated man. Open circles indicate data from right lung, and closed circles, from the left lung.

centimeter descent down the lung. In Table 2–4 this value is shown for a number of body positions.

It should be noted that as a consequence of the effect of gravity and the shape of the pressure–volume curve of the lung, in the normal tidal volume range in a young subject, the distribution of ventilation is preferential to the dependent lung zones and is not profoundly influenced by inspiratory flow. Since blood flow in the resting state is also and more markedly preferentially distributed to the lower zones (*see* page 48), this matching of ventilation to perfusion in different body positions ensures efficient gas exchange under a variety of physiological conditions.

TABLE 2–4 INCREASE IN VENTILATION PER ALVEOLUS* PER CENTIMETER DESCENT DOWN THE LUNG IN NORMAL YOUNG MEN IN DIFFERENT BODY POSITIONS

POSITION	NUMBER OF SUBJECTS	INCREASE IN VENTILATION PER ALVEOLUS PER CM DESCENT
		Mean (Range)
Seated	9	2.3 (1.9–3.6)
Supine	3	2.3 (2.0–2.6)
Prone	3	2.0 (1.9–2.1)
Left lateral	3	2.2 (1.9–2.7)
Right lateral	3	3.1 (3.0–3.2)

*Ventilation per alveolus has been computed as a percentage of the predicted value assuming uniform distribution of ventilation throughout the lung.

If breathing takes place at lung volumes lower than FRC, the distribution of ventilation is quite different. As indicated in Figure 2–19, when the lung volume is reduced below FRC, the slope $\Delta V_r/\Delta V$ increases progressively in all regions until the regional volume reaches a value of about 20 per cent of TLC_r, which corresponds to the regional minimal volume. In a young subject, this minimal volume is reached in the lowest zones when the lung is at about 40 per cent of TLC and in the midzones when the lung is at about 30 per cent of TLC. With loss of elastic recoil in older subjects,[2380] these minimal volumes will be reached at higher fractions of the TLC.[2432, 2455] It appears likely that minimal volume is caused by closure of airways, and it can be shown that ^{133}xenon is still evolved into dependent lung zones when it is delivered into them in saline via the pulmonary artery and when the breath is held with an open glottis at residual volume, indicating that the alveoli are air-containing. The progressive increase in the slope $\Delta V_r/\Delta V$ of the curves in Figure 2–19 is thus to be explained on the basis of airway closure, commencing in the most dependent parts of the lung, which are exposed to more positive pleural pressure, and progressing upward in the lung until the subject reaches residual volume.[2431, 2432] It may be computed that in young, normal, seated subjects the airways begin to close at 30 to 46 per cent of TLC, i.e., below FRC, and the extent of airway closure increases progressively with further decreases in lung volume, until at RV airway closure, it affects about half of all the units in the lung. This is shown graphically in Figure 2–22, which also shows that about 750 ml of gas will be trapped behind the airways at residual volume.

If a slow inspiration is started from RV, the upper lung units start to fill first, and thus the pattern of ventilation is in a sense the reverse of what occurs when all airways are open.[2431] If a fast-velocity inspiration is taken, distribution is more uniform;[2446] in other words, there is less proportionate delay in opening closed airway units. When a small breath is taken from RV, the trapped units receive none of the inspired air until transpulmonary pressure

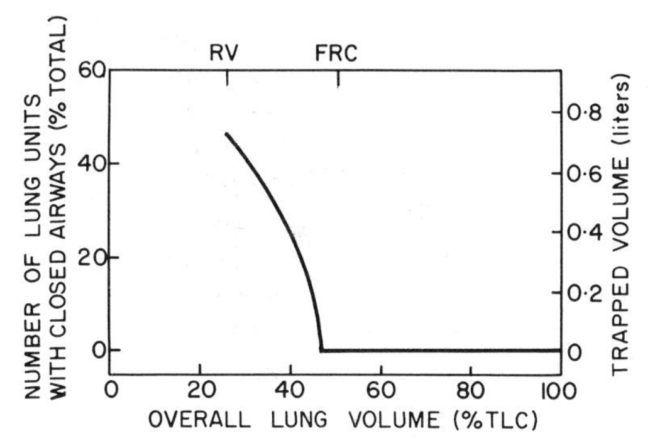

FIGURE 2–22. Number of lung units with closed airways (as a percentage of the total number), and trapped volume (in liters) as a function of overall lung volume (percentage of TLC). Average results for four healthy young men, sitting upright, are shown.

reaches a critical value (opening pressure) sufficient to open the closed airways.[2392, 2432, 2450] This phenomenon is explicable on the same simple model, as shown in Figures 2–23 and 2–24.

The phenomenon of airway closure at low lung volumes has major physiological significance. In conditions in which the lung volume is reduced, as in gross abdominal obesity for example,[2464] airway closure within the tidal volume range appears to be responsible for the low arterial oxygen tension. Abernethy,

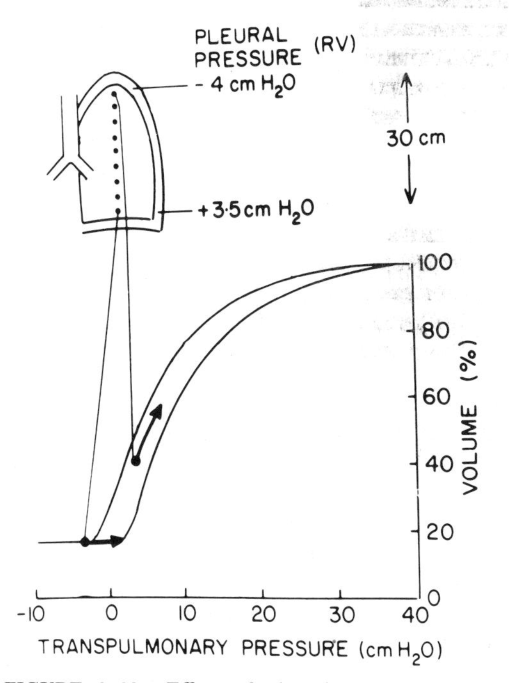

FIGURE 2–23. Effect of pleural pressure gradient on distribution of ventilation. As an inspiration is begun from residual volume, alveoli at the apex will start to fill before those at the base.

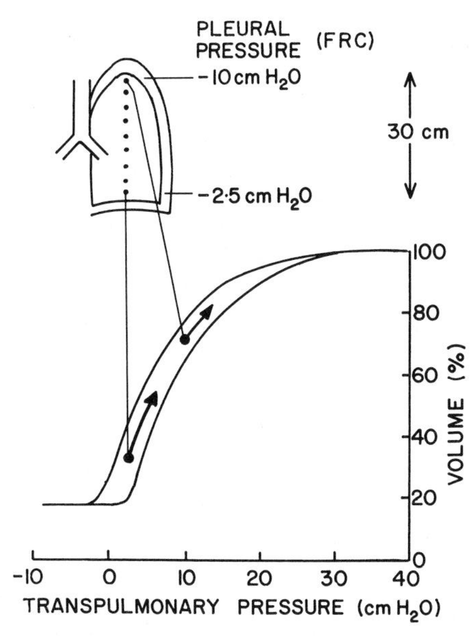

FIGURE 2–24. (*See* also Figure 2–23.) As a tidal volume inspiration is taken from FRC, lower alveoli will receive more gas than upper alveoli, since they are on a steeper part of the pressure-volume curve.

Maurizi, and Farhi[2439] noted that recumbency was associated with a widening of the alveolar-arterial nitrogen difference, indicating the appearance of low $\dot{V}/\dot{Q}$ zones in the lung, and we have observed[2465] that in normal subjects older than 44 years, ventilation is diminished immediately on the assumption of recumbency, presumably as a result of closure.[2466] This phenomenon was further aggravated by a period of shallow breathing in the supine position.[2465] These effects could be reversed by deep breathing and presumably indicate dependent-zone airway closure.

Summary

There is little doubt that regional ventilation distribution plays a major part in determining patterns of lung ventilation non-uniformity in a wide variety of circumstances. It seems likely that in the normal lung, gas distribution is more affected by the regional differences we have described in this section than by diffusion mixing non-uniformity, or by regional differences in airway resistance. The present concept provides a satisfactory basis of understanding and illustrates the fact that the balance of ventilation to perfusion is achieved, under resting conditions, primarily by the shape of the pressure–volume curve, that is by "design" rather than by a control system. A general understanding, if not a detailed one, of this phenomenon is essential if the effects on gas exchange of age, obesity, body position, acceleration, weightlessness, or recumbency are to be understood.

THE PULMONARY CIRCULATION

The regional distribution of pulmonary blood flow

Although it had been suggested for many years that the distribution of blood flow would be less at the apex of the lung than at the base in a man standing upright, the conclusive evidence that this was the case had to await the development of radioactive gas methods of studying the lung. West and Dollery and their colleagues,[342, 343, 344] using ^{15}carbon O_2 and later, in conjunction with us, ^{133}xenon dissolved in saline and injected into an arm vein,[174] found that there was a considerable gradient of distribution of blood flow.

Before this data was available, Banister and Torrance in 1960[2483] had laid the theoretical groundwork for a better understanding of the factors that would determine such a distribution. These concepts were extended by Permutt and his colleagues[2482] and more fully developed by West, Dollery, and Naimark[2467] and ourselves.[2466] As a result of this work, it is now possible to give a reasonably simple description of the regional distribution of pulmonary blood flow and the factors on which this depends.

West and his colleagues[2467] divided the lung into three horizontal zones according to the relative magnitude of the three pressures that determine the flow. At the top of the lung is *Zone 1*, in which the alveolar pressure (P_A) is greater than the pulmonary arterial pressure (P_a), and hence there would be no flow. In a man seated upright and at rest this zone extends about 4 cm from the top of the lung. Below this is *Zone 2*, in which the pulmonary arterial pressure is greater than the alveolar pressure, which in turn is greater than the pulmonary venous pressure (P_v). Since the driving pressure ($P_a - P_A$) increases down the lung in this zone, so would blood flow; and the increase in flow is inversely related to P_a. In *Zone 3*, the pulmonary arterial pressure is greater than the pulmonary venous pressure, which in turn is greater than the alveolar pressure. The pressure gradient in this zone ($P_a - P_v$) would be constant down the zone, but West and his co-workers[2467] postulated that the transmural pressure difference would constantly increase, and part of the vessel would dilate. This would have the effect of causing some increase of flow down Zone 3, but not as great as would exist down Zone 2. More recently, Hughes, Glazier, Maloney, and West,[2477, 3135] and West, Dollery, and Heard[2481] have observed a small zone of reduced flow at the very base of the lung and have attributed this to a possible increase in the interstitial pressure as a consequence of the reduced expansion of the lung parenchyma in the lower zone. This has therefore been called *Zone 4*. There is still some uncertainty as to the cause of the reduced flow in this zone, but the concept of reduction in flow caused by an increased interstitial pressure is almost certainly important in mitral stenosis and may well be initially responsible for the considerable reduction in basal flow observed in that condition. In summary, therefore:

Zone 1: $P_A > P_a$, and therefore no flow.
Zone 2: $P_a > P_A > P_v$, and flow increases linearly.
Zone 3: $P_a > P_v > P_A$, and there is some increase of flow, possibly due to greater vessel distention.
Zone 4: Flow limited by interstitial pressure around small vessels.

To this basic description, several additional points have been added. During exercise in the upright position, there is a proportionately greater increase in blood flow to the upper part of the lungs,[2302] in other words, the increased pulmonary blood flow is largely accommodated by increasing the flow to the upper zones and hence blood-flow distribution becomes more uniform. In different body positions, the vertical zonal distribution is still present, thus causing a greater blood flow in the dependent lung when the subject is lying on his side.[2442] It has been shown that breathing pure oxygen does not affect the blood-flow distribution in the normal subject seated upright.[2479] Most of the observed phenomena can be explained in terms of a Starling resistor model,[2480] but it must be pointed out that the influence of the pulsatile nature of flow on the perfusion of Zone 1 has not yet been analyzed in detail. Nor is there yet a clear understanding of the influence of the critical closing pressure of vessels on the pattern of distribution.

We have studied the effect of different respiratory maneuvers on blood flow in upright man[2466] and have found that similar distributions are observed at FRC and TLC; but if the subject stops breathing at his residual volume, keeping the glottis open, there is a much more uniform blood-flow distribution per alveolus than at the larger lung volumes. This appears to be explained by the finding of a considerable elevation in pulmonary wedge pressure that occurs at residual volume. Glaister[2484] has analyzed the effects of positive centrifugal acceleration on both ventilation and perfusion distribution within the lung and related these to changes in pulmonary arterial and intra-esophageal pressures. The greater blood flow in dependent lung zones has also been demonstrated by use of the macro-aggregated serum albumin tagging technique,[2478] and the same method has been used to demonstrate a shift of blood flow away from a hypoxic lung.[2437] A combination of bronchospirometry and the study of excretion of ^{85}krypton has also been used very effectively to study regional blood flow distribution.[2473]

The greatly increased understanding which has resulted from all these studies has had an important influence on the interpretation of differences in measurements of diffusing capacity, and the techniques that have been used have also found important applications in clinical investigation and research, as is noted in many of the later chapters of this volume.

Factors affecting the pulmonary vascular bed

In the preceding section, the effects of gravity and of the pressures existing within the lung on the distribution of pulmonary blood flow were briefly described. In addition to this, there is a formidable literature on other influences which affect pulmonary vascular reactivity. The book by Harris and Heath[9] provides an excellent starting point, and there are other valuable reviews[1210, 1947, 2323, 2475] of this field. The two volumes on the pulmonary circulation written by Aviado[2470] cover the pharmacological aspects of the circulation through the lung in great detail.

Initially, all relevant data came from animal experiments. The contemporary interest in this field may be conveniently dated from Liljestrand's observations in cats of the effects on the pulmonary arterial pressure of anoxia and of breathing high concentrations of CO_2.[1948] In this paper he prophetically quoted Starling's remark that "the Physiology of today is the medicine of tomorrow." A great deal of careful work with animals followed this,[1949–1956] culminating in the elegant demonstration by Rahn and Bahnson of changes in pulmonary blood flow induced by unilateral hypoxia in the intact dog.[1957] The results of Hall's experiments suggest that the level of alveolar oxygen tension is responsible for production of this effect,[1958] a conclusion supported by the demonstration of significant pulmonary hypertension in residents at altitude.[2267]

The introduction of the cardiac catheter revolutionized the study of this problem, making available for the first time observations of the consequences of breathing high and low concentrations of oxygen, of acetylcholine infusion, and of alterations in acid–base balance in patients and in normal subjects. The enormous contribution made by Cournand and his colleagues to this field of knowledge is well known, and a careful study of their many original publications is obligatory.[1959–1967] Additional information has come from other laboratories.[1968–1975] This work has shown clearly the responsiveness of the human pulmonary bed to disturbances in its normal gas and blood environment, and the relevance of such mechanisms to the control of perfusion distribution in lung disease.

These observations have been supplemented by others of equal importance and interest but concerned with specific parts of the vascular bed. The very important demonstration that blood circulation through the pulmonary bed is probably pulsatile[1976] has been followed by detailed observations that clarify events taking place in the pulmonary capillaries,[1977, 2230] and involving considerations closely linked to measurements of the pulmonary capillary-blood volume.[1993] New techniques have been used to study ion exchanges in pulmonary extravascular water.[1978] A hitherto unknown aspect of pulmonary edema became evident when this condition was produced experimentally in the dog by administration of Gram-negative endotoxin, and it was shown to be a consequence of pulmonary-vein constriction.[1979] Much other work reported is relevant to an understanding of factors controlling perfusion and ventilation in the lung,[1980–1983] from the point of view both of the influence of alveolar hypoxia on flow distribution[1009, 1983] and of the influence of flow reduction on bronchial caliber and ventilation distribution.[1982]

During the past five years, renewed attention has been directed at the problem of the effect of hypoxia on the pulmonary circulation and the mechanism of the response. The shift of blood flow away from a hypoxic lung has been convincingly demonstrated in the intact man,[2437, 2473] and the dependence of this shift on the existence of a lowered alveolar oxygen tension has been elegantly demonstrated by Lloyd,[2471] who has, in addition, made the interesting observation[2468] that the response is dependent on the nature of the lung perfusate, that is, it is present when the perfusate is autologous plasma, but it is much diminished if the lobe is perfused with normal saline. The response to serotonin was also influenced in the same sense by the nature of the perfusing fluid. Dugard and Naimark[2469] demonstrated that an increased hydrogen-ion concentration also produced a more uniform blood distribution, and Haas and Bergofsky[2476] showed that in anesthetized dogs with controlled ventilation, the measured arterial oxygen tension rose during vascoconstriction caused by respiratory acidosis, metabolic acidosis, serotonin, or an elevation of extracellular potassium concentration.

The close relationship between the pulmonary artery pressure and the alveolar hypoxia of altitude, and the apparent dependence of the onset of congestive heart failure in chronic lung disease on abnormalities of gas transfer caused by disturbance of ventilation/perfusion relationships, are both examples of the basic importance of understanding more precisely the reactivity of the pulmonary vascular bed to hypoxia; but it is clear that much remains to be learned.

The Function of the Lung in Relation to Circulating Substances

In his Harvey Lecture of 1953, Comroe pointed out that the lung serves as a major filter,[706] being the only capillary bed through which the whole of the cardiac output passes. It is known to be responsible for trapping the megakaryocytes that contain serotonin, and the lung contains larger quantities of histamine, heparin, and adenosine deaminase in relation to its weight than do most other organs.

More recently, the role of the lung in dealing with a wide variety of vasoactive hormones has been the subject of intensive study.[2485, 2486] Vane, reviewing this field in 1969,[2485] points out that the lung has some role in relation to bradykinin, prostaglandins, angiotensin I, and noradrenaline, in addition to those compounds noted in the preceding paragraph. It seems likely that the full understanding of this important aspect of lung function will be dependent on more knowledge of the biochemical processes within the lung itself, particularly those concerned with the elaboration of surfactant.[2429] At the moment there are far more questions than there are answers.[2486]

THE ARTERIAL BLOOD

Introduction

Although Barcroft[28] and Haldane[2] understood well the general principles underlying gas exchange in the lung, detailed quantitative analysis only became possible following the work of Rahn[234] and his colleagues and Riley and Cournand[413] in the years immediately following 1945. Since then, as a consequence of a considerable volume of work on ventilation/perfusion distribution, on diffusing capacity, and on techniques to measure gas tensions, substantial progress has been made in understanding the various factors that govern gas exchange. This insight has in turn led to a much more detailed understanding of the defects that may impair gas exchange in disease. Unfortunately, however, the whole field of gas transport is a difficult one to follow, largely because of the multiplicity and interdependence of the factors involved. As a result, as Campbell has pointed out,[177] too many physicians abandon the attempt to understand this important field as soon as the realm of complexity is entered.

This section is designed as a guide to methods of measurement, and to those aspects of gas exchange that are critical to an understanding of derangements that are found in various disease processes. A more basic and extensive treatment of different aspects of gas transport and acid–base balance can be found in several excellent reviews and books.[3, 8, 24, 231, 2487–2493, 3454]

Theoretical Considerations

When any liquid is in equilibrium with any gas, the partial pressure in the liquid is proportional to the total ambient pressure and the fractional gas concentration.[10, 13] Thus:

Partial pressure (mm Hg) = Barometric pressure (mm Hg) × Fractional gas concentration

If a gas mixture contains 50 per cent oxygen, and the barometric pressure is 760 mm Hg:

$$Po_2 = (760 \times 0.5) = 380 \text{ mm Hg}$$

This relationship holds for any liquid in equilibrium with any gas, regardless of solubility or any other factors. The solubility of a gas in a simple solution is an expression of the volume dissolved in unit volume of the liquid at some stated temperature and pressure. The relationship between the gas content of a simple solution, such as distilled water, and the gas tension in the fluid is linear at any particular temperature; but it is not linear if the solution contains buffer systems or special methods of gas transport such as are contained within the red blood cell.

The relationship between the oxygen content and the oxygen tension of whole blood under normal physiological conditions is shown in Figure 2–25. An understanding of the importance of the unusual shape of this curve is relevant to many physiological and practical issues of importance to the physician:

1. Since the top of the curve is flat, there may be a considerable fall in oxygen tension at the top end of the curve, with a relatively small change in oxygen content; thus a fall in arterial Po_2 from its normal value of about 95 mm Hg to 60 mm Hg results in a fall in oxygen content of less than 10 per cent. This is of major assistance in maintaining the oxygen content of arterial blood after ascent to a moderate altitude.

2. For the same reason, hyperventilation with a consequent elevation of alveolar Po_2 will result in only a very small increase in the amount of oxygen taken up by the blood

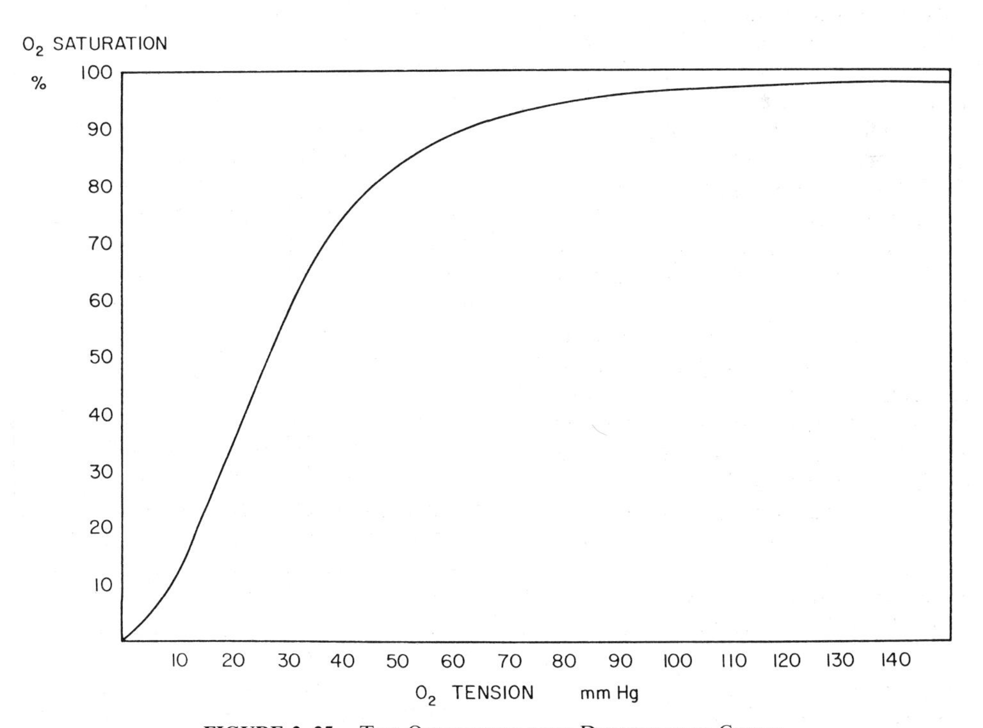

FIGURE 2–25. The Oxyhemoglobin Dissociation Curve

This normal dissociation curve illustrates the relationship between oxygen saturation and oxygen tension for whole blood of normal hematocrit and at a pH of 7.4.

under normal circumstances. Therefore, hyperventilation in one part of the lung cannot compensate for reduced ventilation in other parts.[3]

3. The shape of the dissociation curve is altered by changes in blood pH, P_{CO_2}, and temperature, and by the presence of carbon monoxide (*see* Fig. 2–27). It is also modified in some blood diseases, in cyanotic congenital heart disease,[1526] and in chronic obstructive lung disease with hypoxia.[3459] Recent work has also shown that the shape of the curve is modified by alterations in the constituents of red blood cells.

4. The shift of the dissociation curve with pH means that, as arterial blood enters the capillary of a working tissue and CO_2 diffuses into the blood, the consequent fall in blood pH assists the unloading of oxygen into the tissue. A parallel process occurs at the other end of the capillary, when the increased amount of reduced hemoglobin in the red cells increases the volume of CO_2 that the blood can carry. This mechanism assists the removal of CO_2 from metabolically active tissue.

In Table 2–5 a comparison between the O_2- and CO_2-carrying power of blood and water is shown to emphasize the importance of the physiological properties of blood in the delivery of oxygen to working tissue and the removal of CO_2 from it. In addition, red cells contain a special enzyme system, carbonic anhydrase,[2492] that enables CO_2 to be released quickly enough during the short passage of blood through the pulmonary capillary.

The physician should have a good knowledge of the acid–base field if he is to understand the principles underlying the clinical management of a variety of clinical conditions. In the past there has been little agreement about the criteria by which respiratory and nonrespiratory changes in the acid–base status of the body should be recognized. This confusion was in part semantic and in part physiological in origin.[2495] The semantic confusion arises from the ambiguous use of the terms "acidosis" and "alkalosis" to refer either to a physiological disturbance or to a resultant chemical change in the blood. At a meeting in New York[2499, 3454] there was general agreement that these terms would henceforth be used in a physiological and not a chemical sense. They should therefore be used to indicate a disturbance of mechanism, whatever the resultant pH. The physiological source of confusion arises from the fact that *in vitro* the titration characteristics of the blood are different from what they are *in vivo*. Accordingly, by manipulating whole blood *in vitro* it is not possible to disentangle the respiratory from the nonrespiratory changes in acid–base status which occur *in vivo*. When the P_{CO_2} of blood is altered *in vitro*, the changes in pH and HCO_3^- that occur are not the same as those that are found when the P_{CO_2} of the whole animal is raised or lowered.[3456–3458] In view of this, it is not surprising that much confusion was caused by the use in many laboratories of the "CO_2 combining power," involving the equilibration of the patient's serum with a known concentration of CO_2 and the subsequent measurement of the CO_2 content.[29] This method will reveal the presence of a metabolic acidosis; the CO_2 combining power may well be normal in a patient with acute CO_2 retention (Pa_{CO_2} of 80 mm Hg, for example, and a normal bicarbonate). It is for this reason that the great clinical importance of elevations of CO_2 tension was not recognized until direct tension measurements became possible on a routine basis.[29]

TABLE 2–5 Comparison between Gas Content of Water and of Whole Blood

	Gas Content of 100 ml of Water	Gas Content of 100 ml of Blood	Factor
At a P_{O_2} of 50 mm Hg	0.15 ml of O_2	16.8 ml of O_2	x 110
At a P_{CO_2} of 50 mm Hg	3.8 ml of CO_2	50 ml of CO_2	x 13

Methods of measurement

Oxygen content and capacity, and CO_2 content

The amount of oxygen in the blood may be reported as the content in volumes per cent, or as saturation, which is the content expressed as a percentage of the capacity. The latter is determined by analysis of the amount of oxygen in blood exposed to a high tension of oxygen, making an allowance for the volume of oxygen dissolved in blood. At an oxygen tension of 100 mm Hg this value will be 0.3 ml per 100 ml of blood, and at a tension of 700 mm Hg it will be (7 × 0.3) or 2.1 ml per cent. The capacity of blood for oxygen is directly related to the concentration of hemoglobin, 1 gm of hemoglobin combining with 1.39 ml STPD of oxygen. This coefficient, recently reported by Kelman,[3461] is slightly higher than the traditional value of 1.34 deduced from earlier work.

The Van Slyke method[2494] of determining the O_2 and CO_2 content of blood remains the standard by which other methods are evaluated. The method is too time-consuming for routine work, but it should remain part of the basic equipment of respiratory laboratories, and the staff must still be trained in its use. In skilled hands this method has a random error in a single analysis of about 0.2 volumes per cent of oxygen. The CO_2 content of blood may also be measured accurately on the Van Slyke apparatus, but its tension in blood cannot be deduced from this value without knowledge of the pH. Since the tension of CO_2 in arterial blood is the more informative parameter, the measurement of CO_2 content is now rarely made in patients with lung disease.

Oxygen and CO_2 content of blood can also be measured using a gas chromatograph to record the gas concentrations of samples obtained by extraction in a Van Slyke apparatus,[214] or in a specially designed cuvette,[214] or using a recirculation system.[3512] This technique has also been used to measure the carbon monoxide content of blood.[3468, 3469] Farhi and his colleagues have described a gas chromatographic method of determining the nitrogen content of blood,[1800] a measurement important in the study of alveolar–arterial nitrogen tension differences. Other reviews and articles have appeared on different aspects of gas analysis by gas chromatography.[3470, 3471, 3472, 3480]

Similar extraction methods with gas analysis by infrared gas analyzers have been found very satisfactory for the measurement of carbon monoxide[216, 217, 3515] and carbon dioxide[3473] in blood samples. In the case of carbon monoxide, this method is considerably more accurate than spectrophotometric techniques at very low saturations. Analysis of equilibrated alveolar gas is also an accurate method to use for small carboxyhemoglobin concentrations.[2198, 3514]

The oxygen content of blood can also be measured using oxygen tension electrodes.[3474–3480] The general principle of this method is to dilute a blood sample with acid ferricyanide solution, measure the increase in oxygen tension resulting from the dissociation of oxygen from hemoglobin, and calculate the oxygen content of the sample from the solubility coefficient. The hemoglobin-bound O_2 can also be released by carbon monoxide.[3479] These techniques are quick, relatively simple, and require only small-volume blood samples. They are particularly useful when many determinations of oxygen content are required in a brief period of time.

Spectrophotometric methods for oxyhemoglobin percentage determination

This method of analysis depends on the difference in spectral absorption between oxygenated and reduced hemoglobin. When first introduced, the technique was not a simple one, since the blood had to be hemolyzed anaerobically, but it was greatly simplified when Nahas[178, 179] introduced a cuvette specially designed for this purpose. Several subsequent developments of this technique have since been described.[180, 2238, 3462, 3464]

The spectrophotometric methods are not accurate when applied to hemolyzed blood *in vitro*. The Nahas method enables the saturation of arterial blood samples to be estimated with an accuracy of about 2 per cent. Each estimate takes about 12 minutes, and it is therefore a much faster technique than the Van Slyke, for which at least this much time is required for the determination of content, and a further 12 minutes is required for the estimation of capacity. Abnormal pigments such as methemoglobin may cause erroneous results, and carboxyhemoglobin also interferes with spectrophotometric determinations of blood saturation, but not to as great an extent as does methemoglobin.[3463]

Spectrophotometric methods have also been used for *in vivo* measurements of hemoglobin saturation, but the accuracy is less than when hemolyzed blood is used. Both the Millikan type of oximeter[13] and the Kipp reflection oximeter[222] have been used for these determinations. The real problem of all these instruments is their accurate and individual calibration, and although many are well suited to follow changes in saturation, few provide reliable measurements of saturation in the upper range. Several pulmonary function test procedures have been based on their use.

Fowler and Comroe[219, 221] described a test based on the rate of increase in arterial saturation during the inhalation of 100 per cent oxygen. Woolf, Gunton, and Paul have suggested that the observation of desaturation time would be a more valuable measurement.[223] Perkins, Adams, and Flores[220] devised an original approach wherein the arterial oxygen saturation was compared continuously with the alveolar oxygen tension while this was altered by changes in inspired oxygen concentration. By this means, some quantitation of venous admixture and diffusion defect was possible. Others have used similar methods to compute the "equivalent shunt" component using low inspired oxygen mixtures.[3507] Some assessment of cardiac output is also possible using resaturation curves.[3465] Earpieces designed for the recording of dye-dilution curves have also been described[2238] and are extensively used for the detection of left-to-right shunts.[3466, 3467]

We have found ear oximetry useful in the study of patients thought to have primary alveolar hypoventilation. In such studies, the ear oximeter can be set to 100 per cent while the patient is breathing oxygen and can then be unobtrusively observed over the course of several minutes when he is breathing air and is undisturbed. Enson and his colleagues[224] have been able to accommodate a reflection oximeter at the end of a cardiac catheter.

Since the physician can almost always maintain full oxygen saturation by having the patient breathe oxygen, measurement of the resting oxygen saturation is relatively unimportant compared to the great importance of knowing the $P\text{CO}_2$. When for diagnostic or management purposes it is important to know the resting oxygenation of arterial blood, a direct tension or saturation estimate on an arterial sample should always be preferred to an ear oximetric reading.

Direct O_2 and CO_2 tension measurements

Tremendous advances have been made in these techniques in recent years, and the general introduction of instruments suitable for routine use has led to recognition of important clinical syndromes, particularly involving hypoxemia, that were not previously documented–, for example, the demonstration that significant abnormality of arterial oxygen tension may exist in asthma without any concomitant hypercapnia. The tension of oxygen and CO_2 in blood can be determined several ways, each of which has a standard deviation of approximately ± 2 mm Hg in skilled hands.

In 1945, Riley, Proemmel, and Franke[192] introduced the bubble equilibration technique for measuirng the $P\text{O}_2$ and $P\text{CO}_2$ of blood. This can be seen in retrospect as a turning point in the history of respiratory research. Various modifications of this method have been described[193–196, 197, 199, 200] and its accuracy has been critically measured.[198] However, it has now been made obsolete by the advent of electrode and polarographic methods, which possess the great advantage that they, in contrast to the bubble method, can be used for oxygen tensions up to 700 mm Hg.

The first direct oxygen-tension measurements became possible with the use of the polarographic technique. This method was still in the experimental stage in 1950,[3] but five years later a great deal of excellent analytical work was being accomplished by Bartels and his group.[201, 202] Individual blood samples required separate calibration, but in skilled hands the technique yielded excellent results. In 1957 Connelly[203] reviewed contemporary methods of direct measurement of oxygen tension, and this paper marks the transition from the polarographic method to the design of electrodes based on the use of a membrane between the blood and the platinum tip. Several authors have published modifications with different types of electrodes based on the Clark cell,[204–209, 2292] the results showing some variation in accuracy but being generally satisfactory. Polgar and Forster used a Mylar membrane[210] in front of the platinum cathode.

This material is relatively impermeable to oxygen, and by using it they were able to dispense with the necessity for stirring the blood in contact with the cathode, a requirement previous investigators had met in a variety of ingenious ways. Using this electrode, Polgar and Forster reported a coefficient of variation of ± 2 per cent, which, they pointed out, was comparable to the best results reported by users of the stirred electrode systems.[206]

The oxygen electrode originally designed by Clark, and described by Severinghaus and Bradley,[211] consisted of a silver reference anode and a platinum cathode covered by a polyethylene membrane, which they consider superior to membranes of Teflon or Mylar. The accuracy of reading the output of this electrode can be improved by direct recording on a millivolt full-scale writer with a paper width of at least six inches, and the optimal assembly should include this type of equipment, which inevitably costs a great deal more than the electrode itself.

In the same paper, Severinghaus and Bradley[211] described an electrode for the measurement of CO_2 tension. This incorporates a Teflon membrane lying over a cellophane membrane which retains a 0.01 M solution of $NaHCO_3$ and 0.1 NaCl in front of the cathode—an arrangement that has produced very satisfactory stability and accuracy in performance. It is important to note, however, that a first-class electrometer is necessary if the maximal capability of the electrode is to be realized. Both oxygen and CO_2 electrodes require careful heat stabilization, meticulous maintenance, and routine calibration checks against blood or water of known gas tension. We have found it convenient, for routine calibration purposes, to place three flasks in the same water bath as the electrode, containing distilled water continuously equilibrated with room air, pure oxygen, and pure nitrogen. Although it may be convenient in some situations to mount both electrodes and a pH electrode in the same water bath,[211] for other applications it may be better to mount them individually.

There is no doubt that the electrode measurements of oxygen and carbon dioxide tension have now moved out of the experimental and developmental stage and are suitable for routine laboratory use.[2320] Although it might be thought that speed of determination was their greatest asset over other methods, their major advantage lies in the fact that gas tensions up to 600 mm Hg for oxygen and up to at least 300 mm Hg for CO_2 can be measured with the same facility as those at the lower end of the scale. The necessity for scrupulous calibration is obvious, however, and it is to be feared that in some hands these electrodes may be used without proper precautions. It has been pointed out that, in the clinical management of patients, knowledge of the P_{CO_2} alone often is not sufficient, since the pH also must be determined. For this reason the Astrup technique may be preferred for routine use, but the combination of a CO_2 electrode and a pH electrode offers an alternative certainly capable of the same level of accuracy.

During the past few years, several important developments in electrode design and calibration technique have been reported.[3481–3486] The performance of commercially available microelectrodes has also been extensively tested.[3487–3490, 3508] Electrodes for arterial blood have been fitted through the lumen of thin-walled needles[212, 2287] and on catheters,[3491] permitting *in vivo* measurements of P_{O_2}, though some difficulty has been encountered in ensuring satisfactory stability of these devices over a period of time. Useful correction factors and nomograms for the correction of blood P_{O_2} and P_{CO_2} for time and/or temperature have been published.[1797, 3492–3494, 3509] An extensive description of the theory and practice of electrodes in biology and medicine was published in 1968.[3496] In children, and in situations in which repetitive blood samples might be difficult to obtain, the arterialized capillary blood may be collected and analyzed with microelectrode systems for P_{CO_2}, pH, and P_{O_2}. Several reviews of this technique have appeared, and there seems little doubt that for most clinical purposes, provided the sample collection is carefully done, the results are close enough to those found by simultaneous analysis of arterial blood.[3510]

Recently, Woldring, Owens, and Woolford have described a promising method for continuous *in vivo* recording of partial pressures of O_2 and CO_2 in blood by mass spectrometry.[3495]

Measurement of pH

Until recently[181] the accurate measurement of blood pH presented technical problems. This laboratory determination now can be performed routinely without difficulty to at least ±0.02 unit. This has been made possible by three developments: the substitution of the vacuum tube voltmeter or "reed electrometer" principle to record small potentials, in place of the older null point methods; the general availability of hydrogen electrode standardized buffers or laboratory-prepared buffers of greater reliability than those available previously;[182] and the provision of convenient apparatus for the determination of blood pH without contact of the sample with room air, and with satisfactory temperature stability, using a thermostat-controlled water jacket.[183, 184] Satisfactory micro methods capable of measuring the pH of a drop of blood in a capillary tube also are commercially available.[185, 188] The chief remaining technical difficulty is the glass electrode, which may become unstable with repeated use in blood, almost certainly because of blockage by plasma proteins of the porous porcelain plug which is an inevitable feature of its design. Careful routine standardization with freshly prepared buffer standards will enable any error to be detected quickly and the electrode replaced.

The routine measurement of arterial pH is essential to the proper management of many patients with combined respiratory and metabolic problems. In our experience it is particularly important in the management of postoperative patients and patients with both respiratory and renal failure, and in the treatment of cardiac and respiratory disorders when these coexist.

Astrup technique for measurement of pH, P_{CO_2}, and standard bicarbonate

Astrup and his colleagues have described a new approach to the laboratory study of problems of acid–base imbalance and disturbances of CO_2 elimination. In a series of papers[184–187] recently summarized in convenient form,[188] they base their analysis on accurate determination of the difference between the pH of arterial blood measured at 37° C without contact with air, and the pH of plasma or whole blood after equilibration with a known concentration of CO_2 at the same temperature.

Knowing the pH and P_{CO_2} of the equilibrated sample, one can calculate its bicarbonate from the latter value and from the whole-blood pH, the P_{CO_2} of the whole blood can be calculated. Two of the advantages of this technique are that the accuracy of the P_{CO_2} value is not dependent upon the *absolute* accuracy of the pH determination but upon the accuracy of the difference between two pH measurements; and the P_{CO_2} can be measured when anesthetic gases are present in the blood. In six years of daily experience with it, we have found this to be an ideal laboratory method, and we cannot agree with those who criticize the technique on the grounds of complexity.[189]

Astrup and his co-workers recently have described a development of their original apparatus,[188] using a capillary electrode which requires only about 100 μl of blood. In this technique, no separation of plasma is required, the micro blood sample being equilibrated with two known CO_2 concentrations. Although this method requires more laboratory skill in its use, for purposes of clinical management measurements on arterialized capillary blood may safely be substituted for those on an arterial sample.[190, 191] It is particularly suited to the management of children with respiratory failure, and is unquestionably the laboratory method of choice for newborn infants with respiratory distress (*see* page 426). Arterial or capillary blood analysis by the Astrup technique enables the acid–base status of the blood to be plotted on a nomogram. Many such nomograms have been devised,[189] but that recommended by Siggaard-Andersen and Engel,[600, 1798] shown in Figure 2–26, seems to us to be particularly useful.

Very recently, a three-dimensional visual model has been devised for the analysis of acid–base information, and this is of considerable value in teaching this aspect of respiratory physiology which students and physicians usually find confusing.*

Indirect O_2 and CO_2 tension measurements

As noted earlier, the shape of the oxyhemoglobin dissociation curve is such that the oxygen tension can only be deduced with any precision from the saturation over the steep part of the curve, which is at tensions between 20 mm Hg and 70 mm Hg.[3460] An indirect estimate of the mixed venous gas tension may be obtained by a rebreathing technique, and in recent years much attention has been devoted to this method. It was, in fact, suggested more than 40 years ago by Burwell and Robinson,[3497] but gained momentum only since 1956 when Collier[225] modernized it by using a rapid response infrared CO_2 analyzer in a rebreathing circuit in which the lung is used as a tonometer. He found that the mixed venous CO_2 tension so determined seldom varied by more than 6 mm Hg from that of a blood sample withdrawn by cardiac catheter. Assuming a constant arteriovenous P_{CO_2} difference of 6 mm Hg, he demonstrated that the arterial CO_2 tension could be computed from the mixed venous P_{CO_2} with a mean error of only 0.2 mm Hg and an SD of 2.9

*Available from Acid–Base Inc., 2222 E. 18th Ave., Denver, Colorado 80206

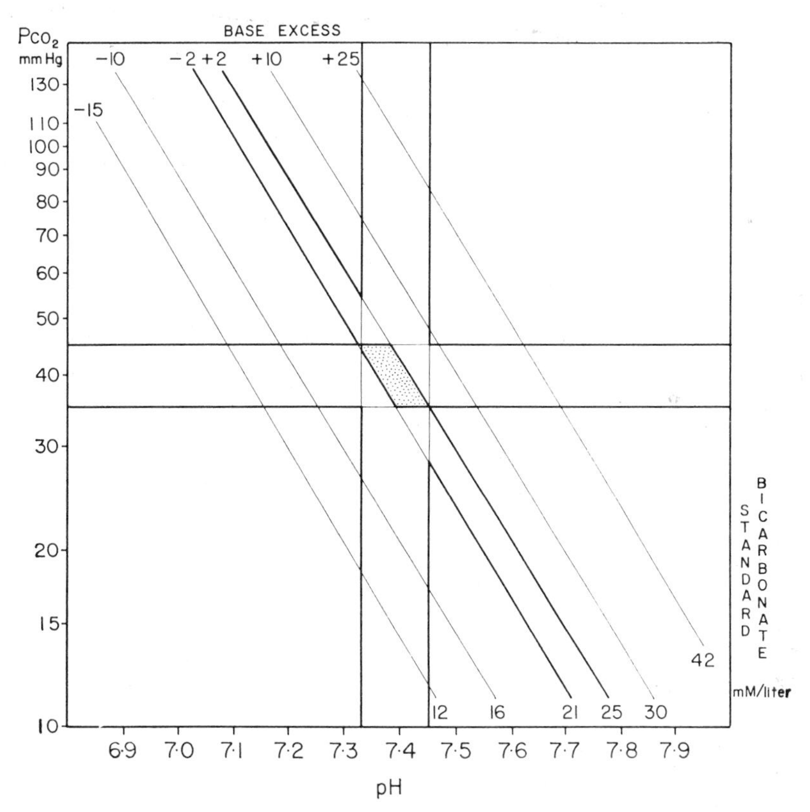

FIGURE 2–26. ACID-BASE DIAGRAM

This illustrates in convenient form the interrelationship between standard bicarbonate, pH, and $P\text{CO}_2$, and enables the physician to follow changes in these values without difficulty. (Adapted from Siggaard-Andersen and Engel.[600])

mm Hg in a series of 60 consecutively studied patients. Since the maximal likely error of a single determination by this method would be 5.8 mm Hg, the accuracy is quite adequate for clinical management. Campbell and Howell[227, 228] later reported on a similar procedure, except that the CO_2 concentration of the equilibrated sample was measured by a simpler gas analysis, and they showed that this technique was very valuable in many clinical management problems. The method has been used to measure the mixed venous $P\text{CO}_2$ in children[2357, 2498] during exercise,[1842, 3499, 3501] and also forms the basis of some methods of measuring cardiac output.[1793, 1794, 3498, 3499] During exercise, however, it has been found that the rebreathing estimate of $P\text{CO}_2$ tends to be higher than that measured directly in blood,[3498, 3503, 3504, 3505] and this difference must be taken into account in computing the cardiac output. Appraisals of this "Bloodless" method for measuring mixed venous blood-gas tensions and cardiac output have recently been published by Farhi and Haab,[3500] Jones and his colleagues,[3501] and other authors.[3503, 3504] Kim, Rahn, and Farhi[3502] have described another "bloodless" method for estimation of the venous and arterial $P\text{CO}_2$ by gas analysis of a single breath, but their ingenious method is probably only applicable to normal subjects.

Collection and storage of blood

When an arterial puncture is performed, it is important to wait until there is no further discomfort before withdrawing the blood sample, since a painful puncture results in overventilation. This may be important if some degree of chronic hypoventilation is suspected.

The white cells in the blood continue their metabolism after removal from the body; on this account at 37° C the arterial oxygen tension falls and that of carbon dioxide rises by 3 to 10 mm Hg per hour, depending on the initial values. Thus, the measurements of arterial $P\text{O}_2$ and $P\text{CO}_2$, as well as the hydrogen

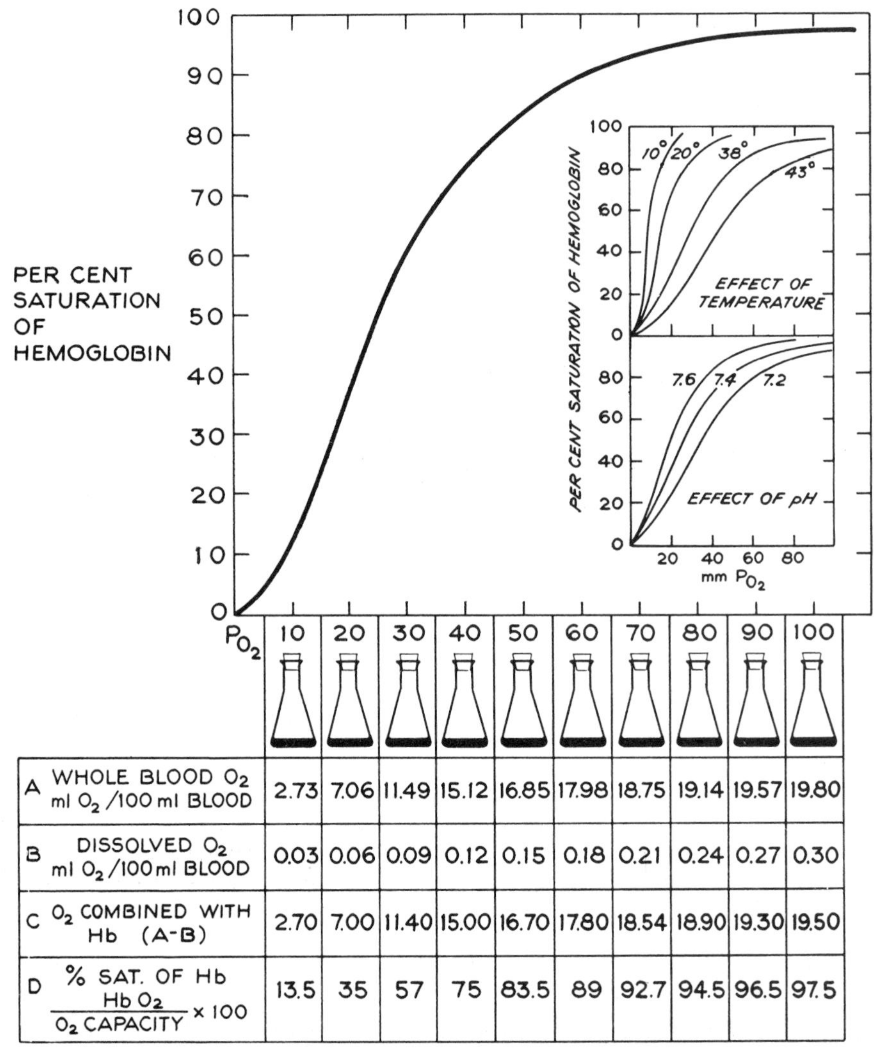

P_{O_2}	10	20	30	40	50	60	70	80	90	100
A WHOLE BLOOD O_2 ml O_2/100 ml BLOOD	2.73	7.06	11.49	15.12	16.85	17.98	18.75	19.14	19.57	19.80
B DISSOLVED O_2 ml O_2/100 ml BLOOD	0.03	0.06	0.09	0.12	0.15	0.18	0.21	0.24	0.27	0.30
C O_2 COMBINED WITH Hb (A-B)	2.70	7.00	11.40	15.00	16.70	17.80	18.54	18.90	19.30	19.50
D % SAT. OF Hb $\frac{HbO_2}{O_2 \text{ CAPACITY}} \times 100$	13.5	35	57	75	83.5	89	92.7	94.5	96.5	97.5

FIGURE 2–27. HbO_2 dissociation curves. The large graph shows a single dissociation curve, applicable when the pH of the blood is 7.40 and temperature 38° C. The blood O_2 tension and saturation of patients with CO_2 retention, acidosis, alkalosis, fever or hypothermia will not fit this curve because the curve shifts to the right or left when temperature, pH, or P_{CO_2} is changed. Effects on the HbO_2 dissociation curve of change in temperature (*upper right*) and in pH (*lower right*) are shown in the smaller graphs. A small change in blood pH occurs regularly in the body; e.g., when mixed venous blood passes through the pulmonary capillaries, P_{CO_2} decreases from 46 to 40 mm Hg and pH rises from 7.37 to 7.40. During this time, blood changes from a pH of 7.37 dissociation curve to a pH of 7.40 curve. (From Comroe, J. H., Jr.: Physiology of Respiration. Chicago, Year Book Medical Publishers, 1969.)

ion concentration, should be made without delay; or, alternatively, correction for time can be made by the use of appropriate nomograms. An immediate analysis of blood is important particularly when pure oxygen is breathed. In this connection, it should also be noted that when the arterial oxygen tension is being measured during oxygen breathing, it is also essential to ensure that pure oxygen is indeed being inspired.

When the temperature of the equipment (usually 37° C) differs from that of the blood at the time of collection, the measured tensions also differ from those which obtain in the body; a corrective factor for this temperature difference effect may be made by use of a nomogram devised by Kelman and Nunn.[3492]

Normal Values of Arterial O_2 and CO_2 Tension

In quiet, steady-state breathing, the alveolar

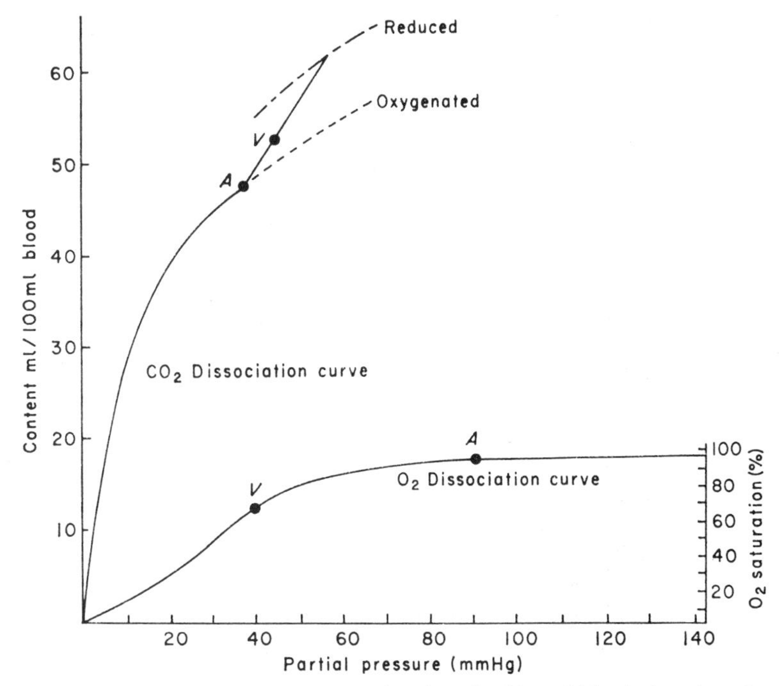

FIGURE 2–28. The dissociation curves for oxygen and carbon dioxide and blood plotted on the same scale. (From Campbell and Dickinson, Clinical Physiology, after Barcroft.). V = mixed venous blood; A = arterial blood.

$P\text{CO}_2$ is about 4 mm Hg higher when the subject is recumbent than when he is standing.[231] When he is sitting upright, the corresponding value is between those for the supine and standing positions. These data were secured by Fenn and Rahn by means of end-tidal automatic sampling, which in normal subjects probably provides a better indication of mean arterial $P\text{CO}_2$ over a period of time than can be obtained from analysis of "spot" samples of arterial blood.[252] The higher $P\text{CO}_2$ in recumbency is associated with a lower minute ventilation due to a decreased frequency of breathing.

It is of interest that during natural sleep the arterial $P\text{CO}_2$ rises a few millimeters as a consequence of a fall in ventilation.[1873, 1874] There is also some evidence that sensitivity to CO_2 is decreased in sleeping subjects.[30] These observations are of interest in relation to the syndrome of primary alveolar hypoventilation, in which considerable arterial desaturation may be noticed when the patient falls asleep (*see* Chapter 16).

In normal, seated subjects at sea level the arterial $P\text{CO}_2$ averages about 38 mm Hg (±2.9 SD) and shows no significant variation with age.[3526] The arterial $P\text{O}_2$, on the contrary, decreases significantly with increasing age. According to Mellemgaard,[3526] in *seated* subjects the regression of arterial $P\text{O}_2$ with age is:

$$\underset{(\text{mm Hg})}{\text{PaO}_2} = 104.2 - 0.27 \times \underset{(\text{years})}{\text{age}}$$

This study was done on 80 subjects whose ages ranged from 15 to 75 years. Sorbini and his co-workers,[3513] in a study on 152 normal, *supine* subjects aged 14 to 84 years, found the following regression:

$$\underset{(\text{mm Hg})}{\text{PaO}_2} = 103.5 - 0.42 \times \underset{(\text{years})}{\text{age}}$$

Thus, the rate of decline of the arterial $P\text{O}_2$ with advancing age appears to be greater in the supine position (0.42 mm Hg per year) than in the sitting position (0.27 mm Hg per year). This is supported by a recent study by Wood and his colleagues.[3634] They measured the arterial $P\text{O}_2$ in a group of elderly subjects in both the sitting and supine positions, and found that the arterial $P\text{O}_2$ in any given individual was almost invariably lower when the subject was supine. This difference is probably caused by the fact that in the supine position airway closure in the dependent lung zones occurs at an earlier age than it does in the sitting position.

A decrease in partial pressure of oxygen in arterial blood is a common feature in patients with cardiorespiratory disease. Although its specific causes are multitudinous, a lowered arterial oxygen tension is due basically to four chief mechanisms: hypoventilation, impaired diffusion, true shunt, and ventilation/perfusion ratio inequality. The first is invariably accompanied by increased arterial CO_2 tension and can be regarded as a disturbance of the control of ventilation system. The last three mechanisms, on the other hand, can be considered as imperfections of the actual lung as a gas exchanger. Hypoventilation, in essence, causes an exaggeration of the normal fall in Po_2 which occurs when air is inspired into the alveoli, whereas the last three mechanisms cause an alveolar–arterial difference for Po_2. The latter mechanisms will be discussed in some detail in the next section, while the causes of hypoventilation will be dealt with in Chapter 3.

Summary

The tremendous technical advances that have occurred in the field of arterial blood analysis have already led to an important understanding of the more profound aspects of gas exchange than was hitherto possible. Simultaneously, the general availability of gas tension measurements in the management of respiratory failure and in the study of such disorders as acute asthma has added a dimension to the study of these problems that can hardly be overstressed at the present time.

Nevertheless, although many commercially available instruments are capable of excellent performance, the physician in charge of such estimates must have good practical training in the methodology and must ensure that routine calibration and tonometric checks are carefully done if accuracy is to be maintained at a high level. For example, an analysis of a measurement of the arterial oxygen tension when a patient is alleged to have been breathing 100 per cent oxygen, in which the administration of the oxygen was not very carefully supervised, in which there was an unknown delay between withdrawal of the sample and its analysis, and in which the routine calibration checks of the oxygen electrode system at high oxygen tensions have not been standard practice, gives rise to puzzling results that defy physiological interpretation and may even form a basis for an erudite discussion at a chest conference; however, they are not worth a great deal.

GAS EXCHANGE WITHIN THE LUNGS

Introduction

A large proportion of the early work on respiratory gas exchange centered around the important advances in blood-gas measurement techniques that were made in the 1920's. For this reason, Meakins and Davies in 1925[1] sought to explain most of the known derangements of respiratory function in terms of disorders of the blood gases.

Although knowledge of the composition of blood gases and the factors that influence this can still be regarded as crucial, the proper evaluation and management of many patients may require not only the determination of the blood gas tensions *per se*, but the consideration of these in conjunction with other measurements. Thus, the simultaneous determination of alveolar as well as arterial partial pressure of gases can provide information of greater value than measurements on blood alone. If the lung were a perfect gas exchanger, the partial pressure of gases in the arterial blood would always be exactly the same as that in alveolar gas, and, therefore, the presence of differences in partial pressure between alveolar gas and arterial blood indicates inefficient gas exchange within the lungs.

Impaired gas exchange in the lungs is caused by three main mechanisms: inequality of the ratio of ventilation to perfusion, right-to-left shunts, and impairment of gas diffusion in the lung. These mechanisms not only cause an increase in alveolar-arterial tension differences, but also contribute to a wastage of ventilation and of blood flow. The reader should note that a *difference* may exist between alveolar-gas mean tension and arterial-blood mean tension for a gas, although the *gradient* that exists between alveolar gas and blood leaving the pulmonary capillary is not widened. It is better to reserve the word "gradient" for circumstances in which there is a widening of this pressure, and to use the word "difference" when only a measured difference between alveolar and arterial gas tensions is to be understood.

This section is designed as a guide to the many methods of measuring such alveolar–arterial gas tension differences and of deducing the cause of abnormality of gas exchange within the lung. Although the general principles are not complex, there are many methods of studying these factors, and the physician commonly finds it a difficult task to unravel them. His reward is the ability to interpret correctly the functional significance of altered blood-gas tensions in conjunction with other measurements of pulmonary function in a wide variety of clinical syndromes.

SYMBOLS

The adoption of a standardized set of symbols to indicate various respiratory parameters has done much to clear the field of confusion. These symbols, first suggested in 1950,[87] and presented in convenient form in *The Lung*,[3] are based on the following general practice: V represents a static volume; $\dot{V}$ indicates the first derivative of volume with respect to time; P indicates a pressure; $\bar{P}$ or any bar over a letter indicates a mean value; F indicates fractional concentration.

Subscripts:

I = inspired gas	E = expired gas
T = tidal gas	D = dead-space gas
B = barometric	A = alveolar gas
c = capillary	a = arterial blood

R indicates respiratory quotient or ratio

$$\frac{\dot{V}CO_2}{\dot{V}O_2}$$

The physician may be reminded, perhaps, that it is impossible to acquire a full understanding of problems of alveolar gas composition without the use of these and other symbols. However, the major concepts in this field can be grasped without the ability to manipulate complex equations. It may be as well to reassure him that this chapter contains no complex mathematics.

ALVEOLAR–ARTERIAL DIFFERENCES IN GAS TENSION

Direct measurement

The alveolar $P\text{O}_2$ and $P\text{CO}_2$ can be measured simultaneously with a mass spectrometer[3636] or separately with an infrared CO_2 analyzer[253, 254] and a rapid paramagnetic, polarographic, or thermal conductivity oxygen meter.[3637, 3638] The changes in these gas tensions measured at the mouth during quiet breathing are illustrated in Figure 2–29. First, gas from the anatomical dead space is exhaled; next, alveolar gas tensions contribute more to the expired gas as the dead space is progressively cleared; and finally, undiluted alveolar gas is sampled.

Although there is a continuous change in $P\text{CO}_2$ and $P\text{O}_2$ during the latter part of expiration (the so-called "alveolar plateau") in the normal subject these changes are small, and the end-tidal $P\text{CO}_2$ and $P\text{O}_2$ can be taken as a good approximation of the "average" mixed alveolar-gas composition when measured at rest. Such end-tidal gas samples can also be collected by a mechanical sampler for later analysis.[251, 252] Arterial blood should be drawn simultaneously and its gas tensions measured, as described previously in this chapter. From these measurements, the *mixed alveolar–arterial* O_2 and CO_2 differences may be obtained.

An increase in the alveolar–arterial difference for oxygen may be due to a variety of factors, as discussed later, and it is therefore, in effect, a nonspecific indicator of impaired gas exchange. The alveolar–arterial CO_2 difference is mainly attributable to ventilation–perfusion inequality; in particular, it is related to the presence of significant volumes of the lung in which the ratio of ventilation to perfusion is raised (an increase in alveolar dead space such as that which occurs, for example, as a consequence of pulmonary embolization).

Impaired gas exchange within the lungs not only causes differences in $P\text{O}_2$ and $P\text{CO}_2$ but also results in differences in nitrogen tension ($P\text{N}_2$).[3639] This is also a fairly specific indicator of impaired gas exchange, since it is mainly influenced by $\dot{V}/\dot{Q}$ inequality, in particular, the presence of areas of low $\dot{V}/\dot{Q}$ ratio. The reason for this is shown in Figure 2–30. Alveoli with a $\dot{V}/\dot{Q}$ ratio of less than 1.0 can be seen to contain an increasing percentage of nitrogen, caused in turn by the sharp fall in oxygen tension in these regions. It is this elevation of nitrogen tension in the blood, as compared to the mean alveolar gas composition, that elevates the alveolar–arterial nitrogen difference in these circumstances. It should also be noted that the (A–a) N_2 difference is unaffected by right-to-left shunts because the

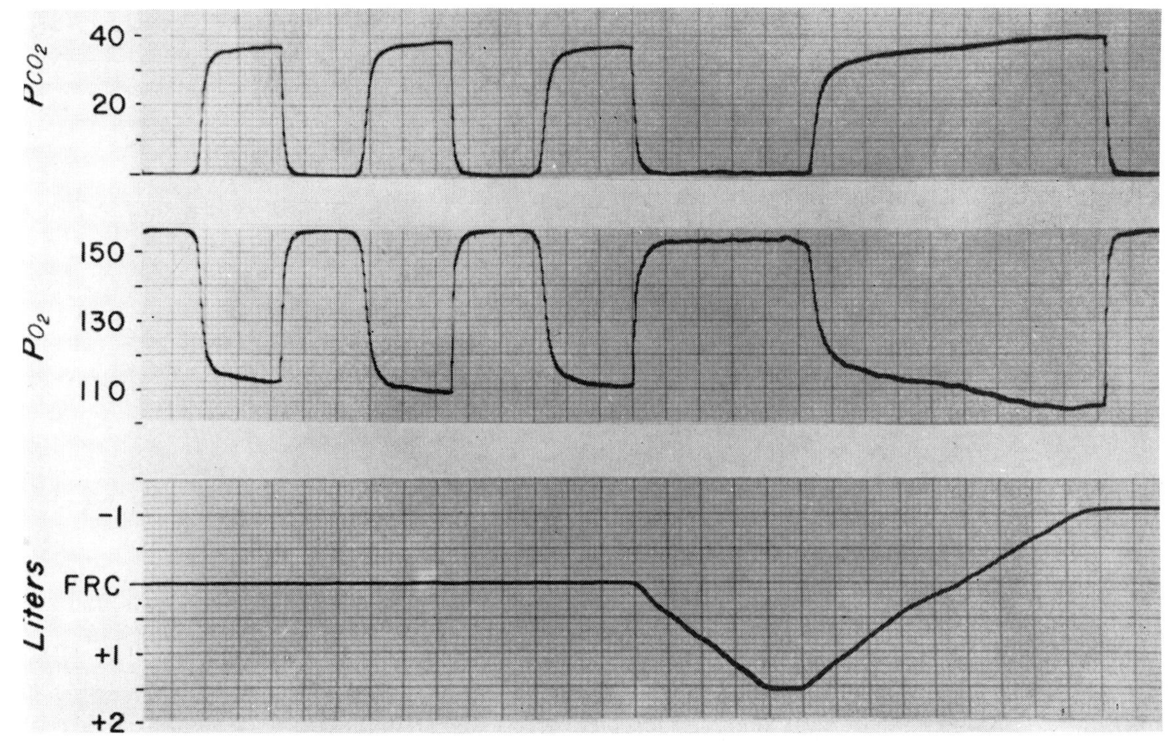

FIGURE 2–29. Continuous recording of expired O_2 and CO_2 tensions in a normal subject. The first three curves show normal expiration values and the last one is a forced expiration. Proceeding with the last inspiration the changes in lung volume were also recorded. Note the continuous change in CO_2 and O_2 during the latter part of each expiration, which makes it difficult to define the alveolar composition. Time: 1 sec between major vertical lines. [Courtesy of Dr. K. T. Fowler, University of Sydney (17).] (From Rahn, H., and Farhi, L. E.: Ventilation, perfusion and gas exchange—the $\dot{V}_A/\dot{Q}$ concept. In Rahn, H., and Fenn, W. O.: Handbook of Physiology. Washington, D.C., The American Physiological Society, 1964.)

venous P_{N_2} is equal to the arterial P_{N_2}. Measurements of this difference are not easy to make. The P_{N_2} of blood can be most easily measured by gas chromatography,[1800] though manometric methods can be adapted for this purpose.[3671] In general, it is not necessary to measure the alveolar P_{N_2} because this value can be assumed with little error.[3639] An earlier suggestion[3644, 3645] that nitrogen-tension measurements on freshly voided urine might be a satisfactory alternative to blood determinations has unfortunately not been confirmed.

The end-tidal gas composition does not always provide a good approximation of the "average" alveolar gas composition. This is the case in many patients with lung disease such as chronic bronchitis, emphysema, and asthma. In such patients, relatively well-ventilated units empty early and poorly ventilated units empty late during expiration, so that any spot sample is unrepresentative of the average gas composition. This is illustrated in Figure 2–31, from which it can be seen that in the patient with pulmonary emphysema there are pronounced changes in P_{O_2} and P_{CO_2} throughout expiration. In such circumstances, it is not at all easy to determine what constitutes the average alveolar gas composition or, indeed, whether the concept of an average alveolar gas concentration has any real meaning when such gross inhomogeneities exist. This problem of obtaining a representative value for "average" alveolar air in different circumstances has plagued the work in this field since it was begun.[230, 247, 248] The definition of such alveolar values, let alone their sampling, presents formidable problems, since alveolar gas composition is in a continual state of flux. Some of these points are considered in the next section.

Variations in alveolar gas tensions and alveolar RQ

With an insoluble gas such as helium or hydrogen, the uniformity of its alveolar concen-

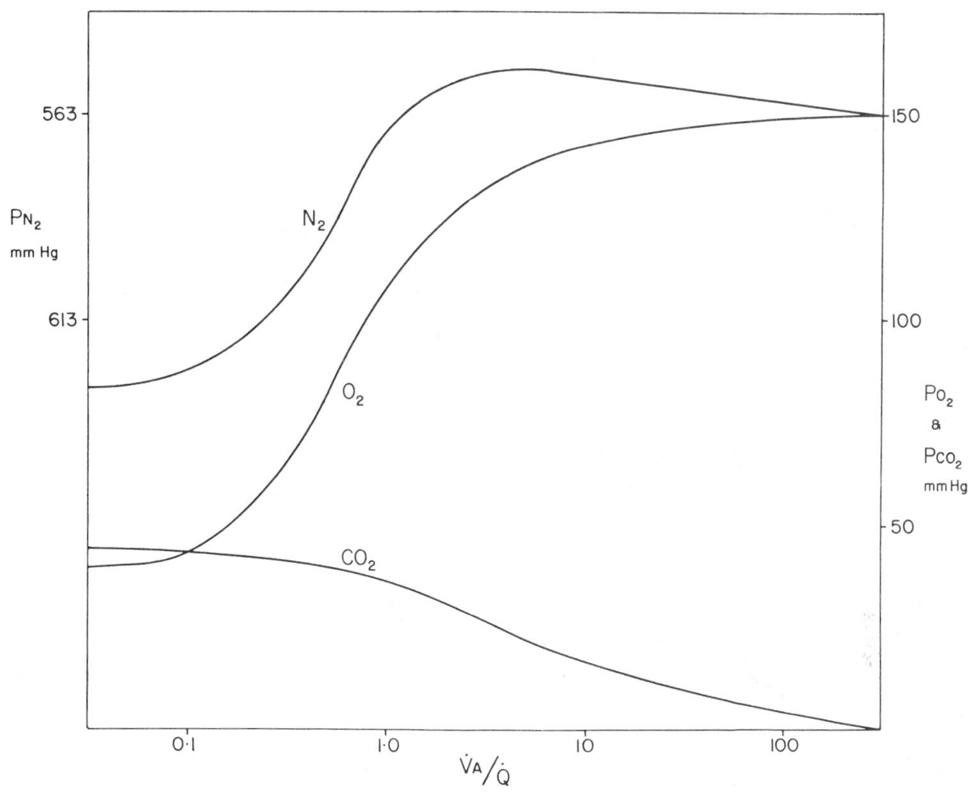

FIGURE 2-30. Effect of Variations of Ventilation and Perfusion Ratio on the Oxygen, Carbon Dioxide, and Nitrogen Tensions in Alveoli

The left-hand ordinate refers to nitrogen tension and the right-hand to tensions of oxygen and carbon dioxide. Note that the nitrogen tension varies most in regions of low $\dot{V}_A/\dot{Q}$ ratio, whereas changes in CO_2 tension are more affected by high $\dot{V}_A/\dot{Q}$ regions. (Diagram from Dr. Leon Farhi.)

tration is principally determined by the evenness of distribution of inspired gas. The uniformity of alveolar oxygen or carbon dioxide tension is, however, by contrast, greatly influenced by the distribution of perfusion in the lung—a factor not so relevant to the alveolar concentration of insoluble gases. Thus the problems of defining a true mean alveolar concentration for oxygen and CO_2 are more complex than for helium or hydrogen.

Within a single alveolus (or group of alveoli) the tension of the respiratory gases, O_2 and CO_2, will fluctuate *in time* from values nearer atmospheric air during inspiration to values approximating the tensions of arterial blood during expiration.[256, 257] The use of a rapid-response CO_2 analyzer enabled DuBois[253, 254] to define the variation in alveolar P_{CO_2} that must occur during quiet breathing at rest, bringing quantitative measurements for the first time to augment the brilliant deductive thinking of Barcroft.[247] Furthermore, during moderately severe exercise, when the tidal volume is large and the amount of CO_2 being evolved is considerable, the fluctuation in alveolar CO_2 is even greater.[259, 260] The demonstration by Suskind[251] that in the normal subject end-tidal gas collected at rest corresponds closely to arterial blood in its CO_2 tension, marked an important step forward. The validity of this observation has been amply confirmed by later work.[24, 252] Many other studies of alveolar gas composition in normal subjects followed, some measuring the consequences of different techniques of sampling,[255, 258] and others more concerned with analysis of the alveolar plateau into its component parts and the relation of its slope to mixed venous and arterial tensions.[256, 257, 1793, 1794] However, on exercise, end-tidal CO_2 values deviate from arterial values, a result foreseen by Aitken and Clark-Kennedy in 1928.[259] Asmussen and Nielsen[260] have com-

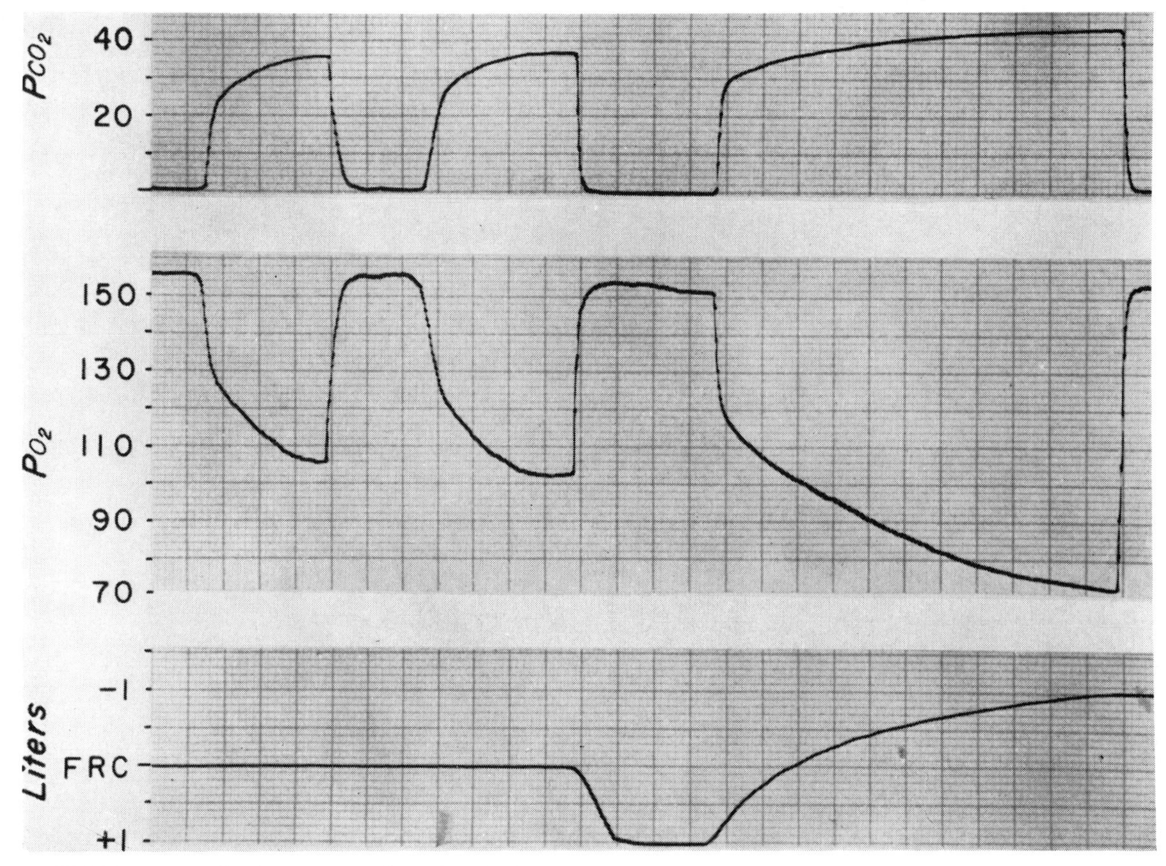

FIGURE 2–31. Continuous recording of expired O_2 and CO_2 tension in an emphysematous subject. This record shows 2 normal expirations followed by a forced expiration. Compare with Fig. 9 and note here that the changes in alveolar gas composition are far more pronounced. (Courtesy of Dr. K. T. Fowler, University of Sydney.) (From Rahn, H., and Farhj, L. E.: Ventilation perfusion and gas exchange—the V_A/Q concept. In Rahn, H., and Fenn, W. O.: Handbook of Physiology. Washington, D.C., The American Physiological Society, 1964.)

pared arterial and end-tidal CO_2 tensions during exercise and have shown that, when the tidal volume exceeds 1.5 liters during exercise, the arterial P_{CO_2} is about 3 mm Hg lower than the alveolar P_{CO_2} collected by an end-normal expiration technique. In these circumstances, the arterial P_{CO_2} may be more reliably calculated using an assumed V_D volume in the Bohr equation (*see* page 18).

Roelsen was one of the first workers to show that even greater variation in expired-gas composition occurs in patients with lung disease.[134, 135] After an inspiration of hydrogen, he analyzed the subsequent expiration so as to show the changing concentrations of hydrogen, oxygen, and carbon dioxide, and from his results he deduced correctly that the distribution of ventilation *vis à vis* perfusion must be deranged in emphysema. Thus he directed attention to the fact that, in addition to the variations of respiratory gas tensions *in time* which occur within a single alveolus, there are also variations *in space* between one alveolus and the next. Similar studies were reported by Gad,[138, 139] who concluded correctly that patients with pulmonary tuberculosis were better able to maintain "the normal interaction between ventilation and circulation than is the case in emphysema."

Subsequent workers using a variety of techniques have fully confirmed the even greater spatial variations in alveolar gas tensions that exist in disease. Thus, using a time-consuming method in which 100-ml fractions of alveolar gas could be collected and analyzed, Marshall, Bates, and Christie[261] measured the changes in expired alveolar gas CO_2 concentration and RQ that occurred in normal subjects and 26 patients with emphysema. The results are shown in Figure 2–32.

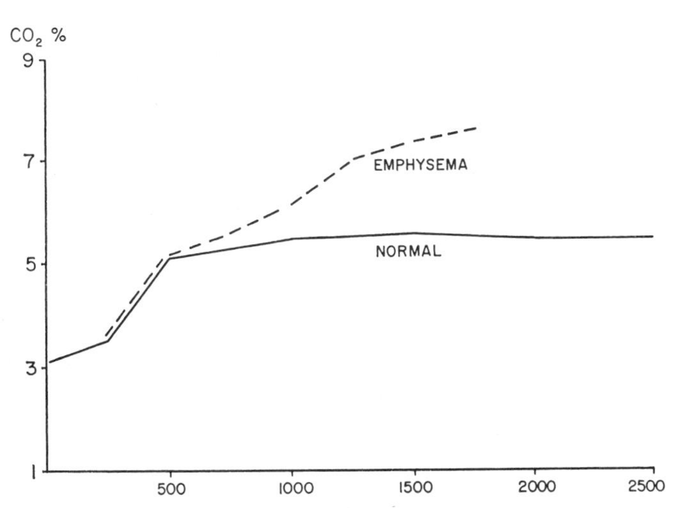

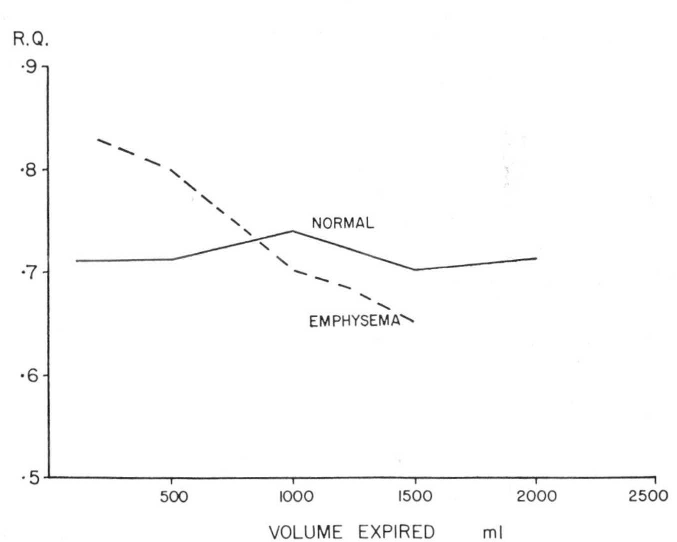

FIGURE 2–32. Slopes of Changing CO_2 Percentage and RQ during a Single Fast Expiration in Normal Subjects and in Patients with Emphysema

These curves have been calculated from data contained in Marshall, Bates and Christie.[261] Note the steeper rise in CO_2 and fall in RQ as expiration proceeds in emphysema compared to normal. As the slope of the CO_2 and RQ lines depends not only on the uniformity of the $\dot{V}/\dot{Q}$ relationships but also on the pattern of emptying of the lung, and is influenced also by the total duration of the measured expiration, this test is of little diagnostic value.

Sivertson and Fowler[257] reported similar experiments, and the method has been refined by West and his colleagues[262–264] and by Read,[265] using a mass spectrometer for continuous and simultaneous recording of gas concentrations. By the simultaneous use of a nitrogen meter and CO_2 analyzer, Martin and Young have demonstrated[266] that variations in these gas concentrations occur from samples drawn from one lobe of the lung.

Although it is clear that a greater than normal change in CO_2 and RQ during the course of an expiration must indicate a wider than normal range of ventilation–perfusion ($\dot{V}/\dot{Q}$) distribution, there has been considerable disagreement in interpretation of these results in terms of lung-emptying patterns and the relative $\dot{V}/\dot{Q}$ of different regions. Recently evidence has been obtained[244, 265] that the uniformity of $\dot{V}/\dot{Q}$ distribution decreases with advancing age. This point is discussed in more detail in Chapter 3. Of considerable interest is the recent demonstration that the uptake of carbon monoxide is pulsatile in the human lung,[3573] and it has been known for some years that the uptake of nitrous oxide is pulsatile.[1976] When this information is added to the recent new concept that airway closure may commonly occur, particularly in the older subject, as he breathes down to residual volume, it becomes evident that an exact computation of fluctuant changes in alveolar gas composition under all circumstances is a most complex task.

Indirect determination of (A–a) D_{O_2}: Ideal alveolar gas

The physician is now in a position to realize some of the difficulties associated with the measurement of the "average" composition of alveolar gas, particularly in patients with lung disease. Even if it were possible to sample gas directly in the lung, its variability from alveolus to alveolus and the time factor would constitute a major obstacle to obtaining what could be reasonably considered a representative or average value.

The possibility of deriving such an average value indirectly was explored more or less simultaneously by Riley and his colleagues in the U.S.A.,[413] and by Rossier in Switzerland.[280–282] The assumption was made that the tension of the most soluble of the respiratory gases (CO_2) in arterial blood approximates the *ideal* alveolar P_{CO_2}, i.e., the alveolar P_{CO_2} which the lung would have if there were no ventilation–perfusion imbalance and if the lungs continued to exchange at the same respiratory exchange ratio. Because of the shape of the blood dissociation curves the error introduced in using the arterial P_{CO_2} is generally very small. As noted in an earlier section (*see* page 18), knowing the arterial P_{CO_2} (P_{aCO_2}), the ideal alveolar P_{O_2} can be computed from the alveolar gas equation:

$$(\text{Ideal})\ P_{A_{O_2}} = P_{I_{O_2}} - \frac{P_{a_{CO_2}}}{R} + 0.209\ P_{a_{CO_2}} \frac{(1-R)}{R}$$

Thus it becomes possible to calculate an "average" alveolar oxygen tension from a knowledge of the inspired oxygen tension ($P_{I_{O_2}}$), of R which is the respiratory quotient, and of the arterial CO_2 tension ($P_{a_{CO_2}}$) which can be directly measured. The need for direct alveolar sampling is thus bypassed.

It must be stressed that the mean alveolar oxygen tension so derived is an "ideal" one, aptly named by Riley and his colleagues[413] because it represents the value which would obtain *if the $\dot{V}/\dot{Q}$ ratios were equal throughout the lung and there was no diffusion limitation.* Comparison of the alveolar P_{O_2} so calculated with the measured arterial P_{O_2} enables an "alveolar–arterial difference" to be computed which will reflect distributional and diffusion impairment.[1807] In describing such differences, however, the word ideal should precede the word alveolar; that is, one should write "ideal alveolar–arterial oxygen difference" to distinguish it from the mixed expired alveolar–arterial oxygen difference obtained from direct measurements of expired gas.[2488] Such a distinction is necessary because the ideal alveolar–arterial difference does not take into account alveolar–arterial differences caused by alveolar dead space, whereas such differences are included when mixed expired alveolar air is used instead.

The problem of using the alveolar air equation to compute a mean alveolar concentration of another gas, such as carbon monoxide, is discussed in detail later in this chapter.

Normal values for alveolar–arterial gas tension differences

In normal young subjects breathing air while seated at rest, the mixed expired alveolar–arterial differences for P_{O_2}, P_{CO_2}, and P_{N_2} average 6.8, −0.4, and −4.0 mm Hg respectively. The (A–a) D_{O_2} has been shown to be larger in older subjects compared to younger ones.[1804, 2260, 2268] According to Mellemgaard,[3526] the regression of ideal alveolar-arterial oxygen tension difference with age is:

$$\underset{(\text{mm Hg})}{(\text{A–a})\ D_{O_2}} = 2.5 + 0.21 \times \underset{(\text{years})}{\text{Age}}$$

This study was performed on 80 healthy, seated subjects whose ages ranged between 15 and 75 years. The increase in (A–a) D_{O_2} was due almost entirely to a decrease in the arterial P_{O_2}, the alveolar P_{O_2} showing no significant variation with age. As noted later, these phenomena are probably to be explained by terminal airway closure in elderly subjects during resting breathing,[2432] and by the lower cardiac output in older people (*see* page 99).[616]

Hesser and Matell[3565] have measured the alveolar–arterial tension difference on moderate exercise and have reported that it decreased under these conditions. However, for reasons not altogether clear, their subjects showed unusually high levels of the (A–a) D_{O_2} at rest (14.7 mm Hg). In newborn infants, the (A–a) D_{O_2} appears to be greater than the Mellemgaard regression would predict.[2540, 3649]

Riley and his colleagues[286] found that the (A–a) D_{O_2} was greater in a normal subject standing than when supine, but others have not confirmed this observation.[287, 1799] Recent work indicates that in elderly subjects the O_2 difference should be greater when the subject is supine than when sitting.[3513, 3634]

Prolonged recumbency was shown by Cardus[3646] to result in an average increase of 10 mm Hg in seven young men after 10 days of bed rest. One hour of recumbency causes an increase in the (A–a) D_{N_2},[2439] and we have found that a measurable decrease in ventilation occurs in dependent lung zones, particularly in older subjects, on recumbency.[2465] Cyclic oscillations of (A–a) D_{O_2} occurring within relatively short periods of normal resting breathing have also been reported.[3647]

It is now clear that the alveolar–arterial gas-tension differences for oxygen, carbon dioxide, and nitrogen that may be observed are mainly influenced in normal people by the uniformity of lung perfusion as a consequence of the cardiac output and by terminal airway closure on a basis of diminished lung recoil.

"WASTED" BLOOD FLOW: VENOUS ADMIXTURE EFFECT

Impairment of gas exchange in the lungs may be expressed in terms of "wasted" pulmonary blood flow (synonyms: venous admixture, right-to-left shunt). Venous admixture, or the addition of mixed venous blood to arterial blood, is, by analogy, the "dead space" of the blood perfusion of the lungs. It may be computed as follows:

$$\frac{\dot{Q}_{va}}{\dot{Q}_t} = \frac{C_{a_{O_2}} - C_{i_{O_2}}}{C_{\bar{v}_{O_2}} - C_{i_{O_2}}}$$

where $\dot{Q}_{va}/\dot{Q}_t$ is the ratio of venous admixture to total flow; $C_{a_{O_2}}$ and $C_{\bar{v}_{O_2}}$ are the arterial and mixed venous oxygen content respectively, and $C_{i_{O_2}}$ is the *ideal* oxygen content of arterial blood, i.e., the content that would obtain *if* the arterial P_{O_2} were equal to the ideal alveolar P_{O_2} (*see* earlier discussion).

Except during pure oxygen breathing, the venous admixture so determined is an expression of both true shunts and of shuntlike effects. The former represent contributions to the arterial blood which have not been through ventilated areas of the lungs, and the latter are an expression of the effect of regions with a low ventilation/perfusion ratio. Although low $\dot{V}/\dot{Q}$ areas do not really contribute mixed venous blood, the arterial blood changes as if venous blood were being added. By giving a patient pure oxygen to breathe, a true shunt can be distinguished from the $\dot{V}/\dot{Q}$ effect because the arterial oxygen tension will be the same in low and high $\dot{V}/\dot{Q}$ regions (or nearly so) when pure oxygen is breathed, and thus a true shunt remains the only cause of arterial hypoxia. It should be noted, however, that the arterial P_{O_2} will rise appreciably in a patient with a true shunt when pure oxygen is breathed, since the unshunted blood will pick up more dissolved oxygen at the higher tension. In some instances, this factor may raise the arterial oxygen saturation to nearly 100 per cent on pure oxygen, even in the presence of a true shunt, but a widened alveolar–arterial oxygen tension difference will still be demonstrable if a shunt exists.

The true shunt contains components from right-to-left intracardiac shunts, bronchial veins, abnormal communications between pulmonary arteries and veins, and alveoli which are perfused but not ventilated. Strictly speaking, such alveoli represent an extreme example of ventilation–perfusion inequality (i.e., a $\dot{V}/\dot{Q}$ ratio of nil), but for convenience these unventilated alveoli are regarded as a true shunt because their effects on gas exchange are indistinguishable from those of other true shunts.

In healthy, seated individuals at rest, the total shunt, in general, amounts to less than 5 per cent of the total cardiac output, and the true shunt is of the order of about 1 to 2 per cent.[3526] Normally, therefore, relatively little of the blood flow is wasted (about 5 per cent), as compared to wasted ventilation (about 30 per cent).

"WASTED" VENTILATION: PHYSIOLOGICAL DEAD SPACE

As noted earlier in this chapter, the physiological dead space represents wasted ventilation, and its magnitude can be used to express one aspect of impaired gas exchange. The difference between anatomical dead space measured with an insoluble gas such as helium and the "physiological dead space" measured with an exchanging gas reflects the component of wasted ventilation. It has been called the "alveolar dead space" by Severinghaus and Stupfel.[246] Measurement of the physiological dead space was first described by Rossier,[280–282] and it is commonly measured by substituting the arterial P_{CO_2} for the alveolar P_{CO_2} in the Bohr Equation, as follows:

$$V_{D_{CO_2}} = \frac{V_T(P_{a_{CO_2}} - P_{\bar{E}_{CO_2}})}{P_{a_{CO_2}}}$$

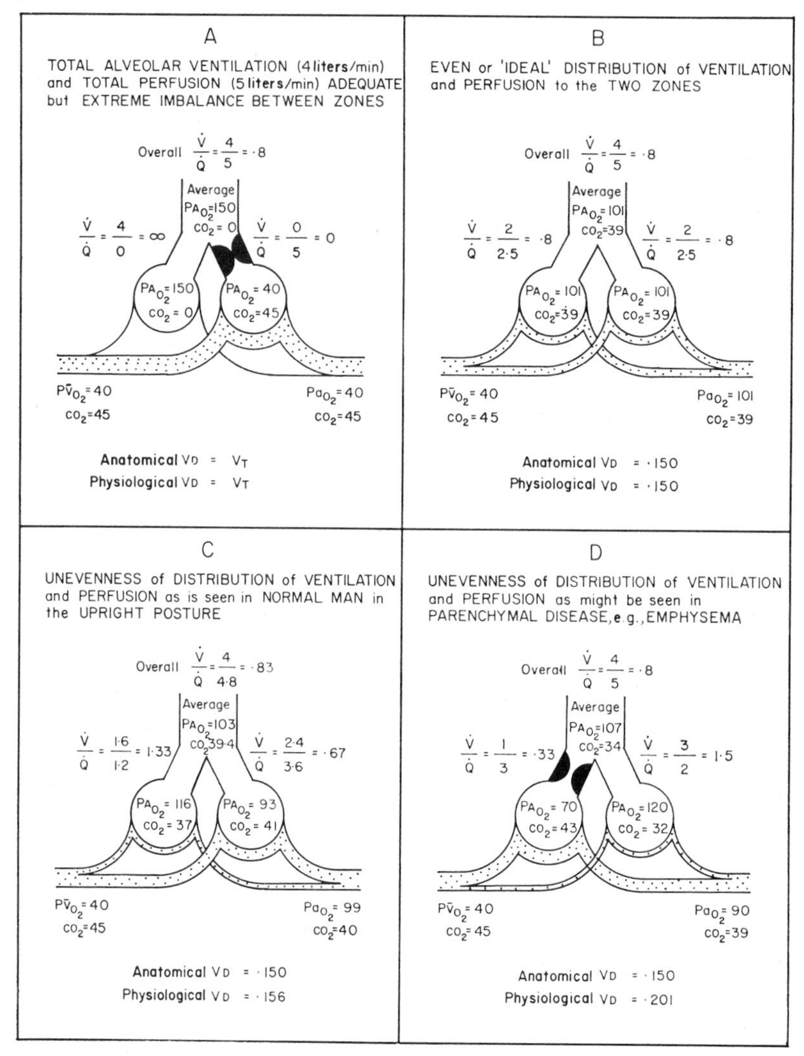

FIGURE 2–33. Consequences of Uneven Distribution of Ventilation in Relation to Perfusion in Different Zones of the Lung

In this model, the lung consists of two zones of equal volume. "Average" alveolar gas tensions are computed from the gas expired from each zone and mixed. Similarly, mixed arterial blood gas tensions are calculated from known gas tensions of blood coming from each zone and mixed.

A, In this extreme example, total alveolar ventilation and total perfusion are both adequate, but since ventilation is wholly distributed to one zone and perfusion wholly to the other there is no gas exchange.

B, In this example, ventilation and perfusion are uniformly distributed. Note that in this circumstance: (1) The "average" alveolar gas tension represents the correct tension existing in both zones. (2) There is no difference between alveolar and arterial gas tensions. (3) The inert-gas dead space (anatomical V_D) is the same as the physiological dead space computed from the arterial P_{CO_2} tension.

C, The degree of uneven distribution of ventilation and perfusion in this example is similar to that existing in the normal man sitting upright at rest. The left-hand zone receives slightly less ventilation and much less perfusion than the right-hand zone; thus the left-hand zone represents alveoli in the upper part of the lung, and the right-hand zone represents alveoli with a lower $\dot{V}/\dot{Q}$ ratio at the lung base. Note that: (1) Although the over-all ratio of ventilation to perfusion is 0.83, that in one zone is 1.33 and that in the other is 0.67. (2) The tensions of oxygen and CO_2 are different in the two zones. (3) The gas tensions in "average" alveolar gas represent those in *neither* zone, being weighted by the gas tensions in the right-hand zone, which contributes more gas to the expirate than the left-hand zone. (4) The gas tensions in arterial blood also represent those in *neither* zone, being weighted by blood coming from the better-perfused right-hand zone. (5) There is a difference in gas tension for oxygen and for CO_2 between "average" alveolar gas and arterial blood, although complete gas equilibration is assumed to occur in both zones. (6) The physiological dead space now exceeds the inert-gas dead space (anatomical V_D).

D, In this example, there is severe imbalance between ventilation and perfusion of a degree encountered in emphysema. Total ventilation and perfusion are the same as in the other examples. The zone with lowered ventilation on the

(Legend continues on opposite page.)

where V_T is the tidal volume and $P_{E_{CO_2}}$ the tension of CO_2 in mixed expired gas.

The physiological dead space is often expressed as a ratio of the tidal volume. In normal young subjects, it is, on the average, a little less than a third of the tidal volume, and it tends to decrease during exercise.[194, 260, 287, 2294, 2484, 3526, 3650] With advancing age, the V_D/V_T ratio increases.[1799, 2294, 3526] According to Mellemgaard,[3526] the regression of the physiological dead space/tidal volume ratio with age in seated, normal subjects at rest is given by the following expression:

$$\underset{\text{(per cent)}}{V_D/V_T} = 24.6 + 0.17 \times \underset{\text{(years)}}{\text{Age}}$$

Strang has made the interesting observation[288] that the ratio of physiological dead space to tidal volume is greater in newborn infants than in adults, indicating some nonuniformity of $\dot{V}/\dot{Q}$ ratios in the lung immediately after birth. Koch[3649] has more recently found that by the age of 24 hours the V_D/V_T ratio is of the same order as in adults.

An increase in the V_D/V_T ratio indicates a loss of efficiency in terms of CO_2 elimination per unit of total ventilation.

ALVEOLAR VENTILATION

The definition of effective alveolar ventilation has already been mentioned in this chapter. Total ventilation, or minute volume in liters, can be measured easily by collecting expired gas over a known period of time. Some fraction of this represents gas wasted in ventilating the anatomical and the alveolar dead spaces and, hence, not contributing to gas exchange. The alveolar ventilation can be computed if the volume of the total dead space is known, since:

$$\begin{aligned}\text{Alveolar ventilation} &= \text{Total ventilation} - \text{Dead space ventilation}\\ &= (V_T \times f) - (V_D \times f)\\ &= f(V_T - V_D)\end{aligned}$$

In practice, since the arterial P_{CO_2} has to be measured to estimate the total dead space, the level of the arterial P_{CO_2} is customarily taken as the prime indicator of the level of alveolar ventilation. This is reasonable, since alveolar ventilation can be considered adequate only if it maintains within physiological limits the tension of the respiratory gases in the blood leaving the lung.

THE O_2–CO_2 DIAGRAM

The accumulating experimental data relevant to the problem of alveolar gas composition were fortunately accompanied by brilliant theoretical analyses of the determinants of this parameter by Fenn and Rahn.[231–234] The graphic presentation by these authors[231] of the O_2–CO_2 diagram provided workers in this research field with an invaluable reference of great use in the solution of many problems of gas exchange.

The diagram is based on the fact that the variables concerned in gas exchange are interdependent. Thus, the tensions of the three gases O_2, CO_2 and N_2 in the alveoli must equal barometric pressure less water-vapor pressure, and if two are known the third can be derived (Fig. 2–30). In its usual form the O_2–CO_2 diagram has oxygen and CO_2 on its axes, the third, N_2, being implicit. Isopleths can be superimposed representing different values for the ventilatory RQ, so that if the value for one gas tension only is known, but the ventilatory RQ also is known, the other two gas tensions can be derived. Similarly, isopleths for arterial oxygen content and saturation, arterial CO_2 content, pH, and alveolar ventilation/100 ml O_2 uptake or CO_2 output also can be superimposed, and can be used in the same way. Thus, if any two of these many variables are known, values for all others can be derived. Finally, if the mixed venous and inspired oxygen tensions are known, then the $\dot{V}/\dot{Q}$ ratio responsible for the observed alveolar gas tensions can be derived. (The values for alveolar gas tensions in Figure 2–33 were all calculated by use of the O_2–CO_2 diagram.)

FIGURE 2–33. *Continued.*

left-hand side now has more perfusion than is received by the better-ventilated right-hand zone. The $\dot{V}/\dot{Q}$ ratio is 0.33 in one zone and 1.5 in the other. Directionally the effects are similar to those described in example *C*, though greater in degree. The alveolar–arterial tension differences are wider, and there is now a 51 ml difference between the anatomical dead space and the physiological dead space.

This simplified description gives little indication of the remarkable development of these concepts so clearly set forth by their originators, and of the power of the graphic solution which made the interrelationship of these factors apparent to physiologists in a way that was not evident from their mathematical solution.

Causes of increased alveolar–arterial differences and of impaired gas exchange within the lung

Ventilation/perfusion ratio inequality

Introduction. Appreciation of the fact that variations in alveolar gas tensions are to be found in different parts of the lung and that these variations might be attributable to differences in the balance of ventilation and perfusion in these different parts opened a new horizon for the chest physician. He could now perceive that, for the lung to perform its respiratory function of gas exchange, the distribution of ventilation *vis à vis* perfusion must be balanced, and that even though the overall amounts of ventilation and perfusion might be adequate, respiratory function would be impaired if they were not appropriately matched throughout the lung.

The extreme example of such imbalance is shown in Figure 2–33*A*, in which an adequate total alveolar ventilation (4 liters/min) reaches half of the alveolar volume exclusively, whereas a similarly adequate total volume of perfusion (5 liters/min) is directed to the other half of the alveolar volume exclusively. Such a situation results in no gas exchange and is, of course, incompatible with life. It is of importance to note that this hypothetical situation is characterized by extreme variation in the alveolar gas tensions, particularly $P_{A_{O_2}}$, in the two lung zones, although a sample of alveolar gas taken at the mouth would not reflect this unevenness because no alveolar air is expired from the nonventilated lung.

By contrast, if the same total volume of ventilation and perfusion is distributed equally to both lungs (*see* Figure 2–33*B*), gas exchange would be complete, alveolar gas tensions in both lungs would be similar, and alveolar gas sampled at the mouth would correctly reflect the "average" alveolar gas tensions. Of course, variations in the alveolar gas tension of the respiratory gases in both lungs would still occur in time with the respiratory cycle, since respiration is not a continuous process.

It is now known, however, that even in normal subjects this ideal situation is not attained; and, in the sitting position at rest, considerably more perfusion occurs in the lower than in the upper parts of the lung (*see* page 48). In Figure 2–33*C* are shown two lung compartments which reflect the uneven $\dot{V}/\dot{Q}$ distribution believed to exist in these circumstances. This relatively slight degree of unevenness results in a difference of 4 mm Hg of oxygen pressure between the mixed alveolar value of 103 mm Hg and the arterial value of 99 mm Hg.[653] The precise quantitation of the magnitude of distributional effects on the alveolar–arterial oxygen difference was first formulated by Farhi and Rahn.[1808]

The presence of adaptive mechanisms to divert blood flow to the best-ventilated regions of the lungs was postulated by Barcroft,[271] Anthony[128] and Haldane[2]; more recent work has in general confirmed their suppositions and suggests also that similar mechanisms operate to redirect ventilation away from nonperfused areas.[1084, 1210, 3642] The normal lung appears to be potentially equipped to deal with imbalance in the distribution of perfusion *vis à vis* ventilation.

The more marked variations in alveolar gas tensions in disease, already referred to, are the result of greater degrees of imbalance between ventilation and perfusion (i.e., greater variation in $\dot{V}/\dot{Q}$ ratios throughout the lungs). This may be the consequence of direct destruction of the lung parenchyma or of disturbance of its adaptive mechanisms. The situation depicted in Figure 2–33*D* might reflect that occurring in emphysema, and its effects upon alveolar gas tensions in the two areas are apparent. In this instance the differences in alveolar O_2 tensions between the two areas represented are more marked and the difference between alveolar and arterial gas tensions is greater than in the other examples.

Rahn and Fenn[231] have shown that, besides a wide disparity of $\dot{V}/\dot{Q}$ ratios among the lung units, two other factors contribute to tension differences between alveolar gas and arterial blood—namely, any diffusion limitations that may exist between alveolar gas and pulmonary capillary blood, and any admixture of venous blood into the left side of the heart from bronchial veins, or direct shunts in the lung allowing blood to bypass alveolar gas. The proportional contribution of these three factors to the total A–a differences in man is shown in Figure 2–34, devised by Farhi and Rahn.[231] From this, it may be seen that the diffusion factor becomes of any importance only at low oxygen tensions, when the effect of direct venous admixture is minimal.[2294] (Riley made use of the minimizing effect of a low inspired oxygen concentration on the influence of the venous admixture component in devising a technique to measure the oxygen-diffusing capacity of the lung.[3]) The venous admixture effect becomes maximal at an inspired tension of oxygen of about 150 mm;[2268, 2271, 2294] the contribution of disparity in $\dot{V}/\dot{Q}$ ratios on the total (A–a) O_2 difference, however, is relatively little influenced by changes in the ambient O_2 tension. Cole and Bishop[3457], however, have recently reported that there is a significant drop in the (A–a) D_{O_2} when the alveolar Po_2 is increased from 291 to 653 mm Hg. This is possibly caused by a change in the magnitude of the true shunt, but it might also indicate that at values of alveolar Po_2 greater than 150 mm Hg, the contribution of the $\dot{V}/\dot{Q}$ ratio effect to the total (A–a) D_{O_2} is greater than had previously been thought. Lenfant[3640, 3641] has pushed the analytical methods one step further and measured simultaneously the A–a differences for O_2, CO_2, and N_2. He concluded that 75 per cent of the (A–a) O_2 difference in normal, resting subjects breathing room air is attributable to distribution effects, and this is supported by the calculations of West, based on regional measurements of ventilation and perfusion (*see* page 74).

The A–a difference for CO_2[2268] (the difference in Pco_2 between mixed alveolar air and mixed arterial blood) is much influenced by the presence of alveoli that are ventilated but poorly perfused (i.e., have high $\dot{V}/\dot{Q}$ ratios) but is virtually unaffected by diffusion (CO_2 is very readily soluble and therefore diffusible) or by shunts of blood (i.e., venous admixture; *see* Figure 2–34). Rahn has used the A–a difference for CO_2 to enable an estimate to be made of the amount of ventilation being "wasted" in the areas with high $\dot{V}/\dot{Q}$ ratios, or what he has called the "air shunt."[26]

The difference between end-tidal CO_2 and arterial CO_2 that may be observed after the occurrence of multiple pulmonary emboli (*see* page 321) depends upon this phenomenon. The more alveoli there are that are ventilated but no longer perfused (high $\dot{V}/\dot{Q}$ ratio), the larger will the difference become.[246]

The presence of disparity in $\dot{V}/\dot{Q}$ ratios throughout the lungs will also cause a difference for N_2 between mixed alveolar air and mixed arterial blood. Though not enumerated in Figure 2–33, this can be calculated, since

		(A−a)D_{O_2} on air	(A−a)D_{O_2} on 100% O_2	(A−a)D_{O_2} on low O_2	(a−A)D_{CO_2}	(a−A)D_{N_2}
Venous admixture		+ +	+ + + +	+	◌	○
Diffusion limitation		+	◌	+ +	◌	○
Uneven $\dot{V}_A/\dot{Q}$	High $\dot{V}_A/\dot{Q}$	+ +	+	+	+ + + +	+
	Low $\dot{V}_A/\dot{Q}$	+ +	+	+	+	+ + + +

FIGURE 2–34. Effect of various disturbances on alveolar-arterial differences. The various disturbances are listed in the first column, and the effects on (A-a)D appear at the proper boxes. The effects are graded from ○ (no effect), through ◌ (theoretically present, but too small to be measured) to ++++. (A-a)D or (a-A)D values which are specific for a given disturbance are indicated by shaded background. (From Farhi, L. E.: Recent Advances in Respiratory Physiology. Ventilation–perfusion relationship and its role in alveolar gas exchange. London, W. H. Arnold, 1965.)

the tensions of O_2, CO_2, and N_2 in blood or gas must equal atmospheric pressure less water-vapor pressure (*see* Figure 2–30). Thus, in Figure 2–33*D*, the "average" alveolar N_2 tension ($P_{A_{N_2}}$) = 574, while the arterial nitrogen tension (P_{aN_2}) = 586 mm. Since this difference is insignificantly affected by diffusion limitations and not at all by venous admixture, Rahn has used it to quantitate the amount of perfusion being wasted in areas of lung with low $\dot{V}/\dot{Q}$ ratios, or what he has called the "blood shunt."[26] The existence of abnormally high alveolar–arterial nitrogen differences in emphysema has been demonstrated by Briscoe and Gurtner.[272, 3645]

Thus the presence of variations in $\dot{V}/\dot{Q}$ ratios in different regions of the lung can be deduced from the differences for O_2, CO_2, and N_2 between "mixed" alveolar air and "mixed" arterial blood, and the proportional contribution of high $\dot{V}/\dot{Q}$ areas and low $\dot{V}/\dot{Q}$ areas can be derived from the differences for CO_2 and N_2 respectively.[2268]

No better summary of the basic concept of the $\dot{V}/\dot{Q}$ ratio has been written than that by Rahn and Farhi[62]: "The lung is an organ with millions of units each having a finite ventilation–perfusion ($\dot{V}/\dot{Q}$) ratio. Normally this ratio averages about 1 but may theoretically vary from zero to infinity. This ratio determines not only the oxygen and carbon dioxide tension in each unit, but allows one to determine the 'total flow requirements' (the total ventilation and perfusion) for exchanging equal units of oxygen and carbon dioxide. At a ratio of about 1 the oxygen and carbon dioxide tensions are 'normal' and the 'total flow requirements' at their lowest. At higher or lower ratios the flow requirements increase rapidly and the gas tension becomes abnormal." Thus the most economical condition for lung performance is when the ventilation/perfusion ratios are uniform throughout the lung and have a value close to unity.

A more detailed treatment of $\dot{V}/\dot{Q}$ ratio inequalities and of their effect on gas exchange can be found in several excellent reviews.[2488, 2489, 2490, 3633] The recent advances in knowledge on regional lung function are described earlier in this chapter.

METHODS OF MEASUREMENT OF $\dot{V}/\dot{Q}$ INEQUALITY. It may be convenient to summarize the many methods that may be and have been used to provide an indication of the presence of $\dot{V}/\dot{Q}$ inequality in the lungs. These have been arranged in the following approximate order of increasing complexity:

1. By measuring the gradient of change of CO_2 concentration and RQ in a single expiration.[257, 261, 264, 3523]
2. By combining the measurement of the arterial P_{CO_2} with observations of CO_2 exchange, computing the physiological dead space, and comparing it with the measured tidal volume.[17]
3. By analyzing alveolar–arterial gas tension differences.[26, 272] The P_{N_2} difference, being unaffected by true venous admixture or diffusion impairment, is a virtually specific index of low $\dot{V}/\dot{Q}$ regions within the lung. Farhi has recently described a sophisticated analysis of $\dot{V}/\dot{Q}$ distribution based on simultaneous measurements of the CO_2 and N_2 differences.[2489] The (A–a) D_{O_2} is not a specific index of impaired gas exchange as ordinarily measured. However Overfield and Kylstra[3651] have recently reported a new method based on respiration of pure oxygen in a high altitude chamber which does permit quantitation of the fraction of the oxygen difference caused by $\dot{V}/\dot{Q}$ imbalance.
4. By combining the measurement of the physiological dead space with determinations of venous admixture according to the classic analysis of Riley and Cournand.[413]
5. By analyzing the elimination of non-radioactive inert gases of different solubility.[2489, 3544, 3655, 3657]
6. By obtaining estimates of the volume of the "poorly ventilated space," using nitrogen clearance data, with computations of the relative perfusion of these spaces that must exist to satisfy the observed arterial blood gas tensions. Such an analysis has been developed by Briscoe and his colleagues,[26, 146, 289, 653] and by Klocke and Farhi.[3654] More recently, Briscoe has extended this method to enable calculation of the diffusion component and to involve a three-compartment analysis,[2540, 2872, 3643] and Lenfant and Okubo[3656] have described a method to determine the distribution function of $\dot{V}/\dot{Q}$ ratios in man.
7. By using radioactive krypton (^{85}Kr) without external counting over the lungs but involving simultaneous analysis of arterial blood and expired gas.[1811, 1828, 3581]
8. By methods employing differential lobar sampling and gas analysis.
9. By recently developed techniques of external radiation detection using radioactive

CO_2 or ^{133}Xenon. These techniques have been described earlier in this chapter.

An important contemporary question is whether the results obtainable by these different methods are in accord or discrepant. In particular, it is not at all clear that the methods involving external radiation detection can be reconciled with the gas tension data.[2644] A detailed discussion of this problem cannot be undertaken here, but it seems clear that regional pulmonary function studies using radioactive gas have to involve continuous study of gas clearance from lung zones in two separate studies if any meaningful $\dot{V}/\dot{Q}$ distribution is to be calculable.[2894] It is not acceptable in disease to measure ventilation distribution with a single breath, and perfusion distribution by clearance into alveoli of xenon dissolved in saline, and then describe "V" divided by "Q" as the $\dot{V}/\dot{Q}$ ratio.

We have applied the continuous gas clearance technique to patients with pulmonary embolism[3184] and with chronic bronchitis of mild degree,[2532] but even with these more elaborate methods the total $\dot{V}/\dot{Q}$ picture in patients frequently does not correspond with estimates based on gas-tension methods. It seems clear that although a failure of any external counter to reflect a distribution of varied $\dot{V}/\dot{Q}$ ratios within its field is a likely cause of such a discrepancy, there are other possible reasons. It should be noted that gas-tension methods may express as a disorder of $\dot{V}/\dot{Q}$ distribution a failure of gas tension equilibration due to a fast capillary transit time, or some complex arrangement of a series dead space by which one part of the lung is ventilated after passage through another: It is clear that more work will have to be done in this field before all existing methods can be reconciled.

It may be concluded that the development of understanding of the consequences of uneven distribution of ventilation and perfusion in the lung represents a major field of advance in respiratory physiology and one that is directly relevant to many problems of lung disease and environmental physiology. An appreciation of the problems involved in definition and measurement of alveolar gas and a full understanding of the classic dispute between Haldane and Krogh, concerning the meaning of the measured dead space of the lung, are both necessary if the physician is to understand why a simple biological measurement of gas transport *in an uneven system* cannot be equated with a precise physical measurement. In this field, measurements are now easier to make than they are to interpret in complex problems of disease; the whole of this section underlies the problem of interpreting the meaning of a simple measurement of carbon monoxide uptake, as noted in the section on diffusion.

EFFECT OF NONUNIFORM $\dot{V}/\dot{Q}$ RATIOS ON TOTAL GAS EXCHANGE. Due to the inherent complexity of the task, it has not been easy to assess the quantitative effect of an abnormal $\dot{V}/\dot{Q}$ distribution on total gas exchange in any kind of rigorous way. West[3633], however, has achieved this with the aid of a computer program, dividing the lung into a varying number of compartments and expressing the distribution of $\dot{V}/\dot{Q}$ ratios as a logarithm of the standard deviation of the assumed $\dot{V}/\dot{Q}$ ratios. (*See* Figures 2–35, 2–36, 2–37, and 2–38.) This important study has illuminated a number of previously obscure points. First, the analysis

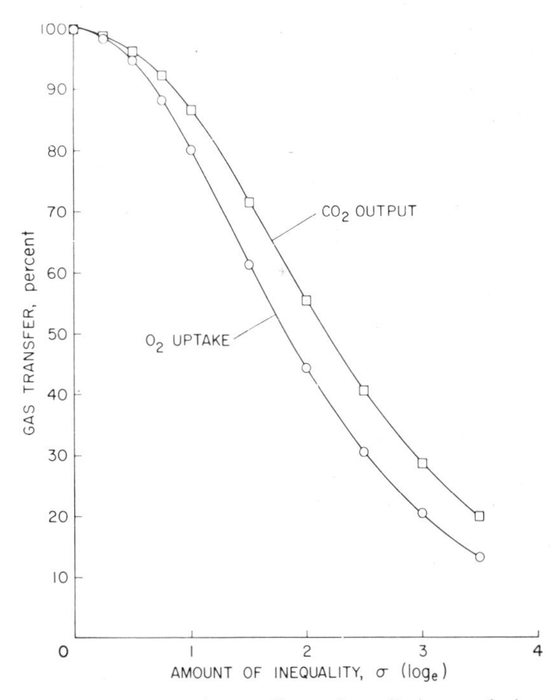

FIGURE 2–35. Acute effects of ventilation–perfusion ratio inequality on the oxygen uptake and carbon dioxide output of a lung model. In this figure, the composition of the mixed venous blood is held constant and the gas transfer is shown as a percentage of its value for no inequality (300 ml/min and 240 ml/min for oxygen and carbon dioxide respectively). The abscissa shows the log S.D. of ventilation or blood flow; both give identical results. Note that the interference with carbon dioxide transfer is almost as great as oxygen. (From West, J. B.: Respiration Physiology, 7:88, 1969.)

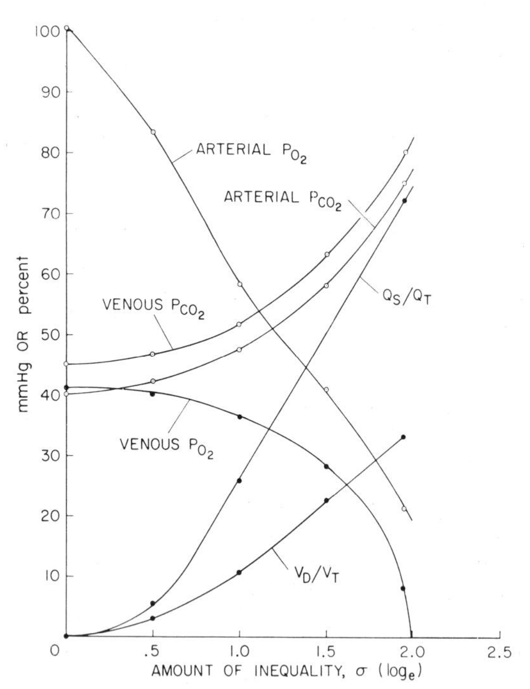

FIGURE 2–36. Effect of increasing ventilation-perfusion ratio inequality on gas exchange in a lung model in which oxygen uptake and carbon dioxide output are maintained at 300 and 240 ml/min respectively (steady-state conditions). Note the rapid fall in arterial and mixed venous P_{O_2} and the corresponding rise in arterial and mixed venous P_{CO_2}. (From West, J. B.: Respiration Physiology, 7:88, 1969.)

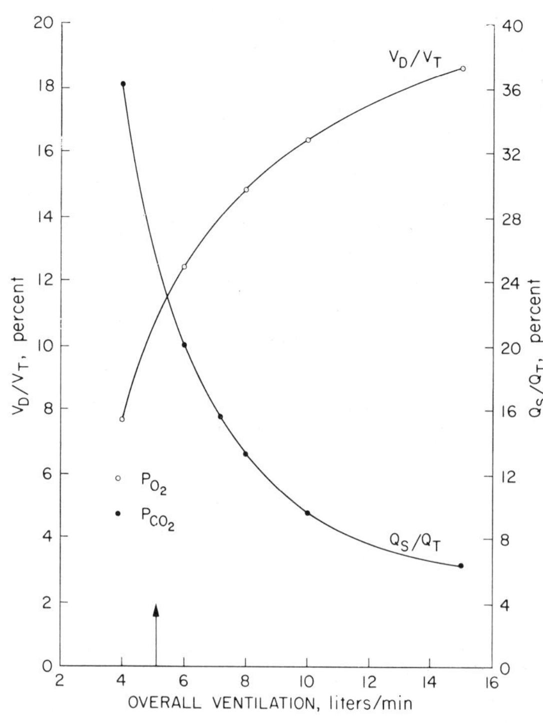

FIGURE 2–37. Example of the sensitivity of the commonly used indices of ventilation-perfusion ratio inequality, alveolar dead space/tidal volume (VD/VT) and venous admixture/total flow (QS/QT), to overall ventilation. Log S.D. 1.0; other parameters. The normal ventilation is shown by the arrow. (From West, J. B.: Respiratory Physiology, 7:88, 1969.)

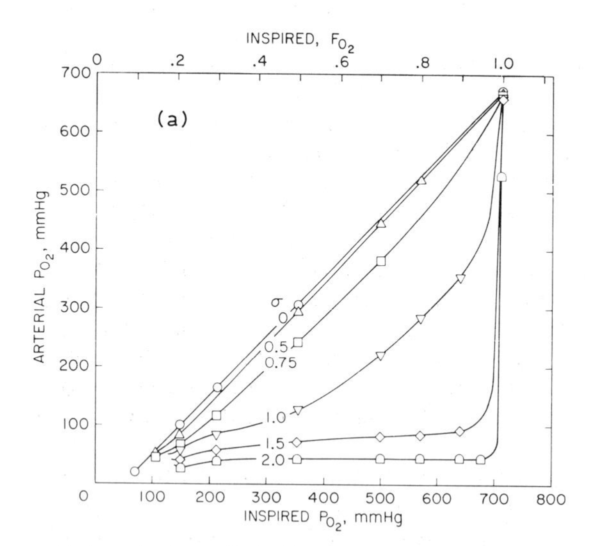

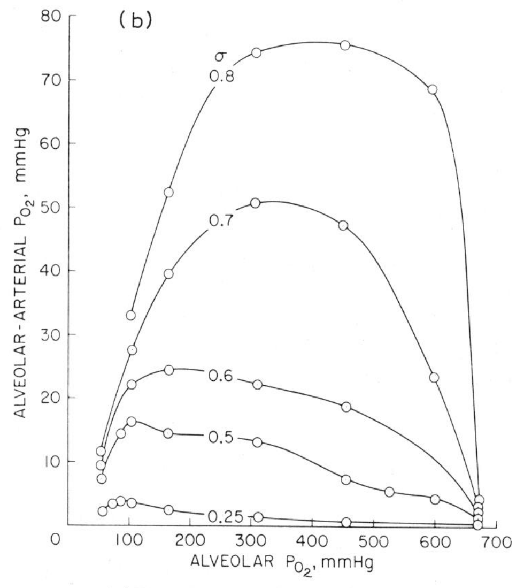

FIGURE 2–38. Effect of increasing inspired oxygen concentration on arterial P_{O_2}. Barometric pressure 760 mm Hg, ventilation 5.1 l/min, blood flow 6 l/min; other parameters as in 2–36. Note the degree of hypoxemia when ventilation-perfusion ratio inequality is severe even for very enriched oxygen mixtures (*a*). The mixed alveolar-arterial oxygen difference (*b*) has a maximum at an alveolar P_{O_2} of less than 100 mm Hg when the log S.D. is small, but when more inequality is present, the maximum value occurs at a higher P_{O_2}. (From West, J. B.: Respiration Physiology, 7:88, 1969.)

of the effects on gas transfer is relatively little affected by increasing the number of assumed pulmonary compartments above 10, and 6 would seem to be the minimum for an analysis of this kind. Second, the study has shown that the interference with CO_2 elimination is almost as great as with O_2 uptake, with an increasing degree of inequality (*see* Figure 2-35). Third, there is a surprising degree of hypoxemia even when the inspired oxygen tension is increased if there is gross non-uniformity of $\dot{V}/\dot{Q}$ distribution (*see* Figure 2-38). These important conclusions provide, for the first time, a quantitative estimate of the effects of $\dot{V}/\dot{Q}$ nonuniformity on total gas exchange.

The diffusion of gases in the lung

DEFINITIONS. Although the importance of the process of gas diffusion between the alveoli and pulmonary capillary blood has been known for 50 years, this aspect of respiratory function has been clarified only since 1945. Yet, despite the enormous volume of published work on the diffusing capacity over the last 15 years, there are still many unsolved problems.

In physical terms, it is helpful to relate the expression of gas diffusion to other transfer equations concerned with three variables. Thus, in electrical terms, the resistance (R) in a circuit is related to potential difference (V) and the current flowing (I) by Ohm's law, as follows:

$$R = \frac{V}{I} \qquad \textit{(Equation 8)}$$

In hydraulic terms, the orifice resistance (R) is related to the pressure drop across it ($P_1 - P_2$) and the total flow (F), as follows:

$$R = \frac{P_1 - P_2}{F} \qquad \textit{(Equation 9)}$$

The latter is an expression used by the cardiologist whenever he calculates the resistance of the pulmonary vascular bed. Thus, if a volume of gas ($\dot{V}_X$) is transferred through a membrane (y) from a pressure (P_{AX}) on one side into a capillary of mean pressure $\bar{P}_{CX}$, the resistance of the membrane, R_y, can be described as follows:

$$R_y = \frac{P_{AX} - \bar{P}_{CX}}{\dot{V}_X} \qquad \textit{(Equation 10)}$$

The diffusion constant of the membrane for the gas (x) is the reciprocal of the resistance in the equation above, which therefore may be rewritten:

$$D_{(X)} = \frac{1}{R} = \frac{\dot{V}_X}{P_{AX} - \bar{P}_{CX}} \qquad \textit{(Equation 11)}$$

In the case of carbon monoxide, which because of its particular properties is often used to measure this aspect of gas transfer, the diffusing capacity of the lung (D_{LCO}) is the rate of uptake of CO for the lung as a whole per minute ($\dot{V}_{CO}$) divided by the mean pressure gradient for CO that exists between alveolar gas and capillary blood. The units of expression of the diffusing capacity, therefore, are ml/min/mm Hg. Forster,[346] in a review of pulmonary diffusing capacity published in 1957, which is a model of its kind and obligatory reading for anyone concerned with this problem, discusses the relationship of this measurement to others characterized by different terms and characteristics, such as "the specific diffusivity of a membrane"; "the coefficient of diffusion"; "the diffusion constant of Krogh"; and "the specific diffusing capacity of Henderson."

The physical definition of the diffusing capacity is straightforward, but the details of its measurement and the interpretation of the results obtained are far from simple, particularly in clinical conditions in which no homogeneity of alveolar gas exists. Furthermore, recent work on the kinetics of combination of hemoglobin with carbon monoxide and oxygen have indicated that this factor, previously unconsidered, may indeed play a major part in determining the rate of gas transfer.[403, 1346]

Since the principles of diffusion measurement are easier to understand in terms of transfer of carbon monoxide than of oxygen, methods using CO will be discussed first. Seven methods of measuring the diffusing capacity with CO have been described, excluding those involving the use of radioactive CO. During the discussion that follows, it is essential to be able to refer to these techniques by symbols, and these are listed in the accompanying table.

METHOD	SYMBOL
Single-breath method using helium and CO. Modified Krogh technique.	$D_{Lco}SB$
Steady-state CO uptake with alveolar CO computed from measured arterial Pco_2. Filley technique.	$D_{Lco}SS_1$
Steady-state CO uptake with alveolar CO measured from an end-tidal sample of gas	$D_{Lco}SS_2$
Steady-state CO uptake with alveolar CO computed from an assumed V_D.	$D_{Lco}SS_3$
Steady-state CO uptake with alveolar CO computed from estimate of mixed venous CO_2.	$D_{Lco}SS_4$
Steady-state CO uptake during rebreathing of CO.	$D_{Lco}RB$
Steady-state CO uptake and analysis of CO and Helium clearance.	$D_{Lco}SSHe$

Even in normal subjects, none of these techniques can be claimed to measure precisely the true physical D_{Lco}, rigorously defined to be the D_{Lco} for each alveolus independently measured and summed together. For this reason it has been suggested that the term "apparent diffusing capacity" should be used. In our view, all contemporary methods succeed in measuring only an "apparent" diffusing capacity of one sort or another, though the factors that modify the result with any particular technique are not necessarily the same. The constant use of the word "apparent" therefore serves little more purpose than to assure the reader of the sophistication and perception of the writer. For this reason, the results obtained by any existing method will be referred to as diffusing capacities, although every such expression must be thought of as having a distinguishing / mark in relation to the true physical measurement.

It may be of value to summarize those factors that clearly influence the rate of gas diffusion in the lung, considered, first, in relation to the single-alveolus model, and second, in relation to the inevitable limitations imposed upon all methods by the fact that nonuniformity exists between alveoli in respect to the relationships between their volume, ventilation, the diffusing characteristics of their membrane, and their perfusion. The rate of diffusion of CO will not be directly influenced by flow except in extreme circumstances.[346]

The factors affecting diffusion in a single alveolus are several:

1. Thickness of alveolar lining membrane.
2. Thickness of protoplasm of alveolar lining cell.
3. Permeability of capillary wall.
4. Thickness of layer of plasma between capillary wall and red blood cell.
5. Permeability of red-cell membrane to CO or oxygen.
6. Reaction rate of hemoglobin with CO and O_2. (a) If this were delayed, a local back-pressure of CO would build up in the layer of plasma, causing a reduced rate of transfer from alveolar gas into plasma. (b) The combination of hemoglobin with CO is affected by the co-existing oxygen tension, and therefore the measured CO-diffusing capacity is influenced by the mean capillary Po_2 level that existed during the experiment (*see* Figure 2–38).
7. Presence of COHb in the pulmonary artery blood, which will diminish rate of CO transfer.

The diffusing capacity of a multiple alveolar system (which may be visualized as the rate of transfer of CO when each alveolus contains CO at a tension of 1 mm Hg and when $\bar{P}c_{co} = O$) inevitably is directly dependent upon the number of alveoli present. For this reason an understanding of the meaning of a single figure for D_{Lco} is dependent upon knowledge of the lung volume of the system being measured. In addition, the factors affecting diffusion in a multiple alveolar system include, of course, all of those mentioned above for a single alveolus, *plus* the complicating factor of the added effect of variation in different parameters from alveolus to alveolus—or, in other words, the nonuniformity of the lung. Such variations of alveolar CO tension will be similar in consequence to the effect of variations in $\dot{V}/\dot{Q}$ ratios on alveolar O_2 tension. Thus it becomes increasingly difficult to define the "mean" alveolar CO tension, and thus to determine the "correct" value to use in the denominator of the D_{Lco} equation.

To the earlier analyses of factors affecting CO uptake of which mention has already been made, must be added an elegant discussion of this problem by Filley and his colleagues,[3556] and valuable analytical reviews, referred to in later sections, by Piiper and Sikand,[3577] Anderson and Shephard,[3538] Armstrong and his co-workers,[3519] and Johnson and Miller.[2472] Menkes and his colleagues have recently shown[3573] that CO uptake in the human lung is pulsatile, and their paper deals at length with detailed aspects of CO transfer at the capillary level.

Modified Krogh technique ($D_{Lco}SB$). Although the introduction of this method of measuring the diffusing capacity often is dated from the paper by Marie Krogh in the *Journal of Physiology* in 1914,[348] the work that led to its development was described by the Kroghs four years before that date.[347] The earlier paper should receive as much attention as the later, because it reveals that these remarkable investigators experimented with a steady-state technique before they adopted the single-breath method for later use. The single-breath technique (their Method B[347]) overcame the difficulty of computing the mean alveolar CO concentration, and was simple to perform. A single deep breath of a mixture of CO in air was taken into the lungs, and a first expiration of about 1 liter was made, the alveolar portion of this being collected.

After a period of breath-holding, a further complete expiration was made, and the alveolar CO concentration was calculated from this. The mean CO concentration was taken as the average of the CO concentrations in the two samples, and the rate of CO uptake could be computed from the same data. The lung volume was measured separately by a hydrogen dilution method.

Results obtained by Harrop and Heath in 1927[352] and Bøje in 1933,[353] using the original Krogh technique, have been supplanted by the data accumulated since 1954 by use of the modified methods. Kety[13] and Forster[346] and his colleagues,[349] among others, have published detailed reviews of the theory underlying the computation of diffusing capacity from this type of experiment. Fowler, realizing that gas distribution even in the normal subject is not uniform, and that therefore the initial alveolar CO in the Krogh method could not be assumed to be a representative initial value for alveolar gas, suggested that the inspired gas mixture should contain helium as well as CO.[350] This modification obviated the necessity for collecting the first bag in the original Krogh method, since the initial alveolar CO concentration could be calculated from the dilution of helium recorded from the sample collected after the period of breath-holding. This technique, later described in more detail by Ogilvie and his co-workers,[38] has come to be known as the modified Krogh method ($D_{Lco}SB$). As it may be assumed that helium and CO are distributed similarly after a single breath, the initial alveolar concentration in the expired alveolar sample will equal the inspired CO concentration multiplied by the fraction shown in Equation twelve. Diffusing capacity can then be computed from a rearrangement of Krogh's equation, from the relationship shown in Equation thirteen, the diffusing capacity then being in terms of ml/mm/CO STPD/mm Hg CO tension. The expired alveolar gas sample will contain carbon dioxide, which will interfere with helium analysis if a katharometer is used for this determination, but if the carbon dioxide is removed before passage through the gas analyzers,[351] no elaborate correction factors need be used. Further simplification of equipment has resulted in the development of a bedside method, suitable for application to sick patients.[364]

A number of contributions have been made to the methodology of this technique. De Graff and Romans[3550] have described a programed valve sequencer and automatic alveolar gas sampler; Meade and his colleagues have also developed an automated method,[3572] and the method has been carefully studied to give maximal reproducibility under normal conditions, so that variations of only 1 per cent can be measured.[3546]

A number of factors affect the single-breath carbon-monoxide diffusing capacity,[345] appreciation of which is necessary for the intelligent interpretation of results. As with the single-breath N_2 wash-out, certain procedural details such as inspiration and expiration times[359, 360] should be controlled. Variations in values from individual to individual may be

$$F_{Ico} \times \frac{\text{He\% in expired alveolar sample}}{\text{Inspired helium percentage}} = F_{Aco} \qquad (\textit{Equation 12})$$

$$D_{Lco} = \frac{\text{Alveolar volume STPD} \times 60}{\text{Seconds of breath-hold} \times P_B - 47} \times \begin{matrix}\text{Natural}\\ \text{log}\end{matrix} \left[\frac{F_{Ico}\text{alv}}{F_{Eco}\text{alv}}\right] \qquad (\textit{Equation 13})$$

the result of size differences (as reflected in body surface area[355] or height; or age differences.[355] Results on a single subject vary somewhat with the lung volume during the breath-holding period when the measurement is being made.[355, 357] Indeed, the sensitivity of the measured value to lung volume and the difficulty in controlling lung volume from experiment to experiment have led some workers to suggest that the diffusion constant (the "k" of Marie Krogh, or D_{Lco}/lung volume) is a more reliable index of diffusion.[366]

Despite these factors that may introduce variation, the method has been applied successfully to a wide variety of situations, including the normal state, at rest and on exercise, in relation to lung expansion,[1839] in animal preparations,[368] after pneumonectomy,[363] and in many types of disease, including heart disease,[361, 362] acute pulmonary tuberculosis,[364] anemia,[365] asbestosis,[366] and emphysema.[38, 367] Daly and Roe have recently reported serial measurements of $D_{Lco}SB$ in a group of men employed in an iron foundry.[1835] They found that the average coefficient of variation in this test was 4.2 per cent. Using this technique, it has been shown that there is apparently a diurnal variation in diffusing capacity. The $D_{Lco}SB$ falls throughout the day at a rate of 1.2 per cent per hour between 9:30 A.M. and 5:30 P.M. and at 2.2 per cent per hour between 5:30 P.M. and 9:30 P.M.[3546] Guyatt and his colleagues showed that immersion in water increased the $D_{Lco}SB$ by 16 per cent, the increase being mainly due to an increase in pulmonary capillary blood volume.[3564] The method has also been used to study athletes,[3529, 3580] though breath-holding methods are less easy to apply during heavy exercise than are steady-state techniques.

It should be noted that the use of some measurement of alveolar volume is essential to the calculation of a diffusing capacity from the observed rate of fall of alveolar CO with time. Much of the discussion of the validity of measurements of diffusing capacity hinges on uncertainty as to error introduced by values of alveolar volume obtained by different procedures. As helium and CO can be assumed to be similarly distributed within the lung after a single breath, it was initially thought (and is still occasionally repeated) that this method was unaffected by uneven gas and blood perfusion in the lung. It is now realized that this is not the case.

Since the pulmonary blood flow at rest in a normal man is relatively reduced in the upper part of the lung, it is to be assumed that the single-breath D_{Lco} method will be sensitive to the extent of this perfusion—indeed, it is possible that the much better perfusion of the upper lung is mainly responsible for the difference in $D_{Lco}SB$ between the resting state and light exercise conditions. Smith and Rankin[3588] have found that the measurement is affected by Valsalva and Müller maneuvers, and they account for their observations by phasic changes in right and left ventricular output. Piiper and Sikand[3577] have shown that "the characteristic feature in the presence of unequal distributions of the diffusing capacity is a decrease of the apparent D_{CO} with increasing times of apnea." Johnson and Miller[2472] concluded that the $\dot{V}/\dot{Q}$ ratios that are now known to be present in the lungs on a regional basis in a normal, seated subject are not of sufficient magnitude to account for the differences between steady-state and single-breath measurements. They suggested that blood flow or transit times or both must be very unevenly distributed to explain the differences. This technique has been very successfully applied to experimental studies of the diffusing capacity of dogs,[3543, 3544, 3571] and Cree and his colleagues have even been able to measure the diffusing capacity of the right and left lungs of the dog independently.[3548]

STEADY-STATE CO METHODS. Although one of Haldane's earliest published experiments[2] was a study of the effect of breathing carbon monoxide, it was a subsequent study in 1910 by the Kroghs[347] that made possible the first measurement of diffusing capacity in man. The rate of CO uptake during continuous breathing was observed, using a mouthpiece and valve box, with the subject respiring about 8 liters of 1.0 per cent CO from one spirometer into another; from this, the numerator of the equation for D_{Lco} (i.e., uptake of CO) was calculated. The denominator of the D_{Lco} equation (mean alveolar CO concentration) was calculated from Bohr's equation, using an assumed value of dead space of 140 ml. Diffusing capacity so calculated was found to be extremely sensitive to the value of dead space chosen, and the Kroghs concluded[347]: "All diffusion determinations made according to the present and similar methods and with shallow respirations are so uncertain as to be practically valueless, so long as the volume of the dead space in the subject experimented on is not exactly known." With Marie Krogh as the subject, $D_{Lco}SS_3$ was found to be 79 if V_D was assumed to be 140 ml, and 26 if the V_D was taken as 100 ml. This phenomenon was confirmed in our laboratory in 1955.[371] It results from the undue sensitivity of F_{Aco} calculated from the Bohr equation to the value of V_D when the ratio of V_D to V_T is large.

The basic method of measuring the steady-state diffusing capacity has not changed since then, although subsequent work has been made easier by the introduction of faster methods of gas analyses. Other workers subsequently were concerned mainly with understanding the interrelationship between inspired concentration, minute volume, and the build-up of COHb.[372–374, 376] Certain significant advances in the understanding of gas transfer in the lungs have resulted from work in this field, however. Thus, Lilienthal in 1946 observed the effect of different alveolar oxygen tensions on the rate of CO uptake,[375] a method of study which was to prove of great value 15 years later. Using values for diffusing capacity calculated from steady-state exercise data, Roughton was able to make a remarkable calculation of the average time spent by the blood in the human lung capillary.[377] Forster and his co-workers[349] in 1954 were able to derive theoretical equations for the parameters involved in CO transfer during steady-state conditions. All workers have recognized that steady-state methods, although more suitable for the measurement of CO uptake and more physiological in some senses than a breath-hold experiment, suffer from the disadvantage that the mean alveolar CO concentration is difficult to measure under steady-state conditions. Six possible methods of mean alveolar CO measurement have been proposed; each of these will be discussed:

1. Steady-state D_{Lco} with F_{Aco} Computed from an Assumed Value for V_D ($D_{Lco}SS_3$). The work of the Kroghs[347] indicated that in normal subjects the computed value for D_{Lco} at rest is particularly sensitive to the value of the mean alveolar CO tension, and thus to small changes in the assumed value of V_D if the mean alveolar CO tension is derived from the solution of the Bohr equation. If V_D is overestimated, computed D_{Lco} will be falsely high; if V_D is underestimated, however, the computed D_{Lco} will be underestimated but not to a comparable degree. As the ratio of V_D/V_T falls, the resulting effects upon computed D_{Lco} diminish. Thus, during exercise, when this ratio is low (V_T increases considerably and V_D minimally), the calculated D_{Lco} becomes relatively insensitive to changes in V_D. In these circumstances the numerator of the equation for D_{Lco} increases to become the chief determinant of the D_{Lco} (*see* Figure 2–37). Thus, the use of an assumed value for V_D to calculate mean alveolar CO tension (and subsequently D_{Lco}) is acceptable for exercise measurements, whereas this procedure cannot be adopted when the tidal volume is small in relation to V_D. In disease, the same arguments hold, and in addition it will be appreciated that the use of an assumed value for V_D, approximating to the "anatomical" dead space, will mean that allowance is made only for the volume of the conducting tubes, which do not participate in CO exchange. It was to overcome this difficulty that Filley and his colleagues[378] devised a method of calculating the mean alveolar CO tension based on measurement of the physiological dead space ($D_{Lco}SS_1$).

Alveolar CO Computed from Measured Arterial P_{CO_2} (Filley Method) ($D_{Lco}SS_1$). In this method, minute volume, inspired and expired CO concentrations, expired carbon-dioxide concentration and arterial CO_2 tension are measured simultaneously. Filley and his colleagues[378] assumed that arterial P_{CO_2} could be taken as representative of mean alveolar CO_2, and showed that the "mean" alveolar CO could be computed from the following relationship, a derivation made in the same way as that of the "ideal" alveolar-oxygen tension, discussed earlier (*see* page 66).

$$P_{Aco} = P_B - 47 \left[\frac{F_{Eco} - rF_{Ico}}{1 - r}\right] \quad (Equation\ 14)$$

$$\text{where } r = \left[\frac{P_{aco_2} - P_{Eco_2}}{P_{aco_2}}\right] \quad (Equation\ 15)$$

It will be appreciated that by this maneuver Filley and his colleagues have used the "physiological" dead space to solve the Bohr equation for "mean" alveolar CO tension in order to obtain the value required for the denominator of the equation for diffusing capacity, thus by-passing the need for direct alveolar sampling. By referring to Figure 2–33, the physician will be reminded that the "physiological" dead space has no volume counterpart; in subjects with similar $\dot{V}/\dot{Q}$ ratios throughout the lung this value approaches the "anatomical" value, i.e., the volume of the conducting tubes. Thus in normal subjects the end-tidal CO can be used as reliably as the arterial P_{CO_2} to compute $F_{A_{CO}}$. However, where $\dot{V}/\dot{Q}$ ratios vary from region to region (as in many diseases), "physiological" dead space will exceed "anatomical" dead space by some undefined amount which increases as the unevenness becomes greater, and so use of "physiological" rather than "anatomical" dead space introduces some undefined "correction" for the unevenness in the computed $D_{L_{CO}}$.

Filley and his colleagues[378] pointed out that, if analytical errors of 2 per cent in expired CO concentration were made at the same time as an error in the opposite direction of 2 mm Hg in arterial P_{CO_2} determination, the measured $D_{L_{CO}}$ at rest by this method might be as much as 40 per cent in error. They pointed out also that, for the same circumstances on exercise, the error would be less than half this amount. Their data for resting normal subjects, together with those published by other authors, indicate that errors of 40 per cent must be rare with this method in practice, since much greater variation in values obtained by its use would have been reported than the literature indicates. The problem of whether the arterial P_{CO_2} can in fact be used to compute the mean alveolar CO tension, any more than it can be used to compute mean alveolar O_2 tension in the presence of wide variation in $\dot{V}/\dot{Q}$ ratio in the lung, is discussed in Chapter 7. The probable validity of this approach has been questioned recently by a number of authors.

The Filley technique for measuring diffusing capacity has been widely and successfully applied, both at rest and on exercise,[379] and in a wide variety of clinical disorders,[381, 382] including mitral stenosis,[380] diffuse interstitial fibrosis,[381, 382] asthma[384] and emphysema,[385] and even in the newborn infant.[388]

A simplified procedure in which the alveolar P_{CO_2} is assumed to be 40 mm, or, if the patient is hyperventilating, alveolar P_{CO_2} and P_{CO} are calculated from an assumed value for V_D (as 40 per cent of tidal volume, V_T), has been described by Williams and Zohman[356] for use in patients without airway obstruction. Results obtained by this modified technique agreed satisfactorily with the standard Filley procedure in 21 patients. The factors affecting the results obtained by computing the diffusing capacity by this technique have been analyzed by Read,[2841] who concluded that it was relatively insensitive to variations in ventilation distribution, but was liable to be falsely high or low if there was considerable nonuniformity of blood-flow distribution. We have found[2843] that in patients with different types of lung disease, measured during exercise, there is a good general correspondence between the $D_{L_{CO}}$ measured using an assumed dead space and the Filley $D_{L_{CO}}$, but the points fall to one side of the line of identity, as shown in Figure 2–39. The careful studies of normal subjects during exercise studied by this method by Holmgren[3566–3568] should be consulted by anyone concerned with the detailed methodology of this method.

Measurement of End-tidal CO Concentration ($D_{L_{CO}}SS_2$). It has been mentioned (page 63) that, in normal subjects during resting breathing, the end-tidal P_{CO_2} corresponds remarkably closely to arterial P_{CO_2}.[252] In the same way in normal subjects the end-expiratory CO value may be used to provide a measurement of mean alveolar CO concentration. Measurements of diffusing capacity using this method are satisfactory at rest, provided the tidal volume is adequate to clear the anatomical and instrumental dead space.[391] In our view the fractional CO uptake always should be calculated at the same time as the $D_{L_{CO}}SS_2$, since errors due to a very low tidal volume are thereby made more obvious.[39] On exercise, however, end-tidal sampling becomes less reliable than a computed alveolar value based on an assumed dead-space value, since the end-tidal portion of an exchanging gas becomes less representative of the mean alveolar gas in these circumstances.[260, 387] It will be recalled that it was this error that misled Haldane into believing that very large increases in dead space in normal subjects occurred during exercise. There is thus little point in collecting end-tidal samples during exercise, particularly if the exercise is strenuous,[387] although they are acceptable during resting studies.

The technical details of a resting end-tidal estimate of diffusing capacity have been fully described.[39] In practice the method is simple, since no helium analysis is required. In contrast to the simplicity of the method, the interpretation of the meaning of the values obtained in the presence of lung disease (discussed in detail in Chapter 7) is neces-

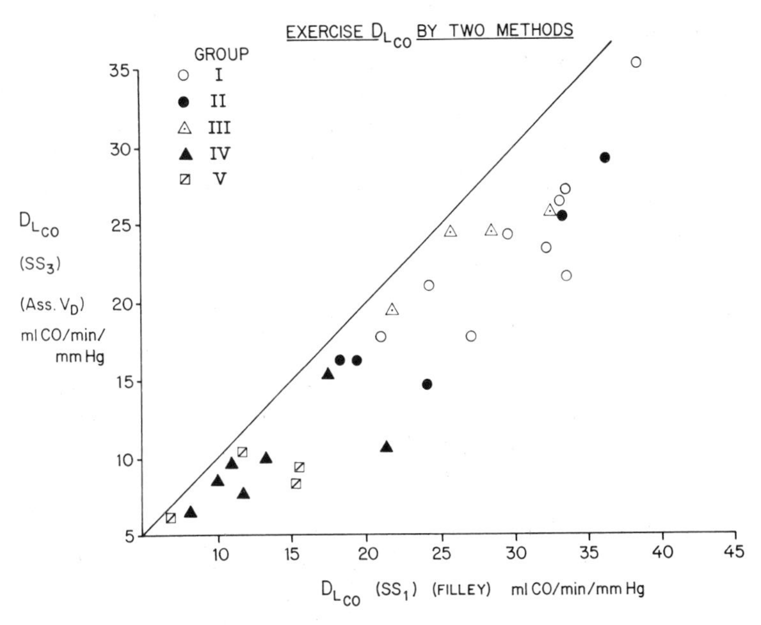

FIGURE 2–39. Comparison between diffusing capacity measured assuming a dead space value (DL_{CO} SS_3) and diffusing capacity calculated from the measured aterial CO_2 tension (DL_{CO} SS_1). All observations were made on moderate exercise, *Group 1:* normal subjects between ages 50 and 60 with no ventilatory defect. *Group 2:* subjects aged between 50 and 60 with slight ventilatory impairment. *Group 3:* four subjects with normal ventilatory function but abnormal electrocardiograms, *Group 4:* patients with severe ventilatory defect and pulmonary emphysema. In 5 of the 6 patients the diagnosis was confirmed pathologically either by subsequent autopsy or by pathological study of part of the lung which was removed at surgery. *Group 5:* four patients with diffuse interstitial fibrosis in all of whom the diagnosis was made pathologically. Notice that the discrepancy between the diffusing capacity calculated by these two methods amounts to approximately 10 units of diffusing capacity but shows little variation as between normal subjects and patients with disease.

sarily far from straightforward. Here it may be concluded briefly that the finding of a normal $D_{Lco}SS_2$ in a patient excludes any severe derangement of the diffusing function of the lung. When the value is lower than normal, however, considerable discretion is required in the interpretation of the result in structural terms. Differences in diffusing capacity between asthma and emphysema have been demonstrated by the use of this method,[370] and it has been applied also to the study of sarcoidosis[56] and after pneumonectomy.[388] We think it is very useful in the routine evaluation of pulmonary function,[389] a conclusion supported by MacNamara and his colleagues,[390] and certainly it is suitable for use in survey work or prospective studies.[39]

Anderson and Shephard[3537] have described a short steady-state method and used this in studies of normal subjects at exercise. Johnson and Miller[2472] have analyzed the difference between the single-breath D_{Lco} and the steady-state D_{Lco} at rest and concluded that regional $\dot{V}/\dot{Q}$ differences are unlikely to account for the observed difference. Piiper and Sikand[3577] have emphasized that it is the mode of distribution of alveolar ventilation in relation to flow (or diffusing capacity) that is critical to the accuracy of this measurement, and that distributions in relation to volume are relatively insignificant.[349] Without doubt the best technique to measure the steady-state D_{Lco} if alveolar sampling is required is to pass the expired gas through a CO meter. The studies of Remmers and Mithoefer[3579] on high-altitude natives made use of this principle to good effect.

Use of Mixed Venous CO_2 Obtained by Equilibration to Compute Arterial P_{CO_2} ($D_{Lco}SS_4$). In 1958 Marshall[395] reported observations on patients in whom the mixed venous P_{CO_2} was computed from an equilibration technique, and more recently Leathart[1814] has used a similar method. This procedure avoids the necessity for arterial puncture, but it may be questioned whether the indirect estimate of arterial P_{CO_2} is likely to be precise enough for use in the Filley equation at rest, and further experience is necessary before this question can be answered with confidence.

Rebreathing Method of Measuring Diffusing Capacity (D_{Lco} RB). This technique was introduced by Lewis and his co-workers[396] in an attempt to overcome the objections to other methods when gross disturbance of $\dot{V}/\dot{Q}$ ratios may be present in the lungs. The subject rebreathes into a bag containing a helium–CO mixture, and the concentrations of these gases are measured continuously. An important precaution is the computation of COHb by a rebreathing experiment before and after the determination, with subsequent correction for this factor. As Lewis points out, some uncertainty is introduced into interpretation of the data by the presence of considerable hyperventilation during the procedure, and the variation in alveolar P_{O_2} and P_{CO_2} that unavoidably occurs. In normal subjects, the method gives calculated values of D_{Lco} slightly higher than steady-state data and somewhat lower than single-breath determinations. Lewis and his colleagues advance some theoretical calculations which indicate that in some situations the D_{Lco}RB may be a more accurate estimate of the true physical D_L than can be obtained by either of the other main techniques. The equilibration method of measuring diffusing capacity has been shown to be a convenient technique for making these measurements in the dog.[1834]

Sølvsteen has published a number of papers on the use of $C^{14}O$ in a closed system to measure diffusing capacity.[2828, 2851, 2861, 2871, 2893] Though less affected by nonuniformity of $\dot{V}/\dot{Q}$ distribution than are the steady-state or single-breath techniques, the method may be too complex for routine use in the pulmonary function laboratory.

Mittman has published a detailed study of a new technique of measuring the diffusing capacity, involving measuring simultaneously the steady-state CO uptake, and then the combined CO and Helium wash-out.[3575] There has not yet been any considerable body of data evolved with this technique, and it seems likely that the data would have to be handled using a computer, since the computation is complex; nevertheless, the method might well be excellently suited to a research protocol. At the present time, it may be stated that this technique probably provides the nearest estimate to the true physical D_L that can be obtained in an uneven system. In Table 2–8 we have designated this method as D_{Lco}SSHe.

Measurements of Actual CO Uptake and Fractional CO Removal. The difficulty of interpreting measurements of diffusing capacity and the uncertainty of the relationship any such determinations bear to the true physical diffusing capacity in lung disease lead to the obvious suggestion that all such attempts should be abandoned. In 1952, we reported measurements of CO uptake and fractional CO removal in normal subjects and in patients with emphysema,[397] concluding that both values were reduced by this disease. The uptake of CO must be expressed in terms of a standardized inspired concentration, conveniently 0.1 per cent CO. The fractional CO uptake may be computed from the expression:

$$\text{Fractional CO uptake} = \frac{\dot{V}_E(F_{Ico} - F_{Eco})}{\dot{V}_E \times F_{Ico}} \quad (\textit{Equation 16})$$

where the numerator represents the uptake of CO and the denominator the volume of CO inspired, no correction being made for RQ. It is apparent that the minute ventilation ($\dot{V}_E$) can be crossed off both numerator and denominator, to leave the fraction:

$$\left[\frac{F_{Ico} - F_{Eco}}{F_{Ico}}\right] \quad (\textit{Equation 17})$$

which may be left as a fraction,[39] or multiplied by 100 and expressed as a percentage. Forster and his colleagues[359] analyzed these expressions in terms of the diffusing capacity, and derived equations to express the interrelationship between fractional removal and D_{Lco}.

The difficulty of using the fractional uptake as an index of diffusing capacity is that it is dependent upon the minute volume respired. In the presence of hyperventilation, the fractional removal falls,[397] although the diffusing capacity is unchanged. In spite of this limitation, however, several workers have found it to be a useful indicator of normality.[358, 382, 390] It is of particular value when compared with the end-tidal diffusing capacity obtained simultaneously, as sampling error of end-tidal gas may lead to a falsely low diffusing capacity in some instances, whereas the fractional removal may be normal.[39] Kreukniet and Visser[1818] have shown recently that normality of fractional CO removal almost certainly indicates normality of pulmonary diffusing capacity, even in lungs that are grossly uneven in respect to ventilation, diffusion, and perfusion distribution. There have been fewer reports of use of the actual CO uptake, although, as pointed out, this may be computed easily from much of the data in the literature. It would be of interest to know whether a simultaneous comparison of oxygen uptake and CO uptake during exercise might be a useful measurement suitable for survey work. Predicted values of fractional CO removal at rest may be found on pages 93 and 94.

Particular mention must be made of the remarkable observations of steady-state CO uptake made by West[398] during a period of several months spent at an altitude of 19,000 feet. Using only the sampling of inspired and expired gas during exercise with very high ventilation rates, he was able to show that no increase in D_L occurred under the strain of residence and work at this altitude. West pointed out that, in the circumstances of his measurement, the calculated diffusing capacity becomes relatively insensitive to changes in the dead-space–tidal-volume ratio, a fact used by other authors, including ourselves.[371, 387, 399] The interrelationships between diffusing capacity, minute volume, V_D/V_T ratio, and extraction ratio for CO are shown in Figure 2–40, taken from West's paper.[398] In an exercise experiment, F_{Ico} may be 0.125 per cent CO; F_{Eco} may equal 0.09 per cent CO; and the fraction $1 - \left[\frac{F_{Eco}}{F_{Ico}}\right]$ will be only 0.28. It can be seen that the V_D/V_T ratio may be taken as 0.1 or 0.4 without any major consequence to the value of D_L that will be computed.

In our view, the measurement of the fractional CO uptake is a most useful index of normality. In a group of patients with mild chronic bronchitis, we found an unexpectedly good correlation between the CO extraction and the computed scatter of $\dot{V}/\dot{Q}$ values, as assessed by the regional wash-out of ^{133}xenon after infusion. There seems little doubt that the extraction ratio is certain to be abnormal if any considerable extent of diffusing surface has been lost from the lung.[2524] While admitting therefore that this single ratio cannot be used to discriminate between developing $\dot{V}/\dot{Q}$ abnormality and loss of surface area, it remains true that the demonstration of a normal or a falling extraction ratio provides an indication of change within the lung not given by ventilatory or mechanical measurements. There are reasons for supposing that changes in this would occur before the gas tensions would be significantly altered. If the minute volume, tidal volume, and respiratory frequency can be duplicated on successive studies, the CO extraction ratio can be used as a sensitive indicator of change.[1679]

MEASUREMENT OF MEMBRANE-DIFFUSION COEFFICIENT (D_M) AND PULMONARY CAPILLARY BLOOD VOLUME (V_c). The very considerable interest in factors determining the rate of CO transfer in health and disease has led, through the work of Roughton and Forster, to a new method of study of this aspect of pulmonary function. In this section no more than a brief outline can be given of the principles of the method and the data so far obtained by its use.

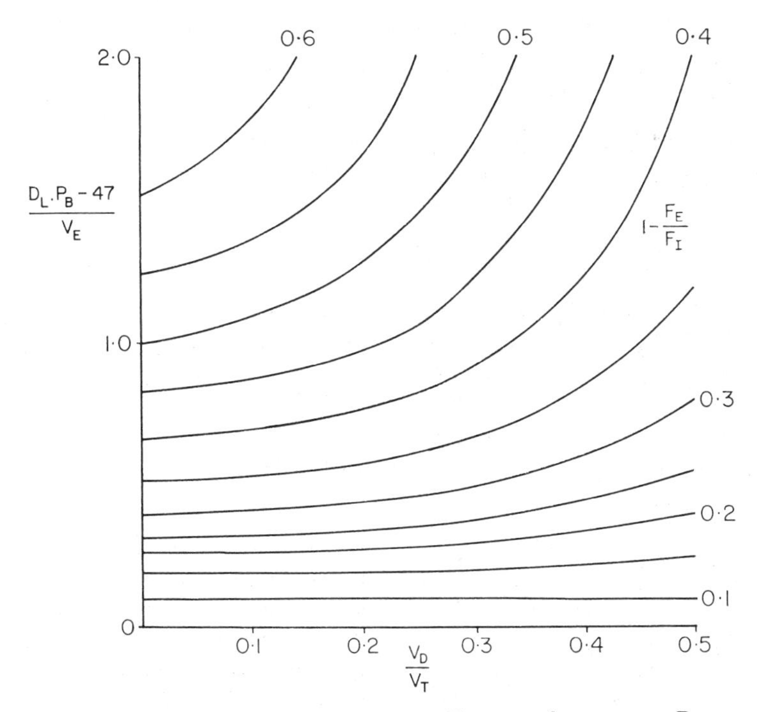

FIGURE 2–40. FACTORS INFLUENCING ERROR IN CALCULATED D_{Lco}

P_B = Barometric pressure; F_I = inspired CO concentration; F_E = mixed expired CO concentration; V_D = assumed value for dead space; V_T = tidal volume; V_E = minute volume.

Note that when the ratio (V_D/V_T) is small and the factor ($1 - F_E/F_I$) is small, the calculated D_L is insensitive to changes in the ratio V_D/V_T. (Diagram from Dr. J. B. West.)

Although the effect of inspired oxygen tension on the rate of elimination of carbon monoxide was well known to Haldane,[2] the first systematic study of the effect of oxygen pressure on the uptake of CO appears to be that by Lilienthal and Pine in 1945.[375] In the same year, Roughton used data on CO uptake at rest and exercise, obtained by Forbes, Sargent and himself,[374] to perform one of the outstanding feats of deductive calculation in the whole field of respiratory physiology. This astonishing paper[377] should be read in the original by anyone concerned with problems of CO exchange. Using recently derived kinetic data on the rate of combination of CO with O_2 Hb, and making reasonable assumptions concerning cardiac output and respiratory dead space, and with a careful assessment of the probable errors of these and other parameters, he calculated that the time spent by blood in the average capillary of the human lung was of the order of 0.73 sec at rest and 0.34 sec during hard work. As he remarked: "No data have, to my knowledge, existed heretofore as to the magnitude of this physiologically important time interval." Roughton also calculated that the total volume of blood in the pulmonary capillaries must be about 60 ml at rest and 95 ml during hard physical work. Roughton and Forster[400] have shown since that the interrelationship between various factors that determine the total diffusing capacity may be expressed by the following equation:

$$\frac{1}{D_L} = \frac{1}{D_M} + \frac{1}{\theta V_c} \quad (\textit{Equation 18})$$

where D_L is the total diffusing capacity of the lung; D_M is the diffusing capacity of the membrane separating the alveolar gas from the blood; V_c is the total volume of blood in the pulmonary capillaries exposed to alveolar gas; and θ is the volume of gas (in ml) which will be taken up by the red cells in 1 ml of blood per minute per mm. Hg gradient of pressure between the plasma and the red cell. D_M is defined as being equal to the fraction:

$$D_M = \frac{Ad}{y} \quad (\textit{Equation 19})$$

where A is the total area of the lung membrane (in square cm); d is the diffusion coefficient for unit area and unit thickness; and y is the average thickness of the membrane (in cm). The numerical value of θ will depend upon the oxygen tension present, and this will influence the rate of uptake of CO by the red cell. By using recently gained kinetic data on CO reaction rates with human red cells, Roughton and Forster were able to calculate probable values for $\frac{1}{\theta}$ for different values of oxygen tension. It follows from the equation given above that, if D_L is measured at two levels of oxygen tension, and $\frac{1}{\theta}$ is known for both oxygen tension values, the simultaneous equations can be solved for the two unknowns, D_M and V_c.

In Figure 2–41 are shown data for three subjects exercising at 3 mph, with the relationship between measured D_L and mean capillary O_2 tension ($P_{\bar{c}_{O_2}}$) plotted against each other. V_c averaged 150 ml, with considerable variation between individuals but with an SD of only about ±12 ml in repeated studies of the same subject.[399]

Since the original paper by Roughton and Forster,[400] referred to earlier, a considerable volume of work has been published concerning the kinetics of various reactions between hemoglobin solutions and red blood cells with oxygen and carbon monoxide,[402–407] too technical to be summarized here. It has become apparent, however, that some of the observed differences between diffusing-capacity measurements made with CO and those using oxygen probably can be explained on kinetic factors. Forster[26] stresses the fact that diffusion resistance due to membrane change cannot be distinguished by any method from delay imposed by a slowed reaction rate. Further, Staub, Bishop, and Forster[403] have shown that values of V_c and D_M commonly obtained from the CO technique are not compatible with gas-tension data used in the Bohr integration procedure. These complicating factors are mentioned here to remind the physician that, in the present state of knowledge, it is premature to visualize D_M as a definitive measurement of membrane thickness, and very considerable discretion must be exercised in explaining observed differences in presumed structural terms.

Since the validity of any method of measuring D_L in an uneven system is open to doubt, it is not possible to use this technique satisfactorily in patients with advanced lung dis-

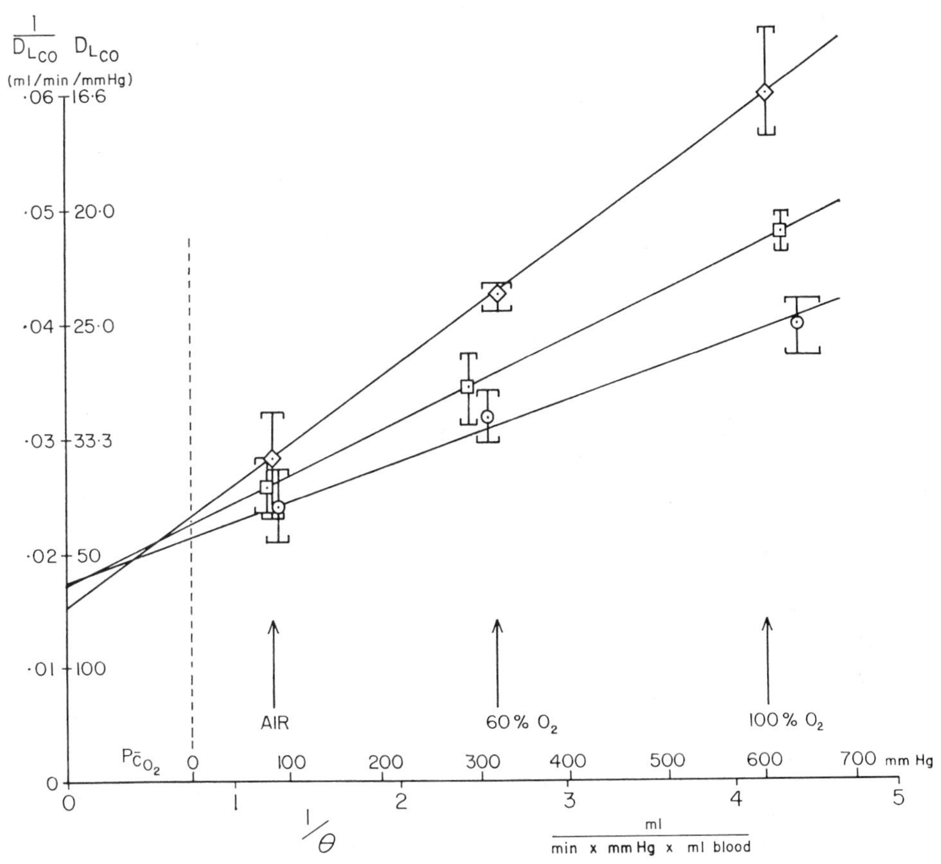

FIGURE 2–41. MEASUREMENTS OF D_{Lco} IN THREE NORMAL SUBJECTS EXERCISING AT 3 MPH BREATHING AIR, 60 PER CENT OXYGEN, AND 100 PER CENT OXYGEN

The ordinate shows both the actual D_{Lco} and its reciprocal. The abscissa shows the calculated mean capillary oxygen tension ($P_{\bar{c}_{O_2}}$), and the kinetic constant θ computed with knowledge of this. The slope of this relationship represents the pulmonary capillary blood volume (V_c) component of the diffusing capacity, and the intercept the other factors expressed as the membrane component (or D_M). Note that considerable precision is required in the measurement of the diffusing capacity on 100 per cent oxygen if errors in both of these estimates are to be minimized. The vertical and horizontal bars around each mean point show the range of variation in three estimates. (Data from Bates, Varvis, Donevan and Christie.[399])

ease. In addition, any change in D_L distribution within the lung, as a consequence of increasing the oxygen tension of inspired gas, will produce errors in the computed values of D_M and V_c. In normal subjects, the method has recently yielded interesting data however. Danzer, Cohn, and Zechman have confirmed that it is changes in V_c that account mainly for the increased D_L on exercise; Guyatt and his colleagues[3564] have shown that V_c increases when men are immersed in water; and Smith and Rankin found that it was changes in V_c that accounted mainly for D_L changes during the Valsalva and Müller maneuvers[3588] and postulated that the pulmonary capillary blood volume was being altered by variations in phase of output of the two ventricles.

MEASUREMENT OF OXYGEN-DIFFUSING CAPACITY ($D_{L_{O_2}}$). Although the problems involved in the measurement of pulmonary diffusing capacity with oxygen were clearly understood after the work of Bohr in 1909,[1817] the technical difficulties were not circumvented until 40 years later. Many reviews of the Bohr integration procedure have appeared in recent years.[3, 1827]

The formula for calculating the diffusing capacity of the lungs for any gas (*see* page 75) is the uptake of the gas in unit time by the lungs, divided by the driving pressure or pressure gradient of the gas between an alveolus and the capillary blood. Thus, for oxygen, the

$$D_{L_{O_2}} = \frac{\dot{V}_{O_2}}{P_{A_{O_2}} - \bar{P}_{C_{O_2}}}. \qquad (Equation\ 20)$$

The crux of the problem was the exact quantitation of the denominator of the equation, i.e., the mean gradient of pressure of oxygen that exists between the alveolar gas and the blood traveling through the pulmonary capillary, whose oxygen tension changes continuously and nonlinearly with this passage.

A fair estimate may be made of the alveolar oxygen tension ($P_{A_{O_2}}$), but the computation of the mean tension of the pulmonary capillary blood ($\bar{P}_{C_{O_2}}$) poses a major problem. Bohr[1817] showed how this might be found by an integration procedure, but the calculated mean capillary oxygen tension is extremely sensitive to the final tension difference that exists between alveolar gas and pulmonary end-capillary blood, a consideration that led Kety[13] to doubt that it could ever be computed in normal circumstances. Some of the difficulties were overcome by Lilienthal, Riley, Cournand and their collaborators in a major series of contributions to this field published between 1946 and 1951.[412–416] The physician would be well advised, however, to start by reading one of the summaries of the technique which sets out the method steps in a simple sequence; Comroe and his colleagues[3] have devised one of the most lucid of these presentations.

The essential measurements required to calculate the $D_{L_{O_2}}$ are the oxygen and CO_2 exchange, the arterial oxygen and CO_2 gas tensions, and the minute volume during breathing of oxygen and nitrogen mixtures designed to produce a level of oxygen saturation of about 95 per cent and 82 per cent. From these data, a mean or "ideal" alveolar Po_2 is calculated by substitution of arterial for alveolar Pco_2 as discussed on page 67. The mixed venous oxygen tension, if not directly measured, can be computed from the arterial value; an error in this estimate contributes little to the error of the method. The levels of arterial, mixed venous, and alveolar Po_2, therefore, are known for two levels of oxygen breathing. The observed difference between alveolar and arterial oxygen tension is assumed to be due to two factors: (1) a difference between the oxygen tension in the pulmonary capillary as it leaves the alveolus and the oxygen tension in the alveolar gas, due to diffusion delay and termed the "membrane component"; and (2) a difference between the end-capillary oxygen tension and the arterial oxygen tension due to addition of unoxygenated blood to that which has traversed inadequately ventilated alveoli, termed the "venous admixture component." (*See* Figure 2–34 for consequences of unequal $\dot{V}/\dot{Q}$ ratios on A–a difference for O_2.) The originators of this technique made skillful use of the fact that, at a low level of oxygen saturation, the venous admixture component has a proportionately much smaller effect on the arterial Po_2 than at higher levels of saturation.[3] Assuming that $D_{L_{O_2}}$ and the ratio of venous admixture to total perfusion are the same at the two levels of oxygenation, and making use of graphs published by Riley and his colleagues,[415] it is possible to compute the unique values for these two parameters that are compatible with the measured gas tensions and computed mean alveolar Po_2.

Armstrong and his colleagues[3519] have recently reported a restudy of the $D_{L_{O_2}}$ in four normal men who had previously been studied with this technique ten years before. They concluded that the technique was capable of measuring the diffusing capacity with an error of about 3 units when the mean alveolar–mean capillary gradient was 10 mm Hg or less. Interestingly, they found no evidence of a significant change in the $D_{L_{O_2}}$ in the subjects they studied over the ten-year interval.

An important new development in the computation of the diffusing capacity for oxygen in the presence of nonuniform $\dot{V}/\dot{Q}$ ratios has been pioneered by Briscoe and King,[2525, 2530] and further developed by Arndt in conjunction with them.[3539] By analysis of the $\dot{V}/\dot{Q}$ distribution in conjunction with the measured blood-gas tensions, and computing the Bohr isopleths that would apply to different phases of the lung, they have been able to separate the effects of $\dot{V}/\dot{Q}$ distribution from D_L in nonhomogeneous lungs. Using this method, they found that in 4 of 8 patients with the capillary alveolar block syndrome whom they studied, the major function disturbance was in the total $D_{L_{O_2}}$ or its distribution.[3539] This much more

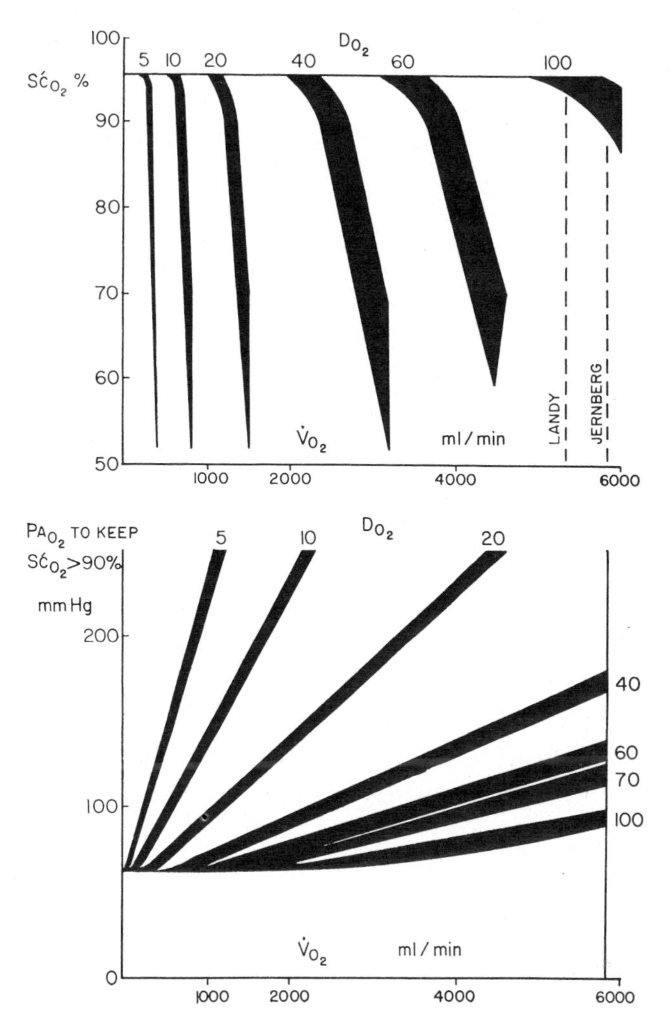

FIGURE 2–42. Relationship between Oxygen Diffusing Capacity, Oxygen Saturation and Oxygen Uptake on Exercise

The upper diagram shows the interrelationship between arterial oxygen saturation (Sc_{O_2}), the oxygen diffusing capacity (D_{O_2}) and the oxygen uptake (V_{O_2}). Note that no fall in saturation occurs initially, but that when desaturation begins, the fall is precipitous as the oxygen uptake increases. The lower diagram illustrates the level of alveolar oxygen tension needed to keep the arterial saturation above 90 at different levels of V_{O_2} and D_{O_2}. The notations "Landy" and "Jernberg" refer to values that prevail at peak performance of these trained athletes. (Diagram from Dr. R. H. Shepard.)

detailed study outdates that of Finley, Swenson, and Comroe,[426] which was widely interpreted as indicating that arterial hypoxemia was *invariably* to be attributed to $\dot{V}/\dot{Q}$ abnormality and not to changes in gas transfer capability. The paper by Arndt, King, and Briscoe will be discussed in a later chapter.

Relationship between diffusing capacity and oxygen saturation: Indirect methods. In 1956, Perkins, Adams, and Flores[220] outlined a method of measuring venous admixture and diffusion defect in the lung by comparing the measured arterial oxygen saturation with the alveolar oxygen tension. The arterial saturation was recorded from an ear oximeter, and the alveolar gas measured with a Rahn end-tidal sampler. In effect the method consisted in the plotting of an *in vivo* saturation/tension curve, and the authors showed that in dogs, under a variety of conditions, the curve so plotted lay slightly to the right of an *in vitro* oxygen dissociation curve. A similar idea has been used by Rinck and his colleagues[424] in studying patients with mitral stenosis, by following the oximetric saturation as the level of oxygen in inspired

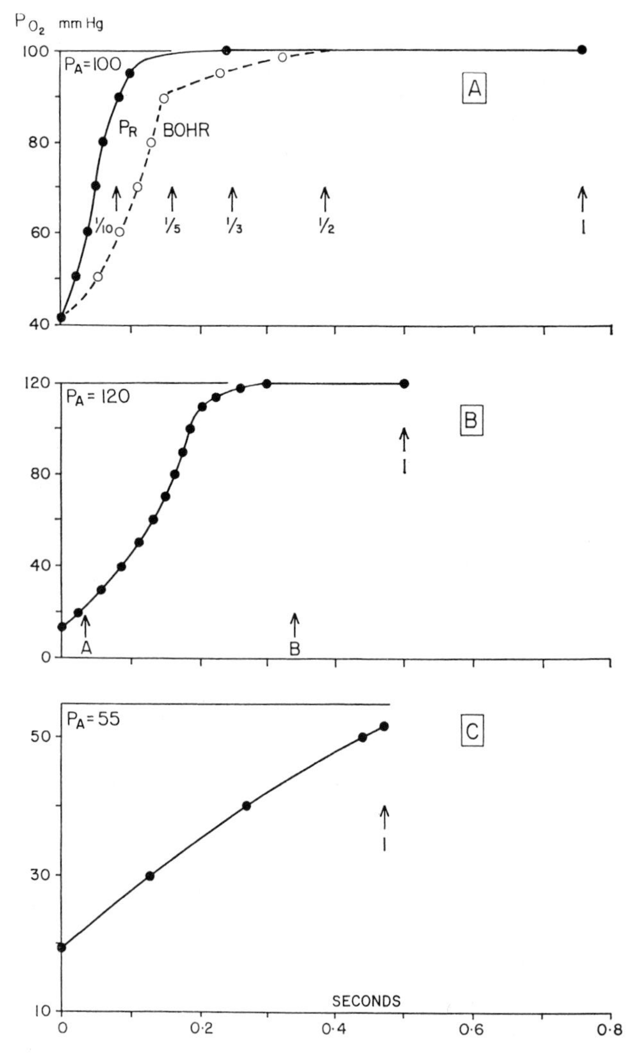

FIGURE 2–43. PROBABLE TIME COURSE OF CHANGES IN ERYTHROCYTE OXYGEN TENSION DURING PASSAGE THROUGH A PULMONARY CAPILLARY

A, Time course of erythrocyte Po_2 rise (P_R) in pulmonary capillaries of normal subject at rest and breathing air. Arrows marked 1/2, 1/3, 1/5 and 1/10 show the end-capillary point for corresponding decreases in transit time in any given lung compartment. The dotted line is the Bohr integration calculated by using data on V_C/D_L ratio to the same end-capillary gradient.

B, Time course of erythrocyte Po_2 rise in a normal subject performing heavy exercise ($\bar{V}_{O_2}$ = 3.0 liter/min) and breathing air.

C, Similar data calculated for a normal subject at lower exercise (V_{O_2} = 1.5 liter/min) but breathing a low-oxygen mixture so that the mean alveolar Po_2 (P_A) is only 55 mm Hg. In this instance, the blood fails to reach equilibrium with alveolar gas within the transit time. (Diagram from Dr. N. C. Staub.)

gas is diminished from 20 to 10 per cent. Although this method revealed a clear distinction between normal subjects and patients, it is difficult to express the difference in meaningful terms. However, the results indicated a reduced diffusing capacity in mitral stenosis, an observation that is in agreement with those made by the direct oxygen and CO methods.

In a useful theoretical study, Shepard[425] analyzed the relationship between the diffusing capacity and the resultant level of oxygen saturation that would follow from impairment of this aspect of function at different levels of work. This relationship is shown in diagram form in Figure 2–42. It is obvious also that, when the saturation begins to decrease as a result of diffusion limitation, the rate of fall becomes, as it were, catastrophic, and a few hundred ml difference in oxygen uptake needed will produce a completely disproportionate fall in saturation. It may be noted from this diagram that the $D_{L_{O_2}}$ has to fall below about 12.0 units (D_{Lco} = 10.0) before the oxygen saturation will begin to fall during performance of exercise such as walking on the level, which requires a $\dot{V}_{O_2}$ of 1 liter/min. It is of particular interest that the validity of this diagram has been strikingly confirmed recently by West and his co-workers[427] in observations of the level of oxygen saturation during physical work at an altitude of 19,000 feet.

CIRCUMSTANCES IN WHICH DIFFUSION LIMITATION LEADS TO A SIGNIFICANT GRADIENT BETWEEN ALVEOLAR AND END-CAPILLARY BLOOD. It has been noted already (*see* page 84) that Staub, Bishop, and Forster[403] found that existing values for the pulmonary capillary blood volume, and other

TABLE 2–6 COMPARISON OF DIFFERENT METHODS OF MEASURING CARBON MONOXIDE EXCHANGE

METHOD	METHODOLOGY	AFFECTED BY	MAIN ADVANTAGES	MAIN DISADVANTAGES	USEFUL FOR
Single-Breath $D_{Lco}SB$	Relatively easy. Requires He and CO analysis and control of timing can be made automatic.	Ratio of D_L to V_A throughout the lung.	Ease and standardization. Insensitive to COHb back pressure.	Serious overestimate of D_L possible in some cases.	Screening. Especially lung fibrosis and infiltrations.
$D_{Lco}SS_1$ (Filley)	Requires estimate of P_{aCO_2} synchronously with measured CO uptake.	Uneven $\dot{V}/\dot{Q}$ ratios in the lung, to a variable extent.	Less affected by V/Q differences than $D_{Lco}SS_2$.	Necessity of P_{aCO_2} estimate.	Exercise studies in which it may be added to other gas exchange measurements.
$D_{Lco}SS_2$ (End-tidal)	Requires automatic end-tidal sample. V_T must be large enough to clear dead space.	Ratio of D_L to ventilation distribution. Magnitude of V_T.	Simplicity. Spirometer record of minute volume and breathing pattern.	D_L may be falsely low due to nonrepresentative alveolar sample.	Screening. Normality of this index excludes significant lung change.
$D_{Lco}RB$ and $D_{Lco}SSHe$	Requires breath-by-breath analysis.	Theoretically *not* affected by nonuniform V/Q or V/V_A distribution.	Relatively unaffected by V/Q. Closest approximation to true summed D_L.	Complexity of method and computation.	Research studies and check on other methods.
Fractional CO Uptake $\left(\frac{F_I - F_{EX}}{F_I}\right)$	Requires only measurement of inspired and mixed expired CO.	Affected by V/Q distribution (V_T/D_L ratio). Lowered by hyperventilation.	Simplicity of measurement and calculation. No helium analysis.	Sensitivity to minute volume.	Screening. If normal, unlikely to be either lung change or severe V/Q disturbance.

parameters related to diffusing capacity, are incompatible with older data of the alveolar and end-capillary gradients that had been reported. In a very important paper,[1346] in which he started from the assumptions that values for V_c and D_M and for the kinetic exchange between oxygen and red blood cells (θ_{O_2}) are correct, and using available measurements of oxygen uptake and cardiac output under varying conditions of rest and exercise, Staub concluded that end gradients would not exist in normal subjects except under conditions of low-oxygen breathing and exercise (*see* Figure 2–43). He points out that apparent increases in gradient would be caused by uneven distribution of diffusing capacity in relation to other parameters, and it is of interest that Piiper and his colleagues[1813] considered that such unevenness undoubtedly contributed to the measured alveolar–arterial pressure difference for oxygen in anesthetized dogs.

A full discussion of the data relating to oxygen exchange at the pulmonary capillary is not possible in this volume. The rapidity of reaction of hemoglobin contained within red cells is critical to this process, as is a knowledge of the mean transit time available for gas exchange to occur. The reader is referred to recent data on these problems,[3557] and to theoretical discussions of $\dot{V}/\dot{Q}$ and diffusing capacity interaction in addition to those already quoted.[3592, 3593] It is important to understand, however, that gas transfer by diffusion is inevitably a "time determined" phenomenon. The question is whether full equilibrium between alveolar gas and pulmonary capillary blood can be achieved in the time available. While it is clear that at sea level in a uniform normal lung the diffusing capacity is not a factor limiting gas transfer, it is equally clear that it becomes important in the following circumstances :

1. When ambient oxygen tension is lowered (even at an altitude of 5000 ft) or when ventilation is restricted during exercise.
2. When the lung is not uniform, leading to abnormally short transit times in some part of the capillary bed, possibly caused by blockage of other parts.
3. When, as a result of $\dot{V}/\dot{Q}$ ratio disturbance, there are low $\dot{V}/\dot{Q}$ regions in which the alveolar P_{O_2} will be low as a mean figure and very low at the end of each expiration.
4. In the presence of some types of lung disease, particularly those causing interstitial edema or alveolar wall thickening.

CHOICE OF METHOD OF MEASUREMENT. The complexity of the interpretation of any measurement of CO transfer (indeed the risk of being thought "unscientific" if any measurement of this kind is made in patients with lung disease) may deter the physician from using any of the methods routinely. We feel that such a decision is unwise. Provided that he understands the limitations of the interpretation, and the reasons for them, it seems clearly established that the routine use of CO transfer methods gives the physician additional information about the patient not easily obtainable by any other means. The follow-up data on the men with chronic bronchitis (*see* Table 2–7) provide one example of the many that might have been chosen. In Table 2–6 are shown the methods available for measuring CO transfer, with a brief note of their characteristics as a guide to the suitability of each for different purposes.

EXCHANGE OF INERT GASES ACROSS THE ALVEOLI. The term "inert" is used to describe gases which are chemically inert in the lungs; this includes all gases except oxygen, carbon monoxide, and carbon dioxide, which combine with hemoglobin and/or the buffer systems of the blood. Examples of inert gases are helium, nitrogen, nitrous oxide, and the like.

The relative rate of diffusion of two different gases between a liquid and a gas phase is related to their solubility in the liquid (α) and their molecular weights. Thus the relative rates of diffusion of oxygen and carbon monoxide may be calculated as shown in Equation 21.

$$\frac{D_{O_2}}{D_{CO}} = \frac{\alpha O_2}{\alpha CO} \times \sqrt{\frac{\text{mol wt CO}}{\text{mol wt } O_2}}$$

$$= \frac{0.024}{0.018}\sqrt{\frac{28}{32}} = 1.23 \qquad (\textit{Equation 21})$$

A similar calculation for CO_2 in relation to oxygen shows that it must diffuse at about 20 times the rate of oxygen through a presumed water membrane.

Forster,[346] in a more modern version of an earlier calculation by Krogh, using recently obtained values for the membrane diffusing component (D_M) and the capillary blood volume of the lungs (V_c), shows that the "tension of dissolved nitrogen in the blood of the capillary will equal 99 per cent of the alveolar tension in about 0.01 second" after the blood is in contact with alveolar gas. This calculation assumes that the solubility of the gas is similar in blood, water, and the membrane itself—a reasonable assumption in the case of most inert gases, although possibly erroneous in some circumstances if a gas is exceptionally soluble in fat. Forster shows also that, even with sulfur hexafluoride, which has a molecular weight of 146 and is the heaviest gas that has been used in respiratory studies, the time required for 99 per cent equilibrium is still only 0.02 sec, a short interval in relation to the period of 0.3 to 0.7 sec in which contact between blood and gas occurs.

The problem of CO_2 release in the lung is complicated by the fact that, were it not for the presence of carbonic anhydrase, the rate of the reaction:

$$CO_2 + H_2O \rightleftharpoons HCO_3 \quad (\textit{Equation 22})$$

would be much too slow for release of CO_2 from the blood.[32]

Dubois and his colleagues have recently restudied the problem of the factors involved in CO_2 exchange at the alveolar level[1820, 1821] and have shown that Diamox, a carbonic-anhydrase inhibitor, slows the reaction to a point where evolution of CO_2 cannot be completed in the time the blood spends in the capillary. In experiments with dogs, this effect can be demonstrated to cause a reduction in total CO_2 evolution of considerable magnitude.[1822] Dubois has shown also that, in dogs, the bicarbonate ions spend an average of 2.2 sec in contact with the gas-exchange surface, a much longer period than the erythrocyte-transit time in the capillaries. The implications of this and other very interesting work on the pulmonary capillary bed[1823–1825] cannot be discussed in detail in this volume.

It is evident, therefore, that with inert gases, in all alveoli there must be a complete tension equilibrium between blood and gas during almost the whole period the blood is in contact with the gas. Thus, there cannot be any end gradient of pressure difference between alveolar gas and pulmonary capillary blood at the end of the capillary. It follows that the rate of uptake of a gas such as nitrous oxide depends upon the pressure gradient between alveoli and blood, the solubility of nitrous oxide in blood, and the volume flow of blood/min past the alveoli. In a recent application of nitrous oxide to the measurement of pulmonary flow,[430] a technique originated by Krogh and Lindhard in 1912,[431] this relationship was expressed as in Equation 23, where α equals 0.474 and is the solubility coefficient for nitrous oxide in blood (i.e., ml of N_2O dry at 37° C, which will dissolve in 1 ml of blood when equilibrated at 760 mm and 37° C).

Many physicians experience difficulty in understanding the different factors that determine the rate of transfer of inert and biologically active gases. A full treatment of these problems, such as those by Jacobs,[432] Kety,[433] or Forster[346] is out of place in this text, but we have found of value a descriptive analogy originally devised by Barcroft. The lung is envisaged as a subway station; prospective travelers represent inspired gas molecules; continuously arriving trains represent pulmonary capillary blood flow; and a turnstile before the platform represents the diffusion limitation of the lung. With this model we can picture the different factors determining gas transfer. In the case of CO, the affinity of hemoglobin for this gas is so large that it is as if every seat in the arriving trains is empty; hence, all people arriving at the platform can step straight to a seat and be carried away. Since the rate of gas diffusion is represented by the turnstile before the platform, in the case of CO it will be the rate of passage through this barrier that determines the rate of removal of the travelers. In the case of oxygen, in addition to this barrier, some of the seats are occupied as the trains come in; if all were full, no net exchange of oxygen would occur, since no passengers could board. With inert gases, there is no turnstile, since diffusion is very fast, and the passing trains are empty (at least until recirculation occurs); in this instance the number of passengers removed

---

$$\dot{Q}_c\,(\text{liters/min}) = \frac{\dot{V}_{N_2O}\ \text{uptake of } N_2O \text{ per minute}}{\alpha\,[F_{A\,N_2O}]\ \dfrac{P_B - 47}{760}} \qquad (\textit{Equation 23})$$

depends upon the pressure from the crowd on the platform, greater crowds on the platform (increasing $F_{A\,N_2O}$) forcing more people into the trains. Comroe and his colleagues have devised an excellent series of diagrams[3] illustrating the same factors pictorially.

Shunts

In the normal lung, a small quantity of venous blood traverses anatomical channels to bypass the gas-exchanging surfaces of the lungs, thereby decreasing the oxygen partial pressure of peripheral arterial blood. This is a *true* shunt which has diverse anatomical origins: bronchial veins, thebesian veins, anterior cardiac veins, and pulmonary arteries. In the normal lung, the volume of shunted blood is generally considered to be less than 2 per cent of the cardiac output.[202, 3661] The small anatomical shunt in the normal state is to be compared to the considerable magnitude which may exist in this component in certain clinical conditions, such as congenital right-to-left intracardiac shunts and pulmonary hemangiomatosis.[423, 3664] Appreciable shunting via portopulmonary[3665, 3666] and intrapulmonary [1740, 3445] communications have also been demonstrated in some patients with liver cirrhosis. In addition, in many disease states the true shunt may be increased because some of the pulmonary alveoli may be perfused but not ventilated. Although strictly speaking the latter represents an extreme example of ventilation–perfusion inequality (i.e., a $\dot{V}/\dot{Q}$ ratio of nil), for convenience the nonventilated lung units are regarded as true shunt because their effects on gas exchange are indistinguishable from those of the other shunts described above.

The total true shunt may be determined by giving a patient pure oxygen to breathe (ensuring that there is no possibility of a leak), and analyzing the arterial blood as soon as it has been drawn.[3661] As noted earlier, it amounts to between 1 and 2 per cent of the cardiac output in normal people. Recently, tritium and ^{85}krypton have been used to measure right-to-left shunts.[423, 3667–3669] The shunt determined by the use of these inert gases does not include contributions through areas of the lungs where gas is trapped behind closed airways, i.e., alveoli which contain gas but are not ventilated. Thus, by simultaneous determination of the right-to-left shunt with pure oxygen breathing and with the inert-gas technique, it is possible to assess whether the increased shunt is due to passage of blood through gas-filled or gas-free areas. Mellemgaard and his colleagues,[3669] using this differential method, concluded that the increased right-to-left shunt in patients following upper abdominal surgery is chiefly a result of the passage of blood through nonventilated but gas-filled alveoli, that is, through areas of lung where gas is trapped.

Direct measurement of the contribution from the thebesian veins to right-to-left shunt has been attempted by Bartels and his coworkers[3662] in patients with normal lungs, and by Bjork and his collaborators in patients with mitral stenosis.[3663] To our knowledge, direct measurements of the contributions of the other anatomical channels to the total right-to-left shunt in man are lacking.

SUMMARY

It is not surprising that the physician finds the task of sorting out all the factors that bear on intrapulmonary gas exchange a complex and confusing task. During the past ten years, this aspect of respiratory physiology has become much better understood, and the general availability and application of methods of arterial blood-gas tension measurement in a wide variety of clinical situations has meant that many physicians have become skilled in the interpretation of abnormalities in these measurements. A full understanding of all the factors that contribute to the measured alveolar–arterial gas-tension difference inevitably requires a detailed understanding of lung function at the alveolar level; the complex task of defining the meaning of an alveolar gas tension is the major factor making complex the interpretation of such measurements as those of diffusing capacity, and the chest physician in command of the basis of his own discipline certainly needs to have at least a "defensive" knowledge of both of these areas.

PREDICTED NORMAL VALUES FOR PULMONARY FUNCTION

In Tables 2–7 and 2–8 are given values for the predicted results of certain pulmonary function tests in men and women of different heights and ages. There are now many sets of values in the literature from which data such

TABLE 2–7 PREDICTED VALUES FOR PULMONARY FUNCTION TESTS: MEN

1	2	3	4	5	6	7	8	9	10	11	12	13
HT (cm)	AGE (yrs)	VC	FRC	RV	TLC	$FEV_{0.75}$ ×40 (l/min)	$FEV_{1.0}$ LITERS	MMFR (l/sec)	$D_{Lco}SS_2$	$\frac{F_{Ico}-F_{EXco}}{F_{Ico}}$	$D_{Lco}SB$	ME%
155	20	3.97	2.72	1.13	5.10	136	3.6	4.3	23.8	.56	26.7	70
	30	3.65	2.72	1.30	4.95	121	3.3	3.9	21.0	.52	23.7	65
	40	3.35	2.72	1.45	4.80	106	3.0	3.5	18.2	.49	20.7	60
	50	3.04	2.72	1.61	4.65	91	2.7	3.1	15.4	.45	17.7	55
	60	2.73	2.72	1.77	4.50	76	2.4	2.7	12.6	.42	14.7	50
	70	2.42	2.72	1.91	4.35	61	2.1	2.3	9.8	.39	11.7	45
160	20	4.30	2.98	1.27	5.57	141	3.8	4.4	24.1	.55	29.0	70
	30	4.00	2.98	1.42	5.42	126	3.5	4.0	21.3	.52	26.0	65
	40	3.70	2.98	1.57	5.27	111	3.2	3.6	18.6	.48	23.0	60
	50	3.40	2.98	1.72	5.12	96	2.8	3.2	15.8	.45	20.0	55
	60	3.10	2.98	1.87	4.97	81	2.5	2.8	13.0	.41	17.0	50
	70	2.80	2.98	2.02	4.82	65	2.2	2.4	10.1	.39	14.0	45
165	20	4.62	3.23	1.42	6.04	145	3.9	4.5	24.5	.55	31.3	70
	30	4.32	3.23	1.57	5.89	130	3.7	4.1	21.7	.52	28.3	65
	40	4.02	3.23	1.72	5.74	115	3.3	3.7	18.9	.48	25.3	60
	50	3.72	3.23	1.87	5.59	100	3.0	3.3	16.1	.44	22.3	55
	60	3.42	3.23	2.02	5.44	85	2.7	2.9	13.3	.42	19.3	50
	70	3.12	3.23	2.17	5.29	70	2.4	2.5	10.6	.38	16.3	45
170	20	4.94	3.48	1.57	6.51	150	4.1	4.6	24.9	.54	33.6	70
	30	4.64	3.48	1.72	6.36	135	3.8	4.2	22.1	.50	30.6	65
	40	4.35	3.48	1.86	6.21	120	3.5	3.8	19.3	.47	27.6	60
	50	4.05	3.48	2.01	6.06	105	3.2	3.4	16.5	.43	24.6	55
	60	3.74	3.48	2.17	5.91	90	2.9	3.0	13.7	.40	21.6	50
	70	3.44	3.48	2.32	5.76	75	2.6	2.6	10.9	.37	18.6	45
175	20	5.26	3.74	1.72	6.98	155	4.3	4.7	25.2	.53	35.8	70
	30	4.96	3.74	1.87	6.83	140	4.0	4.3	22.4	.50	32.8	65
	40	4.66	3.74	2.02	6.68	124	3.7	3.9	19.6	.47	29.9	60
	50	4.36	3.74	2.17	6.53	110	3.4	3.5	16.9	.43	26.9	55
	60	4.06	3.74	2.32	6.38	94	3.1	3.1	14.1	.39	23.9	50
	70	3.76	3.74	2.47	6.23	79	2.8	2.7	11.3	.36	20.9	45
180	20	5.58	3.99	1.87	7.45	159	4.5	4.8	25.6	.52	38.1	70
	30	5.28	3.99	2.02	7.30	145	4.2	4.4	22.8	.49	35.1	65
	40	4.98	3.99	2.17	7.15	129	3.9	4.0	20.0	.46	32.1	60
	50	4.68	3.99	2.32	7.00	114	3.6	3.6	17.2	.42	29.2	55
	60	4.38	3.99	2.47	6.85	99	3.3	3.2	14.2	.39	26.2	50
	70	4.08	3.99	2.62	6.70	83	2.9	2.8	11.6	.35	23.2	45
185	20	5.90	4.25	2.02	7.92	163	4.7	4.9	25.9	.53	40.4	70
	30	5.60	4.25	2.17	7.77	148	4.3	4.5	23.2	.48	37.4	65
	40	5.30	4.25	2.32	7.62	133	4.1	4.1	20.4	.46	34.4	60
	50	5.00	4.25	2.47	7.47	118	3.7	3.7	17.6	.42	31.4	55
	60	4.70	4.25	2.62	7.32	103	3.5	3.3	14.8	.38	28.4	50
	70	4.40	4.25	2.77	7.17	88	3.1	2.9	12.0	.35	25.5	45

Subdivisions of lung volume measured in seated subjects.
Ventilatory tests performed with subjects standing.
Diffusing capacity tests performed on seated subjects.
Values in columns 3 to 6 see ref 118.
Values in column 7 from ref 118 plus additional data in ref 39.
Values in column 8 from ref 3520.
Values in column 9 from ref 74 and additional data in ref 39.
Column 12 values calculated from ref 355 in which the $D_{Lco}SB$ is calculated using the residual volume measured from the single-breath helium dilution.
Column 13 refers to the closed-circuit helium index (*see* ref 39).

TABLE 2–8 PREDICTED VALUES FOR PULMONARY FUNCTION TESTS: WOMEN

1 HT (cm)	2 AGE (yrs)	3 VC	4 FRC	5 RV	6 TLC	7 $FEV_{0.75}$ ×40 (l/min)	8 $FEV_{1.0}$ LITERS	9 MMFR (l/sec)	10 $D_{Lco}SS_2$	11 $\frac{F_{Ico}-F_{EXco}}{F_{Ico}}$	12 $D_{Lco}SB$	13 ME%
145	20	2.81	1.96	1.00	3.81	88	2.6	3.6	20.7	.58	19.5	70
	30	2.63	1.96	1.08	3.71	80	2.4	3.3	18.2	.55	16.9	65
	40	2.45	1.96	1.16	3.61	72	2.1	2.9	15.7	.51	14.2	60
	50	2.27	1.96	1.24	3.51	64	1.9	2.5	13.2	.48	11.7	55
	60	2.09	1.96	1.32	3.41	56	1.5	2.2	10.7	.44	9.0	50
	70	1.91	1.96	1.40	3.31	48	1.4	1.8	8.2	.41	6.4	45
150	20	3.08	2.20	1.05	4.13	92	2.7	3.7	21.1	.57	21.7	70
	30	2.89	2.20	1.14	4.03	84	2.5	3.3	18.6	.54	19.1	65
	40	2.71	2.20	1.22	3.93	76	2.2	3.0	16.0	.51	16.4	60
	50	2.53	2.20	1.30	3.83	67	2.0	2.6	13.5	.47	13.7	55
	60	2.35	2.20	1.38	3.73	60	1.6	2.3	11.0	.43	11.1	50
	70	2.17	2.20	1.46	3.63	52	1.5	1.9	8.5	.40	8.5	45
155	20	3.34	2.43	1.19	4.53	95	2.8	3.8	21.5	.56	23.9	70
	30	3.15	2.43	1.28	4.43	88	2.6	3.4	18.9	.52	21.2	65
	40	2.97	2.43	1.36	4.33	79	2.4	3.1	16.4	.49	18.5	60
	50	2.79	2.43	1.44	4.23	71	2.1	2.7	13.9	.45	15.8	55
	60	2.61	2.43	1.52	4.13	63	1.7	2.3	11.4	.42	13.1	50
	70	2.43	2.43	1.60	4.03	55	1.6	2.0	8.9	.39	10.5	45
160	20	3.60	2.67	1.32	4.92	99	2.9	3.9	21.9	.55	26.0	70
	30	3.41	2.67	1.41	4.82	91	2.7	3.5	19.4	.52	23.3	65
	40	3.22	2.67	1.50	4.72	83	2.5	3.2	16.8	.48	20.6	60
	50	3.05	2.67	1.57	4.62	75	2.2	2.8	14.3	.45	17.9	55
	60	2.87	2.67	1.65	4.52	67	1.8	2.4	11.8	.41	15.2	50
	70	2.69	2.67	1.73	4.42	59	1.7	2.1	9.2	.39	12.5	45
165	20	3.88	2.90	1.44	5.32	103	3.1	4.0	22.2	.55	28.1	70
	30	3.68	2.90	1.54	5.22	95	2.8	3.6	19.7	.52	25.4	65
	40	3.50	2.90	1.62	5.12	87	2.6	3.3	17.2	.48	22.7	60
	50	3.32	2.90	1.70	5.02	79	2.3	2.9	14.6	.44	20.0	55
	60	3.14	2.90	1.78	4.92	71	1.9	2.5	12.1	.42	17.3	50
	70	2.96	2.90	1.86	4.82	63	1.8	2.2	9.6	.38	14.6	45
170	20	4.13	3.14	1.58	5.71	107	3.2	4.1	22.6	.54	30.3	70
	30	3.94	3.14	1.67	5.61	99	2.9	3.7	20.1	.50	27.6	65
	40	3.76	3.14	1.75	5.51	90	2.7	3.3	17.5	.47	24.9	60
	50	3.58	3.14	1.83	5.41	82	2.4	3.0	15.0	.43	22.2	55
	60	3.40	3.14	1.91	5.31	74	2.0	2.6	12.5	.40	19.5	50
	70	3.22	3.14	1.99	5.21	66	1.9	2.3	9.9	.37	16.8	45
175	20	4.38	3.37	1.80	6.18	111	3.3	4.1	22.7	.53	32.3	70
	30	4.20	3.37	1.90	6.10	102	3.0	3.8	20.0	.50	29.6	65
	40	4.02	3.37	2.00	6.02	94	2.8	3.4	17.7	.47	26.9	60
	50	3.84	3.37	2.10	5.94	86	2.5	3.1	15.2	.43	24.2	55
	60	3.66	3.37	2.20	5.86	78	2.1	2.7	12.7	.38	21.5	50
	70	3.38	3.37	2.40	5.78	70	2.0	2.3	10.2	.36	18.8	45

Subdivisions of lung volume measured in seated subjects.
Ventilatory tests performed with subjects standing.
Diffusing capacity tests performed on seated subjects.
Values in columns 3 to 6 see ref 118
Values in column 7 from ref 118 plus additional data in ref 39.
Values in column 8 from ref 3555.
Values in column 9 from ref 74 plus additional data in ref 39.
Values in column 10 corrected for smaller FRC in women and calculated from data for men.
Column 12 values calculated from ref 355 in which the $D_{Lco}SB$ is calculated using the residual volume measured from the single-breath helium dilution.
Column 13 refers to the closed-circuit helium index (*see* ref 39).

as these may be compiled, and the reader should refer to articles by Gaensler and Wright,[3559] Sluis-Cremer and Sichel,[3740] Cotes and his colleagues,[3520] and Anderson, Brown, Hall, and Shephard[3517] for much additional data relating to predicted normal values for the subdivisions of lung volume and tests of ventilatory function. In general, there is excellent conformity in such data, but Sobol and Weinheimer have reported somewhat higher values for the maximal midexpiratory flow rate than those we have given in the Tables,[3738] probably due to some population difference.

Anderson and Shephard have published a regression equation for the single-breath diffusing capacity based on age and body weight,[3518] and Sharma and Williams[3344] have also published a regression equation for this measurement, but they used age and height in meters as the two variables. Pyorala and his colleagues have developed a regression equation for the single-breath diffusing capacity based on age and on the measured vital capacity[3529] and used this in a study of former endurance athletes.

Podlesch and Stevanovic have reviewed existing exercise diffusing-capacity data and added their own studies of 79 healthy men at rest and at exercise.[3528] Their regression is close to one we have published,[1816] the steady-state D_{Lco} increasing about 1.5 ml/min/mm Hg per 100 ml/min of increasing oxygen uptake. Anderson and Shephard[3537] have suggested that the maximal D_{Lco} can be computed from an observed value at submaximal exercise related to the difference between the subject's observed maximal oxygen uptake and the oxygen uptake at which the diffusing capacity was measured. Shephard[3530] has compared world standards of cardiorespiratory performance, and there are now many regression formulae to calculate the maximal oxygen uptake. The reader may find that the regression equation relating the maximal oxygen uptake to load, heart rate, and age in years is useful in exercise testing.[3534] (See page 99.)

During the past few years, there has been some controversy as to how the predicted values for pulmonary function should be used. In the first edition of this book, we suggested, as a handy rule of thumb, that a deviation of more than 20 per cent from the predicted value could be used in assessing the probability of a particular figure representing a normal subject, within the necessarily rather poorly defined limits of that concept. Sobol and Weinheimer[3738] have criticized this advice, pointing out that, in general, a range of 2 standard deviations lies outside the 20 per cent value, and noting that, in a particular population they studied, 12 of 171 tests of the forced vital capacity fell below the 20 per cent mark. Anderson and his colleagues,[3517] considering the vital capacity and FEV data, concluded that "despite the use of multiple regressions to predict 'normal' values of VC and $FEV_{1.0}$, the scatter is such that on the average a 20 per cent loss of function must occur before an individual result can be considered of pathological significance."

It is clear that the physician must no more become a slave to normal data for pulmonary function than to any other biometric information. Borderline data invariably provide much of the challenge and not a little of the interest of interpreting pulmonary function information in the light of clinical and radiological information. It is quite clear that for many purposes, but particularly for follow-up studies, the patient acts as his own best control. Nevertheless, it is very helpful to have some general guide to normal values to serve as a reference.

Normal values for pulmonary mechanics measurements and those for arterial oxygen tension and alveolar–arterial gas-tension differences have been discussed in the sections of this chapter concerned with these aspects of respiratory function.

ASPECTS OF APPLIED PHYSIOLOGY OF THE LUNG

CHAPTER

3

EFFECTS OF AGE ON PULMONARY FUNCTION

INTRODUCTION

There are at least three reasons why the study of the effect of age on the lung is of particular interest. It is important in relation to the interpretation of pulmonary function tests; it raises important questions concerning the interrelationship between biochemical and morphological change and pulmonary function; and it brings into question the important contemporary problem of distinguishing between the effects of aging and the consequences of the environment to which the lung is exposed. General discussions of the biology of aging[21, 646] are relevant to these problems, and the reader will find a summary of data up to 1964 in the proceedings of a symposium on lung aging.[3516] In the following sections particular emphasis will be given to some work done since that date that relates to this area of study.

BIOCHEMICAL AND MORPHOLOGICAL AGE CHANGES

It has been known for some years that the elastin content of the human lung is, if anything, slightly increased in older subjects.[648–650, 652] Pierce and his colleagues[2496] have shown that this increase is significant, that the tensile strength of the lung (which is approximately 1.1 kg/sq meter) is not reduced by age,[3527] and that, with age, there are some alterations in the fibrous network of the lung.[2497] Kohn[3535] has suggested that an important element may be the development of cross-linking of fibrils of collagen with age, which would tend to make the structure more rigid.

Morphologically, there is an increase in the size of the small components of the duct system, apparently involving the alveolar ducts in particular,[645, 654–656, 2224] and it has been clearly demonstrated that there is a small reduction in internal surface area with age.[2506] Thurlbeck has recently compared the published data on this important question (*see* Figure 10 of reference 2506), and it may be concluded that the standardized internal surface area of the lung falls from about 75 sq meters at age 30 to about 60 sq meters at age 70. This represents a loss of about 2.7 sq meters per decade. There are important changes in the thoracic wall with age, particularly progressive calcification of the chondral cartilage and development of a slight kyphosis leading to an increase in the anteroposterior diameter; but these changes do not indicate the presence of morphological changes within the lung.[651]

PULMONARY MECHANICS AND VENTILATION

It is now clear that the changes in lung recoil and in the shape of the pressure–volume curve that occur with age play an important part in determining other aspects of function. Pierce and Ebert[649] noted that the entire pressure–volume curve is shifted to the left with age, and the loss of elastic recoil that occurs has been acknowledged for some years.[1908] Turner, Mead, and Wohl[2380] have studied this phenomenon in detail, and their data is combined with observations we have published[2432] in Figure 3–1. This shows that there are three effects of age: loss of elastic recoil, so that lung volume is greater at the same pressure differential in the older lung; shift of the curve over most of its course; and an increase in the volume of air in the lung at zero transpulmonary pressure. The maximal static negative pressure declines considerably with age,[465, 649, 1908, 2380] and, as can be seen from the figure, this change seems to be occurring in a regular manner from the age of 20 onward. Dynamic compliance becomes frequency-dependent with age,[465] but there is little[1908] or no[481] demonstrable increase in airway resistance with increasing age. Some small differences in these reported results are no doubt to be explained by the very real difficulty in selecting old normal subjects for studies of this kind. All observers have documented a progressive fall in maximal ventilatory capability with age, and Anderson and his colleagues[3517] have recently published a comprehensive comparison of this published data.

SUBDIVISIONS OF LUNG VOLUME

It is agreed that the vital capacity declines with age, an observation first made by John Hutchinson in 1846.[89] Both the inspiratory

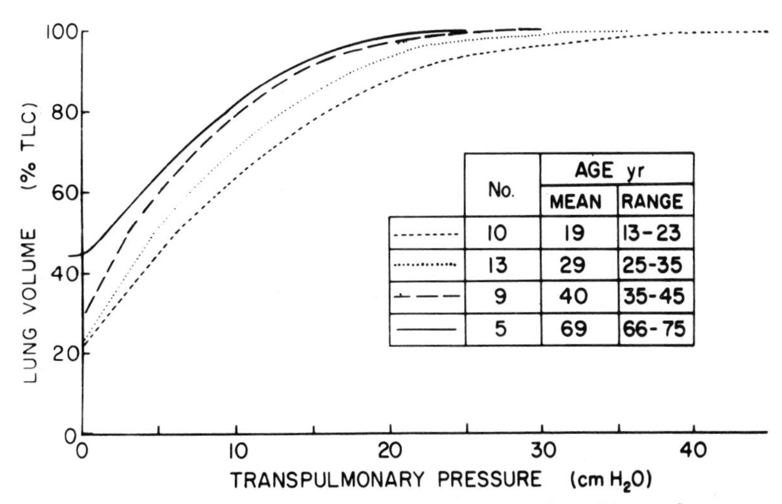

FIGURE 3–1. Changes in pulmonary pressure curves with age. Data for subjects of mean ages 19, 29, and 40, replotted from reference 2380, and for subjects aged 69, from reference 2432. Static deflation curves are shown. The subjects were predominantly male.

capacity and the expiratory reserve volume decline with age. There is some variation in the reported results of measuring the functional residual capacity (FRC) in subjects of different ages, though the balance of evidence shows an increase in this with age. There is general agreement that the residual volume increases, as does the fraction of the total lung capacity that the residual volume occupies. The total lung capacity at age 60 is about 90 per cent of that value at age 20.

Distribution of Ventilation and Airway Closure

It has been known for many years that inert-gas distribution is less uniform in old than in young subjects. This was demonstrated by the single-breath test,[143, 150] open-circuit gas clearance,[153, 154, 1910] and the closed-circuit helium index.[43] There is a definite but small increase in measured anatomical dead space with age,[241] possibly explained by the increased width of the alveolar ducts noted earlier; but this is not likely to be responsible for much of the nonuniformity of ventilation that has been noted.

In a study of a small group of normal men between the ages of 66 and 75,[2432] we found that, as a consequence of the reduced recoil pressure of the lung, airway closure was occurring at the level of the resting FRC. Hence, when the subject took a normal tidal-volume breath, airway units in the dependent part of the lung must have been sequentially opening. By contrast, in the young normal subject, airway closure only occurs as the subject expires from FRC to residual volume. Figure 3–2 shows the reason for the difference. Since the vertical pressure gradient in the intrapleural space is the same in young and old, and since in the older subject the shape of the pressure–volume curve is altered, it follows that in them, in the most dependent regions of the lung at FRC the transpulmonary pressure may be positive and airways may be closed. It is clear that the distribution of ventilation in the older subject is bound to be "unstable" and very much dependent on the actual tidal volume taken. We have quantitated airway closure as a function of age,[2455] and from these experiments it may be computed that the closing volume at age 20 is at a lung volume less than 10 per cent of the vital capacity, but at age 40 closing occurs at about 20 per cent of vital capacity.

These observations accord remarkably well with those published by Edelman and his colleagues.[3522] In a very carefully controlled study of the effect of age and of different respiratory patterns on ventilation uniformity

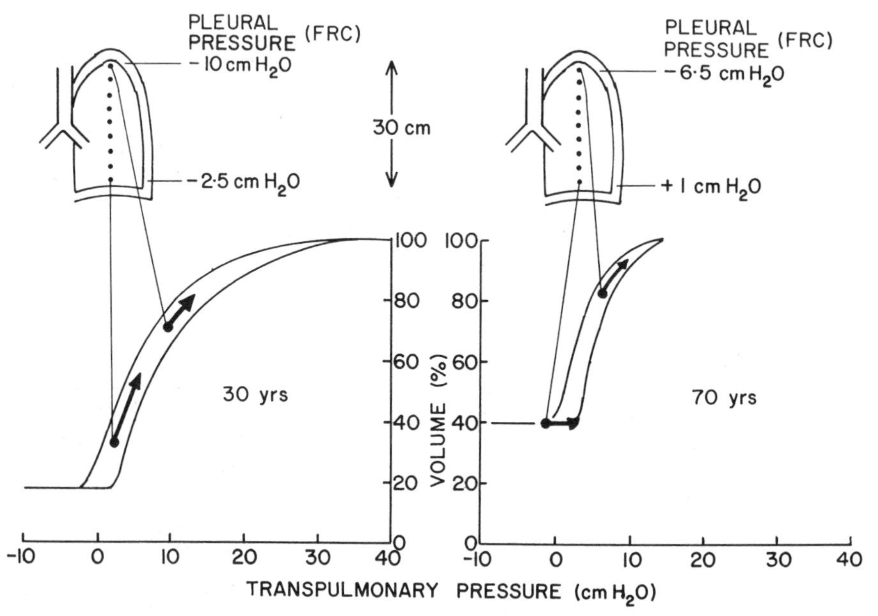

FIGURE 3–2. Aging of the lung is accompanied by loss of recoil (*see* Figure 3–1.) In consequence, the lung of the older subject at FRC has some airways closed in the basal part of the lung, whereas in a 30-year-old subject, all are open at this volume. (From reference 2644.)

as measured by open-circuit clearance, these authors concluded that "ventilation uniformity improved with increasing tidal volume in the older group only," and there were no differences between the age groups if slow, deep breaths were taken.

Thus there seems every reason to suggest that the increased residual volume of age is due to premature closure of airways, due, in turn, to loss of recoil; that ventilation distribution becomes dependent on the magnitude of the tidal volume as the lung loses recoil with advancing age; and that one need not postulate an uneven distribution of age changes within the lung to explain the phenomena observed.[3532]

$\dot{V}/\dot{Q}$ DISTRIBUTION AND DIFFUSING CAPACITY

It has been known for some years that in old subjects, the alveolar–arterial oxygen difference is increased,[1804, 2260, 2268] and more recent work with more precise methodology has confirmed this.[3526] Some of this inequality may be due to the lower resting cardiac output of older people[616] which might lead to an increase in the Zone 1 part of the lung (*see* page 48), but we were unable to demonstrate any decrease in upper zone blood flow in a small group of elderly subjects.[2432] Analysis of expired gas in terms of $\dot{V}/\dot{Q}$ distribution, however, does show consistent age effects[265, 3523] but it is not clear how far these experiments may not have been influenced by the ventilatory factors discussed earlier.

A similar difficulty lies in the interpretation of the decline in diffusing capacity documented by many investigators using the single-breath technique,[355, 3518] the steady-state CO methods,[387, 397, 3528] and the oxygen-diffusing-capacity technique.[421, 3531] However, it is of interest that using the latter method, Armstrong and his colleagues have not found evidence of any significant change in D_{LO_2} in the same individuals over a 10-year period.[3519] The age difference does not seem explicable on the basis of altered perfusion distribution, but whether or not it is to be interpreted as indicating an absolute loss of capillaries, or whether some other change such as an increase in mean red-cell diameter may be partly responsible,[658] is not at all clear.

ARTERIAL BLOOD GASES

The major component in the increased (A–a) O_2 difference with age is a fall in the arterial oxygen tension. Loew and Thews[3524] found an average $P_{a_{O_2}}$ of 95 mm Hg in adults between the ages of 18 and 30, falling to an average of 85 mm Hg by age 35, and again to an average of 75 mm Hg at age 60. Similar data were reported by Sorbini and his colleagues,[3513] and their data show that the decrease occurs almost linearly with advancing age. These two exceptionally careful studies put this matter beyond doubt, and there are other observations which support the conclusion based on measurements made in a hospital population.[3521, 3525] In one of these studies the dependence of the arterial oxygen tension on deep-breathing in older people was particularly noted.[3525] The arterial P_{CO_2} by contrast is not affected by age. Since the altered diffusing capacity could not explain these alterations, it is tempting to suggest that the lowered arterial oxygen tension is a consequence of the presence of low $\dot{V}/\dot{Q}$ regions in the dependent parts of the lung—due, in turn, to the loss of recoil. Ventilation may be occurring in these regions only at the top of a tidal-volume breath. It may well be that this is the explanation, and evidence that we have found that the ventilation of dependent lung regions is less good after an hour of recumbency in older people may well support such an explanation.[2465]

EXERCISE CHANGES

The maximal oxygen uptake falls progressively with age. Von Dobeln, Astrand, and Bergstrom[3534] found that this could best be approximated by the following equation:

$$\text{Max } \dot{V}_{O_2} = 1.29 \sqrt{\frac{L}{H - 60}}\, e^{-0.00884\,T}$$

where L = Load in kilopondmeters per minute at submaximal work;
H = Heart rate after 5 to 6 minutes at L;
T = Age in years.

Between 35 and 65, the Maximal $\dot{V}_{O_2}$ declines from 3.17 liters/min to 2.29 liters/min. It is not completely clear why this occurs, though it seems likely that circulatory factors are mostly responsible for the decline. Dill has noted that his own maximal oxygen intake declined between the age of 38 and 68, so that at the latter age it was only 66 per cent of his original value.[30, 1907]

Summary

This brief account of the effect of age on pulmonary function leaves more questions unanswered than answered. Richards[647] pointed out that there were many documented examples of no apparent disease in people of extreme age. One of the male subjects we recently studied in detail[2432] showed pulmonary function parameters, lung volumes, diffusing capacity, FEV, and lung recoil to be the predicted values for a man half his age. Apart from coming from a long-lived family, there seemed to be no particular reason why his lungs had aged so little as compared to the average. A second unanswered question involves the interaction between aging factors on the one hand (whatever they may be) and environmental factors on the other. In the case of the lung these are particularly hard to separate if the subject has lived in the environment of a modern city. A third consideration is that it is of interest that no coherent explanation can yet be given of the precise reason for the loss of recoil of the lung with age, an effect which seems to have very important consequences for other aspects of lung function. It is not possible to explain this by the loss of internal surface area or actual numbers of alveoli, although some change does occur in these. Nor do the biochemical changes appear to fit in, since the development of cross-linkages of collagen would be expected to lead to a more rigid structure and a fall in static compliance, whereas what occurs is more like the loss of elastic recoil that occurs in aging rubber. Whatever may be the answers to these questions, the continued study of the effect of age on all aspects of lung function still represents an important challenge.

PULMONARY CONSEQUENCES TO OBESITY

Interest in the respiratory consequences of obesity was stimulated by the observation by Burwell and his colleagues[587] that some very fat patients developed full-blown respiratory failure in the absence of lung disease. This syndrome of alveolar hypoventilation is discussed in Chapter 16. Subsequent investigations have revealed that obesity *per se* causes pulmonary malfunction; in most of the studies to be cited, care was taken to exclude obese patients with co-existent bronchitis or emphysema.

Obesity, of course, represents a gross increase in body mass. Because of this, the obese subject's oxygen consumption and carbon dioxide production are higher than normal, both at rest and during exercise.[3741, 3742] Therefore, to maintain normal arterial blood gases in the face of this high metabolic rate, the obese individual must ventilate more than the thin one.

Other major respiratory effects of obesity are due to the fact that a large proportion of the excess body mass is commonly located in and around the thorax. Obesity may be regarded for our purposes as a disease of the chest wall—the term "chest wall" in this context includes both the rib cage and the combination of abdomen and diaphragm. Though measurements of the mechanical properties of the chest wall are difficult to make, most such studies have found abnormalities in obese subjects.[502, 588, 589, 591, 3743, 3744] The compliance of the chest wall is reduced, its inertance is increased and its resistance is increased. Most important, the total work involved in moving the chest wall to expand the lungs is distinctly increased in obese subjects. The most important component of this increased work is elastic, i.e., due to decreased chestwall compliance. This is reflected by the fact that, in response to inhaled CO_2 or exercise, obese subjects increase breathing frequency more and tidal volume less than do normal subjects.[3741]

In addition to these factors, the respiratory muscles of obese subjects may operate less efficiently than those in a normal subject.[503] Thus, because of their high metabolism, fat people must maintain a relatively high ventilation with an increased amount of work demanded per liter of ventilation and perhaps an increased oxygen demand of the respiratory muscles per unit of work done. For these reasons, obese subjects commonly show depressed values for tests involving high levels of effective breathing effort, such as the MBC or MVV, while showing normal values for relative effort-independent tests of expiratory airflow.[3742]

A further effect of the altered thoracic mechanics of the obese subject has been likened to a mass load.[3745] The obese subject is like a normal subject with a weight on his chest wall. The major effect of this mass load is to decrease the FRC; because FRC is reduced and RV is usually not, the expiratory reserve volume (ERV) decreases. This is perhaps the most consistent abnormality found in routine pulmonary function testing of obese subjects.[502, 598, 3741, 3742] Reduction in ERV is more striking when the obese subject lies down and the abdominal mass is applied to the lungs;[593] in many obese subjects in the supine position FRC approaches RV. This change in lung volume has very important consequences. It has been shown in normal subjects that breathing at low lung volumes alters the distribution of inspired gas;[2444] dependent lung regions receive a smaller fraction of the inspirate than do superior lung regions, which is the reverse of the situation at normal (i.e., higher) lung volumes. This maldistribution of inspired gas is very probably due to closure of airways in dependent lung regions.[2444, 2969] The regional distribution of the pulmonary blood flow, however, is probably not greatly changed by lung volume changes, so that in obese subjects, dependent lung regions might be relatively overperfused. Studies of obese subjects using ^{133}xenon have demonstrated the validity of these hypotheses. In obese subjects, upper lung regions are ventilated more than lower lung regions, and lower lung regions are perfused more than upper ones.[2464] Further, in obese subjects at FRC there is evidence of airway closure and gas-trapping in dependent lung regions.[3746] Abnormalities in gas distribution and airway closure correlate with decreases in ERV. These findings afford a rational explanation for demonstrated abnormalities of gas distribution and gas exchange in obese subjects with normal lungs. Abnormalities in the distribution of inspired gas, as deduced from the single-breath N_2 test, have been described.[3742] Abnormally low values of arterial Po_2 have been repeatedly noted in obese subjects,[502, 588, 589, 592] and it has been shown that this is largely due to the presence of units with low $\dot{V}a/\dot{Q}$.[592, 3747] Finally, abnormalities of gas exchange become more striking in the supine position,[592] which would be predicted on the basis of the ^{133}xenon results because of postural changes in FRC.[593]

Care must be taken to distinguish between the changes due to simple obesity and those of the Pickwickian syndrome.[587] The latter occurs in obese subjects, who, while demonstrating the abnormalities just noted, also hypoventilate. Because of hypoventilation, these patients develop severe anoxemia, hypercapnia, polycythemia, pulmonary hypertension, and right heart failure. A similar picture may occur in thin subjects who hypoventilate and it is termed primary alveolar hypoventilation. Whether the Pickwickian syndrome is simply primary alveolar hypoventilation in the obese subject is open to question. It is clear, however, that such hypoventilation occurs much more commonly in fat people than in thin, though among obese subjects the amount of obesity does not correlate with the tendency to hypoventilate. It is reasonable to suppose that obesity predisposes to hypoventilation, since hypoventilation in the presence of normal lungs and a normal neuromuscular system implies abnormal insensitivity to respiratory stimuli, particularly CO_2. It has been shown that the ventilatory response to CO_2 is decreased in the presence of increased mechanical work of breathing;[3748, 3749] the abnormal thoracic mechanics of obesity would therefore be expected to decrease CO_2 responsiveness. It is difficult to demonstrate decreased ventilatory responsiveness to inhaled CO_2 in obese subjects who do not hypoventilate, but the normal range of responsiveness is very wide.[502, 3741] On the other hand, obese subjects with hypoventilation appear to demonstrate more striking abnormalities of thoracic mechanics than do obese subjects who do not hypoventilate.[3744]

ADAPTATION TO ALTITUDE

Introduction

As altitude increases, the barometric pressure falls, and since the fractional concentration of oxygen in the atmosphere is constant, the inspired Po_2 falls. In spite of this difficulty, men frequently go to high altitudes; in the Andes, man has been living at 14,000 to 15,000 feet (barometric pressure 400 to 500 mm Hg) for about 10,000 years.[3598] It has long been clear[3599] that when men go to altitude, a process of acclimatization occurs. The mechanisms of this adaptation are not only of interest to physiologists, but of importance to physicians concerned with the hypoxia that may follow disease of the heart or lungs. The physiological study of men going acutely to altitude began with the observations of Paul Bert on the French balloonists in the latter part of the last century,[2] and continued with the first detailed studies of men on mountain tops in the early years of this century. Since that time a great deal of work has been done, stimulated in recent years by the 1968 Olympic games held at Mexico City (altitude 7340 ft).

A comprehensive review of the altitude literature is beyond the scope of the present volume. In this section, those cardiorespiratory adaptations of clinical relevance will be stressed. Recent reviews of altitude adaptation[3600, 3601] and its specific aspects[3602–3605] are available. The data on altitude indicate levels of hypoxia to which man cannot adapt. Men climbed Mount Everest only with the assistance of oxygen enrichment of inspired air, and men wintering in the Himalayas at an altitude of 19,000 ft lost weight continuously, although their caloric intake was adequate.[3601] Altitude has one minor respiratory consequence not related to the concomitant lowering of oxygen tension, in that the work of breathing is lowered because of the reduction in gas density.[32]

Established adaptations: increased ventilation

When a normal subject is acutely exposed to low inspired-oxygen tensions, minute ventilation increases and the alveolar and arterial P_{CO_2} decreases. This response is mediated by the carotid and aortic chemoreceptors and is quickly reversed when the inspired oxygen is raised to control values. If the same subject is taken to altitude, the same changes are observed acutely, but a further increase in ventilation and decrease in P_{CO_2} is noted if he stays at altitude for the next five to 10 days. Indeed, after the first few days, increasing the inspired-oxygen tension to sea-level values fails to restore either the ventilation or the P_{CO_2} to values found at sea level.

Furthermore, the ventilatory response to an increased alveolar CO_2 tension is altered, in that CO_2 tensions which do not stimulate ventilation at sea level cause considerable hyperventilation at altitude.[2266, 3605] For some time it was postulated that this chain of events could be explained by considering changes in blood-buffering capacity. On initial exposure to hypoxia, the peripheral (carotid and aortic) chemoreceptors caused hyperventilation, but the resulting respiratory alkalosis inhibited the medullary respiratory center, so that the amount of hyperventilation was less than that which would have occurred had the arterial P_{CO_2} remained constant. Over subsequent days, renal excretion of bicarbonate tended to restore the arterial pH to normal, decreasing the inhibitory influence on the medullary center and allowing ventilation to increase as dictated by the peripheral chemoreceptors. Finally, the situation stabilized with a normal arterial pH and with a decreased arterial P_{CO_2} and bicarbonate. In this setting, increasing the arterial P_{CO_2} by a fixed amount would cause a greater change in arterial (and intracellular) pH at altitude than at sea level, and the increased sensitivity to CO_2 at altitude was thus also explained.

The trouble with this hypothesis was that the timing was wrong. Compensatory renal excretion of bicarbonate is a process taking weeks or months, whereas the ventilatory changes were noted to be virtually complete in a few days, well before the arterial blood stopped showing the changes of respiratory alkalosis. An important insight into this problem was offered by Severinghaus and Mitchell.[2266] These workers realized that the medullary chemoreceptors might be more sensitive to the pH of the cerebrospinal fluid (CSF) than to the pH of the arterial blood, and they studied the composition of the cerebrospinal fluid during altitude acclimatization. They found that the CSF bicarbonate decreased much more rapidly than did blood bicarbonate during the first few days at altitude. The speed and magnitude of the decrease were such that they could only be explained by active transport of bicarbonate out of the CSF into the bicarbonate-rich blood. The P_{CO_2} of blood and CSF were always in close agreement throughout their studies, as would be expected from the high diffusivity of this gas.

These findings made possible a rational hypothesis to account for early ventilatory altitude acclimatization. On initial exposure to altitude hypoxia, the peripheral chemoreceptors cause increased ventilation, decreasing the arterial and CSF P_{CO_2}. The resulting increase in CSF pH partially inhibits the peripherally induced hyperventilation and also stimulates active regulation of CSF pH by transport of bicarbonate out of the CSF. Within five to 10 days, this process is complete, CSF pH being the same as it is at sea level. The inhibition of peripheral chemoreceptors therefore ceases and ventilation increases. Because the CSF bicarbonate is low, any increase in P_{CO_2} will now cause a large change in CSF pH and a consequent major change in ventilation. Finally, after 10 days at altitude, the decreased ventilation occasioned by increasing the inspired O_2 tension will be limited by the concomitant rise that will occur in arterial and CSF P_{CO_2}, and because of the low CSF bicarbonate, ventilation will not decrease to sea-level values. These considerations may well explain the changes seen in lowlanders acclimatizing to high altitude. Ventilation is increased and arterial P_{CO_2} is decreased, and these changes increase both with the altitude attained and with the time (up to two to three weeks) at a given altitude.

Are these changes, which have been worked out in altitude sojourners, the same as those seen in people native to high altitude? South American workers[3600] had felt for some time that Andean Indians ventilated less than acclimatized newcomers and therefore maintained higher arterial CO_2 tensions and lower arterial O_2 tensions. This has recently been confirmed in careful studies of two populations native to high altitude, Andean Indians and the Sherpas of the Himalayas.[3606, 3607] Both of these groups have a distinctly higher $P_{a_{CO_2}}$ than do fully acclimatized lowlanders at the same altitude, indicating a ventilatory drive lower in the natives than in the sojourners. The reason for this decrease in ventilatory drive is clearly that both Sherpas and Andean Indians are markedly insensitive to hypoxia.[3608, 3609] They increase their ventilation very little when exposed to low inspired-oxygen tensions. Though knowledge is still somewhat incomplete, there is strong evidence that this respiratory insensitivity to hypoxia is a permanent characteristic that depends on exposure to low arterial oxygen tensions within the first two years of life. Lowlanders who live at altitude for years probably do not lose their sensitivity to hypoxia.[3610, 3611] Highlanders who live at sea level for years remain insensitive to hypoxia.[3611, 3612] North American patients with tetralogy of Fallot have been shown to be insensitive to hypoxia[3613] and it has been suggested that they may remain so for years after their cardiac lesions have been completely corrected.[3614]

Changes in the Blood

Altitude residents, whether long-term sojourners or natives, develop an absolute polycythemia. The red-cell volume is increased and the plasma volume perhaps slightly decreased.[3600] The hematocrit appears to correlate best with the arterial oxygen saturation, which, of course, is dependent on the ambient O_2 tension.[3603] The polycythemia appears to be due to an increase in circulating erythropoietin[3615] and takes months to develop fully. The importance of this adaptation is considerable. The natives of Morococha, in Peru, where the inspired oxygen tension is about 80 mm Hg, have an average hemoglobin concentration of 20 gm per 100 ml, and their arterial oxygen content equals or even exceeds that of a man at sea level.[3600]

In high-altitude natives, the oxygen dissociation curve is displaced downward and to the right, a change which favors the oxygen delivery to the tissues, since a relatively high venous P_{O_2} is maintained for a given arterial P_{O_2} and A-V content difference.[3600] This displacement of the oxygen dissociation curve to the right represents a decreased oxygen affinity of the blood. It has recently been shown by Lenfant and his colleagues[3616] that this change is a property of the hemoglobin itself and that it develops fully within the first 36 hours at altitude and is fully reversible on descent from altitude. These changes in oxygen affinity are accompanied by changes in the red-cell content of 2,3 diphosphoglycerate (2,3 DPG), a substance known to decrease the oxygen affinity of hemoglobin. It is reasonable to postulate that altitude, by imposing a lowered P_{O_2}, triggers an increased production of 2,3 DPG, which, in its turn, decreases the O_2 affinity of hemoglobin and moves the O_2 dissociation curve to the right. Similar changes in oxygen affinity and the red-cell 2,3 DPG content have been demonstrated to occur in patients with cyanotic congenital heart disease, but not uniformly in patients with chronic lung disease and hypoxia.[3617]

Circulatory Changes

Acute altitude exposure is accompanied by tachycardia, but with acclimatization, both the heart rate and resting cardiac output attain sea-level values. Recent data indicate, however, that during exercise, the stroke volume is reduced and the cardiac output is significantly lowered both in residents and in visitors recently arriving at altitude.[3658, 3659] This has been noted in the absence of significant pulmonary hypertension or polycythemia; its mechanism is not known.

The incidence of pulmonary hypertension at altitude is now well-documented. The mean pulmonary-artery pressure in both natives and visitors appears to increase as a parabolic function of altitude or barometric pressure.[3603] In natives at a given altitude, the pulmonary-artery pressure does not relate well to age or hematocrit and tends to increase sharply with exercise or further hypoxia. Although pulmonary-blood volume is probably somewhat increased at altitude, it is clear that the major cause of pulmonary hypertension is an increased precapillary vascular resistance. Since hypoxia at sea level has been shown to cause pulmonary arterial constriction and consequent pulmonary hypertension[1210, 3619, 3660] (*see* page 49), it is likely that this is the initiating mechanism of the pulmonary hypertension at altitude. However, when altitude natives inhale oxygen acutely, the pulmonary-artery pressure decreases but does not reach sea-level values. This is probably due to the fact that in altitude natives, the pulmonary arteries show well-marked hypertrophy of medial smooth muscle, which may explain the fixed high pulmonary vascular resistance during acute transient oxygen breathing. If altitude natives move to sea level, the pulmonary-artery pressure gradually decreases to normal sea-level values, with involution of the medial hypertrophy. Natives of high altitude also have an increase in right ventricular weight and increased elastic tissue in the larger pulmonary arteries. These differences are striking in adults, but much less so in young children, so that it is likely that the involution of the smooth muscle of the fetal pulmonary vascular bed which normally occurs in sea-level residents does not occur in altitude natives, presumably due to hypoxia.[3619]

The question asked by Professor Hermann Rahn at an International Symposium,[3660] namely, "What is the functional significance of the pulmonary hypertension of high altitude?" has yet to receive a satisfactory answer. Grover has suggested that it may be a residual phenomenon arising because of a fetal necessity.

Other changes

It has been shown that the vital capacity decreases as lowlanders go to altitude, but the duration and cause of this change are uncertain.[693, 698] Andean Indians have an increased total lung capacity in relation to their height, owing to an increase in residual volume, the vital capacity being normal.[2266, 3600]

Because of the reduced ambient P_{O_2}, the lung diffusing capacity is a more important determinant of blood oxygenation at altitude than it is at sea level. During vigorous exercise at altitude, the arterial oxygen saturation decreases below resting values, at least in acclimatized lowlanders.[427, 3620] This finding implies a considerable widening of the alveolar–arterial oxygen difference with exercise, and the most likely reason for this is failure of the end-capillary P_{O_2} to achieve equilibrium with the alveolar P_{O_2}. Thus, under the conditions of exercise at altitude, with both a lowered alveolar P_{O_2} and the decreased transit time through the capillary that normally occurs on exercise, the diffusion resistance of the structures between alveolar gas and hemoglobin limits the uptake of oxygen. This limitation appears to begin to be important at an altitude of 5000 ft,[3569] but limitation of maximal oxygen uptake only becomes very significant at altitudes higher than this. The diffusing capacity of lowlanders does not increase with altitude acclimatization,[398] but Remmers and Mithoefer have shown that the membrane component of the diffusing capacity (D_M) is increased in high-altitude natives,[3579] confirming the same earlier observation by Grover,[3660] who could find no corresponding change in pulmonary capillary blood volume.

Measurement of the alveolar–arterial N_2 and CO_2 tension differences have led to the conclusion that there is a greater, and less advantageous, dispersion of $\dot{V}/\dot{Q}$ ratios in the lungs of acclimatizing lowlanders.[3621] Both normal[3608] and large[2312] alveolar–arterial oxygen tension differences have been reported in high-altitude natives.

A great deal of work has been done recently on the effect of altitude on human work capacity.[3563, 3569, 3604, 3605, 3620, 3622] It is clear that in lowlanders the maximal oxygen consumption is decreased shortly after arrival at altitude, and probably by more than it would be during acute hypoxia exposure. During a three to four-week stay at altitude, the maximal oxygen uptake increases gradually, but does not attain sea-level values. It is doubtful whether high-altitude natives are capable of better performance at sea level than are lowlanders.[3563] However, it is clear that at altitude, natives of both the Himalayas and the Andes exhibit maximal oxygen uptakes comparable to those of highly trained lowlander athletes who are fully acclimatized.[3623, 3624] This is particularly remarkable in the light of the fact that these natives ventilate less and therefore have a lower arterial oxygen tension than do the lowlanders. Oxygen transport from the lung to the mitochondria of the working cell is probably more efficient in the highlanders, and this difference cannot apparently be explained, at least in the case of Sherpas, by differences in hematocrit.[3624] It is likely that an increase in tissue capillarity explains this increased efficiency, for if tissue capillaries were closer together, the intercapillary spaces would have a relatively higher mean P_{O_2}.[3660] There are indications that such an increase in tissue diffusing capacity does occur in animals at altitude.[2326]

Diseases of altitude

Acute mountain sickness

When lowlanders ascend rapidly to altitude, they commonly are stricken by a syndrome beginning six to 90 hours after ascent, and characterized by insomnia, headache, nausea, vomiting, dyspnea, and lethargy. Although a problem to physiologists and mountaineers, the general importance of this phenomenon only became apparent during the Sino-Indian border dispute of 1962, when large numbers of Indian troops were quickly moved into the Himalayas. Acute mountain sickness was common, and more severe varieties were described with severe dyspnea, cyanosis, rales in the chest, papilledema, and other signs of cerebral edema.[3625] The cause of these symptoms, whether in minor or major form, is not well understood. A combination of hypoxia and respiratory alkalosis has been blamed, but Singh and his colleagues[3625] felt that fluid retention might play an important part. It has subsequently been shown that the syndrome may be prevented by pretreating the subjects with low doses of acetazolamide.[3626] This has the effect of increasing renal bicarbonate excretion, decreasing the respiratory alkalosis, and thus, by allowing increased ventilation, raising the arterial P_{O_2}.[3627] Whether these changes are crucial or incidental in the prevention of mountain sickness is not yet known.[3628] Indian workers have also succeeded in preventing acute mountain sickness by pretreatment with furosemide, a diuretic with a less specific action than that of acetazolamide.

High-altitude pulmonary edema

Unacclimatized men at altitudes greater than 9000 ft may develop pulmonary edema, which, if untreated, is often fatal.[692, 3603] This can occur in people going to altitude for the first time, or in highlanders who have reascended after as little as two weeks at sea level. Indian workers believe that the pulmonary edema is a variant of acute mountain sickness, but this has been disputed.[3632] High-altitude pulmonary edema commonly, but not invariably, develops in individuals with concomitant symptoms of acute mountain sickness. The clinical picture resembles edema due to left ventricular failure, with cough, dyspnea, cyanosis, rales in the chest, and fluffy infiltrations on the chest x-ray.[3629, 3630] However, it seems clear that left ventricular failure is not a feature of high-altitude pulmonary edema; there is no clinical or radiological venous congestion, and although pressures in the right ventricle and pulmonary artery are very high, the pulmonary wedge pressure is normal.[3603] The chest pain commonly complained of in high-altitude pulmonary edema is probably due to the acute pulmonary hypertension. At autopsy, the left heart is normal, the right heart and pulmonary arteries are dilated, perivascular hemorrhages are seen, and the lungs are full of protein-rich material, often with formation of hyaline membranes. Thrombotic lesions have been noted in pulmonary arteries.

The pathogenesis of this syndrome remains obscure. Most authors feel that the edema results from an increase in hydrostatic pressure in small blood vessels, and that the cause of this increase is an extreme elevation of pulmonary arterial as opposed to pulmonary venous pressure. High-altitude pulmonary edema has been likened to the lung edema that may follow pulmonary embolism.[3603] Edema has been produced in dogs by occluding most of the pulmonary vascular bed,[3603] and rats forced to swim to exhaustion in low oxygen tensions develop perivascular edema in the lung.[3631] Prompt recognition of symptoms, bed rest, oxygen administration, and diuretics usually reverse the edema that occurs at high altitude.

Chronic mountain sickness (Monge's disease)

This disease is seen among long-time altitude residents, usually natives.[3600] It is characterized by the slow onset of fatigue, dyspnea, somnolence, and decreasing mental activity. The patient becomes deeply cyanotic and plethoric, and develops finger-clubbing. The hematocrit is very high, there is considerable pulmonary hypertension sometimes with right ventricular failure, the arterial $P\text{O}_2$ is very low and the $P\text{CO}_2$ higher than in dwellers at the same altitude. All findings return to normal with residence at sea level. When these patients die at altitude, the autopsy findings are only those usually seen in altitude natives but to an extreme degree. The pathogenesis of this illness is not understood, but it seems clear that it develops in those who, for some reason, have lost their respiratory drive and hypoventilate in relation to the altitude at which they are living. The clinical features may be explained as resulting from extreme hypoxia. Severinghaus and others[3597, 3608] have shown that patients with chronic mountain sickness are almost totally without respiratory ventilatory response to hypoxia.

SUMMARY

This brief résumé of what is known of man's respiratory adaptation to altitude clearly indicates the relevance of these studies to clinical questions. Chronic respiratory disease normally leads to a synchronous depression of arterial oxygen tension and elevation of CO_2 tension, whereas at altitude the effects of chronic hypoxia alone are acting on the subject. However, the chronic respiratory patient seems to develop congestive heart failure as a consequence of derangement of his arterial blood gases, with a level of pulmonary hypertension *lower* than that which must commonly occur at altitude and be unaccompanied by right ventricular failure. Thus, although the altitude studies have done much to illuminate the consequences of hypoxia, they do not fully explain the circulatory consequences of chronic respiratory disease.

AN INTEGRATED APPROACH: DEFINITION OF CHRONIC OBSTRUCTIVE LUNG DISEASE

CHAPTER 4

But a theorist is not confronted by just one question, or even by a list of questions numbered off in serial order. He is faced by a tangle of wriggling, intertwined and slippery questions. Very often he has no clear idea what his questions are until he is well on the way towards answering them. He does not know, most of the time, even what is the general pattern of the theory that he is trying to construct, much less what are the precise forms and interconnexions of its ingredient questions. Often, as we shall see, he hopes and sometimes he is misled by the hope that the general pattern of his still rudimentary theory will be like that of some reputable theory which in another field has already reached completion or is near enough to completion for its logical architecture to be apparent. We, wise after the event, may say in retrospect 'Those litigating theorists ought to have seen that some of the propositions which they were championing and contesting belonged not to competing stories of the same general pattern but to non-competing stories of highly disparate patterns'. But how could they have seen this? Unlike playing-cards, problems and solutions of problems do not have their suits and their denominations printed on their faces. Only late in the game can the thinker know even what have been trumps.
– – – PROFESSOR GILBERT RYLE, in Dilemmas (The Tarner Lectures, 1953). Cambridge University Press, 1960, pp. 7–8.

THE DIAGNOSIS OF CHEST DISEASE

An exhaustive account of the different techniques at the disposal of the chest physician to assist him in making a diagnosis cannot be attempted here. It may be useful, however, to stress some aspects of this problem which are particularly relevant to the proper use of the pulmonary function laboratory. In few fields of disease is the taking of a careful history more important than in the case of lung disease. Few medical students graduate with any experience in taking a history of occupation, which includes perceptive questions relating to possible industrial exposures. Even housewives and the suburban "odd-job man" husband may be inadvertently exposed to some substance which may have adversely affected the lung. The dangers of smoke inhalation are not generally recognized, and a history of such exposure may only be elicited on direct questioning.

Forgacs[2823] has published an excellent account of physical signs in the lung and has attempted to provide a morphological correlation for some of them. Unfortunately, it remains the case that most of these signs are difficult to elicit. Fletcher,[709] in 1952, pointed out the inter-observer variability of many of these signs in patients with chronic lung disease. Smyllie, Blendis, and Armitage, in 1965, evaluated 20 chest physical signs assessed by nine observers, and concluded that "inter-observer repeatability of respiratory physical signs falls midway between chance and total agreement." Four years later, Campbell proposed the use of some additional signs to those commonly employed in the examination of the thorax[2820] and, in conjunction with Godfrey and three others,[2819] evaluated these and the older signs in a group of patients. There appeared to be little difference between the "classic" and "unfamiliar" signs, and their conclusion was similar to that reached by Smyllie and his colleagues. It seems that the physician, if armed with only a stethoscope, has to reconcile himself to the equivocal position of suspense between a "totally random" physical examination and one that is 100 per cent precise.

Detailed radiographic study of the lung is such a powerful tool that the opinion of the radiologist is commonly accepted without further question. Yet the diagnostic capability of the radiologist varies inevitably with different types of lesions. In some diseases with plain films alone, the diagnostic capability is very good; in others, more detailed studies will be needed. There can be little doubt that the diagnostic capability of the radiologist has been greatly sharpened in the past 10 or 15 years, partly as a result of a great deal of careful correlative work which that discipline has undertaken in the field of chest disease.[3688] Yet there remain examples of demonstrable function impairment without radiological change, of radiological resolution without function restitution, and of considerable variation of function impairment in the presence of relatively little radiological change in a disease such as chronic bronchitis.

In what way, then, does the pulmonary function laboratory contribute to diagnosis? There is little doubt that tests are required in the early diagnosis of most forms of industrial lung disease, and they play an increasingly important role in following progress over a period of years; they are integral to an evaluation of a man with chronic bronchitis and possible emphysema, though simple and sensitive tests to be used routinely in early cases have yet to be perfected. Some physicians refer to different techniques on occasion, as if these were in some sense competitive, though by their nature they fulfill such different roles that they are bound to be complementary. The paradox, however, is that until a chest physician, in his everyday work, has had available to him the services of a pulmonary function laboratory, he is not in a position to evaluate what contribution the information he derives from it can make to his management of patients.

We have observed very striking differences between different countries, and even between different cities in the same country, in the extent to which pulmonary function laboratories are used effectively and do contribute to a high standard of clinical care. No doubt some of these differences are accidental and related primarily to the training of the local chest physicians, or to the method of financing inpatient and outpatient care. In some instances, some financial formula seems to have been developed which has frozen all laboratory methods at the level at which they existed some years ago, thus making it acceptable to provide the physician with a laboratory service for measuring the blood urea, but not providing the FEV or the P_{CO_2}.

In spite of considerable geographical variation in the extent to which pulmonary function tests are used, there seems little doubt that they will continue to play an increasing role in the early diagnosis and management of chronic lung disease. During the past five years, the limitations of the simple test of expiratory flow rate, have become apparent, and much has been learned of the factors affecting the measured rate of gas uptake. The wider use of measurements of arterial blood-gas tensions has meant that a dangerous degree of hypoxia is now known to exist in situations in which it had not been expected on clinical grounds. (Mithoefer and his colleagues have carefully documented the impossibility of relying on a clinical evaluation of alveolar ventilation.[3724]) It may be hoped that the next few years may see complex methods of regional assessment of the lung made simple and applied to patients with early disease; there is no reason to suppose that such new methods will not increase, by an order of magnitude, the usefulness of the pulmonary function laboratory to the chest physician.

THE DEFINITION OF CHRONIC OBSTRUCTIVE LUNG DISEASE

During the past 15 years a great deal of attention has been devoted to the vexing and controversial problem of the definition of chronic respiratory disease. It cannot be said, however, that these efforts have yet been wholly successful, nor have the systems of differentiation and classification proposed by any investigator or group of investigators proven universally acceptable. In spite of this, much progress has been made, and the key issues involved in this problem can now be much more clearly delineated. It has generally been agreed that pulmonary emphysema can be realistically defined only in morphological terms[24, 815, 2508, 2509, 2517, 2548] and that chronic bronchitis is best defined on clinical criteria,[2500, 2523] at least in the first instance. In Britain and America the differentiation of spasmodic asthma from these two entities does not seem to present a special problem, but in countries where it is taught that there is a considerable "allergic" component to chronic bronchitis, these two diseases are not regarded as sharply distinct.

The presently unresolved problems can be enumerated as follows:

1. Can the clinician differentiate between irreversible airways obstruction due to chronic bronchitis alone and that due to morphological emphysema? It has been suggested that it is not worth attempting this differentiation,[2550] but we feel that although this endeavor may, on occasion, lead to an erroneous conclusion, the attempt should certainly be made, since there are correlations among patterns of function-test defect, radiological appearance, and morphology which are far from negligible.[2524, 2556] The question of whether patients with chronic obstructive lung disease can be divided into "Type A", with predominant morphological emphysema, and "Type B", without morphological emphysema but with severe chronic bronchitis, is considered in detail later (*see* Chapter 6). Scadding has pointed out that it is important for the physician to try to form some estimate of the extent and severity of emphysema during life,[2523] and this seems to us an attempt not just of academic interest but with important implications for therapy and management.

2. Should the same term (chronic bronchitis) be used for the clinical diagnosis based on a history of chronic productive cough, and the severe irreversible airways-obstruction syndrome that may lead to abnormal arterial blood-gas tensions and cor pulmonale in the absence of morphological emphysema? That this severe form of the disease may occur has been known for some years,[903, 934, 958, 998, 1628, 2295] but the use of the same term may give rise to confusion of thought, as Gough[2531] has recently pointed out. Little is yet known of the natural history of chronic bronchitis in these patients, nor of what distinguishes them from the much larger majority of patients in whom chronic bronchitis does not develop into such a malignant disease, though various hypotheses have been advanced to explain it (*see* Chapter 6).

3. To what extent is severe $\dot{V}/\dot{Q}$ imbalance produced by the morphological changes of emphysema and the lesions of chronic bronchitis, respectively? There is not yet a large enough body of evidence on this matter to justify an authoritative opinion, though much lively discussion of it has occurred.[2520]

Although these questions are lurking in the wings whenever problems of definition are discussed, they do not strictly affect the definition of these problems in didactic terms. They are indeed "wriggling, intertwined and slippery questions" (to use the words employed by Professor Ryle in the quotation at the beginning of this chapter), and they engender animated exchanges of opinion; but the three diseases can be defined apart from them.

In this text we have therefore adopted the following broad definitions:

Spasmodic asthma refers to a syndrome characterized by atopy, in which the degree of bronchial obstruction is variable; the subject is abnormally sensitive to inhaled allergens or histamine aerosol; the criteria of emphysema are not constantly present; and evidence of attacks of wheezing dates from early adult life or childhood. The word "asthma" should not be used interchangeably with the word "bronchospasm."

Chronic infective asthma refers to a condition in which the primary condition is believed to be chronic bronchitis, but attacks of respiratory infection are characterized by unusually severe bronchospasm. This disorder was first clearly recognized as an entity by Rackemann who wrote in 1947, "When asthma begins after the age of 40 it should be considered as due to factors other than allergy until proved otherwise."[830]

Chronic bronchitis, as noted by the Ciba Symposium,[815] refers to "the condition of subjects with chronic or excessive mucous secretion in the bronchial tree," the diagnosis being clinical and based on chronic or recurrent cough not attributable to other conditions. The words "chronic or recurrent" were defined as "occurring on most days for at least three months in the year during at least two years." The syndrome may be further subdivided into categories dependent on the purulent nature of the sputum or its quantity,[2500] but it is questionable whether the latter categorization can be rigorously used, since the volume of sputum is not constant.[2555] It is, however, of unquestioned value to accompany a diagnosis of chronic bronchitis with a measurement of the degree of airway obstruction or with a categorization of the concomitant presence of $\dot{V}/\dot{Q}$ disturbance (Type B disease[2510, 2526, 2552]).

Emphysema is a morphological classification; usually it is possible to describe the changes in precise structural terms, and there is now a much larger measure of agreement between pathologists on this matter than used to be the case (*see* Chapter 7). When the clinician says of a patient "I think that there is considerable pulmonary emphysema present," or "I think there is likely to be severe panlobular emphysema, particularly in both lower lobes," he is not defining the condition, but forming a judgment of the morphology. The criteria that may help him to do this are discussed in Chapter 7.

Although Lynne Reid has proposed a classification system of these diseases in some detail,[2508] it seems to us premature to classify emphysema in terms of the degree of airway obstruction it is presumed to cause.

We feel that it is important to stress that it is most necessary for authors to indicate as clearly as possible the detailed state of the patients on whom they are reporting the results of investigations or clinical trials. Little can be made of papers in which the patients are all included under one heading (often "chronic obstructive lung disease" or even simply "chronic bronchitis") and are not further described; and the use of the term "chronisch - asthmatoiden - Emphysem - Bronchitis" by one author,[2545] although solving the difficulty, does not do much to enlighten; yet every chest physician can feel some sympathy with him.

SPASMODIC ASTHMA

CHAPTER 5

"If a man will begin with certainties, he shall end in doubts; but if he will be content to begin with doubts, he shall end in certainties."
———FRANCIS BACON (1561–1626), in Advancement of Learning, I, 8.

DEFINITION

It is unfortunate that, over the years, the word "asthma" has acquired a wide variety of meanings. In some countries it is employed to denote the physical signs of bronchial obstruction and thus is used synonymously with "bronchospasm." This leads to "asthma" being described as a feature of any disease in which rhonchi are audible, including bronchiolitis of all kinds, emphysema, thoracic deformity—and even acute pulmonary edema, still called "cardiac asthma" by some physicians. It seems to us important to rescue the word "asthma" from this connotation, and to try to insist that it be used to denote a condition of usually intermittent episodes of bronchospasm, with symptom-free periods, in a subject with a history or family history of an allergic condition. In some patients the spasm may be chronic and may not respond to any bronchodilator treatment; in others, an acute attack is associated with such extensive plugging of bronchioles with sticky opalescent mucus that life is endangered by asphyxia. When bronchospasm occurs only in association with the development of bronchitis, the condition should be regarded as a variant of chronic bronchitis rather than a type of asthma. In all except the third group the history of intermittent attacks of bronchospasm usually dates from childhood. Only when infection becomes a prominent feature does the asthmatic process lead to the loss of lung parenchyma that is a characteristic feature of emphysema.

Although it used to be widely taught and believed that spasmodic asthma very commonly led to emphysema with irreversible changes, this view is no longer held either by physicians[24] or by pathologists who have studied the lung inflated.[715]

The confusion that may be caused by the use of "asthma" in place of terms such as "bronchial obstruction" or "bronchospasm" can be illustrated by many examples. The very interesting syndrome of bronchospasm apparently caused by an atmospheric pollutant in Japan was described as "air-pollution asthma," although almost all of the sufferers were shown not to have any allergic diathesis.[738] Although it has been shown repeatedly that in established emphysema the response to aerosol bronchodilators often is no greater than in normal people, many papers refer to patients with "emphysema and coexistent asthma"; all that is implied in this connotation is that there is audible evidence of bronchial obstruction. The literature contains many references to patients who develop bronchospasm after some exposure to a potentially harmful substance, such as oxide of nitrogen fumes or oxides of sulfur, or, as noted later, to certain processes involving aluminum. Very few such patients have any history of allergy, either familial or personal, yet they may be clinically classified with typical asthmatics. It is fully realized that there are borderline cases, yet it does seem essential to us to distinguish such patients, who are often suffering from a chronic or unresolved bronchiolitis, from those showing all of the features of spasmodic asthma; the only way to achieve this appears to be by use of the term "bronchospasm" or "bronchial obstruction" in such instances.

PATHOLOGY

The clinical confusion between asthma and chronic bronchitis is reflected in the disparate morphological descriptions of asthma, particularly in reference to the presence of emphysema. If only those patients dying in status asthmaticus are considered, a clear picture emerges, and such examples presumably represent spasmodic asthma. The lungs are found to be voluminous, often meeting in the midline of the chest. They retain air after removal from the body. However, areas of atelectasis are demonstrable in nearly half of the cases.[784] The bronchi and bronchioles are occluded by characteristic tenacious mucous plugs that can be removed only with great difficulty.[1996] Histologically the plugs are slightly basophilic and stain brilliantly with PAS;[785] they contain richly cellular spirals composed of eosinophils and detached respiratory bronchiolar epithelium. Numerous Charcot-Leyden crystals are present.[786] Very characteristically there is extensive detachment of the bronchial epithelium,[784, 785] leaving behind only the basal cells, which may show signs of regeneration. Evidence of bronchial muscle spasm and constriction is equivocal, the fatal bronchial obstruction being due largely to the mucous casts. The surviving bronchial epithelium may be edematous, and the bronchial and bronchiolar walls show an infiltrate of eosinophils, but this does not extend to the respiratory bronchioles.[787] The basement membrane of the epithelium is greatly thickened, but the bronchial mucous glands show no significant hypertrophy,[784, 785] in contrast to the usual findings in patients with chronic bronchitis.[775] It is of interest that identical changes to those just described were seen in bronchial tissue contained in a teratoma in a woman dying of status asthmaticus.[786] Recent evidence has indicated that considerable mucous gland hypertrophy may be present in this syndrome,[3681] and it is clear that much depends on the selection of the material for study.

The muscular layer of the small bronchi and bronchioles may be hypertrophied. Although the lungs are grossly hyperinflated destructive emphysema does not occur more frequently than in the random population.[787, 788] Cor pulmonale is absent. Bronchiectasis, often of the upper lobes, is observed in a quarter of the cases,[784] presumably a result of mucous impaction occurring in previous attacks. Patients with bronchial asthma dying of other causes show slight thickening of the basement membrane of the bronchioles.[789] Dunnill has extended his series of cases of asthma studied at autopsy[784] and reported on the findings in four asthmatic patients who died of trauma when not in an asthmatic attack.[2558] Mucosal edema and separation of the mucosal cells was a common finding, and "the exudate in the bronchial lumen may be seen as an occluding plug in any or all of the bronchial branches down to the level of the terminal bronchiole." These observations accord very well with the documented abnormalities of function that occur in symptom-free asthmatic patients.

When the word "asthma" is used to include bronchospasm occurring with intercurrent bronchial infection in patients with chronic bronchitis, inevitably the pathological findings[790] include those of chronic bronchitis, often associated with pulmonary emphysema of varying degrees of severity.

RADIOLOGY

Radiographic and fluoroscopic examination of the chest in patients with spasmodic asthma generally reveals evidence of overinflation as a sign of expiratory airway obstruction, the degree depending upon the severity of bronchial or bronchiolar narrowing. The overinflation is manifested by an increased volume of the thorax, as shown by hypertranslucency of the lung fields, increased anteroposterior diameter of the chest, deepening of the retrosternal air space, and depressed, flattened diaphragmatic domes. The diaphragm is frequently projected as low as the 11th or 12th rib on postero-anterior films of the chest, and shows varying degrees of restricted excursion on fluoroscopic examination or on films made in full inspiration and maximal expiration. Respiratory movements of the thoracic cage are similarly reduced.

The hyperinflation is associated with splaying of the pulmonary vessels, whose angles of bifurcation are thereby increased. The caliber of the pulmonary arteries and veins is seldom altered, however, an observation that is usually better appreciated on tomographic sections of the lungs than on plain films. We have found the maintenance of a normal caliber and tapering of the peripheral vascular bed to be a useful sign in the differentiation of spasmodic asthma and emphysema, the medium-sized and peripheral arteries in the latter being smaller than normal and showing more-rapid tapering as they proceed from the hila distally.[710]

Parallel linear densities that follow the bronchial distribution of the lungs, most commonly to the bases, have been described by Hodson and Trickey as a not-infrequent finding in asthma.[930] We have not been able to confirm this observation in every patient with typical spasmodic asthma on whom both plain films and tomograms have been available for study. In those few in whom these "tramlines" have been visible there has been evidence suggesting that peribronchial fibrosis or chronic bronchitis may play a part in production of these shadows. It is clear, however, that their exact nature and significance are not yet fully understood.

The heart is usually normal in size, although it may appear smaller than normal in relation to the overall size of the thorax.

Bronchography is seldom productive of much useful information in the investigation of a patient with spasmodic asthma. If it is done during a symptom-free period the bronchial tree will generally be perfectly normal in appearance. If the patient has bronchospasm before the procedure is performed, or if instillation of local anesthetic or opaque medium induces an attack of bronchospasm, the bronchial tree from the lobar bronchi distally will have a narrower caliber than normal. Filling of the more peripheral radicles, therefore, is often difficult to accomplish. Splaying of bronchial subdivisions and increased angles of bifurcation due to hyperinflation follow the same pattern as that observed in the vascular bed. The occasional demonstration of dilated mucous glands in the walls of the central bronchi may supply useful evidence for the presence of associated chronic bronchitis. Although Overholt has reported the presence of bronchiectasis as a "trigger mechanism" in some cases of asthma,[931] our experience has shown that, unless there are suggestive changes on plain films of the chest, the discovery rate of bronchiectasis is extremely low, and it is considered that bronchography seldom is indicated for this purpose alone.

Dynamic studies of bronchial caliber by means of cinebronchography when the patient is symptom-free reveal that the bronchial tree behaves normally.[755] Although the maximal inspiratory caliber may be slightly less than normal, particularly in the peripheral segmental bronchi, the reduction in caliber on forced expiration is roughly proportional throughout the length of the visible bronchial tree, and amounts to about 40 per cent of the inspiratory diameter. There is no tendency for the central bronchi to undergo a disproportionate collapse on forced expiration, a change frequently observed in patients with chronic bronchitis and emphysema.

Certain conditions occur with sufficient fre-

(Text continues on p. 116.)

Case 1
Tropical Eosinophilia

Summary of Clinical Findings. This 23-year-old housewife came to Canada from India two years prior to admission in June, 1965. She had been well until two months before admission when she developed a cough, at first paroxysmal and nocturnal, later persistent. In the week before admission she noticed shortness of breath and wheezing associated with the cough, again mainly at night. The cough had become productive of small amounts of white sputum and was associated with central chest discomfort. She described intermittent chills during the same period but denied fever. She was a strict vegetarian.

On examination she appeared well except for a slight expiratory wheeze. Her blood pressure was 118/78; pulse rate was 88; respiration rate was 24; temperature was 98.2°. The positive findings were limited to her chest. She made use of the accessory muscles of respiration and expiration was prolonged. High-pitched expiratory rhonchi were heard throughout and fine end-inspiratory rales at both bases. The heart was normal; the liver and spleen were not palpable.

Urinalysis was normal. Hemoglobin was 13.3 gm per 100 ml; sedimentation rate was 38 mm/hr; white blood count was 24,800; eosinophils totaled 16,300. The eosinophils remained elevated on repeated counts but by the time the patient was discharged it had fallen to 5100, 50 per cent of the total WBC. Creatinine, BUN, and liver function studies were normal. The gamma globulin was markedly increased at 2.71. Parasites were not found in multiple sputum and stool specimens. Examination of sputum for eosinophils was negative. LE preparation was negative. The report for x-rays and pulmonary function studies follow.

The patient was given a six-day course of diethylcarbamazine (Hetrazan). Following this treatment she noted marked improvement, and, on discharge, 10 days after admission, she was asymptomatic and her chest was clear.

Radiology. A postero-anterior roentgenogram (*A*) reveals diffuse involvement of both lungs by small nodular shadows ranging from 2 to 5 mm in diameter. The lower zones are involved to a greater extent than are the upper. In the bases particularly, there is an accentuation of linear markings. A magnified view of the lower portion of the right lung (*B*) reveals the pattern to better advantage. A roentgenogram of the chest 10 days later (not shown) was normal.

Summary. This patient with the characteristic history and manifestations of tropical eosinophilia, showed a marked reduction in all subdivisions of lung volume and a low diffusing capacity.

														EXERCISE				
	VC	FRC	RV	TLC	ME %	MMFR	$FEV_{0.75}$ ×40	pH+	Pco_2	HCO_3^-	Po_2	O_2Hb %	$D_{Lco}SS_2$	CO Ext %	GRADE	$\dot{V}O_2$	$\dot{V}_e$	$D_{Lco}SS_3$
Predicted	3.3	2.4	1.2	4.5	70	3.8	95						21.5	56				
June 10, 1965	1.4	1.0	0.7	2.1	30	0.9	31						7.8	30				
June 17, 1965	1.4	1.0	0.5	1.9	36	1.7	43						9.4	35				

On June 10, 1965, this patient showed severe reduction in all subdivisions of lung volume, marked impairment of flow, and a low diffusing capacity. One week later, after a course of Hetrazan, there had been no significant change in lung volume but a definite improvement in flow was found, and the diffusing capacity had increased slightly.

Tropical Eosinophilia

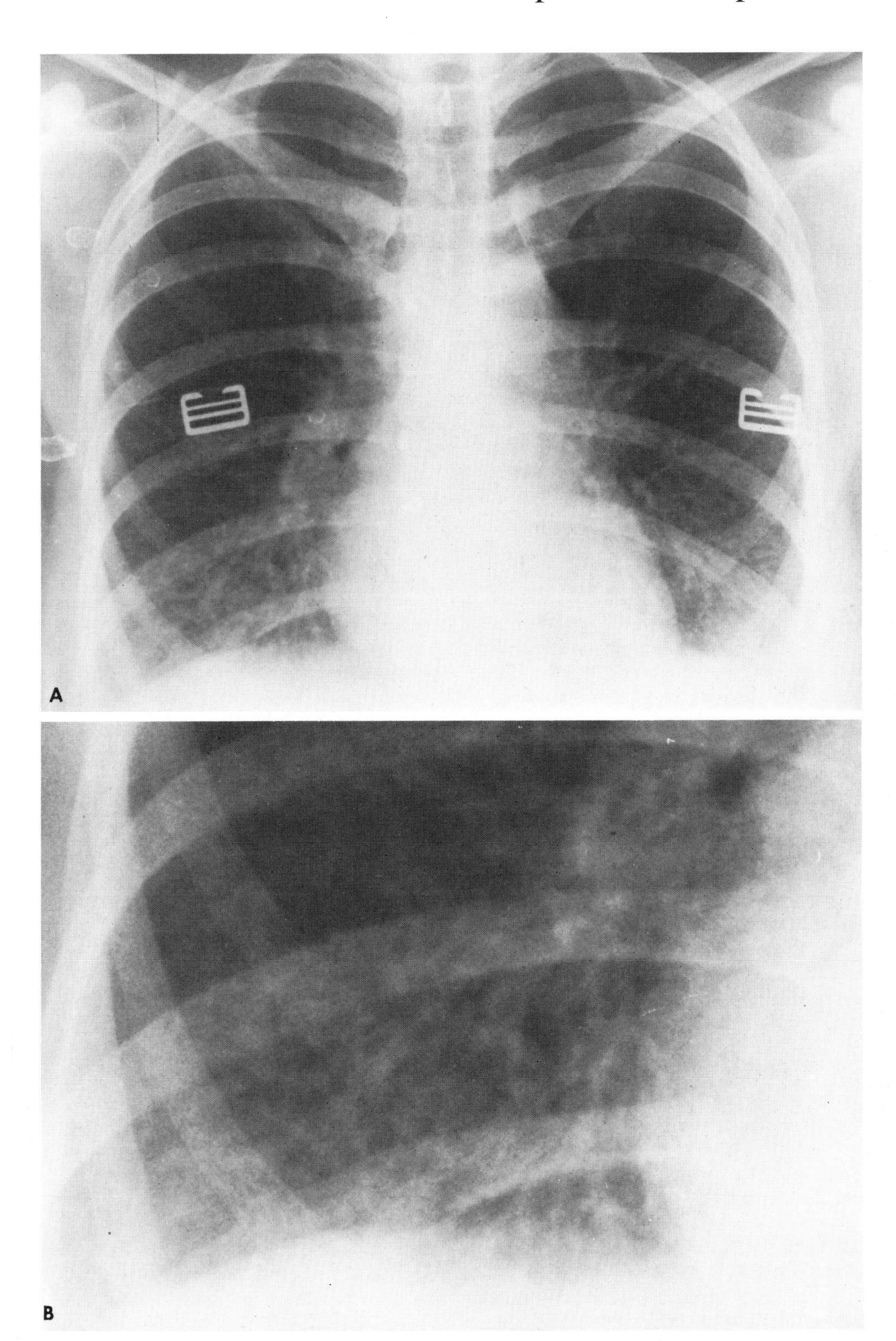

quency in association with spasmodic asthma to be worthy of special note. Atelectasis of varying degrees of severity may result from the plugging of bronchi with thick tenacious mucus, a complication particularly likely to occur in patients in the younger age groups and to involve any portion of the bronchial tree, from a main-stem bronchus to the more peripheral segmental bronchi. Felson and Felson have described a condition peculiar to asthmatics, in which diffuse bilateral parenchymal infiltrations possessing a peribronchial distribution have been associated with signs and symptoms of acute respiratory infection.[932] In one of their patients who came to autopsy, acute bronchiolitis and peribronchitis were associated with patchy areas of atelectasis and bronchopneumonia. This extensive infectious disease, designated by the Felsons as "acute diffuse pneumonia of the asthmatic," has been observed by us in several cases, and is probably related to peripheral bronchiolar obstruction and infection.

The lowered arterial oxygen tensions that have recently been documented to occur commonly in asthmatic attacks of moderate severity (*vide infra*) indicate that peripheral zones of the lung, probably ventilated mainly by collateral drift, must commonly occur, though visible areas of atelectasis on the plain film are only seen in very severe clinical situations as noted by Felson and Felson.

Loeffler's syndrome, which bears a close relationship to spasmodic asthma, is characterized by transient focal pulmonary infiltrations (*see* Chapter 14).

CLINICAL FEATURES

Spasmodic asthma makes its first appearance predominantly in childhood or adolescence; it runs in families, including members who have hay fever, infantile eczema, or urticaria, or who give a history of these conditions or of asthma itself. It may be present for many years in mild form, with occasional exacerbations, and characteristically does not lead to permanent impairment of pulmonary function or parenchymal change. Patients with spasmodic asthma show more bronchial constriction than normal in response to inhalation of inert dust or smoke and are very sensitive to inhaled aerosols of histamine or acetylcholine. During an acute episode they are dyspneic at rest, and often orthopneic; loud rales and rhonchi are often audible in the chest. The number of eosinophils in the blood is usually increased, and these cells are very common in the mucoid sputum produced in the acute stages. Many patients with asthma show abnormal skin reactions following the intracutaneous injection of suitably prepared extracts of commonly encountered airborne allergens and of some common foods. It is not clear what the relationship is between such skin sensitivity and the sensitivity or otherwise of the bronchial tree to these or other substances.[757] Between attacks, or when on suitable treatment, the patient may be symptom-free for long periods. Many asthmatic persons are somewhat unstable, and it is admitted that the course of the disease may be affected by emotional or environmental factors. It is also true that spontaneous improvement and remission are common, often occurring independently of any change in treatment regimen or other factors, although the physician often gets the credit.

In no other common disorder have so many different therapeutic approaches been adopted, and it is suspicious that many of these are credited with improving the condition in these patients. The following excerpt, taken in its entirety from an abstracting journal, demonstrates one approach to the problem:

"The fundamental concepts of existentialism are reviewed. This is followed by the description of a test, based on questions and the symbolic representation by the subject tested of his status in the present, past and future, the near space, the distant space and a number of existential relationships. This test was also used in studying the existence of patients with asthma, defined as a form of life limited in space and time, in which the patient, in an unreal atmosphere of excessive power, spasmodically realizes his dominion over creatures and things. Four illustrations and 18 references are given."

It may be important perhaps to remind the physiologist as well as the physician that therapeutic approaches to the asthmatic, usually defined rather more realistically than in the foregoing excerpt, have included the following, apart from the use of known bronchodilators, steroids, and desensitization procedures: extirpation of the carotid ganglion;[716] pulmonary denervation with[718] or without[717, 726] resection of lung segments; radiotherapy to the brain;[719] removal to high altitude;[720] inhalations of an aerosol of staphylococcus bacteriophage lysate;[721] and hypnosis,[722, 723] which certainly seems to be successful on occasion. Reports on the use of all of these methods have appeared within the past few years. A more detailed scrutiny of the literature would undoubtedly reveal that many other procedures have apparently been successful in the treatment of asthma.

The spontaneous improvement and worsening of the asthmatic state make any carefully controlled trial very laborious and time-consuming. Since many reports give no indication whether the patients studied may or may not have been suffering from emphysema, the presence of which would be certain to diminish the potential response to any treatment, the results become very difficult to assess. The carefully conducted trial by Gandevia and his colleagues is of particular interest, since they found that, although phenobarbitone had no bronchodilator effect, when contrasted with other compounds it was preferred by most of the patients as the compound that had helped them more than any of the others used in this trial.[724]

One of the remarkable clinical features of bronchial asthma is the tremendous variation in severity that may be observed. In an individual patient with a characteristic family history and demonstrated skin sensitivity, the only evidence of bronchospasm may be a slightly diminished FEV and some wheezing on exposure to cold air; in another, severe ventilatory defect may be almost unremitting despite the use of bronchodilators of every kind and long-term steroid maintenance. It is this variability that necessitates a very complete documentation of the patient by the use of function tests when any therapeutic procedure is being studied.

Within the past few years, there has been increasing concern at the increase in mortality from asthma reported in Australia[2617, 2618, 2619] and in Britain,[2615, 2620] but this is probably occurring elsewhere as well. As Gandevia has pointed out, the increase in mortality seems to have been especially marked in the age groups between 5 and 34,[2617] in which cases diagnostic error is unlikely. This phenomenon is not yet explained, but it indicates the need for special attention to be directed to the treatment of status asthmaticus (*see* later discussion).

It is important to note that bronchospasm occurs in relation to some occupations, such as baking,[725] working with cotton (*see* byssinosis, Chapter 17), handling grain, and even in workers with aluminum,[728] or with aluminum soldering flux.[2571] These syndromes illustrate the importance of a careful occupational history in any patient who presents to the physician with unexplained dyspnea, and in whom there is evidence of airway obstruction.

INTERRELATIONSHIP BETWEEN PHYSIOLOGY OF THE BRONCHIAL TREE AND ASTHMA

So much work has been accomplished on the physiology of the bronchial tree, and clinical asthma is such a common disorder, that one might suppose it would be possible to describe the sequence of events in the asthmatic in rather precise terms. This is not true, however. In this section, some of the recent data that have been collected will be reviewed and placed in juxtaposition, but few firm conclusions can be drawn yet with any confidence.

PHYSIOLOGICAL STUDIES

The bronchial tree of the normal adult is highly reactive and exists in a state of maintained tone. It is supplied with a liberal distribution of vagal and sympathetic efferent nerves with many ganglion cells, from which parasympathetic postganglionic fibers are believed to arise. Afferent end organs consist of many subepithelial receptors placed immediately underneath the ciliary layer of the major bronchi, and they are thought to be responsible for the cough reflex. Smooth-muscle endings believed to be responsible for the Hering-Breuer inflation reflex, which is strong in some mammals but very weak in the human,[730] lie in most of the major bronchi.[3829] In addition, some receptors have been described that lie in only the largest bronchi and seem to be confined to the hilar regions. These are particularly noted by some authors as the origins of unusually large nerve fibers.

It is not surprising that the bronchial tree reacts to many stimuli, and that some of the experimental results obtained have been dedetermined in large part by the nature of the preparation used.[3829]

Several reviews of the reactivity of the bronchial tree have appeared,[714, 2563] and some

(Continues on p. 120.)

Case 2
Bronchiolitis; Chronic Inflammatory Disease of Small Airways

Summary of Clinical Findings. This 53-year-old housewife began to suffer from "hay fever" about 25 years prior to admission. This consisted of summer episodes of rhinorrhea and red and itching eyes. Four years later she developed episodes of shortness of breath and wheezing. These attacks became more frequent and were triggered by cold weather, dust, and respiratory infections. During the previous eight years shortness of breath and wheezing had become more constant and her condition had been deteriorating. During the past two years she had been unable to climb stairs and had to walk slowly on the level. She had developed a cough productive of moderate amounts of thick yellow sputum and had frequent upper respiratory infections. She had received bronchodilators, antibiotics, and intermittent steroids, but had not taken the latter during the 1½ years prior to admission. She had never smoked. She was found to be allergic to dust, feathers, and tobacco. Her father, a brother and a sister, and one son suffered from asthma. She was admitted in May, 1968, because of a change in her chest x-ray.

On admission she was noted to be in moderate respiratory distress but not cyanosed. Her temperature was 99°; pulse rate was 140; respiration rate was 28; blood pressure was 140/90. The chest was not enlarged, expiration was prolonged, and there were scattered inspiratory and expiratory rhonchi. Fine rales were noted at both bases. There were no other significant findings. The hemogram was normal. There was no eosinophilia. Urinalysis and biochemical studies were normal. The electrocardiogram showed a right-axis deviation. Descriptions of x-rays and pulmonary function follow. An open-lung biopsy was performed on June 5. She was subsequently treated with bronchodilators, steroids, and antibiotics, and on discharge the patient had markedly improved. Her cough had disappeared, there was no wheezing, and she could climb stairs without difficulty. She has been on prednisone since discharge and has been well except for one mild exacerbation of symptoms associated with an upper respiratory infection. She is able to do her housework and claims normal activity for a woman of her age.

Pathology. There is extensive, severe inflammation of the small airways, with some dilatation and slight mucous plugging (*D*), and unfolding of the mucous membrane (*E*). Focal nodular, nonspecific, subacute pneumonitis is present. There is obvious pulmonary arterial thickening. An old, small fibrotic lesion is also present which may represent an old infarct or healed pneumonitis.

Radiology. A postero-anterior roentgenogram (*A*) in May, 1968, shows a diffuse, coarse reticular pattern, evenly distributed. There is little overinflation and no hilar lymph-node enlargement. There is no evidence of pulmonary hypertension or cor pulmonale. A magnified tomographic section of the lower part of the right lung (*B*) shows tram lines representing bronchial-wall thickening, with or without peribronchial changes.

The roentgenogram in July, 1968, (*C*) shows complete clearing with the exception of the residuum of lung biopsy.

Summary. This patient with longstanding asthma of moderate severity developed the clinical picture, radiological appearances, and biopsy findings of severe bronchiolitis. There was anoxia but no CO_2 retention. The bronchiolitis resolved after treatment with antibiotics and steroids.

Case report continues on page 120

														EXERCISE				
	VC	FRC	RV	TLC	ME %	MMFR	$FEV_{0.75}$ ×40	pH^+	P_{CO_2}	HCO_3^-	P_{O_2}	O_2Hb %	$D_{Lco}SS_2$	CO Ext %	GRADE	$\dot{V}O_2$	$\dot{V}_E$	$D_{Lco}SS_3$
Predicted	2.9	2.5	1.6	4.5	53	2.36	72	7.40	40	25	80	96	11.6	43				
May, 1968	1.8	3.0	2.4	4.2	9	$\frac{0.33}{0.44}$	$\frac{25}{31}$	7.46	35	25	50	86	7.6	31				
Dec., 1968	2.5	2.3	1.6	4.1	41	0.97	58	7.44	38.5	26	61	94	9.8	33				

In May, 1968, this patient showed a low vital capacity and air trapping (increased FRC and RV), with a normal total lung capacity. Flow rates were severely reduced, improving only slightly with bronchodilators, and the diffusing capacity was low. She was severely hypoxemic. Seven months later lung volumes were normal. Flow rates had improved but were still moderately reduced, and the diffusing capacity was nearly within normal limits, although the fractional CO uptake was still reduced. The P_{O_2} had risen.

Bronchiolitis

		Predicted	Feb. 1968	Sept. 1968	April 1969
Resistance at FRC cm H_2O/l/sec		1–2	7.5	4.2	2.6
COMPLIANCE l/cm H_2O	STATIC	0.112	0.073	0.106	0.128
	DYNAMIC		.073(22) .050(38) .038(43)	.110(20) .095(26) .050(45)	.155(11) .138(21) .094(27) .065(36)

In February, 1968, the resistance was moderately increased and the compliance reduced and frequency-dependent. Although subsequent studies showed marked improvement, the compliance remained frequency-dependent. The respiratory frequency is shown in brackets after the dynamic compliance value. The static deflation pressure-volume curve was normal.

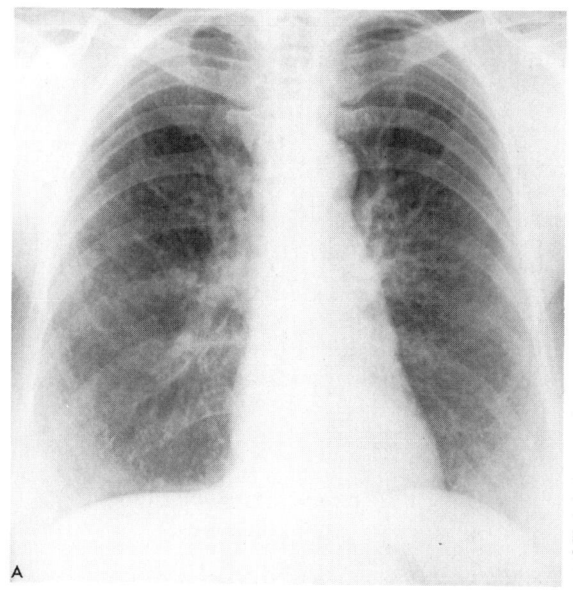
A

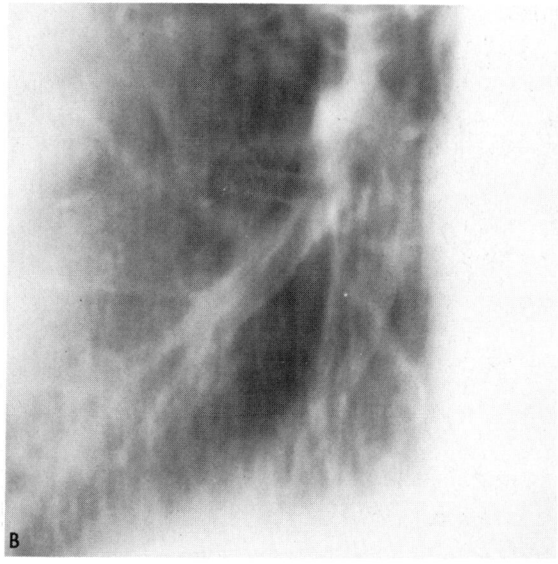
B

Bronchiolitis (Continued)

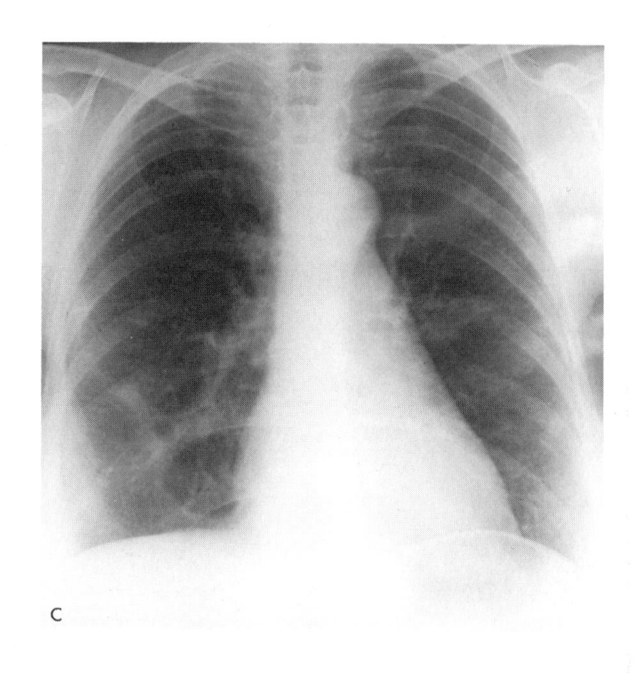

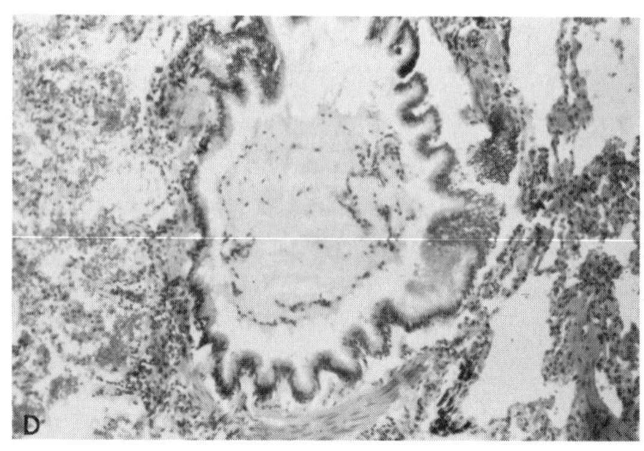

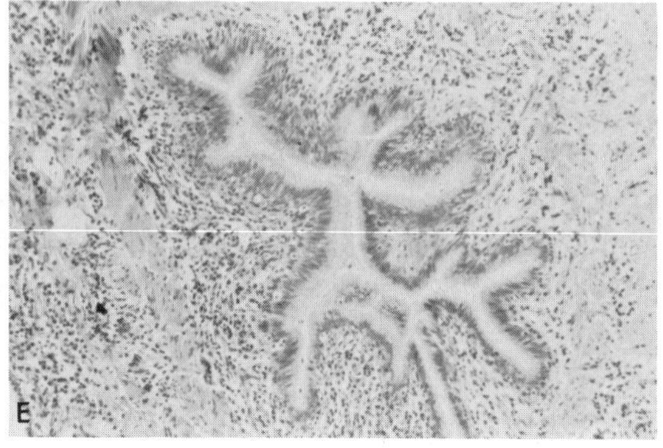

conclusions from the very large body of work that exists in this field can now be drawn with confidence:

1. Normal man responds to the inhalation of inert dust by a prompt increase in airway resistance.[482] Aerosols have a similar effect.[3677] Cigarette smoke increases airway resistance,[483] and Widdicombe, Kent, and Nadel[731] suggested that this response was dependent on the integrity of the cervical vagosympathetic nerves and was not a purely local irritative phenomenon. This conclusion is supported by recent work in man by Sterling,[2570] who has shown that the bronchoconstriction consequent upon inhaling cigarette smoke in both smokers and nonsmokers was blocked by a prior injection subcutaneously of atropine sulphate. Thus the vagus nerve is almost certainly involved in this mechanism. There is considerable individual variation in the magnitude of the effect both of dust and of smoke between different normal subjects.

2. Histamine inhaled as an aerosol narrows all airways from alveolar ducts to bronchioles 600 μ in diameter in the cat.[2563] It is clear that such an aerosol may act on large airways if particle size is large,[2258] or may produce alveolar duct constriction,[791] an effect that explains the decreased pulmonary compliance noted by some authors after its in-

halation. The effects of histamine infusion in normal subjects are complex,[2559] but there appears to be a fall in pulmonary vascular resistance concomitant with an increased cardiac output.

3. Sulphur dioxide stimulates cough receptors in the upper airway and also acts via efferents in the vagus to cause bronchoconstriction.[2569] Mechanisms of response to formaldehyde and ozone in the guinea pig seem essentially similar to the response to histamine.[2566] Cold air at $-20°$ C was found by Millar and his colleagues[2567] to have no effect on the FEV_1 of 5 normal subjects, but it produced a significant reduction in 4 of 10 patients who had asthma.

4. Vagal stimulation in dogs constricts either central or peripheral airways or both, the responses being different in different dogs. The reason for the variability among dogs is not known, but it may be related to differences in distribution of vagal fibers. In those dogs in which central airway constriction is the primary response to vagal stimulation, the increase in total pulmonary resistance was much greater than it was in those dogs in which the peripheral airways were the principal site of constriction. This is because the central airways contribute most to increase the pulmonary resistance. It is conceivable, therefore, that hyper-reactivity could be the result of a difference in site rather than in degree of bronchoconstriction.

5. Sympathetic nerve endings protect against constriction, and, in the dog at least, this effect is principally in airways smaller than 2 mm internal diameter. β-adrenergic blockade removes this protective mechanism and results in a much greater degree of bronchoconstriction and much greater increases in total pulmonary resistance. Thus, β-adrenergic blockade may cause bronchial hyper-reactivity.

Clinical observations

Some clinical observations are of particular interest in relation to this physiological information:

1. Most patients with spasmodic asthma have been found to be very sensitive to aerosol inhalations of acetylcholine or histamine, and Tiffeneau[732, 733] showed that for a given effect on the FEV, the asthmatic requires a minute fraction of these substances, as compared with the dose needed in a normal subject to produce equivalent airway obstruction.

2. It has become increasingly clear that bronchospasm and bronchial obstruction in many asthmatic patients is not at all uniformly distributed throughout the lung,[734, 735, 2572] and reductions in perfusion occur to those parts of the lung that are underventilated.[2572, 2580, 2581, 2583] Aminophylline and Adrenalin may relieve the airway obstruction, at least partially, but there may be a concomitant fall in arterial oxygen tension,[2560, 2561] probably indicating that a "release" has occurred in the previously reduced perfusion to poorly ventilated regions of the lung.

3. The effect of epinephrine (Adrenalin) is almost always additive to that of steroids[736] and other compounds,[737] so that a further improvement from epinephrine can be obtained in patients already receiving these drugs. Although steroids reduce the incidence of spontaneously occurring attacks of asthma, improvement in FEV may not be maintained. It has been suggested also that, in the asthmatic, the abnormal response to histamine or to challenge by an inhaled aerosol containing an allergen is not modified by steroid administration. Several authors have suggested that steroids act by reducing edema in bronchiolar walls and thus increasing the initial lumen of the airway, and that they do not directly influence the response of the tracheobronchial tree to challenge.

It will be apparent that the interrelationship between clinical asthma and known mechanisms that affect tracheobronchial reactivity is very far from being obvious or settled. The chronic unrelievable asthmatic state cannot be duplicated in animal experiments, which therefore have been concerned mainly with acute anaphylaxis or with the response of the normal bronchial tree to different stimuli; all of these are of interest but may have little relevance to the derangement of the lung in chronic asthma. In status asthmaticus, the main danger to the patient arises through plugging of bronchi and bronchioles with thick, gelatinous mucus. Very little is known of the factors that control secretion of this material. Normal mucus increases greatly in viscosity as it loses water, but whether the increased viscosity found in status asthmaticus is the consequence of stagnation, or how it arises, is quite uncertain.

PULMONARY FUNCTION IN SPASMODIC ASTHMA

Patients with spasmodic asthma are seen in one of the following five stages: complete remission, partial remission, moderate bronchospasm, severe bronchospasm, and status asthmaticus. These five subdivisions will be referred to in the following paragraphs.

Complete Remission

There is no doubt that complete remission may occur in patients with asthma, and all tests of pulmonary function, including measurements of pulmonary mechanics and of regional ventilation distribution, may be completely normal. However, the bronchial tree remains abnormally reactive in these patients and will respond to dust, cold air, or histamine with a greater rise in pulmonary resistance than occurs in the normal nonasthmatic person.

Partial remission

Pulmonary function tests have shown that the patient with asthma may be completely asymptomatic, and be regarded by his physician as in complete remission, yet there are measurable defects in pulmonary function. There may be found in such patients ventilatory defect,[741, 745, 747] abnormal inert-gas distribution,[742, 748, 2572] frequency dependence of compliance,[3675] considerable regional variations in ventilation[735, 2572] and in perfusion in the lungs,[2572, 2580, 2581, 2583] and some degree of pulmonary overinflation as measured by the functional residual capacity. Such patients may show some degree of pulmonary hypertension on exercise,[384] but this is not likely to be marked at rest.[2591] Patients in partial remission may show a significant fall in FEV after exercise—a phenomenon discussed in detail later.

Moderate and severe bronchospasm

Ventilatory function

Since airway obstruction is the essential feature of an asthmatic attack, it is not surprising that measurements of ventilatory ability are sensitive indicators of the degree of abnormality present. It is probable that when moderate bronchospasm is present, there is a general diminution in caliber of major airways, and the maximal midexpiratory flow rate and FEV are sensitive indices of such a change

TABLE 5-1 Stages in Spasmodic Asthma

Stage	Clinical Observations	FEV	FRC and TLC	Gas Distrib.	Regional Distrib. $\dot{V}$	Regional Distrib. Q	Arterial Pa_{O_2}	Arterial Pa_{CO_2}
I	Complete remission	N	N	N	N	N	N	N
II	Partial remission (asymptomatic)	N or ↓	N or ↑	ABN	ABN	ABN	N or ↓	N
III	Moderate bronchospasm (rhonchi)	↓ or ↓↓	↑	ABN+	ABN+	ABN	↓	N
IV	Severe bronchospasm	↓↓	↑↑	ABN++	ABN++	ABN+	↓↓	N
V	Status asthmaticus							
	a. Initial	↓↓	↑↑	ABN++	ABN++	ABN++	↓↓	N
	b. Terminal	↓↓	↑↑	ABN++	ABN++	ABN++	↓↓	↑

Possible State of Lungs:

I : Normal, apart from increased bronchial reactivity.
II : Airway resistance of major bronchi increased: Dynamic compliance is frequency dependent. Small airway blockage?
III : II + beginning atelectasis: altered lung recoil.
IV : Obstruction in major bronchi and bronchioles + atelectasis. Beginning mucous plugs.
V : Extensive mucous plugs; atelectasis; fatigue, severe acidosis, and danger of cardiac arrest.

(*see* Chapter 2). The maximal breathing capacity,[740, 742, 1999] FEV_1,[733, 736, 739, 743–746, 1997, 2573, 2594] maximal midexpiratory flow rate,[384, 583, 735, 1988] and peak flow rate[79] have all been used in different series of studies. It is of interest that the maximal midexpiratory flow rate may be shown to be abnormal in an asthmatic patient when there is no evidence of abnormality of regional gas distribution.[2572] On occasion, the inhalation of a bronchodilator aerosol may produce a dramatic improvement in FEV_1 (*see* Figure 5–1).

Pulmonary mechanics

The expiratory difficulty in asthma is associated with an increase in flow resistance, and even in subjects in remission this value is often elevated.[753] In patients with a moderate degree of spasm (causing a reduction in FEV to 86 per cent of predicted values) flow resistance in one series[583] averaged 5.9 cm H_2O/liter/sec, i.e., an increase of two- to threefold above normal; whereas, with more severe reduction of FEV, to 57 per cent of predicted values, the average flow resistance in 9 subjects was 7.4 cm/liter/sec. Much higher values than this have been reported by other investigators. Thus, Campbell[751] found an average value of 16.1 cm H_2O/liter/sec in three asthmatics, and Wells[752] recorded air-flow resistances of 25.0 to 56.5 cm H_2O/liter/sec in patients studied during or immediately after an acute attack. The detailed studies on one subject reported by Petit and his colleagues,[478] in which air-flow resistance and FEV were measured before and after administration of acetylcholine and histamine aerosols, are of particular interest in illustrating the relationship between these parameters. They showed that an increase of air-flow resistance from about 2.5 to 3.5 cm H_2O/liter/sec was accompanied by a minimal decrease in FEV. When air-flow resistance reached about 4.0 cm H_2O/liter/sec, the FEV was reduced to about 70 per cent of the normal value, and when the air-flow resistance reached 6.0 cm H_2O/liter/sec after histamine inhalation, the

(Text continues on p. 126.)

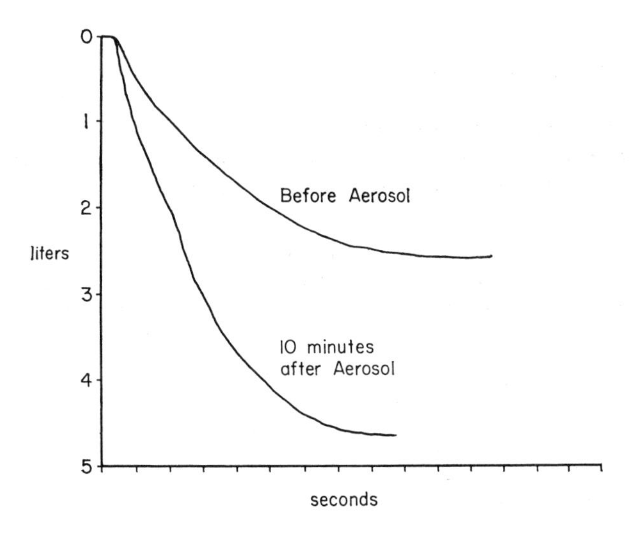

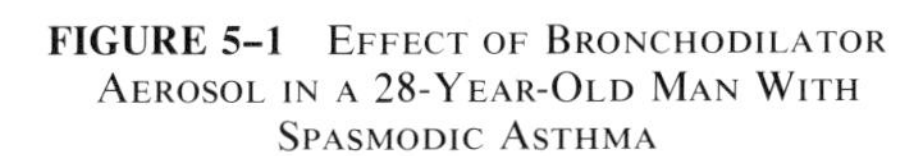

FIGURE 5–1 Effect of Bronchodilator Aerosol in a 28-Year-Old Man With Spasmodic Asthma

This patient was referred to the pulmonary function laboratory, and the first test performed was the FEV. The curve obtained is shown on the top graph. The subdivisions of lung volume, mixing efficiency (ME %) and resting diffusing capacity ($D_{Lco}\,SS_2$) were then measured, after which he was given several breaths of a bronchodilating aerosol. Five minutes after this the FEV curve was retested. Only one of the FEV curves is shown for the initial and post-aerosol studies, although four were recorded on each occasion. Note the absence of overinflation and the slightly, but not grossly lowered diffusing capacity and fractional CO uptake $\left(\frac{F_I - F_{EX}}{F_I}\right)$.

	BEFORE AEROSOL	AFTER AEROSOL	PREDICTED	
EXP. VOL.	2·50	4·68	4·90	liters
$FEV_{.75}\times 40$	42	104	140	liters/min
MMFR	0·74	2·00	4·30	liters/sec

Results of other tests before aerosol, with predicted values in brackets:–

ME %	: 35	(65)	%
FRC	: 3·4	(3·6)	liters
TLC	: 6·0	(6·4)	"
$D_{L_{CO}}\,SS_2$	: 16·6	(23·0)	ml CO/min/mm Hg
$\frac{F_I - F_{EX}}{F_I}$	: 39	(51)	%

Case 3
Spasmodic Asthma

Summary of Clinical Findings. This young man was first seen in 1952 at the age of 19. He complained of periodic attacks of dyspnea and marked wheeziness occurring predominantly in spring and summer, from the age of six years until two years before admission, when dyspnea became more constant and was associated with cough and slight mucoid expectoration. He had had eczema since infancy and hay fever from the age of 7.

On examination at that time there was a marked increase in the AP diameter of his chest, which was hyperresonant and on auscultation revealed diffuse sibilant rhonchi. Skin tests showed positive reactions to several inhalants and foods. On two occasions the differential white-cell count revealed eosinophilia of 8 per cent and 12 per cent.

Because of the persistent dyspnea and failure of conventional treatment, in 1953 he was placed on cortisone therapy. Before this was started, function tests showed the VC to be 2 liters, the FRC 5.7 liters, RV 5 liters and MBC 28 liters/min. The response to cortisone was excellent and 5 weeks later, on 200 mg of cortisone daily, his VC was found to be 5.5 liters, FRC 3.6 liters, RV 1.7 liters and MBC 101 liters per minute. When last seen, in 1963, this patient had been on corticosteroids for 10 years. Episodes of acute dyspnea occurred from time to time, usually in association with lowering of maintenance dose. On such occasions the ventilatory function became markedly impaired, but the diffusing capacity always remained within the predicted normal range. The table below illustrates the changes in pulmonary function during an acute asthmatic episode in 1957.

Radiology. *A* and *B*, Postero-anterior and lateral views of the chest in full inspiration show a very large thoracic volume possessing all of the usual signs of severe and symmetrical hyperinflation of both lungs. Fluoroscopic examination revealed limited diaphragmatic excursion bilaterally. This appearance of severe hyperinflation could be produced by either spasmodic asthma during an attack of bronchospasm or by diffuse emphysema, although the state of the pulmonary vasculature would favor the former.

C, A logEtronic reproduction of a midsagittal tomogram of the right lung of this patient (left) compared to a similar section of a normal control (right) reveals no significant difference in the number or caliber of the pulmonary vessels in the two subjects. This normal peripheral vasculature indicates that parenchymal lung destruction is unlikely to be present.

Summary. A case of spasmodic asthma showing severe ventilatory defect and tremendous overinflation of the lung at the time of moderately severe bronchospasm. The normal appearance of the lung vessels on tomography and the normal diffusing capacity may be taken as evidence against the presence of morphological emphysema—a conclusion supported by the finding, after a previous episode, of a maximal breathing capacity of 101 liters per minute.

	VC	FRC	RV	TLC	ME %	MMFR	$FEV_{0.75}$ ×40	pH	P_{CO_2}	HCO_3	O_2Hb %	$D_{Lco}SS_2$	COExt%
Predicted	5.9	4.2	2.0	7.9	70	4.9	163					25.9	53
May, 1957	3.4	5.4	4.7	8.0	24	0.2	13					26.1	52

Bronchial obstruction with air-trapping is shown by the greatly reduced air-flow rates and increased functional residual capacity and residual volume. The vital capacity is reduced, gas distribution poor, and the steady-state diffusing capacity normal.

Spasmodic Asthma

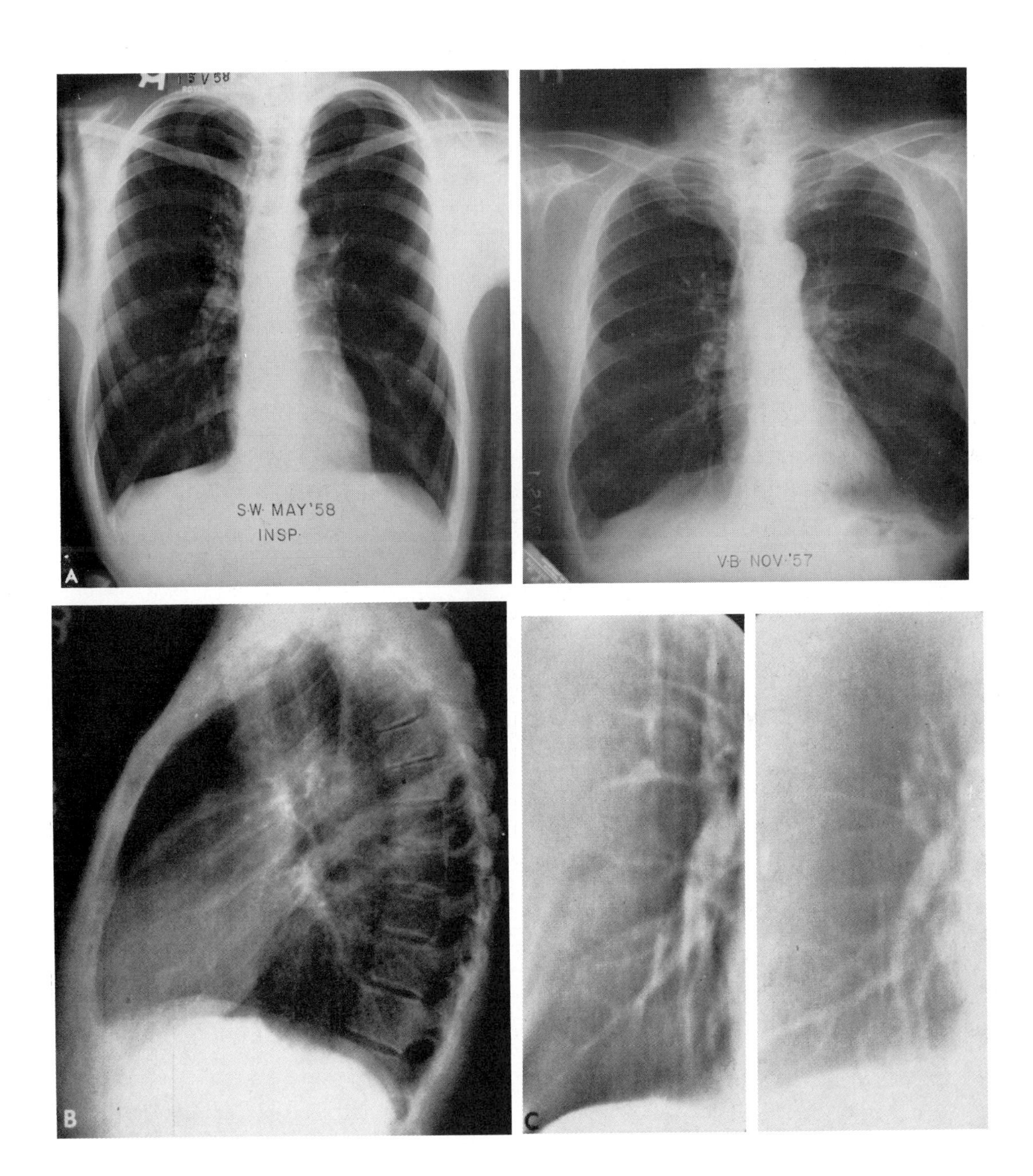

FEV was about half its previous value. These findings accord well with those reported by us in asthmatics studied without aerosol provocation.[583] Several other studies of air-flow resistance in asthma have been reported; Jaeger[477] showed that the interrupter method of measuring alveolar pressure was probably unreliable, a conclusion in conflict with some earlier work[473] but now generally accepted.

Graham and his colleagues[2584] have measured the constancy of change of airway conductance in a group of normal and asthmatic subjects in response to a constant dose of a bronchoconstrictor drug (carbamylcholine). They found little difference in variability of response between the two groups, and hourly measurements of airway conductance in both groups showed less variation than over the longer-term study. In asthmatic subjects, the FEV correlates better with the measured lung compliance than with the airway resistance, whereas in patients with emphysema the correlation between airway resistance and FEV_1 is very close.[2587] Consequent to the increase in flow resistance, the work of breathing is inevitably increased in asthma, often being five to ten times greater than normal.[754]

There has been much discussion as to the site of air-flow obstruction in patients with bronchial asthma. When spasm is not severe, it is not possible to demonstrate any major airway narrowing by bronchography,[755] though there is no doubt that the caliber of major bronchi is reduced during an attack.[758] Campbell, Martin, and Riley[756] concluded that it was predominantly the larger airways that were the site of major obstruction in asthma, and there has been recent confirmation of this from the work of Gayrard.[2588] With more prolonged and more severe spasm, it must be assumed that many bronchioles are obstructed.

In one series of patients with asthma which we studied,[583] the maximal negative static intrathoracic pressure was found to range from 21 to 26 cm H_2O, and similar values have been reported in other series.[752, 2590] The dynamic compliance is usually found to be reduced in patients with asthma,[754, 2575, 2589] a finding presumed to reflect the presence of uneven time constants in the lung[147] and consistent with the demonstrated regional nonuniformity of gas distribution documented to occur in asthma even in remission. Acute bronchoconstriction in animals is also accompanied by a fall in dynamic compliance.[2000] The administration of a bronchodilator to an asthmatic is often accompanied by an increase in dynamic compliance.[2589]

The observation by Woolcock and Read of the state of lung inflation in patients with asthma (*see* later discussion) prompted Gold, Kaufman, and Nadel to restudy the elastic recoil of the lungs in patients with chronic asthma in more detail than previously had been attempted.[2585] They showed that the lung elastic recoil was decreased at the time that there was a considerable degree of overinflation. Relief of the bronchospasm was followed by an increase in lung elastic recoil toward more normal values. They point out that the decrease in recoil can account for the persistent hyperinflation found by Woolcock and Read even after the FEV_1 had improved greatly. They also found that the altered recoil could not be duplicated by inducing bronchoconstriction in either healthy subjects or treated asthmatic patients. These important observations taken together with the measurements of severe hyperinflation reported by Woolcock and Read indicate that there may very well be more complexity to the problem of the measured lung compliance in asthma than has hitherto been supposed. Finucane and Colebatch[2381] have recently produced additional evidence that the elastic recoil is reversibly altered in patients with asthma. There is, as yet, no indication of the manner or mechanisms whereby the lung recoil can be abruptly changed in this disease.

Subdivisions of lung volume

The vital capacity is usually reduced in patients with asthma, but it may be relatively normal in patients with moderate hyperinflation and diminution in maximal midexpiratory flow rate or FEV_1.[2577] The vital capacity has been used to follow changes in patients with asthma,[747] but it is much less sensitive for this purpose than dynamic ventilatory tests. In most of the papers reporting studies on patients with asthma, elevation of FRC was noted in some of the subjects.[154, 370, 583, 710, 735, 740, 742, 748] Sonne and Georg reported that the FRC became more elevated in asthmatic patients after the administration of histamine.[749] However, in 1965, Woolcock and Read[2573] reported much larger increases in FRC and even in TLC than had hitherto been observed, using a helium closed-circuit apparatus. In a subsequent paper[2577] these observations were extended. They documented the fact that treatment might lead to considerable symptomatic relief, accompanied by a fall in FRC and reduction in the work of breathing before much change has occurred in the FEV_1. The total lung capacity was often increased above the normal value for the patient by more than a liter. In one patient, gross changes in lung volumes were demonstrated in an acute episode of asthma with recovery in less than an hour. Similar observations, though of somewhat smaller magnitude, have been reported by others,[2585, 2592] and similar major increases in TLC and FRC have been noted when these volumes were measured by body plethysmography rather than by gas dilution.[2586] These striking findings were probably not previously found because the limitations of gas dilution methods were not appreciated and because patients with only a mild degree of bronchospasm were studied as representative patients with asthma.

There is little direct information on the relationship between increased airway resistance and hyperinflation in asthmatics. Petit, Melon, and Milic-Emili conducted a series of carefully controlled studies in patients with asthma, and concluded that airflow resistance may be doubled without the occurrence of any significant change in FRC.[478]

Uniformity of ventilation

Nonuniformity of gas distribution has been demonstrated to be commonly present in patients with asthma. The single-breath technique,[742, 1789] open-circuit clearance methods,[154, 740, 750] and closed-circuit equilibration techniques[735, 748] have all been employed. More recently, using radioactive gases, it has been possible to demonstrate considerable regional variation in gas distribution and to follow the shifting of these zones of impaired ventilation over a period of time.[735, 2572] That the lung contains "autonomous" units was demonstrated by Arborelius and his colleagues[734] who showed that bronchospasm could be induced within one lung when an allergen was administered through a bronchospirometric catheter.

Uniformity of blood flow

There seems little doubt that the asthmatic lung retains the capability of reducing perfusion to zones that are poorly ventilated. Regional abnormalities of perfusion have been demonstrated with ^{133}xenon and by use of injected MAAI aggregates.[2580, 2581, 2583] Repeat studies in the same patient have shown that these zones of reduced perfusion may disappear with treatment, but in some patients may also be demonstrable during apparent remission.

Pulmonary diffusing capacity

It has proved very difficult to establish reliable conclusions concerning the changes that may be observed in the measured pulmonary diffusing capacity in patients with asthma,[759] because of four main factors: (1) difficulty in selection of patients and their differentiation from those with emphysema and bronchospasm, (2) variability in degree of bronchial obstruction present in patients studied by different observers, (3) differences in methods used to measure the diffusing capacity and technical differences between similar basic methods, and (4) uncertainty as to how relevant results obtained after histamine inhalation may or may not be to studies in patients with asthma.

1. There can be no doubt but that the steady-state diffusing capacity, whether an end-tidal sample ($D_{L_{CO}}SS_2$) or the arterial P_{CO_2} ($D_{L_{CO}}SS_1$) is used, may be normal or very nearly so in asthma, although there may be demonstrable impairment of gas distribution and moderate impairment of ventilation. Using end-tidal samples, we have demonstrated this in four studies reported separately on different groups of asthmatics.[370, 583, 710, 735] Using a somewhat different method of end-tidal sampling, Lorriman[760] found lower values (11.7 ml CO/min/mm Hg), which rose to 12.3 ml in association with an increase in the FEV × 40 from 34 liters/min to about 49 liters/min after isoprenaline. Using arterial sampling to determine the $P_{A_{CO}}$ in 15 asthma patients with an average MMFR of only 0.86 liters/sec, Williams and Zohman reported resting values of 13.9, increasing to 18.7 ml CO/min/mm Hg on exercise.[384] Using the same method in resting subjects ($D_{L_{CO}}SS_1$) Kreukniet and Visser have reported normal or higher than normal values in asthmatics.[1818]

2. Using the single-breath modified Krogh technique ($D_{L_{CO}}SB$), Kanagami and his colleagues reported an average value of 33 ml CO/min/mm Hg in five asthmatics with an average MBC of 71 per cent of the amount predicted.[761] Burrows and his co-workers reported generally similar values,[429] and, more recently, Meisner and Hugh-Jones have docu-

Case 4
Spasmodic Asthma and Status Asthmaticus

Summary of Clinical Findings. This 6-year-old girl had been having frequent attacks of asthma since the age of six months, usually preceded by a respiratory infection. There was a strong family history of allergy. Allergy skin tests were positive for various inhalants. She had been on bronchodilators and steroids, on occasion, for acute attacks. She had been previously admitted to The Montreal Children's Hospital in June, 1968, for an acute attack of asthma at which time she developed only mild respiratory acidosis. She was treated then with intravenous steroids and isoproterenol by inhalation. She recovered and was discharged after a five-day hospitalization.

She was readmitted on October 2, 1968, in severe respiratory distress, with marked supraclavicular, subcostal, and intercostal indrawing, marked prolongation of expiration, poor air entry, and rhonchi bilaterally. The chest x-ray (*A*) showed severe hyperinflation. She was pale but not cyanosed. Her progress in the hospital is summarized in the Table. After 10 hours of positive pressure controlled ventilation, and 16 hours of intravenous steroid and antibiotic therapy she was well enough to maintain normal alveolar ventilation. Her recovery was complete and she was discharged from the hospital on October 9, 1968, with a normal chest film (*B*).

She subsequently was admitted on four occasions for severe attacks of asthma. On two of these admissions she developed mild respiratory failure. None of these episodes was severe enough to require assisted or controlled ventilation.

DATE	TIME	Po_2	Pco_2	HCO_3	pH	CLINICAL STATE
October 2	4:45 p.m.		51	19.0	7.25	Admitted: respirations 64 per minute, pulse 170 per minute, pale, marked indrawing. Rhonchi.++
	5:45 p.m.		77	20.0	7.18	
	7:15 p.m.		99	22.8	7.14	
	7:45 p.m.	108	102	22.8	7.13	Assisted ventilation (bag and mask). Drowsy. Oxygen administered.
	9:45 p.m.		99	22.5	7.13	
	11:15 p.m.	266	194	20.6	6.97	Intubated under sedation with Nembutal, controlled ventilation, positive-pressure (Bird) started under general muscle relaxation with Laudolissin – Some $NaHCO_3$ administered.
October 3	1:00 a.m.	225	62	25.7	7.32	
	2:50 a.m.		71	22.6	7.24	
	5:00 a.m.		48	25.6	7.38	
	9:30 a.m.		45	26.5	7.41	Bird respirator assistance stopped. Child awake.
	12:00 p.m.		45	28.0	7.43	
	4:05 p.m.		44	26.5	7.42	Extubated.
	10:40 p.m.		38	26.5	7.46	
October 4	1:50 p.m.		33	24.3	7.46	Ventilating spontaneously, indrawing markedly decreased. Improving.
October 9						Discharged.

The blood gas values illustrate the extreme severity of the ventilatory failure which developed in this girl, even though it was possible to maintain adequate oxygenation with the administration of increased oxygen in the inspired air. Assisted manual ventilation without intubation was unsuccessful in relieving this severe respiratory acidosis. Controlled ventilation with a positive pressure respirator (Bird respirator) after intubation was successful in reestablishing normal ventilation. This was discontinued after 10 hours and the patient ventilated well spontaneously from that moment onward.

Spasmodic Asthma and Status Asthmaticus

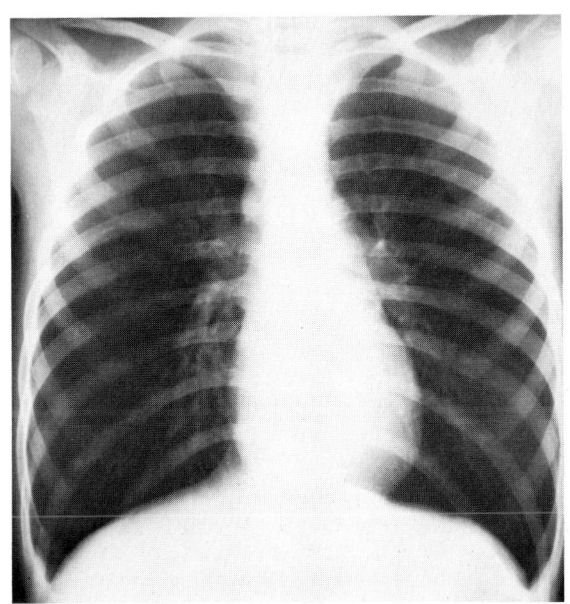

A: Chest x-ray during acute phase.

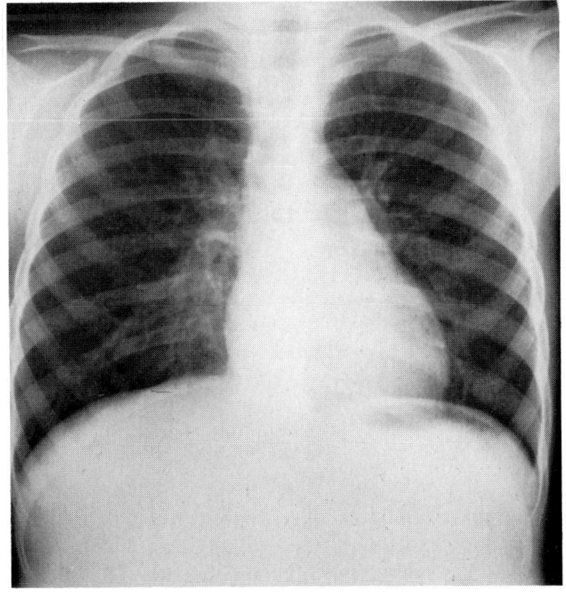

B: After recovery.

mented generally normal values of $D_{Lco}SB$ in spite of wide variations in the FEV_1.[2586] In a study of 72 patients with asthma, Palmer and Diament found mean values of 21.2, 18.5, and 16.2 ml CO/min/mm Hg in patients with mild, moderate, and severe bronchospasm respectively. The main value of this measurement in patients with asthma is that a normal value is of assistance in excluding severe emphysema in the presence of airway obstruction.

3. When very severe bronchospasm is present and there are many areas of atelectasis in the lung, the steady-state D_{Lco} may be low.[763] This stage is reached only rarely, however, and it is more common for the D_{Lco} and the fractional CO removal to remain normal in the presence of a lowered FEV_1.[384, 583, 748, 760, 1818]

4. Histamine inhalation appears to be generally accompanied by a fall in diffusing capacity, however this is measured.[762, 764] Bjure, Soderholm, and Widimsky have shown, however, that infusion of histamine causes an increase in diffusing capacity as a consequence of the increased cardiac output that results.

5. Stanescu and Teculescu have recently shown that acetylcholine aerosols administered to asthmatic subjects cause a lowering of both the single-breath diffusing capacity and of the "K"-permeability constant of the lung.[3678] These effects are presumably attributable to alterations in the distribution of D_L in the lung to the alveolar volume (V_A).

6. In an important study, Kreukniet and Visser have shown that the steady-state diffusing capacity may be erroneously high in bronchial asthma,[1818] though more usually the fractional CO uptake is normal.

Arterial blood-gas tensions

During the past four years, there has been an important advance in knowledge concerning the arterial blood-gas derangements that result from moderately severe bronchospasm in patients with asthma. Although instances of a lowered arterial oxygen saturation in asthma had been noted previously,[384, 740] no systematic study of the arterial oxygen tension had been undertaken. In the first edition of this text we noted, on page 145, "We are unaware of studies in any extensive series of patients with uncomplicated bronchial asthma in which the arterial oxygen has been measured; it seems very likely, however, that a lowered arterial oxygen tension, not sufficient to cause unsaturation, might commonly be encountered in these patients with only a moderate degree of ventilatory impairment." This remark has been fully justified by the many observations on the arterial oxygen tension in asthma that have been reported by different groups of workers since that time. It has now been fully established that a dangerous level of hypoxia may exist with no concomitant rise in arterial P_{CO_2}.[2592, 2593, 2594, 2595, 2596, 2598] Furthermore, both aminophylline[2560, 2568] and Adrenalin, either by injection[2561] or by aerosol as isoprenaline,[2562] may relieve the ventilatory obstruction, at least in part, without causing a rise in arterial oxygen tension; indeed, this may fall further. It has also been shown that oxygen may worsen the $\dot{V}/\dot{Q}$ distribution, as shown by an increase in (A–a) O_2 difference and an increase in physiological dead space in relation to tidal volume.[2565, 2574] The lowered arterial oxygen tension usually occurs without radiological evidence of atelectasis,[2576] and the appearance of the patient may give little warning as to the severity of the hypoxemia. In a major study of exceptional interest, Rees, Millar, and Donald have followed the clinical course and blood-gas tensions of a number of patients with severe bronchial asthma[2598] and have shown that a rise in arterial P_{CO_2} occurs late and may be a terminal event, following days or hours of hypoxemia unaccompanied by hypercapnia. Similar findings have been reported in asthmatic children; in one series, the arterial oxygen tensions varied between 42 mm Hg and 75 mm Hg on admission, and, in the same group of 21 children, the arterial P_{CO_2} ranged between 25 mm Hg and 62 mm Hg.

These studies have established the important facts that hypoxemia, often of dangerous degree, may be present in asthmatic patients; that it is not usually accompanied by severe hypercapnia except terminally; and that the clinician may be unaware of its degree and the rapidity with which it may deepen and become threatening to life. This considerable body of work, together with its important clinical implications, is an impressive attestation of the impact of the introduction of simple gas-tension measurements on clinical practice.

Pulmonary circulation

Williams and Zohman reported cardiac catheterization studies in seven asthmatic patients,[384] finding small elevations at rest but larger increases during exercise. Since asthma itself rarely gives rise to cor pulmonale, sustained pulmonary hypertension is unlikely to be a common occurrence in this condition. Helander and his colleagues have also found very small increases in pulmonary vascular resistance in a group of patients with asthma.[2579]

Status asthmaticus

In spite of traditional aphorisms to the contrary, status asthmaticus has always been a serious and life-threatening condition, and, in our experience, there are few other medical emergencies which can impose such a severe strain on the responsible physician as can a patient with severe status asthmaticus. Many of the papers documenting the hypoxemia of asthma, noted earlier, refer to cases of borderline status asthmaticus; it seems clear that the mortality from this condition has recently increased considerably,[2615–2620] although it has not yet proved possible to establish the reason for this. During the past four years, there have been many papers from a number of different centers on the treatment of status asthmaticus.[2606–2614] Many of these have stressed the crucial importance of repeated monitoring of the arterial blood in proper management,[3674] and the necessity of using muscle relaxants and full ventilation control has been stressed by many authors as the final step in management when more conservative measures have not been effective; by 1966, the Lancet, in an annotation, had given cautious approval of this therapy.

The sequence of events in status asthmaticus involves hypoxemia, fatigue and lactic acidosis, ventilatory failure and progressive hypercapnia, worsening hydrogen-ion accumulation, and sudden cardiac arrest. It seems clear from several detailed case reports[2598, 2608, 2611] that this sequence represents a common but not invariable cause of death in asthma. Other cases seem to suffer cardiac arrest before any significant degree of hypercapnia has developed, and in a number of cases the patients were conscious within half an hour or so of collapsing with cardiac arrest. The mechanism of death in these patients is far from obvious, though in some cases possibly cardiac arrhythmia due to an increased vagal sensitivity together with hours of untreated hypoxia may be responsible. In a recent report, sudden mucus plugging, following more chronic change, appeared to have been the cause of death.[3679]

Mithoefer, Porter, and Karetzky[2621] have found the infusion of sodium bicarbonate to be valuable in the treatment of intractable asthma, and it seems likely that the value of this therapy lies in breaking the vicious circle of acidosis that may develop in the course of deepening status asthmaticus.

In 1968, the Lancet[2620] noted that "... many unexpected deaths from asthma can be attributed, at least indirectly, to inadequate clinical and laboratory assessment." It is important for the physician to realize that the clinical appearance of the patient may actually appear to be improving at the time when hypercapnia is developing, and that the downhill course may be remarkably swift in status asthmaticus. In few other medical conditions are close observation and first-class laboratory facilities more essential to proper management than in this condition. (*See* Case 4, p. 128.)

EFFECTS OF EXERCISE ON AIRWAY RESISTANCE

In 1966, McNeill and his co-workers reported that exercise maintained for about 8 minutes in a number of patients with asthma resulted in a fall in FEV_1, a rise in airway resistance, and impairment of gas distribution.[2599] These effects were maximal 15 minutes after the end of the exercise, and recovery usually took place over the course of the next half hour. Adrenalin administered before the exercise prevented the phenomenon, and hyperventilation, with the patient at rest and breathing carbon dioxide, failed to elicit it. They postulated the release of some substance with a bronchoconstricting effect during the exercise. Since then a number of other studies of this interesting syndrome have appeared. It has become clear that in some asthmatic patients, ventilatory function may improve on exercise,[2601] and significant falls in FEV_1 were observed in only 3 of 23 patients studied by Itkin and Nacman,[2600] and in 14 of 101 patients reported on by Irnell and Swartling.[2601] Jones and Jones[2603] found a significant fall in FEV_1 in a number of symptom-free adults who had had an attack of asthma within the past four years; eleven such patients showed significant falls in FEV_1 after exercise, and isoprenaline administration prevented the phenomenon. One patient, studied by Rebuck and Read,[2605] had a past history of asthma and abnormal subdivisions of lung volume and pulmonary mechanics at rest. Exercise produced a fall of FEV_1 from 2.8 to 0.3 liters, and this fall could be reproduced at rest by voluntary hyperventilation and repeated forced expirations, and prevented by orciprenaline or CO_2 administration. A 40-year-old, somewhat obese asthmatic patient studied by Crompton[2604] was found to have a fall in FEV_1 similar to this case, but the phenomenon was not prevented by isoprenaline, was inhibited by atropine, and occurred also after CO_2-induced hyperventilation as well as after voluntary hyperventilation, and these changes in FEV_1 were also prevented by atropine administration. Atropine sulphate, administered routinely, kept the patient symptom-free. We have observed this syndrome in a woman of 28 whose resting function tests and chest x-ray were normal, and who gave a clear history of chest wheezing which would occur after she had sat down in the train following a five-minute walk to the station every morning. Five minutes of treadmill exercise reduced the maximal midexpiratory flow rate to less than a third of its previously normal value, and the bronchospasm was audible without a stethoscope. No definitive explanation of this syndrome can yet be given. We have reported significant falls in capillary blood pH after exercise in some asthmatic children,[2602] and it seems possible that the bronchial tree might be sensitive to this change of pH or possibly to an increase in lactic acid in these patients; in others, possibly the syndrome represents an exaggeration of the bronchoconstriction that follows hyperventilation on air in the normal subject, and which seems to be related to a lowering of the end-tidal CO_2 tension.[1084] Davies[3676] has recently reported a case of this syndrome in which the post-exercise fall in FEV was prevented by the prior administration of disodium cromoglycate.

SUMMARY

During the past five years, a number of important advances have been made toward understanding the disturbances of pulmonary function that occur in asthma. The documentation of the occurrence of regional abnormalities of ventilation and perfusion; the recognition of the importance of hypoxemia; the more detailed analysis of pulmonary mechanics and lung volumes which has indicated that the asthmatic state may be characterized by some reversible change in lung recoil; the documentation of the lowering of ventilatory capability and increased airway resistance following exercise in some asthmatics—all these advances have broadened our understanding of this condition but still leave many important questions unanswered. A summary of the stages of bronchial asthma together with a note of the possible state of the lungs corresponding to each clinical and physiological stage of the disorder is presented in Table 5-1.

CHRONIC BRONCHITIS AND CHRONIC INFECTIVE ASTHMA

CHAPTER

6

"There are different sorts of conflicts between theories. One familiar kind of conflict is that in which two or more theorists offer rival solutions of the same problem. In the simplest cases, their solutions are rivals in the sense that if one of them is true, the others are false. More often, naturally, the issue is a fairly confused one, in which each of the solutions proffered is in part right, in part wrong and in part just incomplete or nebulous. There is nothing to regret in the existence of disagreements of this sort. Even if, in the end, all the rival theories but one are totally demolished, still their contest has helped to test and develop the power of the arguments in favour of the survivor."

———PROFESSOR GILBERT RYLE, in Dilemmas (The Tarner Lectures, 1953). Cambridge University Press, 1960, p. 1.

DEFINITIONS

CHRONIC BRONCHITIS

Many authors have pointed out the difficulty of arriving at a satisfactory definition of chronic bronchitis,[6, 7] and a good deal of confusion has resulted from the use of the term in different senses in different countries. The Ciba symposium on terminology, among the participants in which were many with considerable experience of survey work on chronic respiratory disease, included a section on definition of chronic bronchitis.[815] In our view, this represented a very considerable advance over anything that had gone before, and accordingly we quote the paragraphs in full:

" 'Chronic bronchitis refers to the condition of subjects with chronic or recurrent excessive mucous secretion in the bronchial tree.' The diagnostic criterion is clinical, and is chronic or recurrent cough with expectoration which is not attributable to conditions excluded from chronic non-specific lung disease.

"Infection of the bronchi is frequently but not necessarily present.

"Not infrequently subjects who produce sputum deny cough. Such subjects are included as having bronchitis. Subjects who habitually swallow sputum should also be included as having chronic bronchitis.

"Opinion is divided concerning the significance of 'dry' chronic bronchitis without hypersecretion, which is excluded by the proposed definition. Population surveys in Great Britain suggest that a persistent cough without expectoration is uncommon.

"The words 'chronic or recurrent' may be defined as 'occurring on most days for at least three months in the year during at least two years.' "

In some epidemiological surveys the criteria for diagnosing chronic bronchitis do not precisely fit this definition, although the Ciba proposals have been followed in most survey work conducted since 1958.[39, 796]

In 1965, a special committee concerned with the etiology of chronic bronchitis reported to the Medical Research Council in Britain[2500] and proposed a division of categories on the basis of volume and infection of the sputum. It seems important to us to emphasize some different terminology to avoid the danger of equating the clinical condition classified by these criteria as "chronic bronchitis," with the much more severe syndrome much more rarely encountered. Gough[2531] has drawn attention to the confusion of thought that may occur when this differentiation is not made; we have attempted to clarify this point in the summary at the end of this chapter.

Chronic infective asthma

It has been recognized for several years that some patients with chronic bronchitis may suffer from such a severe degree of bronchospasm, particularly during exacerbations of infection, that they appear clinically similar to those with spasmodic or extrinsic asthma. Rackemann, writing in 1947, stated: "When asthma begins after the age of 40 it should be considered as due to factors other than allergy until proved otherwise."[830] In the same paper, after a sentence discussing differentiation of asthma from emphysema, he wrote:

"Mention of the disease 'asthma' is included here because it happens not infrequently that patients with structural emphysema are put through the asthma routine, with skin tests to many different substances and sometimes treatment with dust extracts and other materials. The fact that such treatment does no good is not surprising; it reflects the lack of training and insight of the attending physician."

Provided that the nature of the disease is recognized, it is perhaps useful to distinguish patients with the syndrome of chronic infective asthma from the general population of patients with chronic bronchitis, though, as far as we are aware, specific sensitivity to *H. influenzae* has yet to be shown.

It is important to distinguish between the undoubted existence of chronic infective asthma just defined and the possible role of allergic factors in patients with chronic bronchitis. This issue has been the subject of much discussion. Several series of studies of chronic bronchitis show a high frequency of a family history of allergy in the patients evaluated,[2628] and other investigators have noted characteristics in chronic bronchitis which they have interpreted in terms of an important allergic component.[2629, 2634] On the other hand, Charpin and his co-workers[2630] and Fletcher[2635] have been unable to confirm this hypothesis. In view of the non-specificity of the bronchial reactivity in chronic bronchitis, it seems unlikely that allergic factors play any major role in the majority of cases of chronic bronchitis.

PATHOLOGY

Lung morphology

Accepting the definition of chronic bronchitis as a chronic productive cough, the essential morphological change is hypertrophy of the bronchial mucous glands. Normal bronchial glands are compound mucous and serous in type, and their maximal thickness is about one-third that of the bronchial wall measured between the epithelium and the cartilage. In chronic bronchitis[775] the glands increase in size and may occupy two thirds of the distance between the bronchial epithelium and the cartilage; the individual acini of the glands increase in size; there is preponderance of mucous to serous acini; and the ducts of the glands are often dilated. These greatly enlarged ducts may be visible bronchographically as pits in the bronchial wall.[771] The goblet cells of bronchi and bronchioles become prominent, although this development is often patchy. Excess mucus is present in the tracheobronchial tree, and may even be seen in some alveoli. Characteristically, bronchioles occluded by mucus show a sharply demarcated, square-ended filling defect in bronchograms.[771]

The changes in the bronchial glands can be quantitated by calculating the ratio of gland to wall thickness (Reid index).[775]

In the original description of this useful measurement[775] this ratio was said to be always less than 0.36 in nonbronchitic subjects, and always higher than this in patients with bronchitis, with no overlap between the groups. We have found, however, considerable overlap between these groups,[897, 2515] and it seems that, in fact, there is a normal bell-shaped distribution curve between the lowest value in the nonsmoker and the highest value in a heavy cigarette smoker. Since the definition of chronic bronchitis by criteria based on the clinical history is inevitably either positive or negative, this morphological finding indicates that there is bound to be a considerable area of discrepancy between the clinical and morphological diagnosis if the latter is based only on mucous-gland hypertrophy. There is no major variation in the Reid index between different parts of the bronchial tree in the same patient,[2507] but, in spite of this, attempted classifications of chronic bronchitis on the basis of bronchial biopsy have not been encouraging.[2636, 2639]

DeHaller and Reid have recently quantitated the degree of distention of the mucous acini of the glands;[2642] it is these rather than the serous acini that enlarge in chronic bronchitis. It has recently been reported that pipe smokers and ex-cigarette smokers have almost as high an incidence of mucous-gland hypertrophy as cigarette smokers,[2643] and it has been stated that hypertrophy of the glands may occur as part of normal aging,[2641] although we have not been able to confirm this. Restrepo and Heard have been unable to confirm earlier reports of extensive atrophy of bronchial cartilage in chronic bronchitis,[2637] and the importance of this aspect of the disease remains controversial.

Dunnill and his co-workers[3681] have recently described another method of measuring the size of bronchial mucous glands which appears to have many technical advantages over the Reid index. Mucous glands measured by their technique show a striking enlargement in bronchitis and also in emphysema and in the lungs of patients with spasmodic asthma. The value of this method in establishing the diagnosis of chronic bronchitis remains to be determined, however, and it may well be that it will present the same problems as does the Reid index (as noted earlier).

In the last few years, some references to the possible importance of bronchiolitis as a complication of chronic bronchitis have appeared,[2542] and the term "distal atrophic bronchitis" has been used in this connection.[2645] It seems to us that there is almost certainly a quantitative loss of small airways in the course of chronic bronchitis, and that when emphysema has developed, this loss may be considerable.[2727] It may be noted too that recent studies of lung mechanics and gas distribution in patients with mild chronic bronchitis point to the small airways as the earliest site of abnormal function,[2644] but the morphological counterparts to these findings are not yet clarified. Mitchell and his co-workers have placed much emphasis on the functional importance of the morphological findings in major bronchi in chronic bronchitis,[2503] yet it is the complications of chronic bronchitis (defined simply in terms of productive cough) that make it a potentially lethal condition.

The foremost of these are intercurrent and often repetitive bronchopulmonary infection, and the development of complicating emphysema. Varying degrees of bronchopneumonia and abscess formation and organization are found in fatal cases, together with bronchial and bronchiolar obliteration, bronchiolectasis,[899] and perhaps weakening of the bronchial walls. As noted earlier, bronchiolitis is a highly important complication,[900, 901, 902, 2542, 2645, 2727] inadequately described and probably diagnosed too infrequently. It is possible for a patient with chronic bronchitis to die from respiratory failure due to bronchiolitis and for autopsy to reveal a relatively slight degree of pulmonary emphysema (*see* later discussion). There can be little doubt that episodes of

Case 5
Chronic Infective Asthma

Summary of Clinical Findings. This 60-year-old male bookkeeper had a history of sinusitis since childhood, treated with nasal irrigations. His father and one brother suffered from asthma. Episodes of shortness of breath were first noticed in 1957 when he was 55 years of age, and were accompanied by a persistent cough productive of a small amount of white sputum. He had smoked up to 15 cigars daily until three years previously.

In April 1958, he was admitted for an exacerbation of his symptoms. Physical examination revealed obesity. Scattered inspiratory and expiratory rhonchi were heard over the chest. Chest x-rays and pulmonary function studies were done on this admission. Sinus x-rays suggested a chronic maxillary sinusitis, and allergy skin tests revealed a slight sensitivity to stock dust. He responded satisfactorily to bronchodilators.

The symptoms continued intermittently, requiring two admissions during the following year, the first because of a left lower-lobe pneumonia which cleared quickly on antibiotics. He later required cortisone for relief of his dyspnea. On the day before his final admission in September 1962 he suffered several attacks of severe, crushing, anterior chest pain. He was admitted to hospital unconscious, in shock, cyanosed and with labored respirations. His rectal temperature was 105° F. Rales were heard over both lung fields, mainly at the bases. ECG showed no evidence of infarction. An arterial blood sample revealed CO_2 retention and O_2 desaturation. He was treated with oxygen, aminophylline, Neo-Synephrine and intravenous cortisone, but never regained consciousness. He died two hours after admission.

Radiology. Postero-anterior (*A*) and lateral (*B*) films of the chest taken in April 1958 show a rather low position of the diaphragm and a greater than normal anteroposterior diameter of the chest. Lung translucency is increased symmetrically and uniformly, and the arterial pattern is normal. The appearance indicates moderately severe air-trapping.

Pathology. No emphysema was present at necropsy (*C*). The bronchial mucous glands were hypertrophied, with a Reid index of 0.60, clearly indicating the presence of chronic bronchitis.

There was widespread mucous plugging of the small bronchi and bronchioles (*D*), which showed striking thickening of the epithelial basement membrane. Bronchitis and bronchiolitis were present with a prominent eosinophil component. This change stopped short of the terminal bronchioles. Death was caused by a lung abscess which had ruptured into the left pleural cavity, also giving rise to acute mediastinitis. The hypercapnea and acidosis were due to extensive mucous plugging, a phenomenon characteristic of death in "status asthmaticus."

Summary. This case illustrates the difficulty of hard and fast distinctions between chronic bronchitis and spasmodic asthma; it might be classified as a case of "chronic infective asthma." The relative preservation of diffusing capacity when ventilatory defect was severe indicated the probability that morphological emphysema was absent or slight in degree, and at autopsy several months later the lung parenchyma showed no emphysematous changes despite the fact that the patient died in respiratory failure.

	VC	FRC	RV	TLC	ME %	MMFR	$FEV_{0.75}$ ×40	pH	P_{CO_2}	HCO_3^-	O_2Hb %	$D_{L_{CO}}SS_2$	COExt %
Predicted	4.2	3.7	2.2	6.4	53	3.3	102	7.4	40	25	97	15.5	39
April 1958	2.6	3.3	2.7	5.3	27	0.3	27					12.0	32
Sept. 1962								7.03	89	20	39		

The vital capacity and total lung capacity are reduced, and the residual volume is increased. Gas distribution is poor and ventilatory function is severely reduced. Diffusion is only slightly decreased. On his terminal admission in September 1962, there was severe carbon-dioxide retention, with resultant severe acidosis, and gross arterial desaturation was present.

Chronic Infective Asthma

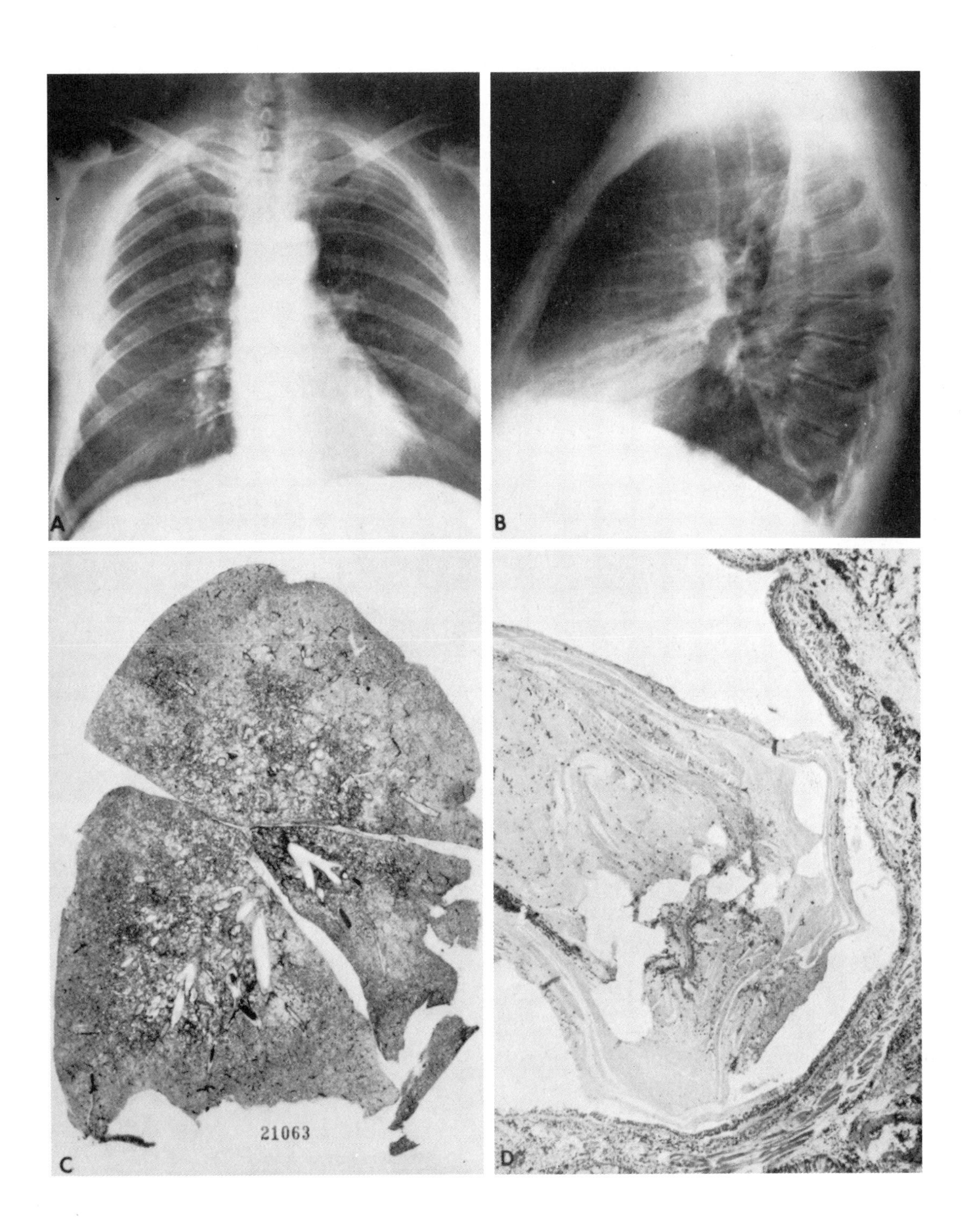

bronchopulmonary infection can be responsible for bouts of respiratory and right ventricular failure in patients with or without morphological emphysema.

The relationship between bronchitis and pulmonary emphysema is not at present completely understood. It seems clear that, in some patients, chronic bronchitis should be regarded as a complication of emphysema (*see* page 207),[904] and that, in others, emphysema should be regarded as a complication of chronic bronchitis. A person with a chronic productive cough is almost twice as likely to have significant morphological emphysematous changes in his lungs as is a person without chronic bronchitis.[905] On the other hand, chronic bronchitis may be present for years without the development of any significant degree of emphysema, a conclusion supported not only by morphological studies,[790] but also by the demonstration of continuous ventilatory impairment in patients with a long history of chronic cough who, in spite of this, have no impairment of carbon-monoxide uptake.[39] It is also possible for patients to have mild or moderately severe grades of emphysema without their giving a history of chronic cough or their bronchi showing a Reid index above the normal limit.

It seems possible that the link between emphysema and chronic bronchitis may be bronchiolitis. This has been shown to be invariably present in centrilobular emphysema,[799] and possibly also in other forms of emphysema.[896, 908] Intercurrent bronchopulmonary infections are more common in, but not confined to, patients with chronic bronchitis. If such episodes represent bronchiolitis, as many of them probably do, this might account for the greater incidence of emphysema in patients suffering from chronic bronchitis. It is also probable that the presence of emphysema may predispose the patient to attacks of bronchitis and bronchiolitis, establishing a vicious circle from which escape is difficult. It should be emphasized that theories of the mechanisms involved in pulmonary emphysema of any type, as a consequence of bronchiolitis, are as yet only speculative.

Sputum volume and composition

Ashcroft[2555] has documented the considerable daily variations that occur in sputum volume in patients with chronic bronchitis. In the Canadian Veterans' Affairs Study of Chronic Bronchitis,[2512] Gordon found that in 14 of 35 men with chronic bronchitis, under strict observation for 24 hours, there was a major discrepancy between the sputum volume estimated by questionnaire and the amount collected—the estimate being an exaggeration.

The mucus secreted in chronic bronchitis appears to have a normal biochemical structure,[2650] the essential components being glycoproteins that include a transferrin of bronchial origin and beta$_2$-globulin, serum albumin and different seromucoids and plasma glycoproteins, mucoids of bronchial origin, and mucopolysaccharide acids. Of all clinical conditions, only alveolar cell carcinoma seems to generate a secretion with characteristics distinctively different from the normal.[2651] Albumin and gamma-A-immunoglobulin are the main plasma proteins in sputum,[2652] and the turnover of albumin is much increased in bronchitic patients with much sputum;[2653] indeed, the protein loss by this route may be considerable. The electrolyte concentrations in sputum appear to be normal,[2654] and the viscosity is related to the DNA content,[2659] measurements of which may be useful in following progress.

Many authors continue to stress the importance of *H. influenzae* in this condition,[2658] but there is much evidence that its role is secondary. Storey and his colleagues[2655] have documented the frequent recovery of *Diplococcus pneumoniae* and *Haemophilus influenzae* from the sputum of 13 patients with chronic bronchitis followed for 40 consecutive days, and the presence of these organisms in the sputum could not be correlated with acute exacerbations of infection. In addition, there is recent serological evidence[2656, 2657] which indicates that it is unlikely that *H. influenzae* is responsible for the initiation of chronic bronchitis, but rather that the damaged bronchial mucosa encourages its proliferation.

RADIOLOGY

Plain films of the chest can contribute little to the definitive diagnosis of chronic bronchitis. Chest radiography serves the essential purpose of excluding other diseases that may mimic chronic bronchitis, or with which bronchitis may be associated,[765] and may be of value in indicating the probable presence or absence of significant emphysema. In a study of 857 patients clinically diagnosed as having chronic bronchitis, Simon and Galbraith concluded that in 59 per cent there were signs of overinflation, and of these, 15 per cent were considered to have undoubted radiological evidence of emphysema; in the remaining 41 per cent the lung fields were completely normal.[765]

Reviewing the plain chest films of 180 of the 216 men in the Canadian Department of Veterans' Affairs study of chronic bronchitis, we found evidence of hyperinflation in about 60 per cent of the films.[2512] These observations are not surprising when one considers the pathological changes already described. Although pulmonary overinflation is frequently observed as evidence of obstructive airway disease, its presence is neither distinctive nor diagnostic, especially in view of the common association of bronchitis and emphysema. Plain-film assessment of the presence or absence of emphysema in a patient with established chronic bronchitis is dependent largely, if not wholly, upon the character of the peripheral vasculature, diminution of which indicates destructive lung disease. Such deficiency may be apparent occasionally on plain films, but it has been shown that accuracy will be significantly improved if additional full-lung tomograms through the midchest are available for assessment.[710, 1866]

The increased thickness of bronchial walls is seldom of sufficient degree to allow for radiological identification, although tomography occasionally reveals parallel lines along the distribution of the bronchial tree in the central and midlung zones which in all likelihood represent thickened bronchial walls. These lines, colloquially referred to as "tramlines," are considered by Hodson and Trickey to be a reliable sign of chronic infective asthma, particularly in children;[930] in adults, however, our experience indicates that they appear with sufficient frequency in normal asymptomatic subjects and in patients with established bronchiectasis that their presence cannot be relied upon as a sign of chronic bronchitis.

The predominantly bronchitic type of chronic obstructive lung disease (classified as Type B or Type BB) is defined by some authors as having a chest x-ray which shows normal, as opposed to increased, translucency of the lungs. In other accounts, the chest x-ray in this type has been said to show evidence of inflammatory change with increased pulmonary markings. We have recently found that this type of x-ray, which we have characterized as "increased marking," is frequently found in patients with chronic bronchitis but often with a considerable degree of associated emphysema, this being particularly centrilobular in type[2524] (see Fig. 7-8, page 171). It is uncertain, therefore, to what extent the radiological appearances should be attributed to chronic bronchitis alone.

Bronchographically, several abnormalities may be found in chronic bronchitis, at least one of which is pathognomonic. The enlarged bronchial glands, which are a distinctive pathological characteristic of this disease,[775] may be wide enough to admit opaque medium; thus the filling of these glands constitutes a reliable sign of abnormality. Such bronchial "diverticulosis," occurring most frequently along the inferior aspects of the larger bronchi, was observed by Simon and Galbraith in one-half of their 90 patients with established bronchitis.[765]

The abrupt termination of bronchioles in a squared or truncated type of ending has been commonly observed,[765] and Reid and Simon[771, 898] have correlated this finding with the blind ends of obliterated bronchioles. Reid has also referred to the similarity of the pathological findings in chronic bronchitis and bronchiectasis, and has suggested that this differentiation may be made by determining the anatomical site of air-way obliteration: in the larger bronchi in bronchiectasis, and in the bronchioles in chronic bronchitis.

An increase in bronchial caliber, either local or general, was reported by Simon and Galbraith as a relatively uncommon finding in chronic bronchitis, occurring in 21 of the 90 patients they investigated.[765] We have been impressed by the frequency with which slight but definite bronchial dilatation is observed in patients with chronic bronchitis. Bronchographic films show a loss of normal tapering of the segmental bronchi down to the sixth- or seventh-stage divisions beyond the lobar bronchi, an appearance that can simulate mild cylindrical bronchiectasis and that often can be differentiated from it only because of absence of parenchymal changes in the adjacent lung. Even more convincing alteration in bronchial caliber has been observed cinefluorographically, some patients with chronic bronchitis without emphysema

Case 6
Chronic Bronchitis (Chronic Infective Asthma)

Summary of Clinical Findings. This 55-year-old machinist had first noticed dyspnea on brisk walking some three years previously. Nine months before admission and following a nasal polypectomy, shortness of breath on exertion became more severe. At the time of admission he was unable to walk more than 100 yards slowly without stopping to catch his breath. He had had a cough with slight purulent expectoration on arising for 10 to 15 years. Cigarette consumption had varied between 20 and 80 per day, but he had given up the habit the year previously. There was no family history of allergy.

On physical examination his chest was hyperresonant. The breath sounds were generally decreased. Expiration was prolonged, with scattered sonorous rhonchi.

Differential white-blood-cell counts revealed 12 per cent and 16 per cent eosinophils. Three stool specimens were negative for parasites. Electrophoresis showed normal values for protein, and allergy skin tests showed no positive reactions.

It was considered that the dyspnea was on a basis of bronchospasm, and the patient was placed on corticosteroids. After only three days of therapy he noticed dramatic improvement in his shortness of breath on exertion.

He continued to suffer episodes of shortness of breath which were treated with steroids. It was finally found necessary to maintain continuous steroids and this was complicated by a gastric ulcer in January, 1969. He now describes mild dyspnea on exertion such as gardening. He has only a slight chronic cough with scanty white sputum.

Repeat function studies are shown.

Radiology. Postero-anterior (*A*) and lateral (*B*) films of the chest show an essentially normal appearance of the lungs, although there is slight hyperinflation. The pulmonary vasculature is unremarkable. Films of the paranasal sinuses (not shown) revealed evidence of chronic pansinusitis.

Summary. This case illustrates chronic bronchitis complicated by a considerable and relievable degree of bronchospasm. Note that, at the time of severe bronchial obstruction, the probable absence of significant morphological emphysema could be inferred from the relatively normal appearance of the pulmonary vasculature on the chest film and the almost normal value for the resting diffusing capacity.

This case illustrates the difficulty of precise separation of individual patients into rigid categories. He might be considered to be suffering primarily from chronic bronchitis with unusually severe bronchospasm (chronic infective asthma) or primarily from spasmodic asthma with secondary chronic bronchitis. It seems unlikely, however, that a significant degree of morphological emphysema is present.

	VC	FRC	RV	TLC	ME %	MMFR	$FEV_{0.75}$ ×40	pH^+	P_{CO_2}	HCO_3^-	P_{O_2}	O_2Hb %	CO Ext %	$D_{LCO}SS_2$
Predicted	4.2	3.8	2.2	6.5	53	3.3	102	7.40	42	25		97	39	15.5
Nov. 5, 1962	3.2	4.2	3.4	6.6	27	0.8	41	7.32	47	23		96	39	14.1
Nov. 8, 1962						1.8	90						45	23.4
Jan. 13, 1969	3.7	–	–	–	–	1.3	64	7.41	39	24		93	31	14.7

On the fifth of November, 1962, the studies showed a slightly increased functional residual capacity, reduced ventilatory flow rates, and impaired gas distribution. The diffusion was, however, only slightly reduced compared to the predicted value, and there was no hypercapnia. After three days of steroid therapy, the ventilatory function, as shown by the MMFR and the $FEV_{0.75} \times 40$, had improved considerably. The diffusing capacity had also increased, and was now above the predicted value. In view of this, it was unlikely that any significant degree of morphological emphysema was present, a conclusion that was tentatively inferred from the finding of a relatively normal diffusing capacity on November 5, 1962, when ventilatory function was seriously impaired. By January, 1969, flow rates were still moderately reduced, and the diffusing capacity had fallen to its original value, although within predicted limits of normal. There was slight hypoxemia but no hypercapnia.

Chronic Bronchitis (Chronic Infective Asthma)

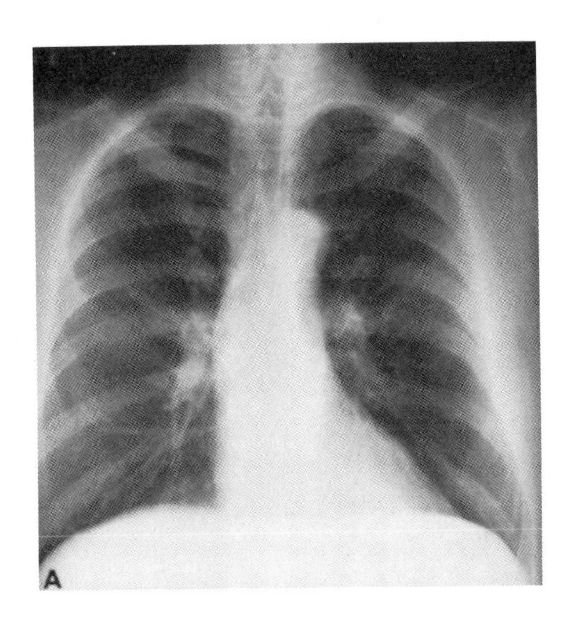

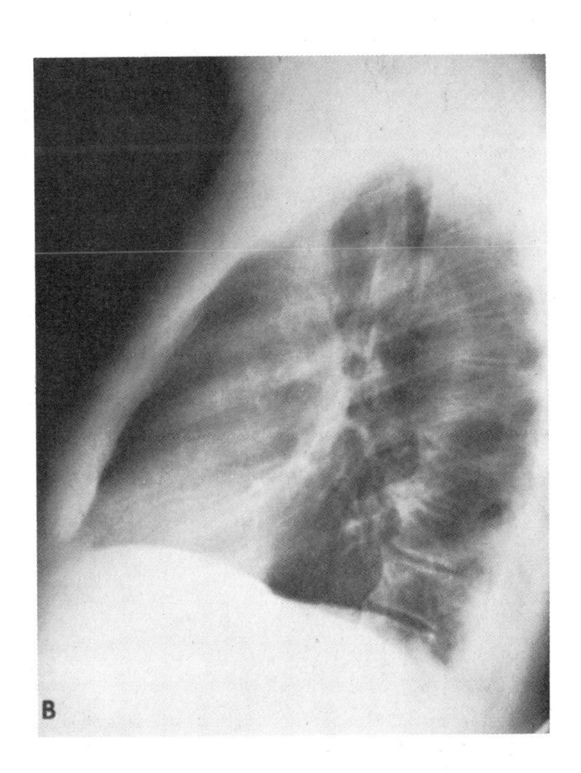

showing an increased inspiratory diameter of all bronchi from the intermediate stem bronchus through the fifth-stage divisions.[755]

These studies have also shown a tendency for the main lower-lobe and middle-lobe bronchi to undergo disproportionate degrees of collapse on forced expiration and cough. Coincident with this collapse, the segmental bronchi distally undergo less decrease in caliber, suggesting that air-trapping occurs as a consequence of central bronchial closure. Manometric studies carried out both independently and simultaneously with cinebronchography have established that, on forced expiration, a high pressure rise occurs distal to the collapsing lower-lobe bronchus, with a large pressure drop across it, confirming the significant role that narrowing of the larger bronchi may play in the causation of expiratory air-flow obstruction in chronic bronchitis.[772]

In disease confined to the bronchial tree, without complicating emphysema, the pattern of pulmonary vessels as seen tomographically or during angiography should be normal.

ETIOLOGY AND EPIDEMIOLOGY

Surveys: comparative incidence

During the past four years, an immense volume of information has been published from many different countries concerning the frequency of chronic bronchitis. In this book we can attempt little more than a brief review to enable the reader to appreciate the universality of this condition and to consult the relevant literature for details. Standard questionnaires,[35] pioneered by Fletcher and his colleagues,[843] have been used by many subsequent investigators. Although some variability in answers has been noted,[844] and there is some inter-observer variability,[845] the method has been very generally established as well repeatable,[2660] provided the questions are carefully standardized.[2681]

There have been many reports of a generally high incidence of chronic bronchitis among male cigarette smokers living and working in industrialized areas in the U.S.A.,[2623, 2660, 2668, 2691] Great Britain,[2670, 2671, 2672, 2702] France,[2679, 2686] Czechoslovakia,[2680] Japan,[2689, 2690] and Poland.[2688] More surprising, perhaps, has been the finding that the incidence is far from negligible in rural areas of Finland,[2662, 2666, 2669, 2684] Norway,[2663] India,[2682] Egypt,[2661] Jamaica,[2684] and Australia.[2713] All these and many other reports have confirmed the original findings of a close association between respiratory symptoms, pulmonary function, as judged by the FEV_1, and cigarette consumption indicated in earlier surveys,[642, 796, 835, 843, 848, 850, 851, 2208] and of a much lower incidence in rural nonsmoker populations.[2273]

Recent work has established more securely the differences between Britain and the United States in terms of chronic respiratory disease in general. Burrows and Fletcher, by their comparison of populations of patients with chronic obstructive lung disease in London and in Chicago, have shown that many patients who in the United States would be characterized as suffering from "emphysema," would in Britain be regarded as having "chronic bronchitis"; but the syndrome is very similar in the two countries.[2504, 2526, 2675, 2728] There is general agreement with Holland and his colleagues,[2721] who concluded that:

1. Chronic bronchitis was more common in London than in rural Britain;
2. Incidence in American cities was closer to that in rural than in industrial Britain;
3. Chronic bronchitis tended to be more severe in Britain, and the incidence of more severely disabled patients with the syndrome was considerably higher in Britain than in the United States in general. This point has been supported by other work.[2674, 2676]

Crofton[2670] has compared the mortality from chronic bronchitis in Scotland with that in England and Wales. He concluded that there was a higher level in England and Wales and suggested that the later spread of cigarette smoking to Scotland might be one of the factors causing the difference. The relationship between chronic bronchitis and specific etiological factors is discussed in more detail later.

In most of the surveys that have been made in recent years, some estimate of a forced expiration has been included. In general, levels of FEV_1 have been found to correlate with the severity of the symptomatology. For reasons mentioned later, it may be misleading to equate the damage caused by chronic bronchitis too closely with the level of FEV_1, which is relatively insensitive to alterations in peripheral airway resistance.

Factors Affecting the Incidence of Chronic Bronchitis

Smoking

The general relationship between cigarette smoking and chronic bronchitis has now been fully established by both epidemiological and morphological studies. It is important to recognize, however, that normal Reid indices may be found in smokers and that non-smokers may have the clinical criteria of chronic bronchitis,[795, 843, 2273] although both of these represent exceptions to the rule. The influence of pipe and cigar smoking on the incidence of chronic bronchitis is much less well-defined, although elevated Reid indices have been reported in pipe smokers.[2643] Ferris[2722] has brought together data on the effect of age and cigarette smoking on the FEV_1, and some investigators have found improvement in the FEV_1 in some patients with chronic bronchitis after smoking has been stopped (*see* following discussion). The effects of cigarette smoking on pulmonary function in the absence of overt chronic bronchitis are discussed in detail later in this chapter.

Air pollution

During the past four years, all industrialized countries have become concerned with the increasing problem of man-made air pollution. The monograph of the World Health Organization;[857] the book on Air Conservation, published by the American Association for the Advancement of Science;[2729] and the recent hearings before a Committee of the U.S. Senate[2732] all provide important information. Technical aspects of air monitoring and control are dealt with in detail in the three-volume book by Arthur Stern,[2730] and many other monographs and publications have appeared that are too numerous to list. There has been much debate on the evidence linking air pollution to disease, and conferences in the United States[2693] and in London[2701] have been devoted to this problem.

The dramatic mortality produced by severe and protracted episodes of air pollution,[857] such as that in London in December, 1952,[35] necessitated more active government recognition of the problem. It is now clear that in many patients severe chronic respiratory disease is made worse by minor episodes of a similar kind, both in London, where Lawther has demonstrated a correlation between exacerbation of symptoms and smoke and SO_2 concentration,[852] and in New York, where a five-day period of heavy air pollution in 1966 produced increased mortality among such patients.[2712, 2726] There seems to us to be reasonable evidence that chronic respiratory disease morbidity is greater among smokers who smoke comparable numbers of cigarettes and live in major urban areas than among those who live in more rural surroundings. In London more bronchitis occurs in regions with higher pollution;[832] in Buffalo,[2692] in Sweden,[2711] and in Genoa in Italy[2715] there are similar relationships. Perhaps the most convincing evidence for the existence of an "urban factor" in the incidence of these diseases is that presented by Holland and Reid.[2678] They compared the frequency of chronic respiratory symptoms and pulmonary function (FEV_1) test results in male postal-van drivers in central London, on the one hand, and those in men of similar age, driving postal vans in and around three country towns in southern England—Gloucester, Norwich, and Peterborough. The London group was shown to have more symptoms and greater phlegm production and considerably more impairment of ventilatory function than the country workers, allowance having been made for individual smoking habits. They concluded: "Of the factors reviewed in this study, differences in local levels of air pollution appear to be the likeliest cause of the difference in respiratory morbidity between men working in central London and those in the three rural areas."

Equally convincing is the study by Douglas and Waller of respiratory disease morbidity among 5000 children followed from birth to the age of 16, in which they found clear evidence of an association between lower respiratory-tract infections and the degree of air pollution in their environment.[2724] Confirmatory data linking air pollution to respiratory disease in children has been published from Sheffield.[2725]

Although the existence of a specific and unique syndrome of "Yokohama Asthma" is now disputed,[2695] there is convincing data of very high levels of chronic respiratory disease in areas of high industrial air pollution in Japan.[2690, 2696, 2697, 2698]

It may be useful to conclude this very brief review by summarizing some other aspects of the relationship between air pollution and chronic respiratory disease.

1. Although the levels of ambient ozone in the photochemical pollution in Los Angeles are nearing concentrations that produce measurable effects in normal humans,[1679, 2703, 2704, 2706] no morbidity from this has yet been demonstrated.

2. Although it is not easy to be certain what concentration of SO_2 reaches the alveoli, since most of it is removed in the nose,[2717, 2718] the levels reached in most cities are not of themselves high enough to produce definite effects. It has been shown experimentally that oxides of nitrogen,[2733] particularly when adsorbed onto carbon particles, are capable of producing lesions very similar to centrilobular emphysema in the rat; but the concentrations needed are higher than those normally encountered. Ozone is also capable of producing a similar lesion. The demonstrated urban factor cannot be linked to any one pollutant and conceivably could be the result of a higher risk of contact with respiratory infection in cities, or even of a potentiating effect of air pollutants on virus or bacterial growth in the air.

3. Trace metals inhaled from polluted air can be found in the lung.[2716, 2734] A chrysotile particle has been identified in an electron microscopy photograph of London air,[2720] and, as noted later (*see* Chapter 17), the lungs of about half the inhabitants of a modern city seem to contain one or more asbestos fibers.

4. Population studies are complicated by the frequent movement of people out of areas of heavy air pollution to country districts. Kelsey, Mood, and Acheson have shown that this movement affected a study of respiratory disease morbidity in rural Connecticut.[2707]

5. In our view, there is ample reason to express concern about present levels of air pollution,[2698, 2720] and concern about acceptable air-quality standards[2719, 2731] should not be based only on proof of increased respiratory morbitidy; it should be enough that the environment in cities should not be unpleasant.[2732] There has been a tendency for the legislators to insist on proof of effect as a basis for legal definitions of acceptable air quality; but it is doubtful whether modern industrial society can afford to wait for much more evidence before legislative action is taken.

Climate

Experimental work on the reactivity of the bronchi to climatic factors includes the observation that the inhalation of cold air can increase airway resistance considerably in certain subjects with chronic disease, in particular those who complain that their symptoms are aggravated on exposure to cold air.[1551] Walker and his associates have postulated that this sensitivity to cold may, in fact, be a failure to humidify inspired air adequately.[1550] As already noted, patients with spasmodic asthma have been shown to respond to cold air with bronchospasm.[2657]

There is, however, little precise documentation of the effect of climatic factors, as opposed to atmospheric pollution, on the incidence of, morbidity from, or mortality of chronic bronchitis. Many patients are convinced of the sensitivity of their symptoms to changes in weather, in terms of both temperature and humidity, and chest physicians in many countries would agree with them. It is of some interest, however, that the pattern of winter exacerbation familiar to the patient and chest physician in London, England,[392] was not apparent in a recent study we conducted on subjects with chronic bronchitis living in Toronto, suggesting perhaps that humidity (high in London) is a more relevant factor than cold (more severe in Toronto). However, in England it is particularly difficult to dissociate climatic factors from pollution, since smoke from domestic fires (a common source of SO_2) is also greater in winter, and the high moisture content of the air may provide a suitable adsorption surface for the fumes: in other words, climatic factors in the winter provide an environment in which air pollutants reach more toxic levels in the lungs. In this connection it is also important to note that seasonal variations have been recorded in the incidence of cor pulmonale in Sheffield, England,[853] and in the deaths from status asthmaticus for England as a whole.[854]

There is some recent evidence that worsening of pulmonary function[2702, 2714] and exacerbations in chronic bronchitis[2699] may be closely related to lowering of ambient temperature. On the basis of comparisons between Australian and British climate, Cullen and his colleagues calculated that the British climate possibly added 20 per cent to the incidence of chronic bronchitis, but such estimates are bound to remain speculative. One study on the effect of a single stay in the High Tatra mountains on chronic bronchitis[2735] unfortunately illustrates the difficulty of having to read papers in translation rather than illuminates the effect of climate on disease, since the final sentence of the abstract reads "a normalization of deviations from normal vegetative tonus and excitability in both plus and minus senses occurred."

The recent experiments of Abernethy[2743] provide direct evidence that water droplets as fog may diminish airway patency in patients with chronic bronchitis. Using water-containing fog at room temperature, he found a mean reduction of 18 per cent in the FEV_1 of seven patients with chronic bronchitis, in contrast to a minimal or absent effect in normal subjects, and postulated that the fog effect might be due to reflex bronchoconstriction. Hsieh, Frayser, and Ross[3680] have studied the effect of breathing cold air (at −40° C) on the FEV and the expired N_2 plateau in patients with chronic bronchitis. Little effect was found in control normal subjects, but a decrease of FEV was documented in those patients who had noted an adverse effect from cold air. The nitrogen slope was diminished by the cold-air breathing, which may thus have caused small airway closure before these regions of the lung could empty at the end of expiration.

Occupation

The incidence of chronic bronchitis in subjects whose occupations involve them in exposure to dust in general appears to be higher than the incidence of this condition in urban populations; representative values range in British collieries from 6 to 43 per cent and reach 33.5 per cent in Pennsylvania collieries.[881] It may be somewhat lower in hardrock mines where the silicosis hazard calls for more-stringent dust control. The higher incidence of symptoms in miners' wives compared with that in women whose husbands worked in dust-free jobs[858] may indicate that associated factors such as location of housing and economic circumstances may contribute in part to the high incidence of the disease among miners, or might also reflect anxiety about respiratory disease in miners and their families.

These data have not proved easy to analyze, however, and Gough[2531] has recently stressed that important differences in severity of "chronic bronchitis" may be concealed by comparison of percentage incidence on an epidemiological basis.

Workers in the chemical industry appear to have an increased incidence of chronic bronchitis,[878] and in a major survey of over 11,000 employees in the gas industry in Britain, Doll and his colleagues[2677] found an increased death rate from bronchitis in some workers in the process of gas production from coal. However, Lowe[2723] concluded that the industrial component of bronchitis was quite small, even in workers in a blast furnace area exposed to high concentrations of SO_2. It seems clear, however, that most, if not all, occupations involving heavy dust exposure carry an increased morbidity from chronic bronchitis.[858]

Income group

The belief that chronic respiratory disease is more common among the lower income population is traditional and some studies have apparently confirmed this opinion.[848] However, the influence of heavier cigarette smoking or work in dustier environments may have been important in relation to this finding. Winkelstein and his colleagues did not find any close relation between economic status and the incidence of chronic respiratory disease in Buffalo,[2692] and Douglas and Waller showed that the incidence of lower respiratory infections in children was related to the air-pollution level of their environment, but was independent of the economic level of the family. In addition, studies of clerical workers in the higher income brackets show a high incidence of chronic bronchitis among cigarette smokers.[642, 2694]

Whether or not the incidence is slightly higher in lower income groups, the social effects on men who have been trained only for manual work, and who become too dyspneic for this, are depressing indeed. We have found a high incidence of chronic respiratory disease in a group of men, between ages 50 and 60, unemployed and dependent on welfare in Montreal.[2249] Neilson and Crofton have studied the social effects of chronic bronchitis on 500 men from three areas of Scotland, and the reports make very depressing reading; their findings are almost certainly relevant to most major industrial cities.[2673] Not only is the mortality from chronic bronchitis and emphysema rising at an alarming rate in the United States, but in 1968 payments made by the Social Security Administration to men and women totally disabled because of these diseases amounted to 90 million dollars, which was 7 per cent of all disability payments, making chronic lung disease second only to heart disease in this regard.[2736] There can be no doubt of the magnitude of the misery caused by these diseases, particularly among lower income groups, regardless of the issue of whether the level of income has or has not much to do with the incidence of chronic bronchitis.

Hereditary predisposition

There is some indirect evidence of a family tendency toward chronic chest infections,[859, 860, 861] and specific instances of this have recently been more fully documented. It has been suggested that there may be a familial sensitivity to tobacco smoke,[2738] and a high incidence of chronic chest disease, extending over 150 years, has been documented to have occurred in one family, including both male and female members.[2739] On the other hand, the familial predisposition to emphysema discovered by Eriksson (*see* Chapter 7) was not associated with concomitant chronic bronchitis; indeed, the relative absence of chronic bronchitis was noted in many of the patients he described. Another syndrome that might be responsible for a familial incidence of chronic bronchitis is mucoviscidosis, but although some reports suggested this as a possibility,[864, 865] and although such patients may survive into adult life,[862, 863] there is little evidence that this disease underlies chronic bronchitis.[866, 2737] Considering the importance of cigarette smoking and environment, including air pollution and occupation, on the incidence of chronic bronchitis, the relative importance of familial factors must be accounted to be small.

Other conditions affecting patency of small airways

It seems clear from recent evidence that in the young, normal subject, small airways are closed at residual volume; that closure occurs at progressively higher volumes as aging of the lung occurs; and that anything that reduces lung volume, such as obesity, has the effect of causing airway closure during tidal-volume breathing that would not otherwise occur. All these phenomena are discussed in detail in the appropriate sections of this text. In addition, there is now evidence that chronic bronchitis affects the patency of small airway units at an early stage (*see* later discussion) and that any elevation of left atrial pressure, as in mitral stenosis, or considerable changes in plasma osmotic pressure may affect terminal airway ventilation, presumably by causing a cuff of fluid to surround the terminal airway (*see* chapters 2 and 21). It may also be mentioned that the ventilation of dependent lung units is impaired after a period of recumbency, as noted on page 67.

These observations, taken together, indicate that a number of clinical circumstances might be described as "additive" to chronic bronchitis in the sense that any compromise of function of the terminal airway units caused by chronic bronchitis is likely to be worsened by them. As far as we know, detailed documentation of this effect does not exist; yet the probability of its occurrence seems to us to justify a preliminary listing of these conditions:

Age
Prolonged recumbency
Obesity; ascites; pregnancy
Increased left atrial pressure { mitral stenosis / left ventricular failure }
Reduced plasma osmotic pressure—cirrhosis hepatitis

Summary of etiological factors

This brief review of the known etiological and aggravating factors in the production of chronic bronchitis would not be complete without additional emphasis on the probability that many of them are, without doubt, additive. The principal cause of the condition is cigarette smoking. The effect of a certain level of smoking is greater if one lives in a heavily polluted atmosphere, and this, in turn, may be more serious if there is much cold and damp weather. As the lung ages and its recoil diminishes, the patency of small airways in the normal range of tidal volume is reduced, and a number of clinical circumstances will at least aggravate the condition. Whatever view is taken of the effect of dust in causing chronic bronchitis, it seems very likely that dust deposition in terminal bronchioles will similarly worsen a pre-existing condition.

As noted later, the question of the primacy of chronic bronchitis in causing ventilation–perfusion disturbances is complex; but there is no doubt that emphysema can legitimately be regarded as a serious complication of chronic bronchitis.[2524]

CLINICAL FEATURES AND EFFECT ON PULMONARY FUNCTION

The correlation between the clinical manifestations of chronic bronchitis and the stage of impairment of function is not very close. One may therefore choose either a classification based on the nature of the sputum or its quantity,[2500] or divide the condition on the basis of the severity of the airway obstruction it has caused. We prefer the latter description, since it appears to us that the physician must employ some measurement of airflow and cannot rely either on the history or the physical signs or chest x-ray to give him this information.

CHRONIC BRONCHITIS WITH A NORMAL FEV_1

It has been shown in many studies that the criteria of chronic bronchitis, based on symptoms elicited by questionnaire, will be found in many subjects in whom the FEV_1 is within normal limits. Of the original group of 44 men with chronic bronchitis whom we have studied in the Department of Veterans' Affairs in Canada, 5 had normal pulmonary function,[39] a proportion that has been approximately maintained in the larger group of 216 men in four centers now under study,[2512] and other surveys have yielded a somewhat higher proportion of normal FEV_1 tests in other populations.

Characteristically, the patient with chronic bronchitis is a man, in early middle age, a cigarette smoker, and probably from one of the lower income groups. When first seen he will complain of a productive cough, the amount of sputum produced being maximal first thing in the morning. He may attribute an increase in amount of sputum to changes in the weather, though it is very likely that this factor varies widely in different countries.[39] He may notice that his chest feels wheezy on occasions, and is very likely to have lost some time from work on account of a chest illness in the past few years. Initially he will have had little dyspnea, though later this may have become troublesome, particularly during the recrudescence of infection. Often, on the advice of a friend or a physician, he will have given up cigarette smoking for a week or two, but, finding little immediate diminution in sputum, resumed the habit.

At the time of his first visit, the only abnormal physical sign may be an expiratory wheeze audible only on a maximal expiration; clinical examination of the chest at rest may well be completely normal. The only physical signs associated with chronic bronchitis uncomplicated by emphysema are those of a variable degree of bronchial obstruction. Usually it is shortness of breath, associated with wheezing, that first prompts the patient to visit a physician, but sometimes it is because he noticed a little blood-streaking of the sputum on one occasion, a symptom that occurs in about a quarter of the patients seen with chronic bronchitis.[7, 39] The importance of this disease as a cause of hemoptysis was confirmed by Johnston and his colleagues in Great Britain, who found it to be the cause in 17 per cent of 324 patients presenting with this symptom.[831] The patient with chronic bronchitis seeking advice because of hemoptysis is often so relieved to hear that he has neither carcinoma of the lung nor pulmonary tuberculosis, that it may be difficult to persuade him to take a serious view of his chronic bronchitis until the condition has been complicated by bronchopneumonia or by emphysema.

Recent work has indicated that it is important for the physician not to equate the finding of a normal FEV_1 with an absence of any changes in the respiratory tract, however. As will be noted later, an increased morbidity from chest infections has been found in young people smoking cigarettes, probably indicating some interference with pulmonary defense or clearance mechanisms. In addition to this, it is now realized that the FEV_1 is relatively insensitive to considerable changes in airway resistance in the peripheral airways, since these normally constitute a small fraction of the total airway resistance.[2744] We have also found that such patients with a normal or almost normal FEV_1 have demonstrable abnormalities of ^{133}xenon clearance from the lung,[2532] and the dynamic compliance may be shown to have become frequency-dependent[2544] and inert-gas distribution may be impaired.[2628] Other tests of function, including the arterial blood-gas tensions, are normal, but the first routine test of lung function to become abnormal may be the elevation of the residual volume. The chest x-ray at this stage is likely to be normal or, at the most, may show some evidence of hyperinflation.

Case 7
Chronic Bronchitis

Summary of Clinical Findings. This patient, a clerk with a railroad company, gave a 30-year history of chronic cough which he ascribed to his consumption of two packages of cigarettes per day. Expectoration, which originally was minimal in quantity and clear, became more copious and, in association with upper respiratory infections, colored yellow or green in the five years before his admission. In recent years he had also noticed shortness of breath on effort and it was this symptom which brought him to the hospital in October 1958 at the age of 52. Coincidental with a return to cigarette smoking, which he had given up some two years before, he had noticed a recent worsening of dyspnea, though he could walk on the flat without stopping. In September 1959, he became worse, with increased sputum, and when admitted on September 7 he was in severe respiratory distress. His blood pressure was 160/90, pulse rate 130/min, and temperature 99.6° F. Many sibilant and sonorous rhonchi were heard over both lungs, and expiration was markedly prolonged. Chest x-ray showed hyperinflation only. White-cell count was 13,800/cmm, with neutrophilia. ECG revealed sinus tachycardia with considerable clockwise rotation. He was treated with intravenous corticosteroids, antibiotics, oxygen and bronchodilators. Over a 3-day period he gradually improved, and during the next two weeks became free from symptoms at rest. Over the total period of observation, now eleven years, his dyspnea has not increased, although there have been occasional exacerbations of his symptoms. He has been maintained on low doses of steroids since 1959. He remains fully at work.

Radiology. A postero-anterior roentgenogram of the chest (*A*) shows an essentially normal appearance of the lungs with the exception of a slight generalized hyperinflation and the calcified lymph node in the right hilum. The midsagittal tomogram of both lungs (*B*) demonstrates a normal caliber and distribution of the peripheral vasculature, indicating the absence of diffuse emphysema. A postero-anterior view of the chest following bilateral bronchography (*C*) shows a perfectly normal appearance of all segments of the bronchial tree. Peripheral radicals are well filled and there are no "pools" or "spikes" to suggest the presence of emphysema. No dilated mucous glands are visible. Cinefluorographic studies of the opacified bronchial tree revealed, however, a disproportionate collapse of the bronchi of both lower lobes on forced expiration and cough, suggesting that these central bronchi were partly responsible for the expiratory air-flow obstruction revealed by pulmonary function tests.

	VC	FRC	RV	TLC	ME %	MMFR	$FEV_{0.75}$ ×40	pH	P_{CO_2}	HCO_3^-	P_{O_2}	O_2Hb %	$D_{LCO}SS_2$	CO Ext %	EXERCISE MPH	GRADE	$\dot{V}O_2$	$\dot{V}_E$	$D_{LCO}SS_3$
Predicted	4.1	3.7	2.3	6.4	60	3.1	94	7.4	40	25	–	97	14.1	39	2	FLAT	1.4	–	28.0
Oct. 1958	4.3	4.3	3.6	7.8	50	1.0	64	7.4	41	25	–	–	11.6	41	2	FLAT	1.4	–	28.8
Jan. 1959	4.1	4.3	3.9	8.0	50	0.9	68	–	–	–	–	–	18.8	–	–	–	–	–	–
Sept. 2/59	3.3	5.4	4.8	8.1	21	0.3	15	–	–	–	–	–	–	–	–	–	–	–	–
Sept. 7/59	–	–	–	–	–	–	–	7.3	55	28	–	–	–	–	–	–	–	–	–
Sept. 23/59	4.7	4.5	3.6	8.3	62	1.0	76	–	–	–	–	–	–	–	2	FLAT	1.6	–	28.1
April 1960	4.5	4.3	3.6	8.1	54	1.4	81	–	–	–	–	–	17.5	42	–	–	–	–	–
May 1963	4.2	5.7	4.9	9.0	46	1.3	72	7.4	37	21	–	98	20.8	50	–	–	–	–	–
Oct. 1966	4.7	4.5	3.6	8.3	49	1.4	72	7.44	43	28	72	91	14.2	42	–	–	–	–	–
June 1968	4.0	5.5	4.4	8.4	56	1.2	73	7.42	34	21	80	96	12.0	40	–	–	–	–	–

When first seen in October 1958, the findings were ventilatory defect with a normal exercise diffusing capacity. January 1959: little change as a result of 4 months of bronchodilator treatment. On September 2, 1959, he had more sputum and considerable dyspnea. On September 7, 5 days later, he was in hospital with severe bronchospasm and definite hypercapnia. Sixteen days later (September 23) function had returned to previous values. In May 1963, he had minimal dyspnea and was still fully employed. Ten years after his first study, function is unchanged. Note the normal diffusing capacity throughout, except for the initial resting value. The CO extraction and exercise tests on that day, however, were normal. The predicted diffusing capacity in 1968 was 12.1.

Chronic Bronchitis

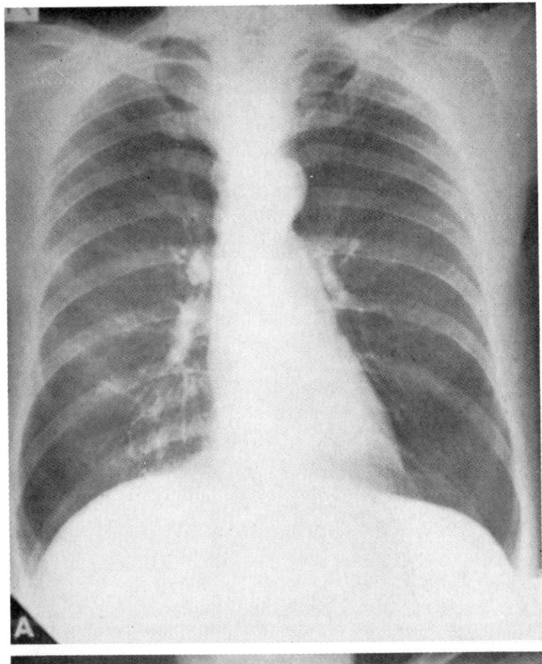

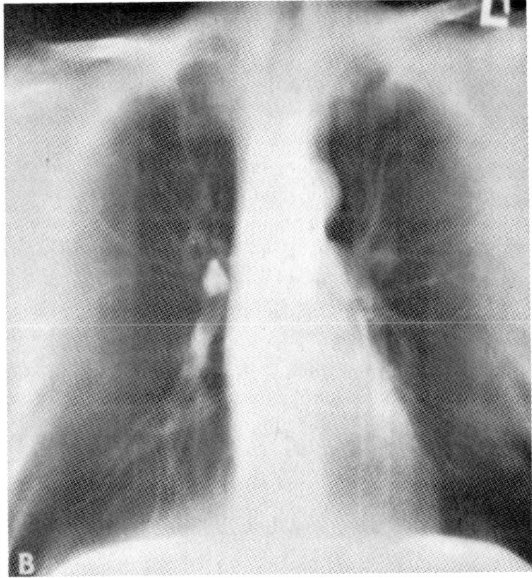

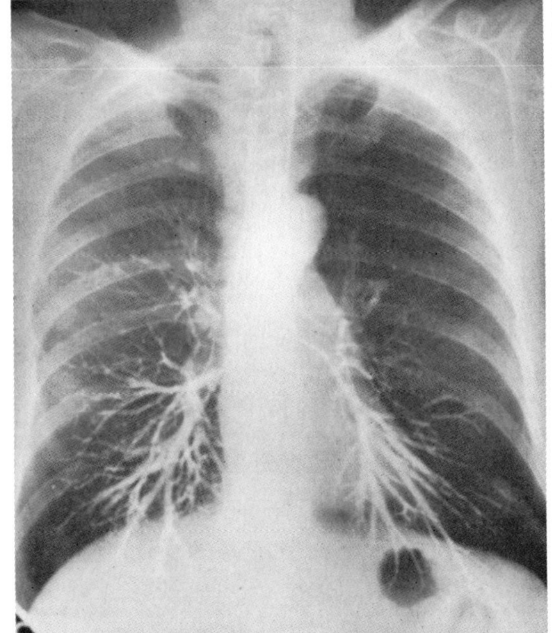

Summary. A middle-aged man with typical chronic bronchitis. The absence of morphological emphysema can be inferred from the normal exercise diffusing capacity and normal tomograms. Note constancy of ventilatory defect, possibly due to collapse of lower-lobe bronchi on forced expiration. Hypercapnia occurred at a time of severe bronchospasm, but is not normally present.

CHRONIC BRONCHITIS WITH AN ABNORMAL FEV_1

Since the prognosis of chronic bronchitis is greatly influenced by whether or not the arterial blood-gas tensions are normal, it is useful to categorize patients with chronic bronchitis and ventilatory defect on this basis. There is a general relationship between the severity of the ventilatory defect and the likelihood of the arterial blood gases being abnormal; but many factors combine to blur the relationship, particularly the presence of hypoventilation or emphysema (*see* later discussion). A further difficulty is that no differentiation can be based on a single observation of the blood-gas tensions, since these may be deranged in an acute exacerbation of infection and subsequently return to normal. In spite of these difficulties, the categorization is useful for discussion and descriptive purposes.

With normal arterial blood gases

Presumably the majority of patients with chronic bronchitis exist for very many years with some diminution of FEV_1, little change in lung volumes, a normal static compliance, some defect of gas distribution, and a normal diffusing capacity and arterial blood gases, although the alveolar–arterial O_2 difference and V_D/V_E may be abnormal. Development of chronic hypercapnia and cor pulmonale without any morphological emphysema probably occurs only in a small percentage of such patients; and although presumably a larger number develop these changes with or without hypercapnia, we still know little of the natural history of this process (*see* later discussion).

It is therefore common to encounter a patient, almost invariably a cigarette smoker in early middle life, with a chronic productive cough; a chest x-ray showing definite overinflation; some physical signs of airway obstruction (which may, however, be evanescent); with none of the criteria the clinician may use to detect the presence of any considerable degree of emphysema, but with a mild or moderate impairment of FEV_1—perhaps this may be between 70 per cent and 40 per cent of the predicted value. Relatively few very detailed studies of patients at this stage have been published, but on the basis of our own experience, such a man may show the following pattern of function change.

The inspiratory capacity, functional residual capacity, and total lung capacity will be normal, but the expiratory reserve volume may well be decreased and the residual volume increased. The ratio of residual volume to total lung capacity will be somewhat increased.[2512] Studies of lung mechanics[2644, 2745] reveal a normal lung recoil or static compliance but a sharp fall in dynamic compliance as respiratory frequency increases, indicating abnormal time constants in the lungs. Tests of inert-gas distribution may be abnormal,[2512, 2628] reflecting the same phenomenon. The uptake of carbon monoxide and the diffusing capacity, whether measured by single-breath or by steady-state methods, will probably be normal. The arterial blood gases at rest will be normal but may become abnormal in exercise. Studies of radioactive-xenon clearance will reveal abnormal zones in the lung, most commonly at the bases, in which there is a discrepancy between clearance of xenon cleared after delivery by perfusion and clearance after equilibration of the lung with xenon in the gas phase.[2532]

These changes taken together indicate interference with function in the peripheral airways smaller than 2 mm in diameter. The reduction in expiratory reserve volume is to be attributed to premature airway closure. The obstruction in peripheral airways accounts for the mechanical and distributional changes which, in turn, results in nonuniformity of ventilation distribution and $\dot{V}/\dot{Q}$ ratios among very small units in the lung rather than on a grossly regional basis. How reversible such changes are cannot yet be stated; one may remark that this is a most important question for study in the next few years.

If this view of the pulmonary function status of patients at an early stage of chronic bronchitis is an accurate one, then it is of great importance that the physician should not underrate the necessity of instituting prompt treatment and of emphasizing to the patient that his disease is at a stage when cessation of smoking and prompt attention to every chest infection may be critical to him in preventing the advance of the disease to the next stage. It is not justifiable to equate a slight diminution in FEV in chronic bronchitis with a similar change in a patient with spasmodic asthma. As we have pointed out,[2532, 2572] in patients with asthma such a change is not accompanied by the changes in peripheral clearance of xenon found in men with chronic bronchitis with only mild diminution in FEV_1, and it is perhaps significant that emphysema is not a common development on a basis of spasmodic asthma.

With abnormal arterial blood gases

In 1949, Baldwin and her colleagues noted presence of severe $\dot{V}/\dot{Q}$ disturbance and cor pulmonale in a patient whose lungs at autopsy showed little morphological emphysema,[934] and since that time others have described similar cases,[26, 958, 998, 2295] and Hentel[903] gave them the name of "fatal chronic bronchitis." Since 1965, much attention has been given to this entity. In that year, Briscoe and Nash[2551] suggested that patients with chronic obstructive lung disease could be divided into two categories on the basis of clinical criteria. Type A patients were considered to have considerable morphological emphysema, whereas patients in Type B were considered to be suffering mainly from severe chronic bronchitis complicated by hypercapnia and often progressing to cor pulmonale.

In a recent study of the function abnormalities in these two groups, King and Briscoe[2530] characterized Type A cases as having not much cough, not much sputum, chronic fixed dyspnea, faint breath sounds, translucent lung fields, low diaphragms, a thin body build, a low cardiothoracic ratio, absence of right ventricular failure, and a hematocrit of less than 50 per cent. By contrast, the Type B case was seen with the reverse of these characteristics. The Type A case had much larger lung capacity, as measured by the TLC or the FRC, than the Type B case.

The work of Burrows,[2504, 2526, 2547, 2675] Filley,[2510] Mitchell,[2503, 2509, 2537, 2546] and Fletcher,[2644, 2728, 2746] independently and in collaboration, has done much to clarify the differences between the two syndromes and to throw light on the prognosis of the two types. However, it is clear that many patients are seen in whom the criteria are mixed; it has not proved to be a simple matter to correlate morphological change with physiological and clinical state. We have discussed elsewhere some of the difficulties inherent in equating either chronic bronchitis or emphysema with specific patterns of function abnormality,[2557] but it may be useful to summarize the issues that can now be seen to lie behind the general question.

(a) Cases of bronchiectasis were included in some of the original papers.[2504] It is clear that severe generalized bronchiectasis is usually associated with bronchiolar obliteration, and there may be severe $\dot{V}/\dot{Q}$ disturbance and cor pulmonale;[2524] but for analytical purposes it is important that these cases should not be considered under the same heading as chronic bronchitis.

(b) McNicol and Pride[2501] have described four patients in detail, all of whom had chronic bronchitis, but in all of whom the clinical presentation with abnormal blood gases was attributable, in major part, to unexplained hypoventilation. Unless these patients are as carefully studied as they were by these authors, there is a real possibility that the abnormal blood gases will be attributed solely to the presence of chronic bronchitis. The problem of CO_2 sensitivity in chronic bronchitis is not a simple one,[2747] and it is not clear what role a reduced central response to CO_2 plays in the development of the Type B syndrome.

(c) It is not clear how important generalized centrilobular emphysema, even of mild degree, may be in causing the abnormal arterial blood-gas tensions. This problem is discussed later (*see* Chapter 7).

(d) The increased markings found in the plain chest x-ray in the absence of hypertranslucency have been considered by some authors to indicate inflammatory change. We have found, however, that this x-ray pattern may be associated with moderately severe emphysema, and it seems likely that many patients will be classified during life as Type B cases who do in fact have quite extensive centrilobular emphysema[2524] (see Figure 7–8); only if the functional consequences of this are denied can the whole syndrome be attributed to chronic bronchitis.

(e) The importance of pulmonary thromboses in this syndrome is very difficult to evaluate either morphologically or clinically.

(f) There are some unresolved differences in the literature between the classifications adopted by different authors. Filley[2510] (who uses the terminology PP and BB to describe the two variants) reported only small differences in steady-state diffusing capacity between the two groups of cases in each of the categories that he studied, whereas Bedell and Ostiguy[2516] found the single-breath $D_{L_{CO}}$ to be reduced in Type A and relatively normal in Type B. Simpson[2529] was unable to show that his patients were divisible into two separate populations. Furthermore, there is considerable difference of opinion concerning the prognosis in the two types. Fletcher[2746] concluded, "It has now been shown that it is the patient with severe obstruction without emphysema who has the worst outlook, though with modern management he may survive several episodes of oedematous cor pulmonale." Davis and McClement,[2533] in a major prospective study of patients at the Bellevue Hospital in New York, found the comparative mortality very similar between Type A and Type B cases, with a higher mortality in cases classified during life as "mixed," and Oswald[2748] found that the death rate was twice as high in patients with radiologic evidence of emphysema in the plain film compared to those with a normal plain film over a five-year period of follow-up in a group of patients with emphysema and chronic bronchitis.

In summary, it seems clear that a valid separation can be made between the two ends of the spectrum of chronic obstructive lung disease. It is not clear how far the different syndromes are influenced by differing sensitivities to CO_2 and by variations in reactivity of the pulmonary vascular bed. Richards, in 1960,[996] pointed out the possible importance of this latter factor, and Mitchell and his colleagues at the Tenth Aspen Conference[2509] brought together these influences in a synthesis of contemporary knowledge. However, we feel that the importance of chronic bronchitis in contemporary industrial societies rests on grounds other than its occasional primary lethal effect, and in the majority of patients who die of chronic obstructive lung disease the presence of emphysema complicating chronic bronchitis has been an important factor contributing to the $\dot{V}/\dot{Q}$ derangement.[2524]

NATURAL HISTORY AND PROGNOSIS OF CHRONIC BRONCHITIS

Many studies of the prognosis of chronic obstructive lung disease have included patients with advanced emphysema, as well as others with moderate or severe chronic bronchitis, and for this reason it has not been easy to determine the course of the disease in milder cases. However, during the past few years a number of studies have been published which permit a better assessment than was formerly the case.

Brinkman and Block in two papers[2749, 2755] have recorded follow-up data on 1317 men between the ages of 40 and 65 who were selected in 1958, when they were working full time, and re-examined in 1964. All except 48 were accounted for at that time. The deterioration in maximal midexpiratory flow rate was not more rapid in the bronchitic than in the normal patients, although the values were consistently lower in those with symptoms of bronchitis, and no appreciable effect of having stopped smoking could be documented. In this study, the rate of change was not greater in 39 of the men whose x-rays were considered to show evidence of emphysema. The overall mortality was slightly higher in the bronchitic patients than in the normal patients, but the difference was not statistically significant. Fletcher[2635] found the mean deterioration of FEV_1 to be −28 ml/year over a five-year period in a large group of men with chronic bronchitis, and the rate of deterioration was unaffected by the purulence, or otherwise, of the sputum and by the frequency of episodes of acute chest infection. In a further series,[2751] he reported that there had been an average decline in sputum volume from 1.9 ml in 1961 to 0.91 ml in 1966, the sputum being measured during the first hour of the morning. A rather higher rate of FEV_1 decline of −46 ml/year was reported by Jones and his co-workers[2691] in a group of men studied in London and Chicago, and in this group the vital capacity declined by −120 ml/year. In a study of serial measurements of peak flow rate in a general practice, Gregg [2752] found that episodes of acute chest infection were seldom followed by a sudden deterioration of function. Davis and McClement,[2533] reporting a prospective study of 600 patients over a period of about 12 years, found that the death rate was four times that predicted for the population as a whole; but these patients were more severe since 83 per cent of them had been hospitalized an average of 2.5 times for respiratory disease before they were admitted into the survey in 1955. They found, however, that patients with "asthmatic" bronchitis had, in general, a better prognosis, which was, however, unfavorably influenced by an elevated arterial CO_2 tension. In a follow-up study of 287 patients over a four-year period in the Veterans Administration Cooperative Study in the United States,

Renzetti, McClement, and Litt[2750] found that for men with an FEV_1 of less than 0.5 liters, the mortality was 89 per cent; when the FEV_1 was between 0.5 and 1.45 liters, it was 44 per cent; and when it was greater than 1.49 liters it was 26 per cent over the period of the follow-up. These investigators also made the interesting observation that the prognosis was adversely affected by the presence of hypoxia and by living at an altitude compared to sea level. Simonsson[2753] found little deterioration of ventilatory function in 57 bronchitic patients over a period of 45 months. Other series of cases have included men with moderately advanced emphysema and have shown a high level of mortality[2758, 2759] often related to the original level of dyspnea.[2748, 2757]

The data we have so far reported from the Canadian Veterans Study of chronic bronchitis[2512] conform to most of these conclusions. Analysis is not yet complete for a ten-year period, but it is evident that there are considerable variations in pulmonary function change between men of similar age and smoking habits in the same city. This conclusion is illustrated in Table 6–1.

It cannot yet be said with certainty what proportion of men, age 45, with mild chronic bronchitis, either continue for the next 20 years in that state, or, on the other hand, develop emphysema or progress to a more severe form of chronic bronchitis with $\dot{V}/\dot{Q}$ disturbance of gross degree and cor pulmonale. Nor can any opinion backed by data yet be

TABLE 6–1 Changes in Pulmonary Function Tests in Three Patients with Chronic Bronchitis

	Year	VC	FRC	TLC	ME%	FEV 1/min	MMFR 1/sec	D_{Lco}	Fractional CO Uptake
PATIENT A	0	4.5	4.7	7.6	48	111	3.8	22.5	0.46
	1	4.9	4.9	7.5	48	136	3.9	21.3	0.46
	2	4.6	4.6	7.3	55	137	4.3	21.2	0.47
	3	4.4	4.4	7.5	42	127	3.8	22.1	0.47
	4	4.7	4.7	7.5	61	135	3.6	24.0	0.47
	5	4.8	4.6	7.7	47	135	4.0	21.4	0.48
	6	4.9	3.9	7.3	33	137	3.9	23.9	0.55
	7	4.5	4.5	7.7	46	133	4.1	19.0	0.49
PATIENT B	0	4.2	4.1	6.6	44	110	3.3	23.6	0.42
	1	4.1	3.8	6.3	46	102	2.7	21.0	0.41
	2	4.0	2.7	5.6	42	115	4.0	26.0	0.38
	3	3.8	3.3	6.1	38	104	4.1	23.8	0.44
	4	3.0	3.4	6.1	45	96	2.9	14.2	0.35
	5	3.9	3.4	6.3	31	102	3.7	19.0	0.34
	6	3.2	3.1	5.9	26	98	3.4	13.0	0.31
PATIENT C	0	2.4	3.8	6.0	25	55	0.7	11.7	0.33
	1	2.4	3.6	5.6	30	54	1.1	12.6	0.31
	2	2.4	3.5	5.6	25	49	0.7	12.7	0.37
	3	2.1	4.2	6.1	26	39	0.6	12.9	0.35
	4	2.2	3.9	5.8	22	38	0.4	9.1	0.30
	5	2.1	3.4	5.4	25	36	0.4	6.0	0.28
	6	1.9	4.1	5.9	17	30	0.3	6.0	0.25

Note: These pulmonary function test data were obtained from three patients under observation in the Canadian DVA Study of chronic bronchitis.[2512] All of these three patients are in the Winnipeg Group; all are cigarette smokers and have continued to smoke over the period of observation. The x-rays of patients A and C were considered to show overinflation but no emphysema, and the x-ray of patient B was considered to be normal at the time of admission to the survey. These data indicate the type of variation that may be encountered between individuals not revealed by average changes in function. In each case, the observations in year "0" are the mean of ten visits to the laboratory. Note that patient A does not appear to have changed, patient B shows little change in ventilatory tests but a significant change in CO transfer; and patient C shows considerable deterioration in all aspects of function

VC = vital capacity; FRC = functional residual capacity; TLC = total lung capacity; ME% = mixing efficiency % (closed-circuit helium distribution index); FEV = forced expiratory volume over 0.75 seconds ×40; MMFR = maximal midexpiratory flow rate: D_{Lco} = resting-end tidal steady state D_{CO}; fractional CO uptake = $\frac{F_I - F_{EX}}{F_I}$ for CO (Data courtesy of Dr. D. P. Snidal of Winnipeg.)

given as to the comparative importance of smoking, environment, and episodes of acute infection in determining the natural history of chronic bronchitis. Since the first two of these factors have already been shown to affect the incidence of the condition, it must be assumed that at least both of them operate to worsen the prognosis.

EFFECTS OF CIGARETTE SMOKING ON PULMONARY FUNCTION

There seems little doubt that cigarette smoking is responsible for an increase in respiratory symptoms and an increased morbidity and absence rate from chest infections even in young people who might not be classifiable as chronic bronchitics. In a group of children, aged 13 and 14, Holland and Elliott found that respiratory symptoms were closely related to smoking,[2771] and others have shown that there is an increased morbidity in adolescents and young adults.[2762, 2763] During the last five years it has become apparent that cigarette smoking causes some changes in pulmonary function without overt bronchitis. Most observers have found a decreased ventilatory capacity,[2004, 2005, 2006, 2766] and there is evidence of slight decrease in vital capacity and residual volume.[2003] However, it must be remembered that the FEV_1 is insensitive to quite considerable increases in airway resistance in the smaller airways, and it cannot be inferred that the lung is normal if this measurement is within the normal range. The specific conductance, calculated from .the measured conductance and the thoracic-gas volume, was found by Pelzer and Thomson to be different between smokers and nonsmokers in a group of 82 adults of widely varying age.[2767]

Using a single breath of oxygen and subsequent comparison of the computed "inert-gas distribution lung volume" and the total lung capacity measured in a body plethysmograph, Ross and his colleagues[2761] found differences between smokers and nonsmokers, indicating impairment of gas distribution related to long-term smoking. This conclusion is supported by the studies of Stanescu and his co-workers who measured the slope of the nitrogen concentration after a breath of oxygen in carefully controlled studies on 87 selected subjects.[2772] Although in both old and young subjects the FEV_1 was not much different, as between smokers and nonsmokers, in the older group, with an average age of about 50 years, the slope of nitrogen concentration was shown to be significantly greater in the smokers. Martt[2007] and Rankin and his colleagues[2774] found differences in single-breath D_{Lco} between smokers and nonsmokers, and this could also be demonstrated by Krumholz and his co-workers[2769] in a matched group of 9 smokers and 9 nonsmokers of comparable age and at rest; it seems likely that these differences may be attributable to a small alteration in $\dot{V}/\dot{Q}$ distribution, no doubt related to the ventilation distribution difference found by Stanescu.

Strieder and Kazemi[2799] have provided interesting data confirming the $\dot{V}/\dot{Q}$ disturbance in young asymptomatic cigarette smokers, by finding an increased alveolar–arterial oxygen tension difference in the smokers, particularly when the subjects were supine.

A number of workers have studied the effect of stopping smoking on pulmonary function. Peterson, Lonergan, and Hardinge[2775] found some improvement in FEV_1 one month after stopping, and after eighteen months of abstinence, the MMFR had increased by 0.6 liters/sec. Although most of these subjects admitted to some cough, they were not definite chronic bronchitics. An increase in ventilatory capacity was demonstrable after six weeks of abstinence in 10 young cigarette smokers studied by Krumholz, Chevalier, and Ross,[2768] who also noted an increased D_{Lco} (single breath) at rest, but not on exercise, after smoking was stopped. These workers have also reported that smoking has a measurable effect on the pulmonary compliance.

A single inhalation of cigarette smoke causes a two- to threefold increase in airway resistance as measured in the body plethysmograph, in both smokers and nonsmokers. This effect[483] is probably due to the irritant effect of smoke particles and is mediated by the vagus nerve, since it is blocked by atropine.[2570] The greater the depth of inhalation, the greater is the effect.[2764] Aviado and Samanek,[2770] in experiments on dogs, have confirmed that cigarette smoke or an aerosol of nicotine to one lung causes initial bronchoconstriction involving the vagus nerve, and that subsequent bronchodilation occurs involving the sympathetic system. There is considerable literature illustrating the adverse effects of cigarette smoke on ciliary activity and lung clearance mechanisms.[909]

All this evidence indicates that the effects of cigarette smoke are far more subtle than just causing mucous-gland hypertrophy. One can ascribe the increased respiratory morbidity to interference with lung defense mechanisms, including ciliary activity, and probably also with the normal phagocytic function of alveolar macrophages. There seems little doubt that uniformity of gas distribution is affected presumably by changes at the terminal bronchiolar level, although these may well be reversible at least in the initial stages. The early involvement of the terminal airway units in chronic bronchitis mentioned earlier[2532] presumably indicates that these are already considerably affected before major changes in large bronchi have occurred and before the FEV_1 has been grossly affected. It needs to be emphasized that these effects underlie the increased respiratory disease morbidity among cigarette smokers, although there is still much to be learned of the exact mechanisms responsible.

In some individuals, heavy cigarette smoking over a period of many years seems to lead to neither mucous-gland hypertrophy[2773] nor to much change in pulmonary function,[39] but these fortunate individuals must be considered exceptions to the general rule rather than the majority.

RELATION TO BRONCHIAL CARCINOMA

It is clear from data published in many countries that, wherever the incidence of lung cancer has risen, the certified incidence of chronic respiratory disease also has increased. This generalization is broadly true, although it is to be expected that there will be discrepancies between different countries, since the criteria determining whether chronic bronchitis and emphysema are notified as causes of death vary greatly from one country to another. Evidence suggesting that patients with chronic bronchitis may be more likely to develop bronchial carcinoma has been excellently summarized by Passey, who concluded that some of the difference in mortality from lung cancer reported from different countries might be explained by a different incidence of chronic bronchitis.[920] He suggests the possibility that the excess of mucoid secretion and its viscidity may interfere in some way with bronchial epithelial cells, making them for some reason more likely to undergo malignant change. It seems very likely that the major factors responsible for chronic bronchitis also play a major part in the incidence of lung cancer,[834] but it is less certain that men with chronic bronchitis are, because of it, more likely to develop lung cancer. This question is by no means closed, however, and more recent studies have found a considerable mortality from lung cancer among men with chronic bronchitis.[2758] The data do not yet appear complete enough for a firm opinion to be given about whether the presence of chronic bronchitis of itself adds to the risk of developing cancer of the lung.

SUMMARY

The advances in knowledge of chronic bronchitis over the past few years have been considerable. Its world-wide importance has been established; there is beginning to be a basis for judgment on the relative importance of different environmental factors in its etiology; the early effects of mild chronic bronchitis on the lung have begun to be disclosed; the occurrence of severe disturbance of pulmonary function with gross abnormalities of gas exchange and consequent cor pulmonale as a nonreversible form of the disease has been documented. The present generation of chest physicians is unlikely to underrate the importance of this disease, as was commonly done only a few years ago. Yet many complicated problems remain to be solved. Among these are the interaction of air pollution and climate; the problem of individual sensitivity or relative immunity from the effects of cigarette smoke; and the difficulty in understanding the natural history of progression of the disease. The physician should bear in mind that the use of one term, "chronic bronchitis," on the one hand to describe mild symptomatology, and on the other to describe the severe form that the disease may take, may lead to some confusion, and that the effects of cigarette smoke and chronic bronchitis are much more subtle than can be measured simply by a test of forced expiratory flow rate.

PULMONARY EMPHYSEMA

CHAPTER 7

DE L'EMPHYSÈME DU POUMON

La maladie que je désigne sous ce nom est fort peu connue, et n'a été jusqu'ici exactement décrite par aucun auteur. Je l'ai cru longtemps trés-rare, parce que je ne l'avais rencontrée ou remarquée qu'un petit nombre de fois. L'usage du cylindre m'ayant conduit à en soupçonner l'existence chez plusiers malades, et l'autopsie ayant vérifie ce diagnostic, j'ai lieu de croire qu'elle est assez commune . . . .

RENÉ THÉOPHILE HYACINTHE LAENNEC, Paris, 1819[2806]

INTRODUCTION

Pulmonary emphysema now attracts so much attention from epidemiologists, pathologists, physiologists, and physicians that it is difficult to realize that until after 1945 very little experimental work had been attempted. Laennec believed he could diagnose emphysema in many patients by stethoscopy, but he was careful to confirm his opinion of the prevalence of the condition by autopsy studies. Thirty years ago, many physicians were confident of their ability to diagnose the condition during life; but at the present time many prefer not to use the word "emphysema" at all, classifying all patients with chronic bronchitis and emphysema as having chronic obstructive lung disease. The present difficulty in defining the disease cannot be attributed to any dearth of consideration of it—and indeed its morphological definition is now relatively clear-cut. Much uncertainty remains, however, in the area of its diagnosis during life, in the question of how much of the observed defect in function during life can be attributed to emphysema and how much to "bronchitis," and the exact pathogenetic basis of the disease remains to be unraveled.

During the past ten years, many books,[6, 7, 11, 2508] symposia,[22, 24, 26, 2509, 2644] and approximately 60 papers a year have appeared on various aspects of the disease. This concern is attributable to four main factors. First, there is evidence of a continuing increase in the incidence of the disease. In heavily polluted industrial areas of Europe, chronic lung disease accounts for 40 per cent of patients with congestive heart failure,[892] and in the United States the reported death rate from emphysema has increased alarmingly. In New York City, the Health Commissioner in 1964 reported that the death rate from emphysema had increased by a factor of ten over the past 10 years, and the mortality for the United States as a whole increased from about 3000 in 1950 to over 20,000 per annum in 1964 from chronic bronchitis and emphysema,[2736] and the present data show that the *rate* of increase of these two diseases is still increasing. Second, every chest physician has become increasingly concerned about the number of patients he sees with emphysema, for many of whom he can do little.[2529] Third, it may be noted that surgery is being undertaken for greater numbers of patients who are over 60 years of age. The incidence of emphysema in random autopsy studies shows that in a cigarette-smoking man of this age, the lungs are unlikely to be free of some degree of emphysema.

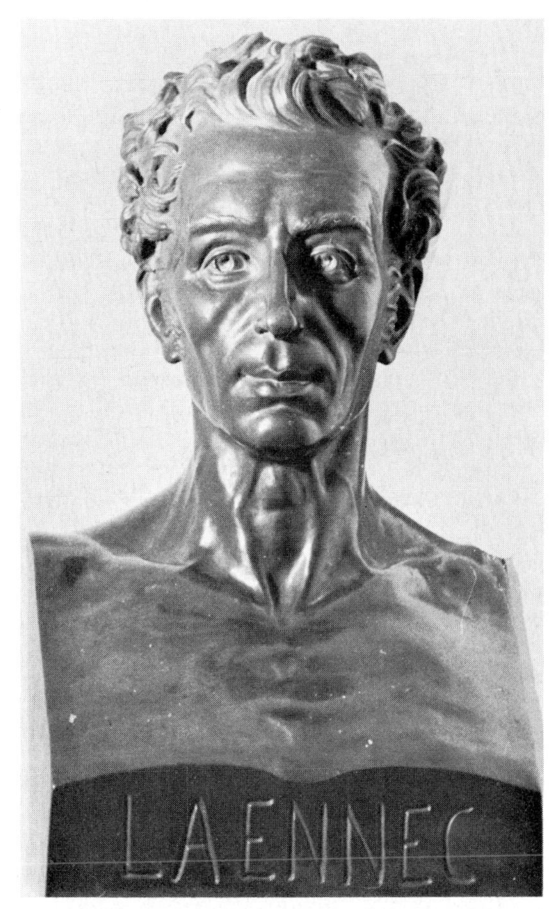

FIGURE 7-1. This striking bust of Laennec is placed close to the amphitheatre of the Charity Hospital in Paris where he taught the art of auscultation. The new Faculté de Medicine building in the Rue des Saint-Pêres in Paris occupies the site on which the hospital stood, but the amphitheatre is preserved. Professor Bargeton of the Department of Physiology in the new building kindly arranged to have this photograph taken.

Finally, emphysema is similar to atherosclerosis in that it is a common and important disease for which many etiological factors are known, but their mechanism and interaction remain to be understood.

PATHOLOGY

Many reviews of the pathology have appeared in the last few years, and the bibliography is extensive.[2012, 2508, 2517, 2548, 2779, 2805] In this section, only the broad outlines of this complex subject will be discussed.

In 1952 Gough[798] described two fundamentally different types of emphysema now known as centrilobular and panlobular, and with Leopold[799] he amplified this description five years later. Until then, as reference to contemporary textbooks will confirm, knowledge of emphysema bore little relation to the facts as they are now understood. In the past fifteen years, as a result of a great deal of work by several groups of pathologists in many countries, a reasonably clear picture of the anatomical pathology of pulmonary emphysema has been established. The reason for the long delay in evolution of accurate knowledge of emphysema is of some interest. In the first half of the nineteenth century there was great interest in the morphology of emphysema, and comprehensive descriptions were documented in the literature. Thereafter, use of the microscope led to concentration of attention at the cellular level, and the overall gross appearance of the lung was neglected. The study of detailed anatomical pathology outstripped clinical understanding of the disease, and accurate pathological recognition of emphysema therefore served little useful purpose. During this period, pathological studies of the lung were used mainly as a basis for speculative thinking on the etiology of emphysema. The pathological diagnosis then became reduced to the microscopical examination of samples taken at random of uninflated and irregularly collapsed lung, a singularly unsuitable technique for the study of a disease concerned with relative air-space size.[2777]

As pointed out in Chapter 4, there is now general agreement that pulmonary emphysema has to be defined in anatomical terms. Two such definitions of emphysema are currently available, and each has its respective advantages and defects. The Ciba symposium[815] defined emphysema as a condition of the lung characterized by increase beyond the normal in the size of air spaces distal to the terminal bronchiole, either from dilatation or destruction of their walls. Both the American Thoracic Society[2013] and the World Health Organization[2014] limited the use of the term emphysema to enlargement of these air spaces accompanied by destruction, enlargement without destruction being termed "overinflation." This is the definition we prefer, although it does not define what is meant by "destruction." For instance, the aging lung shows an increase in size of air spaces together with an increase in the size of the alveolar pores, and it is not clear whether this should be termed "emphysema" or "overinflation." However, apart from this special case, the destructive changes are easily recognized, and to a great extent are independent of minor differences in the degree of inflation of the lung.

It is difficult to make a satisfactory classification of all types of emphysema on the basis of either of these definitions, although some of the difficulties can be resolved by listing the known types of emphysema and overinflation, as we have done recently,[2012] without any attempt at classification. It then becomes apparent that possible sources of disagreement, terms of definition, and classification segregate themselves into relatively unimportant categories, which may then be designated by appropriate alternative terms.

CENTRILOBULAR EMPHYSEMA (SYNONYMS: BRONCHO- AND BRONCHIOLOSTENOTIC OBSTRUCTIVE EMPHYSEMA)

This is a primarily destructive lesion occurring in the region of the respiratory bronchioles. The destroyed and enlarged bronchioles tend to become confluent and form enlarged spaces situated toward the center of the lobules; this change is shown in Figures 7–2 and 7–3*B*. There is usually a rim of intact parenchyma between the destroyed zones and the lobular periphery, the lobule being the smallest discrete portion of the lung surrounded by lobular septum (synonym: secondary lobule of Miller[561]). The changes of centrilobular emphysema appear to occur more frequently and more severely in the upper zones of the lung.[645, 2518] In any given area, the respiratory bronchioles in individual lobules are characteristically unequally involved, and there is variation from lobule to lobule. The walls of the spaces frequently are pigmented, but this is perhaps no more than the pigment that occurs normally in this location. Evidence of old inflammation of distal bronchioles and of the bronchiole supplying the emphysematous spaces is always found. In the majority of instances these bronchioles are narrowed but appear patent, although inadequate support of the wall of the bronchiole may result in some kind of flap valve. During life, broncho-

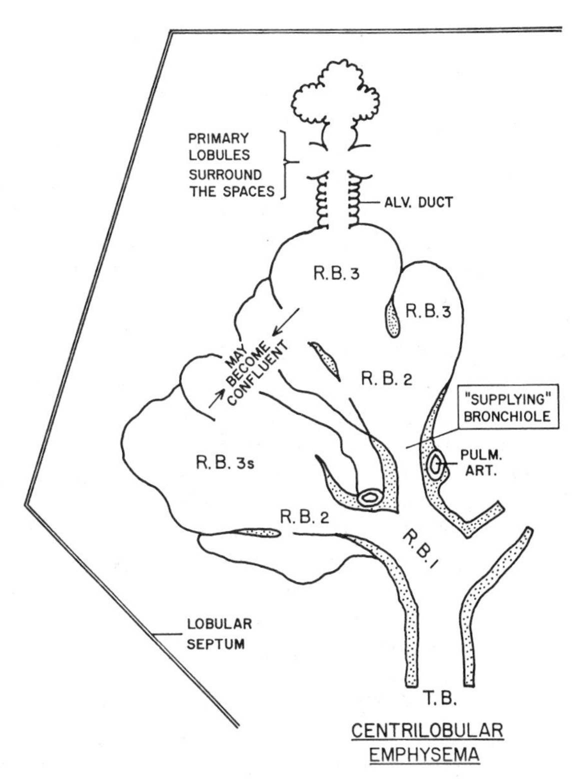

FIGURE 7-2. Schematic representation of a centrilobular emphysematous space, formed by enlarged destroyed respiratory bronchioles that have become confluent. (Reprinted from Thurlbeck, W. M.: Pathology Annual. Chronic obstructive lung disease. Edited by Sheldon C. Sommers, New York, Appleton-Century-Crofts, Inc., Division of Meredith Corporation, 1968 with the permission of the publisher.)

graphic medium may fill the enlarged centrilobular spaces, leading to the characteristic appearance of peripheral pooling. A considerable proportion of patients with a clinical diagnosis of emphysema and chronic bronchitis show these centrilobular changes, and it is very tempting to suppose that this lesion is the link that connects chronic bronchitis with emphysema. Gough[26] has pointed out the vulnerability of the terminal bronchiole to inhaled irritant substances, and this, together with recurrent infection, may well be responsible for the changes of centrilobular emphysema. It is in this region that the lesions of experimental emphysema produced in rats by the inhalation of oxides of nitrogen adsorbed onto carbon particles first appear.

The parenchyma distal to the emphysematous spaces, namely alveolar ducts, alveolar sacs, and alveoli, is often preserved, and in a classic case the picture is one of neatly punched-out holes separated by relatively normal alveolar structures (*see* Figure 7-3).

Another characteristic feature is the variable severity of the lesion from one part of the lung to another and even within the same lobule. Microscopically there is virtually always evidence of inflammation in the walls of the spaces and the supplying bronchioles.[2548] The latter are quite often narrowed but may be normal.[799] There may be a considerable loss of small airways,[2727] however. In advanced cases the peripheral parenchyma is abnormal; it may be compressed and distorted, and even destroyed. Thus there follows a stage in which arbitrary decisions have to be made concerning the type of emphysema, and, as in many other diseases, atypical forms are encountered about as commonly as classic examples. This difficulty of classification may explain the disagreement that exists concerning the functional significance of the lesion.

Centrilobular emphysema is much more common in males than in females,[2780] and it is usually associated with chronic bronchitis and hardly ever found in nonsmokers.[2524, 2789] Horsfield and his colleagues[2521] have illustrated the effect of centrilobular emphysema in three dimensions by the use of casts, but estimates of the volume of lung involved in the volume of the centrilobular spaces have shown considerable variation in different lungs and when different techniques of quantitation have been used.[2524, 2776, 2778, 2805, 2872] There seems little doubt, however, that in

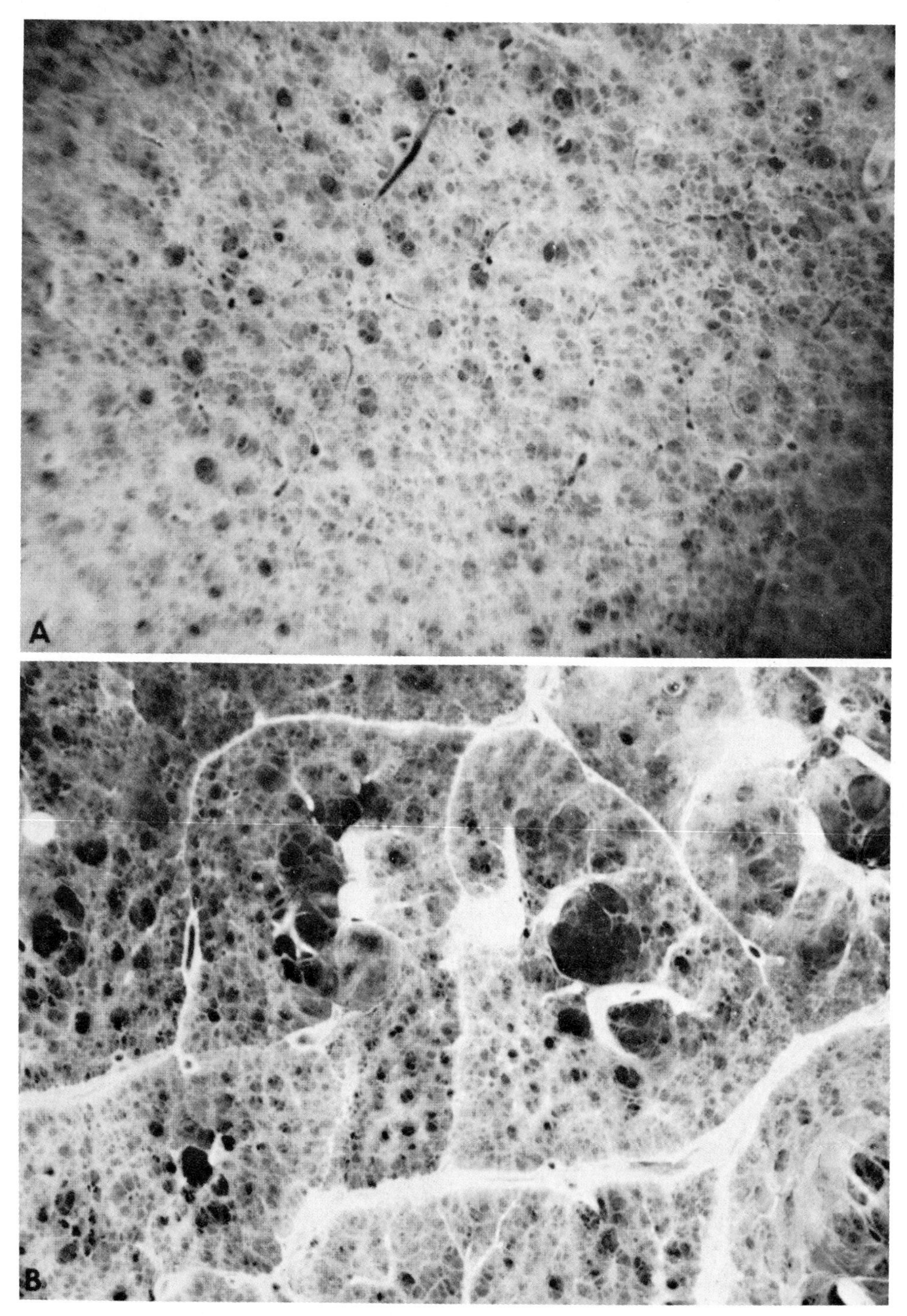

FIGURE 7-3. *A*, Normal lung as viewed through a dissecting microscope after fixation: magnification × 10. *B*, Centrilobular emphysema: magnification × 5.1. (The pulmonary arteries contain a barium-gelatin injection mass.)

severe cases much of the tidal volume must enter these spaces and may diffuse only with difficulty into the more normal parenchyma around them[2520] (a phenomenon to which we drew attention in the first edition of this book).

PANLOBULAR EMPHYSEMA (SYNONYMS: DESTRUCTIVE PANACINAR EMPHYSEMA, PANACINAR EMPHYSEMA, DIFFUSE EMPHYSEMA, GENERALIZED EMPHYSEMA, PRIMARY ATROPHIC SENILE EMPHYSEMA)

In this condition the entire acinus is involved, without selective involvement of any particular component, the acinus being that part of the lung distal to a terminal bronchiole. Such a definition might be interpreted to include examples of centrilobular emphysema that have progressed to involve an entire acinus or lobule, but these cases can usually be recognized by the presence of readily recognizable centrilobular emphysema in adjacent areas. The term "panlobular emphysema" should be reserved for a destructive process unselectively involving the lobule, in which the remaining tissue is attenuated, pale, and relatively unpigmented. Inflammation and distortion of bronchioles is inconspicuous, as compared with the finding in centrilobular emphysema. Strict interpretation of the terms "panlobular" and "panacinar" would imply that every part of the acinus or lobule should be demonstrated to be involved (see Figure 7–4). This can be established only by serial section of every suspected lesion, which is impracticable. The term is therefore applied to the characteristic morphological appearance.

The earliest stage of panlobular emphysema is best recognized on thick sections or on examination with a dissecting microscope of inflated lungs. There is coarsening of the honeycomb structure of the lung, with dissolution of the alveolar walls (*see* Figure 7–5*A*). Loss of parenchyma may be so extensive as to lead to the development of a cotton-candy appearance (*see* Figure 7–5*B*), and the remaining bronchi and blood vessels project above the cut surface of the lung as the parenchyma falls away. Panlobular emphysema appears to be more or less randomly distributed in the lung, with a tendency for more frequent occurrence in the anterior basal segment and the tip of the lingula and the middle lobe. It often becomes more severe in the lower zones of the lung, in contrast to centrilobular emphysema. It is rarely uniformly distributed throughout the lung.

There is some evidence that the mean age of patients who have predominantly panlobular emphysema may be higher than that of

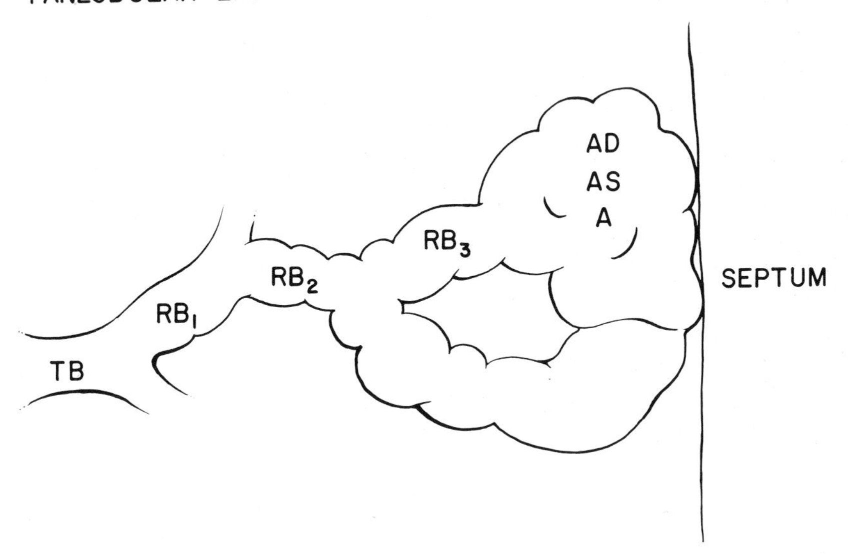

FIGURE 7–4. Diagramatic representation of panlobular emphysema, showing that all structures in the acinus are involved. (Reprinted from Thurlbeck, W. M.: Pathology Annual. Chronic obstructive lung disease. Edited by Sheldon C. Sommers, New York, Appleton-Century-Crofts, Inc., Division of Meredith Corporation, 1968 with the permission of the publisher.)

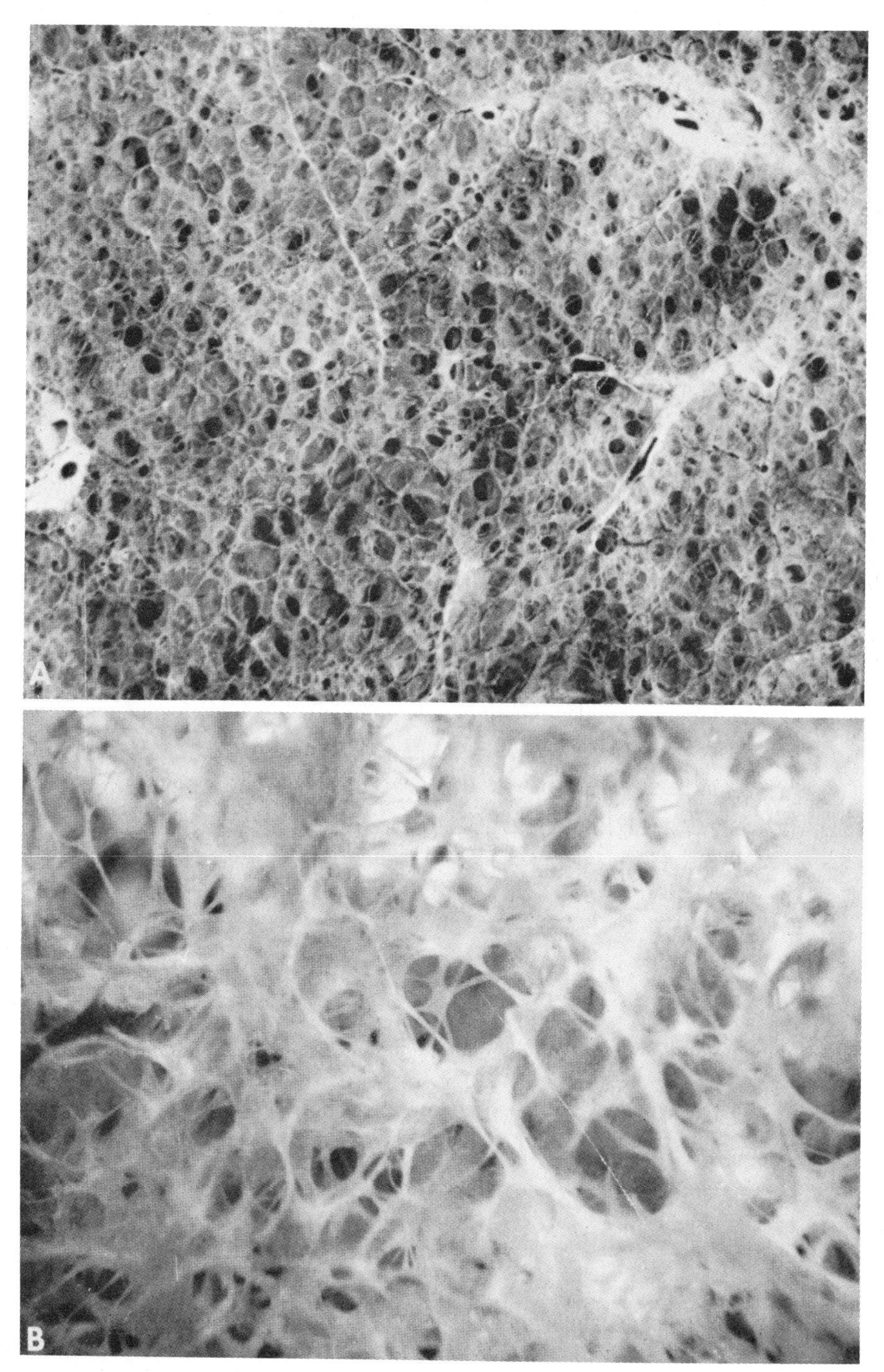

FIGURE 7–5. *A*, Mild panlobular emphysema: magnification × 6. (Compare with normal lung structure, as shown in Figure 7–3 *A*.) *B*, Severe panlobular emphysema: magnification × 10.

patients with predominantly centrilobular emphysema. Panlobular emphysema appears to be commoner than centrilobular in women, though it is clear that both types of emphysema are commoner in men than in women. The two forms are frequently mixed, particularly when the emphysema is severe in degree. Most observers implicitly or explicitly agree with Gough's contention that they represent two fundamentally different types of emphysema, though their frequent co-existence suggests that they have one or more common pathogenetic factors. A minority of pathologists feel that panlobular emphysema represents an end stage of centrilobular emphysema. Panlobular emphysema occurs in the type of emphysema related to deficiency of $alpha_1$ antitrypsin in the serum, and it is also found in unilateral emphysema (McLeod's syndrome). Both of these entities will be discussed later.

Paraseptal emphysema

If the periphery of the acinus is selectively involved, the emphysema is described as "paraseptal," since it was originally described in relation to the lobular septa.[654] These form the peripheral boundary of lobules, and hence the periphery of acini, composed of alveolar sacs and alveoli, abuts upon them. Since lobular septa are inconstant, paraseptal emphysema may be seen, occasionally in gross degree,[2785] around vessels and bronchi, and subpleurally. Because of this, some prefer the terms "periacinar,"[2508] "linear," or "superficial" emphysema, the last term being used when it occurs subpleurally. Paraseptal emphysema, particularly when subpleural in type, may be gross in degree but cause remarkably little interference with pulmonary function.[2508, 2785]

Irregular emphysema

Emphysema which shows no particular localization within the acinus is termed irregular emphysema, since the acinus is irregularly involved. It is most classically seen in relation to scarring, and thus is often termed paracicatricial or scar emphysema. However, the two are not really synonymous, since scar emphysema may involve a particular part of the acinus as in paraseptal emphysema. It is not clear whether the term irregular emphysema could be used to describe severe emphysema that is not otherwise classifiable. However, such emphysema is more appropriately termed "unclassified" or "end stage" emphysema.

Incidence of emphysema at autopsy

It is very difficult to assess the autopsy incidence of emphysema, since if the emphysema associated with small scars is included, emphysema is almost invariably present.[645] McLean, in Melbourne, Australia, estimated that emphysema was the primary cause of death in 2.6 per cent of 2000 patients at autopsy and a contributory cause in a further 4.1 per cent.[821]

It has been our experience that about 50 per cent of random autopsies show well-defined centrilobular or panlobular emphysema or both and about two thirds of males and one quarter of females will have one or both of these types of emphysema. Figure 7–6 illustrates the age distribution of emphysema in two teaching hospitals combined (Royal Victoria Hospital, Montreal, and the Massachusetts General Hospital, Boston). The populations from the two hospitals were so similar with regard to the frequency of emphysema that they may be representative of many teaching hospitals.

The age and sex distribution of the necropsies is also typical; the majority are in the 6th, 7th, and 8th decades, males predominate overall (54 per cent), but females predominate in the 8th and 9th decades. In Figure 7–6, "emphysema" represents the incidence of centrilobular, panlobular, and unclassified emphysema, the last forming about 3 per cent of the total. "Centrilobular emphysema" includes examples of pure CLE, and examples where CLE was thought dominant, or equally mixed with PLE. Even allowing for this mixture, CLE is the commonest type of emphysema up to and including the 7th decade, but in the 8th and 9th decades PLE predominates.

These general conclusions on the autopsy incidence are similar to those of Heard and Williams,[929] who reported that CLE or PLE was present in half of 50 patients examined at autopsy consecutively in London, England, and similar data have recently been reported by others from different parts of the world,[2780,

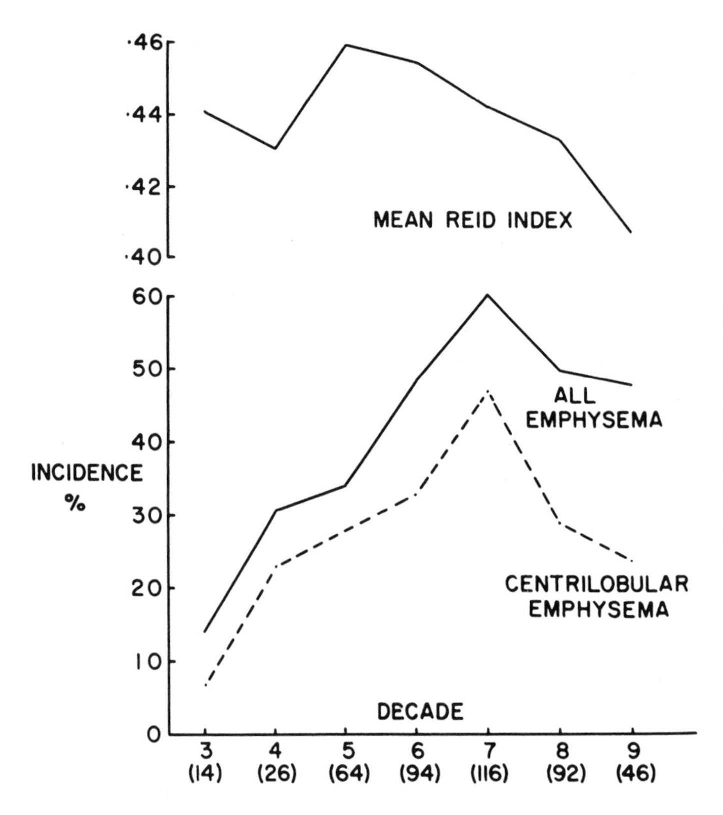

FIGURE 7–6. The mean Reid Index, incidence of emphysema, and incidence of centrilobular emphysema (alone or dominant) in a group of random necropsies. The number of cases in each decade is shown in parentheses. Emphysema reaches a peak incidence in the 7th decade and then declines, but the incidence of panlobular emphysema increases in the 8th and 9th decades. By contrast, the highest mean Reid Index is found in the 5th decade.

[2788, 2800] Australia, Florida, and Texas. Precise comparisons of relative geographic incidence must await the careful standardization of methods of assessment,[2528] but collaboration between two groups of pathologists in Cardiff, Wales, and in Erlangen, Germany, has recently enabled Gough and his collaborators[2801] to establish the higher frequency of emphysema at autopsy, by a factor of approximately three, in the Welsh population.

Otto, Orell, and Guettich[3686] have recently shown that the incidence of emphysema in 691 unselected autopsies in Stockholm is identical to that in Erlangen and thus similarly less severe than in Cardiff. Ishikawa and his colleagues[3682] have compared the autopsy incidence of emphysema between St. Louis, Missouri, and Winnipeg, in Manitoba. They found that the incidence of emphysema in the patients in St. Louis, with similar cigarette smoking history, was four times higher and that the emphysema was not only more frequent but was more severe earlier in life and apparently had progressed more rapidly. This study is of particular interest, since two of the authors had worked as pathologists in both of the cities about which they report, and hence the pathological criteria are very likely to have been uniform. They ascribe the difference largely to the very different air-pollution levels between the two cities.

Associated abnormalities

Cor pulmonale and vascular changes

The relationship of emphysema to cor pulmonale is complex, and we have recently presented a detailed discussion of the problem.[2524] Although all observers agree that there is a close association between blood-gas disturbances and the development of cor pulmonale, the literature contains many conflicting findings concerning the relationship between the extent of anatomical emphysema and the weight of the right ventricle at autopsy.[2794] In the series of patients we have described,[2524] there was a good general relationship between evidence of right ventricular hypertrophy and the extent and severity of emphysema, and we believe this to be the true state of affairs rather than the negative correlation claimed by some. Structural alterations in the pulmonary vessels have been considered by most authors to be inadequate to account for cor pulmonale, though Hicken, Heath, and Brewer, in a series of papers,[2793, 2794, 2802] have described morphological changes in the small pulmonary arterioles which they feel are specific only in cases in which hypoxia had been the factor precipitating pulmonary hypertension.

Thromboembolism is occasionally implicated as a cause of cor pulmonale in emphysema, though the importance of this during life is very difficult to assess. The bronchial arteries are often enlarged and more numerous than normal, but these changes are not nearly as striking as in bronchiectasis and probably are of little significance. Of greater importance is the often considerable size of the bronchial veins, which may be responsible for shunting deoxygenated blood to the left atrium. In some patients with pulmonary hypertension, significant pulmonary arteriovenous shunts have been demonstrated by arteriography.[2740] Some degree of left ventricular hypertrophy has been noted to be present in patients with emphysema and chronic bronchitis, both by ourselves[2524] and by others;[2807] the reason for this is obscure.

Bronchial changes

Since chronic bronchitis is very commonly associated with emphysema, the pathological changes in the bronchi characteristic of that condition are usually found. In addition to these, in the lungs of many patients with severe emphysema, particularly of the panlobular type, the medium-sized bronchi are thin-walled and almost translucent,[656, 2804] with a diminution in the size and number of cartilaginous plates. There is some controversy over whether there is an absolute loss of cartilage, however, and Restrepo and Heard[2637] were recently unable to confirm that this had occurred.

Alveolar fenestrae

Rainey,[2015] who made the first microscopical observations of emphysema, described fenestrations in the walls of air spaces in emphysema, a finding confirmed by subsequent observers; and it has been suggested that this finding may be the best criterion for the diagnosis of emphysema. The fenestrae have been regarded as enlarged pores of Kohn or as new tears; in support of the latter view is the observation that fenestrae are not only much larger than alveolar pores but also occur more frequently.

Changes in lung constituents

Pierce and his colleagues measured the collagen and elastin content of emphysematous lungs[2017] and concluded that, "The presence of emphysema was not associated with any significant alteration in collagen or elastin, or the ratio of these substances." Fitzpatrick[2796] has recently reported that in emphysematous lungs the content of neutral amino acids was strikingly reduced, and he suggested that this might indicate a genetic disorder involving elastic protein synthesis underlying the condition.

RADIOLOGY

General features

Up to about five years ago, there was much uncertainty surrounding the radiological diagnosis of pulmonary emphysema, and the correlation between the presence of morphological change and the radiological appearance was poorly understood. There were a number of studies that illustrated these difficulties,[1232, 2016] During the past few years, however, considerable advances in understanding have been made. It is clear that the correlation between the radiological assessment and the autopsy appearance is generally good,[2524, 2647, 2648, 2649, 2816] though there are still some areas of controversy. In general, the diagnosis of emphysema depends on the recognition of hyperinflation, the assessment of the state of the pulmonary vasculature, and the detection of a pattern of change that we have termed "increased marking pattern";[2524] these aspects will be discussed separately. We have recently published a detailed discussion of the radiological changes in emphysema, of which the following is a summary.[3688]

Hyperinflation

Since an increase in total lung capacity commonly occurs in emphysema, increase in lung size must be a major criterion of emphysema; however, since it occurs in other conditions, notably spasmodic asthma, its presence is not in itself sufficient for a definitive diagnosis.[1235] Moderately severe emphysema can also occur

(*Text continued on p. 169.*)

Case 8
Emphysema (Panlobular; Bilateral)

Summary of Clinical Findings. In 1956, this 41-year-old real-estate agent began to notice shortness of breath which was at first episodic and exertional but which gradually increased in severity and became continuous. Six weeks before his first admission, in November 1961, he developed a cough productive of about a cup of heavy yellowish sputum per day with occasional blood-streaking. He had lost 50 lbs in weight over the previous few years. His past history was noncontributory; he smoked a package of cigarettes a day.

On examination, the patient was not cyanosed and the respiratory rate was 20 per minute. His chest was enlarged in the AP diameter, with hyperresonance and decreased breath sounds over both lower lung fields. Investigations included various x-ray and pulmonary function studies Right heart catheterization and pulmonary angiography also were performed. The mean PA pressure was 18 mm Hg at rest, and on moderate exercise rose to a systolic of 48 mm Hg and diastolic of 28 mm Hg with a mean of 32 mm Hg. A sweat test was normal. He was considered to have emphysema localized to the lower half of both lungs, with bronchiectasis involving the left lower lobe. In February 1962, the right middle and lower lobes were removed.

The patient was readmitted for assessment in April and again in July of 1962. Although his general health had improved and he had gained weight, his dyspnea persisted with no diminution in severity and his cough had recurred. The left lower lobe was removed in September 1962.

Following operation he was slightly less short of breath and his cough and his sputum almost disappeared.

Over the next four years he gradually deteriorated, requiring several admissions for exacerbations of dyspnea. In 1966 he was again reevaluated. X-rays suggested bullous change in the left lower lung field. Radioactive scanning and pulmonary angiography revealed an absence of vasculature in the lingula, which was felt to be hyperinflated and compressing the left upper lobe. In April, 1966, the bronchus to the lingula was divided and ligated. At operation the lingula was noted to be hyperinflated and bullous.

He was readmitted in January, 1968. He had noted no improvement following operation. Cough was no longer a problem, but he was dyspneic after climbing ten stairs. Pulmonary function studies are shown.

Radiology. Postero-anterior (*A*) and lateral (*B*) projections of the chest reveal evidence of marked hyperinflation of both lungs, the deep retrosternal air space being particularly notable. The markings

	VC	FRC	RV	TLC	ME %	MMFR	$FEV_{0.75}$ ×40	pH	P_{CO_2}	HCO_3^-	O_2Hb %	$D_{Lco}SS_2$	CO Ext %	EXERCISE MPH	GRADE	$\dot{V}O_2$	$\dot{V}E$	$D_{Lco}SS_3$
Predicted	4.7	3.7	2.0	6.7	60	3.9	124	7.40	40	25	97	19.6	47					23.0
Nov. 1961	2.8	3.6	3.0	5.8	31	0.4	24	7.40	41	24	98	13.5	37	2	FLAT	0.83	22.2	11.3
Aug. 1962	2.3	3.7	3.2	5.5	32	0.4	28	7.40	37	22	99	11.9	35	1	FLAT	0.80	27.6	12.7
July 1963	2.1	3.7	3.1	5.2	31	0.4	25	7.38	36	22	90	11.8	37	2	FLAT	0.85	25.4	11.1
Jan. 1966	1.9	3.2	2.7	4.6	49	0.2	18	7.38	43	22	100	12.5	39	1	FLAT	0.55	18	10.2
Feb. 1969	2.1	3.9	3.3	5.4	33	0.4	25	7.44	36	24	95	6.6	34	1	FLAT	0.60	18	12.4

In November 1961, the vital vapacity was decreased and the residual volume 1 liter more than the predicted value. The mixing efficiency was reduced, and ventilatory function grossly impaired. The diffusing capacity was reduced at rest, but, more significantly, did not increase with exercise. There was no hypercapnia. Studies of mechanics revealed a reduced elastic recoil and an airway resistance of 7.0 cm H_2O/l/sec on inspiration. Xenon-133 studies showed severe reduction in both ventilation and perfusion over both lower zones and a normal rate of clearance from both upper zones. In August 1962, 6 months after removal of the right middle and lower lobes, there had been essentially no change in function. Xenon distribution showed good perfusion and ventilation over the right upper lobe, which had expanded considerably. In July 1963, after removal of the left lower lobe in November 1962, practically no change in function either for better or for worse had occurred, though the maximal negative intrapleural pressure had become more negative as a result of the removal of the lower lobes.

In January, 1966, prior to lingular divorcement, there had been a fall in the flow rates with a further reduction in vital capacity. The resting Dco was unchanged and did not rise with exercise.

In February, 1969, volumes and flow rates have not returned to their original values; although the diffusign capacity has fallen by half, it rises with exercise.

Blood gases have never shown hypoxia or hypercapnia.

Emphysema (Panlobular; Bilateral)

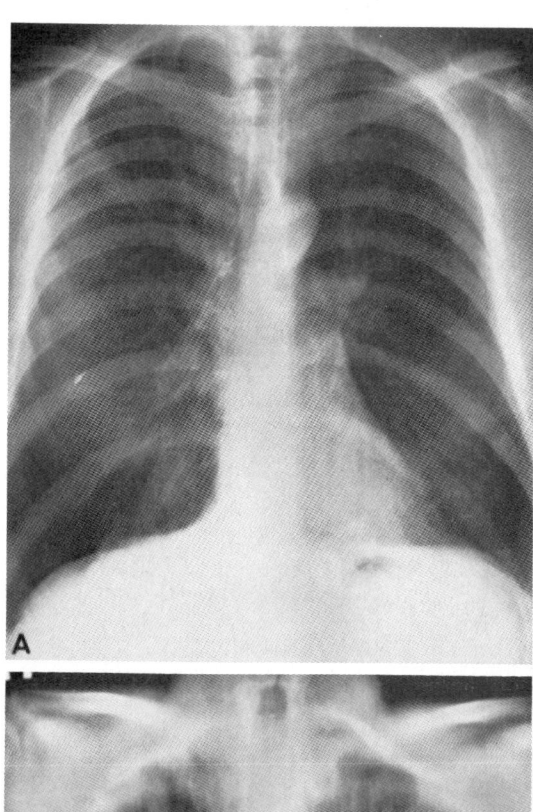

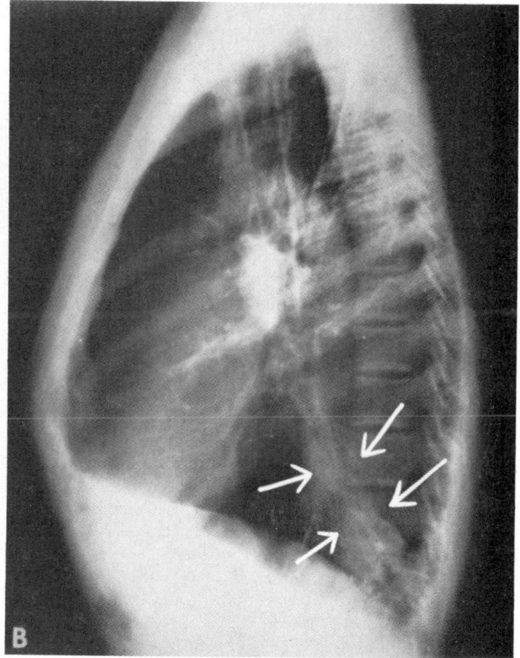

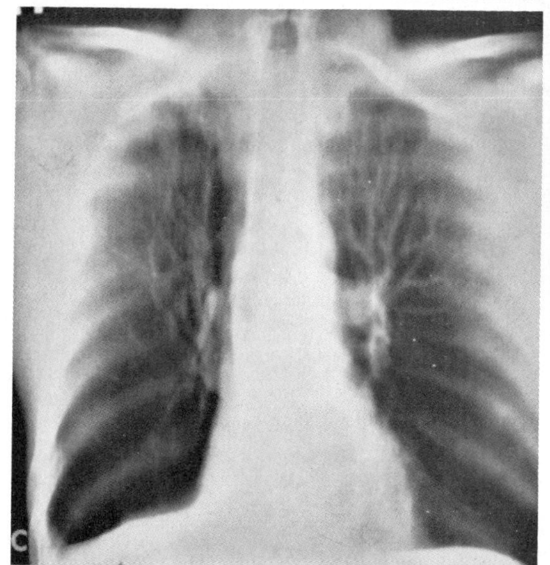

to the basal segments of the left lower lobe show increase in size and loss of definition, and are crowded together (*arrows*). The original films suggested a relative deficiency of the vasculature to the lower lung fields compared with the upper, a change which is difficult to reproduce. A presumptive diagnosis of emphysema was made, predominantly involving the lower lungs, with the additional findings of bronchiectasis of the basal segments of the left lower lobe. A tomogram (*C*) of both lungs confirmed the discrepancy in the size of the vessels to the upper lungs compared with those to the lower and supported the diagnosis of localized lower-lobe emphysema.

A pulmonary angiogram (*D*), exposed 1 second after the rapid injection of 40 ml of contrast medium into the main pulmonary artery via a cardiac catheter, demonstrates a larger size and greater number of arteries to the upper lobes than to the lower. The arteries to the right middle lobe

(Case report continued on page 168.)

Case 8
Emphysema (Panlobular; Bilateral) (Continued)

and lingula are affected in a manner similar to that in the lower lobes. The series of films made at half-second intervals following the beginning of the injection showed significantly earlier filling of the peripheral radicals of the upper lobes than of the lower, indicating less resistance in the former.

Pathology. The right lower lobe (*E*), middle lobe and basal segments of the left lower lobe were destroyed by severe panlobular emphysema. The apical segment of the left lower lobe showed mild to moderate panlobular emphysema. The bronchi showed irregular thinning of their walls, with slight cylindrical dilation in the right lung. Varicose and cylindrical bronchiectasis was present in the basal segments of the left lung. The bronchial mucous glands were hypertrophied (Reid index 0.52) and chronic bronchiolitis was present.

Summary. This 41-year-old man had bilateral panlobular emphysema in both lower lobes, with a slight degree of cylindrical bronchiectasis. Little improvement in symptoms followed removal of the right lower lobe, but a considerable decrease in sputum was noticed after the left lower lobe was removed. Note the remarkable constancy of pulmonary function measurements in spite of removal of both lower lobes.

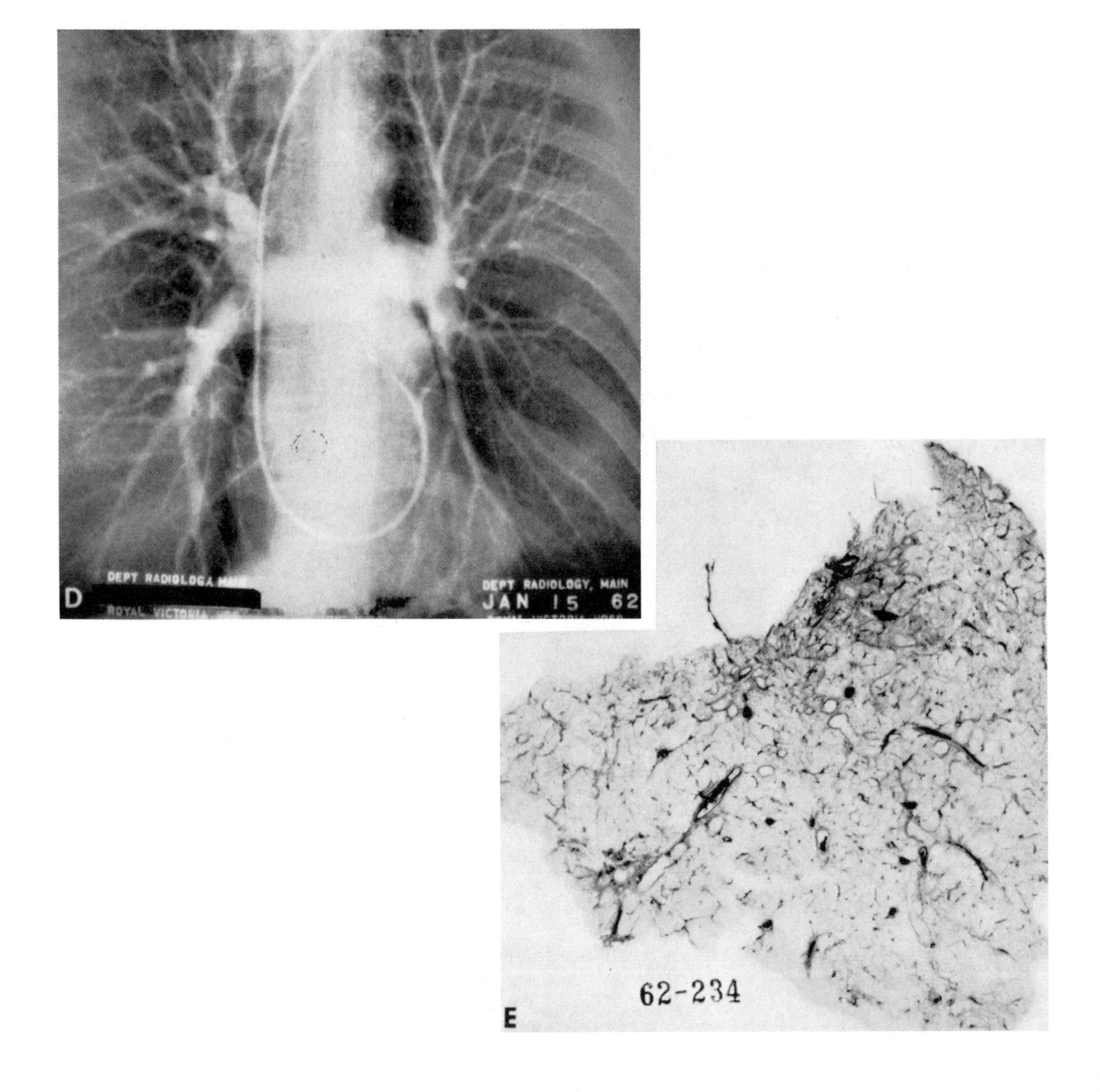

without a striking degree of hyperinflation being present, and this circumstance appears to occur most frequently if centrilobular emphysema is present.[2524, 2808] Probably the most dependable single piece of evidence of pulmonary hyperinflation is a flattening of the diaphragmatic domes. It is important to realize that the level of the diaphragm in relation to the rib cage may be misleading, since a full inspiration in a normal subject will commonly depress the domes to the level of the 11th rib posteriorly, a point below which it is uncommon to see the diaphragm even in advanced emphysema. Flattening of the domes, especially as viewed in lateral projection, is almost always found in the presence of severe emphysema, and serration of the diaphragm is also of some diagnostic value.[2808] An actual concavity of the domes downward, although uncommon, is almost pathognomonic of emphysema; it has rarely been observed by us in other diseases in which air trapping occurs, no matter how severe the distention (except in children with severe asthma).

Other signs of hyperinflation that should be looked for include increase in the antero-posterior diameter of the chest, particularly of the retrosternal air space, anterior bowing of the sternum, and accentuation of the thoracic kyphosis. The heart shadow is generally narrow and long,[2810] largely due to diaphragmatic depression.

A number of studies have shown that the total lung capacity can be reliably calculated from planimetry of the chest x-ray, and there is good evidence that this volume may be more accurate than estimates based on gas dilution methods,[2539, 2817] since they agree closely with total lung capacities measured by body plethysmography.

In addition to these static changes that may be observed on simple postero-anterior and lateral films made in full inspiration, the presence of "air trapping" may be more readily assessed by observing alterations in movement of the chest wall and diaphragm. By viewing films taken in both inspiration and expiration, or preferably by observing deep respirations fluoroscopically, the normal approximation of ribs on expiration may be seen to be reduced or absent in emphysema; the excursion of the diaphragm, normally 3 to 6 cm, may be restricted to one interspace or less; the reduction in translucency of the lungs that occurs normally on expiration may not occur at all.

State of the pulmonary vasculature

It has been recognized for some years that the presence of areas of diminished vasculature is very suggestive of the presence of morphological emphysema. Such areas can be shown to better advantage tomographically,[710, 1866] and angiography in addition is not often indicated. Studies with radioactive isotopes, both using ^{131} iodine-tagged serum albumin[2811, 2880] or ^{133}xenon dissolved in saline,[1684, 2812, 2815] have shown that these areas are regions with greatly diminished perfusion, and the correlation between the measured perfusion and the pulmonary vasculature, as viewed by tomography and angiography, has been good. There is little doubt that such areas are most commonly the site of localized emphysema or of emphysema more severe than that elsewhere in the lungs.[2524, 2647] It is useful, therefore, to describe this as "the arterial deficiency (A.D.)" pattern of emphysema.[2524] Abnormalities of vascular pattern may be demonstrable in the absence of significant hyperinflation,[2813] but it must be remembered that inconstant abnormalities of pulmonary blood flow have been demonstrated to occur in patients with severe bronchospasm with spasmodic asthma, in whom the pattern disappears after the attack is over (*see* Chapter 5). It cannot be stated that the arterial deficiency pattern is diagnostic of panlobular emphysema; its presence seems to depend less on the type of morphological emphysema present than on its severity and distribution.

Pattern of increased markings (I.M. type)

We have drawn attention recently[2524, 3688] to the correlation between a radiological appearance of increased markings without evident arterial deficiency and without hyperinflation that occurred in a number of patients whose lungs were later studied in detail at autopsy. They had, in addition to chronic bronchitis, considerable emphysema, predominantly centrilobular in type but often consisting of mixed panlobular and centrilobular emphysema. Other observers have commented on similar cases in the recent literature. Mori and his colleagues noted that, on occasion, moderately severe emphysema occurred without radiological signs of hyper-

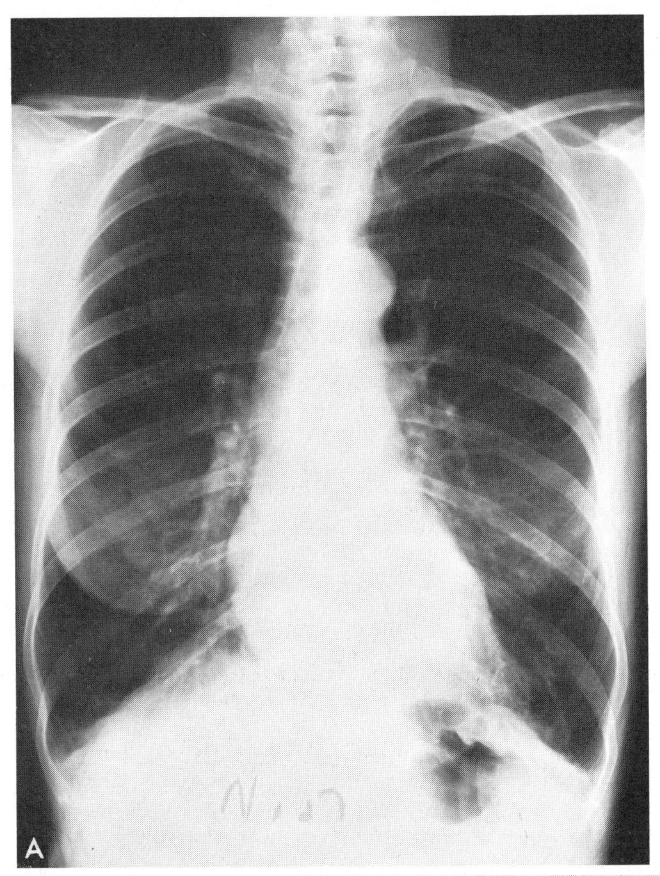

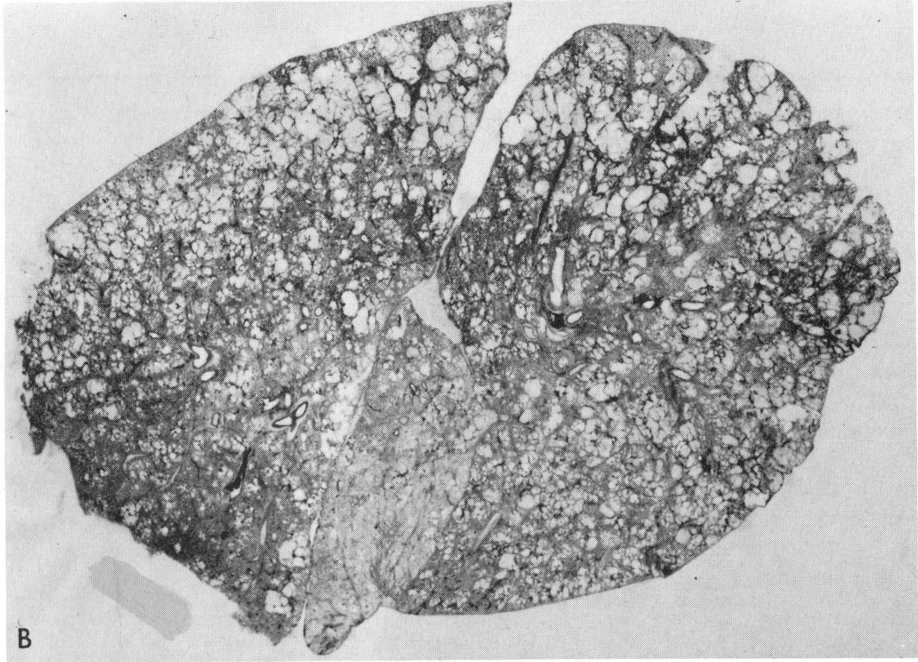

FIGURE 7–7*A*. Typical arterial deficiency emphysema (PA projection). *B*. Paper-mounted, whole lung section of patient whose roentgenogram is shown in Figure 7–7*A*. There is severe emphysema, interpreted as being centrilobular in type.

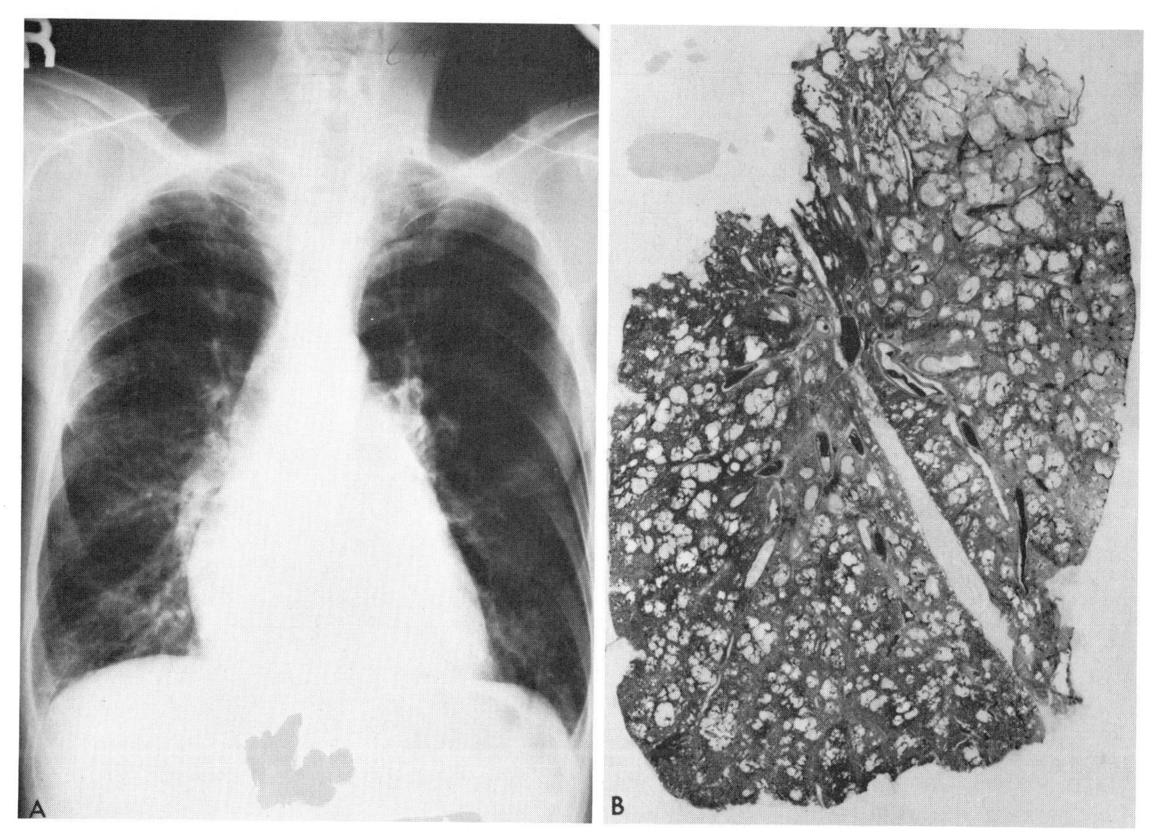

FIGURE 7–8*A*. Typical "increased marking emphysema" (PA projection). *B*. Paper-mounted section from the patient whose roentgenogram is shown in Figure 7–8*A*. Obvious severe centrilobular emphysema is present; despite this, the classic roentgenographic arterial deficiency pattern of emphysema was absent.

inflation;[2808] and Katsura and Martin[2816] in a study of 75 consecutive autopsies observed similar cases, some of them complicated by the coexistence of pulmonary tuberculosis or other infiltrate.

If the condition is complicated by severe $\dot{V}/\dot{Q}$ disturbance with alteration of the arterial blood-gas tensions and cor pulmonale, the radiological appearance is characteristic. The main pulmonary trunks are enlarged, there is rapid tapering of the vessels in the mid-lung, and the lungs show increased markings. Such a film, if accompanied by evidence of irreversible airway obstruction, is very suggestive of the presence of moderately severe centrilobular emphysema together with chronic bronchitis.

It seems likely to us for reasons that we have discussed in detail elsewhere[2524, 3688] that this type of patient gives rise to particular difficulty in correlating the radiological appearance with the morphological state of the lung. If the radiological criteria of "emphysema" are so described that patients with the "I.M." pattern are considered, as a matter of clinical definition to be suffering *only* from chronic bronchitis, considerable confusion is bound to result. For this reason it seems preferable at this juncture to recognize that the pattern of change described as an "increased marking" type may be commonly associated with moderately severe and usually generalized centrilobular emphysema. In the first edition of this volume, we described these patients (on page 184) but had not at that time been able to study a sufficient number with autopsy correlation to separate them into a distinct category; this now appears to be possible.

Other vascular changes

A number of authors have described detailed angiographic studies in patients with chronic lung disease,[2813, 2818] and greater

Radiologic Diagnosis	EMPHYSEMA GROUP						Bronch-iectasis	Asthma
	O	I	II	III	IV	V		
No Emphysema	OOOOO	MMMPCC	UCC	CC			M	OO
AD		MPC	MU	MMMPPPC	MUC	MMPPC	M	
AD/IM				M	MPCC	M		
IM		M	CC	P	CC	MUCCC	PC	
?IM				P				

FIGURE 7–9. The radiologic diagnosis of emphysema compared to the severity and type of emphysema. AD = arterial deficiency emphysema. IM = increased marking emphysema. AD/IM = mixed AD and IM. ? = doubtful. C = centrilobular emphysema, P = panlobular emphysema, M = mixed emphysema, U = unclassified emphysema, and O = no emphysema. (From reference 2524.)

vascular detail can be observed by selective peripheral angiography than with tomography. Jacobson and his colleagues[2740] have found evidence of pulmonary arteriovenous shunts in 4 of 46 patients studied by this method and found evidence that these might be of functional significance.

BRONCHOGRAPHY

Bronchography may reveal both morphological and dynamic abnormalities of the bronchial tree in emphysema. The morphological changes are dependent to some extent upon the presence or absence of chronic bronchitis, which is frequently associated with emphysema and which in itself will cause distinctive bronchographic changes (*see* Chapter 6). In emphysema, the generalized hyperinflation is reflected in splaying of the radicles of the bronchial tree, whose angles of bifurcation will be wider than normal. Not infrequently one encounters some difficulty in filling the more peripheral bronchial radicles, possibly because of a reduction in the ability of the emphysematous patient to aspirate bronchographic medium on inspiration as efficiently as a normal subject. In the absence of chronic bronchitis, the caliber of the segmental bronchial divisions is usually normal.[755]

In a technically satisfactory bronchogram in which good peripheral filling has been accomplished, one commonly sees certain abnormalities that are highly suggestive of emphysema, with or without chronic bronchitis. In 1953, Simon and Galbraith[765] first described certain patterns of bronchiolar deformity, the precise nature of which was subsequently established by Reid pathologically.[771] They described three basic bronchographic abnormalities:

1. *The termination of small peripheral bronchioles in small "berry-like" opacities* measuring 1 to 3 mm in diameter, for which the name "peripheral pools" was suggested. These were shown by Reid and subsequently by Leopold and Seal[1240] to represent the collection of opaque medium in a dilated bronchiole and more specifically in a centrilobular emphysematous space.

2. *The abrupt ending of bronchioles by squared, rounded, or tapered extremities.* Although Simon and Galbraith stated that this appearance of incomplete filling could occasionally be due to technical error, they felt that it generally represented evidence of bronchiolar disease, particularly when the ending was tapered. This conclusion was subsequently confirmed pathologically by Reid, who demonstrated that these abrupt endings represented opaque medium outlining the blind end of a bronchiole that was surrounded by collapsed lung.

3. *A "spiked" or "spider" deformity of distal bronchioles* in which several thin blind

bronchioles appear to extend outwards from a single point. By pathological–bronchographic correlation, Reid showed these to represent opaque medium outlining the blind endings of some terminal bronchioles.

Although these structural changes in the peripheral bronchiolar radicles are commonly seen in emphysema, they are hardly more striking than the alteration in the dynamic activity of the bronchial tree that may be observed fluoroscopically and recorded cinefluorographically.[755, 1242] In normal subjects, the first five divisions of the bronchial tree, beginning at the main-stem bronchus, react to forced expiration or cough in a uniform manner, showing a reduction in caliber from maximal inspiration to forced expiration that is proportional in all divisions. In emphysema, with or without chronic bronchitis, there has been observed repeatedly a disproportionate collapse of the central bronchi, particularly the main lobar bronchi, the segments distal to this collapse showing *less* reduction in caliber than normal. By measurement of the transverse diameter of several bronchial divisions cinebronchographically, it has been shown that in emphysema the lobar bronchi reduce their caliber by 67 per cent compared with 49 per cent in normal controls. Simultaneously, the fifth-stage divisions reduced in caliber by only 32 per cent in patients with emphysema compared with 45 per cent in the normal subjects.[755, 1242] These observations suggested that the central bronchi might make a greater contribution to expiratory airway obstruction in emphysema than had been thought formerly. That this is in fact true in some patients with emphysema has, we feel, been established by us,[772] using a combined manometric-cinefluorographic technique, in which intrabronchial pressures at various points in the bronchial tree, pleural pressure and air flow at the mouth were recorded simultaneously during cinebronchography. Whereas in normal subjects the pressure drop along the bronchial tree from the alveolus to the mouth is gradual and progressive, in some patients with emphysema a large pressure drop occurs across the lower-lobe bronchus coincident with the collapse observed cinebronchographically. At the moment of bronchial collapse, air flow at the mouth drops sharply while pressures within the bronchi distal to the obstruction remain high despite a rising intrapleural or driving pressure.

Variants

The radiological changes in three other varieties of emphysema deserve brief mention.

1. *Bullous emphysema,* discussed in some detail later in this chapter (*see* page 203) presents radiological features that are generally distinctive.[1239] The bullae may be single or multiple, and may vary in size from 1 to 2 cm up to the volume of a whole hemithorax. They tend to be located predominantly in the upper lung fields but may be so extensive as to involve three-quarters of the total volume of both lungs. Serial roentgenograms will frequently reveal their progressive enlargement. Their walls are usually of no more than hairline thickness and, without the aid of tomography, it may be difficult to distinguish them from the adjacent uninvolved parenchyma. This is particularly true when the bullae occur as part of a generalized panlobular emphysema, but here the diagnosis of bullous emphysema is surely semantic; cystic spaces measuring up to 1 cm in diameter are not uncommon in severe panlobular emphysema, and whether they should be considered as bullae or merely large emphysematous spaces becomes a matter of opinion or preference.

2. The radiological findings in *unilateral emphysema* will be described in the appropriate section, but they differ in no fundamental respect from those of localized emphysema occurring, for example, in the lower portions of both lungs, at least insofar as the vascular pattern is concerned. The radiological manifestations of hyperinflation and failure to empty observed in unilateral emphysema are striking because of the mediastinal shift and remarkable asymmetry of lung radiolucency that becomes obvious on full expiration; although identical physiological changes are occurring in bilateral localized emphysema, their appreciation is more difficult because of their symmetry.

3. So-called *senile emphysema* is by far the commonest form of "emphysema" seen radiologically. The typical configuration of an anteriorly bowed sternum, with an increased thoracic kyphosis but an otherwise apparently normal thorax, is seen many times by every radiologist. The diaphragm is generally normal in position and curvature, and lung markings are either normal or slightly more prominent than usual. In essence, the thoracic-wall changes represent the effect of slightly

Case 9
Pulmonary Emphysema and Chronic Bronchitis

Summary of Clinical Findings. This 66-year-old insurance salesman complained of a productive cough of 20 years' duration and increasingly severe dyspnea over a two-year period. The sputum averaged about ½ a cupful a day and was usually mucoid. When he was first seen he was smoking 20 cigarettes per day, but admitted a previous daily consumption of about 60.

The chest appeared to be held in a somewhat expanded position, and there was considered to be a generalized decrease in breath-sound intensity. Rhonchi, together with a prolongation of audible expiration, could be heard over all regions of both lungs. His blood pressure was 150/80, pulse 100/min; no signs of congestive heart failure were found. The hemoglobin was 16 gm per 100 ml, and the white-cell count 9500 per cmm. Repeated sputum cultures failed to grow any pathogens.

He was regularly seen over a two-year period, during which time he had a number of acute respiratory infections. His dyspnea progressed until he was short of breath even at rest. Signs of airway obstruction were constantly present over both lungs. There was no finger clubbing. Serial electrocardiograms revealed the development of tall P waves in lead 2, a large terminal S wave in V 6, and R wave in lead AVR.

The final admission was in December of 1962. He was severely dyspneic and too weak to expectorate. Although the arterial blood revealed some retention of CO_2, respirator treatment was not used in view of his age and because he was believed to be suffering from a severe degree of morphological emphysema.

Radiology. The postero-anterior roentgenogram of the chest (*A*) reveals some degree of pulmonary hyperinflation, better demonstrated in the lateral view (not reproduced) by a low, flattened diaphragm and a deep retrosternal air space. The lung fields are more translucent than normal. The plain films thus indicate the presence of generalized air-trapping. The pulmonary vasculature appears somewhat reduced in the left lung compared with the right, suggesting that, if emphysema is present, it may be more severe on the left.

The tomogram (*B*) made through the midlung zone demonstrates a sparsity of vessels in the peripheral lung fields, with rapid tapering of vessels as they proceed distally from the hila. The changes appear more or less symmetrical. This finding supports a diagnosis of diffuse pulmonary emphysema.

Pathology. At autopsy the lungs were very voluminous and were noted to collapse only slowly. As can be seen from the whole-lung section, severe emphysema was present on both sides but was more severe on the left (*D*). The least involved portion of the lungs was the right middle zone. The emphysema was mixed, being predominantly centrilobular in the upper zones and panlobular in the lower, with the left lower basal segments particularly severely involved. Extensive mucus was present in the bronchial tree, and there was hypertrophy of the bronchial mucous glands, the Reid Index being 0.56. Postmortem angiography of the left lung showed pruning of the small pulmonary arterioles, but no major regional differences could be demonstrated. Only mild changes were present histologically in the arterial tree. The right ventricle showed slight but definite enlargement; it weighed 75 grams, and there was a ratio of left ventricle and septum to right ventricle of 3.2.

These lungs are typical of severe emphysema of mixed type, with rather more asymmetry than is often encountered.

Summary. The radiological appearances and radioactive-xenon studies suggested that the left lung would be more extensively destroyed by emphysema than the right. At autopsy, this was confirmed, though both lungs were involved by severe emphysema of mixed type.

	VC	FRC	RV	TLC	ME %	MMFR	$FEV_{0.75}$ ×40	pH	P_{CO_2}	HCO_3^-	O_2Hb %	$D_{Lco}SS_2$	CO Ext %
Predicted	3.6	3.5	2.3	5.8	47	2.8	83	7.4	40	25	97	12.3	37
March 1961	2.8	3.9	3.2	6.0	30	0.5	22	7.4	35	21	98	8.2	24
Dec. 1962	–	–	–	–	–	–	–	7.35	54	27.8	88	–	–

The increased residual volume, lowered vital capacity, impaired gas distribution and reduced steady-state diffusing capacity, with the marked ventilatory impairment, are characteristic of pulmonary emphysema. When first seen, the blood gases were normal, but on the last admission there was some CO_2 retention and a fall in oxygen saturation. Radioactive-xenon studies performed in March 1961 showed slow ventilatory equilibration over all regions, particularly severe over the left middle- and lower-lobe regions. It was noted that the left side was relatively less well perfused than the right.

Pulmonary Emphysema and Chronic Bronchitis

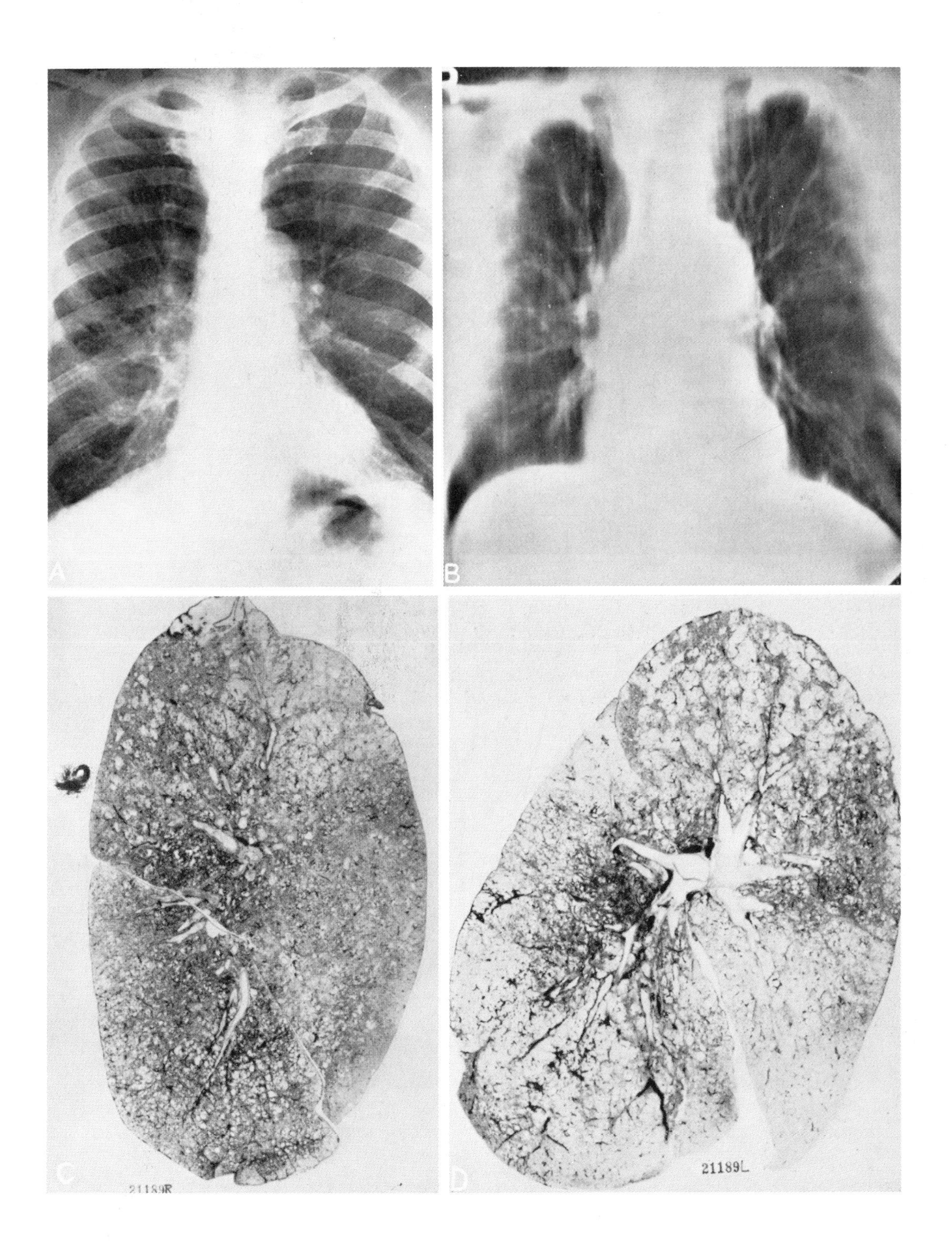

increased lung volume but there are few of the usual manifestations that categorize emphysema radiologically.[2809]

CLINICAL FEATURES AND CLINICAL DIAGNOSIS

It is important for the physician to realize that the clinical diagnosis of emphysema must be based on the assessment of clinical, radiological, and laboratory evidence and does not depend on any one criterion. We agree with others[2523] that the physician should attempt to assess the morphological state of the lung during the patient's life, and we do not believe that he should be content to classify all patients with signs of bronchospasm and dyspnea as having "chronic obstructive lung disease" and let the matter rest there. Nevertheless, any description of the clinical features of emphysema—as distinct from chronic bronchitis—is not easy. Criteria which have been used to separate the two conditions are discussed later.

It is very remarkable that the average age of men disabled with pulmonary emphysema seems to be constantly about 55 years, irrespective of the country from which the author writes. Thus, in our own series of 59 patients in London, England, 57 were men, of average age 57.5 years.[392] The 27 patients with chronic obstructive lung disease studied by Shepard and his colleagues in Baltimore averaged 53 years of age, and included only one woman.[420] Hammond's series of patients from Sheffield, England, were of average age 56 years;[940] the patients studied by Prime and Westlake in London, England, averaged 54.6 years;[945] a group studied by Holland and Blacket in Australia averaged 59 years of age;[945] and the patients with chronic pulmonary emphysema studied in the USA by Borden and his colleagues were aged 33 to 70, averaging 55 years.[2030]

In our pulmonary function laboratory in Montreal, the average age of patients with the changes characteristic of moderately severe emphysema is 55 years. Most of them give a 10- to 15-year history of cough antedating the onset of dyspnea. Often, sputum production has been inconspicuous, the patient seeking advice only when his activities become limited by exertional dyspnea. Initially the shortness of breath is noticed to be variable, depending upon climatic and other conditions, but later it is constant. Most characteristically the patient has been a cigarette-smoker for many years. It is essential that the physician learn to take a careful and painstaking history of the chronology of the onset of cough and dyspnea in these patients and establish whether or not the dyspnea is constant or remittent. Some patients date the onset of this symptom from a particular episode of pneumonia, or inadvertent contact with smoke or some other irritant. The more variable the severity of dyspnea, the more likely it is to be due to the reversible changes of chronic bronchitis or chronic infective asthma. To differentiate between the dyspnea of chronic bronchitis and that of emphysema may be very difficult.

The description of the physical signs associated with and attributed to emphysema is usually quite clear-cut in most textbooks of medicine. These books do not usually find space to tell the student how unreliable they have been shown to be. Although this unreliability was stressed many years ago[927] and repeated by others,[651] the first "observer-error" experiment on signs of chronic lung disease was carried out by Fletcher in 1952.[709] During the past five years there have been further studies of the same problem. In 1965, Smyllie and his colleagues[2822] evaluated the reliability of detection of 20 signs by 9 observers and concluded that "inter-observer repeatability of respiratory physical signs falls midway between chance and total agreement." In the same year, Schneider and Anderson conducted a similar study[2821] and concluded that "as was suspected, the present investigation demonstrated serious limitations in the ability of physicians to diagnose obstructive lung disease by physical examination." In 1969, Campbell described eight physical signs associated with airways obstruction and lung distention in addition to those commonly used,[2820] but he, in association with four colleagues, also found that these were, in general, no more repeatable than the more familiar signs.[2819] These authors also concluded that the repeatability of all the signs fell "about midway between that expected by chance and the maximum possible." It seems that the chest physician must resign himself to sitting in this rather insecure position; certainly he cannot afford to ignore the radiological and laboratory evidence with which he is presented.

In our experience, the clinical diagnosis of

emphysema is particularly difficult in four clinical situations: first, when the history of chronic bronchitis is, even on close questioning, unconvincing, and sputum production has been negligible; second, in patients in whom the vital capacity is relatively well preserved and the chest contour is normal; third, in patients who are known to have another cause of dyspnea, and in addition have mild chronic bronchitis; and fourth, in patients who are obese. In all of these circumstances, which are commonly encountered, unaided clinical diagnosis is often very difficult. Many physicians have emphasized that a carefully taken clinical history of unremitting dyspnea in a patient who has chronic bronchitis is the main clinical criterion of the presence of emphysema, and this diagnosis should at least be suspected, even if the physical signs are unconvincing.

The probability of making a correct prediction of the extent and severity of morphological emphysema during life, is, we believe, reasonably good if a careful assessment is made of all available information in each patient. We have come to this opinion after reviewing clinical, radiological, and laboratory data in relation to the autopsy appearance of the lung.[2524] Many physicians, however, still place too much confidence either in their own skill in physical examination or in the opinion of one radiologist who has studied only a single PA film and is unaware of the importance of the I.M. pattern of radiological change.

PULMONARY FUNCTION IN CLINICAL PULMONARY EMPHYSEMA

In the following subsections an attempt is made to provide an overall view of the commonly encountered disturbances of pulmonary function in emphysema.

VENTILATORY DATA

The quiet resting ventilation of patients with emphysema usually differs little from that recorded in normal subjects of equivalent age. Spirometer tracings taken at rest show an average respiratory rate of about 16/min. The minute volume, at about 10.0 liters/min, is not significantly different from normal, and consequently the tidal volume at rest is usually within the wide range encountered in normal subjects. The respiratory tracing may show some variation in base line—indicating considerable shifts in functional residual capacity—but in our experience this is much less commonly observed in patients with emphysema than in those with spasmodic asthma, in which condition it occurs quite commonly. The resting oxygen uptake is customarily within normal limits.

It has been shown that the resting level of ventilation can be slightly increased in patients with emphysema when they listen to simulated breath sounds.[2310]

MAXIMAL VENTILATION AND EXPIRATORY FLOW RATE

By contrast, the maximal ventilatory capability is invariably reduced in the presence of pulmonary emphysema. A constant impairment of air flow, uninfluenced to any considerable extent by treatment, is the single most constant and important functional defect associated with the disease. In the presence of moderately severe emphysema, the maximal breathing capacity may be reduced from a predicted level of about 100 liters/min to 20 or 30 liters/min and the maximal mid-expiratory flow rate from a predicted value of 3.4 liters/sec to 0.9 liter/sec, or less; these values will be found to increase by only 10 to 15 per cent on inhalation of a bronchodilator aerosol. Indeed, the constancy of the ventilatory defect is one of the remarkable features of clinical emphysema. No doubt in every pulmonary function laboratory, in common with our own, there have been patients in whom the ventilatory tests have shown the same degree of impairment over a five- or six-year period.

Fuleihan andAbboud have recently shown that the diurnal variation in FEV_1 in patients with emphysema is small.[2834] The improvement in maximal breathing capacity noted by Friend[933] in 12 patients studied initially in the winter and later in the summer might well have been related to seasonal bronchitis; for obvious reasons the expiratory flow rate of the patient with emphysema is sensitive to episodes of infection.

It is clear from the very considerable volume of function-test data in the literature that the persistent finding of a low ventilatory capacity is important in the diagnosis of emphysema. How nearly normal may this be

Case 10
Centrilobular Emphysema

Summary of Clinical Findings. This 66-year-old engineer was first admitted to hospital because of respiratory symptoms in November, 1958. He had undergone a subtotal gastric resection for gastric ulcer in 1956. He stated he had been "wheezy" for about 20 years but denied frequent colds or respiratory infections. In the preceding year he had become severely short of breath, tolerating only mild exertion, and was orthopneic. Over the same period he had developed a cough productive of thick yellowish sputum. Neither hemoptysis nor chest pain had ever been present. His ankles had been swollen for one week before admission. He smoked about 6 cigarettes daily.

On examination his temperature was 98° F.; blood pressure 180/120 mm Hg; pulse rate 90/min and regular. He was slightly confused and cyanotic, and dyspneic when lying flat. Jugular veins were distended. Chest movements were limited, with use of accessory muscles during respiration. The chest was hyperresonant and breath sounds were distant. Expiratory musical rhonchi were heard over the chest and inspiratory rales at the bases. Clinically the heart seemed enlarged. The liver was tender and palpable two finger-breadths below the costal margin and pitting edema of the ankles was noted.

On investigation Hb was 12.1 gm/100 ml; ESR 19 mm/hr; white-cell count 10,600/cmm (67 per cent mature neutrophils). Sputum culture revealed a light growth of *Haemophilus influenzae.* Chest x-rays were done, and pulmonary function studied (*below*). ECG showed peaked P waves in lead 2, which suggested right atrial hypertrophy. He improved quickly on a regimen of antibiotics, bronchodilators and digitalis and was discharged.

He was re-admitted in January and March, 1959, each time because of respiratory infections with exacerbation of his symptoms of shortness of breath and ankle edema. He responded quickly to treatment on the first occasion but on the last admission, after an initial improvement, gradually lapsed into confusion and drowsiness and died April 10. A chest x-ray had shown bronchopneumonia of the right lower lobe which did not respond to antibiotics.

Radiology. Postero-anterior (*A*) and lateral (*B*) roentgenograms of the chest reveal evidence of severe hyperinflation of both lungs, with a low flat configuration of the diaphragm and an increased anteroposterior diameter of the chest, particularly of the retrosternal space. The linear markings through the lower half of both lungs are widely spaced and diminished in number and caliber, although those to the upper lung fields appear fairly normal. Enlargement of hilar arteries is equivocal. The picture suggests diffuse emphysema more marked in the lower lobes.

A tomogram (*C*) of both lungs through the mid-sagittal plane reveals a remarkably normal appearance of the pulmonary arterial tree, both hilar and peripheral. The arterial deficiency suspected on the plain films is not substantiated. The radiological evidence for the presence of emphysema is thus equivocal.

Pathology. Widespread centrilobular emphysema was present throughout both lungs. The process was strikingly uniform throughout both lungs with no zonal accentuation. Every lobule appeared involved. The lesions were punched out, heavily pigmented, and fairly uniformly 4 to 6 mm in diameter (*D*). Altogether, the emphysematous spaces occupied 33 per cent of the lung parenchyma.

Summary. A 66-year-old man with generalized and severe centrilobular emphysema. Note the relatively normal appearance of the pulmonary vasculature although the pulmonary function, including the resting diffusing capacity, was considerably impaired.

	VC	FRC	RV	TLC	ME %	MMFR	$FEV_{0.75}$ ×40	pH	P_{CO_2}	HCO_3^-	O_2Hb %	$D_{L_{CO}}SS_2$	CO Ext %
Predicted	3.4	3.5	2.3	5.8	45	2.6	75	7.40	42	25	97	10.9	37
Nov. 1958	1.6	5.1	4.6	6.2	36	0.2	19	7.35	58	29	97	7.1	27
March 1959								7.44	56	35	90		

The function studies in November, 1958, were obtained two days before admission. The vital capacity is halved and there is hyperinflation (RV twice normal). Mixing is only slightly inefficient, but ventilatory function (MMFR and FEV) is grossly impaired. Diffusing capacity is reduced. The blood gases were measured two weeks later after the dyspnea had improved and the heart failure had cleared. Both the P_{CO_2} and bicarbonate are raised and the pH is at the lower limit of normal. He is fully saturated.

The last (March, 1959) arterial blood sample was drawn during the terminal admission shortly before he showed signs of confusion and drowsiness. The P_{CO_2} and bicarbonate are raised, the latter so much that the pH is well within the normal range. There is slight arterial unsaturation.

Centrilobular Emphysema

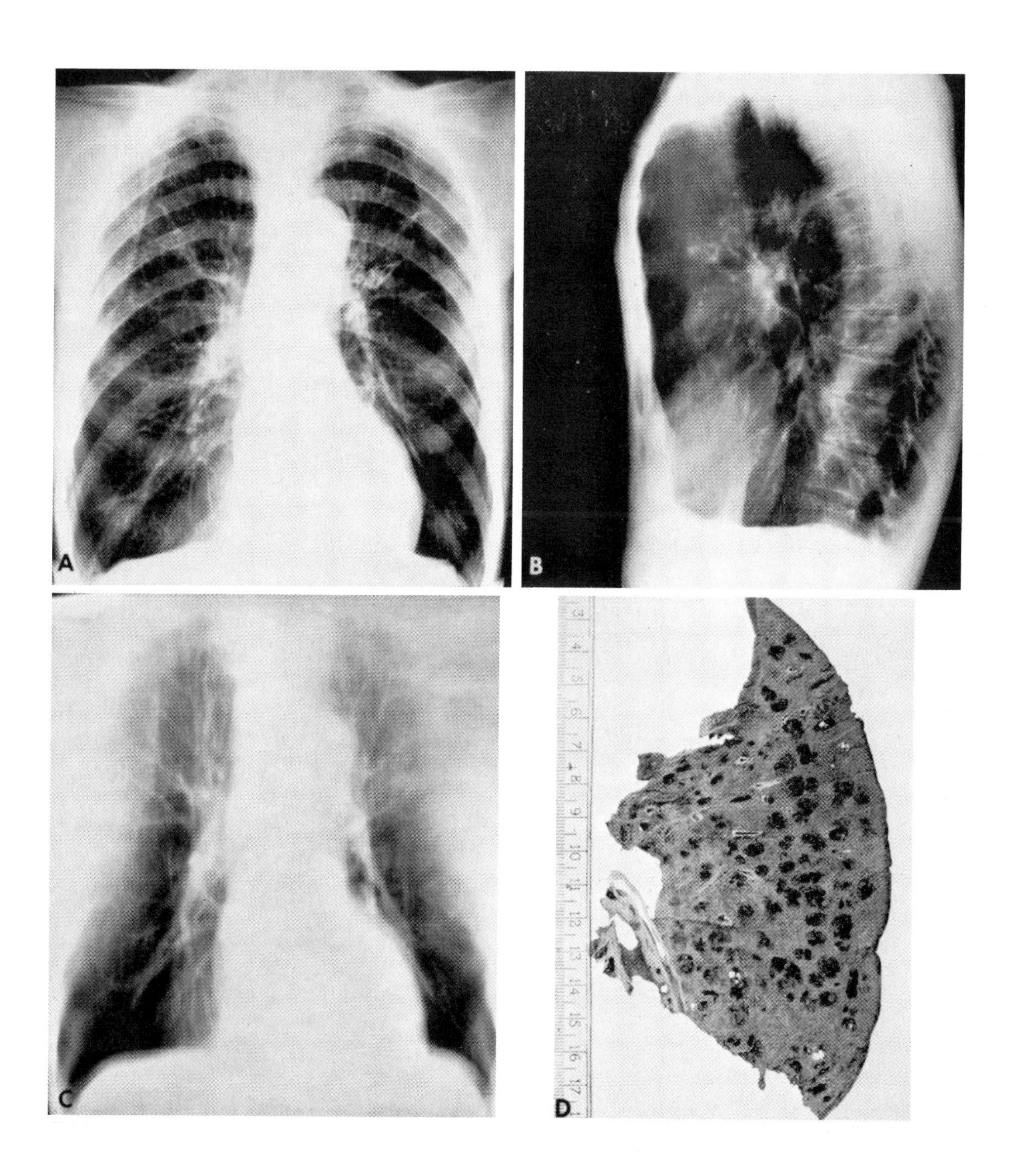

in patients in whom a diagnosis of clinical emphysema is made? Different authors have accepted different criteria in regard to this problem. For example, individual patients classified as having pulmonary emphysema and studied by a variety of techniques have been included in this category with maximal breathing capacities of 64 liters/min,[628] 65 and 81 liters/min,[416] 63 liters/min,[978] and 50 liters/min.[392] In the last instance, reported in one of our own papers, we noted that it had increased in this patient to 90 liters/min a year later, and concluded that the case had originally been wrongly selected as one of emphysema. In many series, the ventilatory-flow data show gross impairment,[710] as for example in the study by Baldwin and her colleagues,[934] in which many of the function-test changes in emphysema were precisely delineated for the first time, and that by Williams and Zohman,[385] in which the maximal midexpiratory flow rate in the 22 patients with pulmonary emphysema studied was only 0.42 liter/sec as a mean for the group, and the highest single value recorded was 0.80 liter/sec. More recently, Filley and his colleagues described the characteristics of 66 patients with what they considered to be Type A (their Type PP) or predominant emphysema disease. In these patients, the mean maximal breathing capacity was 27 per cent of predicted, and the mean maximal midexpiratory flow rate was 0.40 liter/sec.

It is not yet possible to correlate the extent and degree of morphological emphysema unassociated with severe chronic bronchitis with a particular level of ventilatory impairment. Our own observations suggest that moderate or severe emphysema is always associated with a ventilatory flow rate of less than a third of the predicted value, except in paraseptal or unilateral emphysema.[2524] We have been unable to confirm Lynne Reid's view[2508] that generalized centrilobular emphysema may be found with normal ventilatory function.

For the reasons discussed in Chapter 2, we feel that routine measurements of this important aspect of function are best made by recording a fast expiratory tracing, with subsequent analysis of both the FEV and the maximal midexpiratory flow rate. It seems to us very important that, when a detailed investigation of some other aspect of function is being undertaken in patients believed to have clinical emphysema, as for example studies of cardiac output or exercise studies, only those patients who show severe or moderately severe air-flow impairment on every occasion on which they are studied should be included.

There is a generally good correlation between the ventilatory capability and the measured airway resistance in patients with emphysema,[2849, 2866] and the arterial P_{CO_2} also bears a relationship, with some scatter, to the FEV_1 or similar measurement.

Clark and his colleagues recently found that patients with emphysema could sustain about 88 per cent of their measured maximum voluntary ventilation (MVV) when they exercised,[2534] a rather higher level than that previously recorded.[1039]

Subdivisions of Lung Volume

The vital capacity is commonly reduced in emphysema, but even in severe cases the average is still about half the predicted normal value.[385] It is not uncommon, however, to see patients with a severe degree of parenchymal destruction in whom the vital capacity may be 3 liters. In one recent study,[2824] 10 patients with emphysema had a vital capacity between 131 and 166 per cent of that predicted; and another laboratory has reported that 10 per cent of 170 patients with emphysema had vital capacities ranging from 90 to 130 per cent of that predicted.

As mentioned in Chapter 2, there is reason to presume that many published measurements of residual volume, functional residual capacity, and total capacity may be too low, since the use of the body plethysmograph has revealed that the nitrogen- and helium-clearance methods of measuring these parameters are not infrequently in error in patients with advanced emphysema, in whom gas replacement takes many minutes to complete. In spite of this reservation, the majority of the patients with advanced morphological emphysema are found during life to have an increase in residual volume, both absolute and expressed as a percentage of total capacity. The functional residual capacity is usually increased—occasionally being as much as double the predicted value—and a slight increase in total lung capacity is often encountered. In general, all these volumes are found to increase as the morphological emphysema becomes more severe.[2524]

The diminution in vital capacity occurs because of a reduction in both the inspiratory capacity and the expiratory reserve volume. Typically, therefore, the patient with clinical emphysema will be found to have a vital capacity reduced by about half, a residual volume about 1 liter more than predicted, a functional residual capacity about 2 liters more than predicted, and a slight increase in total capacity compared with the predicted value. The residual volume expressed as a percentage of total capacity—a fraction in which Hurtado and his colleagues[935] and others[659, 817, 934] have placed much reliance as an indicator of emphysema—is almost always increased, averaging about 58 per cent instead of a predicted value of about 33 per cent in a 50-year-old man.

The ratio of residual volume to TLC cannot be simply interpreted in this way, however, since it is altered by any condition that restricts total lung capacity, as, for example, in thoracic deformity. For this reason, it is important for the physician always to look closely at the absolute values of residual volume, FRC, vital capacity, and TLC and for the laboratory always to report the actual numerical values of these volumes.

Although this general picture has been so extensively documented that its outlines are no longer disputed, it is still difficult to give definitive answers to some of the questions raised by the observations. In particular, the relative preservation of the vital capacity in some patients but not in others has not been satisfactorily explained. And all the factors causing the increased residual volume are not clearly understood. There is some indication that loss of elastic recoil may be an earlier manifestation of emphysema than airflow obstruction; whether this is so or not, the loss of recoil of itself will have the consequence of causing premature closure of airways during expiration, with a resultant increase in residual volume.

In our experience, a clinical diagnosis of emphysema, unless it is unilateral in type, can seldom be made when values for the subdivisions of lung volume are completely normal; but the clinical diagnosis cannot be made on these indices alone, since the volumes that constitute the subdivisions are affected by bronchial obstruction or thoracic deformity which, of themselves, are independent of morphological changes in the lung parenchyma. Relatively complex classifications of respiratory disease based on variations in the subdivisions of lung volume or on the vital capacity measured before and after various respiratory maneuvers have been proposed,[936] but these do not seem to us to form a satisfactory basis for the classification of types of bronchitis or emphysema.

If the value of the measured subdivisions of lung volume is thus limited, it may be asked whether they contribute to the diagnosis of emphysema. Besides being confirmatory and providing useful base-line data, the chief use of volume measurements is to enable the physician to interpret other measurements that are volume-dependent, e.g., diffusing capacity and pulmonary compliance. Sweet and his colleagues[817] suggested, on the basis of autopsy studies, that in emphysema the residual-volume–total-capacity ratio correlated better than the maximal breathing capacity or nitrogen clearance with the morphological findings. However, in only 9 of the 31 cases studied was emphysema the sole diagnosis, and this seems too small a number from which to draw reliable conclusions.

In our own series of autopsied cases,[2524] there was a general increase in lung volumes as the extent of morphological emphysema increased. This relationship might be even more striking if all the lung volumes were measured by body plethysmography rather than by helium-dilution techniques.

Inert-Gas Distribution and Anatomical Dead Space

Those who have studied inert-gas distribution either by the single-breath technique (*see* page 23), or by observing the rate of equilibration with a closed circuit (*see* page 26) or rate of nitrogen clearance (*see* page 24) have all reported the largest abnormalities of this distribution in patients with emphysema. With the single-breath index, the rise of nitrogen percentage between the 750- and 1250-ml points, normally about 1.8 per cent, has been noted to be as high as 12.0 per cent,[142] and there is little if any overlap between the most abnormal normals and the most normal of the patients thought to have emphysema. The demonstration by Fowler[241] that the inert-gas dead space was normal in patients with emphysema marked an important step forward; previously the impairment of gas distribution in this disease had been thought of in terms of

Case 11
Infantile Lobar Emphysema

Summary of Clinical Findings. This infant was admitted to the Montreal Children's Hospital for the first and only time on October 23, 1961, with a history of two previous admissions to another hospital for high fever said to be "cured" by penicillin.

The mother had noticed that the child had some respiratory difficulty, especially while crying or breathing very deeply, since birth. The difficulties were of insidious onset, characterized by rapid breathing and subxiphoid indrawing, and without causing cyanosis.

Physical examination revealed a two-year-old white boy in no distress. The only positive finding was that of inspiratory indrawing at the lower rib cage. The weight on admission was 12.69 kg.

The hemoglobin, white-blood-cell count and urinalysis were normal.

Bronchoscopy, performed on November 3, showed a tracheobronchial tree within normal limits except for an orifice of the secondary bronchus to the right upper lobe, which was considerably reduced in size.

A right thoracotomy and lobectomy was performed on November 8. At operation the right upper lobe was distended and failed to collapse normally. It was removed without difficulty and the postoperative course was uneventful.

Radiology. The plain film of the chest (*A*) shows hyperinflation apparently involving much of the right lung, but particularly its upper lobe. On the bronchogram (*B*) the hyperinflation is shown to involve mostly the right upper-lobe apical and subapical segments, the middle and lower lobes being displaced inferomedially. The right middle-lobe bronchus shows narrowing which is greater than average and which suggests mild bronchomalacia. In the upper lobe, filling of the involved apical and subapical segments was not achieved in spite of adequate use of contrast medium and positioning. The uninvolved anterior segment of the upper lobe appears essentially normal. Thus, the plain films and bronchograms showed selective hyperinflation of two of the upper-lobe segments, but the etiology of this hyperinflation—bronchomalacia—could not be convincingly demonstrated radiologically.

Pathology. Bronchi were dissected out as far as eighth or tenth generation, opened and stained with toluidine blue, differentiated, cleared and mounted (*C*). The bronchial cartilages (shown in purple) are of normal size and shape in the anterior and posterior segmental bronchi. Cartilages of the apical segmental bronchus (*see arrow*) are hypoplastic and, although normal in number centrally, do not extend out as far as in the other segments. They are also approximately only half the thickness of normal, on average. In circumference, this bronchus is slightly but definitely wider than the others. On histological examination the alveoli of all segments were normal. The posterior segment showed microscars of previous pneumonic infections.

Summary. This case is a somewhat unusual variant of the syndrome of infantile lobar emphysema in that only the cartilages of the apical segment of the right upper lobe were defective; normally a lobar bronchus is involved. The lung parenchyma was normal, although the apical segment was grossly overinflated at operation.

Case 11
Infantile Lobar Emphysema

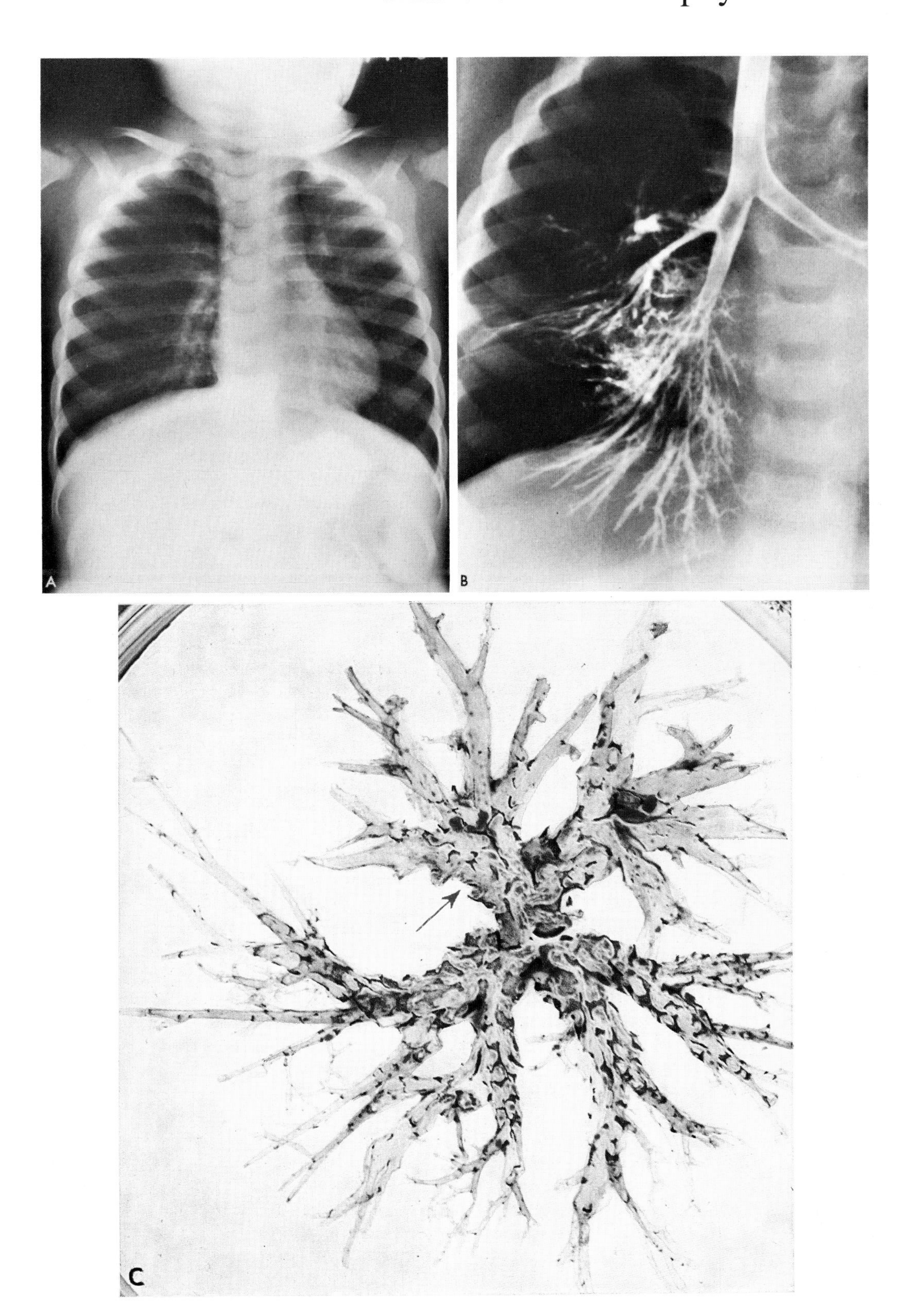

an increase in dead space. In a recent study Birath[1836] has confirmed the normality of inert-gas dead space in patients with emphysema, and by an ingenious model experiment has shown that Fowler's method of measurement may be used to obtain a reliable estimate of this space even when there is no alveolar nitrogen plateau. Similarly, the closed-circuit index using helium[114] separates normal subjects from patients with emphysema, and gross prolongation of the time taken to achieve equilibrium has been noted in many patients with emphysema. It is accepted that impairment of gas distribution is an inevitable consequence of the parenchymal distortion and destruction that are features of widespread morphological emphysema.

Of great interest is the use of a technique of analyzing the nonuniform gas distribution found in emphysema into discrete computed volume compartments, each with a particular volume and proportion of total ventilation. This approach was pioneered by Fowler, Cornish and Kety[154] and by Briscoe.[26, 167] The nonlinear semilogarithmic fall in nitrogen percentage as this gas is cleared by oxygen breathing may be resolved into two phases, and, as Briscoe has pointed out, the washout from poorly ventilated spaces fits one slow exponent within the limits of experimental error, so that these spaces can be regarded as homogeneous.[26] In an average case of emphysema, between two thirds and three quarters of the FRC constitutes this poorly ventilated space, and appears to receive as little as one fifth to one tenth of the total alveolar ventilation. This expression of the unevenness of inert-gas distribution enabled Briscoe to compute some important data concerning ventilation and perfusion distribution in the emphysematous lung, discussed later (*see* page 191). Fowler and his colleagues calculated the "pulmonary nitrogen-clearance delay" to express impaired gas distribution on nitrogen clearance in one number.[154] They showed that, in emphysema, the abnormality of gas distribution demonstrable with the single-breath test was closely paralleled by that derived from the much more complex open-circuit studies, although the latter yielded more information on the pattern of distribution present.

Nakamura and his colleagues have recently analyzed open-circuit helium wash-out data by a new method[2850] which has enabled the clearance curve to be expressed in terms of the distribution function of the clearance time constant of the lung. The defect in gas distribution in emphysema can, by this method, be expressed in terms of a flattening of the distribution curve of time constants within the lung. The application of methods of "compartment analysis" in emphysema to the analysis of the ventilation/perfusion defect is discussed later.

As a result of studies of regional ventilation in patients with emphysema, it has become clear that uneven tidal volume distribution may occur on a grossly regional basis,[1684, 2812, 2815] so that, for example, one zone representing only a quarter of the lung volume may be receiving three quarters of the tidal volume, and also may occur on a basis of disturbed gaseous diffusion due to the abnormal architecture.[2521, 2859] In many patients, no doubt, both factors are operative in causing impaired ventilation distribution. Williams and Park have recently[2836] found that the nonuniformity of the expired gas invariably lessened in 79 patients with chronic obstructive pulmonary disease if the breath was held for 20 seconds between inspiration and expiration, a phenomenon presumably due to inadequate diffusion gas mixing when expiration immediately followed maximal inspiration.

The single-breath nitrogen test has been shown to correlate with measured pulmonary conductance.[2881] In general, these tests of gas distribution seem to be of more value in detecting early changes (*see* page 154) than in indicating the severity of morphological change.

The merit of measuring the unevenness of gas distribution lies in the fact that the abnormality demonstrated is entirely independent of the patient's voluntary effort. It must be realized that chronic bronchitis, asthma (*see* page 127), and many other conditions produce uneven gas distribution; thus it is of no value in the differential diagnosis of these conditions. In our experience, its usefulness lies in the demonstration of undoubted abnormality when the ventilatory flow rates are slightly but not grossly impaired.

Mechanics

The application of recently developed methods of studying pulmonary mechanics to patients with pulmonary emphysema has led to a better understanding of the effect of this disease on pulmonary function and a better, though still incomplete, comprehension of the cause of the dyspnea that is its most characteristic and troublesome symptom. In the paragraphs that follow the many contributions that have been made have been necessarily abbreviated and summarized.

Loss of recoil

The basic observation that, at a given lung volume, the intrathoracic pressure was less negative in a man with advanced emphysema than in a normal man was documented by one of us (R. V. C.) in 1934,[438] using a direct recording of intrapleural pressure, and subsequently by Dayman, in 1951, in a patient with emphysema and pneumothorax[939] and in 1952 by Stead and his colleagues.[938] The implication of this observation is that, for a given degree of distention, the emphysematous lung has less recoil than a normal lung.

The loss of recoil is best demonstrated by plotting absolute elastic recoil pressure against lung volume expressed as percentage of predicted total lung capacity (*see* Figure 7–10). This reveals the shift of the static pressure–volume curve upward and to the left. Several indices have been suggested as an expression of this loss of recoil, such as the elastic recoil pressure at total lung capacity,[583] this pressure divided by total lung capacity,[2865] and the resting end-expiratory pressure divided by the functional residual capacity. All of these

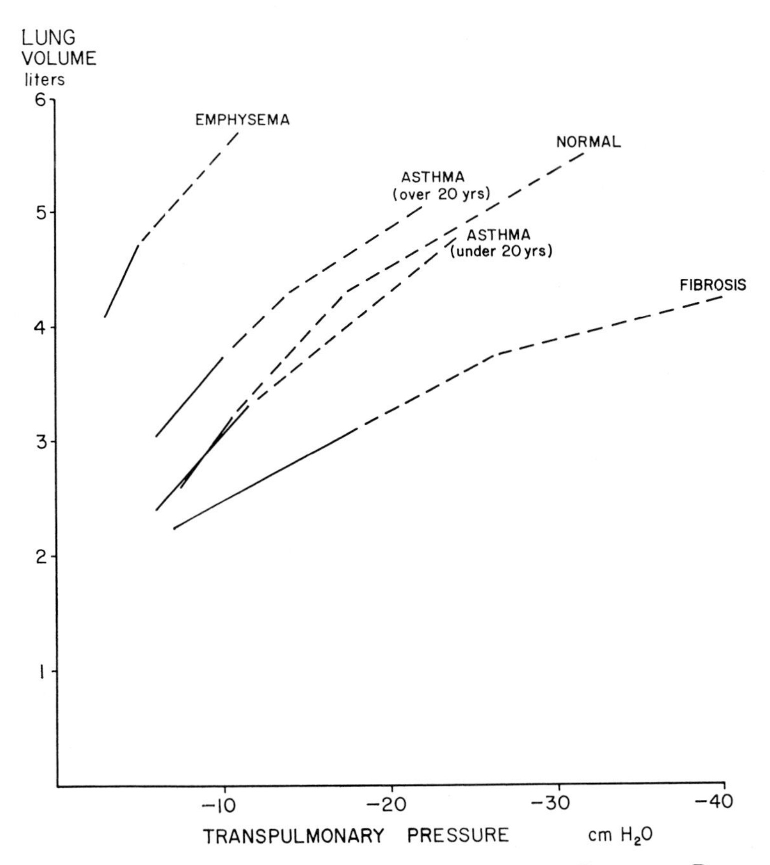

FIGURE 7–10. STATIC-PRESSURE–VOLUME RELATIONSHIPS IN DIFFERENT DISEASES.

The slope of the solid lines over the tidal-volume range, which represents the compliance, is not grossly dissimilar in normal subjects and in patients with asthma or emphysema. However, when total lung volume is related to transpulmonary pressure at full inspiration the differences between these conditions become apparent. At the same lung volume, as for example 5 liters, the transpulmonary pressure is much less negative (minus 9 cm H_2O) in emphysema than in patients with asthma (minus 22 cm H_2O). In patients with diffuse interstitial fibrosis the transpulmonary pressure is more negative at an equivalent lung volume. These data (from Macklem and Becklake[583]) illustrate the limited value of a single figure for pulmonary compliance in the tidal-volume range as a description of the mechanical features of the lungs.

Case 12
Unilateral Emphysema (McLeod's Syndrome)

Summary of Clinical Findings. This man, aged 36 at the time of study, gave a history of having had an attack of pneumonia at the age of 26. This quickly resolved and he was free of all symptoms of chest disease. He was referred for study after routine chest x-ray had been reported as abnormal. He had no history of childhood chest trouble and had never noticed any exercise limitation. Physical examination showed him to be a normally healthy-looking man, the only abnormal signs being decreased tactile and vocal fremitus over the left chest, which was more resonant on percussion than the right side. There was no finger-clubbing.

Radiology. PA films in inspiration (*A*) and expiration (*B*) show considerable asymmetry of radiolucency of the two lungs, the right lung being of greater density in both films. The sparsity of vascular markings throughout the left lung is clearly seen and is in contrast to the slight increase in size of the vessels on the right. On expiration, the left lung undergoes little change in volume, while the right shows an average decrease in size, so that the mediastinum has shifted to the right. A pulmonary angiogram (*C*) shows to excellent advantage the contrast between the size of the arteries in the two lungs. The vessels on the left are sparse and of very small caliber, whereas those on the right reflect a slight plethora. Tapering of the arteries in the right lung is normal so that there is no evidence of arterial hypertension. A left bronchogram (*D*) shows an abrupt termination of all visualized bronchi of the left lung at about their 8th-stage divisions. Although not well shown on this reproduction, all segmental bronchi are slightly dilated and bronchiectatic. The local collections of contrast medium in the upper lung presumably represent filling of large emphysematous spaces.

Summary. This case illustrates the common findings of unilateral translucency in a patient complaining of no cough or dyspnea. Total pulmonary function is good, and both ventilation and perfusion are carried out predominantly by the normal lung.

													EXERCISE				
	VC	FRC	RV	TLC	ME %	MMFR	$FEV_{0.75}$ ×40	pH	P_{CO_2}	HCO_3^-	O_2Hb %	$D_{Lco}SS_2$	MPH	GRADE	$\dot{V}O_2$	$\dot{V}_E$	$D_{Lco}SS_3$
Predicted	4.0	3.1	1.4	5.4	65	3.8	115	7.4	40	25	97	21.1					28.0
Feb. 1961	2.4	3.4	2.0	4.4	33	3.5	68	7.4	38	24	98	17.2	3	5%	1.1	34	23.2

There is a diminution is vital capacity and in total capacity and some impairment of inert-gas distribution, presumably due to slow helium equilibration in the left lung. Resting diffusing capacity is nearly normal. Radioactive-xenon studies, reported elsewhere on this patient,[1684] showed gross impairment of ventilation and perfusion to the left middle and lower zones, with relative preservation of perfusion to the left upper zone. Xenon clearance from the right lung was normal.

Unilateral Emphysema (McLeod's Syndrome)

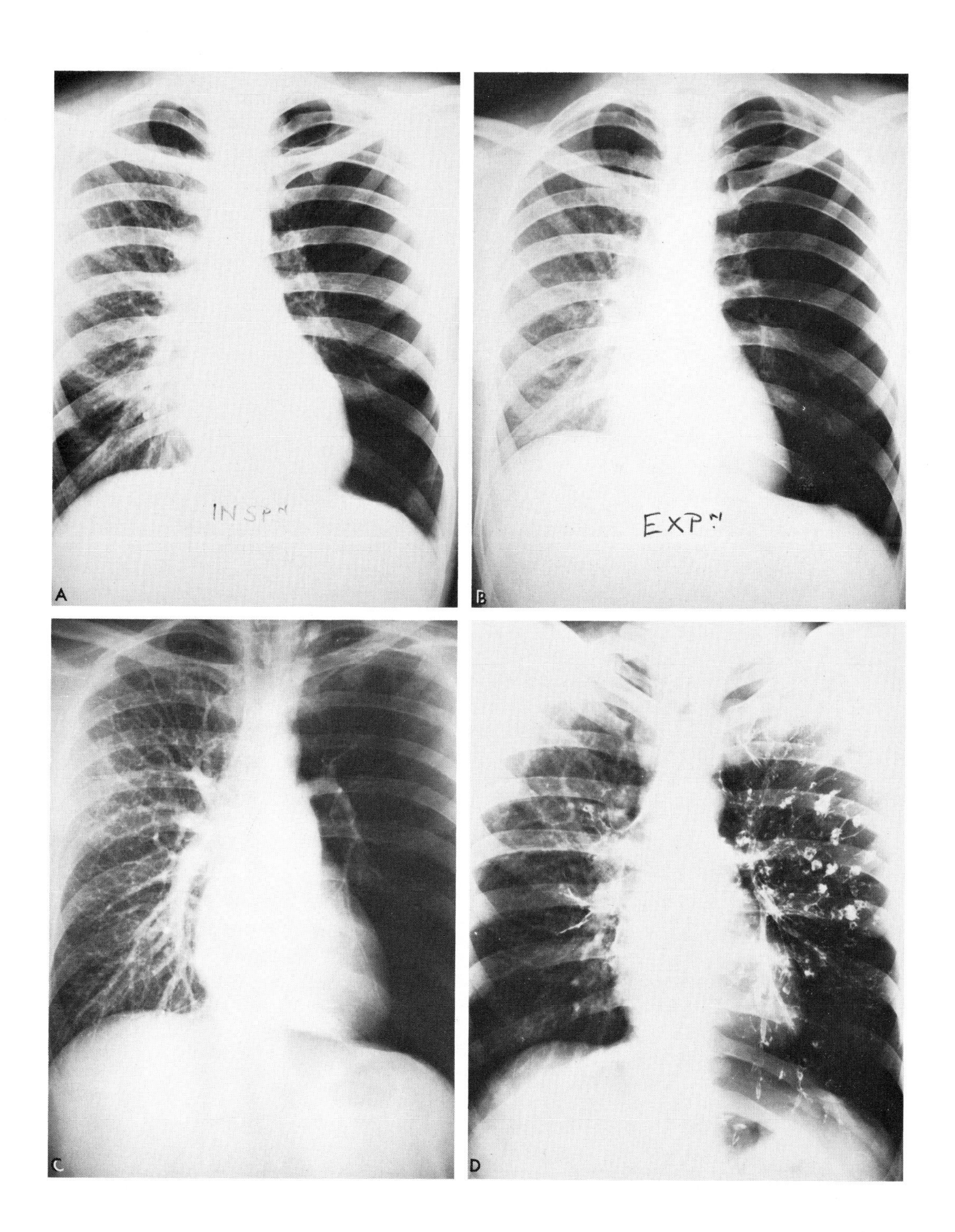

are useful and more valuable than measurements of either static or dynamic compliance, but there can be no doubt that the best assessment of the elastic properties of the lungs is the whole static pressure–volume curve.

Compliance

Although static compliance is increased in emphysema,[583] values as high as 0.600 liter/cm having been reported,[941] there is significant overlap between patients and normal subjects.[583] The value for dynamic compliance, on the other hand, is usually considerably lower than for static compliance, is often lower than the normal range, and is frequency-dependent. As Otis and his colleagues pointed out,[147] in a lung in which resistances and compliances vary between the different zones, equilibrium time for the different zones will vary, with the result that, as frequency increases, progressively more of the tidal volume will be distributed to the units with the shortest time constants, and fewer and fewer units will receive the tidal volume (*see* page 38). Thus, effective ventilation will be restricted to a relatively small volume of the lung.

In the presence of right ventricular failure in emphysema, the dynamic compliance is even lower,[940, 941] and static compliance also may be reduced.[941] The higher respiratory frequencies occurring during heart failure may account for part of this further fall, but it also seems very possible that the presence of infection in the part of the lung being predominantly ventilated might well be another factor.

Airway resistance

All observers have noted very considerable increases in airway resistance in almost every case of emphysema they have studied. If the average normal flow resistance is taken to be about 1.5 cm H_2O/liter/sec, patients with emphysema are commonly found to have values six times as large as this,[583] although in the occasional patient resistance may be only minimally increased.

The airway obstruction is even more apparent when specific resistance or specific conductance is measured. Because in normal individuals, resistance is inversely and hyperbolically related to lung volume, the product of resistance and lung volume is nearly constant. This product or its inverse, specific conductance, permits comparison between individuals of different size, and of measurements made at different lung volumes. Because the FRC is usually greatly increased in emphysema, the specific conductance is a good discriminatory test to detect obstruction at a stage when resistance is not markedly increased.

Airway resistance is frequency-dependent in patients with emphysema, falling with increasing respiratory frequency in the same manner as dynamic compliance and for the same reasons. Because of this, the measurement of resistance at ordinary breathing frequencies yields somewhat higher values than those obtained while panting. This may make the former test somewhat more sensitive, but it requires the passage of an esophageal balloon. One of the characteristic features of the obstruction in chronic bronchitis and emphysema is that, by comparison with that found in asthma, it may be little changed by the administration of bronchodilators.

The major site of obstruction in emphysema is in the peripheral airways smaller than 2 mm in diameter. Normally the resistance of these airways is in the neighborhood of 0.1 to 0.2 cm H_2O/liter/sec, but in advanced emphysema their resistance may be increased 50 to 100 times, a much greater degree of obstruction than is commonly visualized.[2544]

The combination of loss of elastic recoil and peripheral airway obstruction results in a grossly abnormal MEFV curve, with a marked reduction in maximal expiratory flow rate at all lung volumes.

Much time and effort have been expended in determining which airways are responsible for limiting expiratory flow. There is little doubt that lobar and larger airways may collapse dramatically during a forced expiration in some patients with chronic bronchitis and emphysema,[2837, 3688] and lobar bronchi may be flow-limiting in a large number of such patients. In others, flow-limitation may occur in more peripheral airways or at both levels of the tracheobronchial tree. Regardless of the site of flow-limitation, a distinction must be made between those airways which narrow and limit flow, and the value for flow through them. Although the distinction is a subtle one, it is important because the principal determinant of maximal expiratory flow is the elastic recoil of the lung, and the resistance of small airways and the site and characteristics of the flow-limiting segments have a relatively much smaller effect.

The profound disturbances in mechanics of

the lung that occur in emphysema may be responsible for impeding venous return to the thorax;[2838] this phenomenon is discussed below in relation to circulatory changes.

Thoracic-cage compliance

It has been suggested by Ting and Lyons[942] that, in some patients with emphysema, a decrease in thoracic-wall compliance may play some part in the overall increase in elastic resistance of the total respiratory system. These measurements were difficult to make, however, and it does not appear certain that the chest wall can be incriminated with certainty since the data obtained are very dependent upon the ability of the patient to execute the necessary relaxation pressure, and might possibly have been influenced by the fact that the studies were made with the subjects in the supine position. Using a different technique, Cherniack and Hodson also found evidence of a reduction in chest-wall compliance in patients with chronic bronchitis and emphysema;[1282] thus the important possibility remains that thoracic-cage changes, particularly in patients who acquire a severe mid-dorsal kyphosis, may play a part in increasing the work of breathing, and hence the dyspnea.

Krumholz and Albright have reported data from 8 patients with emphysema supporting this view.[2884] They found that the mean chest-wall compliance was about one third of that found in normal subjects, and the magnitude of the change appeared to be independent of the functional residual capacity.

The work of breathing

It follows from the foregoing observations that, since air-flow resistance is greatly increased and dynamic compliance reduced in emphysema, the work of breathing must be considerably increased in patients with this disease. This increase has been documented by several authors,[497, 499, 504, 2888] and Hammond has shown that it is still further increased when right ventricular failure is present.[2018] There can be little doubt that this increased work is related to dyspnea,[17, 495, 943] although in these patients the sensation of dyspnea is related more closely to the force exerted on the lung[520] and the oxygen cost of breathing[520] than to the mechanical work of breathing. It also appears likely that the respiratory muscles may be relatively inefficient in emphysema.[517]

The high oxygen cost of hyperventilation in patients with emphysema appears to be due not only to the increased work of breathing but also to an increased oxygen cost of unit work, possibly incurred as much by the abnormally inflated chest position as by any inherent abnormality of the muscles themselves. Riley, in a characteristically instructive essay, has discussed the implications of these mechanical factors in emphysema, in terms of alterations of alveolar ventilation and arterial gas tensions.[944] Briscoe and Cournand[26] noted that a patient with advanced emphysema increased his oxygen consumption from 277 ml/min to 319 ml/min when attempting to hyperventilate, but when the same level of hyperventilation was attained with the assistance of a positive-pressure respirator, the oxygen uptake rose only to 296 ml/min—a remarkable illustration of the fact that some of these patients with advanced emphysema are caught between the desirability of increasing their ventilation to lower the arterial P_{CO_2}, and the greatly increased CO_2 production that, because of the increased work of breathing, such hyperventilation will cause. It has been pointed out that normal subjects, when exercising, may settle for an elevation of arterial P_{CO_2} if the airway is obstructed, rather than increase still further the level of ventilatory work;[24, 962] it seems clear that this type of balance must be of constant concern to the patient with advanced pulmonary emphysema,[966, 2332] though its appraisal is presumably subconsciously controlled.

Jaeger and Otis showed that compression of alveolar gas may occur in patients with emphysema, and this factor may have to be considered in relation to the work of breathing during attempted hyperventilation.[2265]

ARTERIAL BLOOD-GAS TENSIONS

It has been known for many years[1] that many patients with emphysema have a reduced arterial oxygen saturation, usually with concomitant increase in P_{CO_2}. The availability of gas-tension electrode systems and the improvements that have been made in techniques of arterial blood sampling have both led to a much more general appreciation of the variations that may be found in the tensions of CO_2 and O_2 in chronic respiratory disease. Some investigators have suggested that the disturbance of $\dot{V}/\dot{Q}$ usually responsible for the abnormal gas tensions in these conditions is most commonly to be attributed to chronic bronchitis rather than to emphysema; this problem is dealt with in a later section. Certainly it is now realized that many factors may contribute to the resulting arterial gas tensions—it is the difficulty of establishing which of these mechanisms is mainly responsible in any given patient for the observed arterial gas tensions that accounts for present uncertainties.

There are many papers on this aspect of chronic respiratory disease;[947, 948] in the following paragraphs some of this information is summarized.

1. In patients with severe pulmonary emphysema and longstanding ventilatory defect the arterial blood-gas tensions may be normal.

2. Severe changes in blood-gas tensions may occur in some patients with comparatively little morphological emphysema, though we do not regard this syndrome, uncomplicated by bronchiectasis or alveolar hypoventilation due to CO_2 insensitivity, as particularly common[2524] (*see* later discussion).

3. Persistent changes in blood-gas tensions indicate a poor prognosis,[947, 2877] and the onset of right ventricular failure is more closely related to disturbances in blood-gas tensions than to any other factor. The mechanism of this relationship is obscure.[2892] The importance of the level of arterial oxygen tension in relation of prognosis is also shown by the fact that the mortality from emphysema is worsened by living at altitude—this exceptionally interesting observation was reported by Renzetti, McClement, and Litt in 1968.[2750]

4. There is a general but not a very close relationship between the maximal breathing capacity and the arterial P_{CO_2}.[945] The arterial saturation is poorly correlated with the maximal expiratory flow rate.[385]

5. In general, the worsening of ventilatory function is associated with a worsening of the $\dot{V}/\dot{Q}$ distribution.[2554]

6. The daily fluctuations in arterial P_{CO_2} in patients with emphysema is about 8 mm Hg,[2842] and the value is usually at its maximum early in the morning.

7. In patients with severe respiratory failure as yet untreated by the administration of oxygen, the arterial P_{CO_2} will not be found to be above about 80 mm Hg, since levels above this would inevitably be accompanied by a level of hypoxemia incompatible with survival. This point is discussed in Chapter 22. Refsum[2827] has pointed out that the plasma bicarbonate increases with the P_{CO_2} increase up to a level of about 70 mm Hg when this occurs chronically. At this level of P_{CO_2}, the bicarbonate will be between 35 and 39 mEq/liter, and the hydrogen-ion concentration little increased. Beyond this level, if the P_{CO_2} rises further, the hydrogen-ion concentration increases markedly.

The factors related to the alterations in blood-gas tension will now be discussed in detail.

VENTILATION/PERFUSION ($\dot{V}/\dot{Q}$) ABNORMALITIES

It should be clear from the discussion in relevant sections of Chapter 2, that the presence of an abnormality of distribution of $\dot{V}/\dot{Q}$ ratios in the lungs of patients with emphysema can be inferred from many lines of evidence. The finding of an elevated level of arterial P_{CO_2} in the presence of a normal level of minute ventilation is, by itself, presumptive evidence of nonuniformity of distribution of ventilation *vis-a-vis* perfusion. Other simple methods include the demonstration of an abnormally large difference between the RQ of expired gas at the beginning and end of an expiration,[261] and the finding of a greater CO_2 rise than normal;[2848] the finding of a large value for physiological dead space;[17] the demonstration of large alveolar–arterial oxygen differences[2862] not caused by shunts; the demonstration of an increased alveolar–arterial nitrogen-tension difference, indicating an increase in units with a low $\dot{V}/\dot{Q}$[26, 2878]—all of these methods have provided evidence that a disturbance of ventilation and perfusion is a common if not an invariable accompaniment of emphysema. Recently there have been a number of attempts to express the abnormality in more quantitative terms or to compare the lung function to a compartmental model. These more complex techniques include the following analytical methods based upon computation from measurable parameters:

1. By analyzing the function of the lung in terms of "equivalent shunts." This memorable advance was made by Riley and Cournand in 1949,[413] and subsequently was applied and extended by them and by other investigators. It involves the expression of an "ideal alveolar gas," and quantitates the departure from this in terms of a "venous-admixture" or "blood-

shunt" component expressed as a percentage of total cardiac output, and a "dead-space" component expressed as a percentage of the observed tidal volume. In many patients with emphysema both of these are found to be increased.

2. By analyzing the same equivalent-shunt components in slightly different terms, making use of observed differences for oxygen, CO_2, and, particularly, nitrogen. This approach has been described recently by Rahn and Farhi, with illustrative data from a patient with advanced emphysema.[26] In this patient, the results could be expressed by saying that, of the total ventilation, 30 per cent went to the "ideal" alveoli, 30 per cent to anatomical dead space and 40 per cent to alveoli that were virtually unperfused; in the same patient, 50 per cent of the pulmonary blood flow went to the "ideal" alveoli, 30 per cent to alveoli that were barely ventilated, and 20 per cent went through totally nonexchanging tissues or shunts. It is important to realize that this method must be viewed as an attempt to describe the continuous statistical distribution of alveoli between those with a very high and those with a very low $\dot{V}/\dot{Q}$ ratio.

3. In a series of papers published over a 10-year period, Briscoe has developed a method of compartmental analysis originally using the analysis of nitrogen-clearance curves combined with measurement of arterial and mixed venous-gas tensions and cardiac output[26, 146] and most recently combining this approach with the use of Bohr isopleths to compute the diffusing capacity in separate "compartments" of the nonhomogeneous lung.[2530, 2540, 2868, 2872] In general, in emphysema, the poorly ventilated space commonly constitutes three quarters of the FRC, yet receives only one tenth of the total alveolar ventilation, but is perfused by half of the cardiac output.[26] In the Type A (emphysema) patient, a low transfer factor (diffusing capacity) in the less-ventilated lung spaces appears to contribute materially to the arterial hypoxemia.[2530] Lenfant and Pace[2554] have studied the $\dot{V}/\dot{Q}$ disorder in patients with chronic obstructive lung disease analyzing lung function into three rather than two compartments, and they have shown that a worsening of total ventilatory function, as judged by the FEV_1, is accompanied by a worsening of the $\dot{V}/\dot{Q}$ distribution. There is some uncertainty as to how far recirculation of a gas as soluble as nitrogen may interfere with these methods of analysis, and Giuntini and his colleagues, on the basis of experiments using tritium,[2870] have produced evidence that this source of error may be considerable.

4. Gurtner, Briscoe, and Cournand combined the use of radioactive krypton with earlier techniques[1811] and generally validated the compartmental results. Gurtner[2878] has recently described a method of analysis combining helium clearance and krypton and compared these results to the $\dot{V}/\dot{Q}$ abnormality deducible from the alveolar–arterial nitrogen-tension difference. Using radioactive krypton and helium, Cellerino and his co-workers concluded that the cardiac output was almost evenly distributed between two compartments, one of which had about five times the fraction of tidal volume per unit of lung volume distributed to it more than the other.[2875]

5. The distribution of ventilation to a lung zone and the relative perfusion distribution to it may be measured with ^{133}xenon or with isotopes of CO_2. These methods have revealed that there are marked zonal abnormalities of ventilation and perfusion in many patients with emphysema.[26, 174, 342, 1684, 2812, 2815, 2873] It is unlikely that the full effect of the disturbances of $\dot{V}/\dot{Q}$ that are occurring at lobular level can be demonstrated by these methods which essentially treat ventilation and perfusion as dissociated phenomena, and Pain and West[2815] have emphasized the limitations of this type of external counting technique in attempting such an analysis, quite apart from errors introduced due to the solubility and recirculation of xenon.[2831] Nevertheless, these methods are valuable in showing regions of the lung with very grossly different distributions of tidal volume and blood flow.

6. We have recently published a new technique using ^{133}xenon that depends on comparison of the clearance of xenon delivered to the lung in solution via the pulmonary artery to clearance after lung equilibration with gaseous ^{133}xenon. The technique is not simple,[2894] but it has revealed interesting differences in the behavior of the lung in patients with asthma,[2572] chronic bronchitis,[2532] and emphysema.[2873] In the latter condition, there are often gross disparities between xenon clearance in the two experiments, illustrating that each scintillation detector is viewing a non-homogeneous population of functional units. The technique overcomes some of the difficulties of interpretation of external count-rate data and confirms

Case 13

Lobar Emphysema (Lobar Pulmonary Transradiancy: Obliterative Bronchitis and Bronchiolitis)

Summary of Clinical Findings. This 28-year-old Air Force ground-crewman was admitted to a Veterans Hospital in May 1959 after a routine x-ray had revealed a localized translucency of the right lower lung field. The history is perhaps colored by the fact that the patient subsequently claimed a pension for his disability. His main complaint was cough which he stated began with an attack of tonsillitis in 1951 while in the army in Korea. A tonsillectomy was performed in 1957 and his cough had been worse since then and had become productive of moderate amounts of grayish sputum. In 1958 he began to notice shortness of breath on exertion. He denied any respiratory illness before his enlistment in the army in 1950. He smoked about 25 cigarettes per day. The physical findings of interest were restricted to the chest. The percussion note was resonant over the right base posteriorly and breath sounds and vocal resonance were diminished in this area. There were high-pitched inspiratory rhonchi scattered over the chest but no rales. There were no signs of congestive failure. There was no clubbing or cyanosis.

Investigations included x-rays, pulmonary function studies, pulmonary angiograms and bronchospirometry (*opposite*).

In September, 1959, the patient underwent a right middle- and lower-lobe resection. At operation the middle lobe appeared to be excessively distended, compared with the upper and lower lobes, and after inflation remained distended while the others gradually collapsed.

Postoperatively he continued to complain of cough and expectoration. After discharge the patient did not return for follow-up.

Radiology. A full inspiratory film of the chest (*A*) reveals a subtle but definite asymmetry of the vascular pattern to the lower half of the two lungs, that on the right being distinctly reduced. The reduction in number and caliber of vessels on the right is reflected in a slight difference in radiolucency of the lung bases. A film made in full expiration during bronchospirometry (*B*) shows a striking degree of air-trapping in the region of the right middle and lower lobes, with corresponding shift of the mediastinum to the left and lack of elevation of the right diaphragmatic dome.

A pulmonary angiogram (*C*) confirms the presence of severe reduction in arterial supply to both the middle and lower lobes of the right lung, vascularity elsewhere being normal.

Pathology. The middle lobe when sectioned after fixation in inflation showed moderate panlobular emphysema (*D* and *E*) with few remaining normal alveoli. In the lower lobe the emphysema was more patchy and often appeared to be adjacent to bronchioles. No abnormalities of branches of the pulmonary artery could be found, and the major bronchi appeared to be normal. In both lobes, however, there was extensive obliterative bronchiolitis, the obliterated bronchioles being represented by stellate-shaped scars often pigmented. Scattered foci of bronchiolectasia also were observed in both lobes.

Summary. This is a case of obliterative bronchitis and bronchiolitis localized to the right middle and lower lobes.

The almost normal function results indicate that the remaining lung must be free of disease.

														EXERCISE				
	VC	FRC	RV	TLC	ME %	MMFR	$FEV_{0.75}$ ×40	pH	P_{CO_2}	HCO_3^-	O_2Hb %	$D_{LCO}SS_2$	MPH	GRADE	$\dot{V}O_2$	$\dot{V}_E$	$D_{LCO}SS_3$
Predicted	4.0	3.0	1.4	5.4	65	4.0	126					21.3					38
June 1959	4.0	3.0	1.8	5.8	64	2.5	112					15.3	3	FLAT	1.12	21.6	23.0

In these studies preoperatively, flow rates are slightly reduced and diffusing capacity is lower than predicted at both rest and exercise.

By bronchospirometry, 40 per cent of the ventilation and 35 per cent of the oxygen consumption are achieved by the right lung as compared with normal values of 55 per cent (*F*).

Lobar Emphysema (Lobar Pulmonary Transradiancy: Obliterative Bronchitis and Bronchiolitis)

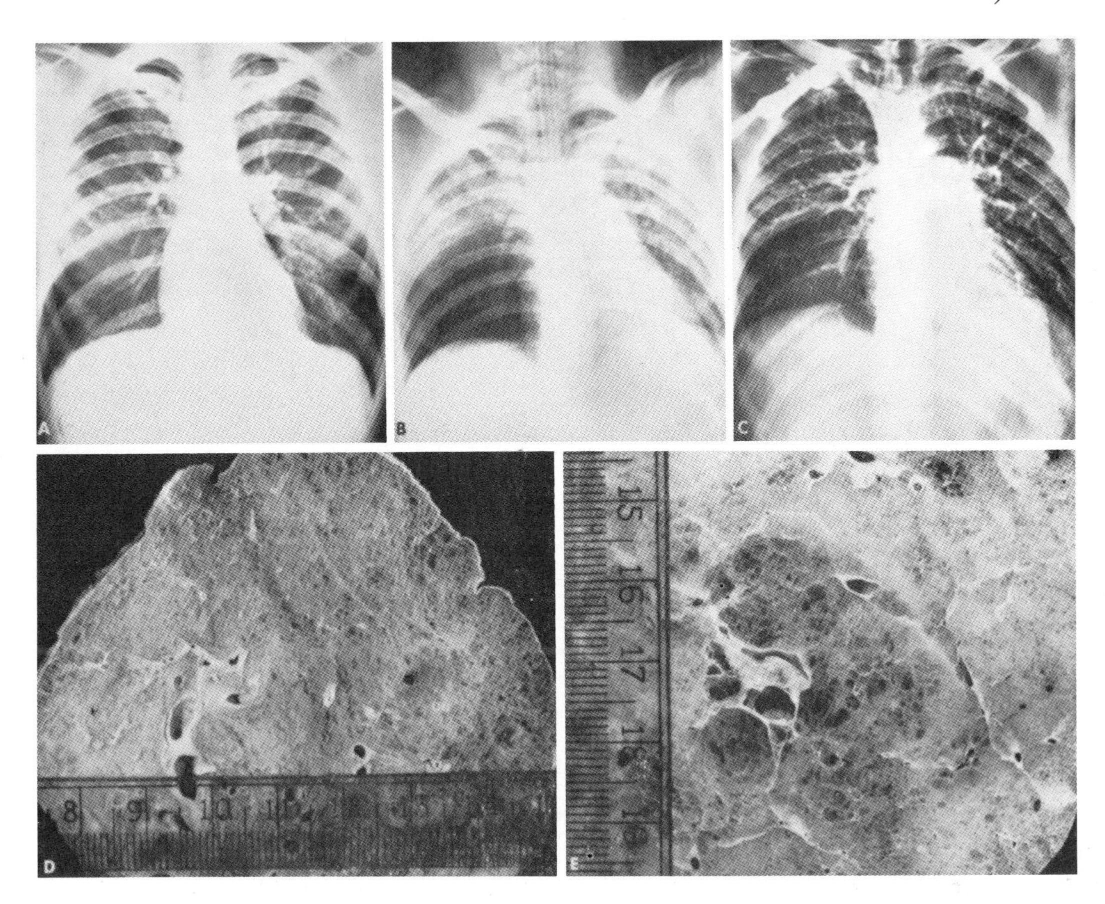

MR H.W. AGE 28 JUNE 1959		
	RT	LT
VENTILATION liters/min	1·78 (40%)	2·65 (60%)
O_2 UPTAKE liters/min	0·10	0·19
VITAL CAPACITY liters	1·34 (41%)	1·91 (59%)

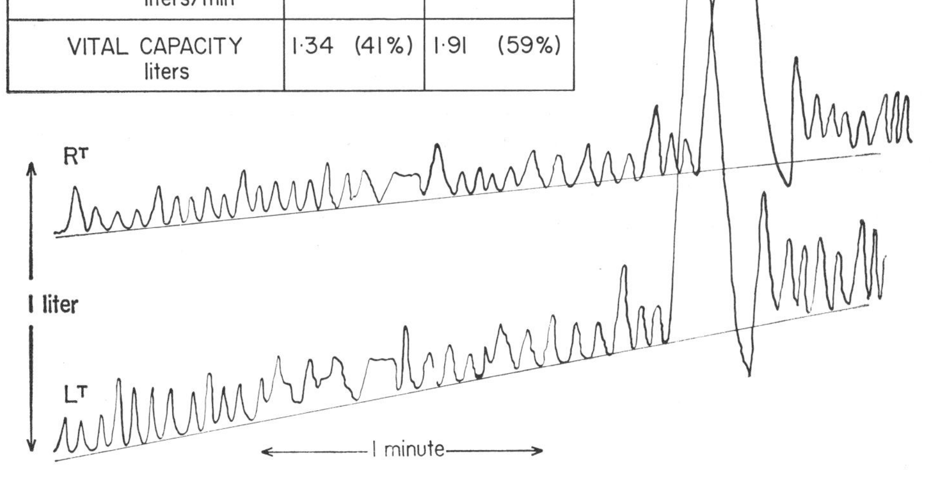

the fact that the abnormal $\dot{V}/\dot{Q}$ distribution in emphysema is a composite of many different factors (*see* following section).

This brief summary of techniques will serve as an introduction to the complex problem of measurement of the distribution of $\dot{V}/\dot{Q}$ ratios in emphysema. It is not surprising that much attention has been devoted to this problem, since the disturbance in arterial blood-gas tensions is mainly due to this factor and is critical in determining prognosis. For this reason, an attempt is made in a later section to interrelate the factors that may be responsible for arterial hypoxemia in this condition.

DIFFUSING CAPACITY

Since measurement of pulmonary diffusing capacity inevitably requires that some single figure be used to represent the mean alveolar CO pressure that exists in the lung, it follows that there must be considerable difficulty in making the measurement at all in emphysema, in which condition there is bound to be variation between gas concentrations in different alveoli. The problem deserves serious attention, however, since if morphological emphysema, by definition, involves loss of alveoli, some measurement related to the internal surface area of the lung should play an important part in its assessment and diagnosis. The complexity of understanding the interpretation of the results of diffusing-capacity measurements obtained by different techniques in this disease has, unfortunately, led many physicians and physiologists to believe that such measurements are not worth attempting. It is our view, however, that the whole problem can now be viewed in perspective, since a considerable volume of data which is not contradictory exists on this problem. All measurements of diffusing capacity are potentially influenced by the qualitative characteristics and surface area of the internal membrane and the effective hemoglobin surface area exposed. All methods involving steady-state breathing are bound to be influenced by the total membrane and blood surface area of the predominantly ventilated region. Thus, if one lung were to receive 1 per cent of ventilation and 1 per cent of perfusion, even though it contributed half of the FRC and had a normal membrane, internal surface area and blood volume, under steady-state conditions its contribution to the measured diffusing capacity would inevitably be negligible. Furthermore, all steady-state determinations are influenced by the uniformity of distribution of diffusing capacity in relation to ventilation. The single-breath method is theoretically insensitive to ventilation distribution but is affected by the uniformity of distribution of diffusing capacity, in relation to alveolar volume.

During the past few years, there have been many useful contributions to the understanding of the factors that influence the value of the diffusing capacity of the lung, which may be calculated from different types of measurement in patients with emphysema. It may be useful to discuss these contributions in relation to the separate techniques that have been employed.

1. The diffusing capacity for oxygen (D_{LO_2}), which was the original method developed by Riley and Lilienthal,[416, 420, 955] has been restudied by Fruhmann[2883] using Thew's technique. Values found in a group of patients with emphysema were only about 50 per cent of the values in normal patients. The author points out that the reduction in arterial oxygen tension does not correlate with the measured reduction in diffusing capacity but rather with the degree of "venous admixture" or $\dot{V}/\dot{Q}$ component. This method is difficult technically and does not appear to yield any more information than do methods using carbon monoxide.

2. The single-breath modified Krogh method ($D_{LCO}SB$) may give low values for diffusing capacity in patients with emphysema,[38, 361, 429, 761, 958, 959, 961, 2491, 2516] but on occasion a normal value is found in patients in whom the steady-state value is low.[267, 395] Part of this effect may be explained by the value used for the alveolar volume in the single-breath technique.[960] In spite of reservations expressed about the diffusing capacity calculated by this method in patients with emphysema[759] many investigators have found it to be of value in indicating the probable degree of morphological emphysema that is present.[2491, 2516, 2867] Piiper and Sikand[2852] have published a detailed theoretical analysis of the method and the effects of different $\dot{V}/\dot{Q}$ patterns on the computed value of D_L. They also noted that a characteristic feature of the presence of unequal distributions of diffusing capacity would be a decrease of the apparent D_{LCO} with increasing times of apnea.

3. Read and his colleagues have published

a similarly useful analysis of the effects of nonuniformity on the D_{Lco} computed from the measured arterial $P\text{CO}_2$ (Filley method). Different patterns of abnormality can produce over- and underestimations of the true physical D_L, and the method is particularly sensitive to gross changes in blood distribution and rather less affected by ventilation changes. They noted that a low value of D_L might be found in patients with a normal arterial $P\text{O}_2$—a result predicted from their theoretical analysis. Lim and Brownlee[2825] have pointed out that this measurement may be a more sensitive indicator of change than is the arterial blood, and argue that the theoretical objections to the method that have been raised do not diminish its usefulness in indicating early change. Using this technique to study differences in gas exchange between the Type A (emphysema) and the Type B (bronchitic) patient with chronic obstructive lung disease, Filley and his colleagues[2510] noted that the technique on exercise gave generally higher values than the end-tidal method. The differences in D_L between the two groups were (rather unexpectedly) not striking. (*see* Fig. 2–39.)

4. The end-tidal sampling technique is much simpler to perform than the Filley method. Although its computed alveolar CO tension is inevitably suspect, the results run below but parallel to those obtained by simultaneous arterial CO_2 analysis.[2843] At rest, the technique, if used in conjunction with the fractional uptake of carbon monoxide, is certainly very useful in indicating relative normality of function.

5. Some reports of diffusing capacity data in emphysema have appeared, based on closed-circuit equilibration with CO or with radioactive ^{14}CO. Sølvsteen has published a detailed analysis of the theory of this technique[2828] and a number of experimental studies of its application.[2851, 2861, 2893] The method is less liable to be influenced by nonuniformity of $\dot{V}/\dot{Q}$ distribution than are the steady-state or single-breath methods; low values for D_L have been recorded for emphysema by use of this method. The equilibration technique is not without its difficulties, and some incredibly high values of D_L in emphysema recorded by its use must presumably be attributed to experimental error.[2887]

6. There is general agreement that a more reliable estimate of diffusing capacity by steady-state methods may be made during exercise than at rest (*see* Fig. 2–39.) If the arterial blood is sampled continually ($D_{Lco}SS_1$), in patients with emphysema the exercise diffusing capacity increases compared with resting values,[385, 945] though this increase may be small in some patients. Williams and Zohman noted changes from 6.7 to 9.2, 12.0 to 12.7, and 8.5 to 9.1 ml CO/min/mm Hg in three of their patients with emphysema on transition from rest to exercise.[385] If the diffusing capacity on exercise is calculated using an assumed value for dead space, in some patients there is very little increase on exercise.[392] This finding, apparently discrepant, would be inevitable if the increased respiratory frequency of exercise, and the uneven time constants in the lung in patients with emphysema, had led to a worsening of gas distribution. As a result of this mechanism, an even smaller volume of lung might be effectively ventilated during exercise than at rest. It is of interest that Bedell and Adams, using the single-breath method ($D_{Lco}SB$), reported recently that in some of these patients there may be little or no increase in diffusing capacity on exercise.[361]

Detailed computer-calculated data will be required before we can achieve a complete understanding of the influence of different patterns of distribution of ventilation, alveolar volume, perfusion and diffusing capacity in lungs in which the ratios between these are not uniform. Nevertheless, despite absence of proof for some of the comments that follow, it seems to us that certain statements can be made concerning the use and interpretation of measurements of diffusing capacity in patients thought to have emphysema. Marshall suggested that such measurements should not be expressed in terms of diffusing capacity, since they are not true physical measurements.[391] However, it now seems clear that no method can be proved to approximate the diffusing capacity that would be present if the system were totally uniform, and further, that if such a number were obtainable, it might not be relevant to the surface area available to the patient for gas exchange, and therefore have little functional meaning.

In our opinion it is short-sighted to dismiss as valueless all measurements of CO transfer in emphysema because none can approximate the true physical D_L. We have shown that there is a highly significant correlation between CO uptake and the extent of morphological emphysema in the lungs at autopsy.[2524] Although in life it would be unwise to assume such a correlation, the $\dot{V}/\dot{Q}$ abnormality which lowers CO transfer in the absence of such morphological change, as on occasion it may do, can be more sensitively detected by the use of CO than by any other simple technique, and the detection of this—and particularly its observation over a period of years in individual patients—is undoubtedly valuable.

It is therefore important that the physician learn the limitations of interpretation of whatever technique he chooses to establish in the pulmonary function laboratory—and there are points to be made in favor of both the single-breath and the steady-state methods. In general, if the steady-state methods are normal, he can be assured that there is no serious $\dot{V}/\dot{Q}$ abnormality, no severe loss of internal surface area, and no qualitative change in alveolar membrane.

The question of the role played by the diffusing capacity in relation to the arterial oxygen tension in emphysema is discussed later.

Mechanisms Responsible for Impaired Gas Exchange in Emphysema

Although much attention has been directed to the problem of identifying the prime factor in impairment of gas exchange in emphysema, only the bare outlines of the problem are yet visible. It seems to us that some authors have taken too superficial a view of this problem and, on occasion, have failed to take account of the interaction between different defects of function. Thus, if there is a zone or region in a particular lung in which the $\dot{V}/\dot{Q}$ ratio is low due primarily to ventilation reduction, then the arterial oxygen tension of blood leaving that zone may be critically dependent on the velocity of blood flow through it, or on its internal surface area available for diffusion, since the mean alveolar oxygen tension within the region will be low.

Some of these factors are noted in Table 7–1. It is to be supposed that in the lung grossly damaged by emphysema, many of these factors are operative; no doubt there will continue to be much discussion of their importance in the generality of cases. One problem, however, deserves special mention, since it is of importance in relation to the classification of chronic bronchitis and emphysema and the differentiation during life between Type A (emphysematous) patients and Type B (bronchitic) patients. The problem is whether a mild or moderate degree of centrilobular emphysema in which less than 25 per cent of the internal surface area has disappeared is capable, by the nature and site of the lesion, of producing marked changes in

TABLE 7–1 Mechanisms Responsible for Impaired Gas Exchange in Emphysema

A Producing regions of low $\dot{V}/\dot{Q}$ ratio	1. Impaired ventilation	– Regional differences in compliance – Morphological small airway change – Reduced lung recoil and instability leading to premature small airway closure
	2. Slowed diffusion in the gas phase	– ?Effect of centrilobular emphysema and disordered architecture
	3. Collateral ventilation	– ?Gas exchange in patent alveoli before inspired gas reaches collaterally ventilated spaces.
B Factors influencing normality of gas tensions of blood leaving a low $\dot{V}/\dot{Q}$ region.		
	1. Adequate time for capillary gas exchange – Normality of $\dot{V}_A/\dot{Q}_C$ ratio – Restriction of parts of vascular bed may cause abnormally fast transit times elsewhere – Loss of internal surface area will reduce D_L – Widening of remaining capillaries may lead to slow equilibration of oxygen	
	2. Possible direct A-V shunts (not major)	

arterial gas tensions; or whether these can be ascribed to the almost invariably concomitant lesions of chronic bronchitis. In the first edition of this volume (page 200) we suggested that the centrilobular lesions might well be responsible for severe $\dot{V}/\dot{Q}$ disturbance, and Horsfield,[2521] Cumming,[2859] and Williams and Park[2836] have all produced evidence that diffusion impairment within the gas phase in the centrilobular spaces of emphysema may well be an important mechanism. The point has been made eloquently by Dunnill:[2520] "Each centrilobular space is served by a terminal bronchiole; the respiratory bronchiole in the normal lung is approximately 500 μ in diameter. If this dilates to four times its diameter, to form a centrilobular space, its volumes will increase 64 times. If each of the 64,000 terminal bronchioles leads to a space, the volume of 'emphysema' in the lung will only be of the order of 15-20% of the total lung volume, but every single gas molecule going to or coming from the alveolar membrane will have to pass through one of these spaces. I do not think that we can say categorically that such a state of affairs will occur without very profound pathophysiological consequences."

In their complex compartmental analysis using calculated Bohr isopleths, Briscoe and King[2525, 2530] concluded that in both Type A and Type B patients the total diffusing capacity was reduced. In the Type A patient, the major barrier to diffusion appeared to be in the slowly ventilating space, whereas in the Type B case it was in the well-ventilated space. It is tempting to suppose that in the slowly ventilated space, the defect might have been due to relative loss of internal surface area, and in the well-ventilated space to the shortened capillary transit time that may exist in such a region. Rossier[17] proposed that this mechanism might be important, and certainly it can be shown that there is great variation in capillary transit time in cases of emphysema (Figure 7–12) illustrates one such study indicating this). Whether or not this plays a major part cannot yet be considered proven. A recent morphological study of the pulmonary capillaries in patients with emphysema shows that the mean diameter of these capillaries may be substantially increased—perhaps to a degree that would prevent full oxygenation of blood within them.[2847]

RESPONSE TO INHALED CO_2

In 1925 Meakins and Davies noted that patients with advanced emphysema responded to inhaled CO_2 with a smaller increase in ventilation than did normal subjects.[1] Since that time several other workers have studied this phenomenon in an attempt to elucidate the cause of the reduced response.[963, 1038] Cherniack and Snidal showed that the response could be still further reduced by added respiratory resistance, which caused a fall in maximal breathing capacity and a diminution of the response curve.[962] Donald and Christie suggested that the delay in response to CO_2, as well as its total reduction, might be

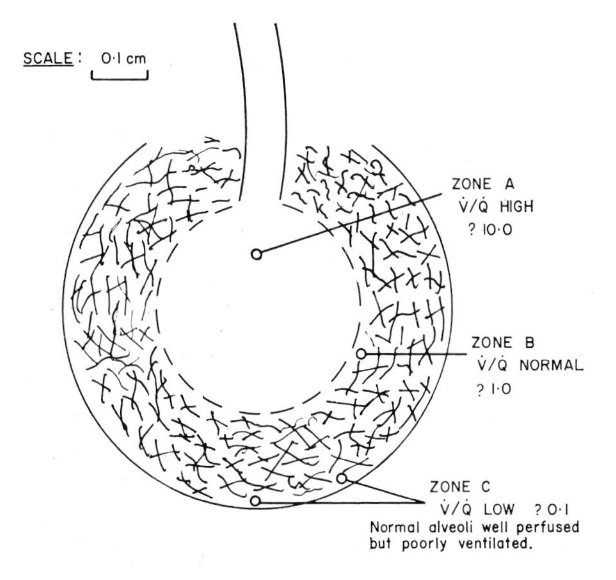

FIGURE 7–11. This diagram was published in the first edition to suggest a possible mechanism to account for the severe defect in gas exchange that may be seen in centrilobular emphysema, disproportionate to the loss of alveolar surface area. Several recent observations referred to in the text indicate that impaired diffusion in the gas phase might be important in relation to the lesions of centrilobular emphysema.[2521, 2859, 2836, 2520]

ascribable in part to the increased bicarbonate in the blood of many of these patients.[963] In two very elegant pieces of work published in 1954, Tenney[964] and Prime and Westlake[945] showed beyond reasonable doubt that the response in patients with emphysema could be correlated with the degree of pre-existing CO_2 retention, diminishing with increasing levels of resting arterial P_{CO_2}, a conclusion confirmed recently by Clark[2891] in a study of 36 patients with chronic obstructive lung disease. The response to CO_2 correlated best with the resting pre-existing mixed venous P_{CO_2}, and was judged to be independent of the amount of emphysema present. Other investigators have reached similar conclusions,[2747] but the precise reason for diminished response remains unclear. Flenley and Millar[2864, 2888] do not believe that mechanical factors account for the diminished response, nor that it can be attributed to the increased buffering power of the blood, and others have concluded that a diminished respiratory-center response must be the principal causative factor.[2882]

Tenney suggested that this paradoxical adjustment might serve to diminish the distress of dyspnea.[966] As several authors have pointed out, the progressive accumulation of CO_2 in pulmonary emphysema should perhaps be viewed as a series of steps, producing bicarbonate increase, leading to reduced ventilatory response, followed by more accumulation, and so on, with, at each step, an increase in the total CO_2 stores of the body.

It has been suggested that the response to CO_2 should be used as a test of emphysema.[965] Quite apart from the inherent undesirability of giving CO_2 to any patient with emphysema, it seems very unlikely from published data that such information is of more value than the maximal breathing capacity or arterial P_{CO_2} levels.

A paper from the USSR on this topic describes the results of giving a 5 or 6 per cent CO_2 mixture to 28 patients with emphysema, measurements being made of minute volume together with recordings of the bioelectric potentials from respiratory muscles.[980] A sharp increase in the electrical activity of the respiratory muscles and a diminished respiratory response were noted. The author suggests that the reason for the diminished response to CO_2 in patients with emphysema and hypercapnia may be not an adaptation of the respiratory center but some adaptation of the peripheral respiratory apparatus.

Effects of Aminophylline and Oxygen Administration

The problem of oxygen administration to patients with emphysema and respiratory failure is discussed in a later chapter, but some note is appropriate here since an understanding of the effects is relevant to the problem of the $\dot{V}/\dot{Q}$ distribution in emphysema. The administration of oxygen has been shown to worsen the $\dot{V}/\dot{Q}$ distribution in this disease,[2844, 2856] and part of the increased arterial P_{CO_2} is the result of this effect rather than the consequence of a reduced minute ventilation. Furthermore, in a study of 58 patients with chronic obstructive lung disease, Pain, Charlton, and Read[2858] found that the administration of 250 mg of aminophylline intravenously over a three-minute period led to a fall of arterial P_{aO_2} of 4 mm Hg or more in 20 of the patients. They attribute this phenomenon to the release by aminophylline of control of perfusion of poorly ventilated regions, with a consequent increase in blood flow through these units. These results, of both oxygen administration and aminophylline administration, confirm the existence of vasoconstrictor mechanisms reducing perfusion to poorly ventilated lung in these patients.

Pulmonary Hypertension, Cardiac Output, and Venous Return

Although it had been generally believed that the loss of pulmonary parenchyma in emphysema led to pulmonary hypertension,[927] it was the advent of cardiac catheterization that for the first time enabled changes in the pulmonary circulation to be studied in detail. This work, together with much more knowledge of the abnormal blood gas tensions in emphysema, has led to the idea that blood gas tensions may, in themselves, cause changes in the pulmonary vascular resistance. These may be independent of or additional to the fixed increase in resistance that may result from loss of total capillary bed. This evidence is summarized elsewhere (*see* Chapter 2), but it may be stated at this juncture that there is every reason to assume that the responses of the pulmonary vascular bed to changes in arterial pH and to alveolar gas tensions are relevant to an understanding of the genesis of pulmonary hypertension in emphysema.

The original observations of cardiac output in patients with pulmonary emphysema suggested that, in some patients with cor pulmonale, this might be elevated above the normal value.[967] However, subsequent studies have indicated that, although occasionally higher than normal, the cardiac index at rest and on exercise is more commonly normal or low.[2895] Recent evidence suggests that in extreme hypoxemia in emphysema, the cardiac output may not uncommonly be considerably lower than normal.[2877]

Ebert, in a useful review of this aspect of emphysema, suggested that cor pulmonale secondary to emphysema should be regarded as failure with a normal output.[968] There have been many careful serial studies of hemodynamics in a total of more than 100 patients with emphysema,[385, 624, 969–976, 979] from which the following generalizations can be made:

1. Some elevation of pulmonary artery pressure is commonly, though not invariably, found at rest. This bears little relationship to the maximal breathing capacity, although the elevation is greater in the presence of arterial desaturation and an elevated P_{CO_2}.

2. Pulmonary vascular resistance is increased during acute episodes of infection in the presence of blood gas disturbances;[2023] it may decrease after successful treatment.[969]

3. Some elevation in pulmonary artery pressure on exercise is almost invariable.[385, 2025] These patients can increase their cardiac output on exercise, but only at the expense of a rise in pressure. However, Charms and his colleagues have reported the surprising observation that, in patients with emphysema, occlusion of one pulmonary artery with consequent doubling of flow through the contralateral lung produces little elevation of pressure.[2024] The discrepancy that exists in relation to these observations cannot yet be satisfactorily explained.

4. The increase in pulmonary artery pressure is moderate and does not approach the systemic pressure levels seen in patients with postembolic or idiopathic pulmonary hypertension.

5. Administration of oxygen to such patients during resting or exercise conditions usually causes a small reduction in pulmonary artery pressure,[2025, 2026] but not to normal values unless the administration is continued for a long time. Hyperventilation also may be followed by a lowering of pulmonary vascular resistance.

Harvey and Ferrer suggested that the pulmonary hypertension of emphysema should be regarded as partly reversible and partly irreversible.[977] It has been pointed out (*see* page 165) that the morphological changes in the arterioles in emphysema are not adequate to account for the elevation of pulmonary pressure and the right ventricular hypertrophy commonly seen in patients with pulmonary emphysema. Furthermore, severe and protracted pulmonary hypertension may occur in patients with only a slight degree of morphological emphysema (*see* page 151). Combination of these data with many of the recent physiological findings on the effect of alterations in gas tensions on the pulmonary circulation suggests the inescapable conclusion that the mechanism of pulmonary hypertension in emphysema is closely linked to the gas-tension disturbances, or to the failure of effective alveolar ventilation that led to these; such effects will be aggravated by the general reduction in capillary bed that occurs, rather than be directly ascribable to this factor alone.

Although the effects of acute hypoxia and CO_2 retention on the myocardium itself have been extensively studied in animals, it is not clear to what extent the effect on the myocardium of sudden hypoxia and respiratory acidosis determines the onset of frank congestive heart failure. It is not known whether the increased blood viscosity that results from the polycythemia secondary to anoxia in emphysema of itself results in pulmonary hypertension. Although phlebotomy is recommended in the treatment of such patients,[977] Whitaker[970] did not consider that increased blood viscosity was an important factor in causing the pulmonary hypertension.

Nakhjavan, Palmer, and McGregor[2838] have recently documented the occurrence of significant obstruction to venous inflow into the thorax in the inferior vena cava in 6 patients with emphysema. This mechanism was found when the lungs were grossly hyperinflated and the diaphragm position was low. It is of interest and importance, since it is likely to be the mechanism responsible for leg edema and hepatomegaly in a patient with emphysema in whom the arterial blood-gas tensions are normal.

MEASUREMENTS DURING EXERCISE IN PATIENTS WITH EMPHYSEMA

Although there are technical reasons why exercise studies may be of more value than observations made at rest in the assessment of patients with emphysema, some of the physiological measurements are more difficult to make under these conditions. Thus, collection of arterial blood, recording of intraesophageal pressure, and measurement of cardiac output may all be done more simply in the resting subject.

However, in our experience it is often of very considerable value to observe the patient closely when he is exercising, since this affords a better impression of the degree of incapacity than can be obtained from the history.

Gilbert and his colleagues have shown that exercise tolerance in emphysema is broadly correlated with the FEV_1, but they emphasize that the variation is great enough between these two measurements that an exercise test is important in assessing effort capability.[2826]

During exercise, in patients with emphysema and abnormal arterial blood gases at rest, there is commonly a further worsening, the drop in arterial saturation often being proportionately greater.[385] There are some discrepancies in the results of studies of Type A (emphysematous) patients as compared to those in the bronchitic or Type B group. Jones[2505] found that on exercise the arterial $P{O_2}$ fell an average of 11 mm Hg in the Type A group, but rose 6 mm Hg in the bronchitic patients. Filley and his co-workers, however, noted little difference in the effect of exercise on the $P{CO_2}$ in arterial blood between two groups of patients with Type A and Type B disease. Emmanuel and Moreno[2855] concluded that in patients with only mild hypoxemia at rest, exercise produced an increase in arterial oxygen saturation, whereas in those with more severe resting hypoxemia, it usually produced a considerable further fall. Cohn and Donoso[2860] reported a difference between treadmill exercise and step-test exercise in their effect on the changes in arterial oxygen tension; the former produced a rise of 2.3 mm Hg in P_{aO_2}, whereas the latter caused a fall of 10 mm Hg, the level of oxygen uptake being comparable in the two exercise loads. In both groups the CO_2 tension changed relatively little. The reason for this difference was not apparent. Gilbert and his colleagues make the point[2741] that voluntary hyperventilation during exercise in patients with emphysema does not lead to a lowering of arterial $P{CO_2}$, and they conclude that chronic hypercapnia in these patients is not attributable to overall hypoventilation.

As others have pointed out,[385] it seems clear that these observed changes are not due to an increase in true blood shunt, nor to a decreasing alveolar ventilation, but (in general terms) to a worsening $\dot{V}/\dot{Q}$ distribution. It must not be forgotten, however, that present techniques do not permit a precise analysis of the main factor responsible, and, as noted earlier, there is bound to be complex interaction between the various component influences. One may guess that increasing respiratory frequency may worsen ventilation distribution and that increasing cardiac output may increase perfusion of poorly ventilated regions and may shorten an already too brief transit time, as suggested by Rossier.[17]

Other measurements made during exercise may be of value in the assessment of the patient with emphysema. The first of these is measurement of the maximal oxygen uptake during exercise. Sometimes this cannot be measured, but in younger patients it is often possible to increase the work-load and measure oxygen consumption when the limit of effort tolerance has been reached. In patients with emphysema, O_2 consumption is reduced when they reach that limit. The level of ventilation used for any given oxygen uptake differs little from the normal, though it is commonly found that a few patients with emphysema may overventilate in relation to oxygen uptake. In the majority, the normal proportionality between ventilation and oxygen uptake is approximately maintained. Filley pointed out that the oxygen cost of external work in patients with emphysema seems remarkably normal, and the increased oxygen cost of ventilation is not reflected in any observable decrease of external work for a given oxygen uptake.[978]

Secondly, there are advantages in measuring diffusing capacity in emphysema during exercise rather than at rest. The occurrence of considerable increases in diffusing capacity in normal subjects during exercise widens the gap between these people and patients with emphysema on exercise,[361, 370, 385] thus making the measurement more sensitive in discriminating one group from the other; also, as the tidal volume increases, the calculated alveolar CO tension becomes less sensitive to the ratio between the assumed value of respiratory dead space and tidal volume. A reasonable estimate of diffusing capacity may be possible, therefore, even without sampling arterial blood ($D_{L_{CO}}SS_3$).[370, 2843] Thus, when feasible, it is clearly preferable to study such patients during exercise, regardless of which

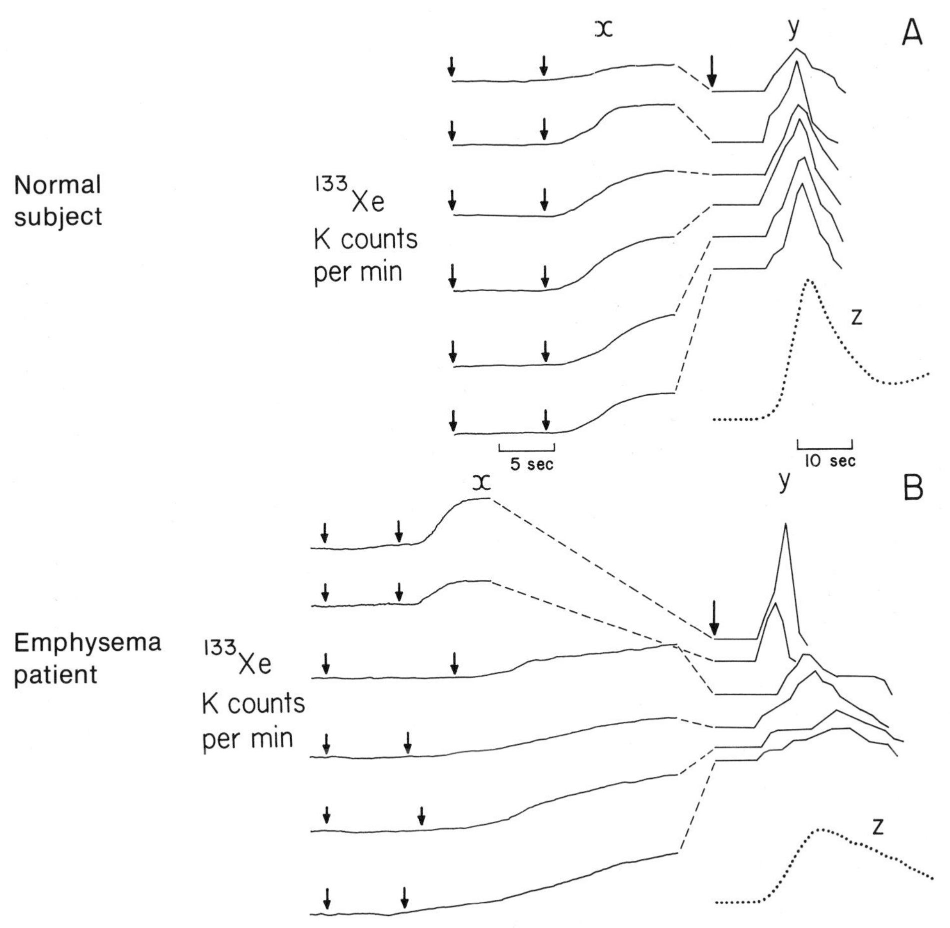

FIGURE 7–12. Variation of transit time through the lung in a patient with severe emphysema compared to a normal subject. *A:* At first arrow a bolus of ^{133} xenon dissolved in saline is injected into brachial vein catheter. At X, six scintillation detectors record arrival of xenon and build-up of gas concentration in the alveoli. Section Y is the computed transit time from the first derivative of the curves measured from the second arrow. Z shows the computed mean transit curve for the lung as a whole. *B:* A similar experiment made on a patient with severe emphysema (mostly panlobular). A very fast transit time is recorded for the top two counter positions, which were over the right upper lobe where the vasculature was relatively well preserved. Very slow transit times occur through the lung under the other four detectors. (Data kindly provided by Dr. M. McGregor and Dr. A. Oriol.)

method is used to measure the diffusing capacity.[361, 370, 385, 2510, 2843] (*see* Fig. 2–39, p. 81.)

There is no evidence that much can be gained from measurements of pulmonary mechanics during exercise in these patients, and the technical problems outweigh any slight advantage there may be in measuring airway resistance or lung compliance during exercise rather than at rest.

VARIANTS OF CLINICAL PULMONARY EMPHYSEMA

Several important variants of the commonly occurring types of emphysema necessitate separate description and emphasis. Not only are these of considerable interest and importance in themselves, but the study of the derangements of pulmonary function that they cause throws light on the relationship between structural change and function in the more common conditions.

Unilateral emphysema (McLeod's syndrome; unilateral transradiancy)

During the past 15 years, the syndrome of unilateral emphysema has been greatly clarified. Eleven major papers, published since

1953, form the basis for the following description of this syndrome, a total of about 60 patients having been described in detail. The pathology of the lung has been described in 5 of these patients.

The abnormalities revealed on chest x-ray may be noted clinically in childhood,[981] and in many of the cases described the patient is below the age of 40.[982] Many of the patients are symptom-free and have noticed no dyspnea.[763] All observers are agreed that it is common to be given a history of a previous, and often severe, attack of pneumonia, either bacterial or viral, in childhood or in adolescence.[983, 2929] After such an episode the patient may produce little sputum or may suffer from frequent chest infections or bronchitis.[984] Plain x-rays of the chest and bronchograms of the affected lung are diagnostic.[342, 763, 981–987] There is a loss of lung markings on the affected side, and a film taken in expiration shows the normal lung to empty, whereas the emphysematous lung remains filled, the mediastinum moving toward the normally emptying side (*see* Case 12). The bronchoscopic appearances are usually normal. Bronchograms reveal normal filling and normal contour of major bronchi; peripherally, however,[763, 983] the bronchi end in irregularities—abrupt endings termed "broken boughs" by Reid and Simon[983]—and many of the branches end in small dilations or pools of contrast medium.[763, 2922] The relative avascularity of the affected lung may be evident on the plain film, and is very strikingly demonstrated by tomography or on angiograms.[763, 985, 986] A pulmonary artery is always visible, however, though appearing narrower than normal, a finding that led to the erroneous suggestion that this entity was due to hypoplasia of the pulmonary artery.[988]

At operation[981] or on pathological study[983, 2928] the pulmonary artery and its branches are normal. Obliteration of bronchi and bronchioles is a striking feature; this appears to have resulted from a previous inflammatory lesion in many instances, since there may be extensive submucous bronchiolar fibrosis. Reid and Simon[983] have noted, however, that distribution of the bronchiolar lesions is irregular, with preservation of enough normal pathways to permit ventilation to the lung as a whole, though it is probable that gas may reach some areas by way of alveolar pores and collateral air drift. The lung parenchyma may show widespread destructive emphysema, probably always panlobular in type since in none of the material has a centrilobular pattern of destruction been noted.

Reid and Simon have also noted that in some cases there may be little destructive emphysema present; they feel that a more usual pathological picture is that of overinflation of the lung with intact structure.[983] The alveolar walls are avascular, and these authors suggest that an episode of pulmonary infection in these patients may have deterred the normal postnatal growth of the lung, resulting in an essentially overinflated hypoplastic lung. If this is correct, the maximal negative intrapleural pressure in these patients should be normal, in contrast to the findings in patients with destructive disease. The recording of an intrapleural pressure less negative than normal in a patient with unilateral emphysema would substantiate the theory that loss of recoil is an essential feature of the condition, but to date there are no reports that this measurement has been made.

The pattern of change in pulmonary function tests fits the pathology satisfactorily. The contralateral lung in these patients is normal. As has been mentioned, there may be no dyspnea even on moderately severe exertion. There is a slight reduction in vital capacity and ventilatory function,[1684] approximating that found in a patient who has undergone a pneumonectomy. Helium closed-circuit equilibration or inert-gas distribution is greatly reduced[763, 986] because of slow movement of gas into the affected lung. The abnormal lung fills more efficiently when a deep breath is taken than during ordinary tidal breathing,[987] a phenomenon that can be observed during helium equilibration as well as quantitated by bronchospirometry or radioactive-isotope studies.[342, 1684, 2896, 2897]

In an interesting study of 10 patients with this syndrome, Weg and his colleagues measured the single-breath diffusing capacity in the two lungs separately, using bronchospirometry.[2897] Their data show that the D_L on the affected side may be reduced to only one fifth of that on the contralateral side.

Using radioactive ^{133}xenon, Nairn and Prime[2896] have made a detailed investigation of ventilation and perfusion distribution in both lungs in 7 patients. All these patients had a history of childhood illness and 5 had chronic bronchitis, according to MRC questionnaire criteria. Major differences in ventilation were observed, being particularly evident on dynamic ventilation clearance experiments, but were also present when a slow deep inspiration was taken.

The arterial blood gases are usually normal,[2897] though some reduction in oxygen saturation has been reported.[984] This finding should always raise the suspicion of abnormality on the apparently normal side.

It is obvious that, when one lung is normal, the patient will not "use" the abnormal lung to any considerable extent. It is possible that perfusion is shifted away from the affected lung as a consequence of its impaired ventilation; or the resistance to blood flow may be greater through it than through the normal lung, for structural reasons. Differentiation of unilateral emphysema from agenesis of the lung[989, 990] depends upon demonstration of the presence of the pulmonary artery, even though flow through it may be greatly reduced. It is also of importance to stress that some patients with generalized emphysema show a preponderant loss of function on one side compared with the other (*see* Case 9), though such examples should be differentiated from the syndrome of true unilateral emphysema.

This entity is of importance for several reasons: first, because it suggests that emphysema may follow a specific episode of infection with apparent resolution, without any intervening period of chronic bronchitis; second, because it supports the view that a chronic bronchiolitis may play an important part in the etiology of emphysema; third, because it illustrates the fact that, although the patient may have half of his lungs destroyed by emphysema, when it is unilateral he may have no dyspnea since he can shift both perfusion and ventilation to the normal side; and fourth, because it raises the interesting question as to what one would call this syndrome if it occurred in both lungs simultaneously instead of in one lung. It seems to us that it might fall into the category of "vanishing lung" as an example of rapidly progressive panlobular emphysema. As noted in the next section, the same pathological process that causes unilateral emphysema occurs, in some patients, in one or two lobes only, a situation noted to occur by Reid and Simon.[983] There seems little reason to doubt, therefore, that it might occur in one lobe or any other part of either lung, though this must be regarded as unproven.

Lobar emphysema

This condition must be distinguished from infantile lobar emphysema, which is discussed in detail in a subsequent section of this chapter. Lobar emphysema differs from the syndrome of unilateral emphysema *only* by virtue of the fact that one lobe has been spared. Case No. 13 demonstrates widespread emphysema occurring in the middle and right-lower lobes of an otherwise healthy young man of 28. It is important to stress that this syndrome can occur in the absence of any history of an episode of bronchial obstruction due to a foreign body or other mechanism, and pathological study of the removed lobe reveals a normal bronchial tree as far as the level of the small bronchioles.[2920]

Emphysema with large bullae

The classification of clinical and functional patterns found in the presence of lung cysts and bullae is discussed in Chapter 8. Although such bullae may occur in otherwise normal lungs or may be associated with a remarkable preservation of ventilatory capacity, in some patients with generalized pulmonary emphysema the degree of lung destruction in one region may be sufficient to give rise to bullae measuring 1 cm or more in diameter. What proportion of patients with generalized emphysema shows them radiologically is not known. Reviewing the radiographs of 299 patients with chronic bronchitis, Simon and Medvei considered that 87 showed radiographic evidence of emphysema, and of these no fewer than 33 were considered to show obvious bullae.[991] In the absence of other evidence it is not possible to be sure of the degree of emphysema in these 87 patients. Our experience has been to see obvious bullae in about 10 per cent of patients with generalized emphysema, but we know of no precise data on this incidence. Those authors who have studied the pulmonary function of patients with bullae have documented examples of large air spaces associated with such marked pulmonary-function impairment that the presence of generalized emphysema is inferred.[992–997] It is the patients in this group who need very careful assessment of function before surgery is undertaken. It may be important to note that, when co-existent with generalized emphysema, the bullae communi-

Case 14
Emphysema, Centrilobular Mild; Severe Bronchitis and $\dot{V}/\dot{Q}$ Disturbance

Summary of Clinical Findings. This 37-year-old man, who had worked for 15 years as a plumber, was first seen in February 1960 when he was admitted to hospital with acute bronchitis and cardiac failure. His illness had begun a year earlier with a febrile episode diagnosed by his family doctor as pneumonia. Since that time he had had cough with moderate amounts of mucoid expectoration. Increasing dyspnea on exertion had occurred over the five-week period before admission and his ankles had begun to swell a week before. He smoked one to two packages of cigarettes per day. On physical examination some rhonchi were noted in the lungs, the jugular venous pressure was increased, the liver was enlarged, and 1+ edema was present in the legs. Bed rest and antibiotics resulted in the clearing of the respiratory infection and of the signs of congestive failure. His clinical diagnosis was acute bronchitis and arteriosclerotic heart disease after this admission. Eight months later, in October 1960, he was readmitted with a similar picture. On this occasion diagnosis on discharge was chronic bronchitis and cor pulmonale. Diminished air entry and prolonged expiration over the lungs were noted and an electrocardiogram revealed definite evidence of right ventricular hypertrophy. A right heart catheterization revealed a mean pulmonary artery pressure of 27 mm Hg at rest. On exercise the pulmonary systolic pressure rose to 90 mm Hg and the diastolic to 45 mm Hg. Pulmonary function tests on this admission are shown on page 216.

The patient was readmitted five times during the next two years. On each occasion he presented a clinical picture of respiratory infection with right-sided heart failure and, latterly, ascites. He was successfully treated with antibiotics, digitalis and diuretics until his final admission, when, despite a tracheostomy for respiratory failure, he died following an episode of ventricular fibrillation.

Radiology. A postero-anterior view of the chest (*A*) made in January, 1960, shows a generalized accentuation of linear markings, with several ill-defined patchy densities scattered throughout both lungs. The heart is broad, with a contour compatible with right ventricular enlargement. The hilar pulmonary arteries are moderately enlarged and there is a discrepancy between hilar and peripheral arterial caliber, due to the increase in hilar size rather than a decrease in the peripheral vessels. It is to be noted that there is little or no evidence of pulmonary hyperinflation to suggest air-trapping. The lateral projection (not reproduced here) showed a normal configuration of the diaphragm and no increase in the anteroposterior diameter of the chest.

The appearance of the pulmonary vasculature is consistent with a moderate degree of pulmonary arterial hypertension: however, the significance of the diffuse parenchymal disease was not recognized. A postero-anterior film made 10 days later (*B*) reveals clearing of the diffuse pulmonary disease. The heart is now much smaller and could be regarded as normal in size. The hilar pulmonary arteries remain large, however, and there is still considerable discrepancy between hilar and peripheral arterial caliber.

The nature of the changes observed earlier (*A*) are now clear. The diffuse parenchymal disease represented an acute diffuse pneumonia or bronchiolitis which was in all likelihood responsible for the development of right heart failure. The chest

(Case 14 continued on page 206.)

														EXERCISE				
	VC	FRC	RV	TLC	ME %	MMFR	$FEV_{0.75}$ ×40	pH	P_{CO_2}	HCO_3^-	O_2Hb %	$D_{LCO}SS_2$	CO Ext %	MPH	GRADE	$\dot{V}O_2$	$\dot{V}_E$	$D_{LCO}SS_3$
Predicted	3.4	2.7	1.6	5.6	60	3.4	100	7.4	42	25	97	18.3	49					30.0
Oct. 1960	1.8	2.5	2.0	3.8	22	0.4	33	7.41	64	33	68	10.4	31	3	FLAT	1.01	25	12.6
Nov. 1961	1.4	2.8	2.5	3.9	25	0.26	16	7.40	64	36	87	9.7	31					
March 1962	1.1	2.9	2.7	3.8	25	0.22	11	7.37	64	33	84	9.0	37					

The total lung capacity was always lower than predicted, with the residual volume proportionately and absolutely increased. A progressive decrease in vital capacity, expiratory flow rates and resting diffusing capacity and an increase in residual volume occurred over a two-year period. Many specimens of arterial blood were studied, and hypoxemia and CO_2 retention were invariably found. The exercise diffusing capacity was less than half the predicted value.

In addition to the above, this patient was found to have a normal static lung compliance but an airway resistance on quiet expiration of 15 cm H_2O/l/sec (normally 2.5). Maximal static intrapleural pressure was −17 cm H_2O, indicating only mild loss of elastic recoil and implying preservation of much of the lung tissue. Xenon studies showed perfusion to both lower zones to be less than normal and grossly delayed clearance of xenon from all lung regions.

Emphysema, Centrilobular Mild; Severe Bronchitis and $\dot{V}/\dot{Q}$ Disturbance

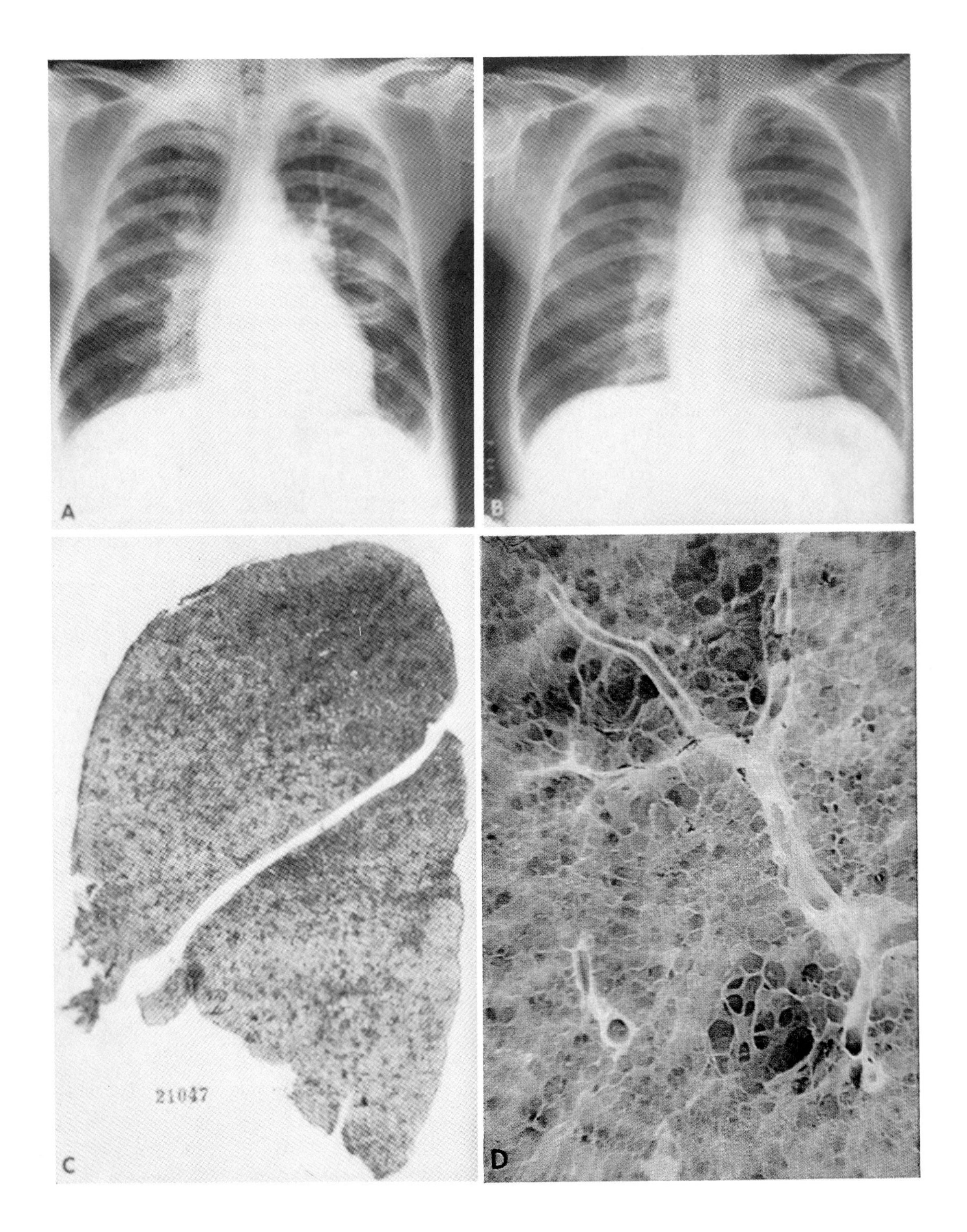

Case 14
Emphysema, Centrilobular Mild; Severe Bronchitis and $\dot{V}/\dot{Q}$ Disturbance (Continued)

film 10 days later (*B*) still shows evidence of pulmonary arterial hypertension, however, despite the return of the heart to normal size.

Repeated chest films over the next two years showed persistent enlargement of hilar pulmonary arteries and relative smallness of the peripheral pulmonary arteries, establishing the picture of pulmonary arterial hypertension.

Tomographic examination of the pulmonary vasculature (not reproduced here) confirmed the normal size of the peripheral vessels and the increased caliber of the hilar arteries. Bronchography (not reproduced here) revealed a normal tracheobronchial tree on both sides.

Pathology. The lungs showed widespread mild centrilobular emphysema which could scarcely be recognized in the gross specimen (*C*). Examination with the dissecting microscope disclosed involvement of the majority of the third-order and many second-order respiratory bronchioles by heavily pigmented destructive emphysema (*D*). The bronchioles themselves were only moderately enlarged and confluence of adjacent respiratory bronchioles was infrequent. The process was more conspicuous in the upper than in the lower zones of the lung, but altogether only 7.7 per cent of the lung parenchyma was involved by emphysematous spaces. The tips of the lingula and anterior basal segment showed mild panlobular emphysema. A severe degree of subacute bronchiolitis, with narrowing of the bronchioles and focal squamous metaplasia, was observed in both lower lobes, more particularly on the right side. Many bronchioles were plugged with mucopurulent secretion. The bronchial mucous glands were hypertrophied, with a Reid index of 0.53.

Severe cor pulmonale was present, the right ventricle weighing 140 g. The pulmonary arteries showed no thrombi or emboli, but microscopically a striking degree of medial thickening was observed. The coronary arteries were normal.

Summary. This is an example of severe and chronic $\dot{V}/\dot{Q}$ disturbance and cor pulmonale with preservation of the alveolar surface. It is not clear whether this was due to emphysema that, though mild and involving only a small proportion of the lung parenchyma, affected the majority of the acini, or whether it was due to unusually severe bronchiolitis complicating chronic bronchitis.

---

cate very poorly with the airways, the volume of intrathoracic gas measured by the plethysmographic technique being much larger than that measured by gas-equilibration methods unless helium equilibration or nitrogen clearance is continued for a very long time.

When large bullae are visible on the chest radiograph, but total pulmonary function is little disturbed, there is an increased likelihood that the emphysema may be paraseptal in distribution.[2508, 2785] This type of the disease appears to be particularly prone to result in large bullae and, since the major part of the rest of the lung may be normal, function may be well-preserved until the bullae occupy so much space that expansion of the normal lung is compromised.

Emphysema secondary to pulmonary fibrosis

Parenchymal destruction and irregular emphysema may occur in association with any inflammatory process in the lung, as for example the apical emphysema in association with a small healed tuberculous lesion. Emphysema may complicate and finally dominate the late stages of progressive massive fibrosis of the lung occurring in pneumoconiosis (*see* Chapter 17). Emphysema may develop in other forms of pulmonary interstitial fibrosis. This occurs in familial fibrocystic dysplasia[1001] (*see* Chapter 17), in scleroderma (Chapter 17), eosinophilic granuloma (Chapter 18), and a variety of other conditions. Such patients have been described as having bronchiolar emphysema,[1000, 1002] though in our view, in all of these examples of various types of interstitial fibrosis with bronchiolectasis and terminally some emphysema often included under the term of "honeycomb lung," the emphysema present is of relatively little importance.

Severe progressive emphysema

Emphysema with minimal chronic bronchitis in young people

This entity, sometimes referred to as "vanishing lung," a term introduced by Burke in 1937[1007] to describe the condition in a patient with severe emphysema causing incapacity before the age of 30, merits separation, not on pathological grounds, but because there is reason to suspect that it may constitute a separate entity etiologically. Burke's patient died six years after onset of dyspnea, and sputum was never a prominent feature. We described the similar, rapidly progressive development of bilateral upper-lobe emphysema in a 49-year-old woman[763] and another variant of this picture (case 16 in ref. 710) in which both lower lobes had been destroyed by panlobular emphysema, with relative sparing of the upper zones; a further example is given in Case No. 8. Several similar cases have been reported.[1037, 2028, 2029] Some have been classified as cystic lung disease. Thus, the 34-year-old patient described by Stanford and Nalle[1008] showed bilateral lower-lobe destruction identical to that observed by others.[710, 1037] Although Stanford and Nalle's paper was entitled "Some Notes on Cystic Disease of the Lungs," the distinguished pathologist who examined the lungs at autopsy noted: "It is our interpretation of this case that it is one of acquired pulmonary emphysema." In the five or six examples of this syndrome in which we have been able to examine the lungs at autopsy or after lobectomy, as in two patients reported[710, 763] and in Case No. 8, the affected parts were destroyed by a process indistinguishable from that found in other patients with advanced emphysema. It is also important to stress that all lobes are involved, although the emphysematous changes are often more severe in some areas than in others. This is in contrast to unilateral or lobar emphysema of the type discussed earlier.

Clinically, it is important for several reasons to distinguish these patients from more-typical and older patients with emphysema. It is our opinion, shared by others,[2029] (and, it must be admitted, lacking rigorous proof) that this type of emphysema occurs in younger people, often at about the age of 30; is as common in women as in men; usually when first seen is not complicated by the presence of chronic bronchitis; occurs in nonsmokers; and is characterized by severe ventilatory disturbance. Several of those patients we have seen had endured psychiatric treatment for dyspnea believed to be psychogenic in origin. Richards[996] has pointed out that chronic bronchitis may occur as a complication of this type of emphysema, and we have seen this happen. When this stage is reached, the patient begins to be indistinguishable from one whose chronic bronchitis has antedated the onset of dyspnea.

It must be repeated that there are no grounds for regarding these patients as pathologically distinct from others with advanced centrilobular and panlobular emphysema; it is on clinical grounds that they appear to fall into a separate group. It has been noted that the average age of many series of patients studied with emphysema from different parts of the world is about 55 years. This mean age implies that, in all series, the patients aged 70 have been balanced by a nearly equal number of those about 40 years of age. If these younger patients are carefully analyzed, it is our experience that many of them will come within the category just described.

It now seems likely that at least some of these patients suffer from what may be examples of emphysema of hereditary type, linked to, or possibly caused by, a deficiency of α_1 antitrypsin in the serum. This syndrome is discussed in detail in a later section (*see* page 231), although its characteristics of early onset, prevalence in women, dissociation from chronic bronchitis, and the fact that pathologically it seems to be panlobular in type certainly conform to the clinical pattern not uncommonly encountered in younger patients.

CORRELATION OF STRUCTURAL AND FUNCTIONAL CHANGE

INTERRELATIONSHIP BETWEEN FUNCTION AND MORPHOLOGY

Observations of the morphological changes characteristic of emphysema may be considered to provide an almost complete explanation of the commonly encountered defects of function. The destruction of alveoli and of lung parenchyma accounts for the decreased negativity of the intrapleural pressure and for the increased resting FRC that results from the outward pull of the chest wall on lungs with less recoil. Airway obstruction at the terminal bronchiolar level results from chronic bronchiolitis, mucous plugging, and possibly loss of surfactant from the inner walls of bronchioles, leading to instability.[2448] Furthermore, the loss of elastic recoil reduces peribronchial and peribronchiolar pressure,

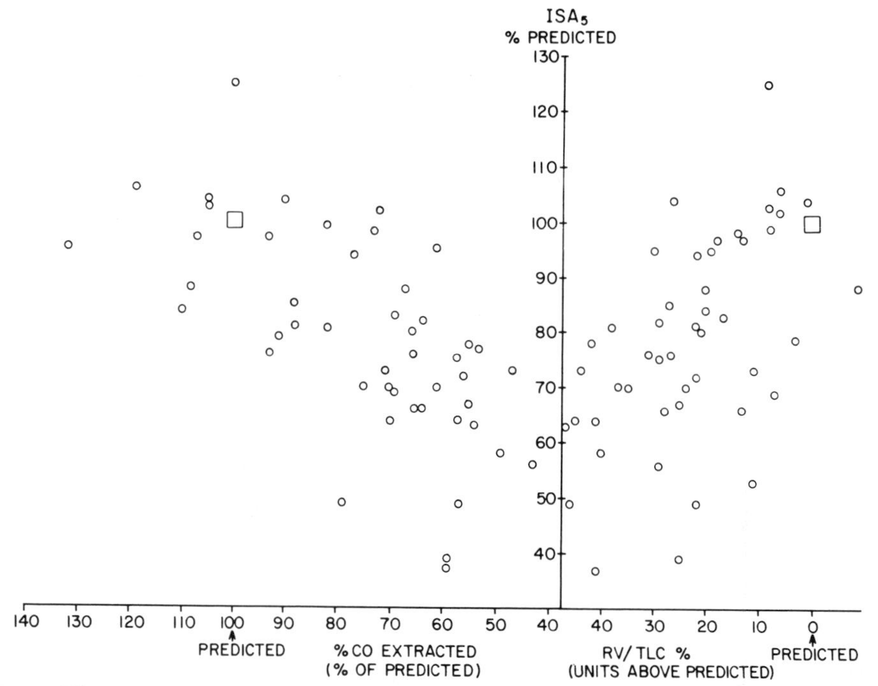

FIGURE 7–13. The measured alveolar surface area at an arbitrary lung volume of 5 liters (ISA_5) is plotted against the fractional uptake of carbon monoxide (% CO extracted) and the ratio of residual volume to total lung capacity. (From reference 2524.)

resulting in a reduction in caliber. In larger bronchi, obstruction may be attributable to collapse of their walls during forced expiration,[2272] as a result of cartilage atrophy consequent upon chronic infection. The grossly uneven gas distribution is caused by variability of the degree of airway change and of alveolar damage in different parts of the lung, with consequent wide variation in time constants. It seems very likely that complete obliteration of terminal bronchioles may occur, leading to drift ventilation into large regions of the lung, with consequent incredibly slow equilibration rates. The emphysematous spaces themselves act as collateral channels, so that the resistance to collateral flow is very markedly reduced in emphysema and may even be less than the airway resistance in this disease.[2440, 3833]

In some cases, the loss of diffusing capacity may be directly related to loss of alveolar surface area and at least a normal CO transfer is not found in the presence of major alveolar loss;[2524] however, all methods of measurement are also affected by abnormality of $\dot{V}/\dot{Q}$ distribution. There is evidence that the lung with emphysema is capable of reducing perfusion of poorly ventilated zones.

THE RELATIVE ROLES OF EMPHYSEMA AND CHRONIC BRONCHITIS IN CAUSING DISTURBANCES OF FUNCTION

As noted in Chapter 6, there is considerable contemporary discussion of the relative importance of chronic bronchitis and emphysema in causing abnormalities of pulmonary function. It is not possible to resolve this matter at the present juncture; the reader may find many lively discussions of the problem.[2509, 2519, 2557, 2644] It is possible, however, to summarize some points about which there is fairly general if not total agreement—and it may be worth attempting this, since otherwise there is little solid ground on which the spectator can safely stand. In addition, some of the discussions have so emphasized points of controversy that points of agreement have been obscured.

1. Chronic bronchitis, as defined, may cause severe $\dot{V}/\dot{Q}$ disturbance. In such patients there are almost certain to be widespread changes in peripheral parts of the lung. It is not known what percentage of patients who fulfill the criteria of chronic bronchitis progress to this severe stage of the disease.

2. There is a general correlation between

TABLE 7–2 THE MEAN VALUES FOR VARIOUS PULMONARY FUNCTION TESTS IN THE VARIOUS GROUPS

EMPHYSEMA GROUP	VC	FRC	RV	TLC	RV/TLC	ME%	MMFR	FEV	DL_{CO}	CO%
0	101.4	93.5	104.75	102.25	0.25	105.7	98.8	110.4	120.8	98.6
I	80.5	108.3	133.4	99.6	13.2	102.2	44.8	72.2	121.6	88.6
II	64.8	122.8	177.4	103.1	23.7	74.8	33.3	41.7	85.7	85.7
III	60.4	126.1	167.6	101.4	24.9	67.8	17.9	30.8	75.9	72.2
IV	53.8	133.0	178.2	102.2	28.2	71.8	16.2	27.3	67.9	65.0
V	47.2	162.4	240.6	116.4	36.3	54.5	9.2	16.2	45.7	56.8
Asthma	77.0	107.0	124.0	95.0	11.0	76.5	18.0	41.5	65.0	71.0
Bronchiectasis	43.4	114.0	172.0	89.0	30.8	47.2	11.0	18.2	55.4	71.2

All are expressed as a percentage of predicted except for RV/TLC which is expressed as a percentage over predicted. VC = vital capacity, FRC = functional residual capacity, RV = residual volume, TLC = total lung capacity, RV/TLC = ratio of RV to TLC, ME = mixing efficiency, MMFR = maximal mid expiratory flow rate, FEV = forced expiratory volume in the first 3/4 second, DL_{CO} = steady-state diffusing capacity for carbon monoxide, CO% = fractional uptake of carbon monoxide.

These results show increasing impairment in relation to degree of morphological emphysema (O-V in ascending severity).[2524] All patients except two had chronic bronchitis.

the defect of pulmonary function—particularly the changes in lung volumes and CO transfer—and the extent of morphological emphysema,[2524] regardless of the coexistence of chronic bronchitis in almost every patient. We have recently documented this phenomenon in detail (*see* Table 7–2) by comparing the impairment of function during life with the extent of morphological emphysema at autopsy. In syndromes of emphysema not associated with bronchitis (particularly alpha$_1$-antitrypsin deficiency) there is considerable disturbance of pulmonary function.

3. No specific test of function, except possibly measurement of lung recoil, is in any sense "specific" for the presence of emphysema.

4. Bronchiectasis may cause a severe disturbance of arterial blood-gas tensions but is to be distinghished from the majority of cases of chronic bronchitis.

5. Unexplained hypoventilation, presumably of central origin, may occur in patients with chronic bronchitis. In such patients the disturbed arterial blood-gas tensions cannot be attributed solely to the presence of the chronic bronchitis.

6. Clinically, a rough division can be attempted between patients in whom there is a high probability of morphological emphysema present (Type A) and patients whose chronic bronchitis is severe and in whom the presence of morphological emphysema is more doubtful (Type B). Many patients, however, are unclassifiable using such criteria, and morphological studies provide little basis for any hard and fast division.[2524] Opinion varies on the exact criteria on which a clinical differentiation should be based.

We feel that it is unfortunate that only one term, "chronic bronchitis," is available to characterize, on the one hand, a man with a chronic productive cough of long-standing, but completely normal pulmonary function; and, on the other, a patient with severe ventilatory defect and $\dot{V}/\dot{Q}$ disturbance. Although no one can claim that the respiratory field has suffered from "under-classification," this does seem to

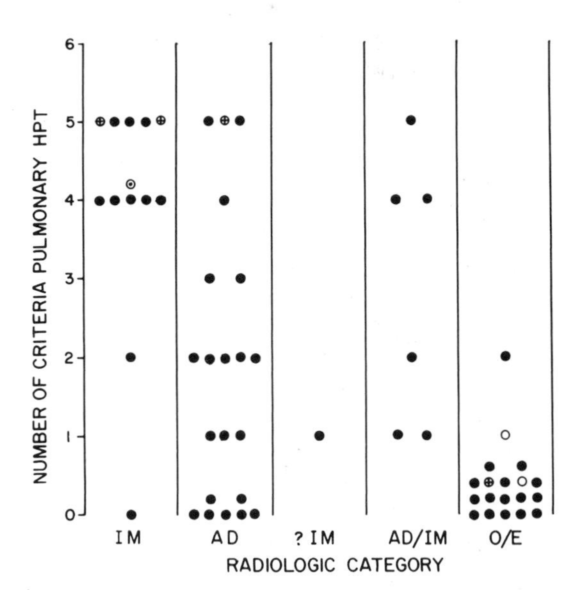

FIGURE 7–14. *Ordinate:* Number of criteria of right ventricular hypertrophy; *abscissa:* radiologic category of emphysema. ⊕ = bronchiectasis; ○ = asthma; ⊙ = multiple pulmonary emboli; ● = cases with varying degrees of emphysema at autopsy. (*See* reference 2524 for detailed description.)

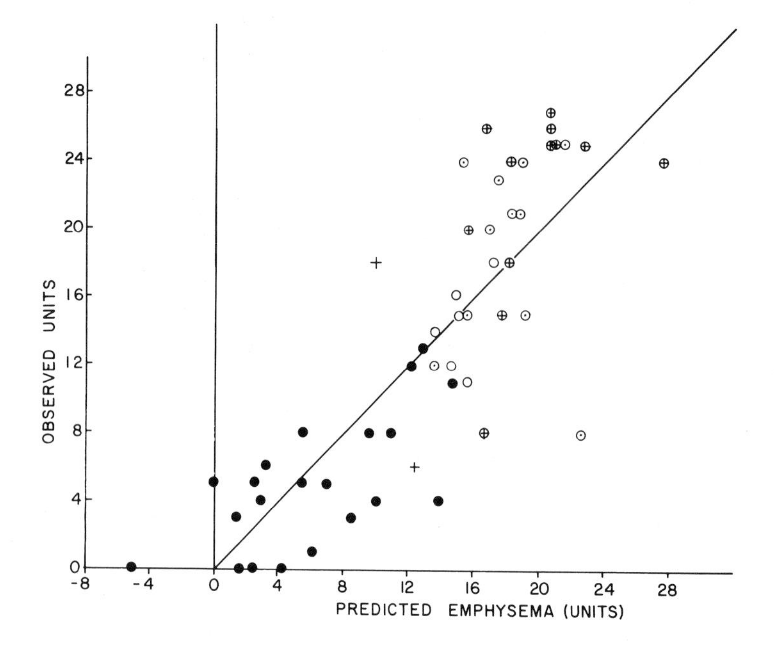

FIGURE 7–15. The actual subjective emphysema score in units (observed units) is compared to that predicted from the multiple correlation coefficient, based on pulmonary function tests. ● = asymptomatic cases; ○ = symptomatic obstructive lung disease; ⊙ = died of obstructive lung disease; + = 4 or 5 criteria of pulmonary hypertension and symptomatic obstructive lung disease; ⊕ = 4 or 5 criteria of pulmonary hypertension and died of obstructive lung disease.[2524]

be an instance in which some additional term would serve a very useful purpose.

We are also of the opinion that a careful study of each individual patient in the pulmonary function laboratory and by the radiologist is most important if proper decisions concerning management and treatment are to be made, and the physician must continuously attempt to assess the morphological state of the lung during life. It is because of this that we have discouraged the wholesale use of the nondiscriminatory term "chronic obstructive lung disease" for all these types of conditions. We are well aware that not all physicians share this view, however, and Filley, Dart, and Mitchell[2519] have recently written: "When the physician observes that chronic productive cough is by far the most common early manifestation of chronic airway obstruction, and considers this part of a disease, 'chronic bronchitis,' he should not be unduly influenced by physiologists who may claim that the patient's disease is really emphysema."

Emphysema and Aging

Several authors, including ourselves,[21] have pointed out that in almost every major aspect of function the changes observed in patients with emphysema are those characteristic of aging in the apparently normal population. This is true of the alterations in the subdivisions of lung volume, decline of ventilatory ability, loss of elastic recoil, less-uniform inert-gas mixing and $\dot{V}/\dot{Q}$ ratios, loss of diffusing capacity (however measured), and loss of maximal oxygen uptake. The airway resistance, however, is not much influenced by age, though Cohn and Donoso have found it to be increased in a group of elderly men.[1908]

The morphological changes that occur in the lung apparently as a result of aging have been discussed (*see* page 96). Principally, these appear to be an increase in the proportionate size of the alveolar duct system, as yet not well quantitated. Thus there seems little basis for ascribing emphysema to aging *per se*, though it is possible that repetitive irritants or infection may play some part both in causing the changes of age in the lung and in the genesis of emphysema. It is not easy to establish how far alterations in function or morphology are a consequence of environmental exposure; and it certainly seems probable that continued inhalation of dust or more-noxious materials is one factor that may link together the phenomena apparently ascribable to age and those that result in morphological emphysema.

Recent advances in understanding of the effects of the loss of recoil of the lung with age are relevant to the problem of the interrelationship between aging and pulmonary emphysema (*see* page 98). Loss of recoil, whether due to age or to emphysema, results in "premature" small-airway closure; this, in turn, will impair ventilation, particularly in dependent lung zones, with a consequent worsening of the $\dot{V}/\dot{Q}$ distribution, particularly during shallow tidal breathing.

THE NATURAL HISTORY OF EMPHYSEMA

It is conventional to discuss the natural history of a disease entity at the beginning; in the case of emphysema, however, we have preferred to describe the various ways in which this disease may present itself before discussing problems of etiology and prognosis.

THEORIES OF ETIOLOGY

The morphological study of emphysema has not provided conclusive evidence concerning its etiology and pathogenesis, but there is no shortage of theories. Since there are several forms of emphysema, it is to be supposed that each may have its own particular etiology. A number of facts can be readily observed, but often it is not clear whether these are primary or secondary; even in a single emphysematous locus, it may well be that several processes are at work simultaneously. Theories of etiology may be divided into three categories, each with several variations; thus, emphysema has been regarded as primarily inflammatory, degenerative, or obstructive in origin.

Inflammation

In random autopsy cases, about double the incidence of pulmonary emphysema is found in those patients believed to have suffered from chronic bronchitis, and mucous-gland hypertrophy is greater in lungs which also show emphysema, though it does not increase in degree with increasing degrees of emphysema.[2524] However, emphysema may be absent despite a long history of chronic bronchitis, and it may be present in lungs which show no mucous-gland hypertrophy or in patients who produced no sputum.[2503]

It has also been noted that although the Reid Index may be fairly uniform throughout the lung,[2507] the distribution of emphysema is commonly not uniform at all. Greenberg, Boushy, and Jenkins, in a recent study, concluded: "The discrepancy in the interlobar distribution of emphysema as opposed to chronic bronchitis lends no support to the frequently assumed cause and effect relationship between the two conditions."[2511]

These findings suggest that emphysema results from a condition that is frequently but not invariably a complication of chronic bronchitis. Bronchiolitis certainly meets these requirements; and recently more evidence has appeared which indicates to us that it may be the state of the small airways—rather than the mucous-gland hypertrophy in the larger bronchi—which provides the link between chronic bronchitis and emphysema. This idea is not new, since McLean[906] suggested that the primary lesion was obliterative bronchiolitis, and Reid[7] proposed that bronchiolar ulceration might be important in the genesis of emphysema. Bronchiolitis is universally present in centrilobular emphysema, and all types of emphysema are accompanied by a diminution in number of terminal bronchioles.[2727] Furthermore, there is recent evidence that the first lesion in cigarette smokers may well be at the terminal bronchiolar level (*see* Chapter 6).

The incidence of intercurrent bronchial infections is high in patients with chronic bronchitis, though prognosis in that condition seems to be independent of the purulence of the sputum (*see* page 152). These episodes of infection may well represent attacks of bronchiolitis. On occasion such an attack may be seen as producing a miliary pattern on the chest x-ray (*see* Case 2). Individual patients have been reported in whom an attack of acute bronchiolitis has been followed by chronic obstructive lung disease,[2907] and we believe we have seen at least one patient in whom an acute miliary episode of short duration was apparently followed by severe emphysema in the absence of chronic bronchitis.[763] Cullen and his colleagues have documented emphysema occurring after granulomata associated with terminal bronchioles.[2904]

It must be admitted that this kind of evidence is far from definitive; but there is little doubt that infection of one form or another is of importance in the etiology of most cases of emphysema.

Atrophy

Three atrophic changes have been implicated in the etiology of emphysema. All have been known and discussed for many years, and each has received renewed attention recently. These are the formation of alveolar fenestrae, obliteration of the capillary bed, and disruption and destruction of elastic tissue. Since they occur together, the problem is one of priority. A primary disorder of elastic tissue is perhaps the least likely, since this tissue is relatively indestructible, and chemical assays do not reveal any loss of elastin in emphysema.[2017] It may be important to point out that destructive emphysema is not a disease of extreme old age (*see* page 176), and there is little evidence to support the idea that generalized atrophy of lung tissue of a type recognizably distinct from the ordinary forms of emphysema occurs in the very elderly. The strongest evidence of a primary capillary origin is the experimental production of so-called emphysema in rabbits by obliteration of the capillary bed,[2033] though this lesion appears to have little in common with emphysema in man.

Probably of more importance has been the demonstration that various chemical irritants, when adsorbed onto carbon particles which are then inhaled, may be capable of producing a circumscribed area of destruction that resembles the lesion of centrilobular emphysema.

Obstruction

Since obstruction to air flow not only is present in emphysema but also is characteristic of chronic bronchitis, it is not surprising that the genesis of emphysema has been attributed for many years to the effects of this obstruction. Reading one of the more recent articles advocating this theory,[1010] one is left with the impression that the pathogenesis of emphysema presents no problems to anyone who has ever inflated a bicycle tire. However, as has been pointed out frequently, when the lung parenchyma is normal, a flap valve in the bronchus that opens on inspiration but closes on expiration may lead to overinflation, but this is not the same as morphological emphysema.

The observation that severe repeated attacks of spasmodic asthma, when unaccompanied by infection, do not result in development of emphysema (*see* Chapter 5) weakens the postulate of obstruction alone as the primary cause of this disease. It has been shown recently that some patients with emphysema and chronic bronchitis may experience severe localized collapse of major airways during expiration.[772] This narrowing may be a source of obstruction at the point of entry of the bronchus into the parenchyma, and this result of chronic infection of the bronchus may play a part in causing the development of bronchiolitis. The cough mechanism is seriously impaired in airway obstruction because the maximal expiratory flow rates are reduced. Excessive dynamic compression of lobar and stem bronchi results in the equal pressure points being located there rather than further upstream (*see* pages 34–39). If the equal pressure points were further upstream, the segment of the bronchial tree that is compressed would be longer and the cough more efficient, since it is only in the part of the airway that is dynamically compressed that cough will be effective. Thus, excessive compression of lobar bronchi will impair mucous elimination from smaller airways, leading to retention of secretions in this region.

FAMILIAL EMPHYSEMA

The literature contains sporadic references to a familial predisposition to emphysema, and there are a number of reports of emphysema occurring in several members of the same family.[24, 1030] Recently, Larson and Barman[2738] have described a family in which 6 out of 11 members had severe disease, and the remaining 5 had significant abnormalities of pulmonary function. As noted earlier, Hole and Wasserman[2739] have traced a family pedigree, with a high incidence of respiratory disease, back over 150 years and have suggested that a familial predisposition of sensitivity to cigarette smoke may be the responsible factor. We have also noted emphysema occurring in three pairs of brothers.[3685] Some of these reports may, in fact, be instances of an inherited deficiency in serum $alpha_1$ antitrypsin (*see* later discussion). Other cases may indeed reflect sensitivity to environmental factors; but in general, considering the frequency of the condition, inherited factors seem unlikely to play a major part in the etiology.

SERUM $ALPHA_1$-ANTITRYPSIN DEFICIENCY AND EMPHYSEMA

The recognition by Eriksson in 1965[2898] that a deficiency of this enzyme was associated with an unusually high incidence of respiratory disease and, in particular, of emphysema unassociated with chronic bronchitis

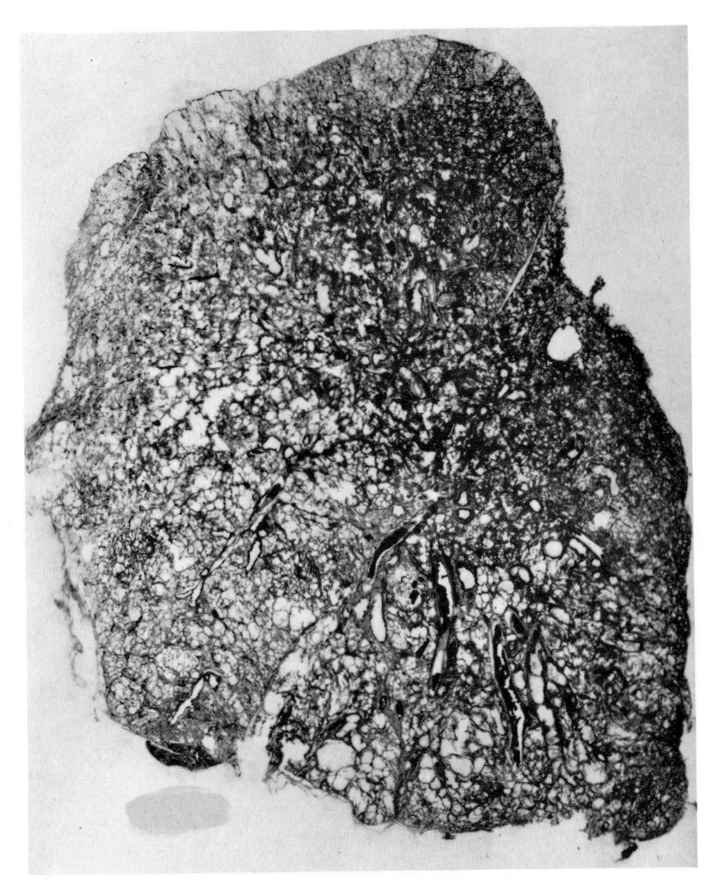

FIGURE 7–16. An example of almost pure, severe panlobular emphysema from a patient with familial emphysema associated with $alpha_1$-antitrypsin deficiency. This patient had a very large right ventricle at necropsy, together with clinical evidence of cor pulmonale. (Reprinted from Thurlbeck, W. M.: Internal surface area and other measurements in emphysema. Thorax, *22*: 487, 1967, with the permission of the Editor of Thorax, British Medical Association.[2506]

represents a major step forward in contemporary understanding of these diseases. It is believed that the type of emphysema is panlobular,[2900] the onset is at an early age, there is a high incidence in females, and a lack of clinical bronchitis, which may occur as a dangerous complication.[2901, 2918] Subclinical cases with abnormalities of pulmonary function may occur in heterozygotes.[2918, 2918] In a typical group of patients with emphysema, the deficiency was found by Brun and his colleagues[2916] in 13 of 143 patients screened; and by Briscoe and his co-workers[2899] in 1 out of 99 patients surveyed. Normally, 1 ml of serum inhibits more than 0.80 mg of trypsin; the serum of heterozygotes inhibits between 0.80 and 0.40 mg of trypsin; and the serum of homozygotes who may have lung changes inhibits less than 0.40 mg of trypsin.[2901]

Erkstam and his co-workers have reported 5 patients in whom the serum levels of antitrypsin were only 25 per cent of normal; 4 of these had chronic bronchitis combined with emphysema, and the 5 cases constituted 3.1 per cent of the 149 patients with chronic bronchitis and emphysema admitted to their department during the same period. We have recorded this condition in brothers of the same family,[3685] and Guenter and his colleagues have recorded it in 7 patients in three families.[3684] In their group, 2 patients were described as asymptomatic, but had abnormal pulmonary function tests with a lowered diffusing capacity and arterial oxygen tension. There was decreased vascularity at the lung bases in these patients, and the authors concluded that they probably had panlobular emphysema in the lower lobes.

Although this syndrome does not appear to account for any very large percentage of patients with emphysema, its importance is considerable, since it provides a clue to the biochemical state necessary for lung integrity. It is not yet clear exactly how the lung may come to be damaged in the absence of a sufficient level of the enzyme,[2902, 2903] and clearly much more remains to be learned. The examination of young patients who appear to have unusually severe panlobular emphysema without much antecedent history of chronic bronchitis should clearly henceforth include an examination of the blood to establish the normality or otherwise of the serum antitrypsin-enzyme level. Such data may well throw new light on etiological factors relating to this form of the disease. Perhaps it should be emphasized that centrilobular emphysema and panlobular emphysema very frequently coexist in the same lung; for this reason, if for no other, the complete understanding of etiology is likely to be complex.

Factors relevant to prognosis in emphysema

Although little further knowledge of the etiology of emphysema has accrued in the past few years, except indirectly through increasing information on the problem of chronic bronchitis, there is now a much better understanding of the factors that may determine prognosis. These fall under two main headings.

Role of disordered gas tensions

Campbell performed a very useful service by suggesting that disordered arterial blood gas tensions determine the onset of cor pulmonale.[953] There is little doubt that these changes are closely related to prognosis,[947] and there has been ample documentation of the importance of cor pulmonale in determining the long-term outlook in emphysema.[392, 892] Insofar as the diffusing capacity reflects both the uneven $\dot{V}/\dot{Q}$ distribution that underlies these disturbances and the loss of total alveolar surface, it is not surprising that, even when crudely measured, the steady-state CO uptake is found to be related to prognosis.[392, 2022] In the group of patients with "chronic obstructive lung disease" studied by Shepard and his colleagues,[420] considerable variation in diffusing capacity (D_{LO_2}) was found, but the relationship of this value to prognosis was not assessed. One may predict, however, that both the degree of $\dot{V}/\dot{Q}$ disturbance and the extent of reduction in the alveolar surface area are related to prognosis.

Vulnerability of remaining functioning lung

It seems quite clear that, in some patients, most of the remaining function is confined to a lobe representing the least damaged portion of the two lungs. In such patients, one of whom we described in considerable detail,[174] one lobe may be responsible for five-sixths of ventilation and perfusion. Such a patient may continue for many years with severe ventilatory restriction but with a normal arterial P_{CO_2} and without developing cor pulmonale. If, however, he is unfortunate enough to get an acute infection in his remaining functioning zone or acquires acute bronchiolitis as a result of smog, he is immediately thrown into very severe anoxia. Many of the severe anoxic episodes documented in the literature, accompanied by CO_2 retention and the swift development of cor pulmonale,[951, 1012, 1013] probably have been cases of this type. In such instances, prognosis is determined entirely by the freedom from intercurrent infection of the part of the lung upon which the patient has become completely dependent, the remainder of the lung being virtually destroyed. Some studies indicate that the prognosis of patients with chronic bronchitis, though suffering from an undetermined degree of emphysema, may be poor in urban areas.[991, 1011] It may be inferred from the association of episodes of smog with the worsening of symptoms in patients with emphysema[392, 852] that the prognosis in such patients must be adversely affected by atmospheric pollution.

SECONDARY EFFECTS OF EMPHYSEMA

The development of pulmonary hypertension and cor pulmonale as a consequence of emphysema has been noted already, as has the phenomenon of impaired filling of the right heart. The disease has, however, other secondary effects involving the body as a whole. It is not possible to distinguish whether these effects are due to the abnormalities in arterial gas tension in every instance; certainly most of them occur both in chronic bronchitis and in emphysema.

General systemic effects

Most physicians have seen patients with severe progressive emphysema, often in the younger age group, who note much loss of weight at the time of onset of their dyspnea. There may appear to be considerable loss of muscle tone, appetite and libido, and increased fatigue, well in advance of chronic respiratory failure, though such changes are most commonly seen in patients with chronic anoxia and retention of CO_2. Although occasionally these may appear clinically to be possible cases of thyrotoxicosis or adrenal insufficiency, we have never been able to demonstrate either of these disorders in them by laboratory tests.

As noted in Chapter 6, attention has recently been drawn to the possibility that in some patients with chronic bronchitis there may be a significant loss of protein in the sputum, with consequent general systemic effects.[2653]

SECONDARY CHANGES IN THE BLOOD

There have been many studies of the effects of chronic anoxia on the hemopoietic system in patients with emphysema.[392, 967, 979] Some authors have recorded a blood volume greater than normal in these patients, particularly in those who have had an episode of cor pulmonale,[979] and an increase in size of the erythrocyte[1031] with a decrease in mean corpuscular hemoglobin concentration[1032] and an increase in red-cell water[1034] have all been noted. More recently, Hume and Goldberg have compared patients with chronic bronchitis and emphysema to a group suffering from polycythemia rubra vera, as well as to normal subjects. They have concluded[2912] that in the patients with lung disease, there is a significant reduction in plasma volume associated with hypoxia; the red-cell volume was twice as great in the patients with primary polycythemia as in those with polycythemia secondary to the lung disease. The increased buffering power of the red cell in patients with emphysema, found by Platts and Greaves,[950] is probably related to the increased cell water.

There has been some variation in the correlation found between the secondary polycythemia and the hypoxic stimulus. Some investigators have found no relationship,[1031, 1034] and others have noted some proportionality.[1033] Hume[2917] has reported that the percentage increase in the red-cell volume in patients with chronic bronchitis was inversely related to the logarithm of the arterial $P\text{O}_2$, and was similar to the altitude effect on normal subjects. The plasma of patients with emphysema but without secondary polycythemia has been shown to contain more erythropoietin than normal.[2031] Massaro and his colleagues noted a good general relationship between the arterial oxygen tension and the erythroid response,[2910] and documented the fact that in patients with polycythemia and chronic hypercapnia due to lung disease, venesection was not followed by any fall in the arterial $P\text{CO}_2$.[2911] Finley and his co-workers have noted no variation in $P\text{CO}_2$ in spite of considerable differences in hematocrit in different groups studied at altitude.[2913]

SECONDARY CHANGES IN THE CEREBROSPINAL FLUID

Several interesting studies of the CSF in patients with chronic bronchitis and emphysema have appeared within the last few years,[2886, 2889, 2914, 2915] including one major thesis on the subject.[2885] It appears that the CSF $P\text{CO}_2$ generally follows the arterial level, but the bicarbonate is usually lower; consequently, the hydrogen-ion concentration is commonly increased. There is no significant increase in CSF lactate concentration,[2886] but some increase in calcium content has been reported.[2914] In patients with chronic hypercapnia, there is believed to be an increased ammonia production in the central nervous system, leading to an increase in glutamine concentration in the CSF of these patients.[2915] The significance of all these deviations from normal, in relation to ventilation control in emphysema, is unfortunately still quite uncertain.

SPECIAL ENTITIES

INFANTILE LOBAR EMPHYSEMA (CONGENITAL LOBAR EMPHYSEMA)

For many years this important condition has attracted attention as a potentially dangerous illness usually requiring operative intervention. The usual symptom is respiratory distress noted during the first few days or weeks of life or as late as three years or so after birth. The chest x-ray reveals overinflation, usually of one of the upper lobes, with displacement of the trachea and mediastinum away from the abnormal side. Lung markings can be seen in the diseased lobe, but are sparse. Fluoroscopic examination reveals that the affected lobe fails to empty on expiration, and the lesion may be most dramatically demonstrated, as in unilateral emphysema in adults, by exposure of a film on expiration. The respiratory distress, particularly severe if pneumonia occurs elsewhere in the lung, usually necessitates lobectomy. Typical cases are reported in the world literature each year.[1014–1018, 2923, 2924, 2926] Several useful reviews of collected cases have been published,[1019–1021] and recently there has been considerable clarification of the pathogenesis of this condition. In the majority of infants seen with this condition, the essential lesion is a failure of development of the normally concentrically arranged cartilages in the wall of the upper-lobe bronchus. Cottom and Myers noted that this anomaly had been intermittently recorded in the literature since 1944 and that expiratory collapse of the bronchus had been observed during bronchoscopy; in their six cases the bronchial cartilage anomaly was the dominant lesion.[1020] Joseph and his colleagues reviewed 62 reported cases and concluded that the bronchus was abnormal in 31.[1019] It should be stressed that cases with this anomaly must often have been missed, since the surgical clamp during lobectomy often mutilates the exact region where the lesion is, and very careful reconstruction of the bronchus may be necessary to detect the abnormality. In few of the reported cases has the lobe been fixed in inflation and critically examined for the presence of morphological change, presumably because the inflation of the lobe at operation is taken to justify the diagnosis of lobar emphysema.

Several additional cases of this syndrome, recently reported, have added to the general description. A case has been described in which the condition persisted into adult life;[2921] another case, in infancy, presented a problem in diagnosis because the lobe was filled with fluid;[2927] and a third case was studied by angiography, which revealed very sparse filling of the vessels in the affected lobe.[2925] It appears from the literature that at least four distinct syndromes may seem clinically and radiologically to be identical, as follows:

1. Infantile lobar emphysema due to an anomaly of bronchial-wall cartilage development, not associated with any alveolar abnormality: this is probably the commonest syndrome.

2. Congenital cystic abnormality, a relatively rare phenomenon, clinically indistinguishable from the first syndrome. Several examples have been described in which alveolar spaces are lined by abnormal epithelium and the architecture of the parenchyma is destroyed.[1022–1025]

3. Associated hypoplasia or anomaly of the pulmonary artery; often the lobe is noted to be cystic, in addition to the arterial-supply anomaly.[988, 989, 1026]

4. The occasional case in which careful pathological study, by an observer accustomed to looking specifically for bronchiolar and bronchial-wall abnormality, fails to disclose any primary lesion at this site, as in the single case reported by Myers.[1027] In some of the reported cases (case 2 in ref. 1023) fragmentation of alveoli has been noted that gives rise to a pathological appearance of alternating areas of destruction and atelectasis. These may be considered as definite examples of morphological emphysema, although in some of them, as Ehrenhaft and Taber have pointed out, prolonged and forceful resuscitative measures had had to be employed, which may have caused destructive changes.[1023]

It may be questioned whether the term "emphysema" should be used for a syndrome in which the disorder is either bronchial, with overinflation of the parenchyma only, or developmental, with failure of formation of adult alveoli. However, the term "congenital" or "infantile" lobar emphysema is so well established in all countries that it seems pointless to suggest it should be changed. Furthermore, until many more cases have been described in which the affected lobe has been studied while inflated after lobectomy, one cannot be completely sure that disruption or actual destruction of alveoli may not have occurred in some cases.

The syndrome is of considerable general interest, since it illustrates the importance of the concentrically arranged bronchial cartilages in maintaining the patency of the large airways even at an early age. There is, too, no doubt that this anomaly is congenital, and the bronchomalacia cannot be blamed on infection. That a clinically similar and radiologically identical lesion may follow an attack of pneumonia with resultant bronchial damage has been suggested by Campbell and his colleagues, who describe a typical case in the right lower lobe of a 26-year-old man.[1028]

From the point of view of function, the presence of an overinflated lobe on one side of the chest, altering little in volume between inspiration and expiration and with no possibility of collateral ventilation into the lower lobes, considerably impairs ventilation of the remainder of the lung. Presumably the mediastinal displacement causes further respiratory embarrassment to the uninvolved side, the expansion of which also is impeded. Certainly the dramatic relief that follows lobectomy indicates the potential seriousness of the lesion in the small infant.

Overinflation after pneumonectomy

The consequences upon the remaining lung of removal of the other are discussed fully in Chapter 11. It may be noted here that the commonly observed changes in function can be ascribed to overinflation of the lung and do not of themselves indicate that the morphological changes of emphysema have occurred. As noted later, the question of whether such overinflation may or may not predispose to the development of emphysema has not been decisively settled.

Focal emphysema of coalworkers

This condition is discussed in Chapter 17. It consists essentially of extensive deposits of coal dust, with minimal fibrosis occurring around the respiratory bronchioles, which are dilated. The problem of the relationship of this condition, usually unaccompanied by any significant impairment of function, to centrilobular emphysema is discussed later.

Senile emphysema

For many years it was thought that the progressive kyphotic changes and development of a barrel-shaped chest that occur in elderly people were associated with some form of atrophic emphysema occurring in the absence of airway obstruction or chronic bronchitis. It has been shown by Pierce and Ebert,[651] however, that these changes[1029] are not associated with any of the alterations in pulmonary function that occur in established morphological emphysema of any significant degree. It has been pointed out in Chapter 3 that some morphological changes in the lung, probably ascribable to age rather than to other factors, have been described since Laennec's day, and the changes in pulmonary function that occur with age are well-documented. There seems no reason to establish senile emphysema as a separate or distinct entity, and it is to be hoped that the term will disappear from use.

PULMONARY FUNCTION TESTS IN THE EVALUATION OF TREATMENT OF EMPHYSEMA

The careful evaluation of patients with chronic bronchitis and emphysema by the pulmonary function laboratory is essential if the effect of any therapeutic measure is to be assessed. During the past few years, some useful studies of this type have appeared, and these may be briefly summarized. A full discussion of treatment of these conditions is beyond the scope of this volume.

Carefully graded physical training may be of considerable help to patients with emphysema, and although this does not increase the FEV_1, the minute volume at maximal work levels may be improved.[2905] A study of 100 patients with chronic bronchitis and emphysema, about half of whom were thought to have radiological evidence of emphysema, on a carefully controlled plan, failed to reveal any objective improvement as a consequence of breathing exercises;[2906] this study therefore confirms previously negative results reported by others.

Goldberg and Cherniack[2908] could find no evidence of a difference between the effects of a nebulized bronchodilator delivered with and without intermittent positive pressure in a group of patients with emphysema.

Several reviews have appeared of the effects of surgical treatment of emphysema, and Hugh-Jones and his colleagues showed that in a limited number of cases, objective improvement could follow the resection of the more heavily damaged parts of the lung.[2909, 3689] The selection of those patients for operation who are most likely to benefit from it remains a major and unresolved problem.[3689]

SUMMARY

It is now beginning to be generally recognized that chronic bronchitis and pulmonary emphysema are major health problems. In retrospect, one may distinguish several factors that may have played a part in delaying a clearer understanding of these extremely important conditions, though the extent to which each of them was important was different in different countries. However, the absence of striking early radiological change; the uncertainty of physical diagnosis; the unfamiliarity—and some would say the outlandish—nature of the laboratory tests (in contrast, for example, to those of liver function); the disinterest in respiratory physiology; the absence of an easily understood diagnostic criterion, such as the electrocardiogram; the few pathologists trained to assess these conditions critically at autopsy; and, not least, the absence of any effective treatment in the final stages of the condition—all of these may have been partly responsible for the initial lack of concern with these conditions.

Although in many respects contemporary understanding of chronic bronchitis and emphysema is much improved compared to that of only five years ago, there are a number of important areas of uncertainty to which attention may be drawn. There is no certainty regarding the relative importance of chronic bronchitis on the one hand and emphysema on the other in causing disturbances of function. The intermediate steps in the relationship between chronic hypercapnia and hypoxia and right ventricular failure are still poorly understood. Although it is clear that the discovery of a link between an enzyme deficiency in the serum and the early development of panlobular emphysema without concomitant chronic bronchitis is a very important clue as to etiology, it is far from clear, at this point, what conclusions should be drawn from it. Indeed the whole question of the etiological factors important in the genesis of emphysema independent of chronic bronchitis remains quite unsolved.

However these questions may eventually be answered, there is every reason for the contemporary physician to have a comprehensive understanding of these diseases and their manifestations and differential diagnoses. It is now quite unnecessary to stress, as we felt it necessary to do six years ago, the contribution that the pulmonary function laboratory could make to the practical, day-to-day work of the chest physician. So much has been published illustrating the importance to the chest physician of ventilatory tests, arterial blood-gas measurements, and so on, that he has every reason to press for these laboratory facilities to be established and made available to him. It is remarkable that in many hospitals in which it is regarded as normal for the physician to be able to follow the course of chronic renal disease with electrolyte estimations, or to follow the changes in blood diseases with repeated blood counts, it is still regarded as unnecessary for the chest physician to be able to have available measurements of ventilatory status, or arterial blood gases, or the mixed venous equilibrated P_{CO_2} during routine outpatient visits of patients with chronic bronchitis and emphysema.

PULMONARY CYSTS AND BULLAE

CHAPTER

8

DEFINITION

The term "cyst" or bulla" of the lung is generally used to denote an intrapulmonary air sac larger than 1 cm in diameter. The remainder of the lung may or may not be normal. Bullae sometimes become very large, so that they occupy most of one side of the chest. Conventionally, the designation "cyst" carries an implication that the air space was developmental in origin, but this distinction is not observed closely.

PATHOLOGY

As many authors have pointed out,[1045, 2034, 2035, 2930, 2932] the pathological classification of these "air spaces" in the lung is extremely complex. Indeed, even when the specimen has been subjected to close study, it may be impossible to be sure whether it was congenital or the result of infection or other acquired mechanism.[1040] There can be no doubt that some of these cysts are congenital, since they have been found in a one-day-old infant;[1024] in such instances it is usual to assume some failure of bronchial development as the cause of the cyst.[2934, 2935] There is equally no doubt that large bullae in the lung may be acquired, apparently as a local gross extension of a generalized emphysematous process, as a consequence of infection, or *de novo* with no recognizable antecedent factor.

RADIOLOGICAL FEATURES

Careful radiological examination plays an essential part in the study and evaluation of any patient with a bulla or cyst in the lung. It is important to assume that there may well be multiple cysts, and when necessary to make a tomographic examination of both lungs to define the extent of the lesion. Fluoroscopic studies in inspiration and expiration, with particular emphasis on mediastinal movement, will help to establish the differential ventilation of different parts of the lung. Bronchography is often of value in mapping the bronchial tree on the side affected by a large bulla; this may show on the affected side a poorly inflated lobe in which the bronchi are crowded together. Studies of pulmonary vasculature by tomography or angiography may well be necessary to ascertain the state of the apparently uninvolved areas of the lung; this may be an important precaution if surgery is contemplated.[2931, 2937]

CLINICAL FEATURES

Many authors have noted that cysts occupying most or all of one side of the chest may give rise to little apparent disability. They may be very poorly ventilated, and their blood supply may be scanty, so that they act as a physiological "plombage;" but they may embarrass the ventilation of normal lobes on the same side, and it is customary to find some reduction of ventilatory ability when a cyst is larger than a grapefruit. The discovery of the solitary cyst may be a chance finding on routine x-ray, or the examination may have been occasioned by respiratory infection. Occasionally, the patient first presents with a spontaneous pneumothorax, a complication somewhat commoner with the cysts that follow various types of diffuse interstitial fibrosis than with those in which the rest of the lung is normal.

The symptoms referable to the cyst or bulla are a consequence, first, of its size and, second, of the state of the remainder of the lung. Absence of noticed incapacity generally indicates that the remainder of the lung probably is normal, but this is not a wholly reliable guide, since in some patients multiple bullae may be associated with considerable diffusion defect even though ventilatory ability is well preserved; such patients usually notice little dyspnea until diffusing capacity has fallen to very low levels (*see* Case No. 15 for an example of this situation).

Physical signs will be determined by air entry into the cyst, whether or not it has compressed surrounding lung tissue; and by whether or not the surrounding lung tissue is normal or is the seat of disease (e.g., emphysema or bronchitis).

CLINICAL DIFFERENTIATION AND EFFECT ON FUNCTION

Baldwin and her colleagues in 1950[995] pioneered the study, from the point of view of pulmonary function, of patients with large air cysts in the lung. The differentiation of such patients in terms of pulmonary function plays an important part in their assessment and is critical to an understanding of operative indications and hazards. Patients with large air cysts and bullae may be broadly classified in four principal groups, and the physician will be assisted in his approach to these patients by a knowledge of these more or less distinct entities.

SINGLE BULLAE IN OTHERWISE HEALTHY LUNGS

These patients were classified by Baldwin *et al.* [995] as Group 1; by Laurenzi and his colleagues more recently[997] as Group I; and by Ogilvie and Catterall[992] as Group B. There are four distinct clinical variants within this heading, as follows:

1. Patients with a large bulla in the lung after antibiotic treatment of tuberculosis,[1006, 1041, 1042] either as a result of previous cavitation or from some unknown mechanism.

2. Patients having one of the well-known apical blebs (no larger than a grape) that are responsible for recurrent pneumothoraces. When the lungs are re-expanded, it is usual to find that pulmonary function is normal in these patients.

3. Patients with a single large cyst of unknown origin. These patients constitute an important group. In general, the function of the lung is as good as could be expected in someone in whom a considerable intrathoracic volume is playing no part in either ventilation or perfusion. If bronchial communication is very poor, as it often is, the measured lung volume may be falsely low on gas-replacement techniques, since it may take very many minutes to reach equilibrium in the cyst. Thus the degree of impairment of gas distribution by the nitrogen or helium methods cannot be taken as reflecting the state of the uninvolved lung. Maximal ventilation may be normal in relation to the amount of lung being effectively ventilated; and the same may be true of the diffusing capacity, as pointed out by Laurenzi and his co-workers.[997] Although there may be a very slight degree of arterial unsaturation, an elevated P_{CO_2} is not found in these patients; the probability that there may be extensive generalized lung disease immediately suggests itself if such an elevation is present. It often happens that the bulla has displaced a normal lobe so that this is unable to expand normally; when such a bulla is removed, there may be a spectacular improvement in ventilatory ability.[993, 994, 1043]

4. Laurenzi and his colleagues[997] have documented an example of lung cysts with normal

intervening lung in a patient with Marfan's syndrome. Chisholm, Cherniack, and Carton[3710] have recently described pulmonary function studies in five cases of Marfan's syndrome, finding normal values; it appears that the pulmonary and skeletal abnormalities in this condition are not linked. Lung cysts may be found also in association with anomalous pulmonary arteries,[1026] sequestration of the lung, and von Recklinghausen disease.[2933]

The criteria enabling the physician to decide that his patient indeed has a single bulla in an otherwise healthy lung are not easy to define with any precision. In general, the pulmonary function, usually best studied on exercise, has to be sufficiently normal for him to judge that the degree of abnormality can be fully accounted for by the extent of the cyst. The arterial blood should be normal both at rest and on exercise, and the maximal ventilatory ability and the diffusing capacity should be commensurate with the volume of the apparently normal lung. In their excellent study of pulmonary bullae, Laurenzi and his colleagues[997] make the point that some patients with single cysts may acquire chronic bronchitis or other chronic infections, and in this circumstance it may be very difficult indeed to decide whether the lung cyst is or is not part of a generalized process.

Patients with multiple bullae but with no bronchitis initially, with well-preserved ventilatory function, and with a normal or occasionally reduced diffusing capacity

Ogilvie and Catterall classify such patients as group A.[992] Laurenzi and his co-workers describe a case (V. C., in Table IV of ref. 997), and Bedell and Adams give further examples;[361] another is shown in our Case No. 15. These patients also overlap with those in whom there is, in addition to the cystic process, considerable interstitial fibrosis, which may indeed be the primary lesion (*see* page 270). In 1958 McKusick and Fisher published extensive pulmonary-function data on a man aged 32 believed to have congenital cystic disease of the lung with progressive pulmonary fibrosis, in whom the maximal breathing capacity was 92 liters/min and oxygen saturation only 89 per cent.[1003] The patient's brother, aged 37, had a similar lesion; his MBC was 179 liters/min and the oxygen diffusing capacity ($D_{L_{O_2}}$) was only 7.0 compared with a predicted value of 33 ml O_2/min/mm Hg/sq m body surface area. These brothers, as will be noted later (*see* Chapter 12) probably represent examples of the entity of familial fibrocystic dysplasia. They illustrate, however, the occasional finding of extensive cystic change with a normal ventilatory ability but impaired diffusion. It is important to recognize, therefore, that patients with multiple bullae may have normal ventilatory ability and normal diffusing capacity or a reduced value, presumably dependent upon the state of the remaining lung tissue in terms of both remaining surface area and interstitial alveolar change.

Bullae as part of generalized emphysema

As noted in Chapter 7 (page 203), some patients with generalized morphological emphysema may also have large bullae. These are classified as Group 3 by Baldwin and her associates,[995] Group II by Laurenzi and his co-workers,[997] and Group C by Ogilvie and Catterall.[992] They are usually found to have severe ventilatory impairment, a low diffusing capacity, and, not infrequently, abnormal arterial blood-gas tensions. From the practical point of view, the severity of the functional disturbance is usually taken to indicate that surgical excision of the larger bullae is contraindicated, though in some of these patients it may be that such procedures may lead to some clinical improvement, as has been claimed.[1044, 2936] Fain and his colleagues have reported an improvement in exercise tolerance in their patients greater than was to be expected from function-test changes.[2936]

Cysts and bullae as a sequel of other lesions

This last clinical group is of patients sometimes described as suffering from "bronchiolar emphysema"[1000] or "honeycomb lung,"[1046, 1047] in whom the cystic degeneration of the lung is secondary to or part of some other process. These diseases are discussed in detail in the appropriate sections. Here it may be noted

Case 15
Pulmonary Cysts and Bullae; ? Septal Emphysema

Summary of Clinical Findings. This 67-year-old man was first seen in hospital in 1960 for investigation of gastrointestinal complaints. A chest x-ray at that time showed abnormal lung fields, and he was referred to the pulmonary function laboratory for investigation. He gave a history of having been told several years before that he had a cyst or "balloon" in his lung. He had had a chronic cough for the past four years, productive of about an ounce of sputum per day. He denied any shortness of breath, though for a man of his age he was physically very active. He had smoked 20 cigarettes a day for many years.

On physical examination, blood pressure was 140/80 mm Hg. The fingers were not clubbed. The only findings of note over the chest were a decrease in breath sounds at the right apex, and at the right base compared with the left. An electrocardiogram showed a pattern of myocardial ischemia, and he was considered to be suffering from some degree of peripheral arteriosclerosis since he had had mild intermittent claudication and the peripheral leg pulses were difficult to feel. When seen in 1963, he again denied noticing any effort dyspnea.

Radiology. Postero-anterior (*A*) and lateral (*B*) roentgenograms of the chest show a moderate degree of generalized hyperinflation of both lungs which is more severe on the right than on the left, as evidenced by a lower position of the diaphragm on the right side. Whereas the hyperinflation is diffuse and uniform throughout the left lung, it is interrupted on the right by large well-defined cystic areas in the apex and base. These bullae appear unilocular and possess no vascular or other markings within them. Their walls are formed by compressed lung parenchyma, probably with some scarring.

A midsagittal tomogram (*C*) of both lungs demonstrates the bullae in the right apex and base to better advantage. The vasculature of the lungs is normal elsewhere, suggesting that there is no generalized emphysema. The walls of bullous spaces are commonly much thinner than are seen in this patient, and it is probable that considerable post-infection scarring in the lung forming these walls has occurred.

Summary. This is a case of considerable bullous change in the lung with preservation of ventilatory function and vital capacity. The lowered diffusing capacity can best be demonstrated on exercise, during which the patient has slight hyperventilation in relation to oxygen uptake. It may be postulated that this pattern of change represents primary alveolar loss without any concomitant airway obstruction, and it is of particular interest that this patient had suffered no pulmonary incapacity. Cases of this type illustrate the fact that considerable loss of alveolar surface may occur, and the lungs may be overinflated, but if no airway obstruction occurs, symptoms are insignificant.

1970: This patient has been lost to follow-up.

	VC	FRC	RV	TLC	ME %	MMFR	$FEV_{0.75}$ ×40	pH	P_{CO_2}	HCO_3^-	O_2Hb %	$D_{Lco}SS_2$	EXERCISE MPH	GRADE	$\dot{V}O_2$	$\dot{V}_E$	$D_{Lco}SS_3$
Predicted	4.1	4.0	2.6	6.7	45	2.7	83	7.4	40	25	97	11.6					22.0
May 1960	4.9	4.4	2.8	7.7	44	2.0	112					6.8					
July 1963	4.4	4.7	4.0	8.4	31	1.8	93	7.43	36.8	23.2	98	10.5*	3	FLAT	0.9	31	12.2

The total lung capacity is significantly above predicted value, and the vital capacity is normal. The residual volume increased to an abnormal value between the two studies. Ventilatory function shows normal $FEV_{0.75} \times 40$ values, but slight reduction in MMFR. In May, 1960, the resting diffusing capacity was reduced but it was normal in July, 1963, probably as a consequence of a much higher minute volume during this second study.* It increases little on exercise, however, and the diminution in D_{Lco} is clearly shown by the low value on moderate exercise. There was some hyperventilation in relation to oxygen uptake on exercise, the $\dot{V}O_2/\dot{V}_E$ ratio being only 2.9, whereas this is normally 3.5 or higher. The resting arterial blood gases are normal.

Pulmonary Cysts and Bullae; ? Septal Emphysema

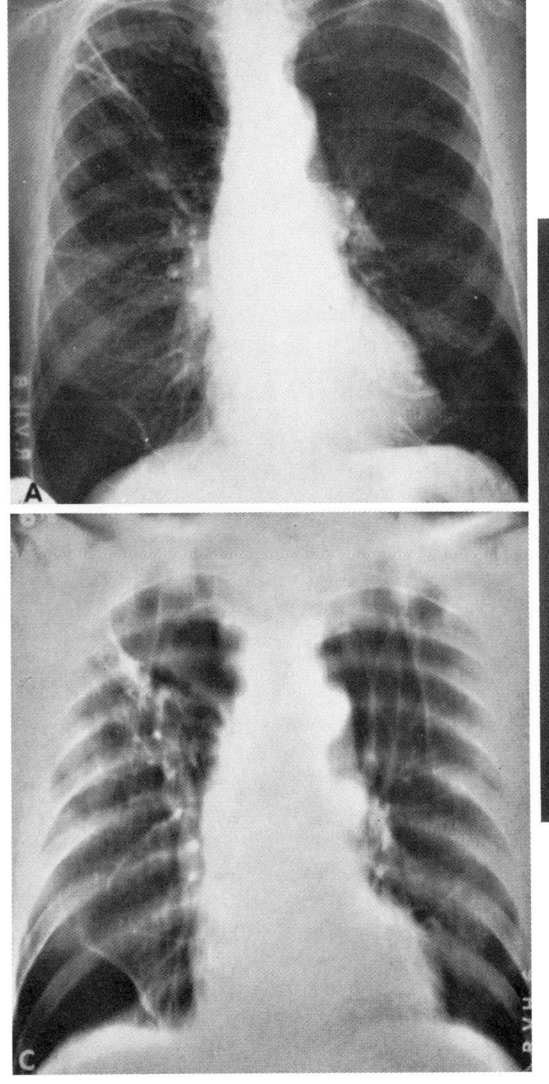

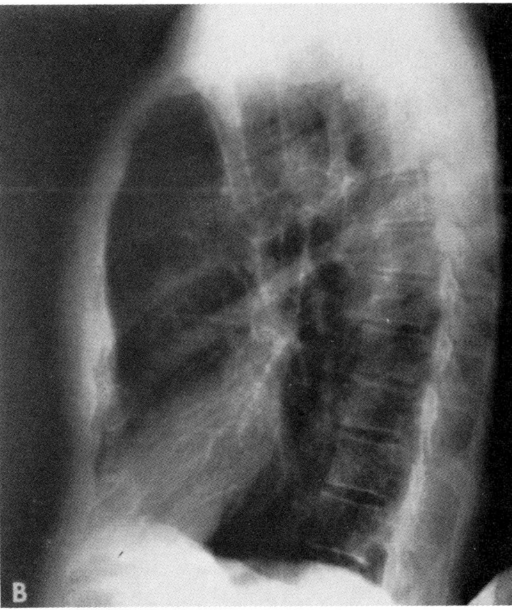

that they include the entities of familial fibrocystic dysplasia, scleroderma, eosinophilic granuloma, tuberous sclerosis, Hamman–Rich syndrome or chronic diffuse interstitial fibrosis, and, this type of degenerative change can be a consequence of histoplasmosis. Although these lesions may progress to cause recurrent spontaneous pneumothoraces, the bullae or cysts often are not very large, but invariably are multiple. In most instances the defect of function produced is a consequence of the severity of the underlying lesion. It is probably safe to say that excisional surgery is never indicated in these patients, though lung biopsy may be required to establish the diagnosis.

THE INTERPRETATION OF FUNCTION TESTS IN THE PRESENCE OF CYSTS AND BULLAE

It should be clear from the foregoing paragraphs that the evaluation of patients with a single cyst or multiple cysts in the lung is, on occasion, a difficult problem. The question that has to be answered is whether the changes in function can be explained on the basis of the space occupied by the cyst, remembering that, if it is large enough, it may interfere with the ventilation and even perhaps perfusion of normal lung tissue on the same side of the chest. Measurements of lung volumes by gas-replacement methods may well be in error in these patients if the cyst communicates very poorly with the airways. Such patients are found to show considerable discrepancies between the lung volume measured by these techniques and the intrathoracic gas volume measured in a body plethysmograph, a phenomenon demonstrated by Bedell and his colleagues.[121] It must be remembered also that intrapulmonary gas-distribution indices may be grossly abnormal because of slow mixing of gas into the cyst, and demonstrated abnormality of this aspect of function does not necessarily indicate that the remaining lung must be abnormal.

In our experience, which is similar to that noted by Laurenzi and his co-workers,[997] the finding of a comparatively normal ventilatory ability, normal blood gases and an exercise diffusing capacity normal for the volume of functioning lung can be taken to indicate that most of the lung tissue is normal. On the other hand, impairment in all of these aspects of function, when severe, is highly suggestive of a state in which the bulla is in fact only part of a generalized process. It must be admitted, however, that the condition of many patients lies between these two extremes, and the final decision as to the probable state of the lung parenchyma becomes a matter of intelligent guesswork rather than precise measurement. Laurenzi and his colleagues showed that the measurement of diffusing capacity plays a major part in this evaluation.[997] We consider that this aspect of function should be measured during exercise in all patients with large bullae who are being considered for resectional surgery. It might be thought that bronchospirometry or the radioactive gas methods could play an important part in decisions about surgery. However, although one can demonstrate by bronchospirometry the low ventilation and oxygen uptake on the side with the cyst or bulla, the relatively normal findings on the contralateral side are no guarantee that this lung may not be affected by emphysema. When bullous lesions are visible on both sides, the technique is of value in showing which of the two lungs is contributing more to resting function.

It is too early to forecast whether the radioactive gas techniques will play a major part in evaluation. Our limited experience[174] with the use of radioactive xenon in such patients suggests that the main contribution of these studies is to measure the rate of gas clearance from the apparently uninvolved portions of the affected lung and from the normal one. Gas clearance occurring normally from these regions provides some assurance that they are unlikely to be the seat of morphological emphysema.

A review of the results of resectional surgery does not permit delineation of any precise criteria for selection of patients for operation. Apart from saying that there is no contraindication to surgery when function is normal and that surgery may be hazardous or unsuccessful if the bulla is part of generalized disease, it is difficult to make any firm recommendations. It may be noted, however, that many authors have reported considerable improvement in some of these patients after the bulla has been resected.[993, 994, 1043, 2936] Capel and Belcher[994] found that, of 21 such patients undergoing operation, 9 showed considerable improvement (several showing a 50 per cent increase in vital capacity, FEV and effort tolerance); in the remaining 12, there was either very little improvement or a worsening of function postoperatively. This study emphasizes the importance of careful preoperative evaluation of these patients, in which, as noted earlier, exercise studies including observations of arterial blood gases and diffusing capacity are obligatory. The physician may be reminded that, however carefully these studies are performed, he will still on occasion be surprised at the degree of improvement that follows resectional surgery, and in other patients he will be disappointed that improvement in function and effort tolerance is not greater.

BRONCHIECTASIS

CHAPTER 9

DEFINITION

Bronchiectasis is a condition in which one or more bronchi are chronically dilated. This definition excludes those examples of bronchial dilatation occurring in the course of an acute pneumonia,[1049] in which the bronchi return to normal caliber after a few months.[1050]

PATHOLOGY

Bronchiectasis may on occasion be the sequel of bronchial obstruction caused by tumors or foreign bodies, but in the vast majority of cases no such obvious cause is demonstrable. More than half of these patients seen with bronchiectasis have had an episode of bronchopulmonary infection in early childhood, often following pertussis or measles.[1051, 1052] In the latter condition, characteristic bronchiolar and parenchymal lesions in the lungs have been described in some patients.[1053] Some cases of bronchiectasis may be developmental in origin, and a very few, of which Case No. 48 is an example, may develop after inhalation of a chemical irritant or corrosive compound. It is usually a disease of childhood, most patients having symptoms before the age of 20. It is a common condition, though believed to be decreasing in incidence, and its presence has been reported in 0.4 to 4.0 per cent of necropsies.[1054] The lower-lobe bronchi are much more commonly involved than the upper,[1052, 1055, 1056] and the left side more commonly than the right;[1052, 1056] about half of the cases with left lower-lobe involvement show diseased lingular bronchi.[1052] Both lungs are involved in roughly one-third of all cases. Bronchiectasis of the upper lobe is usually the result of old pulmonary tuberculosis and may be present in unusual situations in patients with asthma.[784]

Classification of bronchiectasis is unsatisfactory. The customary one, into cylindrical and saccular bronchiectasis alone, is inadequate, since the majority of cases do not fall into either category.[1057] Detailed classifications by radiologists of the lesions as seen on bronchograms lead to cumbersome terms, as, for example, "tubular," "early fusiform," "late fusiform," "fusiform commencing saccular," "fuso-saccular," and "?congenital."[1057] Pathologists experience even more difficulty in classification on the basis of morphology of the dilated bronchi, and the pathological classification may relate poorly to the radiological appearance.[1052]

A reasonable compromise is that proposed by Reid.[769] This is satisfactory to radiologists and is meaningful in terms of bronchial and bronchiolar obliteration. She classifies bronchiectasis into three types:

1. CYLINDRICAL. The bronchi are dilated,

with regular outlines. Six to ten orders of the bronchial tree are visible on bronchograms, and the ends may terminate squarely because of obstruction by mucus or mucopus. Several more orders of bronchioles can be found on dissection and microscopy of the lung. There is some obliteration of distal bronchioles although these are only slightly fewer in number than in a normal lung.

2. VARICOSE. The ectatic bronchi are irregular in form and size, and are deformed by irregularly placed areas of relative constriction. The ends of the bronchial tree are bulbous and distorted. Two to eight bronchial generations are visible on the bronchogram, and a further three or four may be found on dissection and microscopy. There is microscopical evidence of obliterative bronchitis and bronchiolitis.

3. SACCULAR. The bronchi increase in diameter progressively and end in large blind sacs. Three or four generations are seen on the bronchograms, and no further divisions can be found on dissection. No trace of the remnants of destroyed distal bronchi can be recognized microscopically. This form of bronchiectasis has the most severe impairment of function and the worst prognosis.[1051]

Microscopical examination shows destruction of the walls of the dilated bronchi, with disappearance of cartilage, elastic tissue and muscle. In saccular bronchiectasis the destruction is complete; the wall is composed of fibrous tissue alone, usually with squamous metaplasia of the lining epithelium.[1052] In other forms of bronchiectasis, destruction of the normal components of the bronchi is often focal. Lymphoid-follicle formation occurs frequently, and in such cases the destruction of the wall is often related to the follicles. It has been suggested that these deserve special recognition, and that the term "follicular bronchiectasis" be applied.[1052] Edema, inflammation, and peribronchial fibrosis may result in focal thickening of the bronchial wall. Mucous-gland hypertrophy is irregular,[775] and may occur in nonectatic bronchi.[907] Histologically the disease is often more widespread than the bronchograms indicated.[1059, 2524] There is always some change in the pulmonary parenchyma;[1050] this is extremely variable, not only from case to case but also in different parts of the same specimen. Varying degrees of atelectasis, pulmonary fibrosis, and pneumonitis occur. Emphysema is found uncommonly.[1060] However, some examples of saccular bronchiectasis may show almost complete disappearance of the parenchyma: in this type of bronchiectasis extensive anastomoses may be found between greatly enlarged bronchial arteries and the pulmonary circulation.[24, 1061] Turner-Warwick has shown that there is a significant correlation between the hypertrophy of the bronchial arteries and the presence of finger-clubbing.[2038]

As shown in Case No. 19, bronchiectasis may occur in association with situs inversus[1062] (Kartagener's syndrome[1063, 2940]), and is usual in cases of fibrocystic disease of the pancreas.

Bronchiectasis of varying degree occurs in other conditions in which it is not the primary diagnosis. Thus, cylindrical dilatation of bronchi[808] occurs in patients with panlobular emphysema no exact distinction between cylindrical bronchiectasis and the ectasia associated with this type of emphysema has yet been attempted. Bronchiectasis and bronchial and bronchiolar obliteration are usual in the syndrome of unilateral pulmonary emphysema or transradiancy[983] (*see* Chapter 7, page 201), indeed, some of these cases have been described in the literature as "bronchiectasis without atelectasis."[1064] Bronchiectasis may occur also in pulmonary sequestration, a condition in which a bronchopulmonary mass, situated within the lung, may be dissociated from the normal bronchial tree and supplied by an abnormal systemic artery.[1065–1068]

Finally, in some instances bronchiectasis may be associated with chronic atelectasis; this most commonly involves the middle lobe, where it is characterized as the "middle-lobe syndrome."

RADIOLOGY

Bronchiectasis due to a specific cause, such as chronic pulmonary tuberculosis, although not uncommon, will not be considered in this section. Attention will rather be directed toward the type of bronchiectasis in which etiology is not clear and usually is remote and which comprises the majority of cases of significant disease seen clinically and radiologically.

The morphological characteristics of the three main varieties of bronchiectasis have already been described. Although the classification suggested by Reid[769] is useful in general

Case 16
Bronchiectasis (Saccular: Bilateral)

Summary of Clinical Findings. At the age of 2 years this 42-year-old patient had severe bronchopneumonia. During her childhood she had a chronic cough and expectoration, and suffered frequent febrile episodes, during which the color of the sputum would change from white to green and increase from a tablespoonful to 1/2 cupful per day. Slight hemoptysis had occurred on two occasions. Dyspnea, present from childhood, had been attributed to "asthma" despite the fact that it occurred only on effort. At the time of her admission to hospital, shortness of breath was precipitated by the slightest exertion.

On physical examination there was noted to be a moderate dorsal kyphosis, hyperresonance over both lungs, prolonged expiration and a generalized decrease in breath sounds. After coughing, coarse moist rales could be heard over both lung bases. Moderately severe clubbing of the fingers was present.

Urinalysis was negative. The hemoglobin was 13.5 g per 100 ml, white cells totalled 8,300 per cmm, with a normal differential count, and the erythrocyte sedimentation rate was slightly increased. The sputum grew *H. influenzae* on culture. X-rays of the sinuses revealed pansinusitis. A medical regimen of bronchodilators, postural drainage and courses of antibiotics has served to control the patient's symptoms.

Radiology. The postero-anterior plain film projection of the chest (*A*) shows extensive bilateral pulmonary disease, more severe in the right lung than in the left. The linear markings throughout most of the right lung and lower half of the left lung are increased in size. Numerous saccular or cystic spaces of variable size are present in the bases bilaterally. In some of these, air–fluid levels can be identified. The left upper lobe appears to have been spared this bronchial disease, but is somewhat hyperinflated. This combination of changes strongly suggests the presence of advanced bronchiectasis.

Three views of the chest, (*B*) postero-anterior, (*C*) left anterior oblique, and (*D*) right lateral projection following bilateral bronchography, demonstrate severe deformity of all opacified bronchi except those of the left upper lobe. The bronchiectasis is more severe in the right lung. The generalized hyperinflation, particularly in the presence of crowding of bronchi in the involved portions of the lungs, suggests that emphysema may be present. Measurement of the diameters of various bronchial segments during cinebronchography revealed collapse of both lower-lobe bronchi on forced expiration and cough, whereas the saccular spaces underwent little change in diameter.

Summary. This 42-year-old woman has had extensive bilateral saccular bronchiectasis since childhood. There is severe impairment of every aspect of pulmonary function, and considerable secondary parenchymal damage is almost certainly present in the lungs.

	VC	FRC	RV	TLC	ME %	MMFR	$FEV_{0.75}$ ×40	pH	P_{CO_2}	HCO_3^-	O_2Hb %	$D_{LCO}SS_2$	CO Ext %
Predicted	3.0	2.4	1.4	4.4	60	3.1	79	7.4	40	25	97	16.4	49
July 1962	1.4	3.0	2.8	4.2	18	0.2	14	7.37	47	25	89	8.7	35

The vital capacity is reduced, but the residual volume is twice the normal value; hence the total lung capacity is at the predicted level. Inert-gas distribution is grossly abnormal, and there is severe ventilatory defect. The resting diffusing capacity is reduced, and the arterial blood shows definite hypoxia and a slight degree of hypercapnia. These changes probably indicate secondary parenchymal change in the lungs.

Case 16
Bronchiectasis (Saccular: Bilateral)

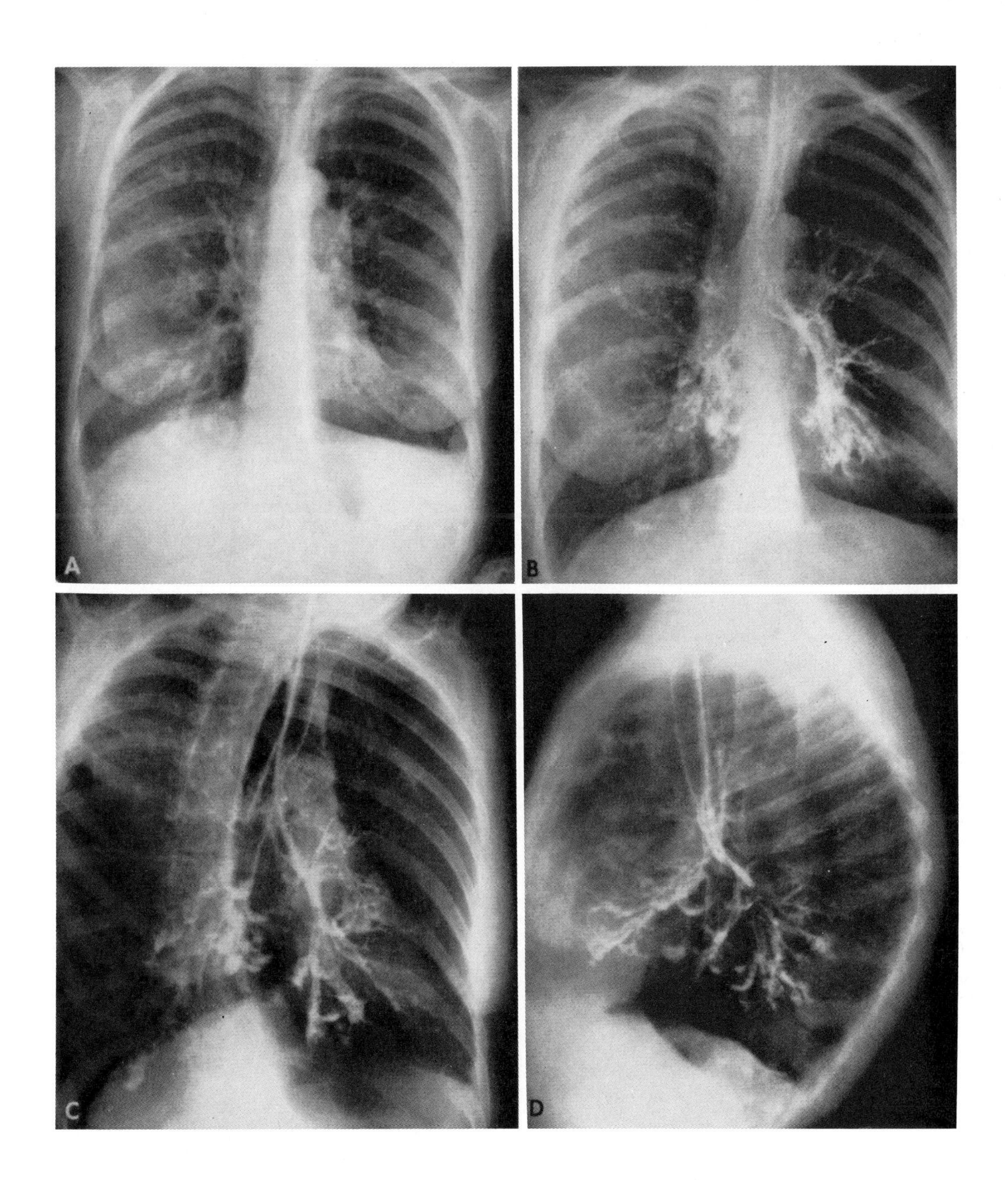

terms, overlap of types is frequent: it is not uncommon, for example, to find varicose and saccular or cylindrical and varicose deformity coexisting in the same lobe or in different lobes in the same patient. It is apparent, however, that division into these three broad categories on a basis of severity of dilatation serves more than a superficial descriptive purpose.

As will be pointed out in the section on pulmonary function in this chapter, a rough correlation exists between the degree and extent of bronchial dilatation and the severity of derangement of function. Some support for this observation has been found in a study of the dynamic activity of the bronchial tree in a number of patients with bronchiectasis. In cinebronchographic studies made during various respiratory maneuvers we have found significant differences in degree of collapse of the main lobar bronchi and bronchiectatic spaces on forced expiration and coughing. In cylindrical bronchiectasis, the caliber of the lobar and bronchiectatic bronchi reduces normally. Since efficiency of cough depends largely upon ratio of tube diameter to particle size, and since no collapse occurs in the outflow tract of these bronchi, coughing rids them of secretion, a fact that has been observed repeatedly in these patients through their ability to cough up the medium after bronchography. In contrast, patients with varicose and saccular bronchiectasis show disproportionate collapse of their lobar bronchi on coughing, with little or no change in the caliber of the bronchiectatic spaces. These patients are unable to cough up the medium after bronchography, and for a similar reason are presumably unable to rid their diseased bronchi of pus and retained secretions. A rough correlation exists between the dynamic activity of the bronchi in these patients, the severity of their bronchiectasis, and the derangement in certain parameters of pulmonary function, particularly the ventilatory tests.[2945]

Contrary to general belief, in most cases the presence of this disease may be strongly suspected from plain films of the chest. In a survey of 112 cases, Gudbjerg found the plain films to be abnormal in 104; even in retrospect, however, those of the remaining 7 per cent could not be interpreted as being abnormal.[1904] These figures are in general agreement with our experience, and it may be concluded that the plain films are usually abnormal in cases of significant bronchiectasis. The changes apparent radiologically are obviously dependent upon the extent and severity of the disease. Cylindrical bronchiectasis characteristically manifests itself by an increase in size and loss of definition of the vascular markings to the area of lung involved. The markings are hazy and indistinct and often closer together than normal, indicating some loss of volume. The normal lobes of the involved lung often show a degree of overinflation and increased radiolucency consistent with the degree of atelectasis in the bronchiectatic region. The more severe forms of varicose and saccular bronchiectasis are generally associated with considerable atelectasis, at times amounting to almost complete collapse of a lobe. In such circumstances, the presence of air–fluid levels in dilated bronchiectatic spaces within the collapsed lung indicate the true nature of the underlying disease and help to differentiate the collapse from such causes as obstructing neoplasm. Although tomography has been advocated as a useful technique in assessing deformity in certain diseases of the bronchial tree, it is doubtful whether it contributes sufficient information in bronchiectasis to warrant its use except in unusual circumstances when obstructing lesions or enlarged lymph nodes may be suspected.

Although the presence of bronchiectasis should usually be suspected from plain-film analysis, bronchography is the essential diagnostic examination, both for accurate assessment of distribution and for determination of severity. It is generally advisable to vary the technique of bronchography by insisting on a regimen of postural drainage for at least two or three days before the examination; otherwise, the presence of abundant secretion and pus frequently prevents adequate filling of the diseased bronchi by bronchographic media; only thorough drainage beforehand will allow complete visualization. Care must be exercised in ordering bronchograms, since bronchography produces considerable regional impairment of ventilation[2945] and hence may cause a dangerous reduction of function for several hours, particularly when the more normal parts of the lung are being filled with radiopaque medium.

In most cases it is necessary to perform complete bilateral bronchography, especially if surgery is contemplated. Involvement of even one segmental bronchus of an upper lobe in a patient with advanced disease of a lower lobe may necessitate further assessment before surgical resection is performed, and incomplete visualization before operation may lead to an unexpectedly poor result after resection if pre-existing disease was not detected.

CLINICAL FEATURES

The symptomatology of bronchiectasis is inevitably very variable, since it depends upon the extent of the lesion, the chronicity of infection, and the degree of associated bronchospasm and chronic bronchitis. It is not uncommon to encounter patients with large areas of lung destroyed by saccular bronchiectasis who have remarkably few symptoms of any kind. Much more often, however, this severe form of the disease is attended by chronic infection, and leads to the production of fetid sputum, severe constitutional disturbance, and on occasion secondary amyloidosis. Similarly, patients with cylindrical or varicose bronchiectasis may have a greater or lesser degree of chronic infection; their lives may be endangered by severe hemorrhage from the bronchi or they may never have hemoptysis. These hazards, together with repeated episodes of bronchopneumonia and the common finding of bronchospasm in more-normal lung regions, occur in all types of bronchiectasis.

It is true to say that the diagnosis of bronchiectasis can be made only radiologically, the perceptive physician becoming suspicious of the possibility of this underlying disease because of repeated infections or occasional hemoptyses, and by eliciting evidence of bronchiectasis on auscultation. Physical signs are variable, and there may be none even in the presence of extensive disease; they depend mainly upon the amount of secretion and upon the degree of involvement of adjacent lung parenchyma.

The advent of vaccines that have reduced the severity of both whooping cough and measles and the prompt treatment with antibiotics of the bronchopneumonia that may complicate these conditions have been responsible for a very considerable decrease in the number of cases now encountered in children.[2942] The onset of the disease, in most of the adults now seen with it, antedated these therapeutic advances.

We have recently drawn attention to the severe impairment of function, leading to marked $\dot{V}/\dot{Q}$ disturbance and cor pulmonale, that bronchiectasis may occasionally cause.[2524]

PULMONARY FUNCTION IN BRONCHIECTASIS

Although observations of pulmonary function, often of considerable complexity, have been reported in individual cases of bronchiectasis, the data in the literature permit only broad generalizations concerning correlation between defects in function and the extent or type of lesion. It is obvious that bronchiectasis confined to the middle lobe, for example, will not lead to significant impairment of function if no other region is involved and there is no bronchitis. It is equally clear that a lung destroyed by saccular bronchiectasis can be expected to contribute little to total function. But between these limits there are insufficient data for securely founded statements on pulmonary function in this disease.

The problem may best be approached by describing the status of pulmonary function commonly existing in patients with easily recognizable patterns of bronchiectasis, and then considering the variations of these situations encountered in practice.

SACCULAR BRONCHIECTASIS OF ONE LUNG

When one lung is virtually destroyed and the other is normal there is very little oxygen uptake from the diseased side. The vital capacity in such patients is reduced to about one half to two thirds of the predicted value, the FEV is lower than predicted, inert-gas distribution is very considerably impaired because of slow gas equilibration in the affected lung, and the total diffusing capacity measured by steady-state methods is reduced to about three quarters of the normal value. In such patients, studies by bronchospirometry reveal that the affected lung may be receiving about one third of the ventilation and may be responsible for less than 10 per cent of the total oxygen uptake.[307] In a remarkable study that included observations on six patients with extensive bronchiectasis, Roosenburg and Deenstra showed that the arterial saturation of blood collected from pulmonary

Case 17
Mucoviscidosis (Fibrocystic Disease of the Pancreas)

Summary of Clinical Findings. This child, born in October 1952, was first admitted to the Montreal Children's Hospital on November 27, 1953, with a history of a persistent cough since he had had a "very bad cold" when aged 2 months. Three weeks before admission, the cough had increased and the child had begun to vomit and to have some diarrhea.

On admission he seemed acutely ill, with a dusky color and with moderate indrawing of the chest wall, very rapid respirations, and a severe dry cough. Fine inspiratory rales were present in the lower two-thirds of the right lung field and there was increased resonance to percussion throughout both lung fields. Chest x-ray showed bilateral peripheral pneumonia. There was absence of trypsin in the stools and in the duodenal juice. The diagnosis of fibrocystic disease of the pancreas was made, therefore, and the child was treated with antibiotics and pancreatic granules. Treatment with digitalis also was started, since the ECG showed right ventricular preponderance and the liver could be palpated 7 cm below the right costal margin. This therapy produced clearing of the chest x-ray and improvement in the ECG tracing. He was discharged December 19, 1953.

The child was followed-up in the Medical Clinic and he was readmitted to hospital in October 1956 with an exacerbation of his respiratory symptoms. At that time a sweat test was done and revealed a sodium concentration of 124 mEq/l and chlorides of 102 mEq/l. He was discharged October 30, 1956, after a course of antibiotic therapy, humidity and postural drainage. One sibling also was diagnosed as having fibrocystic disease of the pancreas. The patient had two admissions in 1957 because of acute respiratory symptoms, and was readmitted in April 1959 for a seven-day intensive program of aerosol treatment and physiotherapy, and for respiratory function assessment. In October 1959 his symptoms increased, and on October 26 he was in severe respiratory distress. With intensive therapy, his condition improved slightly and on discharge his hypercapnia had disappeared but his ventilatory ability was very poor.

His final admission was in May 1960, in a very poor physical condition and in extreme respiratory difficulty. By this time he was emaciated and stunted in growth, and had a barrel-shaped chest, very severe wheezing, cyanosis and very severe clubbing of the finger tips. His condition deteriorated throughout this hospital stay. He developed cor pulmonale and a paralytic ileus. A tracheostomy was performed on June 4 in an attempt to facilitate his bronchial toilet and ventilation. He died on June 7, 1960.

Radiology. Frontal (*A*) and lateral (*B*) projections of the chest show characteristic changes of fibrocystic disease of the pancreas. The lungs are moderately overinflated, as shown by increase in all diameters, increase in retrosternal air space and flattening of the diaphragm. There are multiple opacities, approximately in the distribution of the bronchi, scattered throughout both lungs, and involving all lobes about equally. Many of them represent tiny abscesses. The bronchial walls are thickened, particularly in the lower lobes and in the perihilar areas. There is probably some bronchiectasis, as shown by increase in the diameter of the bronchial lumina, particularly in the lower lobes. Each hilum shows moderate lymph-node enlargement. There is undernutrition, as shown by almost complete absence of subcutaneous fat. Osteoporosis is present in mild degree.

	VC	FRC	RV	TLC	ME %	MMFR	$FEV_{0.75}$ ×40	pH	P_{CO_2}	HCO_3^-	O_2Hb %
Predicted (1959)	1.2	0.7	0.34	1.6	50+	1.50	34	7.40	35	25	97
April 21, 1959	0.9	1.7	1.29	2.2	21	0.21	11				
Oct. 25, 1959	0.8	1.9	1.61	2.4	13	0.19	9	7.32	74	37	65
Nov. 2, 1959								7.43	46	30	90
March 22, 1959	0.8	1.5	1.28	2.1	13	0.38	11				
May 3, 1960								7.24	80	30	

The severe overinflation of the lung and chronic ventilatory defect are apparent. Two episodes of acute respiratory failure with severe hypercapnia followed acute respiratory infections. Death occurred in June of 1960 in such an attack.

Mucoviscidosis (Fibrocystic Disease of the Pancreas)

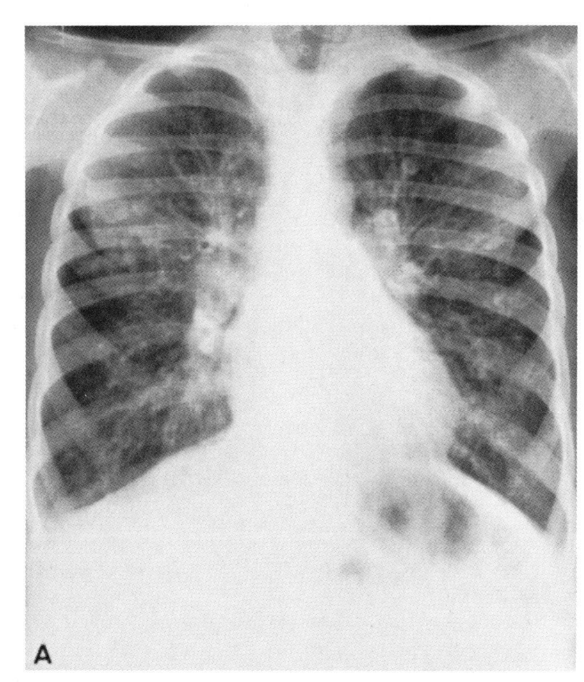

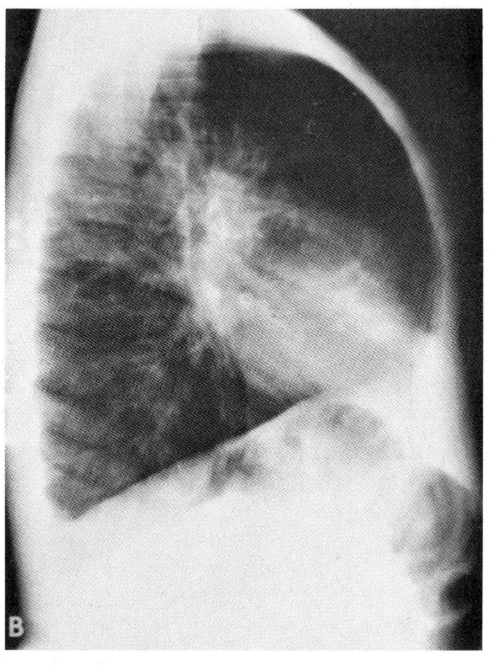

arteries in the involved segments was substantially higher than that in the main pulmonary artery or the right ventricle.[1069] Furthermore, in some of these studies the pressure was higher in the catheter wedged into the involved segment than it was in the pulmonary artery. The authors concluded from these observations that an extensive bronchial arterial blood supply must be shunting into the pulmonary circulation in many of the bronchiectatic segments. This is in keeping with the demonstration by Fritts and his co-workers[2239] that the left ventricular output exceeds that of the right in bronchiectasis, and with the postmortem demonstration of dilated bronchial vessels communicating with the pulmonary artery in cases of saccular bronchiectasis.[24, 2036, 2946] If such segments are to be visualized as being perfused mainly through the bronchial arteries, the very low oxygen uptake observed without a proportionate diminution in ventilation is readily explainable; it is to be expected that such a lung would be capable of some CO_2 elimination from the bronchial artery blood.

Such a mechanism may explain the discrepancy between the severity of some aspects of function derangement in bronchiectasis and the often normal values for oxygen saturation. Although the arterial blood is not normal in the patient with saccular bronchiectasis shown in Case No. 16, it is not remarkably deranged in view of the very severe abnormalities in other tests of function that she demonstrates.

Bilateral lower-lobe bronchiectasis

In our experience it is not uncommon to see patients with bilateral lower-lobe bronchiectasis known to have been present since childhood and chronically infected, in whom the maximal breathing capacity and diffusing capacity are almost normal; vital capacity may be slightly reduced, but impairment of function is minimal and there is no dyspnea. This situation is shown in Case No. 18. In these patients sometimes the inert-gas distribution, as studied by a helium closed-circuit technique, may be abnormal; in two such cases, using a radioactive-xenon technique, we found reduction in ventilation to the involved lobes. When this combination is encountered the physician can be confident that the uninvolved parts of the lung are not diseased. This type of conclusion may be an important contribution to management of the patient and may influence decisions on treatment. For instance, two patients, each with bronchiectasis apparently localized to the lower lobes, may have very different values for pulmonary function; one may be almost normal, whereas the other may have an FEV only 30 per cent of normal, considerable reduction in vital capacity, and even some loss of diffusing capacity. In the latter case, the statement can be made that the degree of impairment of function is greater than would occur if the abnormality were confined to the lower lobes and the remainder of both lungs were completely normal. Useful interpretation of such function-test data can be accomplished only when the physician knows the details of the clinical history and physical examination and is fully conversant with the radiological appearances and the apparent extent of the disease. Cherniack and his colleagues[2943] have recently documented the deterioration of function that follows episodes of acute chest infection in patients with bronchiectasis.

In a second study of pulmonary function in this disease, Cherniack and Castor[2942] followed 32 cases closely for three years and showed that general deterioration of function occurred as the disease became more extensive. Regional studies of function also demonstrate the close relationship between generally impaired function and the number of involved segments.[2945]

It is of interest that patients similar to the one in Case No. 18 can cough up chronically infected sputum from the lower lobes for many years without developing generalized disease in the lung.

Complex problems of evaluation

Case No. 21 (*see* page 258) depicts an example of very extensive saccular bronchiectasis in which a decision whether to remove diseased parts of the lungs could not be made without bronchospirometric evaluation of the proportionate contribution of the two lungs to total function. This procedure is of particular use when removal of a lung is contemplated, but when removal of two lower lobes, for instance, is proposed, more relevant information may be obtained in the future by the use of radioactive-gas methods.[2945]

If it can be shown that one lung is responsible for the sputum production and is not contributing to total function, there is every reason to advise its removal, although respirator care may be needed to carry the patient safely through the postoperative period. Such patients, as for example those with severe bilateral disease, require a careful function assessment with consideration of all data obtained by general function tests and special methods. In some, additional information of value can be secured by testing during temporary obstruction of one pulmonary artery, a method of study pioneered by Hanson.[308]

In patients in whom the severity of function defect is greater than can be accounted for by the apparent extent of the bronchiectasis, it may be of value to assess pulmonary function after a period of careful medical treatment involving clearing of infection, use of bronchodilators, and, most important, a two- to three-month course of postural drainage under proper supervision and instruction. We have seen many such patients in whom these measures have resulted in considerable improvement of function. It must be remembered that bronchography causes impairment of ventilation,[2945] and care and judgment must be exercised in its use in some of these patients. The objective evidence is of great value in assessing the results of such periods of medical treatment; the procedure may be an important preliminary to any decision on operative treatment. It is to be supposed that these measures diminish the chronic bronchitis and attendant bronchial obstruction in other parts of the lung.

In some patients, however, usually those with severe bilateral bronchiectasis, there is considerable destruction of parenchyma combined with chronic pneumonitis and atelectasis. These patients appear terminally with severe blood-gas changes and cor pulmonale, and from the point of view of pulmonary function resemble those with advanced pulmonary emphysema, except that the total lung capacity is usually reduced.[2524]

We have recently reported[2945] the results of studies of regional function in bronchiectasis using ^{133}xenon. Reduction of ventilation to the affected zones appeared to be of similar magnitude in lesions of differing radiological type and severity, and impairment of ventilation appeared to be of greater extent than the extent of radiologically demonstrable disease.

Bronchiectasis in Children

The bronchiectasis that may occur in fibrocystic disease of children is considered on page 240. In an interesting study that included eight children with bronchiectasis, Cook and Bucci[1071] assessed pulmonary function after lobectomy. These patients were considered to have residual disease in their lungs. The observed maximal breathing capacity was 33 to 92 per cent of predicted value, averaging 59 per cent; taking account of the volume of lung that had been removed, vital capacity was about 70 per cent of predicted, and diffusing capacity was normal.

Although there is little difficulty in deciding what course of treatment to follow when pulmonary function in children is relatively normal, any resectional surgery in those who have considerable function impairment should be undertaken only after the most careful consideration in each individual patient, a point emphasized by these authors.[1071] The extensive literature on the relative merits of medical and surgical treatment of bronchiectasis has been well reviewed by Strang, with an analysis of the results in 61 children treated medically and 163 treated surgically.[2042] Other reviews[2039, 2040] have stressed different aspects of this often difficult decision, but it seems clear that the results of surgery are usually excellent in all patients in whom the bronchiectasis is localized to one lobe. It is in those whose lesions are more extensive that the difficulties arise.

A review of the remote results of pneumonectomy for bronchiectasis during adolescence on pulmonary function several years later has been published from the U.S.S.R.[2941] but the translated abstract is inadequate for critical analysis.

EFFECT ON PULMONARY FUNCTION OF SURGERY IN BRONCHIECTASIS

In 1958 Kamener and his colleagues reported studies on 21 patients with bronchiectasis, including results of pulmonary function tests preoperatively and at varying

Case 18 Bronchiectasis

Summary of Clinical Findings. This 31-year-old man was referred to the outpatient department in November, 1962. He had been treated in another hospital for fever and chronic cough thought to be on a basis of pneumonia and bronchiectasis. He stated that a diagnosis of bronchiectasis had been made eight years previously.

At the age of 1½ years he had suffered an attack of whooping cough complicated by pneumonia which left him with a dry hacking cough. His chief complaint of left anterior chest pain began after a second attack of pneumonia at the age of 18 years. The pain was only slightly aggravated by lifting but completely relieved by a bandage strapped around his chest. It increased on breathing or coughing. He had no further history of chest infection until the recent pneumonia. For several years his cough had been productive of a moderate amount of white sputum (about an ounce) every day. He had never noticed hemoptysis and was not short of breath. Physical examination did not reveal any abnormal findings.

Pulmonary function and x-ray studies shown below were obtained at this time. He has not returned to the clinic.

Radiology. Postero-anterior (*A*) and lateral (*B*) films of the chest reveal changes localized to the left lung. The basal markings show an increase in size and a loss of definition and are crowded together. Equally important but more subtle changes are those indicating loss of volume of the lower lobe, including an elevation of the ipsilateral diaphragmatic dome, particularly posteriorly, and a greater translucency of the left lung field compared with the right, suggesting compensatory hyperinflation of the upper lobe. The combination of findings is strongly suggestive of bronchiectasis.

A bronchogram of the left lung in PA projection (*C*) shows cylindrical dilatation of all basal segments of the lower lobe and of the inferior segmental bronchus of the lingula. The involved bronchi end rather abruptly, with little peripheral filling. Measurement of the bronchi on cine film recorded during deep inspiration and forced expiration and cough revealed a normal degree of variation in bronchial diameter and no regions of abnormal collapse. The bronchi of the left upper lobe and of the right lung were normal.

Summary. This patient had left lower lobe cylindrical bronchiectasis with chronic sputum production that caused no interference with pulmonary function.

	VC	FRC	RV	TLC	ME %	MMFR	$FEV_{0.75}$ ×40	pH	P_{CO_2}	HCO_3^-	O_2Hb %	$D_{L_{CO}}SS_2$	CO Ext %
Predicted	5.0	3.7	1.9	6.9	65	4.3	140	7.4	40	25	97	22.4	50
Nov. 1962	4.1	4.8	2.6	6.7	47	5.2	127	–	–	–	–	23.8	48

Aside from an increased functional residual capacity and slight impairment of gas distribution, pulmonary function is normal.

Bronchiectasis

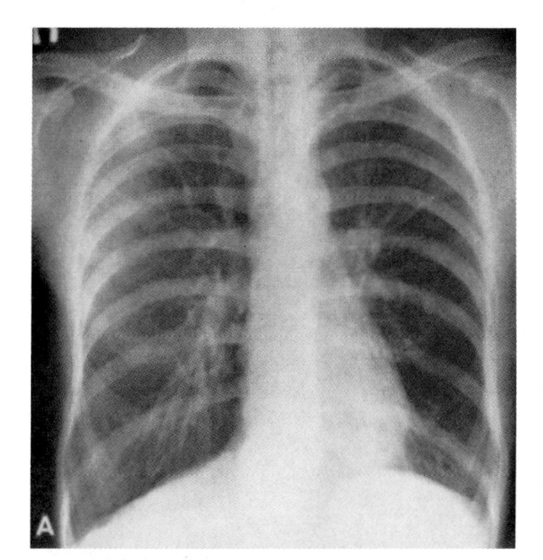

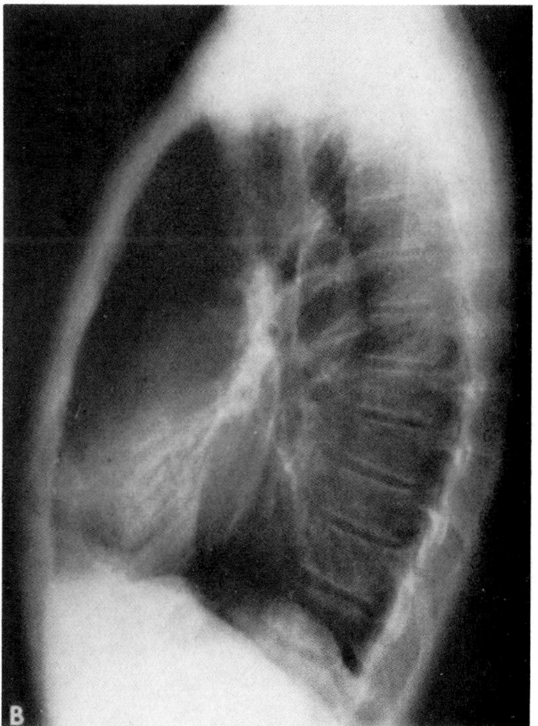

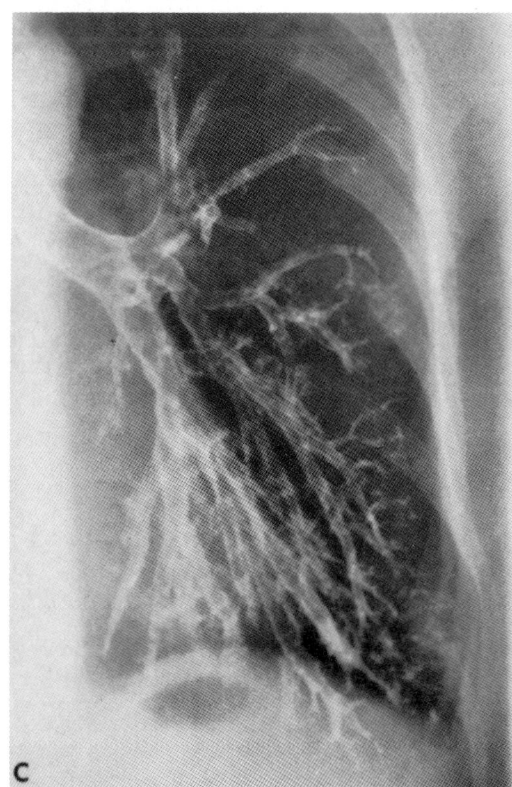

Case 19
Kartagener's Syndrome

Summary of Clinical Findings. This 14-year-old girl had had a chronic cough since infancy, which had become productive of mucopurulent material some five months before admission. Two brothers had died of pneumonia in infancy.

On examination, she was well developed and nourished. Temperature, pulse and blood pressure were within normal limits. There was a discharge from the right middle ear and many persistent moist rales were heard at the right lung base. The cardiac apex was noted to be on the right side. There were no heart murmurs. She showed a mild hypochromic anemia, with a hemoglobin of 11.7 g per 100 ml, and a rapid sedimentation rate. Urinalysis was negative. X-rays revealed pansinusitis, situs inversus, and changes suggesting bronchiectasis at the right base.

After adequate treatment of the infection in both ear and sinuses, the lingula and the basilar segments of the "right" lung were removed. Pulmonary function tests were performed before and six months after surgery. She has not returned for follow-up.

Radiology. Postero-anterior (*A*) and lateral (*B*) projections of the thorax show dextrocardia and a right-sided stomach bubble. Subsequent examinations established the presence of complete transposition of the thoracic and abdominal viscera, including the pulmonary lobes. In both projections, the basal markings of the lower lobe of the "right" lung are crowded together and show increase in size and loss of definition (*arrows*). The crowding of markings and slight posterior displacement of the chief fissure are the only signs of loss of volume. In the absence of symptoms of an acute respiratory infection, the appearance is diagnostic of bronchiectasis.

Figure *C* shows a postero-anterior film following instillation of contrast medium into the "right" bronchial tree. There is moderate cylindrical bronchiectasis of all basal segments of the lower lobe and of both segments of the lingula. The involved bronchi end abruptly at the fifth or sixth-stage divisions beyond the stem bronchus.

Films of the paranasal sinuses revealed chronic ethmoid and maxillary sinusitis, completing the triad of Kartagener's syndrome.

Pathology. The right lower lobe and lingula were resected, the segmental anatomy being that of the left side. The bronchi showed cylindrical bronchiectasis and the mucous membranes were transversely rather than longitudinally striated. The bronchial walls were generally thickened, with focal areas of thinning. Many bronchi contained thick mucoid plugs. Except where involved by peribronchial fibrosis, the pulmonary parenchyma appeared undamaged. Histological examination showed an intense chronic inflammatory infiltrate in the bronchi, with formation of lymphoid follicles (*D*), loss of muscle and elastic tissue, particularly related to the lymphoid follicles, and peribronchial fibrosis and collagenization. There was widespread narrowing of the bronchiolar lumina (*E*). An active chronic inflammatory infiltrate was present in their walls, with peribronchiolar fibrosis and some collagenization. The bronchiolar epithelium showed focal squamous metaplasia, and lining cells of surrounding alveoli showed cuboidal metaplasia.

Summary. This case illustrates cylindrical bronchiectasis as part of Kartagener's syndrome. Six months after resectional surgery, there is considerable functional defect, which is more severe than the apparent extent of the lesion might have suggested. Presumably all lobes of both lungs are involved with chronic bronchitis, if not with overt bronchiectasis.

	VC	FRC	RV	TLC	ME %	MMFR	$FEV_{0.75}$ ×40	pH	P_{CO_2}	HCO_3^-	O_2Hb %	$D_{L_{CO}}SS_2$
Predicted	3.2	2.3	0.9	4.2	65	3.9	99					21.9
Dec. 1961	2.0	1.4	0.9	2.9	46	2.1	62					17.8
July 1962	1.5	1.4	0.9	2.4	45	1.1	33					11.0

The preoperative studies in December 1961 showed a significant decrease in vital capacity. The total lung capacity is also lower than predicted, but the residual volume is not increased. There was moderate ventilatory impairment, but a nearly normal diffusing capacity. In January, 1962, the lower lobe and lingula on the right side were removed, and she was referred for reassessment of function six months later. The tests reveal a considerable worsening of most aspects of function, including ventilatory ability and diffusing capacity. These changes cannot be directly attributed to the lobectomy, but presumably indicate a worsening of chronic bronchitis in the remainder of the lung in the interval. The lowered diffusing capacity may indicate alveolar abnormality of the "left" lung or of the "right" upper lobe.

Kartagener's Syndrome

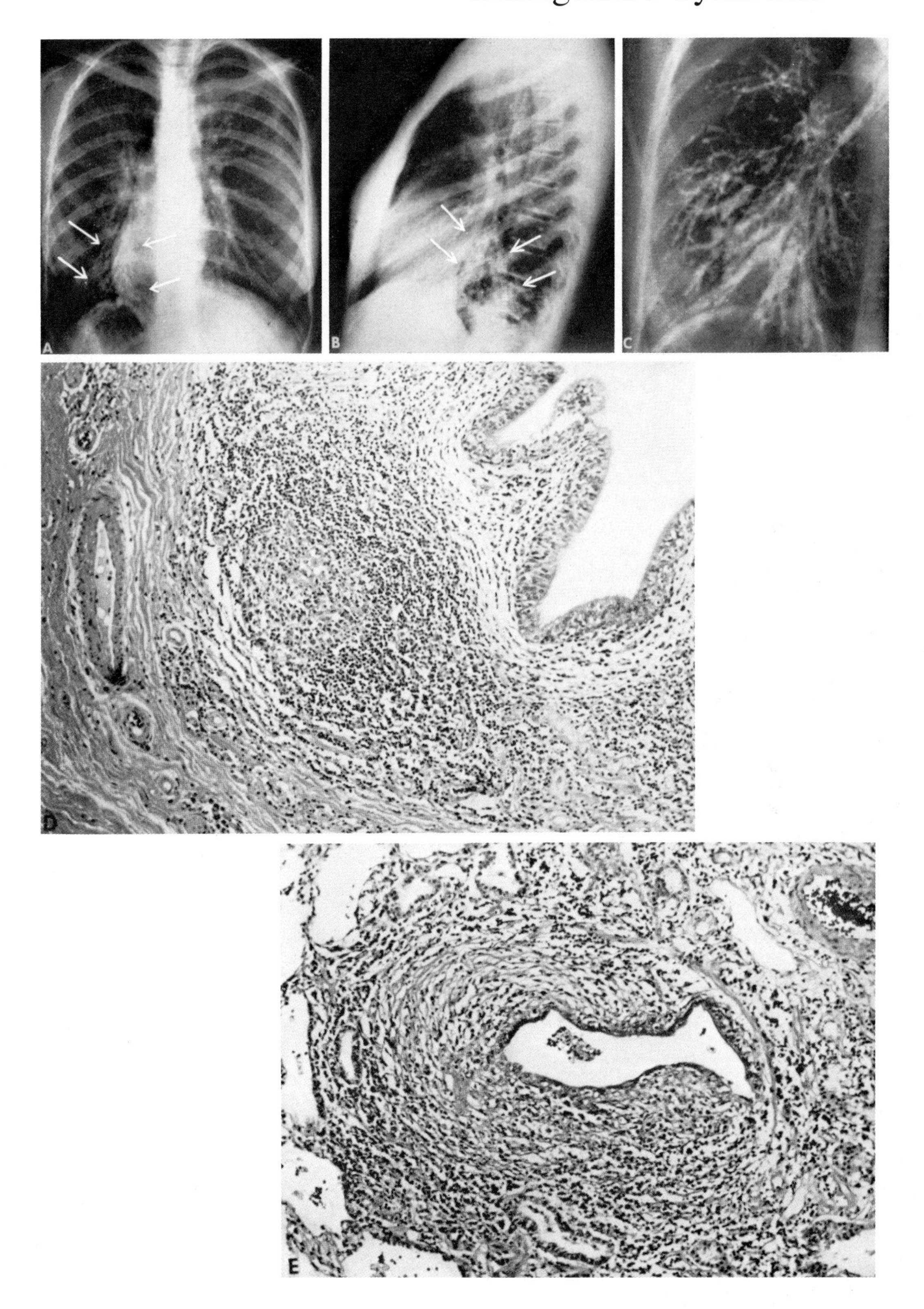

intervals after surgery to remove one to ten lung segments in each patient.[1072] Most of the subjects showed some ventilatory impairment before operation, together with impaired inert-gas distribution as shown by a prolonged lung-clearance index. It was found that the operation did not result in any decrease in vital capacity or maximal breathing capacity; gas distribution was somewhat improved; there was a slight increase in nonelastic resistance and a tendency to increased arterial unsaturation on exercise. Many patients showed progressive improvement for many months postoperatively, an important observation that suggests that any final assessment of the results of surgery in these patients should not be made until at least a year after operation. These findings—which, as the authors point out, conflict to some extent with previous observations[1086, 1125]—suggest that, when bronchiectatic segments are removed, the intervening lung, when normal, takes up the space without loss of function. Hashimoto[2944] has found that although the VC is usually lower after surgery, inert-gas distribution is commonly improved by it. Thus, except in extreme cases, the removal of nonfunctioning chronically infected tissue from the lung will have no adverse effect on function, and the clinical improvement and amelioration of symptoms may be very considerable. As pointed out earlier, however, considerable judgment has to be exercised in this decision, for resection when chronic bronchitis exists elsewhere in the lung can lead to further loss of function; in the absence of chronic bronchitis or generalized lung involvement, however, lobar or segmental resection may be advised. In some instances, removal of the involved segments, by removing the source of chronic expectoration, may well improve total function, and it is to be assumed that this occurred in two patients of Kamener *et al.* in whom operation was followed by improvement in the maximal breathing capacity from 53 to 105 and from 28 to 102 liters/min, respectively. Extensive resectional surgery for bronchiectasis is illustrated by Case No. 21.

CYSTIC FIBROSIS (MUCOVISCIDOSIS)

Basically a hereditary disease usually manifested in infancy or early childhood, cystic fibrosis is a generalized dysfunction of exocrine glands. The triad of chronic pulmonary disease, pancreatic deficiency, and abnormally high sweat electrolytes is present in most patients. Although the basic defect in cystic fibrosis is not clearly understood, it is generally accepted to be an inborn error of metabolism, transmitted as an autosomal recessive trait. Homozygotes for the recessive gene present all or substantially all the manifestations of the syndrome. It is striking in its racial distribution—it is most prevalent in the Caucasian race, in which it occurs approximately once in 2000 births, comparatively rare in American Negroes, and virtually absent in Mongolians and African Negroes.[3692]

May recognized the importance of the pulmonary aspects of this disorder in 1954, and wrote: "The variation in the manifestations and in the course of the disease are largely dependent, in our opinion, upon the circumstances in the lungs."[2115] In North America, it is, in the pediatric age group, one of the main causes of chronic illness and one of the main causes of death. It accounts for most of the chronic nontuberculous pulmonary disease in this age group. The pulmonary involvement in cystic fibrosis varies considerably. The lungs can be completely normal in infants dying with meconium ileus in early infancy.[3693] The cases that come to autopsy at a later age usually show widespread disease characterized by obliterative or acute bronchiolitis, bronchitis, plugs of tenacious yellow-green mucus clinging to the bronchi, widespread cylindrical or varicose bronchiectasis, patchy atelectasis, extensive pneumonitis, and numerous small pulmonary abcesses.[2337, 3694, 3690, 3691] Even though centrilobular emphysema has been observed by ourselves and others,[3695, 3696] it is not a prominent feature of this disease.[3690, 3696] Pulmonary elasticity, as measured by viscous resistance postmortem, is reported to be normal. The pathology is essentially one of bronchial obstruction with infection. The infection is remarkable in that *Staphylococcus aureus* and *Pseudomonas aeruginosa* are so frequently and repeatedly cultured in the pulmonary secretions[3697] that this combination in a child should lead one immediately to suspect cystic fibrosis.

Pulmonary function studies are indicative of obstructive airway disease, varying in degree with the evolution of the disease.[2114, 2119, 3698, 3699] The vital capacity is usually reduced in those showing radiological evidence of the disease. The residual volume is usually increased as is the functional residual capacity.

The total lung capacity is usually normal, but has been reported as reduced in the most severe cases. This reduction is true only of the measurement of total lung capacity done by helium dilution. It has not been confirmed when total lung volume is measured by body plethysmography.[3699] Compliance is reduced and airway resistance increased in most children with marked pulmonary involvement. Inert-gas distribution is commonly impaired, sometimes before other parameters of lung function. In the later stages of the disease, there is no good correlation between indices of gas distribution and other clinical or functional parameters.[3700, 3701] Diffusion capacity is reported as normal.[3699] The forced expiratory volume and maximum midexpiratory flow rate are usually decreased in proportion to the severity of the lung disease.

The partial pressure of CO_2 in arterial blood is usually normal or slightly decreased,[3699, 3702] a sustained elevation of P_{CO_2} occurring in the late stages of the disease and indicating irreversible obstructive airway disease.[3702] In contrast to the usually normal P_{CO_2}, the oxygen tension (and saturation) is often decreased.[3695, 3699] There is evidence of marked ventilation–perfusion ($\dot{V}/\dot{Q}$) abnormality as reflected in the increased arterial–alveolar nitrogen gradient.[3703, 3704] There is little doubt that the resultant hypoxemia leads to hypertension, cor pulmonale, and death.[3695] This pulmonary hypertension may be reversible by the administration of oxygen[3695] or not,[3705] and it may be relieved by the use of tolazoline hydrochloride.[3706] Right ventricular hypertrophy,[3695, 3705, 3706] at least in relation to the thickness of the wall of the left ventricle,[2117] and the medial hypertrophy of the pulmonary arterioles[3707] are changes that can be explained on the basis of prolonged hypoxemia.

An active program of bronchial care, including the judicious use of antibiotics controlled by frequent cultures and sensitivities, and the timely use of oxygen therapy are essential parts of a good therapeutic program for the pulmonary aspects of this disease. The use of prolonged periods of mist therapy has been advocated as essential to the regimen if optimal results are to be obtained.[3708] This widespread use of mist tents still needs confirmation, particularly in view of the recent data on penetration of particulate water in the respiratory tree in man.[3709] In all cases, routine evaluation of pulmonary function is a prerequisite to their proper management.

SUMMARY

Pulmonary function tests are useful in three ways in the management of patients with bronchiectasis. They provide an indication of the functional normality or otherwise of the apparently uninvolved lung tissue; they are useful in evaluating effects of medical treatment; and finally, they are essential for the preoperative evaluation of adults and children in whom any extensive resectional surgery is proposed. Some of these children present the most complex problems of evaluation seen by the physician, which necessitate not only measurements of exercise diffusing capacity and a full battery of resting tests, but also often the use of bronchospirometry to determine the differential function of the lungs. It is to be expected that the new radioactive-isotope techniques, which are much easier for the patient than is bronchospirometry, may contribute much information on the ventilation and perfusion distribution in diseased and healthy segments, and they may eventually permit a more precise statement of operative indications than is currently possible.[2945]

The comparative merits of medical[2947] and surgical[2938] treatment are still discussed in the literature, but there is little doubt that the patient is best served when individual decisions are taken on the basis of all the available information.

It is particularly true of bronchiectasis that an intelligent and useful report of pulmonary function can be written only when the radiographs, clinical findings, and test results have all been studied. When he has considered all of the data collectively, the physician is usually in a good position to understand the probable status of the uninvolved lung; not infrequently, the finding of considerable impairment of function in the presence of apparently localized disease will suggest a more thorough bronchographic examination of the lungs as a whole, or a period of a month or two of medical treatment before any resectional surgery is undertaken.

It cannot be claimed that laboratory tests of pulmonary function are invariably essential to the management of patients with bronchiectasis, but there is no doubt that they are commonly of material assistance to the physician in the management of the patient and in evaluating the results of medical and surgical treatment.

KYPHOSCOLIOSIS; ANKYLOSING SPONDYLITIS; PECTUS EXCAVATUM

CHAPTER 10

DEFINITIONS

The term *kyphoscoliosis* is generally used to indicate any degree of angulation, both in the lateral plane (scoliosis) and forward and backward. Kyphoscoliosis of sufficient degree to impair respiratory function may start as an idiopathic scoliosis during adolescence, later becoming kyphotic to a varying degree. When it is secondary to Pott's disease, with collapse of vertebral bodies, the kyphotic element predominates and the scoliosis is much less prominent. In *ankylosing spondylitis,* which is an acquired and often familial disease of the spine, the sacro-iliac and later the vertebral joints become immobile, with ossification of paravertebral ligaments; rib movement is much reduced, and in a severe case the thoracic cage moves very little on deep respiration. *Pectus excavatum,* "funnel chest" or "Trichterbrust," is a congenital developmental anomaly in which the lower end of the sternum is attached to the spine by a number of fibromuscular bands, causing sternal depression. In severe cases only a few inches may separate the lower end of the sternum from the vertebral bodies. In a sense, this condition is the opposite of "pigeon breast," usually seen as a result of childhood rickets, in which the lower half of the sternum projects forward, making the transthoracic section at the level of the lower sternum triangular in shape. Pectus excavatum is occasionally associated with other developmental anomalies, such as congenital heart disease.

PATHOLOGY

Although the pathological changes that may occur in the lungs as a result of the severe distortion produced by *kyphoscoliosis* are rather poorly documented, Bergofsky, Turino and Fishman have pointed out that there are sufficient data now to permit some valid generalizations.[1087] They reviewed the results of autopsies on 26 patients with kyphoscoliosis, and added 5 carefully studied cases of their own. Some other reports have appeared,[1088–1090] and that of Naeye[1091] includes postmortem studies of the pulmonary vascular bed in 9 cases, yielding information which, as Bergofsky and his colleagues noted, was previously lacking.

Although it is common to find areas of atelectasis and bronchopneumonia in these specimens, morphological emphysema is not usual, being noted only in patients whose illness has been complicated by chronic bronchitis. Bergofsky and his co-workers stress the fact that no thinning of lung substance or bullae can be observed, and note: "Although microscopic examination revealed occasional areas of mild alveolar dilatation, these were taken to reflect the anatomic adaptation of the lung to localized changes in thoracic configuration or to collapse of adjacent segments, rather than to bronchial obstruction."[1087] Liebow, describing the autopsy findings in a patient with severe kyphoscoliosis, stated that the thorax was narrowed like a cone posteriorly in the region of the spinal angulation and remarkably flared anteriorly, leading to compression and atelectasis of the lower lobes, with considerable overexpansion of the upper lobes.[24] He noted also that the unusual contour of the lungs was maintained after their removal from the deformed chest. Although this type of deformity may produce considerable aortic kinking, the distortion of major vessels is usually inadequate to account for the development of pulmonary hypertension and cor pulmonale. However, in one patient described by Abrahamson, the aorta appeared to have been nipped in the spinal angulation, since there was marked left ventricular hypertrophy, and death was attributed to thrombotic occlusion of the left coronary artery.[1090] This patient's lungs appeared to be normal. In his study of the pulmonary vasculature of nine cases coming to autopsy, Naeye concluded that there was marked hypertrophy of the media and general dilatation of the pulmonary arterial system; in all cases the lungs were noted to be small.[1091]

Patients with *ankylosing spondylitis* usually have normal lungs. The recent comprehensive review by Zorab of the lungs in this condition leaves little doubt on this point; he stressed the fact that, on postmortem examination of the lungs of eight patients with severe ankylosing spondylitis, there was no segmental pneumonia, no lobar collapse, and no bronchiectasis.[1092]

In the case of *pectus excavatum,* we know of no evidence to suggest that this deformity leads to any permanent changes in the lung.

RADIOLOGY

A review of specialized methods and techniques of measuring degrees of lateral and anteroposterior angulation of the spine would not be in place in this volume. When the degree of kyphoscoliosis is severe, evaluation by x-ray of the state of the lungs may be difficult. The shape of the chest often presents formidable difficulties to fluoroscopic examination, and it may prove difficult to determine which parts of the lung are being predominantly ventilated. It may be even more difficult to assess the state of the right ventricle of the heart or the pulmonary vasculature. In short, the radiological assessment of the lungs and heart in these patients is seriously handicapped by the often severe degree of thoracic deformity. These problems are much less serious in cases of pectus excavatum or ankylosing spondylitis, in both of which conditions the state of the lungs can be accurately assessed radiologically and the movement of the diaphragm can be measured.

CLINICAL FEATURES

In adult life the commonest causes of kyphoscoliosis are poliomyelitis and Pott's disease. Thus, in one group of 24 such patients, 9 had had Pott's disease, 5 poliomyelitis, and 2 rickets; in the remaining 8 the cause was unknown.[1093] These 8 probably belonged to the group in which idiopathic scoliosis, often of considerable severity, develops during early adolescence, presumably as a result of some developmental error. The gross angulation of the spine that may occur in these unfortunate children has been well described and illustrated by James[1094] and Gucker.[1095] The degree of kyphosis is variable. From whatever cause, there may be considerable respiratory difficulty early in life. Death follows the onset of cor pulmonale, often precipitated by a respiratory infection. It has been noted that the right ventricular failure, once developed, is singularly resistant to treatment by diuretics or digitalis, and for this reason its onset is attended by a very limited prognosis. All authors have noted the young age at which such patients may die. In one of the earlier papers in the English literature on this problem, Coombs, in 1930, wrote an excellent description of four patients with "fatal cardiac failure occurring in persons with angular deformity of the spine;"[1096] they were 19, 23, 29, and 38 years of age. Similar young adults have been reported in other series,[1097, 1098] and Samuelsson,[1099] who reviewed 103 cases from the literature, concluded that the average age at death was about 46 years. Little need be said on the clinical features of the disorder, except perhaps to note that there may be tachypnea, and air entry is markedly variable over different parts of the distorted thorax. Moist sounds and rhonchi are often audible, particularly in advanced cases. Some authors have noted that finger-clubbing is rarely seen. Daley has pointed out that these patients are extremely sensitive to morphine,[1100] and the injudicious use of respiratory depressants, often in routine preoperative dosage before a minor surgical procedure, may cause death. The fact that these patients cannot tolerate any reduction in respiratory activity can readily be understood when the severity of their disorder of ventilatory function is appreciated (*see* Case No. 20).

The clinical features of ankylosing spondylitis call for no special comment. Zorab's recent review[1092] clearly documents the fact that chronic respiratory illness with acute exacerbations is not a feature of this condition. It has been shown recently that the occurrence of rheumatoid lung (*see* page 270) is unusual in patients with ankylosing spondylitis.[2954]

In pectus excavatum, there is displacement of the heart to the left. This gives rise to complex electrocardiographic changes[1101] that, taken with unusual findings on auscultation,[1102] may lead to an erroneous diagnosis of coexistent heart disease. It is only very rarely that this deformity gives rise to respiratory or secondary cardiac impairment.

PHYSIOLOGICAL EFFECTS OF CHEST STRAPPING

Of particular interest in connection with the derangements of pulmonary function that occur in patients with chest deformity has been the recent investigation of the physiological consequences of tight strapping of the thorax in normal subjects. A detailed study of this phenomenon was published in 1960 by Caro, Butler and DuBois,[1103] who applied adhesive tape or wide strips of rubber tubing to the chests of 25 normal subjects. They found that this greatly reduced the vital capacity, inspiratory capacity and expiratory reserve volume; the residual volume was not changed, and consequently the functional residual capacity was reduced. The total capacity fell by about 2 liters. This altered the pressure–volume relationships over much of the vital-capacity range, reduced the tidal volume, increased the respiratory frequency, and caused no change in airway conductance. However, inert-gas distribution as measured by the single-breath technique was impaired as a result of the strapping, and the arterial oxygen tension fell during air breathing (compared with control values) and when 100 per cent oxygen was administered. The arterial oxygen tension did not return to normal immediately after the strapping was removed, but soon rose to its previous value after the subject took a few deep breaths. These ingenious experiments clearly demonstrated that the severe restriction imposed by the strapping caused collapse of some alveolar units and impaired ventilation of others. These findings have been confirmed by McIlroy, Butler and Finley,[1104] who showed, in addition, that the anatomical dead space was reduced and that there was alveolar hyperventilation during the period of strapping: this they considered to be reflex in origin. It was found also that complex alterations in ventilation and perfusion distribution must be occurring to explain the observed changes in arterial gas tension, which could not be accounted for only on the basis of areas of atelectasis in the lungs. There seems little doubt that the findings are to be explained by closure of small airways in the dependent parts of the lung, without the occurrence of radiological atelectasis (*see* page 47).

The prolonged lung compression endured by those with severe kyphoscoliotic disease obviously leads to the same changes in greater degree, and finally to severe disturbances in gas exchange. The experimental chest constriction described by these authors is far from comfortable, and attempts to exercise when the chest is constricted provoke extremely distressing sensations of dyspnea, presumably not unlike those experienced by patients with advanced ventilatory restriction.

PULMONARY FUNCTION IN THORACIC DEFORMITY

KYPHOSCOLIOSIS

Until recently little attention was paid to the pulmonary aspects of kyphoscoliosis. Early reports of pulmonary function[1] contain no exact account of this problem, and standard textbooks of medicine published as late as 1937[1105] make no mention of it. In 1930 Anthony reported the impaired ventilatory capacity of a 52-year-old man with severe kyphosis.[128] Studies of the interrelationship between ventilatory aspects of this condition and its circulatory consequences were first published in 1939, and were carried out by Chapman and his associates.[1097] These have now been superseded by more detailed observations. Kyphoscoliosis produces the same pattern of pulmonary function impairment whether seen in children[1095, 1106] or in adults,[1087, 1107–1109] though the severity of the disorder is very variable in both groups, and disturbances of blood gases are usually found only in adults.

In spite of the deceptively increased anteroposterior chest diameter, there is invariably a considerable reduction in total capacity and in vital capacity. In adults it is usual to find the total capacity reduced below 3.0 liters, from normal values of about 4.5 liters; and figures below 2.0 liters were found in several of the adult patients studied by Hanley and his colleagues,[1093] and in 4 of 21 patients we have studied.[1107] The vital capacity may be less than one-third of the predicted value. Hepper, Black, and Fowler have suggested[3136] that the arm span be used to predict lung volumes in these patients, whose height is usually affected by the disease process and hence unreliable for prediction purposes. Since there is proportionately less reduction in residual volume than in the total capacity, the ratio RV/TLC is raised, a finding that may be wrongly construed as representing "overinflation" or "emphysema" when, in fact, neither is present. The maximal midexpiratory flow rate[1106] or maximal breathing capacity[1087, 1093, 1109] is reduced only in proportion to the reduction in lung volumes, and airway resistance is normal. Most of these patients have demonstrable impairment of inert-gas distribution when studied by a helium closed-circuit method,[1107, 1109] though this is less easy to detect when open-circuit nitrogen techniques are used,[1087] since the latter methods are not optimal for study of gas distribution when the lung volume is very small and when there may be considerable resting hyperventilation. Dollery and his colleagues have reported the results of a study of 10 patients with kyphoscoliosis using ^{133}xenon and determining regional lung function.[2948] In 7 patients younger than 23 years, no abnormalities of ventilation or blood flow were demonstrable; in 3 older patients, ventilation was reduced to lower lung zones, but it was not clear whether this could be directly attributed to the deformity. The diffusing capacity is not reduced when allowance is made for the volume of lung being ventilated, and the fractional CO removal is usually normal or nearly so;[1087, 1106, 1107] it is found to be lower, however, when the patient is in cor pulmonale.[1087, 1107] Shaw and Read have demonstrated that uneven ventilation–perfusion ($\dot{V}/\dot{Q}$) ratios are commonly present in patients with kyphoscoliosis.[1109]

It is almost certainly the disturbances in the blood gases consequent upon both inadequate total ventilation and disturbed $\dot{V}/\dot{Q}$ relationships that determine the prognosis.[1109] Hanley and his co-workers noted that the average arterial P_{CO_2} was 44.0 mm Hg and the arterial saturation 91.5 per cent in 14 subjects without a history of cor pulmonale, and 53.6 mm Hg and 79.3 per cent in 10 with such a history.[1093] The same conclusion can be drawn from other data.[1087, 1108, 1109] Sadoul and Cherrier found hypercapnia and arterial desaturation in 8 of 18 patients with kyphoscoliosis.[2043] These authors reported, however, that in 8 patients with "chronic cor pulmonale" the mean vital capacity was the same as in 10 without evidence of this; in both groups it averaged 1.98 liters. The total capacity of each of these two groups was 3.2 liters. As noted above, it has been our experience that cor pulmonale is rarely encountered in these patients when the vital capacity is as high as 2 liters, a conclusion in conflict with Sadoul and Cherrier's data. It should be emphasized that patients with kyphoscoliosis usually have considerable dyspnea on exertion and limitation of effort for many years before any abnormality of blood gases occurs.

Only one comprehensive study has been

Case 20 Kyphoscoliosis

Summary of Clinical Findings. This 49-year-old woman was admitted to hospital in December, 1957, complaining of swelling of the ankles, shortness of breath and cough. She had had Pott's disease as a child, with resultant kyphoscoliosis that had remained relatively unchanged for years. Over the previous year, however, she had become increasingly short of breath, until now she was dyspneic with the slightest exertion. She had noticed increasing ankle swelling over the previous few weeks. Cough began in 1957 and was productive of small amounts of whitish-yellow sputum. There had never been hemoptysis. Aside from whooping cough and Pott's disease as a child, her past history was negative.

Examination revealed a thin female with severe kyphosis of the upper dorsal spine and a scoliosis in the mid-dorsal region, concave to the left. The anterior chest was prominent. Her blood pressure was 135/90 mm Hg; pulse rate was 128 per minute. The jugular veins were distended to the angles of the jaw. Heart size could not be ascertained, but a gallop rhythm was present. There were no murmurs. Respiratory excursions were severely limited; fine rales were heard at both lung bases. The liver was enlarged three finger-breadths below the costal margin, and 3+ pitting edema was present over the lower extremities.

Investigation included a hemogram, the hemoglobin being 15.2 g per 100 ml and the hematocrit 47.5 per cent, an electrocardiogram, which showed sinus tachycardia and a vertical heart, respiratory function studies and x-rays of the chest. Other investigation was noncontributory.

The edema partially cleared on a regimen of bed rest, low-salt diet, digitalization and diuretics. Her course was complicated by pneumonia, which responded to antibiotics. She died in congestive heart failure after a respiratory infection 9 months after this admission. Autopsy was not performed.

Radiology. There is a severe degree of kyphoscoliosis with resulting deformity of the rib cage and of the intrathoracic structures. It is impossible to assess accurately cardiac size or the presence or absence of pulmonary disease.

Summary. This patient illustrates the very severe defect of function that follows thoracic deformity. The congestive heart failure, present on her admission to hospital, is an extremely serious prognostic sign when it is secondary to severe kyphoscoliosis; as in this patient, it is most often seen when chronic hypercapnia has resulted from the condition.

	VC	FRC	RV	TLC	ME %	MMFR	$FEV_{0.75}$ ×40	pH	P_{CO_2}	HCO_3^-	O_2Hb %	$D_{L_{CO}}SS_2$
Predicted	2.3	2.0	1.2	3.5	55	2.5	64	7.40	42	25	97	13.1
Dec. 1957	0.5	1.1	1.0	1.5	31	0.2	10	7.40	66	37	71	5.5

All lung volumes are markedly reduced. There are impairment of mixing and gross reduction in ventilatory flow rate, as reflected in the MMFR and FEV. There is chronic hypercapnia and considerable arterial desaturation. The low diffusing capacity probably reflects the fact that only a very small volume of lung is being ventilated; in the presence of such severe reduction in lung volume it cannot be taken to indicate the probability that morphological emphysema is present.

Case 20
Kyphoscoliosis

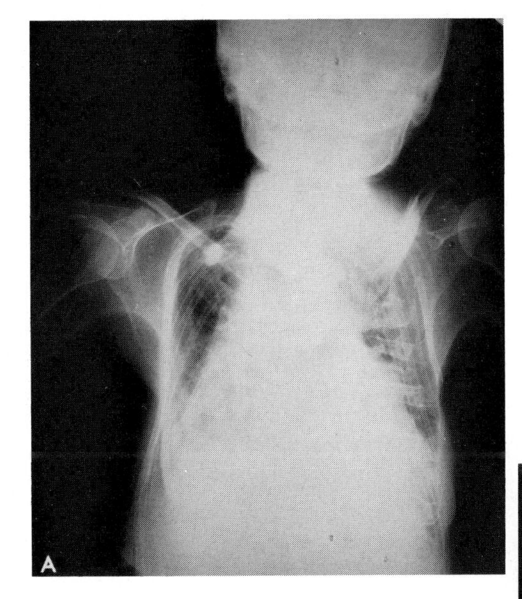

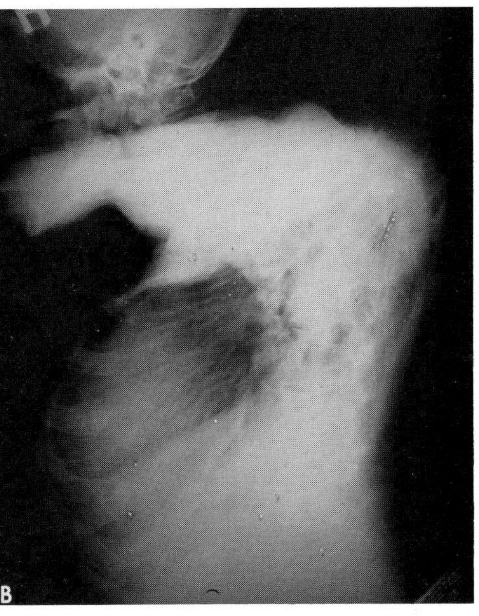

published of the effects on pulmonary function of various therapeutic measures designed to correct the spinal deformity. Using measurements of vital capacity in 49 children, extending over periods of months—or, in a few cases, years—Gucker showed that correction of scoliosis by wedging or localized casts produced a mean loss of vital capacity of 21 per cent in patients with paralytic scoliosis, and 29 per cent in those with idiopathic scoliosis.[1095] A less detrimental effect on vital capacity resulted from use of a frame. The importance of these, and of other observations, led the *Lancet* in 1963 to stress the importance of routine pulmonary function testing in young and adult patients with kyphoscoliosis,[1111] and others have recently re-emphasized this.[2949]

Ankylosing spondylitis

Although the changes in pulmonary function that may occur in kyphosis and ankylosing spondylitis have occasionally been considered together,[1110] it is important to recognize that the effect of spondylitis is much less and somewhat different from that seen in kyphosis.

Patients with ankylosing spondylitis possess very good diaphragm movement,[1112] and their ventilatory ability when considered in relation to their vital capacity is normal.[1113, 2952, 2953] There is some diminution in total capacity,[1092, 1114] although this is not as severe as in kyphoscoliosis. Sharp and his colleagues[2950, 2951] have found a considerable lowering of thoracic-wall compliance in their patients. In 8 control normal patients, this measured 0.214 liters/cm H_2O, whereas in 13 patients with ankylosing spondylitis with reduced TLC it averaged only 0.096 liters/cm H_2O. Pulmonary compliance was also reduced in 6 patients. All authors are agreed that the vital capacity is reduced, the degree of reduction correlating with the severity of the condition.[1092, 1114, 1115] The functional residual capacity has been reported as twice the predicted value;[1115] as increased, but to a lesser extent;[1092, 2950] and slightly lower than predicted.[1114] These differences depend largely upon the prediction data used. In the first of these papers,[1115] the predicted values appear too small for seated normal subjects; in the second[1092] they were similar to those shown in Tables 2-6 and 2-7; and in the third[1114] the predicted value was based on the age and sex of each subject, and not on the height, since it was considered that this would have been modified by the disease. It seems likely that, in general, in this condition the chest is often held in a slightly inspiratory position, although doubtless there is some variation from patient to patient. The ratio of residual volume to total lung capacity tends to be increased in most of the patients.[1092, 1115] There is also some disagreement in the literature concerning gas distribution, some finding that it is little altered[1092] and others that it becomes progressively less uniform with increasing severity of the disease.[1114] The diffusing capacity is usually normal,[1095, 1115] as are the arterial blood gases.[1115] In general, the $\dot{V}/\dot{Q}$ distribution is normal and pulmonary insufficiency does not occur.[2952] It seems unlikely that cor pulmonale could occur as a result of ankylosing spondylitis alone, though such patients may suffer lung damage from radiotherapy directed at the spine, or may acquire chronic bronchitis and emphysema in the same way as those with a normal thorax. In many of these patients, ventilation is carried out entirely, and very efficiently, by the diaphragm; any interference with its action may have serious consequences. For this reason, these patients must be very carefully cared for when any surgical procedure has to be undertaken, particularly if it involves an upper abdominal incision.

Pectus excavatum

This deformity occurs in very variable degrees of severity, so that whereas in most cases there is only some cardiac displacement to the left and little interference with respiratory function, in others there may be more severe consequences. It has been recognized for many years that very occasionally there may even be cor pulmonale secondary to this condition.[1116] Far more commonly, however, the only defects are a slight diminution in vital capacity and total capacity and reduction in the maximal breathing capacity,[1117–1119] but none of these changes is very considerable. Of five children with pectus excavatum whom we have studied, only one showed any such changes that could be considered statistically significant. Pulmonary hypertension must be exceedingly rare in this condition;[1102] its occurrence in the absence of changes in arterial gas tensions might reasonably suggest a cause other than the thoracic deformity itself. There is no defect of gas exchange on exercise.[2955] In general, from the point of view of pulmonary function, such patients should rarely be considered for corrective surgery,[1120] though there may be cosmetic reasons for advising this. It must be a very unusual case indeed in which the physiological derangement of function would necessitate an attempt at operative correction, though it has been suggested in one report that such an indication is commonly present.[1121] Most authors stress the fact that their patients may suffer from serious psychiatric disability as a consequence of this disorder; operative treatment may be justified by this consideration.[2955]

PULMONARY HYPERTENSION AND COR PULMONALE SECONDARY TO THORACIC DEFORMITY

Although in exceptional cases, such as that described by Abrahamson,[1090] kinking of vessels may play some part in the genesis of cardiac failure—the aorta and left ventricle being affected as commonly as the pulmonary artery and right ventricle—it seems true that cor pulmonale and pulmonary hypertension occur only in those patients in whom the arterial gas tensions are abnormal. It would seem reasonable to conclude, therefore, that right ventricular hypertrophy, as observed at autopsy by Kerwin in all of the five cases he described,[1098] results from loss of capillary bed, due to chronic atelectasis; possibly from structural changes in the small pulmonary arterioles;[1091] and finally is aggravated, and cor pulmonale precipitated, by chronic alveolar hypoventilation with disturbance of the normal $\dot{V}/\dot{Q}$ ratio, leading to arterial unsaturation and pulmonary hypertension. Although some data do not wholly support such a simple explanation,[1122, 2043] the generally close relationship between impairment of vital capacity and total capacity on the one hand and arterial gas-tension changes on the other hand,[1087, 1093, 1108, 1114] and the close relationship between arterial unsaturation and hypercapnia with cor pulmonale[1087, 1108] provide evidence suggesting that some such sequence underlies the natural history of severe kyphoscoliosis. Progressive compression of the lung, followed by loss of compliance such as that seen in patients with paralytic poliomyelitis, who are unable to take a deep breath, finally makes these patients dependent for their survival upon a lung volume of less than 2 liters, with a vital capacity of only a few hundred ml. We have found it generally valid to teach that a vital capacity of less than a liter should always indicate the possibility of hypercapnia. If any operative procedure is considered on these patients, the arterial blood should be sampled before anesthesia is induced. If CO_2 retention or unsaturation is found, extreme care is required to see the patient safely through even a minor surgical procedure.

As many physicians have noted, once right ventricular failure has occurred there is small hope of effective treatment; in our view, as discussed more fully in Chapter 22, there is little reason to advise treatment by artificial respiratory assistance once this stage has been reached.

KYPHOSIS SECONDARY TO CHRONIC LUNG DISEASE

It is well known that some, but not all, patients with chronic respiratory disease commonly develop a progressive mid-dorsal kyphosis. Halmagyi measured the angle of kyphosis in 360 men. Some of these had normal respiratory function, but most of them were suffering from advanced coalworker's pneumoconiosis or pulmonary emphysema.[1123] In miners with chronic respiratory disease he found a positive correlation between the angle of kyphosis (carefully measured on lateral radiographs) and age, and also between the measured angle and the maximal breathing capacity. It was not clear how far these two correlations were interdependent.

In practice there is usually little difficulty in establishing whether a patient with a moderate kyphosis has or has not a significant degree of emphysema. It is obvious that the ratio of residual volume to total capacity cannot be used in this differentiation, but the normal total capacity, increased absolute values of functional residual capacity, and severe airway obstruction that characterize emphysema usually serve to distinguish such patients from those with kyphoscoliosis, who have a reduced total capacity and a normal airway resistance, the maximal breathing capacity being well preserved in relation to the available volume. As pointed out by Shaw and Read,[1109] and by Bergofsky and his colleagues,[1087] the occurrence of kyphoscoliosis with bronchitis may raise complex problems of interpretation, and the extent to which associated chronic bronchitis or bronchospasm has contributed to disability and alteration of pulmonary function may become apparent only when the patient is re-evaluated after these conditions have been treated successfully.

SUMMARY

Neither pectus excavatum nor ankylosing spondylitis is associated as a rule with any major disturbance of pulmonary function, since in neither is there any very considerable encroachment on intrathoracic volume, and diaphragm activity is unimpaired.

In kyphoscoliosis, however, the total lung capacity is not uncommonly half of what it should be. When the vital capacity drops below 1 liter, the arterial gas tensions are frequently found to be abnormal; and this abnormality, which is attributable to alveolar hypoventilation and disturbances of ventilation–perfusion ($\dot{V}/\dot{Q}$) ratios, must be regarded as a precursor of cor pulmonale. Since respiratory depression from any cause is a major hazard to a patient with kyphoscoliosis, careful evaluation of pulmonary function, with measurement of arterial gas tensions if the subdivisions of lung volume are much reduced, is essential before administration of an anesthetic. Careful assessment of the effect on pulmonary function of various orthopedic procedures designed to straighten the spine in children, which has already been pioneered,[1095] should be made in all cases.

Although the association between kyphoscoliosis and cor pulmonale has been recognized in the English literature since 1921 at least,[1124] and has attracted more attention in France and Germany, there is still much to be learned about the mechanism of pulmonary hypertension in this condition; some recent studies undertaken on both sides of the Atlantic have provided much valuable data, and excellent reviews of this interesting clinical problem have appeared.[1087, 1093]

ATELECTASIS; PNEUMOTHORAX; FIBROTHORAX; RESECTIONAL SURGERY AND LUNG TRANSPLANTATION

CHAPTER 11

Research—technology—critical evaluation: this is the triad that has radically changed human life in our century. It is this triad that has made modern medicine possible. But it has basically altered the simple relationship that was once the center of social organization of medicine. Today, when a doctor meets his patient, each stands at the apex of a pyramid of complex assumptions that did not exist for the majority of their parents. The doctor's assumptions derive from the complexities of modern medical research, technology, social, economic, and legal considerations. The patient's assumptions are shaped by new and powerful forces. Stimulated by mass media, he—or his employer, or his union, or his lawyer—demands of the physician a degree of technical virtuosity in keeping with the twentieth century. Yet his appraisal of the results achieved by this virtuosity may be darkened by nostalgia for the simple relationship of the past. Of course, a similar nostalgia for the simple relationships of the past is also found among physicians and professional organisations that represent them.

While the social organisation of medicine is thus made complex, it is also immeasurably enriched. . . .[3032]

C. H. KEENE

ATELECTASIS

General features

Acute atelectasis of any considerable volume of the lung is often referred to as "massive collapse." It is usually due to sudden bronchial obstruction from aspirated material, or to a sudden transition from partial obstruction to total obstruction by tumors in the bronchial wall. This is followed by the absorption of air beyond the obstruction, with progressive atelectasis. The physical signs are those that follow the absence of air entry, and displacement of the heart and mediastinum toward the affected side. There may be considerable tachypnea and apparent respiratory distress if the onset is sudden and if most of the lung is involved. Radiologically, the displacement of structures can be seen and displacement of vessels in the noncollapsed lung may be noted.[2960] The lung parenchyma is uniformly opacified. Atelectasis of segments of the lung most commonly occurs as a result of inflammation but also occasionally develops as a result of radiotherapy in patients without primary bronchial obstruction (*see* Chapter 17). Atelectasis may become chronic, and it is remarkable that a lobe may finally re-expand and function normally after a period of collapse lasting up to two years;[1126] although bronchiectasis may follow such episodes, this is by no means invariable.

The changes that occur in the lung after bronchial occlusion have been extensively investigated. In general it is true that any gas trapped in the body is absorbed by the blood. This is because the fall in oxygen pressure in the tissues greatly exceeds the rise in CO_2 pressure, so that the sum of the partial pressure in the venous blood is considerably less than that of the atmosphere.[1865] This pressure difference amounts to approximately 60 mm Hg, which is more than sufficient to remove any gas trapped in the body. The lungs are no exception to this rule. If a bronchus is occluded, the air beyond the obstruction is quickly absorbed, with collapse of the area involved in a matter of a few hours if room air is breathed. If the patient is breathing oxygen, however, the pressure gradient is greatly increased and collapse of the obstructed lobe may take place in a matter of a few minutes, a phenomenon that may be of considerable importance during anesthesia.

When a smaller bronchus is obstructed, the situation may be quite different since, within each lobe, there are openings in the alveolar walls that allow the passage of air from one segment to another (*see* Chapter 2). For this reason, blockage of a small bronchus may not lead to collapse of the area it serves, the air spaces beyond the obstruction remaining in contact with the outside atmosphere through these collateral channels. It is undoubtedly true, however, that collapse of a segment of a lobe is sometimes observed; when this occurs, it is presumably due to the blockage of collateral channels or to local loss of pulmonary surfactant.[2338] Small areas of pulmonary atelectasis may be found in basal regions in some abdominal conditions.[2956]

When a large bronchus is blocked, the blood passing through the lobe involved will not be aerated and the saturation of the arterial blood will fall, sometimes to a level sufficient to cause cyanosis. However, this is only transitory; as the air is absorbed, blood flow through the airless alveoli is so reduced that the arterial saturation may return to normal. In other words, the blood flow through the area of atelectasis is deflected to the healthy and fully aerated lobes. The mechanism of this circulatory readjustment has been in dispute for several decades. It was formerly explained on the basis of mechanical obliteration of the collapsed capillaries, but in recent years reflex vasoconstriction due to the lowering of oxygen tension in the affected alveoli has been favored as an explanation of this interesting phenomenon[1210] (*see* Chapter 3). Whatever the cause, the shunting of blood to healthy areas is on a sound teleological basis, since it maintains adequate oxygenation of the arterial blood.

The effect on pulmonary function of atelectasis due to bronchial obstruction depends very largely upon whether it is acute or chronic. Pulmonary atelectasis occurring in a generalized form postoperatively is discussed in Chapter 22, and that seen in the respiratory distress syndrome also in the same chapter.

Experimental studies

The immediate effect of bronchial occlusion in the dog is an increased blood flow through the region due to mechanical factors; later the blood flow falls.[2957] Some investigators have found that atelectasis is followed by a fall in pulmonary surfactant,[2338, 2958, 2959, 2965] whereas others using different techniques find little reduction.[2964, 2968] One group of workers initially found no reduction of surfactant,[2964] but in a later paper[2967] they showed that with the establishment of increased bronchial artery flow over the next 30 days, surfactant returned and atelectasis diminished.[2967] These variable results may be explained in part by the effect of alveolar hemorrhage,[2968] but occasional large lung inflations seem to be essential for the integrity of surfactant.[2962]

On oxygen breathing, between 5 per cent and 30 per cent nitrogen is needed to prevent resorption atelectasis;[2963] reversible airway closure occurs on oxygen breathing at low lung volumes and may not be associated with true atelectasis.[2969]

Total bronchial occlusion in dogs is followed by hypertrophy of mucous glands distal to the obstruction.[2961]

Acute atelectasis

Knowledge of the effects of acute atelectasis due to bronchial obstruction has been derived mainly from experimental work in animals. Dale and Rahn[1127, 1128] showed in dogs that sudden occlusion of the bronchus to one lung resulted in an immediate increase in tidal volume and total ventilation of the unobstructed lung and an increase in the total oxygen uptake, which they ascribed to an increased oxygen cost of breathing. The mechanism of the hyperventilation was obscure, but there was a prompt fall in arterial oxygen saturation[1128] that might have been partly responsible for the increased ventilation. There were mechanical changes that the authors considered were probably mainly responsible for increasing the ventilation of the open lung. Pump[1129] showed that the same phenomenon occurred in patients in whom he temporarily blocked the bronchus during bronchospirometric examinations. When one bronchus was completely occluded at the end of a normal expiration, there was an immediate increase in tidal volume, respiratory frequency and functional residual capacity of the open unoccluded lung. It was of interest that this did not occur if the bronchus was occluded to a lung that was extensively involved by disease. Berglund, Simonsson, and Birath have recorded unique observations on a patient who suffered acute occlusion of the left bronchus.[1130] The patient was noted to be very dyspneic and cyanosed when walking slowly. At rest her arterial saturation was 92.5 per cent, increasing to 97.7 per cent when she moved into the right lateral position. On exercise it fell to 74 per cent, rising to only 81.7 per cent when she breathed 50 per cent oxygen. Of particular interest was the ventilation on exercise, which was 38.5 liters/min for an oxygen uptake of only 0.75 liter/min, giving a ratio of $\dot{V}O_2/\dot{V}E$ of only 1.95 (normally more than 3.5). This patient was treated by inducing a pneumothorax on the side of the atelectasis, which greatly relieved the dyspnea and raised the resting saturation to 94.5 per cent at rest and to 95.2 per cent on exercise. Ventilation was 18.8 liters/min for an oxygen uptake of 0.63 liter/min on exercise, thus elevating the $\dot{V}O_2/\dot{V}E$ from its previous exercise value of 1.95 to an almost normal value of 3.58.

These studies reveal that the immediate effect of a massive atelectasis is to produce hyperventilation of the contralateral lung, a fall in arterial oxygen tension and a fall in arterial P_{CO_2}. On exercise in the patient studied by Berglund and his colleagues the P_{CO_2} was only 25 mm Hg. The hyperventilation, therefore, as would be predicted, cannot combat the drop in arterial oxygen tension that is an inevitable consequence of the major shunt that occurs, and leads to a fall in the arterial P_{CO_2}. A similar combination of a lowered arterial saturation and P_{CO_2} is not infrequently observed during lung injuries (*see* Chapter 22).

Chronic atelectasis

When one lobe is collapsed as a result of a bronchial carcinoma, there is little subjective evidence of incapacity. Pulmonary function tests reveal a reduced total lung capacity and functional residual capacity, and the vital capacity also is reduced. If the rest of the lungs is normal, there is only a slight drop in ventilatory ability. The diffusing capacity may be noted to be slightly lowered, but often this is within the normal predicted range. If the lobe is completely airless and collapsed, the compliance may be reduced, but only in proportion to the loss of FRC; thus, the specific compliance will be normal.

PNEUMOTHORAX

Clinical, pathological and radiological features

Spontaneous pneumothorax most often occurs in previously healthy young adults, when it is caused by rupture of a small apical bleb; such blebs are usually no larger than grapes, but may be multiple and may occur in both lungs. Acute pneumothorax may occur also as a complication of other lung disease, such as emphysema, cystic lung disease of any type, carcinoma, pulmonary tuberculosis, and many other conditions, including Marfan's syndrome.[2976] The onset is marked by chest pain or discomfort, which is worsened by body movement as well as by attempts to take a deep breath, and some dyspnea. After some hours, this discomfort has usually worn off, and by the following day there is no dyspnea, although the lung may be as far collapsed as it was originally. The air within a pneumothorax is absorbed, the mechanism being similar to that described in atelectasis, but absorption is much slower because the air is not in such intimate contact with the blood. When the lung has fully expanded, pulmonary function in such patients is most commonly found to be normal, though occasionally a slight defect in gas distribution and a somewhat lower value for pulmonary compliance than predicted may be observed.[2971]

When artificial pneumothorax was the accepted treatment for pulmonary tuberculosis, chronic induced pneumothoraces were commonplace in every chest clinic. The popularity of this treatment in the pre-antibiotic era led at an early date[1] to considerable interest in the physiological consequences of pneumothorax. Such chronically maintained pneumothoraces not infrequently were followed by considerable fibrotic change in the visceral pleura and in the parietal pleura, particularly around the diaphragm. These changes led to considerable difficulty in lung re-expansion, or, when re-expansion did occur, to considerable functional defect in the lung re-expanded after an interval of many years.

Spontaneous bilateral pneumothoraces are encountered only in those unfortunate enough to rupture apical blebs on both sides simultaneously, or in patients with widespread emphysema or cystic lung changes. This condition may be rapidly fatal.[2973] In tension pneumothorax, the effort of coughing forces air into the pleural space progressively, causing a very considerable elevation of intrapleural pressure to positive levels, and progressive pulmonary collapse and mediastinal shift. Such a lesion occurs only when air can more easily pass outward into the pleura than it can return into the lung parenchyma and bronchial tree through the tear. It causes severe respiratory distress, rapidly relieved when the pleural space is decompressed. Surgical (or "open") pneumothorax occurs when the chest wall is opened to atmospheric pressure, and is most often seen with penetrating chest wounds. It leads to complete cessation of lung expansion on the affected side. It is important to stress that small pneumothoraces often cannot be diagnosed clinically and on occasion may be overlooked when all that can be seen is a thin pleural line at one apex on the radiograph; and that a useful level of activity can be maintained even when there is a partial pneumothorax of both lungs. This classic illustration is reproduced from textbook to textbook to illustrate that normal subjects possess an "immense pulmonary reserve". There is some interesting recent evidence that the incidence of spontaneous pneumothoraces may be increasing.[2975]

Acute pneumothorax

The first observations of the effect on the arterial blood of acute induction of a pneumothorax seem to have been made in 1925 by Meakins and Davies,[1] whose book contains an excellent summary of what was then known about the consequences of pneumothorax. They found the effects on the arterial blood somewhat variable, a phenomenon easily understood in view of the variable degrees of parenchymal disease in the lungs being collapsed. Using the newly developed method of measuring lung volume,[91] Christie and McIntosh showed that only about 30 per cent of air injected into the pleural space collapses the lung, the remainder being taken up by the outward movement of the chest wall.[1131] They showed also that there was an expansion of the contralateral lung as the pneumothorax progressed,[1131] and that the compliance of the lung was reduced,[1132] probably because of its smaller volume. Several subsequent studies have shown that an acute spontaneous pneumothorax with at least 50 per cent of collapse is accompanied by an immediate fall in arterial oxygen saturation,[1133, 1134] as occurred in one of the patients studied by Meakins and Davies. Over the course of the next few hours, however, the perfusion of the collapsed lung is progressively reduced, so that the patient is usually fully saturated 24 hours after the pneumothorax occurred. Once the perfusion adjustment has occurred, there is relatively little disability. Norris, Jones, and Bishop[2970] have recently documented the increased alveolar–arterial oxygen difference and lowered arterial oxygen tension in patients with spontaneous pneumothorax, and in 4 patients studied after acetylcholine infusion, they demonstrated that active vasoconstriction was present in the affected lung. Riska[1135] found that the acute induction of pneumothorax was followed by a measurable increase in reticulocyte count, which did not occur if oxygen was breathed as the pneumothorax was induced.

In Table 11–1 are shown some observations on a patient, made within 24 hours of a spontaneous pneumothorax that produced almost complete collapse of the left lung, and repeated when the lung had completely re-expanded of its own accord three weeks later. It may be noted that the diffusing capacity of the single functioning lung is about as predicted for one lung, and the reduction in all lung subdivisions are those expected with almost complete collapse of one lung.

The acute effect of pneumothorax in dogs with intact vagi appears to be to induce tachypnea and hyperventilation, with lowering of the arterial P_{CO_2}.[1136] This response is abolished by prior vagotomy, and the induction of pneumothorax in the vagotomized dog, but not in the normal, leads to arterial unsaturation. It is not clear how these results may be applied to the intact adult, nor what part the vagus may play in adaptation to a pneumothorax. The observations reported by Kilburn are of very considerable interest in relation to the mechanism of adaptation to pneumothorax in dogs.[2041] He found that when a pneumothorax was acutely induced in a conscious dog, it was followed by an increased respiratory frequency and reduced physiological dead space, but other changes were minimal. By contrast, induction of the same degree of pneumothorax in a dog anesthetized with pentobarbital was followed by an increase in minute volume and alveolar ventilation, a fall in oxygen saturation, increase in pulmonary artery pressure, and reduction in diffusing capacity. He concluded that the anesthetic had impaired the normally operative adaptive changes in ventilation and perfusion that follow acute induction of pneumothorax.

Pulmonary function tests may be of considerable value in studying patients who have suffered from one or more spontaneous pneumothoraces and in whom pleurodesis is being considered. Assurance that the re-expanded lungs perform normally and that any bullae present are too small to interfere with normal function may be valuable information for such patients, particularly if they are middle-aged and complain of mild bronchitis.[2971]

TABLE 11–1 Pulmonary Function Tests before and after Re-expansion of a Spontaneous Pneumothorax (Mrs. L. F., Aged 39; Height 163 cm)

	Predicted Values	24 May, 1955: Left Lung Two-thirds Collapsed; 24 Hours after Spontaneous Pneumothorax	13 June, 1955: Left Lung has Re-expanded; Normal Radiographic Appearance
Vital capacity (liters)	3.4	1.7	3.1
Functional residual capacity (liters)	2.8	1.9	3.0
Total lung capacity (liters)	5.1	3.2	5.1
Mixing efficiency (%)	60.0	37.0	62.0
Resting $D_{L_{CO}}SS_2$ (ml CO/min/mm Hg)	17.2	8.6	14.0
Exercise (1/2 mph, flat)			
V_E (L/min)		32.4	26.2
$D_{L_{CO}}SS_3$ (ml CO/min/mm Hg)		12.9	33.0

Note the reduced total lung capacity and impaired gas distribution, which was presumably due to slow helium equilibration in the collapsed lung. The diffusing capacity was reduced both at rest and on exercise when the left lung was two-thirds collapsed. Re-expansion of the left lung was followed by a decrease of 6 liters a minute in exercise ventilation at the same level of exercise.

Chronic pneumothorax

As will be noted later (*see* page 262), a patient with one normal lung may be capable of normal walking on the flat without dyspnea and as a rule does not suffer from any troublesome respiratory symptoms. The same is true of a patient with a unilateral chronic pneumothorax. However, when the lung is re-expanded, there may be considerable impairment of function[1137] due to secondary pleural changes and diaphragm limitation.[1138, 1139] In such patients it has been shown that the limitation of maximal breathing capacity and vital capacity after re-expansion is directly related to these changes.[1140] The loss of pulmonary function after re-expansion is often greater than after segmental resection of parts of the lung.[304] The operation of parietal pleurectomy[1141, 1142] is referred to in the section on fibrothorax.

Bilateral pneumothorax

It is remarkable that chronic bilateral pneumothoraces may be compatible with some degree of exercise tolerance. Such a patient, fully documented by Christie,[1132] had 75 per cent collapse of the right lung and 50 per cent collapse of the left. The patient had no dyspnea at rest, "but very mild exercise, such as walking to the bathroom, caused some respiratory embarrassment." His total lung capacity was 1.84 liters, FRC 0.75 liter, and vital capacity 1.19 liters. The arterial blood was 94 per cent saturated, and the arterial P_{CO_2} was 43 mm Hg. It is of interest to compare these findings with those noted in patients with severe kyphoscoliosis. The lung volumes appear very comparable to those commonly seen in that condition, and they are not incompatible with normal arterial gas tensions. The degree of exercise limitation also appears to be similar. It may be, however, that the patient with kyphoscoliosis is less well able to maintain a normal $\dot{V}/\dot{Q}$ adjustment than is the patient with the lungs partially collapsed by pneumothoraces, and lung expansion may be more uniform in pneumothorax compared with the pattern that results from the abnormal intrathoracic contour found in kyphoscoliosis.

As previously noted, acute spontaneous bilateral pneumothorax is a dangerous and often fatal condition.[2973]

Surgical or open pneumothorax

When the chest wall on one side is widely opened, it is obvious that all respiration must stop on that side since there can be no pressure swing around the lung. Moreover, since the mediastinum is mobile, these consequences may not be confined to one side only. Thus, a report from the USSR[1143] indicated that, in patients with an open pneumothorax on one side, the contralateral lung can take up only 45 to 85 ml O_2/min, which is less than its normal contribution when both of the lungs are working. It is not clear from the translated abstract of this paper under what conditions these observations were made, but it seems probable that the ventilation of the contralateral lung was seriously compromised, and its volume decreased, by movement of the mediastinum. Pulmonary artery pressure has been shown to rise considerably (to 16 to 25 mm Hg) when the thoracic cavity is opened before resectional surgery.[1144] However, more information is required before any complete description of the ventilatory and circulatory consequences of open pneumothorax can be given.

FIBROTHORAX

Clinical, pathological, and radiological features

In fibrothorax, the two layers of pleura are adherent, the lung being covered by a thick layer of nonexpansible fibrous tissue, much as an orange is covered by peel. Organization of a traumatic hemothorax and the late results of a tuberculous effusion or healed empyema are the mechanisms most commonly responsible for the development of this condition. If it is consequent upon trauma, the underlying lung may be normal, but if the cause is tuberculous, the clinical picture may be complicated by parenchymal disease in the lung itself in addition to the pleural lesion.

When this condition is advanced in degree its radiological diagnosis offers little difficulty; it is important to recognize, however, that there may be considerable diminution in function of a lung as a result of fibrothorax, with relatively unspectacular radiological changes. A careful study of the parenchyma of the lung on the involved side may be an important examination before the decortication operation, and in many cases it will be necessary to perform tomography, bronchography, and perhaps even angiography,[1145] before complete evaluation is possible.

The physical signs of this condition are characteristic. The extreme fixity and rigidity of one side of the chest, almost total absence of breath sounds, and a very dull percussion note all suggest the clinical diagnosis of fibrothorax.

A recent experimental study by Condon[2974] has revealed that normally a bloodclot is fully absorbed from the pleural space, and fibrothorax occurs only if the integrity of the parietal pleura is impaired, or if the phrenic nerve is sectioned.

Effect on function; results of decortication

All those who have studied patients with fibrothorax have agreed that there is more interference with function on the involved side than one might expect. Some authors have noted that it is the secondary pleural fibrotic change that determines the loss of function after attempted re-expansion of a chronic pneumothorax,[1139, 1141, 1146] and have stressed that pleural fibrosis has a more severe effect on function than do many parenchymal lesions.[1139] Successful "peeling" of the layer of thick fibrous tissue off the involved lung may cause a remarkable improvement in pulmonary function. In the case reported by Petty, Filley, and Mitchell,[1145] the patient had a severe fibrothorax on the right side as a consequence of pulmonary tuberculosis. Preoperatively the vital capacity was 2.4 liters against a predicted normal of 4.4; the maximal midexpiratory flow rate was 0.62 liter/sec (predicted 4.37 liters/sec); and the maximal breathing capacity, predicted to be 150 liters/min, was only 47 liters/min. Bronchospirometry showed no oxygen uptake or CO_2 output from the right lung, which was capable of contributing only 5 per cent of the vital capacity. The arterial saturation was normal at rest and on exercise, although there was moderate elevation of pulmonary arterial pressure on exercise. A repeat of these studies 18 weeks after decortication showed a vital capacity of 3.4 liters, maximal midexpiratory flow rate of 2.6 liters/sec, and maximal breathing capacity of 111 liters/min; and bronchospirometry revealed that the right lung was now contributing 18 per cent of the vital capacity, 37 per cent of the resting ventilation, and 22 per cent of the resting oxygen uptake. Other authors have documented similar, though in some cases less dramatic, examples of improvement,[301, 302, 1147, 1149, 1150] and have stressed the fact that the functional improvement is usually very satisfactory unless extensive parenchymal disease is present. An effort should be made to determine beforehand the likely extent of parenchymal disease,[1148, 1149] but, in view of the major improvement that may result from surgery, it is important that the attitude to this should not be too conservative.

It is not clear why a unilateral lesion should lead to such impairment of ventilatory ability as that shown to be reversible in the case reported by Petty and his colleagues, in which the preoperative maximal ventilation figures were lower than if the right lung had been removed completely; it seems possible that the ventilation of the normal side is hindered in some way by the rigid thorax on the other, though the precise mechanism of this is obscure. When ventilation is much reduced on the involved side, the steady-state diffusing capacity will be mainly determined by the functional integrity of the normal lung. Physiologically, it is of very considerable interest that the circulation can be resumed through a lung in which it had been reduced to negligible amounts for a period of years—a reduction that is adaptive to the reduced ventilation but presumably not accompanied by structural change.

It is important to stress that, although in some patients the increase in maximal ventilatory ability postoperatively may be only of the order of 30 liters/min, operation may result in a much better ventilation and greatly increased oxygen uptake on the involved side, a point well illustrated by Savage and Fleming (*see* case 23 in ref. 301); and also that function may be restored after 20 years of restriction. Restoration of function to the lung is usually accompanied by considerable subjective benefit, but in addition greatly reduces the hazard from pneumonia or other infection in the normal lung, that might otherwise prove overwhelming.

RESECTIONAL SURGERY

Clinical, pathological, and radiological features

With the very considerable increase in incidence of bronchial carcinoma in many parts

Case 21
Bronchiectasis; Resection of All Lung Tissue Except Right Upper Lobe

Summary of Clinical Findings. This woman was first admitted to hospital in 1945 at the age of 14. She complained of chronic cough productive of copious amounts of greenish-yellow sputum, present since an attack of scarlet fever at 1 year of age. Physical examination showed that she was a frail, undernourished girl. Fine, moist rales were heard over both lung bases. An x-ray revealed a right lower-lobe pneumonia, and when this had cleared, bronchograms demonstrated bronchiectasis of both lower lobes. Subsequently the right lower and middle lobes, and later the left lower lobe including the lingula, were resected.

She was readmitted to hospital in 1952. She had had some relief of symptoms immediately after the operations, but soon the productive cough had recurred and, in addition, she had become short of breath on exertion. X-rays revealed loss of volume and multiple cavities of the left upper lobe, whereas the right upper lobe was hyperinflated. Bronchography revealed no evidence of bronchiectasis in the right upper lobe. The vital capacity and MBC were reduced to 1.4 liters and 30.9 liters per minute, respectively.

The patient was readmitted to hospital in 1956, having suffered recurrent episodes of chest infection in the interval, and was now completely incapacitated by cough and dyspnea. Bronchograms revealed cystic and saccular bronchiectasis of the remaining left upper lobe, which was thought to be the source of continuing infections. A bronchospirometric examination showed that this contributed little to function and was grossly bronchiectatic; therefore, it was resected, leaving only her right upper lobe. Her postoperative course was complicated by an empyema but since that time she has required no further hospital admissions. She has been able to live fairly comfortably, but her activities are limited. She is capable of walking on the flat without discomfort, and there is no significant sputum, but she has difficulty in walking up an incline.

Radiology. The left hemithorax shows considerable loss of volume, as indicated by mediastinal shift, diaphragmatic elevation and rib approximation. The right upper lobe, which is the only lung tissue remaining in the thorax, has undergone remarkable overinflation; not only does it occupy a right hemithorax of greatly increased volume, but it has extended across the midline into the left hemithorax so as to fill the anterior half of this side as well (*A* and *C*).

Case report continues on page 260

												CO		EXERCISE				
	VC	FRC	RV	TLC	ME %	MMFR	$FEV_{0.75}$ ×40	pH	P_{CO_2}	HCO_3^-	O_2Hb %	Ext %	$D_{Lco}SS_2$	MPH	GRADE	$\dot{V}_{O_2}$	$\dot{V}_E$	$D_{Lco}SS_3$
Predicted*	3.9	3.1	1.7	5.6	65	3.7	99	7.4	40	25	97	48	20.1					
Predicted†	0.59	0.46	0.25	0.84		0.5	15					–	3.0					
Dec. 1956	1.4	2.2	1.7	3.1	16						93	28	6.7					
May 1962	1.5	2.3	1.7	3.2	32	0.5	22	7.37	42	23	100	38	12.0	1.5	FLAT	0.51	14.3	13.4
Jan. 1968	1.4	2.6	2.1	3.5	33	0.7	32	–	–	–	–	32	6.6	–	–	–	–	–

*Values for normal subject with two lungs.
†Values for a normal right upper lobe in a normal subject calculated as 15 per cent of the normal total value.

The left upper lobe was removed in July, 1956, leaving only the right upper lobe in the thorax, since the right middle and lower and the left lower lobes had all been removed previously. In December, 1956, the right upper lobe was inflated to about four times its normal volume; gas distribution was poor within it, but the diffusing capacity was good for one lobe. Twelve years later, the volume of the lobe is unchanged; gas distribution has improved, and ventilatory tests are about what would be predicted for one lobe. The arterial blood gases are normal, and the exercise diffusing capacity is amazingly good for one lobe of the lung. Mechanics studies at this time showed that the maximal negative intrapleural pressure was −27 cm H_2O. The static compliance was 0.08 and the dynamic compliance was 0.06 cm H_2O/liter. Airway resistance on expiration was 11 cm H_2O/ 1 /sec, this high figure presumably reflecting the paucity of airways through which flow can occur.

Bronchiectasis; Resection of All Lung Tissue Except Right Upper Lobe

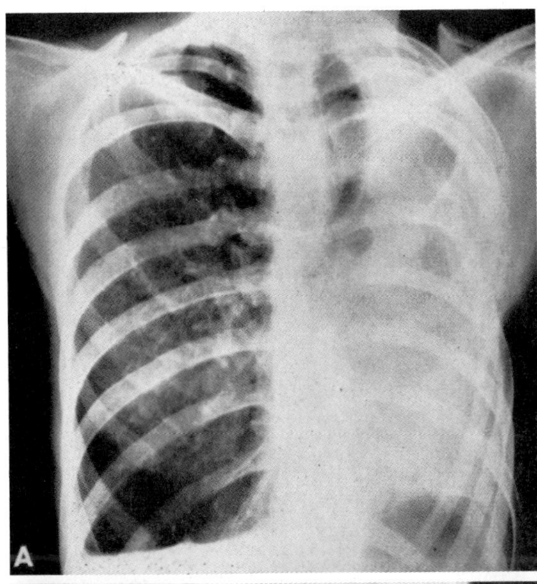

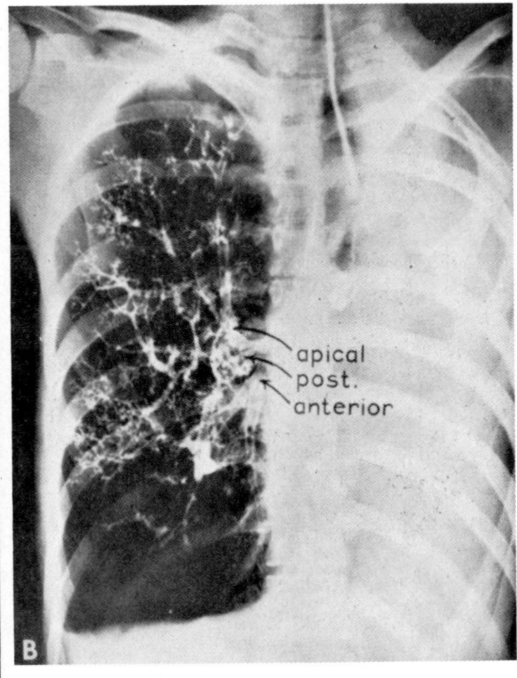

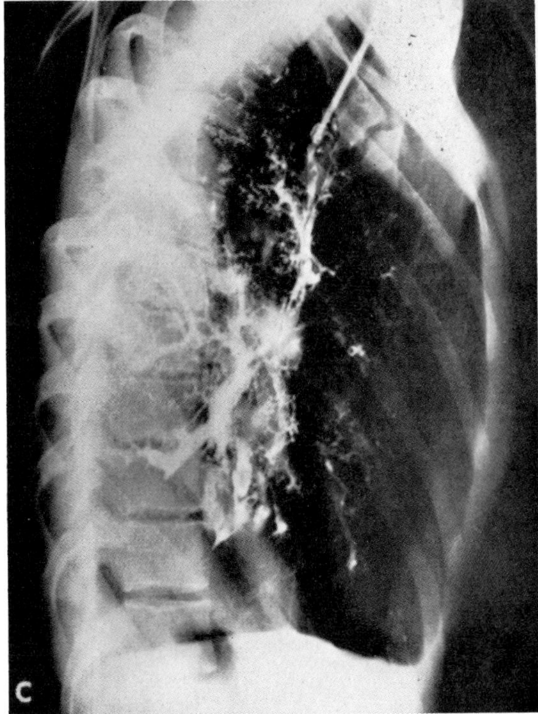

Case 21
Bronchiectasis; Resection of All Lung Tissue Except Right Upper Lobe (Continued)

The size of the pulmonary vessels in the residual right lung is perhaps not as large as one might expect in view of the fact that these vessels are carrying the whole right ventricular output. There are no changes suggesting pulmonary arterial hypertension. Bronchograms (*B* and *C*) in postero-anterior and lateral projections show only three segmental bronchi remaining out of the original 19. The three segmental bronchi of the right upper lobe, appropriately indicated in the PA view, have fanned out so as to be distributed evenly throughout the markedly overinflated lobe. Note in the lateral projection that the heart has been displaced against the posterior chest wall by the overinflated right lobe, which has crossed the midline so as to occupy the anterior half of the left hemithorax; three or four subsegmental bronchi inferiorly show considerable bronchiectasis.

Summary. This patient, now aged 39, has lived for 13 years entirely dependent upon the function of the right upper lobe, all other lung tissue having been removed because of gross bronchiectasis without evidence of cor pulmonale. Pulmonary function tests show that the right upper lobe has overinflated to at least three times its normal volume, but its diffusing capacity is good, and the arterial blood gases are normal. It has a good elastic recoil as shown by a maximal negative intrapleural pressure of -27 cm H_2O. This lobe is grossly overinflated but has presumably not suffered the changes of morphological emphysema.

---

of the world, the operation of pneumonectomy has become a common procedure in many hospitals. In most recent series of patients studied after this operation, carcinoma has been the indication for lung removal, the remainder of the cases being operations for tuberculosis or extensive unilateral bronchiectasis. As will be noted later, there is considerable uncertainty as to whether any specific changes occur in the structure of the lung left behind after pneumonectomy.

Clinically, the patient who has had a lung removed is often physically very well, noticing no dyspnea in ordinary life, though some activities, such as lawn-mowing or snow-shovelling, previously done without consequent symptoms, may now be restricted.

Radiologically, the hyperinflation of the remaining lung generally leads to considerable displacement of the mediastinum to the opposite side, resulting in some tracheal deviation. Some plethora of the remaining lung may be noted, and its pulmonary artery may be somewhat larger than normal.

EXPERIMENTAL WORK ON LUNG RESECTION

Although it has been recognized for many years that the lung left behind after pneumonectomy will often assume a larger volume than it formerly possessed, there has been considerable uncertainty as to exactly what changes take place. This is true not only in man but also in experimental animals. Longacre's experiments on dogs showed that the changes that occurred might be influenced by the age of the animal at the time of pneumonectomy.[1151] Work on rats reported from the USSR[1152, 1153] has been interpreted as indicating that definite lung regeneration may occur in these animals; it has been suggested also that similar changes may be observed in rabbits.[1154] The availability of these papers only in translation or as abstracts prevents any precise evaluation of their contents. Evidence as to whether increased lung growth follows pneumonectomy in puppies is somewhat conflicting. Massion and Schilling[2992] have reported that this does not occur in dogs, but Keszler[1159] has reported evidence of true hypertrophic change in the remaining lung in dogs and has found evidence of it in the lung of a child accidentally killed 1½ years after undergoing pneumonectomy. The experiments of Harrison and his colleagues on dogs clearly show that some adaptive changes occur in the remaining lung after pneumonectomy; after resection of as much as 75 per cent of the total lung volume, there was initially an increase in pulmonary artery pressure measured at rest, but several years later this had fallen to normal levels.[1155] Abnormal elevation of pulmonary arterial pressure on exercise was always observed, however. Other workers have noted an immediate increase in pulmonary artery pressure, with little tendency to return to normal values.[1156] In experiments on dogs, Williams, Canney, and Rayford[1157] found that, after about 68 per cent of lung tissue had been removed by pneumonectomy and lobectomy, a rise in pulmonary artery pressure was invariable. However, there was no disturbance of ventilation–perfusion relationships, and no appreciable gradient between alveolar and end-capillary oxygen tension when breathing room air or 12 per cent oxygen. This observation is of interest, since, if the pulmonary capillary blood volume is reduced, the same total pulmonary blood flow will be possible only if the transit time of blood through the capillary is reduced—a phenomenon that might have led to a fall in capillary oxygen tension. It is clear that tolerance to removal of about half of the lung tissue in dogs is very good, but that reduction to about 20 per cent of the original is associated with very considerable disability and with secondary hematocrit changes presumably consequent upon chronic hypoxia.[1158] Case No. 21 shows an example of very extensive resection in an adult.

Effects of thoracotomy and lobectomy; segmental resection

There is no doubt that thoracotomy alone, without resection of lung tissue, leads to a temporary decrease in vital capacity and maximal breathing capacity, changes that Gorlin and his co-workers found to be present for three weeks after operation, receding rapidly between the fourth and sixth postoperative weeks.[1160] Segmental resection is accompanied by very little loss of vital capacity or ventilatory function;[303–305, 1161 1162, 2977] and, provided the remainder of the lungs is normal, lobectomy does not cause any noticeable disability or dyspnea,[1071 1163–1165] although there may be a loss of 20 per cent of vital capacity and between 10 and 20 per cent of maximal breathing capacity after this procedure.[1166, 1167 2047] It is important to note, however, that much depends upon the function of the area removed as well as the state of the remaining lung.[1125] Although, in our experience, lobectomy is followed by a slight fall in exercise diffusing capacity, this is minimal.

Effects of pneumonectomy

Function of the remaining lung

Although some authors had noted that moderate exercise was possible after a pneumonectomy, the start of investigations into the consequences of this operation in the adult may be dated from the work of Lester and Cournand and their colleagues in 1942. In that year Cournand and Berry[1168] presented pulmonary function data on 12 patients who had undergone pneumonectomy, 7 of them having been tested preoperatively. They found that the volume of the remaining lung was in general larger than that predicted for one lung; that the maximal breathing capacity in those whose remaining lung was normal was about 63 per cent of the predicted value for two normal lungs, a finding subsequently confirmed by others;[1169, 1172] that in the older subjects the ventilation during a given level of exercise and oxygen uptake was greater than normal; that inert-gas distribution, as measured by alveolar nitrogen after 7 minutes of oxygen breathing, was normal; and that arterial oxygen saturation and CO_2 tension were normal at rest and during exercise. A later report indicated arterial unsaturation on exercise in one of these subjects;[1170] and subsequently, using the newly developed oxygen method of measuring the diffusing capacity, Cournand and his colleagues concluded that the diffusing capacity after pneumonectomy in the three young subjects studied was very nearly equal to that of someone with two lungs, but that it was somewhat lower in two older patients.[1171]

In 1956 we extended these observations by measuring the steady-state diffusing capacity and lung mechanics in 10 patients postoperatively.[388] We found that the diffusing capacity was reduced below the predicted levels in every patient, but considered in relation to their postoperative lung volume was usually normal; that inert-gas mixing was normal except in one man; and that the compliance was as predicted for one lung with a more than normally negative end-expiratory pressure in those showing overinflation. The effect of pulmonary resection on compliance was also studied by Frank, Siebens, and Newman,[1173] who produced convincing evidence that the compliance falls in direct proportion to the number of segments of lung removed. It has been pointed out subsequently that intra-esophageal pressure measurements may be erroneous after a patient has had a pneumonectomy,[455] but it seems unlikely that these conclusions need to be modified to any major extent.

For these reasons, it was argued that the state of overinflation could not be equated with clinical emphysema, in which all of these parameters of function are customarily altered. Further support for such a distinction came from the observation that there was no fall in dynamic compliance at increasing respiratory frequencies. The distinction between "overinflation" and "emphysema" had been obscured previously by the fact that the ratio of residual volume to total lung capacity is invariably increased after pneumonectomy, and this had been taken to indicate that the remaining lung must be the site of morphological emphysema. Indeed, it had been argued that space-reducing operations might be indicated to reduce the possibility of emphysema in the remaining lung.

Several authors have confirmed the ventilatory findings noted above,[1175, 1176] and all observers who have studied these patients on exercise have noted that there is an increased total ventilation in relation to oxygen uptake, or that the ratio of $\dot{V}O_2/\dot{V}E$ is reduced.[283, 388, 628, 972, 1165] The diffusing capacity has been found to be reduced in proportion to the amount of lung removed.[363, 1177, 1178, 2985] Using a steady-state exercise method at two oxygen tensions to study three patients who had undergone pneumonectomy, we found that the membrane diffusion component was about half normal, and the pulmonary capillary blood volume in relation to lung volume was variable.[399] In the majority of patients, the arterial blood gases at rest and exercise are normal.[283, 628, 1179]

In a study of seven patients, we found no abnormality of ventilation distribution, and a more than normal uniformity of perfusion distribution.[3827]

Ogilvie and his colleagues compared the function status of 10 patients one year after with that of 12 others 10 years after pneumonectomy.[2044] They found that the mean vital capacity was 2.15 liters in the one-year group and 1.72 liters in the 10-year group. The maximal ventilatory volume averaged 74 liters/min in the former and 40 liters/min in the latter group, but the diffusing capacity ($D_{LCO}SB$) was if anything higher in the latter. Bronchitis was noted to be commoner in the 10-year group, but the authors concluded that the diminution in vital capacity and ventilatory function was probably attributable to changes occurring in the chest wall during the ten years since operation.

Most patients who have led active lives and who have had to have a pneumonectomy undoubtedly notice that their activities are somewhat restricted afterwards. Their consciousness of dyspnea presumably results from the necessity for a high level of ventilation on exercise, which, because of the reduction in lung volume, requires greater respiratory effort. It is doubtful whether their reduced diffusing capacity can in any sense be regarded as a factor limiting physical activity,[628] though it may be partly responsible for the higher level of ventilation in relation to oxygen uptake,[388] and hence may indirectly contribute to a sensation of dyspnea. The degree of lung distention does not seem to depend upon the side of the pneumonectomy, the age of the patient, or the nature of the lung disease for which the operation was performed.[1176] The development of morphological emphysema, which no doubt may occur as readily in a man with one lung as in a man with two, should be regarded as a phenomenon separate from overinflation.[388] In this connection Burrows and his colleagues, who studied 36 patients after pneumonectomy, found that 9 might be considered to have emphysema in the remaining lung; they concluded that in 4 of these it had been present before operation, and in the remainder had developed quite independently of it.[363]

Several more recent evaluations of pulmonary function after pneumonectomy have generally confirmed these findings. Most authors have found evidence of overinflation, with a normal diffusing capacity when this is related to lung volume;[2980, 2983, 2985] however, if one lung is left intact, the reduced maximal oxygen uptake is probably caused by a reduced cardiac output and not by the reduction in internal surface area.[2987] Birath and his colleagues[2986] found some evidence of abnormal inert-gas distribution, but concluded that emphysema did not occur in the remaining lung. They also concluded that thoracoplasty was in general contraindicated.

The problems of whether chronic overinflation leads to or predisposes to later development of emphysema and whether such emphysema might consist of progressive alveolar loss without airway obstruction have not yet been definitely resolved. Nevertheless, the obvious danger of emphysema should lead the physician to watch very carefully for the development of chronic bronchitis in patients who have only one lung, to treat episodes of acute infection seriously, and to advise the patient to stop cigarette-smoking and to leave any dusty atmosphere. It certainly seems likely that chronic bronchitis may be more dangerous in an overinflated lung that has to do the work of both lungs. At the very least, the effects of environmental contaminants might be expected to be more severe.

Resection of more than one lung may be followed by adequate pulmonary function,[2988] a situation illustrated by Case 21.

Pulmonary arterial pressure in the remaining lung

Since the original observations of pulmonary arterial pressure in patients who had undergone pneumonectomy, by Cournand and his colleagues,[1171] there have been other studies in which pulmonary hypertension has been noted to be present at rest,[971, 1180] though more frequently an abnormal elevation was present only, but almost always, during exercise.[363, 971] Denolin has contributed a review of the evidence on this problem and concludes from his own and other data that, on exercise, the mean pulmonary arterial pressure is raised by 10 to 19 mm Hg.[972] He points out that this elevation is a consequence of the doubling of flow the remaining lung must accommodate, and that the pulmonary vascular resistance for one lung is not increased. Adams and his coworkers[1181, 1182] have presented data which suggest that the exercise capability and sensation of dyspnea are mainly determined by the level of pulmonary hypertension, a concept that accords with Linderholm's view that the limitation of exercise in these patients is circulatory rather than being either ventilatory or due to a reduced diffusing capacity.[628] In the erect subject, there is still a gradient of perfusion distribution favoring the lower zones after pneumonectomy, though Martin, Cline, and Marshall[313] noted that the differences in lobar RQ were less than in normal subjects, as would be expected with a higher blood flow through the lung. In a study of seven patients within two weeks after a pneumonectomy, we have recently reported that ventilation distribution in the remaining lung was normal, and the distribution of perfusion was more uniform than in a normal subject; this latter finding is to be attributed to the increased blood flow through the remaining lung.[3827] Recently several authors have documented the increased pulmonary artery pressure on exercise in patients after pneumonectomy,[2981, 2989] together with abnormal exercise electrocardiograms,[2980] and even some increased pulmonary arterial sclerosis at autopsy.[2989, 2990]

Many authors have studied the effect upon the heart of pneumonectomy, and although some have concluded that cardiac effects are seen in at least half of the patients who undergo pneumonectomy,[1183] it seems probable that these include a considerable number in whom the only abnormalities are electrocardiographic changes consequent upon displacement or rotation.[1184] It does not seem that evidence of right ventricular hypertrophy is commonly found, though the data are very limited.

Pneumonectomy in childhood

In contrast to earlier studies indicating that in children the total lung volume is normal after lobectomy, Cook and Bucci have shown that the lung volume is reduced on the average by approximately the amount that would be predicted from the amount of lung tissue removed.[1071] Also in contrast to several authors who suggested that lung removal may be followed in children by hyperplasia of the remaining lung,[1159, 1169] these authors could find no evidence for this in their series of 17 children who underwent resection of one lobe or more of their lungs. A high level of physical performance has been documented to occur in some patients who have to have a pneumonectomy in childhood,[1164, 1185] and it is not considered essential, though undoubtedly desirable, to postpone pneumonectomy until thoracic development is completed.[1186] If pneumonectomy has to be done in childhood, it is important that careful physiotherapy and observation of the child be maintained to prevent the development of later postural defects, since these, if uncorrected, may impair function more than the pneumonectomy itself does.

Effect of space-occupying procedures

At a time when the observed overinflation that commonly occurs after pneumonectomy was thought to be harmful in itself, there was some interest in procedures such as thoracoplasty and plombage that would reduce the volume of the thorax into which lobes of the lung would have to expand. A considerable amount of evidence now exists that these procedures are undesirable after lobectomy or pneumonectomy, partly because they do not significantly diminish the resultant volume of the remaining lung, and also because they may cause even more impairment of function.[306, 1167, 1176, 1187–1190, 2986] Since most of these procedures have now been abandoned, and since the overexpansion of the remaining lung does not of itself impair function, it is not necessary to review this evidence in detail.

Evaluation of patients for resectional surgery

By tests of total function

The increasing incidence of bronchial carcinoma has meant that lobectomy and pneumonectomy are now indicated more often in middle-aged and elderly patients than formerly. Källqvist reported the results of 36 pulmonary resections, including three pneumonectomies, in people over the age of 50,[1191] and there has been an increasing realization that it is the probable postoperative pulmonary function rather than simply the age of the patient that should influence the decision whether to operate.

There is no doubt that considerable assistance in the evaluation of such patients can be obtained from tests of total function, even when it is known that one bronchus may be partially occluded by a tumor. In such circumstances, the physician should ask himself whether the maximal breathing capacity, subdivisions of lung volume, airway resistance, and exercise diffusing capacity can be considered as probably normal in the light of the total pulmonary area available for ventilation. Since partial bronchial occlusion results not uncommonly in very slow helium equilibration on the affected side, this index cannot be taken to refer to the normal lung. Thus, if one lobe is partially collapsed because of carcinoma in a man of 55, and the $FEV_{0.75} \times 40$ is found to be 60 liters/min, the blood gases are normal, and the exercise diffusing capacity is 25 ml CO/min/mm Hg—in such circumstances the physician can be fairly confident that lobectomy or pneumonectomy would be completely safe. If pulmonary function is more seriously impaired, however, and there is good reason to suppose that the patient has chronic bronchitis and some degree of emphysema in the uninvolved lung, the physician may be able to warn the surgeon that, although lobectomy might not seriously impair his effort tolerance, pneumonectomy might well leave him dyspneic on the slightest effort. Zohman and Williams noted the usefulness of the steady-state diffusing capacity in this kind of evaluation by quoting the case of a 49-year-old man with chronic bronchitis who developed a lung carcinoma.[1192] Preoperatively, the vital capacity was 80 per cent of predicted, the FEV was only 53 per cent of normal, and the maximal midexpiratory flow rate was 0.74 liter/sec; the predicted normal would have been about 3.8 liters/sec. There was pulmonary hypertension (30/10 mm Hg) at rest, and this increased to 56/20 mm Hg on moderate exercise. However, the diffusing capacity ($D_{L_{CO}}SS_1$) on exercise was 17.0 ml CO/mm Hg. This relatively normal finding was interpreted to indicate that morphological emphysema was probably only slight in degree. A pneumonectomy was performed "without anesthesia difficulty, postoperative complications, or postoperative pulmonary insufficiency."

Although the measurement of the maximal breathing capacity is an important part in such an evaluation,[1172] the simplicity of this measurement has perhaps led some workers, particularly in Europe, to depend solely on this kind of evaluation. In our opinion, the careful preoperative assessment of many of these problems requires an evaluation of exercise capability, combined with a measurement of the diffusing capacity; some patients will be denied surgery, and in others the resulting disability will be greater than expected, if spirometric tests of function alone are used.[2993, 2994] Laros and Swierenga[2996] have shown that preoperative assessment by unilateral pulmonary arterial occlusion is probably too hazardous a procedure to be used routinely.

By measurements of regional function

In the evaluation of complex surgical problems of fibrothorax, advanced tuberculosis and bronchiectasis, bronchospirometry has made a major contribution to clinical management and to an intelligent and informed approach to surgical resection. Björkman, whose team has been responsible for many contributions to this field of knowledge, has summarized the result of 20 years' experience in the evaluation of patients for thoracic surgery,[1193] and many papers have appeared since his original contribution was published in 1934. Cases 13 and 21 demonstrate the kind of information that may be obtained at bronchospirometry and indicate the importance of measurement of differential lung function before extensive resectional surgery can be undertaken with safety. It is too early to predict what part the new methods of regional study, using radioactive gases, will come to play in the evaluation of such patients.[342, 1194] It seems likely, however, that differential ^{133}xenon measurements of ventilation and perfusion might be most valuable in doubtful cases, though no systematic study has yet been published.

POSTOPERATIVE CARE

In many of these patients who represent a relatively poor risk it is essential that elective respirator care be available for the first few days or weeks after operation. It was noted earlier that ventilatory function after thoracotomy is not restored until between four and six weeks after operation; some patients need respiratory assistance for this period, but later have sufficient respiratory function to lead active and useful lives. It was in such patients[1195, 1196] that the value of positive-pressure respirators in postoperative management was first demonstrated. For the first few hours after resectional surgery, in most patients the arterial oxygen tension during air breathing is reduced from control values.[2045, 2046] Swenson and his colleagues noted that a fall in oxygen saturation values not uncommonly was present for as long as two weeks in these cases.[2047]

LUNG TRANSPLANTATION

Since 1964, a great volume of experimental work has been published on different aspects of lung transplantation; only a small fraction of this literature can be reviewed here. However, since this method of treatment offers the only realistic possibility of aiding patients with a wide variety of chronic lung diseases, it is important that physicians and surgeons be well informed of the present status of some of this work.

A number of papers have dealt with techniques to preserve the lung outside the body,[3005, 3009, 3027, 3028] and most recently it has been reported that the lung may be successfully implanted into the dog after a period of 24 hours of storage under hypothermia and in 2 atmospheres of oxygen.[3029] Postoperative anticoagulation is necessary, but the lungs were shown to have a normal fractional carbon monoxide uptake and were contributing about a third of ventilation and oxygen uptake—in these respects being similar to lungs immediately reimplanted without storage.

After removal and reimplantation, lymph drainage is not restored for about two weeks,[2999] and during this period, edema is frequently observed.[3003] In general, reimplanted lungs show fair but generally not perfect function,[3001] and there is general agreement that the most frequent reason for failure is venous thrombosis and failure of the lung to maintain normal perfusion.[3008, 3010, 3023] It seems likely that surfactant is generally normal seven days or so after reimplantation,[3026] but if for any reason pulmonary perfusion is low, the level of surfactant falls with resulting atelectasis. In one study of three-year-survival in dogs following reimplantation, the authors made the interesting observation that perfusion of the reimplanted lung rose after the contralateral lung had been removed,[3030] which suggests that one of the problems of the reimplanted lung may be that in the presence of a contralateral normal lung in the dog, the higher pressure needed for perfusion of the donated lung is sometimes not reached.

A number of workers have studied the fate of the nerve supply to the lung after reimplantation. There seems no doubt that nerve regrowth appears,[3015] but these nerves do not appear to be sensory fibers since the Hering-Breuer reflex never reappears, and stimulation of the bronchial mucosa of the donated lung does not lead to coughing.[3003, 3004, 3019, 3020]

However, a return of stretch reflexes has been recorded three years after reimplantation.[3019] Some workers believe that it is vagal section that is responsible for the lowering of surfactant that occurs initially, and that the absence of the vagus may also account for the less than perfect function of the reimplanted lung.[3016] In most cases, oxygen exchange is not normal even a year after successful surgery,[3020] and the most likely reason for this appears to be a reduced perfusion through the lung. Two groups of investigators using ^{133}xenon to evaluate postoperative function in dogs were able to demonstrate impaired perfusion in a number of them.[3012, 3023] Division of the bronchial arteries and lymphatics does not appear to be of much consequence in the dog[3016] or in the sheep.[3006] The results of homotransplantation in the dog are much improved by the use of immunosuppressive drugs.[3002, 3014]

There is some evidence that lung function after reimplantation may be more difficult to achieve in the dog than in the baboon,[2997] and it cannot be assumed that human transplantation will face problems identical to those encountered in the dog.

Any review of human lung transplantation is likely to be out of date before it is printed. In Japan, a lobe was transplanted but had to be removed after a period of 18 days; it had, however, served a useful purpose in maintaining a patient with bronchiectasis and intractable hemorrhage.[3010] In a 15-year-old boy in Edinburgh who had inadvertently taken a lethal dose of paraquat, the transplanted lung was probably destroyed by residual paraquat in the blood at the time of transplantation.[2998] It seemed likely that had this not occurred, a very good result might have been achieved. The young man with acute silicosis fully described in Case 44 was operated upon at the Royal Victoria Hospital. Since both his lungs were irreversibly destroyed and since he had become respirator-dependent at a young age, lung transplantation offered him the only hope of any kind of recovery of function. Initially, the transplanted lung functioned well but began to fail after five days, and at the patient's death it was very poorly ventilated and perfused.[3018]

We have heard that another young patient with acute silicosis has been successfully operated upon in Ghent in Belgium, and has survived several months with good function in the transplanted lung,[3031] but we have not yet seen a full published account of this case.

It is too early to claim that the basic problems of lung transplantation in the human have been overcome. Quite apart from the problems encountered in the dog, there are additional difficulties in man. It is far from easy to be sure that the donor lung is free from infection; and in any patient in whom lung transplantation is clinically justified, the pulmonary artery pressure is likely to be elevated, and the high resistance through the contralateral patient's lung means that the donor lung will receive most of the cardiac output as soon as the clamp is removed from the artery. Admittedly a high level of perfusion may be useful in ensuring surfactant production, but it may be difficult to prevent the transplanted lung from becoming edematous. There is little doubt that careful measurement of perfusion and ventilation of transplanted lungs, which has been shown to be useful in the dog,[3012, 3023, 3024] and which we employed postoperatively in a human case,[3018] will be valuable in following patients after these procedures. The preoperative assessment should also include these methods of examination.

Transplantation of lobes and, later, of lungs will eventually become possible. There are certainly many patients with untreatable chronic pulmonary disease for whom this method of treatment offers the only hope of a reasonably active life; and in our view, provided that the patient has been very fully studied and followed for some years if his disease is chronic—or is facing certain death if the illness is acute—then the physician and surgeon are fully justified in considering this method of treatment in spite of the severe hazard involved.[3719] In some ways the indications are easier to define for lung transplantation than for cardiac transplantation.

SUMMARY

It has been in the study of some of the problems with which this chapter is concerned that the techniques of pulmonary function testing have made some of their most dramatic contributions to surgery. The careful preoperative evaluation of patients before thoracotomy; the study of the effects on function of different surgical procedures; the differentiation between overinflation of a lung and the presence of morphological emphysema; the data that exist on the effect of lung collapse and on the ability of a lung immobilized by fibrous tissue to resume normal function after 20 years; and the confidence which the many techniques available can give the physician concerning the probable level of dyspnea after resectional surgery, or the degree of improvement he may expect from it—all of these, one might think, would fully justify the very considerable effort that has been devoted to establishing methods of assessing pulmonary function. As in many areas of the field of medicine, the secret of first-class work lies in the closest contact and cooperation between the surgeon, the anesthetist, the radiologist, and the physician responsible for the assessment of function. Collaboration of these persons in preoperative assessment and postoperative care provides a standard of management undreamt of 30 years ago.

DIFFUSE INTERSTITIAL FIBROSIS

CHAPTER

12

. . . Words strain,
Crack and sometimes break, under the burden,
Under the tension, slip, slide, perish,
Decay with imprecision, will not stay in place,
Will not stay still . . . .

T. S. ELIOT, from "Burnt Norton"

INTRODUCTION

Minor degrees of localized pulmonary fibrosis are commonly encountered in routine autopsies, and a number of conditions may give rise to widespread interstitial fibrosis. In some, the disease has distinctive morphological characteristics, e.g., eosinophilic granuloma, or asbestosis. In others, the clinical history may be the only clue to the etiology of the condition, since the morphological features may be entirely nonspecific, as in the fibrosis sometimes seen in workers with nickel,[1362] or in lung damage due to inhalation of smoke-bomb fumes[2054] and even in sprayers of vineyards.[3715] In yet other cases, extrapulmonary findings may be necessary to establish the complete diagnosis, as in the pulmonary fibrosis found in scleroderma, in which esophageal or intestinal changes may suggest the presence of generalized systemic sclerosis. In perhaps the largest group, however, the etiological factor is never established, and such cases are generally labeled idiopathic, or examples of the "Hamman-Rich syndrome" if the lesions are widespread. It is important to recognize, however, that similar if not identical lesions may be found in the lungs of patients suffering from various diseases; in such circumstances, one can readily understand the perplexity of the pathologist when he is expected to apply an exact diagnostic label on a minute piece of fibrotic lung removed at biopsy. The relationship between the Hamman-Rich syndrome and other forms of diffuse pulmonary fibrosis is shown in Figure 14–1.

PATHOLOGY

Just as the original concept of the clinical entity known as the Hamman-Rich syndrome has changed from that of a relatively acute disease to a more chronic one (*see* page 271), so have the descriptions of the morphology changed from those of acute to chronic lesions. Considerable variation may be found in the histological appearances of tissue in different patients, and striking variations may be noted in the appearance of different regions of the same lung at autopsy. It is not clear whether some of these variations, notably evidence of acute inflammation, represent stages in the pathogenesis of the disorder, or are superimposed acute infection, as has been postulated.[1360]

THE HAMMAN-RICH SYNDROME

Gross pathological examination of typical cases of the Hamman-Rich syndrome shows small firm lungs with pleural thickening and a characteristic "hob-nailed" surface resembling a cirrhotic liver. Some pleural adhesions may be present. The cut surface of the lungs shows thickened interlobular septa, and a cystic pattern of the pulmonary parenchyma which has led to the apt description of "honeycomb lung." These cysts are small, seldom more than 5 mm in diameter, and have fibrous walls. Mucus may be recognizable within them. Cyst formation is usually most marked in the posterior and inferior portions of the lungs. In many areas the gross appearance may be normal, but microscopically the lungs may show evidence of considerable disease.

Microscopically, the essential features are interstitial fibrosis, obliteration of alveoli, formation of epithelial-lined cystic spaces, and varying degrees of interstitial inflammation. The exact nature of the cystic spaces and their pathogenesis are obscure.[2052] They generally appear to represent dilated bronchioles, both respiratory and nonrespiratory, rather than dilated alveoli whose lining has undergone metaplastic change. The bronchioles supplying the cysts are usually patent and the general picture appears to be one of obliteration of the more distal pulmonary structures and dilatation of those more proximal.[3043] The epithelium lining the spaces is variable, and may be cuboidal, columnar, or ciliated columnar in various combinations. Squamous metaplasia is sometimes seen. Intervening fibrous tissue shows varying degrees of maturity, from granulation tissue to dense collagenized scars in which lung structure is hardly discernible. Fat may be present in the fibrous scars, and there may be granulation tissue in the alveoli or deep to the bronchiolar epithelium. Interstitial inflammation, which is variable in severity, is usually mononuclear in type. Scattered foci of irregular emphysema may be seen, but this change is limited in extent and the dominant picture is of pulmonary fibrosis and bronchiolectasis. A severe degree of muscular hyperplasia occurs sometimes, and this finding has led to the description of a separate entity (*see* page 281).

Other changes that have been noted and are regarded as early stages of the disease include acute inflammatory-cell infiltration, eosinophilic infiltration, edema within the alveoli and in the interstitium, necrosis of alveolar walls and bronchiolar epithelium, and formation of hyaline membranes. We have seen these changes in few cases, and only when fibrosis is poorly developed. In these circumstances, the general architecture may be intact, "honeycombing" slight, and capillary proliferation severe. Striking thickening of the pulmonary arterial tree is often present, and cor pulmonale is usual in fatal cases.

An apparently distinctive variant of the Hamman-Rich lung disorder has been termed "desquamative interstitial pneumonitis," probably occurring as a result of an acute viral pneumonitis.[3074] The predominant histological feature appears to be the accumulation of desquamated histiocytes in the air spaces. Interstitial fibrosis is relatively slight, although there may be considerable evidence of interstitial inflammation. It is important to recognize the probable existence of this entity, since it seems that it carries a better prognosis than does the Hamman-Rich syndrome (*see* illustrative Case No. 22). Changes in the lungs similar to those in the Hamman-Rich syndrome have recently been described in association with von Recklinghausen's disease.[3042]

Scleroderma

Varying degrees of interstitial pulmonary fibrosis have been reported in 29 (more than 90 per cent) of a series of 31 cases of scleroderma studied at autopsy.[1351] As will be noted, the almost invariable disturbance of pulmonary function suggests that lung involvement is the rule in this condition. The changes may be widespread throughout the lung, though they appear to be more severe in the basal portions. Honeycombing of the lung is seen frequently.[3043] The pathological changes are probably indistinguishable from those described in the Hamman-Rich syndrome, but are typically chronic, often with dense pulmonary fibrosis, and usually with formation of large cysts. A particular feature of the lung in scleroderma is striking hyperplasia of the epithelium lining the cysts. Malignant change may occur, and bronchiolar carcinoma arising in "honeycomb lung" appears to be a feature of scleroderma but not of the Hamman-Rich syndrome.[1368, 2274, 2348]

Rheumatoid arthritis

The manifestations of lung disease associated with rheumatoid arthritis include pulmonary nodules, pleurisy and pleural thickening, chronic pneumonitis, and diffuse interstitial fibrosis.[3067]

It has been estimated that about one fifth of patients with diffuse interstitial fibrosis reported in the literature have associated rheumatoid arthritis,[1359] but this estimate may be high since many cases of interstitial fibrosis without arthritis are probably seen which are not reported. Scadding noted recently that 15 of 104 cases of fibrosing alveolitis observed by him had rheumatoid arthritis.[3060] He concluded from his valuable review of the data that "a pathogenetic factor common to rheumatoid arthritis and fibrosing alveolitis has yet to be demonstrated." Small necrobiotic granulomata of the rheumatoid type may be seen in patients with rheumatoid arthritis and pulmonary fibrosis,[1369] but in the majority of cases the changes in the lung appear to be in no way distinguishable from those seen in the Hamman-Rich syndrome, except that they are usually less widespread and rarely as severe.[2053, 3059] According to Edge and Rickards,[1370] 43 cases of "rheumatoid lung disease" had been described by 1957, excluding those patients in whom pneumoconiosis also was present (Caplan's syndrome).

It is difficult to give a precise estimate of the incidence of pulmonary involvement in patients with rheumatoid arthritis. One author found no case in 133 patients with rheumatoid arthritis; another diagnosed five cases out of 180 patients;[3064] others have reported a 32 per cent[3065] and a 17 per cent[3035] incidence of thoracic abnormality. Sievers and his colleagues[3063] screened 3500 patients with rheumatoid arthritis and found an incidence of pulmonary involvement of 23 per cent in those patients with high rheumatoid factor titers in their serum. Many atypical cases have been noted;[3069, 3070, 3071] one patient, aged fifteen, studied with particular care, showed severe pulmonary vasculitis and right-sided heart failure.[3072] In general, the syndrome is not common,[3038] and interstitial fibrosis of any severity probably will occur in about 3 per cent of all cases.[3081]

In addition to the changes in the lung that resemble those found in the Hamman-Rich syndrome, various other lesions may be present in the lungs of patients suffering from rheumatoid arthritis. Pleural adhesions are not uncommon,[1527, 1528] and classic rheumatoid nodules may be found in the pleura or the underlying parenchyma.[1529–1531] A striking form of rheumatoid lung disease is Caplan's syndrome,[1532–1534, 3073] in which nodules measuring from 1 cm in diameter to much larger confluent masses are found in the lungs of miners, most frequently coalworkers, who are suffering from rheumatoid arthritis. The nodules are well defined and present a laminated cut surface with concentric black and yellow rings. Microscopically the center of the nodules, which is often necrotic and may cavitate, is composed of collagen, and is separated from the margin of viable tissue by a cleft-like space that contains many polymorphs. The fibroblasts at the periphery of the necrotic center are palisaded in typical rheumatoid fashion. Outside the palisaded layer is a fibrous capsule with a chronic inflammatory-cell exudate.

Dermatomyositis

Only a few cases of pulmonary involvement in dermatomyositis have been described, and we have seen only one case. In this patient, chronic interstitial inflammation was striking, and large numbers of plasma cells were present. The degree of pulmonary fibrosis was not severe, however, and the general architecture of the lung was well maintained. Edema fluid and desquamated alveolar lining cells were seen in the alveoli. This case appeared similar to those reported in the literature, and such an entity may be distinct from the lesions described in other disorders.

Sjögren's syndrome

This syndrome consists of the triad of keratoconjunctivitis sicca, rheumatoid arthritis, and swelling of the salivary glands. The term is sometimes applied in cases that show only two of the three manifestations. Only 11 autopsies in this condition had been reported up to 1959.[1358] The pulmonary changes are not well established; areas of atelectasis are said to be common,[1357, 1358] but pulmonary fibrosis when present appears to be localized rather than generalized.[1356] Bucher and Reid[1358] have stressed the occurrence of arteritis in this condition and described nodular hyaline masses in the pulmonary parenchyma in relation to vessels, as well as an exudative pneumonitis. Because of these changes, together with the atrophy of bronchial glands that they found, the pulmonary changes in Sjögren's syndrome probably should be considered independently from those in rheumatoid arthritis.

We have had an opportunity of studying the pulmonary function in only one case of Sjögren's syndrome. The pattern of derangement was identical to that found in the Hamman-Rich syndrome, and lung biopsy revealed an interstitial fibrosis involving almost all the alveoli in the specimen.

THE HAMMAN-RICH SYNDROME (FIBROSING ALVEOLITIS)

Definition

In 1944 Hamman and Rich published a full account of a syndrome they termed "acute diffuse interstitial fibrosis of the lungs."[1330] They brought together the clinical and pathological details of three patients seen between 1931 and 1933 on whom they had reported briefly in 1935, and two others seen 10 years later. This syndrome, now known to occur in a more chronic form than was characteristic of the original cases, is customarily referred to by the names of these two investigators. Of unknown etiology, it is a condition of severe and generalized alveolar thickening, unassociated with any changes in other organs. As already noted, it is doubtful whether the pathological picture in the lung can be distinguished from that found in scleroderma. For this reason the diagnosis cannot be based solely on morphological criteria. The field of definition has been still further confused by the variability of degree of severity in different patients with this disease.

Scadding and Hinson[3039] and others[3044] have used the term "diffuse fibrosing alveolitis" to include cases of the Hamman-Rich syndrome and diffuse interstitial pneumonia. Future work will be required (and more knowledge about etiology) before a firm opinion can be given as to whether these two conditions should be classified as one. A recent paper by Swaye and his co-workers has described this syndrome, histologically proven, in eight members of the same family, the youngest being only 3½ years old.[3723]

Clinical features

This condition (and its variants, to be described later) has been noted in patients of all ages from childhood[3033, 3034] to the seventh decade, and it appears to affect both sexes equally.

In the original cases described by Hamman and Rich, the course was relatively short, and death occurred within a few months or a year of apparent onset of the disease. Several cases have been described, particularly by Scadding[1331] and others,[1379, 2048, 2296] in which the course was much more chronic, extending over many years. Usually dyspnea is the earliest and most characteristic symptom; in most cases it is unassociated with sputum or any evidence of preceding respiratory infection. It is characteristically slowly progressive, and other symptoms occur only when cor pulmonale has developed or chronic arterial unsaturation is present. On occasion, clubbing

(Text continued on page 276.)

Case 22
Desquamative Histiocytic Interstitial Pneumonitis

Summary of Clinical Findings. This 11-year-old boy was first admitted to hospital in July, 1959, complaining of shortness of breath for 18 months. This first appeared after a bout of Asian influenza from which the whole family had suffered. The other members of the family rapidly returned to normal health but, in the patient, shortness of breath persisted and increased until he could not climb comfortably one flight of stairs. There was no cough. There had been no exposure to fumes or inhalants of any variety and no contact with animals. On examination he was not in respiratory distress or cyanosed. Temperature was 98.3° F. Respiratory rate was 18 per minute. His fingers and toes were clubbed and fine crepitations were heard at the bases of both lungs.

Hemoglobin was 12.8 gm/100 ml. White-cell count was 10,500/cmm with a normal differential. Old tuberculin and histoplasmin skin tests were negative. Total proteins = 6.00 gm/100 ml (albumen, 3.7 gm/100 ml; globulin, 2.3 gm/100 ml).

Bronchoscopic findings were normal and, therefore, lung biopsy was performed (*see* Pathology).

During the next five months the dyspnea increased and in January, 1960, prednisone was started (20 mg three times a day). Following this there was a temporary improvement, both symptomatically and radiologically, but by the summer of 1960 the shortness of breath was increasing, and in September, 1960, it was decided to give him a course of cyclophosphamide. This was administered in a dose of 200 mg daily for six weeks. The prednisone was continued at 60 mg per day. Over the following year he showed remarkable improvement in his symptoms, which was reflected in the pulmonary function studies. He did develop signs of steroid toxicity—cushingoid facies, hypertension and osteoporosis—for which he was readmitted in September, 1961. The steroid dosage was reduced gradually and finally discontinued in January, 1962. He continued to do extremely well, and on readmission in 1962 had no complaints. Another lung biopsy, taken at this time, is described under Pathology.

He was still asymptomatic in October, 1963, even though the chest x-ray showed increased infiltrates in the right lower lung field. One year later he was again complaining of shortness of breath. Fine crepitations were again heard mainly in the right lower lung field. Pulmonary function studies showed a dramatic worsening, returning to levels observed initially. His symptoms persisted in spite of a second course of cyclophosphamide in early 1965 and resumption of steroid therapy later that year. He died in a car accident in 1967. No autopsy was performed.

Radiology. A series of films made over almost three years shows a varying picture indistinguishable from that of pneumonitis. In January, 1959, there was loss of volume of the lower lobe on each side (*A*), affecting particularly the basilar segments, and the vascular markings in the involved lower lobes were increased in number and diminished in definition. The left upper lobe, particularly its lingular segment, shows a similar change which is, however, more variable, being most conspicuous in January, 1960, about two years after onset of the disease (*B*). On the original films it seemed likely that changes present in the lower lobes were also recognizable throughout all lobes, but much less severe and without associated loss of volume. The x-ray appearance in October, 1960, is shown in *C*. There is no evidence of bronchial-wall thickening, hilar lymph-node enlargement, abscess or cavity formation, or cor pulmonale. The final film, in November, 1962 (*D*), shows marked improvement, and, in fact, almost complete resolution of the disease bilaterally.

Pathology. *1. Biopsy, lower lobe of left lung,* ×140; July 17, 1959 (*E*).

Grossly the tissue presented a rubbery, airless, fleshy appearance of *café-au-lait* color. It sank in fixing fluid.

Histologically the lung presents an abnormality characterized by alveolar-wall fibrosis, an alveolar-wall lining composed of cuboidal cells, and plugging of the alveoli by masses of pneumonocytes and histiocytes. The terminal bronchioles show no definite abnormality.

The alveolar walls show a mature type of fibrosis, and the connective tissue contains small numbers, thinly distributed, of plasma cells, lymphocytes, occasional neutrophil and eosinophil leukocytes and relatively numerous mast cells. The epithelial lining gives the alveoli a glandular appearance and is uniform throughout. In some alveoli the epithelial cells are seen to be continuous with the intraluminal masses; this is more obvious in frozen section. Occasional multinucleate cells are present. A few cells contain Oil Red O positive lipid. There is no evidence of phagocytosis or inclusion bodies.

Muscular hypertrophy of the alveolar orifices and respiratory bronchioles is striking. Alveolar elastic content is depleted. Lymph follicles are present in moderate numbers. The pleura is normal except for a few siderocytes. The lesion is compatible with desquamative histiocytic interstitial pneumonia (Liebow).

2. Second biopsy, lower lobe of left lung, ×140; October 17, 1962 (*F*).

Grossly the tissue was rubbery, distinctly fleshy centrally with peripheral honeycomb appearance,

(Case 22 continued on page 274.)

Desquamative Histiocytic Interstitial Pneumonitis

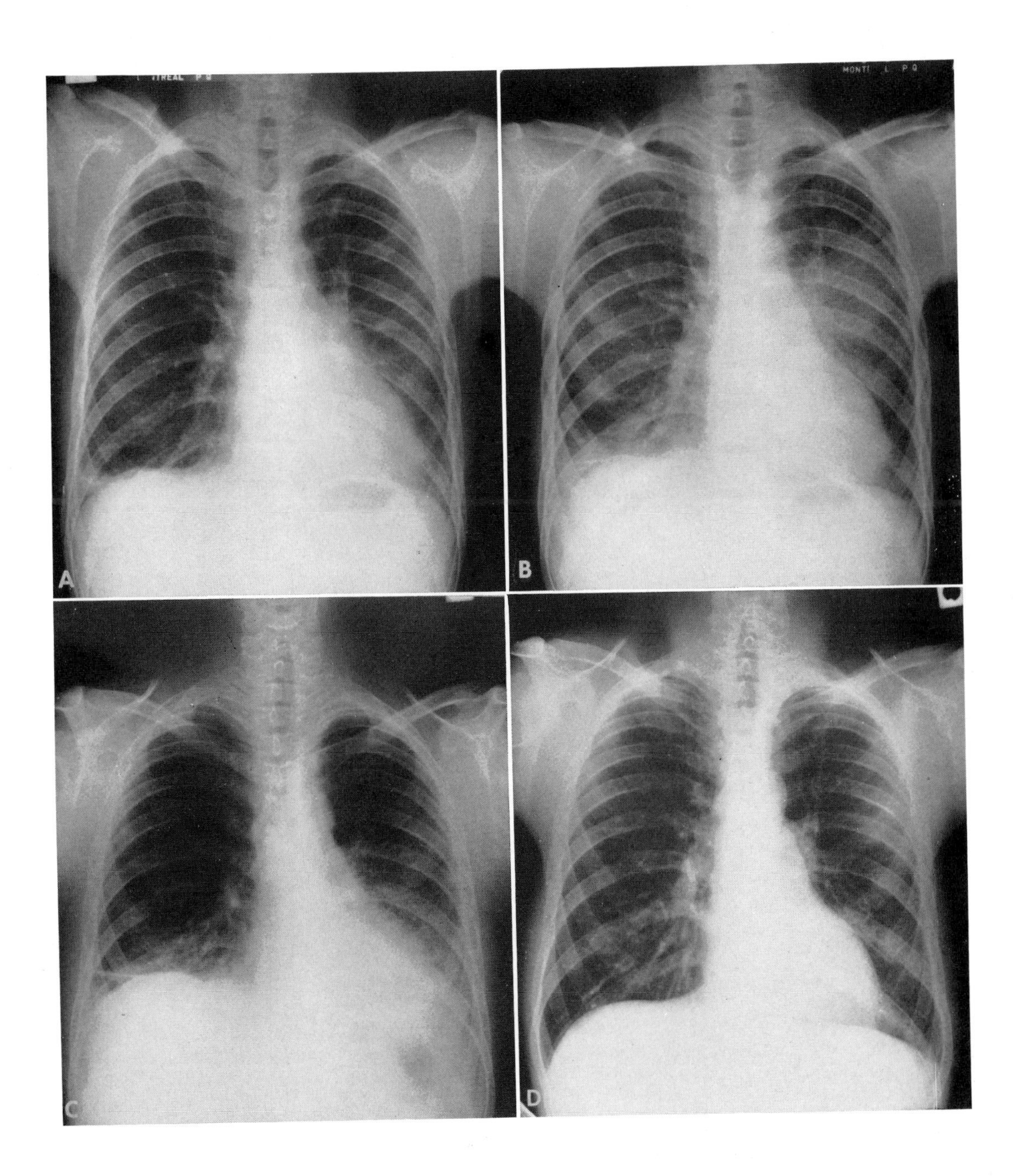

Case 22
Desquamative Histiocytic Interstitial Pneumonitis (Continued)

and of a gray color. In contrast with the 1959 biopsy specimen the tissue floated at the surface of the fixing fluid.

Microscopically much of the central two-thirds of the tissue is collapsed, but this is compatible with the usual collapsed appearance of a lung biopsy specimen. Peripherally the alveoli show patches of collapse with dominant hyperdilatation. In contrast to the first biopsy specimen, the alveoli show little plugging by pneumonocytes and are rarely lined by epithelial cells. Their walls are often densely fibrotic but contain almost no inflammatory cells. Even the walls of the hyperdilated alveoli are fibrosed.

Occasional minute foci of foreign-body granulomata are seen related to acicular crystals of cholesterol. These are probably due to retained secretions, for several atretic bronchioles are present.

In comparison with the first biopsy specimen, there has been considerable improvement as indicated by the decreased cellularity of the lesion.

Summary. This case illustrates the rare event of improvement, documented radiologically, functionally and histologically, in a patient whose initial lesion would generally be classified as due to the Hamman-Rich syndrome. The case illustrates the use of pulmonary function tests to follow the course of the disease and to observe the effects of therapy. The diagnosis is believed to be that of desquamative histiocytic interstitial pneumonitis, which may be tentatively regarded as an abnormal pulmonary response to viral infection.

												EXERCISE					
	VC	FRC	RV	TLC	ME %	MMFR	$FEV_{0.75}$ ×40	pH	P_{CO_2}	HCO_3^-	O_2Hb %	$D_{LCO}SS_2$	MPH	GRADE	$\dot{V}O_2$	$\dot{V}_E$	$D_{LCO}SS_3$
Predicted (In 1959)	3.7	2.3	1.1	4.8	70	4.0	106	7.40	42	25	97	15.0					20.0
July 1959	1.2	1.4	0.9	2.1	49	0.9	35	7.39	48	27		7.3	2.5	FLAT			10.8
Dec. 1959	1.1	1.2	0.7	1.8	46	0.5	29					6.8	2.5	FLAT			8.0
March 1960	3.0	1.3	0.5	3.5	45	2.7	88						2.0	FLAT			9.1
July 1960	2.9	1.6	0.8	3.7	41	2.9	97					9.5	2.0	FLAT			9.8
Oct. 1960	1.9	1.4	0.9	2.8	50	1.2	51										
Oct. 1962	3.9	2.5	1.4	5.3	64	2.9	108					11.5	2.5	FLAT			18.2
Oct. 1963													3.0	FLAT	1.3	24.4	19.2
Sept. 1964	1.9	2.5	1.8	3.7	53	1.4	52										
Nov. 1964	2.0	2.5	1.7	3.7	56	1.6	58	7.39	34	21							
Apr. 1965	1.9	2.0	1.3	3.2	62	2.0	60										
Nov. 1965	1.6	2.0	1.4	3.0	51	1.5	48										
Apr. 1966	1.5	2.0	1.4	2.9	62	1.1	42										
Dec. 1966	1.8	2.2	1.4	3.2	47	1.4	51										

These results show the remarkable changes in pulmonary function that have been observed over a 7-year period. Note the striking improvement in lung volumes, vital capacity and ventilatory flow rate between July, 1959, and July, 1960, unaccompanied by improvement in diffusing capacity. By October, 1962, not only were total capacity and ventilatory function normal, but the exercise diffusing capacity had increased from a low of 8.0 in December, 1959, to 18.2 ml CO/min/mm Hg, both estimates being made at the same exercise load. Treatment with prednisone extended from January, 1960, to January, 1962, and with cyclophosphamide between September and November of 1960. The static compliance doubled between 1960 and 1963. There was a reversal in this improvement to initial levels, unchanged after a second course of cyclophosphamide, followed by a second course of steroids.

Desquamative Histiocytic Interstitial Pneumonitis (Continued)

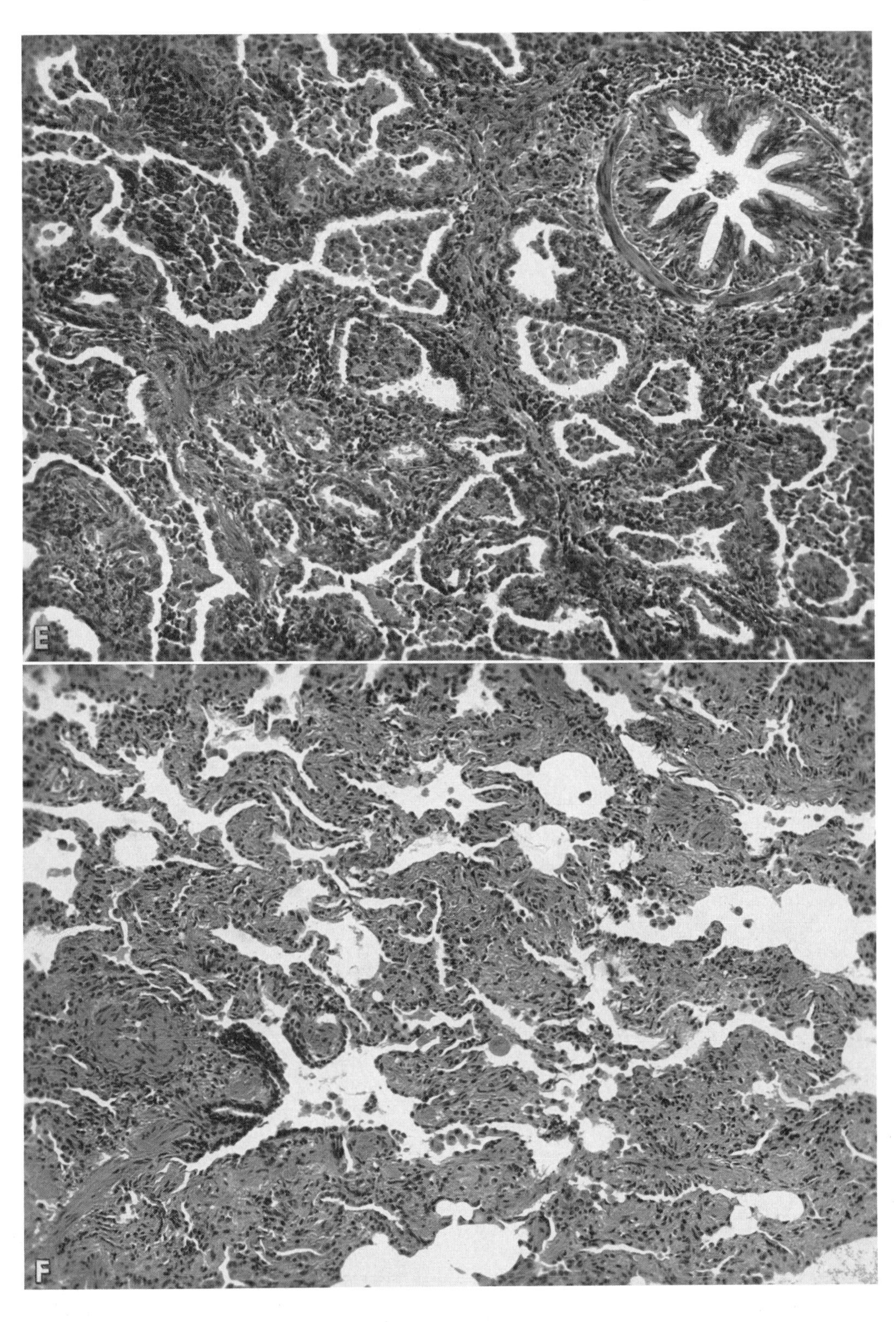

of the fingers develops early; in one of our patients this was the presenting symptom, preceding the complaint of dyspnea by nearly a year. The only characteristic sign—and its finding is important—is the presence of persistent rales over the lungs, usually best heard posteriorly and not accompanied by any alteration in breath-sound quality or evidence of bronchospasm. In an early case there may be no additional history, and all other systems are normal on physical examination. As the severity of the condition increases, cyanosis may be noticed and congestive heart failure may be present. Terminally, cyanosis is often extreme, and severe respiratory distress may be present even at rest.

A precise diagnosis can be made only by demonstration of the characteristic lung pathology and exclusion of other conditions that are similar. Thus, the presence of scleroderma must be excluded by the finding of a normal skin and a normal esophagus, and by the absence of symptoms of Raynaud's phenomenon, which is relatively common in scleroderma but rare, if it occurs at all, in the Hamman-Rich syndrome. Various forms of pneumoconiosis and sarcoidosis also have to be excluded from the diagnosis. The radiological picture is suggestive but not in itself diagnostic between these various conditions. As noted below, pulmonary function tests may be of value in making an early clinical diagnosis by the demonstration of more defect in diffusion than would be predicted from the radiological appearances. In many patients the characteristic combination of clinical features, radiological change and pattern of function impairment enables a confident clinical diagnosis to be made in advance of a lung biopsy. In some patients the later stages may be complicated by the development of cystic changes in the lungs or by the presence of intercurrent chronic pulmonary infection. The literature contains several excellent clinical reviews of the reported cases of this condition, many examples of which have been described in the past few years. In some reports, however, the reader cannot judge whether scleroderma or examples of pulmonary fibrosis in such conditions as rheumatoid arthritis or dermatomyositis have been excluded; nevertheless, more than 100 cases have been well documented. The reader is referred to some of the clinical papers that contain reviews of this syndrome from different points of view.[1331–1336, 2049, 2296, 3037, 3039]

As noted in the preceding section on pathology, the general syndrome of "diffuse interstitial fibrosis" includes a number of related conditions. Until more is known about the cause of the condition these cannot be reliably classified, and it may be argued that the two variants of "familial fibrocystic dysplasia" and "desquamative interstitial pneumonitis" discussed under Clinical Variants (page 280) are essentially manifestations of the same condition.[3039] Yet the familial occurrence of the first of these and the possible etiological and clinical differences of the second seem to us to warrant their provisional separation from the syndrome in general.

X-RAY CHARACTERISTICS IN IDIOPATHIC PULMONARY FIBROSIS AND SCLERODERMA

The radiological changes in the lungs in these two conditions are frequently indistinguishable and are extremely variable. The picture may vary from that of an apparently normal chest x-ray in a patient who has pathologically proved interstitial fibrosis to one in which there is extensive involvement of both lungs by a very coarse reticular and nodular pattern extending from the apices to the bases. Characteristically, the lower portion of the lung fields is more severely involved than the upper, the typical pattern being one of a fine lace-like reticulation which appears to extend along the peripheral vascular distribution; a fine nodular component is seen occasionally. Enlargement of lymph nodes is rare in these conditions, and pleural effusions do not occur except in the presence of secondary malignant change.

PULMONARY FUNCTION

Although Knipping[1337] suspected that certain lung conditions, which he named under the general heading of "die Pneumonose," caused impairment of oxygen transfer across the alveolar wall, it was not until Austrian and his colleagues[428] applied the then recently devised method of measuring the oxygen-diffusing capacity (D_{LO_2}) to patients with scleroderma and diffuse pulmonary fibroses of unknown origin that it became clear that these disorders were characterized by a relative preservation of ventilatory capability and a low (and in some patients, very low) measured diffusing capacity. It took only a few years for a large number of different entities to be classified as belonging to an "alveolar-capillary block syndrome," in which the essential disorder was regarded as a thickening of the alveolar wall and consequent lowering of the diffusing capacity. In the excellent review of the syndrome by Dickie and Rankin,[1338] 28 more or less distinct clinical disorders are classified under this heading. As will be noted, there is some doubt how far the observed lowering of arterial saturation or tension in these patients is ascribable to the lowered diffusing capacity and how far it is caused by ventilation–perfusion distribution abnormalities. Since it seems clear that in most, if not all patients, the two phenomena coexist and ultimately are not really distinguishable from one another,[1339] it may be wiser to recognize the existence of a characteristic disease pattern, in functional terms, without implying that in all such patients arterial desaturation is the direct consequence of the low diffusing capacity that is an invariable feature of this group of disorders. For this reason the term "alveolar-capillary block syndrome" will not be used as a general heading in this text. It seems better to discuss various disease entities as they occur, without parceling them into a category based on a specific disorder of function.

Subdivisions of lung volume

A review of the function-test data published of these patients shows that, characteristically, the vital capacity is reduced, the residual volume is normal or in some patients slightly increased, and the total lung capacity is usually lower than predicted.[399, 411, 428, 583, 761, 1338, 1340] Linderholm reported a patient in whom the vital capacity was still 4.4 liters, although diffusing capacity and working capacity were both very much reduced.[628] In most series, however, the fall in vital capacity is sufficiently large to cause a significant diminution in total lung capacity,[1340, 3039] often to very low values.

Inert-gas distribution

Measurement of inert-gas distribution in patients with the Hamman-Rich syndrome shows either normal values or a slight impairment so that often they are just outside the normal range but are much less abnormal than those found in patients with emphysema or asthma. This generalization appears to be valid whether this aspect of function is measured by open-circuit nitrogen clearance,[428, 1340] single-breath nitrogen plateau,[411] or closed-circuit helium equilibration.[370, 399, 583] It must be remembered, however, that such measurements, particularly those based on the rate of nitrogen elimination, may be misleading if there is resting hyperventilation in the presence of a reduced total lung capacity. Furthermore, the studies of Read and Williams,[1344] using a mass spectrometer to analyze ventilation inequality, suggest that the degree of uneven gas distribution is somewhat larger than would appear from other published data.

Ventilatory and mechanical function

There is a great deal of evidence that the ventilatory ability of patients with this disease is usually normal at the time when dyspnea is first noticed and when there has been a significant reduction in diffusing capacity.[381, 399, 411, 428, 583, 628, 761, 1338, 1340, 1341, 2048, 2049] In the later stages, however, ventilatory capacity may become somewhat reduced. From the point of view of pulmonary mechanics, the pattern of change found in these patients is quite characteristic. As we have pointed out,[583] at a given level of FRC the transpulmonary pressure is abnormally negative, because of the increased recoil force exerted by the lungs (*see* Figure 2–7). There is reduction in both static and dynamic compliance; and total flow resistance is slightly increased. Perrett[1342] suggested that the loss of compliance is an early finding in this condition, as one would expect from the fact that the patient may complain of dyspnea before much striking radiological change occurs. In the series of 19 patients with this disorder studied by Turino and his coworkers[1340] there was no overlap of measured values of pulmonary compliance between the patients and the normal subjects. The severity of gas exchange interference is not closely correlated with the decreased compliance.[3711] It is clear that the decreased compliance means that increased respiratory work will be performed for a given level of ventilation and that this will be most economically managed with a relative increase in respiratory frequency rather than in tidal volume. This aspect is discussed later in relation to exercise data.

Measurements of diffusing capacity

Although it has been suggested by Finley and his colleagues[426] and recently by Hamer,[3041] that the lowered diffusing capacity found in these patients is not the cause of the arterial hypoxemia it cannot be denied that their level of carbon monoxide uptake and rate of oxygen transfer are invariably reduced, regardless of the method of measurement. Thus the diffusing capacity was grossly impaired when the D_{LO_2} was measured,[382, 416, 428] or when using either the single-breath $D_{LCO}SB$[38, 411, 761, 3041] or steady-state CO methods.[381, 399, 628, 1340, 1341, 2296, 3039] In view of such general unanimity with methods subject to very diverse sources of error, it may safely be concluded that this syndrome is characterized by a severe defect in gas transfer, *whether or not this is visualized as a defect in transfer through a thickened membrane, or whether it is thought of as a reduction in available surface area because of virtual obliteration of the affected alveoli.* Measurements of diffusing capacity on exercise accentuate the great reduction in CO transfer in these patients compared with normal subjects[399, 628]—a situation well exemplified by Linderholm's patient, whose vital capacity was 4.4 liters, maximal breathing capacity 97 liters/min, and exercise $D_{LCO}SS_1$ only 8.7 ml CO/min/mm Hg, at which time his arterial oxygen was measured at only 20 mm Hg.[628] It might be expected that studies of diffusing capacity in these patients at two levels of alveolar oxygen tension would reveal that the low diffusing capacity was always and solely due to a fall in the membrane component D_M. It is true that this has been found in the few cases studied by this method,[399, 411, 3041] but in some patients the pulmonary capillary blood volume (V_c) also was reduced.[3037]

The recent studies by Arndt, King, and Briscoe[3539] now permit a more precise delineation of the probable importance of diffusion defect in these disorders. Using a complex technique of compartmental analysis combined with calculation of Bohr isopleths, in a study of 8 patients, they have shown that both $\dot{V}/\dot{Q}$ and diffusion effects were present in two patients with sarcoidosis, in one with diffuse interstitial pneumonitis and in one with eosinophilic granuloma; and that the major disturbance was a diffusion defect rather than a $\dot{V}/\dot{Q}$ disorder in two patients with interstitial edema, in one with scleroderma and in one with sarcoidosis. These detailed studies unquestionably necessitate a re-evaluation of the commonly held concept (based on Finley's data) that an actual defect in gas transfer at the alveolar level is generally of little importance in these and similar diseases.

Problems of interpretation of diffusing-capacity measurements in the light of ventilation-perfusion inequality are discussed under Disturbance of Ventilation-Perfusion Ratio (page 280).

Exercise studies: arterial blood-gas tensions

In many patients with this disorder, the level of resting ventilation is raised and hyperventilation in relation to oxygen uptake may become extreme on exercise. This phenomenon has been carefully studied by Turino and his co-workers,[1340] who showed that 19 such patients could be divided into two groups: the majority, with a high minute ventilation at rest and exercise but with a normal P_{CO_2}, and the minority, who also had a high minute ventilation but in whom the arterial P_{CO_2} was lowered. This general conclusion accords with our own experience that a lowered arterial P_{CO_2} is far from invariable in this condition.

The hyperventilation is associated with lowering of the ratio of oxygen uptake to ventilation ($\dot{V}O_2/\dot{V}_e$), often of marked degree. This may be explained on a teleological basis, by the theory that elevation of the alveolar oxygen tension is necessitated by the low diffusing capacity. However, it seems more likely that Turino and his colleagues[1340] are correct in their conclusion that it is not related to hypoxemia, since it is unaffected by oxygen breathing, and that it may well be related to abnormal proprioceptive impulses from the disordered lungs. The observation that resting and exercise ventilation may be increased in these patients without a concomitant fall in arterial P_{CO_2} means that there must be an increase in physiological dead space, which Holland[1343] found in studies on five patients with this disease. This in turn may be extended to mean that significant $\dot{V}/\dot{Q}$ abnormality must exist in this disorder.

Arterial oxygen tension may fall to very low levels in patients with the Hamman-Rich syndrome or with similar clinical entities. Linderholm reported an observation of an arterial tension of oxygen on exercise as low as 20 mm Hg,[628] Nahmias and his colleagues a reading of 33 mm Hg in similar circumstances,[2049] and Cugell and his co-workers a value of 35 mm Hg Po_2[381] (*see* Case 32). Characteristically, in this disorder the arterial tension and saturation fall during exercise, in spite of the high levels of ventilation reached by these patients. This may be explained by shortening of the time spent by the blood in the pulmonary capillary when the cardiac output increases on exercise. In health, the diffusing capacity of the membrane is sufficiently high to ensure full equilibration between alveolar gas and blood for oxygen when the transit time is reduced from 0.7 sec to 0.3 sec, or less (*see* page 88). If the membrane is thickened, however, a similar reduction in transit time may result in a lowering of end-capillary oxygen tension. Alternatively, it may be argued that the $\dot{V}/\dot{Q}$ distribution in these patients becomes much less uniform on exercise, and this factor is predominant in lowering the arterial oxygen tension in these circumstances. The comparative merits of these two explanations are discussed under the next heading.

Disturbance of ventilation-perfusion ($\dot{V}/\dot{Q}$) ratio

In view of the unanimous finding by all observers that the diffusing capacity is reduced, often to very low values, in patients considered to have the Hamman-Rich syndrome, it is not surprising that initially this was interpreted to mean that impairment of diffusion through the alveolar membrane was the principal functional disorder in this condition. The low arterial oxygen tension was attributed mainly, if not entirely, to this phenomenon, and the "alveolar-capillary block syndrome" was considered to be a relatively homogeneous and straightforward pathophysiological entity. Recently, however, it has been suggested that much, if not all, of the arterial hypoxemia is in reality due to a disturbance in $\dot{V}/\dot{Q}$ ratios. Holland noted that, in five of these patients, the ratio of V_D to V_T was considerably increased because of an increase of physiological dead space.[1343] On this basis he criticized the calculation of diffusing capacity based on an assumed value of $V_D(D_{Lco}SS_2)$. As has been pointed out earlier, however (*see* Fig. 2–40), during exercise the calculated D_{Lco} is relatively insensitive to quite considerable changes in V_D/V_T ratio.[370] Read and Williams studied 17 patients (mostly suffering from asbestosis), using the analysis of expired gas by a mass spectrometer as an indicator of $\dot{V}/\dot{Q}$ abnormality, and found evidence for this in the majority; though it is to be noted that in several of these patients the single-breath $D_{Lco}SB$ was only about half the predicted value although no $\dot{V}/\dot{Q}$ abnormality could be demonstrated by this method.[1344] More recently, Finley, Swenson, and Comroe, in an important contribution,[426] studied 11 patients at rest, using a technique previously described by Finley,[1345] and concluded that the level of arterial hypoxemia that existed in these patients "could be explained on the basis of uneven distribution of ventilation in relation to blood flow and pulmonary artery-to-vein shunting." The technique used consisted of the simultaneous measurement of alveolar nitrogen concentration and arterial Po_2 change during inhalation of 100 per cent oxygen, and the method of analysis was similar to that devised by Briscoe and his colleagues.[289] No observations were recorded during exercise. As has been pointed out in Chapter 7 it appears somewhat doubtful to us that the lung can be divided into two such zones in patients with lung disease; further, it may be noted that when Finley applied this technique to normal subjects seated upright[1345] it led him to conclude: "In normal subjects the ratio of ventilation to perfusion is approximately the same for both the well and the poorly ventilated regions"—a finding not in conformity with recent data on the marked variations in $\dot{V}/\dot{Q}$ that exist under these conditions (*see* Chapter 2, page 46). Said and his colleagues have pointed out that "The physiologic effects of extreme impairment of pulmonary diffusion are predominantly those of a large right-to-left shunt."[1339] The detailed calculations by Staub[1346] on the probable magnitude of the alveolar arterial gradient due to diffusion in a wide variety of circumstances are very relevant to this problem. If these can be taken as correct, it certainly seems to be unlikely that, even in disease, a thickening of alveolar membrane, i.e., a decrease in D_M, can be responsible as a general rule for any significant end-capillary gradient. From Staub's calculations, therefore, it appears that an observed low value for D_L must be due almost invariably to uneven distribution of ventilation, perfusion, and diffusion within the lung, and not to a low D_M. On the other hand, in many patients with advanced

Hamman-Rich syndrome the lesion is generalized and no remnants of normal alveolar wall can be found at necropsy. Thus, it is surprising to be told that the physiological situation is that of no alveolar end-capillary gradient in some alveoli, whereas others are so thickened that they are in fact acting as right-to-left shunts. It seems to us much more likely that many alveoli must exist in which, perhaps because of their low compliance, ventilation is reduced. The alveolar oxygen tension in such alveoli, if perfusion is maintained at a normal level, may be insufficient to ensure a normal end-capillary oxygen tension when D_M has been lowered by the thickening of the alveolar wall. We have observed several of these patients in whom the arterial oxygen tension on exercise was much reduced in the presence of a low diffusing capacity, and in whom we have been unable to demonstrate any significant $\dot{V}/\dot{Q}$ abnormality by the use of radioactive xenon.

At the present it seems wise to recognize the following aspects of this problem:

1. Significant lowering of D_L as measured by any technique occurs in this disorder.

2. It cannot be assumed that this lowering is responsible for the lowered arterial tension that may be noted. In many, uneven distribution of ventilation, perfusion, and the alveolar lesion within the lung is mainly responsible for the hypoxemia.

3. When large areas of the lung are completely obliterated by gross alveolar-wall thickening, so that diffusion can occur in only a small part of the original FRC, the diffusing capacity will be reduced because of the smaller surface area available for diffusion. In a sense, this is comparable to the state obtaining in a man who has had one lung removed. Is he to be described as suffering from a diffusion defect? It is clearly unwise to categorize him as having an "alveolar-capillary block syndrome;" but it is equally important to recognize that the demonstration of a diffusing capacity only half of normal in both of these instances is an important and valid measurement of function, even if no conclusions can be drawn regarding the probable existence of a significant alveolar end-capillary gradient for oxygen.

4. Although it may be correct to conclude that in most patients the fall in arterial oxygen saturation is due to uneven distribution effects,[3041] it is essential to recognize that in terms of gas exchange, a slight lowering of D_L will have more effect on the end-capillary oxygen tension if the region has a low $\dot{V}/\dot{Q}$, since the mean alveolar $P_{A_{O_2}}$ in such a region will be lowered. It is not proven that present methods of study can separate these effects with certainty at the alveolar level, but the studies by Arndt, King, and Briscoe[3539] indicate that an actual defect of diffusion is unquestionably important in some patients.

Summary of data of pulmonary function

Though there is uncertainty of the precise factors underlying the lowered arterial oxygen tension in this condition, the general pattern of pulmonary function defect is clearly demarcated. The fall in vital capacity, relative or absolute preservation of maximal ventilatory ability, low compliance and diffusing capacity, and resting and exercise hyperventilation with or without a lowered arterial P_{CO_2} form a characteristic pattern of function disorder that closely parallels the observed pathology. It is not difficult to appreciate why the sensation of dyspnea occurs early in this condition. The combination of exercise hyperventilation and lowering of compliance results in an increased level of respiratory work and an increased intrapleural pressure swing for any given level of external work, and the patient notices this as dyspnea. Early in the disease, there is no arterial unsaturation at rest, though the diffusing capacity will be found to be lowered. Later, the resting arterial blood becomes abnormal. In our view, the measurement of an exercise diffusing capacity provides the best indicator of abnormality in this condition: if the diffusing capacity is normal, the appearance of some reticulation on the x-ray film is unlikely to indicate that the lesions visible are evidence of the Hamman-Rich syndrome; if the diffusing capacity is abnormal and if the compliance is reduced, a lung biopsy may well be indicated even if the radiological changes are minimal.

Clinical variants of the Hamman-Rich syndrome

Familial fibrocystic pulmonary dysplasia

In 1959, Donohue and his colleagues reviewed all cases of the Hamman-Rich syndrome then reported, and noted the apparent familial incidence in some of them.[1001] They reported several more similar cases in children, and suggested that the disease of "familial fibrocystic dysplasia" should be recognized as a variant of the syndrome. It should be noted that there is no suggestion that this entity is related in any way to mucoviscidosis or fibrocystic disease of the pancreas, in spite of the rather unfortunate use of the term "fibrocystic" in the name. The lung pathology in the reported cases was a combination of diffuse interstitial fibrosis, cystic and emphysematous changes, and ultimately a total disorganization of the normal architecture throughout the lung. There seems no reason to suppose that pulmonary function in these patients would be very different from that in others with the Hamman-Rich syndrome, except possibly that the greater degree of cystic change might lead to an increased airway resistance in some of them. Nevertheless, for clinical purposes it is useful to regard this as a separate variant, for the separation of such cases from those of the Hamman-Rich syndrome may help to clarify the etiological factors involved in that entity.

One can find other cases described in the literature that might be examples of this familial syndrome. For example, it seems probable that the two brothers studied by McKusick and Fisher may well have suffered from this,[1003] and Hughes[3040] has described a mother and two daughters with this condition. Swaye and his colleagues have described eight members of a family with a condition apparently typical of the Hamman-Rich syndrome.[3723]

Desquamative interstitial pneumonitis (DIP)

Liebow and his co-workers[3074] have fully described 18 patients in their first description of such cases, and several other patients have been recorded,[3045, 3046, 3713] including two children who suffered from it.[3047, 3048]

The condition is characterized by masses of desquamated large alveolar cells which proliferate actively in the linings and within the lumina of alveoli; accumulations of lymphoid follicles; absence of necrosis; hyaline membranes; cytopathologic effects of viruses; and relatively slight thickening of alveolar walls, and the monotonous uniformity of the lesion.[3714] Scadding and Hinson[3039] in a detailed review have presented evidence for considering this condition and the Hamman-Rich syndrome essentially the same. Apart from histological differences, however, there may be good reason to separate them, since DIP appears to respond better to steroids and may resolve to a significant degree.[3714] Several authors noted that the onset of dyspnea was preceded by virus pneumonia, and reports of patients diagnosed as having the Hamman-Rich syndrome not infrequently mentioned the occurrence of such an infection, as for example Case 1 in reference 381. Other series of cases and reviews, however, contain little evidence that the syndrome might be preceded by this infection, though the possibility has been discussed.[12, 1371, 2050] Case No. 22 illustrates what might be regarded as a typical case of the Hamman-Rich syndrome, in a 13-year-old boy. He contracted viral pneumonia at a time when Asian influenza was endemic in the area. His subsequent course and remarkable improvement cannot confidently be ascribed to therapy, and it is unlike the unremitting downhill course of most patients with classical Hamman-Rich syndrome. We have seen a similar situation in a housewife of 24, who is alive and active 8 years after her lesion was so severe that there was arterial unsaturation at rest and a diffusing capacity of only 4.0 ml CO/mm Hg.* In this patient, too, there was a clear history of a preceding episode of influenzal pneumonia. Both of these patients should be classified as having DIP rather than the Hamman-Rich syndrome.

Miscellaneous entities

In some cases of diffuse interstitial fibrosis, there has been so much muscle hyperplasia in the lung that they have been described under the heading of pulmonary muscular hyperplasia or muscular cirrhosis of the lung.[1372, 1373] It may be noted that some earlier reports in the European literature contain references to this condition, but it is not easy to be sure from these published accounts whether the cases described represent examples of the Hamman-Rich syndrome.[1336] There seems little reason to consider those patients in whom there is relatively more muscle hypertrophy than in others as in a separate category.[3038] It is of interest, how-

*Reported as Case 1 in reference 2296.

Case 23
Chronic Diffuse Interstitial Fibrosis (Hamman-Rich Syndrome)

Summary of Clinical Findings. This 62-year-old retired superintendent at a paint factory complained of progressively increasing dyspnea over a period of one year. At the time of admission to hospital he was obviously dyspneic on the slightest exertion. He was troubled with a dry cough with minimal expectoration of thick mucoid material. Diabetes mellitus had been diagnosed ten years previously and this was satisfactorily controlled by diet and insulin. There was no history of Raynaud's phenomenon. On physical examination his blood pressure was 115/70 mm Hg, pulse rate 105 and respiratory rate 32 per minute. There was slight restriction of chest movement and a decrease in breath sounds. Fine moist rales were audible over most areas of both lungs, and there was intercostal indrawing at both bases. No rhonchi were heard and expiration was not prolonged. The second pulmonic sound was increased; there were no cardiac murmurs and no signs of heart failure. There was slight finger-clubbing and the skin of the hands and elsewhere was not thickened. The rest of the physical examination was noncontributory.

Investigation revealed a hemoglobin of 17.2 gm/100 ml, a hematocrit of 54 per cent, and a white-cell count of 10,100/cmm with a normal differential. The sputum contained no pathogens or malignant cells. Electrophoresis showed a moderate decrease in albumin and increase in globulin. Skin tests for tuberculosis, histoplasmosis and blastomycosis were negative. An electrocardiogram was interpreted as indicating right ventricular hypertrophy. In view of the radiological findings and the serious impairment of pulmonary function, it was decided that a direct lung biopsy should be undertaken. His recovery from this was rapid and without incident. He was then given corticosteroids, and pulmonary function was reassessed one month later. He has since been lost to follow-up.

Radiology. The normal lung markings are obscured by a very coarse reticulation, which in the bases resembles a "honeycomb" pattern (*A*). No portion of either lung is free of involvement. The hila are indistinct but not enlarged. The heart appears slightly enlarged to the left. The lungs are not overinflated and, in fact, appear to be of smaller volume than normal. Barium examination of the esophagus revealed a small hiatus hernia but no evidence of disturbed peristaltic activity to suggest diffuse systemic sclerosis.

A magnified view of the lower portion of the right lung (*B*) demonstrates the reticulation to better advantage. Note that the altered pattern is purely linear without a nodular component.

Pathology. Biopsy of the lung showed complete disorganization of lung structure with formation of cysts up to 2 mm in diameter, separated by dense, fibrous tissue (*C*). The cysts were lined by goblet cells and ciliated columnar cells, and many contained mucus. Loose myxoid fibrous tissue appeared to impinge on the lumina of large bronchioles, and in these areas the lining epithelium was flattened (*D*).

Summary. An elderly man presenting with clinical, radiological, histological and function-test findings characteristic of the Hamman-Rich syndrome. In our experience a lung biopsy should be advised in all such patients unless they are severely dyspneic, even when the clinical diagnosis seems evident. Otherwise a difficult situation may arise if steroids are administered without a histological diagnosis.

	VC	FRC	RV	TLC	ME %	MMFR	$FEV_{0.75}$ ×40	pH	P_{CO_2}	HCO_3^-	O_2Hb %	$D_{L_{CO}}SS_2$
Predicted	3.1	3.2	2.2	5.3	45	2.5	70	7.4	42	25	97	10.6
July 9, 1963	0.9	1.6	1.3	2.2	27	1.3	31	7.36	41	22	87	5.7
Aug. 7, 1963						1.1	26	7.39	44	25	96	4.7

There is a very considerable decrease in vital capacity and functional residual capacity resulting in a total capacity 3 liters below the predicted value. The expiratory flow rates also are impaired. There is hypoxemia at rest, with a greatly reduced diffusing capacity. The only change noted after a month of steroid therapy is the return of the arterial oxygen saturation to normal. The diffusing capacity is further reduced, however.

Chronic Diffuse Interstitial Fibrosis (Hamman-Rich Syndrome) (Continued)

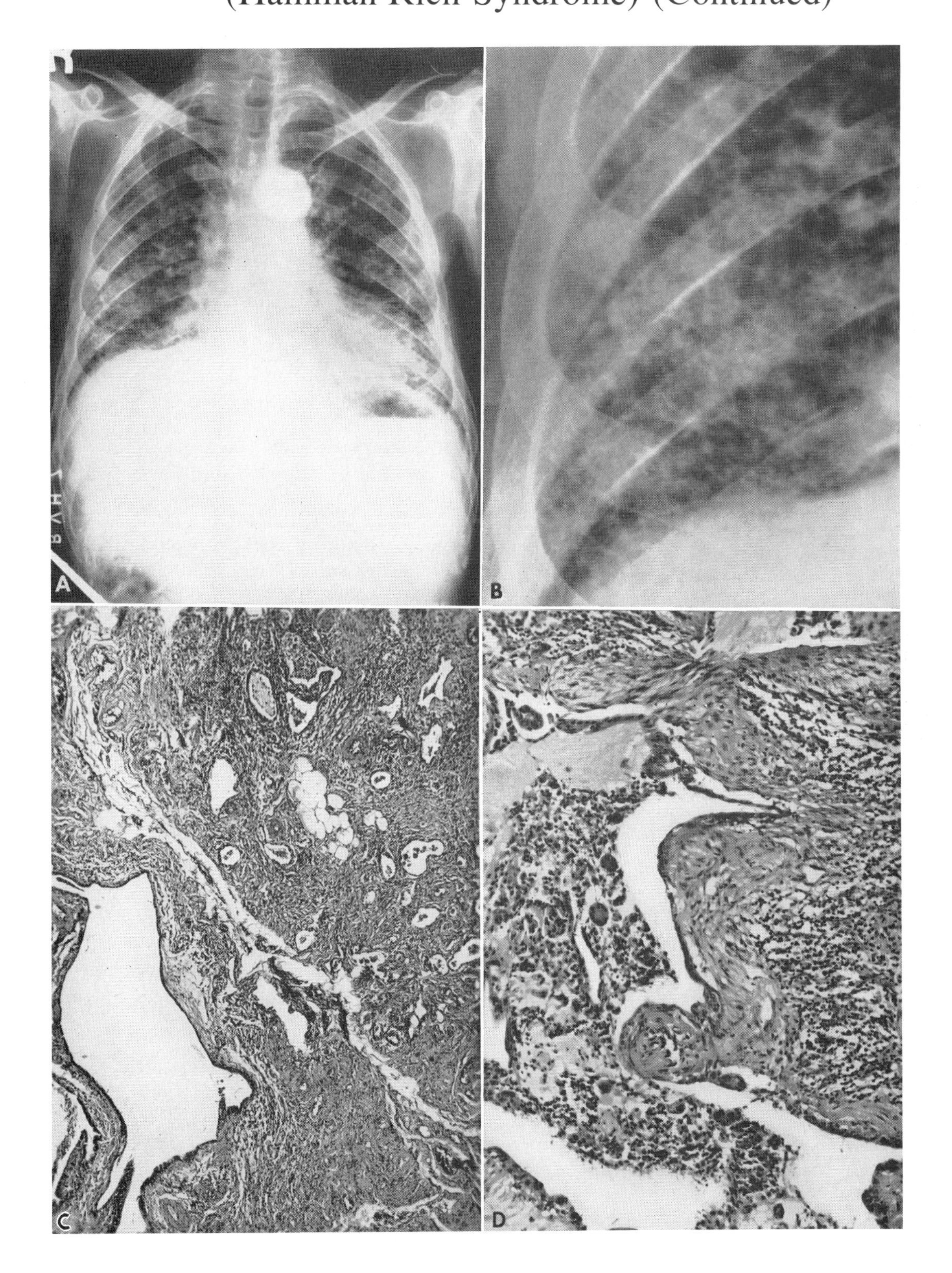

ever, that the increased elastic recoil of the lung, which is a well-documented phenomenon in patients with diffuse interstitial fibrosis,[583] might well be related to the diffuse muscular hypertrophy which in some of these cases is such a prominent feature of the pathological picture.

In 1957, Andrews described five patients in whom the characteristic pathological changes of diffuse interstitial fibrosis had apparently developed after obstruction of the pulmonary veins.[1354] Two of these patients had rheumatic heart disease, the pulmonary veins being blocked by a mural thrombus in one and by a left atrial myxoma in the second. Of unique interest was a third case in which a mediastinal collagenosis had resulted in obstruction of the right pulmonary vein only, and at autopsy only the right lung showed the changes of diffuse interstitial fibrosis. The fourth case showed a similar unilateral pathology as a consequence of tricuspid atresia and obliteration of the left pulmonary vein. In the fifth case, extensive mediastinal fibrosis had produced bilateral changes. Other similar reports have appeared since,[1355, 1361, 1374, 2316] and it seems clearly established that obstruction to one pulmonary vein may produce the histological picture of the Hamman-Rich syndrome. However, relevance of this observation to the etiology of the syndrome in general is far from clear. (see also Chapter 15, page 351.)

The nonspecificity of the lung pathology in this group of disorders has been noted previously. It is not surprising that many individual patients have been described with bizarre clinical or pathological features[1375–1378] that cannot be fitted into any very definite clinical diagnosis.

PULMONARY AND LYMPH-NODE MYOMATOSIS

Only seven cases of this unusual disease have been reported, but one of these, which we have studied in detail,[3720] presented features suggesting that it should be regarded as a different though possibly related entity, not only from the histological point of view, but also on account of an unusual pattern of function abnormality. The patient was a young woman (*see* Case 52), and the increase in pulmonary compliance and loss of elastic recoil (rather than the reverse, which are features of the diffuse interstitial fibroses), combined with severe diffusion defect, were striking features of this one case. (*See* also Chapter 21.)

PULMONARY FUNCTION IN RHEUMATOID LUNG; SJÖGREN'S SYNDROME; DERMATOMYOSITIS

There have been relatively few reports of pulmonary function tests in patients with rheumatoid arthritis, and some excellent clinical discussions have included mention of only a ventilatory test.[1370] The patient described by Cudkowicz and his colleagues,[1369] who had considerable alveolar-wall thickening, was noted to have some reduction in vital capacity and maximal breathing capacity, and the single-breath diffusing capacity ($D_{L_{CO}}SB$) was only 7.7 ml CO/min/mm Hg instead of a predicted value of 25 ml CO/min/mm Hg. However, as far as we are aware, no series of cases with rheumatoid arthritis has been carefully surveyed as to the frequency of pulmonary function derangement. It seems likely that the diffusing capacity would reflect the extent and severity of interstitial pulmonary fibrosis in this condition, and one might expect that considerable function impairment would be demonstrable in some of these patients with little radiological change, as has been shown to be the case in scleroderma. It is to be assumed that the pattern of function disorder in Sjögren's syndrome parallels that in similar conditions.

The single-breath diffusing capacity is lowered in dermatomyositis;[3054] the severity of the pulmonary fibrosis that may accompany this condition was illustrated by a patient reported by Sandbank and his colleagues.[3075] Death from respiratory failure occurred within two years of onset, as a result of rapidly progressive diffuse interstitial fibrosis. The lesions of dermatomyositis appeared six months before death.

SCLERODERMA

Clinical features

Scleroderma is an atrophic and sclerotic disease affecting the skin, viscera, skeletal system, and lung parenchyma, often with Raynaud's phenomenon occurring as an early manifestation of the condition.[1350] The extent and severity of involvement of different tissues is variable from case to case, although, as was noted earlier, the autopsy incidence of pulmonary involvement has been said to be as high as 90 per cent.[1351] Before the frequency of pulmonary parenchymal change in this condition was recognized,[1352, 2055] the pulmonary manifestations were ascribed to the thickening of the skin of the chest wall,[1105] though it is now evident that changes in the pulmonary parenchyma are much more frequently the cause of dyspnea. Clinically, the patient with advanced scleroderma presents a characteristic and distressing picture[1329] that is dominated by the sclerotic changes in the skin known as acrosclerosis. Renal and cardiac involvement may occur,[1350] and changes in the skeletal muscle have been described which are similar, if not identical, to those found in dermatomyositis. The course is slow and progressive, and it is not certain that any agent significantly alters the long-term progress of the condition. There seems little doubt that scleroderma is associated with an increased occurrence of lung cancer.[2274, 2348]

Pulmonary function

During the past decade a number of excellent studies of the pulmonary function in scleroderma have been published, establishing a very clear picture of the characteristic derangements found in this condition.

In most of the reported cases the vital capacity was reduced well below the normal predicted value.[2311] Thus, in a series of 22 patients it was from 15 to 63 per cent of what was predicted;[1347] in another group of 13 patients, values fell between 40 and 90 per cent of predicted normal;[1348] and in the 16 cases studied by Catterall and Rowell it appeared to be reduced in all but two patients.[1329] The residual volume may be normal, however,[1348, 1349] but as a consequence of the reduction in vital capacity the total lung capacity is reduced, often by as much as 2 liters less than the predicted value. Most authors have found but little interference with ventilation,[1348, 2311] and Miller and his colleagues[1347] considered that the diminution in maximal midexpiratory flow rate they observed in some patients was a consequence of the considerable reduction in pulmonary volume and could not be interpreted to indicate airway obstruction. The pulmonary compliance is reduced in most, if not all, of these patients,[2311] and Adhikari and his colleagues,[1348] who reported these measurements, bring forward convincing reasons why neither the alterations in subdivisions of lung volume nor the reduction in pulmonary compliance can be attributed to thickening and sclerosis of the skin of the chest wall; both are almost certainly due to parenchymal change.

Miller and his co-workers observed arterial hypoxemia on exercise in 12 of their 22 cases.[1347] Using the rebreathing technique to measure CO-diffusing capacity ($D_{Lco}RB$), Adhikari and his colleagues found a normal value for diffusing capacity in only 1 of the 13 patients they studied;[1348] they further showed that the predominant defect was in the membrane-diffusing capacity (D_M). They concluded that abnormal pulmonary function in scleroderma was "more common than either symptoms related to the lungs or changes in the chest roentgenogram." The truth of this observation has been strikingly confirmed by Catterall and Rowell,[1329] and Hughes and Lee.[1349] The former found that 8 of their 16 cases had abnormal function but a normal chest x-ray, and in all of these the single-breath $D_{Lco}SB$ was less than the predicted normal value; in 5 it was less than 60 per cent of the normal predicted figure. These authors[1329] pointed out the insensitivity of the FEV in discriminating between patients, and concluded: "The diffusing capacity was impaired in all patients, and the degree of impairment corresponded with the degree of dyspnea and with diffuse fibrosis of the lung parenchyma found at three necropsies: there was no correlation with the radiological findings or with the E.C.G." Ritchie recently reported on the pulmonary function of 22 patients with scleroderma and emphasized the disparity among clinical state, radiological findings, and impairment of pulmonary function in his series,[2311] a feature of this condition to which others have recently called attention.[3057, 3058]

Since 1964, many further studies of pulmonary function have been published, and it is clear that impairment of CO transfer is the cardinal finding.[3049, 3055, 3056, 3057, 3716] There is good histological reason for this as the lesions seem to be closely related to vascular structures,[3049] and may even involve the vessels themselves.

Pulmonary hypertension was found by one group of workers in all of 18 patients studied by right-heart catheterization.[3053] In a major review of the lung in scleroderma, Weaver, Divertie, and Titus[3058] noted the fact that changes in function may precede radiological change, and at this stage physical signs may be scanty. They also documented the occurrence of pulmonary hypertension.

In view of all this evidence, it is surprising to find the statement that "the lungs are involved in only 5 to 10 per cent of cases of scleroderma" repeated even in textbooks that have been written recently.[15] It seems clear that sparing of the pulmonary parenchyma is the exception rather than the rule; and such a view of the infrequent incidence of pulmonary parenchymal involvement springs from a traditional reliance on clinical and radiological methods in pronouncing the lungs free from involvement. Indeed it seems likely that the finding of the characteristic pattern of pulmonary function derangement in a patient with Raynaud's phenomenon or esophageal changes should be regarded as a very important point in making the diagnosis of scleroderma, regardless of the state of the lung parenchyma on x-ray examination.[3055, 3058]

PULMONARY SARCOIDOSIS

The qualities which make for success in research are very elusive. Applied research, which seeks to use scientific knowledge for practical ends, demands judgment and the courage to follow it, a knowledge of economics and affairs, and an organizing ability, which are not required to anything like the same extent by the fundamental scientist whose aim is the gaining of a deeper knowledge about Nature . . . .

Sir Lawrence Bragg[3673]

CHAPTER 13

DEFINITION

At an International Conference on Sarcoidosis held in the USA in 1960,[1395] no short and precise definition of the disease known generally as Boeck's sarcoid was considered possible, though there seemed no reason to doubt that all of the participants had little difficulty in making the clinical diagnosis in most instances. Such a diagnosis is based on the clinical presentation, together with the demonstration of granulomatous changes in lung, liver, skin, or lymph glands. These granulomata cannot be considered as morphologically "specific," however, and it is this fact that makes a precise definition impossible.

PATHOLOGY

Multiple noncaseating granulomata are the characteristic lesions of sarcoid. The granulomata are microscopic in size, but when clustered together may form gray or yellow nodules resembling miliary tuberculosis in gross appearance. Microscopically they consist of groups of large epithelioid cells, with abundant pale, eosinophilic cytoplasm and sharp cell borders, and with little or no surrounding cuff of nonspecific, chronic, inflammatory cells which are so prominent a feature of infective conditions. Multinucleate giant cells are common, and inclusions, such as asteroid bodies, conchoid bodies (Schaumann bodies) or anisotropic fragments, are often seen. These granulomata are not specific, but in certain circumstances, particularly when the lesions occur in scalene lymph nodes or the lung, the monotonous regularity of their appearance and distribution enable one to make the diagnosis of sarcoidosis with a fair degree of certainty.

The lungs are the most commonly involved organ in sarcoidosis, approximated or equalled only by lymph-node involvement.[1399] Although hilar lymph-node involvement without parenchymal disease is described radiologically, it is unlikely that the lung tissue is spared in these cases. The granulomata occur typically in relation to lymphatics—peribronchiolar, subpleural, and along lobular septa—and scattered throughout the interstitium of the lung, lying in alveolar walls but never in alveolar lumina. The intervening parenchyma is normal, and the amount spared is variable between slight and extensive (*see* Cases 24 and 25). Granulomata are seen also in the walls of larger bronchi. Large aggregates may form nodules up to 3 or 4 cm in diameter, and the lung architecture is completely distorted in these regions. From radiological evidence it is clear that the smaller lesions, whether single or in clusters, can resolve and then are pathologically represented by small scars in the lung.

Extensive pulmonary fibrosis ensues in a small proportion of cases.[528] The exact mechanism of this process is obscure, but the end-result is widespread interstitial fibrosis, bronchiolectasis, and distortion of the lung. Some degree of irregular emphysema may be present in such lungs, but it is unlikely that this would cause any significant disturbance of function. Occasionally the bronchial sarcoid lesions and bronchial adenopathy may obstruct or distort bronchi, resulting in lipid pneumonia,[1399] localized emphysema,[794] or atelectasis. Exceptionally, typical centrilobular and panlobular emphysema may follow infiltration with sarcoid granulomata.[3092] Vascular destruction and thrombosis due to sarcoidosis have been described, and it is possible that in some patients this may be the cause of pulmonary hypertension. It may be speculated that peri-arterial sarcoid granulomata play a similar role.

RADIOLOGY

Sarcoidosis may present any one of four appearances radiologically in the thorax.

1. *Lymph-node enlargement without pulmonary abnormality.* The node enlargement is usually localized to the paratracheal, tracheobronchial, and bronchopulmonary groups of nodes, and is generally symmetrical on the two sides. The most obvious radiological abnormality is an irregular nodular enlargement of the hilar shadows. The retrosternal nodes are seldom enlarged, a point which is of considerable value in the differentiation from lymphoma, in which retrosternal and asymmetrical paratracheal node enlargement is the rule.

2. *Diffuse pulmonary disease without lymph-node enlargement.* The pulmonary abnormality is almost always diffuse and evenly distributed from the apices to the bases. The pattern is generally reticulonodular, although reticulation or nodularity may predominate in any one patient. The reticulation may be in the form of a very fine network or may be very coarse. The mediastinal silhouette and pulmonary vasculature are normal, and pleural effusion is rarely, if ever, seen.

3. *A combination of diffuse pulmonary disease and lymph-node enlargement.*

4. *Pulmonary fibrosis,* representing the end result of the diffuse pulmonary changes described in (2) and (3). The scarring, which is generally very coarse and in the form of irregular linear strands extending outward from the hila toward the periphery, does not resemble that seen in the "active" reticulonodular disease described in (2); it is commonly more uneven in its distribution, involving only certain areas of the lungs and leaving others apparently clear. There may be signs of overinflation in the areas of lung not obviously involved. The heart and pulmonary vasculature may develop the changes typical of pulmonary hypertension.

The relationship between these four x-ray manifestations varies considerably from patient to patient. Pure lymph-node enlargement may disappear spontaneously, leaving no radiological residua, and may be the only manifestation of the disease; it may disappear and be replaced by diffuse pulmonary involvement, either concurrently or as remotely as several years later, a situation well illustrated in Case 25; or it may remain, with diffuse pulmonary involvement becoming superimposed upon it. Ring calcification of lymph nodes occurs rarely, but the possibility must be recognized in view of the differential diagnosis from silicosis, in which diffuse pulmonary disease and "eggshell" calcification of lymph nodes are not infrequently seen.

Atypical cases, with unilateral involvement or with large homogeneous foci in the lung, resembling metastatic cancer, have been recorded.[3082] Detailed radiographic studies of the pulmonary peripheral circulation have revealed marked vascular abnormalities in the fibrotic, but not in the granulomatous, stages of the disease.[3088]

CLINICAL FEATURES

As far as pulmonary sarcoidosis is concerned, for descriptive purposes it is convenient to classify patients into the following general groups. This classification has been used by many of those who have studied this interesting condition,[56, 393, 1396–1398] and is in conformity with the radiological grouping.

Group 1: Patients having hilar adenopathy alone, with no radiological involvement of pulmonary parenchyma.

Group 2: Patients with hilar adenopathy, and with mottling or reticular changes in the lung fields.

Group 3: Patients with pulmonary parenchymal changes and without significant adenopathy.

Group 4: Patients in whom pulmonary parenchymal changes are known to have been present for two years or more (pulmonary fibrosis).

This kind of classification is very useful in that the majority of patients are included within the first two groups (88 per cent in one series[1396]). When pulmonary changes have been present for a period of more than two years, resolution is the exception rather than the rule.

The clinical presentation is so varied that it is difficult to draw any general picture of the disease. In many of these patients, complaints of vague malaise or weight loss cause the physician to request a chest x-ray, which reveals hilar adenopathy with or without parenchymal change. In others, these findings are revealed accidentally on a routine film. In a few, systemic manifestations of sarcoidosis in the eyes, skin, or elsewhere lead to the discovery of pulmonary involvement. There is no doubt that pulmonary involvement is extremely common, if not invariable.[1396] Many clinical reports stress the frequency of dyspnea as a symptom,[1396] and an irritative cough may cause some patients to seek medical advice. The disease, as noted by Longcope and Freiman,[1399] is, in many patients, of long duration with remissions that may be mistaken for cures and exacerbations that may reflect progression of the disease or involvement of another organ.

Occasionally pulmonary sarcoidosis occurs in an acute form, and the course may be very rapidly progressive.[3089]

There is some disagreement as to what percentage of patients with pulmonary sarcoid develop irreversible pulmonary changes and become classifiable within Group 4. However, in two series the incidence of "pulmonary fibrosis" was reported as 20 per cent, Smellie and Hoyle finding it in 25 of their 125 patients[1396] and Scadding in 27 of 136 patients.[1397] Other comments, particularly those in textbooks, give the general impression that sarcoid less commonly leads to permanent pulmonary changes, and that there may be considerable variation in this figure in different parts of the world. The reader should consult the Proceedings of the International Conference on Sarcoidosis already referred to[1395] for an exhaustive discussion of every aspect of sarcoidosis except its effect on pulmonary function. Several clinical reviews also provide excellent accounts of the disease from a clinical and radiological standpoint.[1396–1400]

EFFECT ON PULMONARY FUNCTION

Although several useful observations on the effect on the lung of sarcoidosis had been published before 1961, the remarkable studies by Svanborg in that year[393] can be said to have rendered obsolete much previous literature. This monograph of 130 pages represents the most complete study of cardiac and respiratory function in one disease that, as far as we are aware, has ever been undertaken. It is convenient to consider these and other findings in sarcoid in relation to the relevant clinical group of the patients. This clinical classification closely follows the radiological criteria outlined earlier.

Group 1: Patients showing hilar adenopathy alone, with no evidence of pulmonary parenchymal involvement

Svanborg studied 11 patients in this group,[393] Marshall and his colleagues 5,[56] and Coates and Comroe 3;[1401] the two last-named authors found a decreased maximal breathing capacity in one of their cases and a lowered arterial saturation in another. Of Marshall's patients, three had some reduction of ventilatory flow rate, in one case thought to be due to pressure on the bronchi from the enlarged glands; in addition, one of these patients had a reduced diffusing capacity and another a reduction in lung compliance. More recently, several authors have stressed that a low pulmonary compliance may be found in asymptomatic patients.[3083, 3085, 3090] Svanborg reported that cardiovascular function studied during right-heart catheterization was normal in all 11 cases.[393] However, he found that lung compliance was decreased in six, and airway resistance increased in two. In 8 of the 11 patients, the diffusing capacity ($D_{Lco}SS_1$) was decreased at rest or on exercise, which reduction he considered was not sufficient to limit oxygen uptake in this group. It may be important to stress that muscular weakness is a notable feature in many cases of sarcoidosis; this might well be responsible for limitation of

Case 24
Sarcoidosis

Summary of Clinical Findings. This 47-year-old housewife was first admitted to this service in December, 1957. Over the previous two years, she had noticed gradually increasing shortness of breath on exertion, now so severe that she could not do housework. She had a slight nonproductive cough. Her other main complaint was of chronic fatigue. The patient had received no radiotherapy after undergoing left radical mastectomy for carcinoma in 1954.

Apart from the absence of the left breast, no abnormalities were found on physical examination. Investigations revealed Hb, 96 per cent; ESR, 18 mm/hr; WBC, 5,600/cmm, with a normal differential; prothrombin activity, 100 per cent. Urinalysis was normal. Serum cholesterol was 256 mg/100 ml. Old tuberculin testing (1/100) was negative. Biopsy of the left upper lobe of the lung revealed a granulomatous inflammation consistent with sarcoidosis. She was placed on Meticorten and isoniazid, and was discharged to outpatient supervision. When she was reassessed in March, 1958, there had been no improvement clinically or morphologically. Considerable clearing had occurred by January 1959, when steroid medication was discontinued.

By May, 1963, she was complaining of increasing fatigue, and a chest x-ray showed a return of the reticulation throughout the lungs. Steroids were reinstituted and by July she felt improved and the lungs had cleared radiologically.

She was readmitted after an episode of hemoptysis in September, 1968. In the intervening period she had had several exacerbations symptomatically and radiologically and had been treated intermittently with steroids. She had last received steroids in January, 1968, and since then had noted a gradual increase in shortness of breath and fatigue. No cause of the hemoptysis could be found, but x-rays suggested progression of the disease. A Kweim test was performed, and a biopsy performed five weeks later was negative. Function studies are shown. Steroids were not reinstituted. When last seen in September, 1969, she felt well but admitted to mild shortness of breath while doing housework.

Radiology. A postero-anterior roentgenogram of the chest in December, 1957, (*A*) demonstrates considerable asymmetry of radiolucency of the two lung fields because of absence of soft tissue on the left (radical mastectomy for carcinoma of the breast). The lungs are involved in a diffuse disease characterized by a coarse reticular pattern which generally follows the vascular distribution. The hilar and mediastinal lymph nodes show no evidence of enlargement, and the cardiovascular silhouette is normal. With the history of carcinoma of the breast, there is perhaps good reason to implicate neoplastic lymphatic permeation of the lungs as the cause of such a radiological picture. In this patient however, two factors militate against this possibility: (1) the uniform distribution throughout the lungs without the basal predominance which usually characterizes lymphangitic carcinomatosis, and (2) the rather mild respiratory symptoms in the presence of such extensive pul-

	VC	FRC	RV	TLC	ME %	MMFR	$FEV_{0.75}$ ×40	pH^+	P_{CO_2}	HCO_3^-	P_{O_2}	O_2Hb %	$D_{Lco}SS_2$	CO Ext %
Predicted	3.0	2.7	1.6	4.6	55	2.8	75						14.3	45
Dec. 1957	2.1	1.8	1.3	3.4	44	2.9	66						9.1	33
March 1958	1.9	1.5	1.1	3.0	42	2.6	66						6.9	28
Jan. 1959	1.8	1.8	1.5	3.3	46	2.5	58						12.7	32
Feb. 1963						1.7	47						9.8	31
Sept. 1968	1.2	1.6	1.3	2.5	44	1.6	46	39	38	23	74	96	5.1	22
Jan. 1969	1.7	1.8	1.3	3.0	37	2.3	61						6.2	25

On her first admission, there was a loss of pulmonary volume, but no ventilatory defect. Resting and exercise diffusing capacity were below normal. In March, 1958, after steroid therapy and with no improvement in dyspnea or in the x-ray appearance, the resting diffusing capacity had fallen further. The x-ray was still unchanged in January, 1959, but clinical improvement had occurred. In February, 1963, the lung fields were radiologically clear (*see* Figure *C*), but the ventilatory defect had worsened and there had been no improvement in resting diffusing capacity.

In September, 1968, all aspects of function had further worsened, but by January, 1969, without treatment, lung volumes and flow rates had again improved but diffusing capacity remained low.

Sarcoidosis

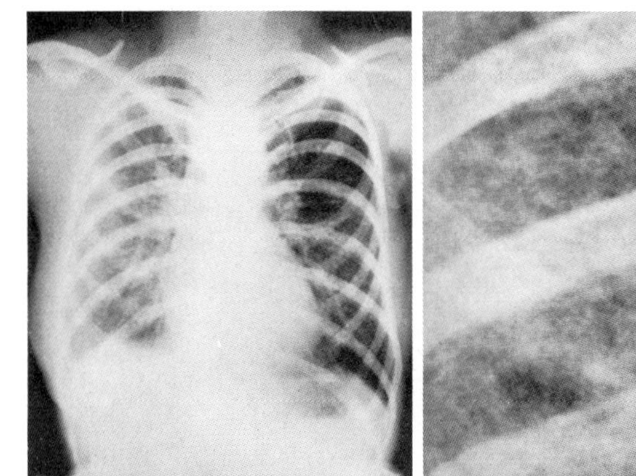

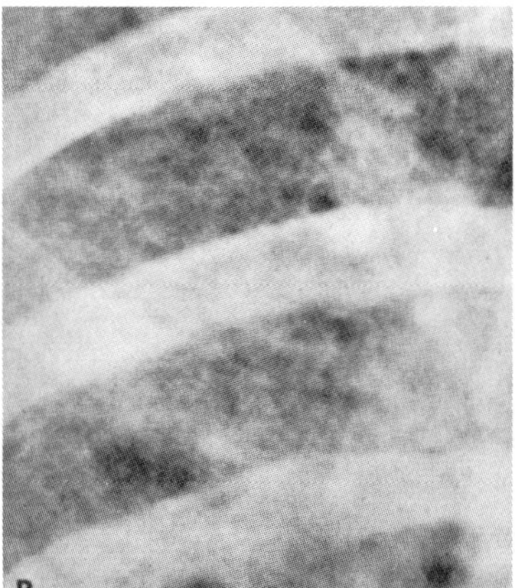

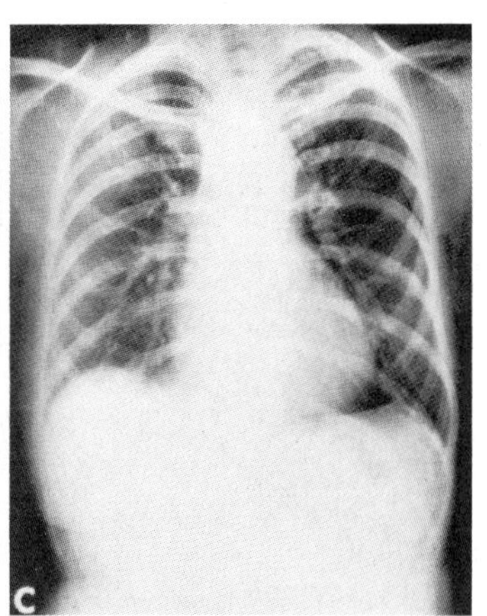

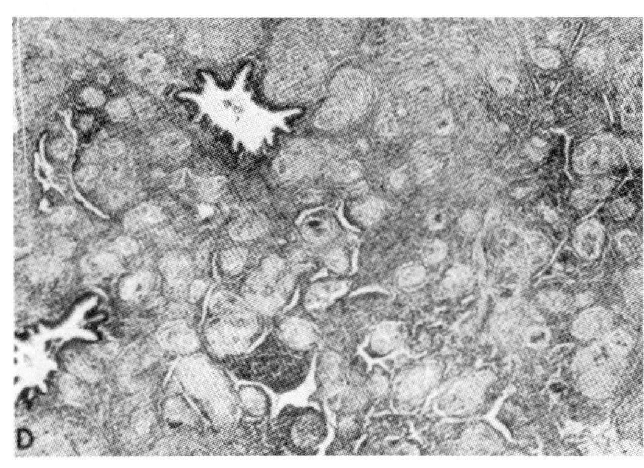

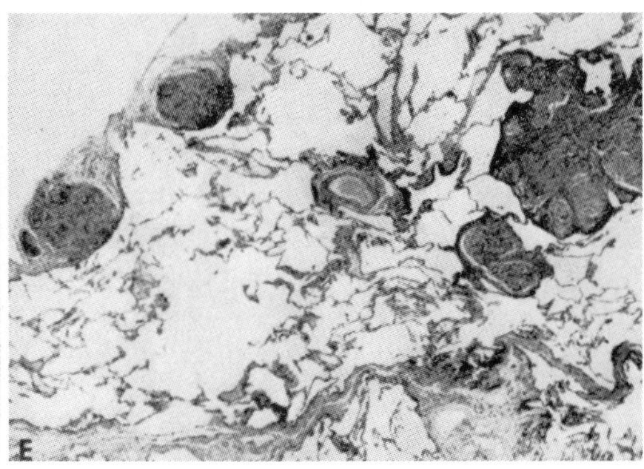

monary involvement. This type of radiological picture, however, presents no features which are in any way pathognomonic, and the differential diagnosis must be extensive.

A magnified view of a portion of the right upper lung field shows the reticular character of the disease (*B*). A postero-anterior view of the chest made in 1963 (*C*) shows almost complete clearing of the diffuse disease. Except for minor residual changes in the right subclavicular zone, the lungs now appear normal.

Pathology. Multiple noncaseating granulomata were seen throughout the lung biopsy specimen, and were situated in the pleura and lobular septa and adjacent to bronchioles. Four large conglomerations of granulomata were present, the largest one being 1.2 cm in diameter, and in these areas lung structure was entirely lost (*D*). Elsewhere the alveolar surface was relatively normal (*E*). Fibrosis was well developed around most of the granulomata, and asteroid bodies were frequently present in giant cells.

Summary. This case illustrates the value of establishing the diagnosis by open lung biopsy. The patient, who had had a radical mastectomy for breast cancer three years previously, was found to be suffering from pulmonary sarcoidosis. Clearing of the pulmonary infiltration on the chest x-ray has not been accompanied by any evidence of improvement in pulmonary function.

the maximal breathing capacity when it is measured over a 15- or 30-second period of maximal effort. Some reduction in vital capacity and in residual volume was recorded by Marshall and his co-workers[56] and by Svanborg,[393] the latter author concluding, however, that alveolar ventilation was in general normal in his cases. Hamer[2060] has recently reported a lowered membrane-diffusing component (D_M) in three cases of sarcoidosis with a normal chest x-ray at the time of study, and Sharma and his colleagues[3089] found a lowered single-breath diffusing capacity in 17 out of 18 patients with hilar-gland enlargement only. Five of the same group also had a lowered pulmonary compliance.

It seems clear from these results that some patients in this group, while possessing apparently normal lung fields, do in fact have some degree of parenchymal lung involvement, demonstrable by abnormal lung mechanics and diffusing capacity, and an abnormal lung parenchyma has been demonstrated to be present by biopsy at this stage.[3087]

Groups 2 and 3: Patients with parenchymal involvement, with or without adenopathy, thought to have been present for two years or less

Svanborg[393] studied 11 patients in this group, differentiating them from those considered to have established pulmonary fibrosis. Marshall *et al.'s* series[56] included 9 patients in this group, and Hamer's group of 30 cases included 13 in this category.[2060] Other authors' series[418, 466, 1341, 1401–1406] contain variable numbers of such patients, often not clearly distinguishable from those with established pulmonary fibrosis (Group 4).

With few exceptions, there is general agreement that patients in this group are characterized by the following pattern of changes, the severity of these being very variable indeed from patient to patient. All static lung volumes are reduced, though the ratio of residual volume to total lung capacity (RV/TLC) may be elevated, since the vital capacity is proportionately more lowered than the residual volume. Intrapulmonary gas distribution is infrequently abnormal, and arterial blood-gas tensions at rest and on exercise are often, but by no means invariably, within normal limits. Recent papers have stressed the usefulness of measurements of this kind in the assessment of lung function in sarcoidosis.[3078] Maximal ventilatory volume is either normal or slightly reduced. Svanborg,[393] in common with most other observers, noted a decreased pulmonary compliance in relation to height. Marshall and his colleagues,[56] however, considered that this decrease was proportional to the diminished lung volume, in contrast to Svanborg[393] and others,[1403, 3083, 3085] who found that, in many of these patients, it was lower than would be predicted on the basis of the measured vital capacity or FRC. The diffusing capacity at rest may be at the lower limit of normal in some of these patients,[56, 393] but it is very commonly reduced even at rest,[3078, 3081, 3085, 3086, 3089] and more often lowered on exercise. Its level may be approximately correlated with the duration of the illness.[3085] In most instances this reduction is still apparent if the diffusing capacity is expressed in relation to the volume of lung being ventilated. In a few cases, the reduction was considered by Svanborg to be sufficient to limit the maximal oxygen-uptake capability. There was little evidence of circulatory or hemodynamic abnormality. Several authors have recently stressed that the arterial oxygen saturation or tension is often lower than normal when these patients exercise, and the A–a oxygen difference is commonly widened.[3078, 3080, 3091]

In a study of sarcoidosis at different stages, using the single-breath D_L (D_{Lco}SB) and partitioning D_L into its components of D_M and V_c (*see* Chapter 2), Hamer has shown that the diffusing capacity is usually impaired in this group of cases.[2060] Accepting his category of "pulmonary infiltration" as including Group 3 cases, he found normal values for D_L, D_M, and V_c in three patients, a reduced D_L and D_M in seven, and a reduction in all three of these measurements in a further three patients in this group.

Group 4: Patients considered to have established pulmonary fibrosis

The changes in this group are similar to those described above, but usually more severe. In addition,[393] some degree of pulmonary hypertension is not uncommon and there may be considerable limitation of maximal working capacity. In a few patients with apparent pulmonary fibrosis, the general level of pulmonary function is found to be surprisingly good.[56] However, Hamer[2060] found no cases with a normal single-breath D_L in this group; all of his eight patients in this category had impairment of D_L and D_M, and in four of them the pulmonary capillary blood volume (V_c) was significantly lowered. At this stage of the disease, the arterial oxygen tension on exercise is commonly abnormal,[3078, 3080, 3091] and the pulmonary compliance is reduced with an increase in the oxygen cost of breathing.[3090]

Some authors who reported earlier studies of sarcoidosis[1401, 1402] noted the presence of an increased residual volume and some obstructive changes in some of their patients. The larger series now reported by Svanborg,[393] Hamer[2060] and Marshall and his colleagues[56] have not confirmed the idea that secondary pulmonary emphysema commonly occurs in sarcoidosis, although this clinical picture is still emphasized by some authors.[3079]

This general picture should not be allowed to obscure the remarkable variations noted by many observers in different patients who would be classified in the same radiological group. In order to discuss the meaning of the pulmonary function status in relation to the pathology of this disease, separate consideration must be given to the interrelationship between the radiological picture and function, and to the reported effects of treatment on both of these aspects in individual cases.

INTERRELATIONSHIP BETWEEN RADIOLOGICAL APPEARANCE AND FUNCTION

In few other diseases is this problem so perplexing as in sarcoidosis. It has been, we consider, clearly established that significant abnormality of function may be present in patients with a normal chest x-ray and, further, that when infiltration has resolved completely, impaired pulmonary function may demonstrate that the lung is far from healed (*see* Case 16 in Marshall *et al.'s* data[56] and Cases J. S. and P. W. reported by Hamer[2060]). It may be presumed, therefore, that significant parenchymal sarcoidosis may and probably commonly does exist in the presence of a normal x-ray, and may be revealed by reduction in static lung volumes, in pulmonary compliance or in diffusing capacity. On the other hand, as indicated in Case No. 26, an apparently severe infiltrative lesion may sometimes be associated with but little impairment in function. When the pulmonary lesion is known to have been present for several years, a more or less severe abnormality of function is usual, as Svanborg's data show very elegantly. Furthermore, several studies[56, 3085] show that, in general, the longer the infiltration is known to have been present the more severe the diffusion defect is likely to be. However, Marshall and his co-workers documented a case in which marked radiological change was known to have been present for several years in a patient whom the clinician considered to have moderately severe dyspnea but in whom pulmonary function was normal (*see* Case 1 in ref. 56). Furthermore, there was considerable variation in function among different patients in Svanborg's group with established pulmonary fibrosis. During the past few years, a number of authors have pointed out that the diffusing capacity commonly remains impaired in spite of clinical or radiological improvement,[3076, 3079, 3081, 3086] and the same is true of the pulmonary compliance.[3085] Turiaf, Basset, and Georges,[3722] in a follow-up study of 35 patients, have recently provided additional evidence of the importance of pulmonary function tests in following the course of the disease in patients who have, on clinical and radiological criteria, completely recovered from it.

It is not easy to make sense of these observations or to be sure of drawing meaningful conclusions from them. However, it may be suggested that a considerable infiltrative lesion of the type illustrated in Case No. 26 in all probability represents predominant change in pulmonary lymphatics, particularly perhaps peribronchial in situation, and further, that the predilection for sarcoid granulomata to form around small vessels in the lung may well have something to do with the observation that diffusing capacity may be much more abnormal than the extent or severity of radiological change would indicate. More correlative work on the pathology of this interesting condition and its effects upon lung function is necessary before these questions can be answered.

EFFECTS OF TREATMENT ON FUNCTION

The discrepancy between the evaluation of function and the radiological picture can be illustrated further by the many reported observations on the comparative effect of treatment (usually by means of steroids), on the x-ray appearances and on function. This

(Text continued on page 298.)

Case 25
Sarcoidosis

Summary of Clinical Findings. This 46-year-old housewife was first admitted to the Royal Victoria Hospital in 1959. Nine years previously she had been discovered to have enlarged hilar glands (*A*), an x-ray one year before that having been reported as normal. At that time she was complaining of fatigue and shortness of breath. Her symptoms lessened and she remained well until the fall of 1958, when she began to notice increasing weakness and fatigue. Her appetite decreased and she lost 20 to 25 lb in weight over the next three months. She was short of breath after climbing one flight of stairs and had a minimal unproductive cough, but had no fever, night sweats, rash or eye symptoms. Physical examination was normal except that breath sounds were harsher over the left upper chest.

Investigations included urinalysis and a hemogram, which were normal; NPN was 2 mg/100 ml; serum calcium was 5.45 mEq/1; the electrophoretic pattern was within normal limits. A right scalene-node biopsy showed "chronic lymphadenitis" and a lung biopsy of the tip of the lingula was performed. Old tuberculin (1/1000) testing was negative. Treatment with oral prednisone was started, together with isoniazid hydrochloride, 400 mg daily.

By June, 1959, she was much improved symptomatically and was able to manage all of her household work without discomfort. Steroid therapy was discontinued in March, 1962, and INH six months later. She was admitted for reassessment in 1968. There were no complaints referable to the respiratory system and the chest roentgenogram was considered normal.

Radiology. A postero-anterior roentgenogram of the chest made in 1950 (*A*) demonstrates bilateral hilar lymph-node enlargement without involvement of the paratracheal or retrosternal areas. The lungs are clear. Such a picture is not pathognomonic, but in a young asymptomatic patient it should suggest sarcoidosis as the first diagnostic possibility.

A chest film made nine years later, in February 1959, (*B*) shows the lymph-node enlargement to have disappeared. However, the lungs are now diffusely involved in a disease which has created a fine reticulonodular pattern evenly distributed from the apices to the bases. There is no pleural effusion and the cardiovascular and hilar shadows are normal. This combination of hilar lymph-node enlargement and diffuse reticular disease of the lungs, despite their separation in time, is strongly suggestive of sarcoidosis.

A magnified view (*C*) of a portion of the right upper lung field shows to better advantage the combined reticular and nodular character of the pulmonary disease.

Chest films made at intervals during the following months showed gradual clearing of the diffuse disease, the lungs returning to a completely normal appearance by June, 1959.

Pathology. Sections of the lung biopsy showed multiple noncaseating granulomata (*D*), generally situated along lobular septa and adjacent to bronchioles, where they were probably related to lymphatics. A few were present in the pleura. In the granulomata there were large numbers of epithelioid cells, a few giant cells and occasional Schaumann bodies but no asteroids. The alveolar walls were generally normal and were rarely im-

														EXERCISE				
	VC	FRC	RV	TLC	ME %	MMFR	$FEV_{0.75}$ ×40	pH	P_{CO_2}	HCO_3^-	O_2Hb %	$D_{Lco}SS_2$	CO Ext %	MPH	GRADE	$\dot{V}O_2$	$\dot{V}_E$	$D_{Lco}SS_3$
Predicted	3.3	2.9	1.7	5.0	55	2.9	79	7.40	42	25	97	14.6	44					22.3
Feb. 1959	1.7	2.4	2.0	3.7	52	2.5	62	7.45	46	27	99	11.6	37	1.5	FLAT	0.72	18.9	17.9
June 1959	1.9	2.5	2.0	3.9	66	3.6	83					11.1	43	1.5	FLAT	0.47	12.5	18.1
April 1963	2.4	2.4	1.7	4.1	59	3.2	83					16.0	51					
April 1968	2.3	2.7	2.1	4.4	57	4.0	88					11.6	42					

In February, 1959, before the start of treatment, there is only moderate impairment of function. There is a reduction in vital capacity and total lung capacity. Diffusion both at rest and exercise is borderline normal. After five months of steroid therapy, in June, 1959, the subdivisions of lung volume are unchanged, but there has been a significant improvement in ventilatory function. The diffusing capacity is unchanged. Four years later, the vital capacity and total capacity have increased further, ventilatory function is normal and the diffusing capacity has returned to normal. There has been little further change in 1968. The diffusing capacity has shown an apparent fall but the predicted level at her present age is 11.7 with a CO extraction percentage of 42.

Sarcoidosis

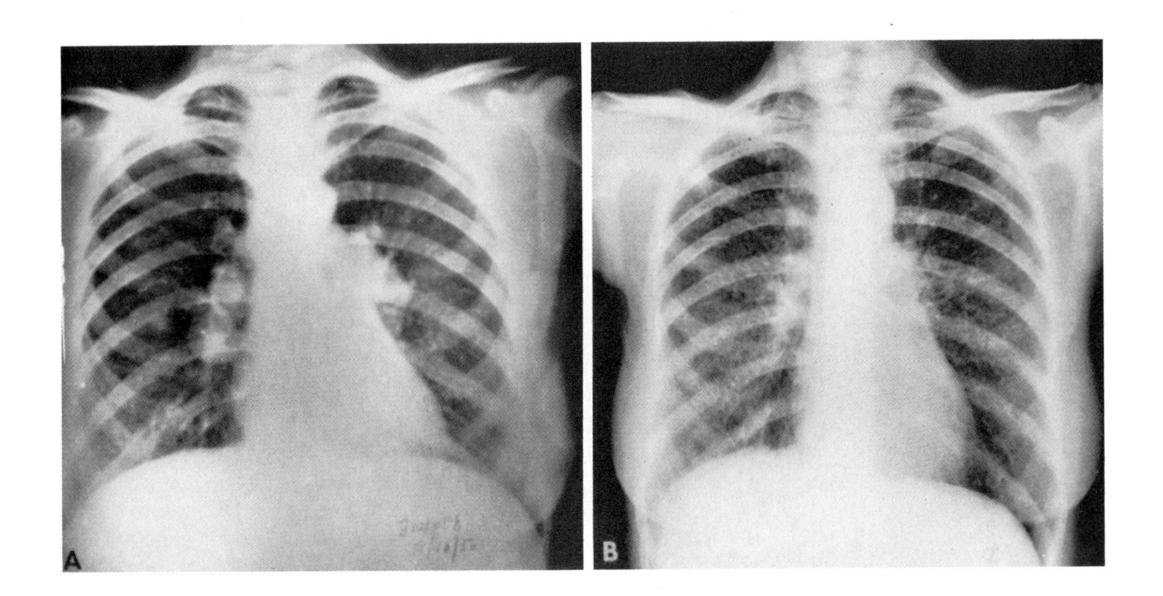

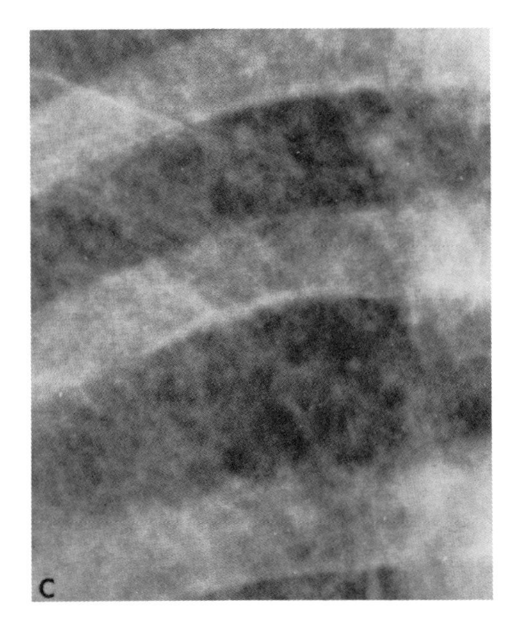

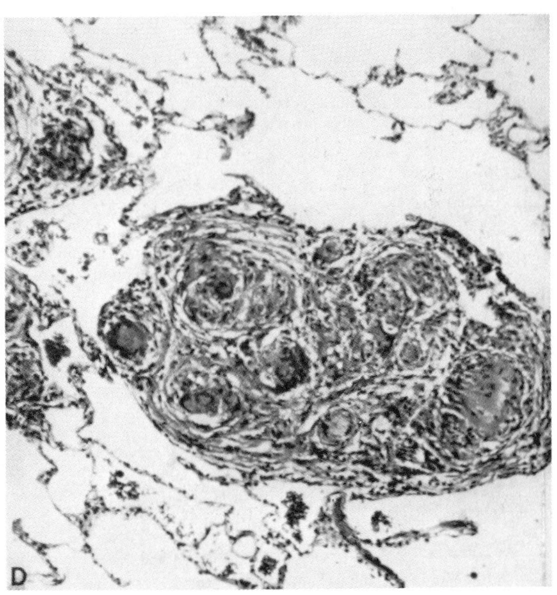

pinged upon by the granulomatous process. The lesions were diagnostic of sarcoid.

Summary. This case of sarcoidosis showed hilar lymphadenopathy without parenchymal lung involvement as judged radiologically, and nine years later diffuse pulmonary involvement without lymph-node enlargement. It is of interest that, during the first six months of treatment, ventilatory function improved but the diffusing capacity was unchanged. Four years later diffusing capacity had increased to normal values and the total lung capacity had increased from 3.7 to 4.1 liters.

Case 26
Sarcoidosis

Summary of Clinical Findings. In September, 1955, a routine chest x-ray of this 30-year-old male physician had shown a diffuse bilateral infiltration. At that time he was asymptomatic except for a rapid pulse rate noted on exertion. The only abnormal findings on physical examination were a few slightly enlarged lymph nodes in the right supraclavicular area and a pulse rate of 100/min. The chest was clear. Hb, WBC and sedimentation rate, urinalysis, plasma proteins and electrophoretic pattern were normal. Tuberculin (1/100) testing was negative. X-rays of the hands showed no abnormality. Three gastric washings were negative on culture. Supraclavicular glands on biopsy showed granuloma compatible with a diagnosis of sarcoid. The patient was treated with rest and started on streptomycin and isoniazid for two months. He remained fairly well except for a mild cough with light morning sputum and dyspnea with exertion.

Chest x-ray one year later (September, 1956) showed progression of the infiltration and he was given a three-month course of cortisone. The cough and dyspnea disappeared but returned with cessation of treatment. The chest x-ray showed no change.

In February, 1957, he began to notice night sweats and his temperature hovered around 99° F. The tuberculin test was repeated and was this time strongly positive at 1/100 dilution. Chest x-rays and pulmonary function studies were obtained (*below*) and he was readmitted in April. The only abnormal physical findings were a few pea-sized glands in the right posterior triangle of the neck. The chest was clear.

Sputum, gastric washings and bronchial lavage all grew *Mycobacterium tuberculosis*. Biopsy of a right supraclavicular lymph node revealed granulomatous inflammation typical of sarcoidosis. Alpha$_2$ globulin was increased on electrophoresis. Serum calcium and phosphorus were normal.

Treatment with PAS and INH was started and he was transferred to a sanatorium, from which he was discharged in May, 1958. The disease showed no further progression and he was able to return to work. His pulmonary function was last studied in 1968. He continues to work full-time as a family physician.

Radiology. In the x-ray taken in March, 1957, (*A*), both lungs were extensively involved by nodular densities which measured 2 to 3 mm in diameter and which were for the most part discrete. The right midlung field was more severely involved than elsewhere, to such an extent, in fact, that the densities were so numerous that they were confluent. The hila were largely obscured by the pulmonary disease so that the presence or absence of lymph-node enlargement could not be positively established. There was no pleural effusion.

By January, 1964, the character of the disease had changed remarkably (*B*). The massive involvement of the right lung had disappeared, but was replaced by a diffuse fine reticulation (not easily reproduced) which now occupied most of both lung fields and suggested diffuse fibrosis.

Summary. This case illustrates severe infiltrative involvement of the lungs by sarcoid radiologically, with evidence of superimposed active tuberculosis, and yet only slight disturbance of function. In fifteen years there has been a considerable improvement in the x-ray appearances but only minor changes in results of function tests.

	VC	FRC	RV	TLC	ME %	MMFR	$FEV_{0.75}$ ×40	pH^+	P_{CO_2}	HCO_3^-	P_{O_2}	O_2Hb %	$D_{Lco}SS_2$	CO Ext %	EXERCISE MPH	GRADE	$\dot{V}O_2$	$\dot{V}_E$	$D_{Lco}SS_3$
Predicted	4.9	3.7	1.9	6.8	65	4.3	140					97	22.4	50					34.2
March 1957	3.4	1.8	1.2	4.6	55	2.5	97					96*	14.7	43	2	FLAT	0.95	22.2	23.4
Jan. 1964	4.0	2.9	1.7	5.7	48	2.8	111						18.6	43					
Oct. 1968	4.2	3.0	2.0	6.2	54	2.6	113						16.6	43					

*Oximetric reading.

In March, 1957, (*see* chest x-ray *A*) the vital capacity was reduced and there was a marked reduction in the FRC. This reduction was associated with the lowered diffusing capacity, which was probably normal for the available lung surface area. For the same reason, while there was a rise in D_{co} with exercise, the value attained was lower than predicted. There was only slight reduction in flow rates as reflected in the MMFR and FEV.

By 1964, all the measurements had shown improvement. Although the resting D_{CO} had increased, the CO extraction was unchanged.

There was no further change four years later.

Sarcoidosis

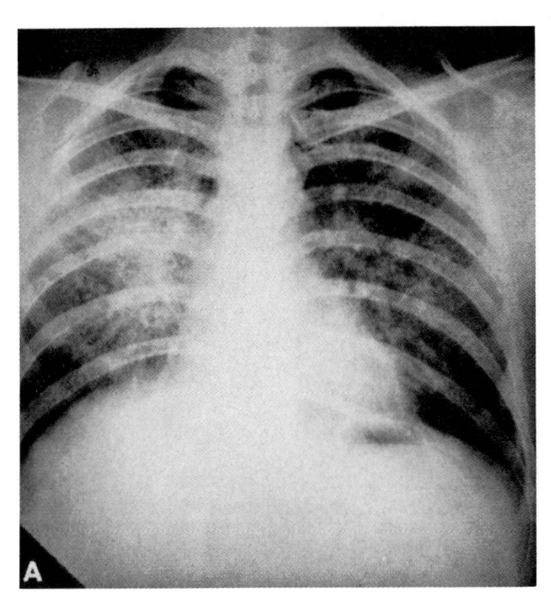

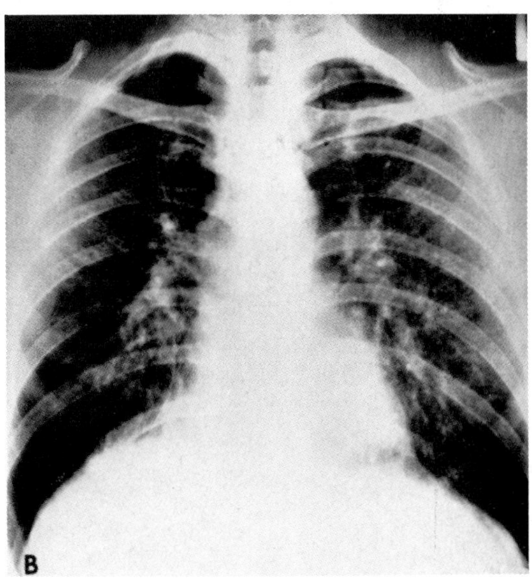

aspect of sarcoidosis has been studied in detail by Smellie, Apthorp and Marshall.[1407] In a study of 11 patients they found that treatment usually produced an improvement in vital capacity and in forced expiratory volume when this was reduced initially; it had little effect on an initially low compliance; and it produced a small increase in diffusing capacity, although not to normal levels. Four patients were shown radiologically to have moderate or considerable clearing with treatment, together with an increase in vital capacity, but there was no improvement in diffusing capacity. It is to be noted that these authors used both a steady-state method ($D_{Lco}SS_2$) as well as a single-breath technique ($D_{Lco}SB$). Wigderson and his co-workers documented a similar case, in which there was a very striking change in the radiological picture, accompanied by an increase in diffusing capacity from an original very low value of 3.9 ml CO/min/mm Hg to one of only 5.1 after almost complete clearing had occurred.[1408] Riley, Riley and Hill in 1952 described the same phenomenon, using the oxygen diffusing-capacity method, and commented on the disparity between the extent of radiological clearing and the minimal improvement in diffusing capacity.[418] An exception to this general pattern was the case of sarcoidosis described in detail by Cournand, in which the oxygen-diffusing capacity rose from 8 to 18 ml/min/mm Hg after treatment with cortisone.[1409]

More recently, Boushy and his colleagues[3076] followed 18 patients for 41 months and documented the common failure of the diffusing capacity to rise to normal levels in spite of clinical improvement. Other authors have made the same observation and have noted that when steroids are discontinued, any improvement in function that may have occurred[3084] commonly disappears.[3086] These factors underlie the comment by Doll and his co-workers that careful following of pulmonary function is obligatory if the effects of steroids in this disease are to be properly assessed,[3081] or if the clinician is to be warned early of a deterioration occurring without radiological change.[3722]

SUMMARY

The evidence, which has been briefly summarized in this chapter, leads to the inescapable conclusion that measurements of compliance and diffusing capacity—the latter preferably during exercise—are essential to the physician if he wishes to know how seriously the lung is involved in sarcoidosis. It has been made quite clear by all who have studied the problem that, in this disease, these objective methods of assessment are obligatory.[3081] Clinical papers, often excellent in their way,[1397, 1398] which discuss the treatment and prognosis of sarcoidosis of the lungs from a purely clinical standpoint cannot but provide an incomplete picture of the disease as a whole.

PULMONARY INVOLVEMENT IN THE COLLAGEN DISEASES

CHAPTER 14

INTRODUCTION

The classification of collagen diseases is both difficult and controversial, as are the relationships among them. There is even controversy about whether they should be called "collagen" diseases, since there is no certainty that they are really primarily diseases of collagen; some would prefer to call them the "group" diseases, a term we do not favor. If the various conditions constituting the collagen diseases are too rigidly defined, there is a danger of their being considered unrelated, which in turn hinders their understanding. Too loose a classification ignores the fact that often the syndromes can be defined precisely, with important therapeutic and prognostic implications. Eponymous diagnoses are often applied to syndromes different from those described originally, and apparently similar syndromes may be described as different conditions.

We have found the classification presented in this text to be useful in practice. It is not intended to be used as a rigid classification, and we recognize extensive overlap among the conditions, as illustrated in Figure 14–1. Interstitial fibrosis and pneumonitis are often related to the collagen diseases, but we have preferred to describe these elsewhere as a separate group (*see* Chapter 12). This has been done because the physiological and pathological features are similar; if, however, we were primarily interested in etiology, this group should be considered here. We have also chosen to include Löffler's syndrome in this chapter, although by our definition it is unrelated to the collagen diseases; this has been done because eosinophilic pneumonitis is often a feature of periarteritis, and early in

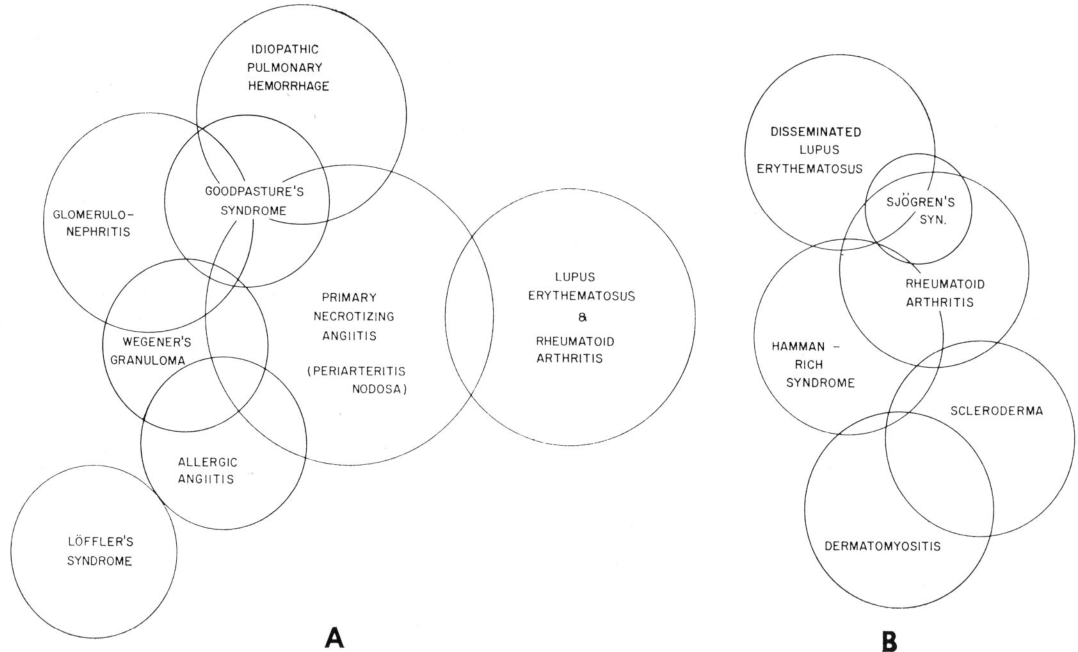

FIGURE 14–1. Diagrammatic Illustration of the Interrelationships of the Collagen Diseases.

A, The vasculitis syndrome.
B, Syndromes associated with pulmonary fibrosis or pneumonitis.

the course of Löffler's syndrome it may not be apparent whether the patient has this benign condition or has a fatal collagen disease.

THE COLLAGEN DISEASES

Periarteritis nodosa (primary necrotizing angiitis)

Widespread necrotizing angiitis without known cause is the dominant lesion in this condition. Rose and Spencer[1412, 1554] in 1957 suggested that patients with this disease might be best classified in two groups: those in whom the lungs were not involved (about two thirds of their cases), and those with lung involvement (about one third). A history of respiratory infection was not uncommon in the latter group, and clinically the main features were bronchospasm (and even attacks of asthma), pneumonia resistant to antibiotic treatment, hemoptysis, and apparent chronic bronchitis. In some patients the lung lesions progressed to severe destruction, individual cases featuring nodular interstitial lesions, hemorrhagic pneumonia, cavities in necrotic lung, extensive infarction and severe bronchiectasis.

Rose and Spencer's classification is useful but perhaps oversimplified. From the pathological point of view, the following subdivisions of this category are useful:

1. *Periarteritis nodosa.*[1555] In this condition, small and medium-sized muscular arteries especially are involved, often at the site of bifurcation or division. Lesions occur commonly in the wall of the gastrointestinal tract near the mesenteric attachment, in the pancreas, kidneys, and striated muscles, and near nerves; they are generally widespread, and in many cases the lungs are spared. Healing and healed lesions are often seen, usually involving only part of the vessel wall; aneurysms may form at this stage. Polyneuritis and involvement of many organs is the rule, and hypertension is commonly present. The illness may last for several months or years.

2. *Hypersensitivity angiitis.*[1555] Widespread necrosis of small vessels—arterioles, venules, and capillaries—occurs in this variant. All the lesions are of approximately the same age. The heart and kidneys are predominantly affected, and necrotizing glomerulonephritis is common. Pulmonary arterioles may be involved, whereas vessels in the pancreas and gastrointestinal tract are usually spared. The

course of the disease is brief, lasting a few days to a few weeks, and may be related to hypersensitivity to serum or sulfonamides or other drugs. This form of necrotizing angiitis is closely related to Goodpasture's syndrome (*see* page 306).

3. *Allergic angiitis.*[1556] In this condition, vessels of any size may be affected, but small arteries and veins are the most usual site. Vessel involvement is widespread, often including the heart and lungs. The lesions are of various ages, typically granulomatous, with a striking eosinophilic infiltration; multinucleated giant cells may be present. Extravascular granulomata of similar appearance are usually observed in serous membranes and connective tissue. Eosinophilic pneumonitis may occur. The clinical course is often of months to years, and asthma and other allergic manifestations are prominent clinical findings. Wanke[3094] has recently studied the pulmonary vasculature in detail in these conditions and has emphasized the importance of early intimal hyperplasia in the elastic arteries.

As with all of the collagen diseases, the x-ray manifestations of polyarteritis are extremely varied, but certain characteristics appear with sufficient frequency that their presence should suggest the possibility of this diagnosis. A changing roentgenographic picture is certainly suggestive, progression and regression of lesions in serial films reflecting the appearance of new lesions and the healing of old.[3095] Increased size in the hilar vascular complex, especially if associated with a pattern of pulmonary edema, is almost pathognomonic of polyarteritis in the collagen group of diseases. Pleural effusions may occur, but are not common, although nonspecific cardiac enlargement probably associated with pericardial effusion is often seen. Small nodular lesions may appear throughout the lung fields. Areas of consolidation in various areas of the lungs may be due to pneumonitis or to infarcts, and patchy, fleeting consolidation of nonsegmental distribution, identical to the pattern of Löffler's syndrome, may occur. Pulmonary lesions of one sort or another occur in about a third of all cases of periarteritis.[3093]

It seems quite evident that severe defects of pulmonary function will be present in many of those patients whose lungs are involved, and it is equally clear that the clinical presentation and the lung pathology may vary very widely from patient to patient and at different stages of the disease. Initially there may be some interference with gas exchange, and we have observed severe cyanosis and hypocapnea with gross hyperventilation in a boy of 14 with an acute allergic angiitis involving the lungs. However, data presently available are inadequate for formulation of a general account of the interrelationship between function and the changes seen on x-ray in this disorder. Rose[1412] comments that in some patients with periarteritis nodosa the lung lesions precede by many years those in other organs, and it may be that the demonstration of abnormalities of pulmonary function, particularly of diffusion, might be of value in diagnosis, especially if this defect appears out of proportion to the change observed radiologically.

LÖFFLER'S SYNDROME (PULMONARY EOSINOPHILIA)

We believe that the diagnosis of the syndrome described by Löffler[1413] should be restricted to those cases in which the radiological shadows of pulmonary infiltration are transient, often shifting from day to day; in which very high eosinophil counts are found; and in which there are few other symptoms, no renal involvement, and almost always full resolution.[1415] It has been suggested that the syndrome is due to migration through the lung of the larvae of *Ascaris lumbricoides,* but it is probable that there are other causes. In our experience the eosinophilia is very variable even from hour to hour, and several blood counts must be made before the absence of significant eosinophilia can be assured. Pulmonary infiltration accompanied by eosinophilia in the blood may occur in periarteritis, particularly allergic angiitis, but it is important to distinguish this disorder from the benign condition, Löffler's syndrome as we have defined it.

The two major radiological criteria of Löffler's syndrome are the fleeting nature of the pulmonary infiltrations and their nonsegmental distribution within the lungs. The densities may be large and are commonly ill defined and of homogeneous density. Associated abnormalities within the thorax, such as pleural effusion or cardiac enlargement, are lacking. The radiological picture should cause little difficulty in diagnosis, especially if serial films are available to allow assessment

(Text continued on page 306.)

Case 27
Löffler's Syndrome; Chronic Bronchitis

Summary of Clinical Findings. This 48-year-old electrician was admitted to hospital in September 1947 complaining of a recent 20-pound loss of weight, night sweats and flushes and general malaise. He denied cough. The only remarkable physical findings were areas of reduced breath sounds and fine rales on deep inspiration, over the right middle lobe and the left anterior chest at the anterior axillary line.

Urinalysis was normal, but a hemogram showed a Hb of 82 per cent; ESR, 41 mm/hr; and a total white-cell count of 22,000/cmm, with 44 per cent eosinophils. Radiographs of the chest revealed scattered areas of increased density over the left midlung field and right middle lobe. Nine days later these infiltrations had disappeared and similar lesions were now present in both lower lobes. A diagnosis of Löffler's syndrome was made and the patient was treated with Pyribenzamine. Since that time he has had several admissions to hospital with similar symptoms accompanied by transient shadows in the lung and an eosinophilia.

In 1957 he began to develop exertional dyspnea and a cough productive of yellow to brown sputum. These symptoms were quite variable in severity. In February, 1959, he had an attack of bronchitis, and at that time the lung parenchyma was radiologically clear. His cough was severe, however, and was accompanied by much wheezing and clinical evidence of bronchial obstruction.

In February, 1960, he was admitted because of dyspnea and on investigation was found to have a high but fluctuating eosinophilia and patchy infiltrations in the lung (*see* Figure *A*). He had little clinical bronchitis at this time, however. By April, 1960, the chest x-ray was clear, the bronchitis was not troublesome and he was symptom-free. He has had no further attacks of bronchitis or of pulmonary infiltration.

Radiology. The film of February, 1960, (*A*) shows numerous patchy, indistinctly defined densities of varying size scattered widely throughout both lungs. None of the densities possesses a specific anatomical segmental distribution, a fact which is particularly evident on the lateral projection (not reproduced). The heart is not enlarged and there is no pleural effusion. Films made during the days immediately preceding and following this x-ray revealed a remarkable change in the distribution of the densities from day to day, large areas of consolidation clearing rapidly and others appearing equally rapidly elsewhere.

Ten days later (*B*), the lungs have almost completely cleared, leaving no significant residue. In April also the chest film was clear.

The combination of large areas of consolidation of indistinct definition, possessing no specific anatomical distribution and undergoing rapid change from day to day is distinctive of transient focal pulmonary eosinophilia or Löffler's syndrome.

Summary. The changes in clinical and functional state in this man who at first had chronic bronchitis with airway obstruction but a normal diffusing capacity, and then Löffler's syndrome with normal ventilatory ability but an impaired diffusing capacity, and finally complete resolution of both lesions illustrate the independence of ventilatory and gas-exchange function in the lung.

	VC	FRC	RV	TLC	ME %	MMFR	$FEV_{0.75}$ ×40	pH	P_{CO_2}	HCO_3^-	O_2Hb %	$D_{Lco}SS_2$	CO Ext %
Predicted	3.7	3.5	2.2	5.9	50	3.0	90	7.40	42	25	97	13.7	40
Feb. 1959	3.8	3.5	2.5	6.3	42	1.0	58	7.45	46	26	95	13.8	38
Feb. 1960	3.0	2.2	1.1	4.1	49	3.1	87	7.43	40	25	96	10.0	28
April 1960	4.0	2.9	2.1	6.1	57	2.5	102					18.1	37

In February, 1959, when he had clinically severe bronchitis, there was considerable ventilatory obstruction, but a normal diffusing capacity. In February, 1960, when there were many patchy pulmonary infiltrations and an eosinophilia (*see* Figure *A*), there was no ventilatory defect, but the FRC and TLC had fallen and the resting diffusing capacity had fallen. The arterial blood was normal, however. Resolution of the infiltration by April of 1960 (*B*) was accompanied by restoration of the diffusing capacity, and the vital capacity and total lung capacity returned to normal. The arterial blood was normal throughout.

Löffler's Syndrome; Chronic Bronchitis

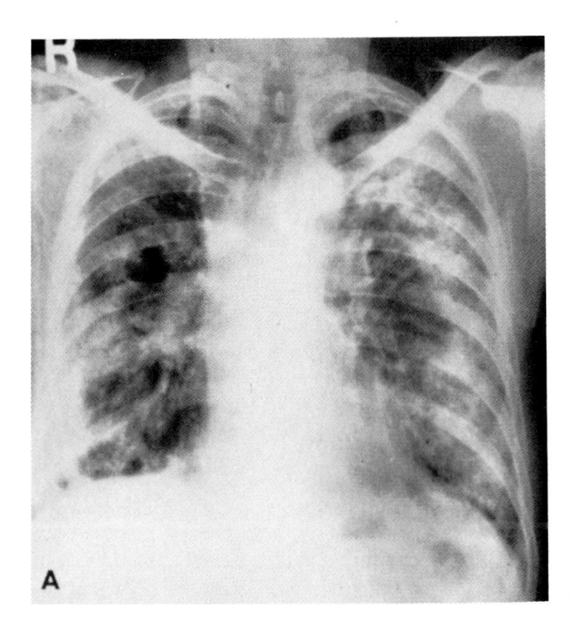

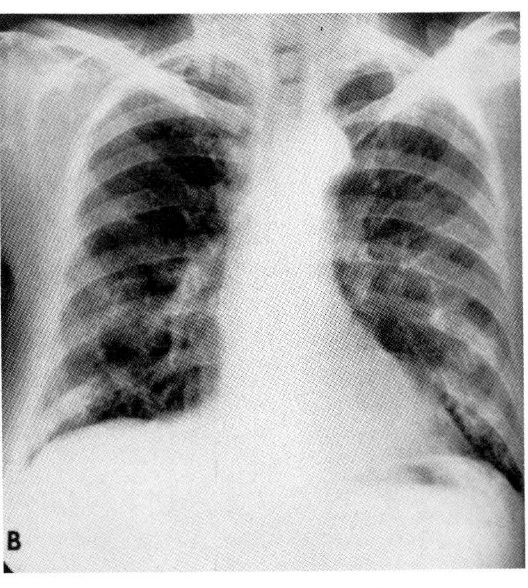

Case 28
Rheumatoid Lung

Summary of Clinical Findings. This 70-year-old spinster was last admitted to the hospital in March, 1969. She had had several previous admissions to hospital for diabetes mellitus and rheumatoid arthritis. The former was diagnosed in 1956 and she had been managed since on insulin and diet. She first complained of joint pain and swelling of the hands in 1961 and since then had had pain and stiffness involving most of her joints. She had also developed nodules at the elbows. Rheumatoid factor has been present in her serum since 1964. LE cells have always been absent. Steroids have been used continuously since 1964 with moderately good control of the arthritis.

During her first admission in 1956 she complained of mild shortness of breath on exertion such as walking six or seven blocks, and chest x-ray revealed increased bronchovascular markings over the lower lobes. By 1961 a "lace-like" pattern was described in the chest x-ray. Her shortness of breath very gradually increased and by 1967 she could only walk a block on the level. On her final admission she felt dyspneic upon any exertion. Pulmonary function had been studied on several occasions and these are reported below. She had smoked 10 to 15 cigarettes for many years and had a morning cough productive of small amounts of white sputum. Clubbing of fingers and toes had been noted since 1964. The final admission was precipitated by recent fever, purulent sputum and increased shortness of breath.

On examination she looked younger than her stated age, but was in moderate respiratory distress. There was no cyanosis. There was clubbing of fingers and toes. Her blood pressure was 130/70; pulse rate was 100; temperature was 100-102; and respiration rate was 36/min. The AP diameter of the chest was increased. Breath sounds were well heard and fine inspiratory and expiratory rales were heard throughout both lung fields. There were no signs of congestive failure. There were soft mobile nodules at both elbows. The small muscles of the hands were atrophied and there was slight ulnar deviation of the fingers. There was tenderness but only mild swelling of the joints of the hands and feet, wrists, ankles, elbows, and knees. There was only slight restriction of movement.

Investigation revealed a white blood count of 15,000, mature neutrophils 75 per cent; hemoglobin was 11.0 gm; hematocrit was 35; sedimentation rate was 42. Urinalysis was negative. Sputum grew staph pyogenes. Rheumatoid factor was again present. Serum electrophoresis showed a severe reduction in albumin and increase in alpha$_1$, alpha$_2$, and gamma globulins. Chest x-ray revealed a right-sided pneumonia superimposed on the diffuse changes described below. She was treated with antibiotics, resulting in gradual resolution of the pneumonia.

Radiology. The roentgenogram (*A*) in December, 1956, shows a fine reticular pattern localized

	VC	FRC	RV	TLC	ME %	MMFR	$FEV_{0.75}$ ×40	pH	P_{CO_2}	HCO_3^-	P_{O_2}	O_2Hb %	CO Ext %	$D_{LCO}SS_2$
Predicted	3.1	3.0	2.1	5.2	46	1.9	67	7.40	40	25	80	96	36	8.9
Feb. 1967	2.0	2.6	1.7	3.7	45	3.1	78	7.46	40	29	61	92	25	5.9
April 1969	1.7	3.0	2.2	3.9	37	1.6	50	7.46	44	31	65	93	9	2.4

In February, 1967, this patient showed a generalized reduction in lung volumes and a low diffusing capacity. The flow rates were higher than predicted. Two years later the flow rates had fallen, although still within predicted levels, but the diffusing capacity was extremely low. Blood gas determinations showed a mild hypoxemia without hypercapnia on both occasions.

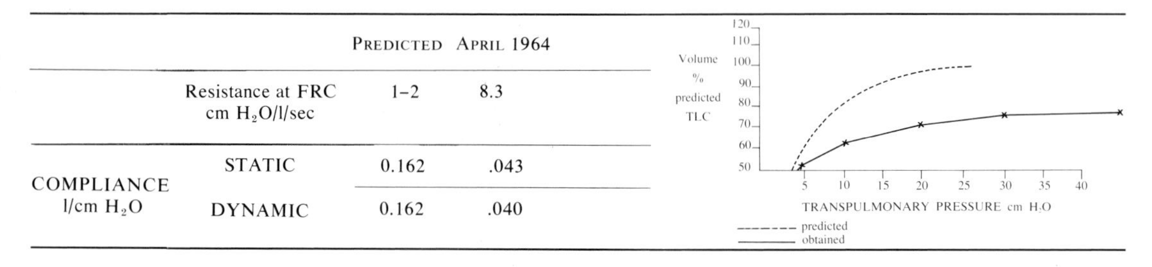

		PREDICTED	APRIL 1964
	Resistance at FRC cm H_2O/l/sec	1–2	8.3
COMPLIANCE l/cm H_2O	STATIC	0.162	.043
	DYNAMIC	0.162	.040

This patient showed increased resistance and decreased compliance, indicating both obstructive and restrictive disease.

Rheumatoid Lung

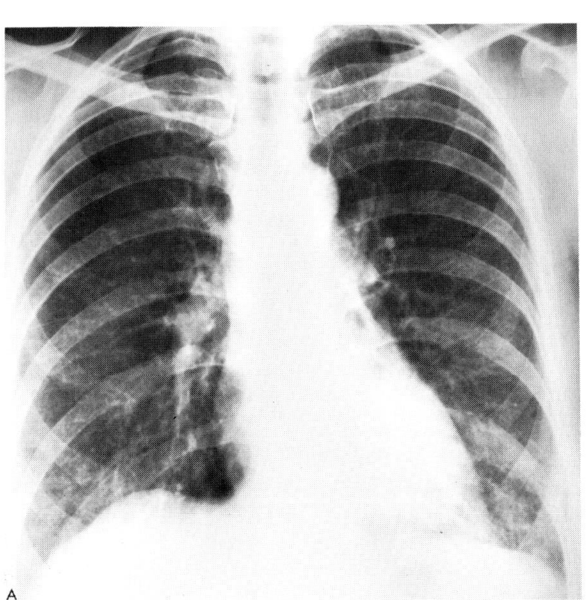

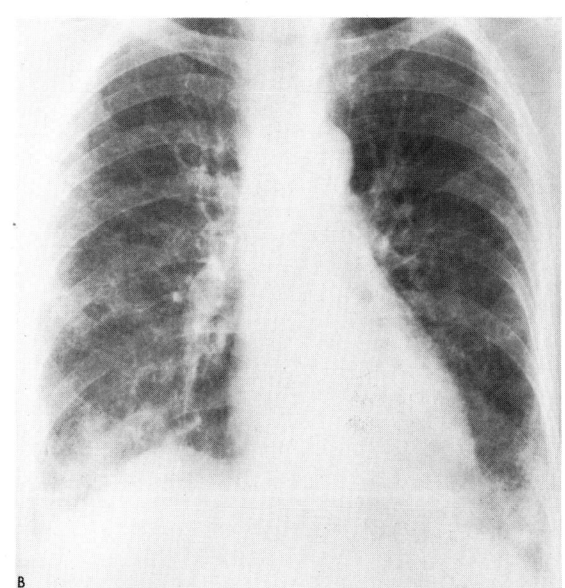

to the lung bases. A diagnosis was not made at this time and no further roentgenographic examinations of the chest were performed until eight years later when the patient first noted the coincident onset of dyspnea on exertion and peripheral arthralgia. At this time, a posteroanterior roentgenogram (*B*) revealed diffuse involvement of both lungs by a rather fine reticular pattern more marked in the bases than elsewhere. Thirteen years after the first roentgenographic study the reticulation has become much coarser and now resembles a small honeycomb pattern (*C*). Note that in this 13-year interval, there has been a progressive loss of lung volume.

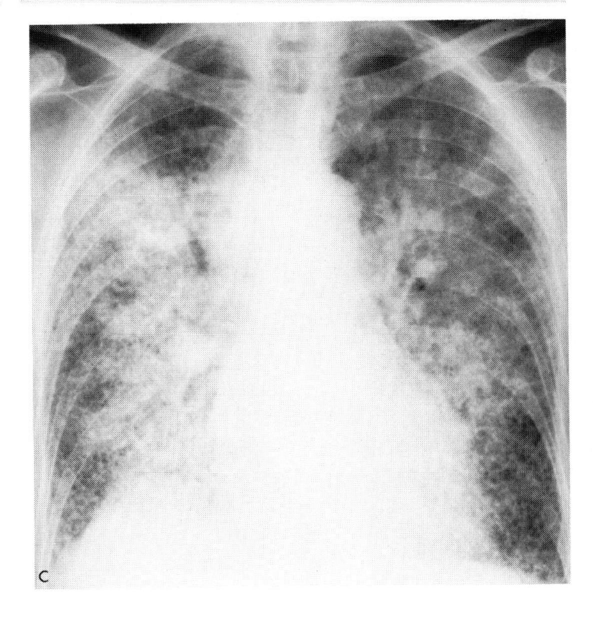

Summary. The onset of rheumatoid arthritis was preceded by the appearance of a reticular pattern in the chest roentgenogram. This became associated with dyspnea on slight exertion and a reduction in lung volumes, with a low diffusing capacity.

of the shifting, fleeting nature of the parenchymal disease.

We are unaware of any studies in which tests of pulmonary function have been reported in this syndrome, with the exception of that of the patient described by Eldridge,[1414] in whom a transient diffusion defect was documented. Our experience in studying two patients, one of whom is presented in Case 27, confirms this observation. It is to be assumed that the fall in diffusing capacity reflects virtual shutting-off of those areas involved in the patchy pneumonitis that is the characteristic feature of this condition.

Pulmonary eosinophilia may also be a presenting symptom of necrotizing angiitis, in which case the pathological findings are those of the underlying disorder. The morphological findings in pulmonary eosinophilia not associated with necrotizing angiitis are poorly described, since the lesion is rarely, if ever, fatal. Von Meyenburg, in a study of four such patients who died of other causes, found an extensive infiltration with eosinophils, particularly in the interstitial tissue, but also in the bronchi and alveolar spaces.[1557] Histiocytic proliferation and foreign-body giant cells also were seen.

GOODPASTURE'S SYNDROME (ACUTE HEMORRHAGIC PNEUMONITIS AND NEPHRITIS)

First described by Goodpasture, in 1919,[1416] the syndrome of glomerulonephritis and clinically apparent intrapulmonary hemorrhage and hemosiderosis generally bears his name. However, it is clear that nephritis and pulmonary hemorrhage may occur at some time in the course of idiopathic pulmonary hemorrhage, glomerulonephritis,[1559] or necrotizing angiitis; indeed, necrotizing angiitis was present in Goodpasture's first case. Any of these diagnoses may be applied to a case of nephritis with pulmonary hemorrhage, and may be dependent upon the relative severity or the time sequence of the two components. Thus, there is reason to question the necessity for recognizing Goodpasture's syndrome as a separate entity.[3103] However, we feel that there are two reasons for using the term. First, some consider that the morphological findings in the lungs are distinctive.[1558] Second, it provides a convenient designation for patients who cannot be adequately diagnosed as having either nephritis or idiopathic pulmonary hemorrhage alone, and in whom there is no evidence of necrotizing angiitis during life.

Recent reviews of published cases[3099, 3105] reveal that the male/female ratio was 89/16 in the 105 cases published up to 1966; that the syndrome has occurred in a nine-year-old child,[3097] and that the course may be fulminating[3107] and, very rarely, a remission may occur.[3098]

At autopsy, the lungs are heavy and dark, with varying degrees of intra-alveolar hemorrhage and hemosiderin deposition. Alveolitis has been described in many of the cases,[1418, 1558–1560, 3104] particularly when hemorrhage predominates over hemosiderosis; it may be widespread or focal and typically occurs in areas of severe hemorrhage. There may be difficulty in differentiating it from reaction to hemorrhage or coincidental infection, but it appears to be a specific condition.[1418] Swelling of the alveolar lining cells, focal hypercellularity of the alveoli and tortuosity of the capillaries have been observed. Electron microscopy studies have revealed that the primary change involves the membrane and the alveolar lining, and the capillary endothelial cells are said not to be abnormal initially.[3100] The typical kidney lesion is that of a focal or diffuse necrotizing glomerulonephritis (the form of nephritis often encountered in necrotizing angiitis) or a fulminating subacute glomerulonephritis. Necrotizing angiitis in other vessels is commonly seen in this syndrome.[1418, 1558–1560]

The radiological signs in the thorax in this syndrome are indistinguishable from those of idiopathic pulmonary hemosiderosis.[3101] They consist of the development of numerous patchy densities throughout both lung fields, varying in size from 2 or 3 mm up to 3 cm in diameter, which appear rapidly and generally clear completely within a period of 7 or 8 days. They are usually rather indistinctly defined and may be partly confluent. In most cases there are no associated changes within the thorax, such as pleural effusions or cardiac enlargement. Atypical cases have been described;[3102, 3105] in one patient the lesions were apparently unilateral.[3096]

We have had an opportunity of studying the pulmonary function in only one such patient, described in Case 31, and we do not know whether our findings are representative of those commonly encountered in this condition. There seems little doubt that partial resolution of the lung lesions may occur, the eventual course being determined mainly by the severity of the renal involvement.

WEGENER'S GRANULOMATOSIS

The distinctive feature of this condition is the presence of aggressive, destructive, granulomatous lesions in the upper and lower respiratory tract. Since the original descriptions of Klinger[1564] and of Wegener[1565] included glomerulonephritis and necrotizing angiitis, these findings are generally considered necessary to the diagnosis. We feel, however, that the lesions in the upper or lower respiratory tract may be so distinctive that the syndrome can be diagnosed in the absence of renal involvement or of necrotizing angiitis. This syndrome has been excellently described and summarized by Walton,[1419] and many useful case reports and reviews have been published.[1561–1563] Varying degrees of sinus involvement occur, from relatively slight symptoms to severe tissue destruction, and there is almost invariable and often severe renal involvement.[1420] Variable respiratory symptoms may be related to the presence of discrete, large, rounded granulomata in the lung[1421] which on x-ray may resemble secondary malignant deposits. In a useful review of the condition, Kuntz and his colleagues collected 132 cases from the literature, with a male/female ratio of 62/38 per cent and a peak incidence between the ages of 40 and 50.[3111]

Typical granulomata show a central area of necrosis surrounded by granulation tissue in which epithelioid cells may be scanty but foreign-body and Langhans' giant cells are commonly found. Nodules in the lung measure less than 1 cm to more than 10 cm in diameter; usually they are scanty and well circumscribed. Necrotizing pulmonary vasculitis has been described as a frequent finding,[3111] but in our experience it is not a constant feature. Changes in the intervening parenchyma are nonspecific, although pulmonary infarcts are frequent. Extensive pulmonary hemorrhage has been described,[1566, 1567] and we have seen this in three cases. Necrotizing glomerulitis is the usual renal finding, and vascular lesions are usually found in other organs.

There is much confusion in the diagnostic criteria of this condition. The lesions and clinical features of Wegener's granulomatosis and allergic angiitis are similar, as can be seen by comparing the published illustrations of these two conditions,[1556, 1561] and by the fact that sinus disease was noted to be present in 10 out of 13 cases of allergic angiitis.[1556] The term "allergic angiitis" as used by Zeek[1555] would appear to include both conditions, as does Rose and Spencer's term "polyarteritis nodosa with lung involvement."[1554] The main distinguishing features appear to be the presence of bronchospasm and extensive tissue eosinophilia in the periarteritis syndrome, and of multiple aggressive extravascular granulomata in Wegener's granulomatosis.

Although the classic appearance in the lungs of solitary or multiple nodules or infiltrations with central cavitation should suggest the diagnosis of Wegener's granulomatosis, especially when associated with sinusitis, the roentgen manifestations of this disease may be extremely varied. The chest film is not uncommonly normal initially and may remain so until death. Nonspecific changes, such as bronchopneumonia, pulmonary infarction, and pulmonary congestion and edema, are not uncommon. The typical nodular lesions vary in diameter from 1 to 8 cm, and may be solitary or multiple, but when multiple are seldom numerous. Cavitation in some of the lesions is also extremely variable; they may increase in size and number or they may remain static; occasionally they may disappear completely, with or without the appearance of new lesions in other portions of the lungs. Chlorambucil has recently been reported to have a favorable effect on the course of the disease.[3109]

We are unaware of any systematic data on disturbances of pulmonary function in Wegener's syndrome, though it appears very probable that little interference would be caused by the pulmonary lesions in some of the reported cases, at least at the stage when these are circumscribed (*see* Case 30). In others, there may be disruption of function as severe as that seen in terminal cases of periarteritis nodosa.

Leak and Clein have recently documented impairment of gas exchange in a patient with Wegener's granulomatosis in partial remission.[3108]

(Text continued on page 313.)

Case 29
Systemic Lupus Erythematosus

Summary of Clinical Findings. This 16-year-old white female was admitted to the Royal Edward Chest Hospital in September, 1967. In July of 1967, on the morning following an afternoon of swimming and exposure to the sun, the patient awoke with fever and pain in both shoulders and anterior chest. She was given antibiotics and the symptoms disappeared in a few days. In August she developed painful swelling of both ankles and an afternoon fever of 102° to 104°. The febrile periods were accompanied by pain in both shoulders and she developed pain and swelling of both knees. She became anorexic, tired and listless, amenorrheic, and had lost 24 lbs. by the time of her admission in September. She had noted increasing exertional shortness of breath during the same period and on admission was breathless after one flight of stairs. She described a vague left anterior chest pain increased by deep breathing. She had had the usual childhood illness. There had been no skin rashes.

On examination she was slightly obese with a dorsal kyphosis. There were no skin rashes. Her temperature was 98.6°; pulse rate was 96 and regular; blood pressure was 110/76. The chest moved symmetrically, air entry was good, and there were no adventitious sounds. The remainder of her examination was normal.

On investigation she was anemic, hemoglobin was 8.3 gm%; hematocrit was 27; reticulocyte count was 3.1%; sedimentation rate was 3.1; white blood count was 4000 with a lymphocytopenia. Urinalysis showed albuminuria, but microscopic examination was negative. Creatinine level was 1.1 mgm%; BUN equalled 8.7 mgm%. ECG showed voltage T wave in all leads. Chest x-rays and pulmonary function are shown below. Three LE cell preparations were positive; anti-nuclear and rheumatoid factor were present.

The patient was transferred to the Royal Victoria Hospital for further study. The above findings were confirmed and pulmonary mechanics investigated. The patient was started on high doses of prednisone, and the fever and joint pain promptly disappeared.

Her course was complicated by the development of a Cushingoid appearance and aseptic necrosis of both hips. Steroids were tapered, and Imuran was started in December. She was admitted for assessment and renal biopsy in 1968. Fever recurred while she was in the hospital, again necessitating steroid treatment. The renal biopsy

	VC	FRC	RV	TLC	ME %	MMFR	$FEV_{0.75}$ ×40	pH^+	P_{CO_2}	HCO_3	P_{O_2}	O_2Hb %	$D_{L_{CO}}SS_2$	CO Ext %
Predicted	3.5	2.5	1.3	4.8	76	3.9	103	7.40	40	25	80	96	19.7	56
9/25/67	0.8	1.3	1.1	1.9	66	1.9	27	7.43	39	26	70	94	7.2	31
3/21/68	1.8	1.1	0.6	2.4	46	2.5	65						7.8	26
9/4/69	2.3	1.6	1.0	3.3	67	3.1	82						8.7	31

In 1967 this patient showed severe reduction in all subdivisions of lung volume with corresponding decreases in flow and diffusing capacity. In 1968 there had been a significant increase in vital capacity with a similar improvement in flow. She was mildly hypoxemic in 1967, without CO_2 retention. In September, 1969, there had been further improvement in lung volume and a slight increase in diffusing capacity. Flow rates were within normal limits.

		Predicted	6/29/67
	Resistance at FRC cm H_2O/l/sec	1–2	3.7
	STATIC	0.10	0.05
COMPLIANCE l/cm H_2O	DYNAMIC	RESP/min 22	0.05
		40	0.047
		54	0.050
		180	0.050

Resistance was increased for a girl of this age. The compliance was reduced but did not fall as the frequency of breathing decreased. The pressure-volume curve indicated increased elastic recoil, even though the maximal static intrapleural pressure was reduced. These results indicate severe restrictive lung disease with some obstruction.

Systemic Lupus Erythematosus

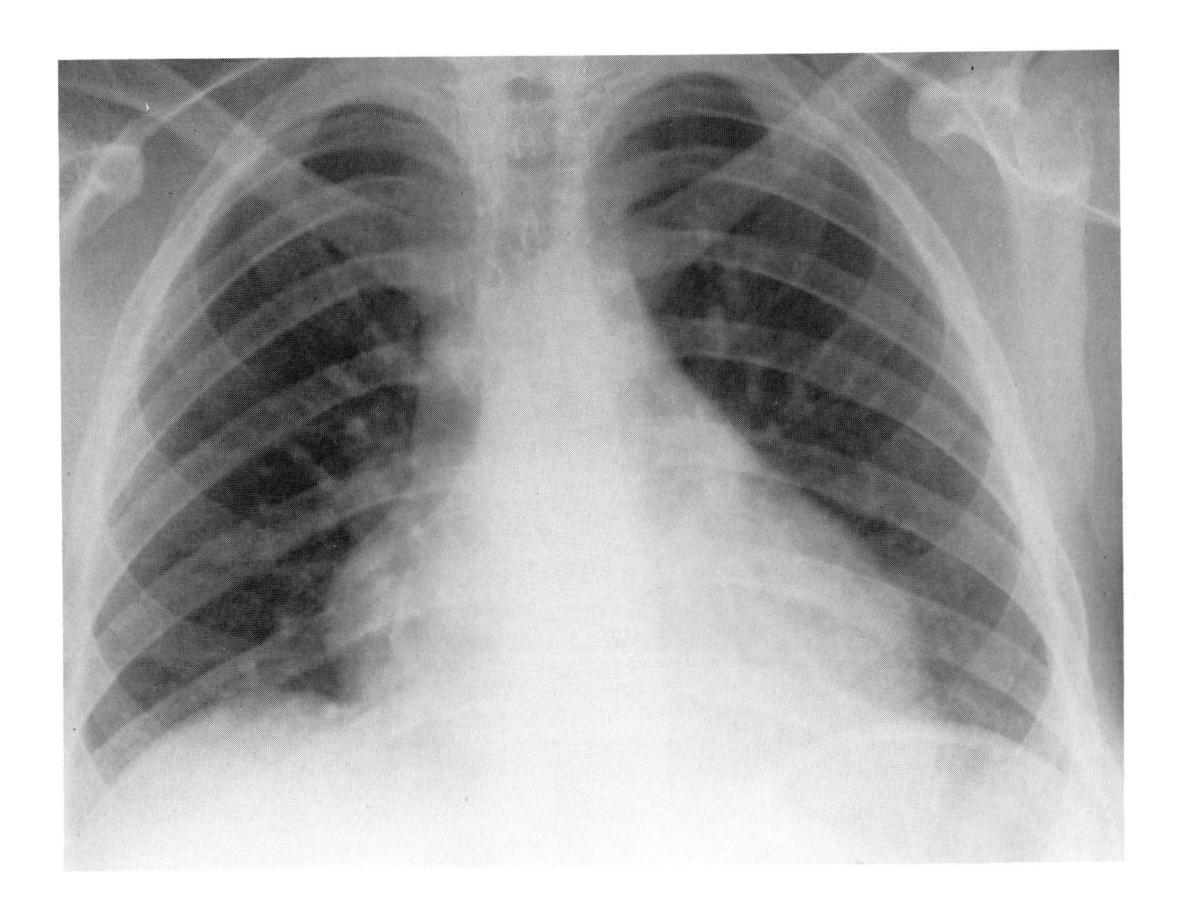

showed focal glomerulonephritis consistent with mild lupus nephritis.

She was admitted because of fever in August, 1969. She still noted dyspnea after one flight of stairs and was bothered by hip pain. Pulmonary function is shown. The fever subsided when steroids were increased and she was discharged early in September.

Radiology. A posteroanterior roentgenogram in September, 1967, shows a very small lung volume but no other evidence of diffuse pulmonary disease.

Summary. This patient with systemic lupus erythematosus and increasing dyspnea on exertion showed a reduction in all subdivisions of lung volume and a low diffusing capacity. The compliance of the lung was reduced. The x-ray confirmed the small lung volume but gave no evidence of diffuse pulmonary disease.

Case 30
Wegener's Granulomatosis

Summary of Clinical Findings. This 71-year-old metal inspector was admitted to the hospital in 1964, complaining of frontal headache and nasal obstruction of about six-months' duration, with recent bloody rhinorrhea. His past history was unremarkable with the exception of a possible myocardial infarction in 1958.

Examination was normal except for nasal mucosal congestion and erosion. The chest was clear.

Hemogram and urinalysis were negative. Microscopic examination of the urine revealed a few hyaline and granular casts but no red cells or red-cell casts. Other biochemical investigations, including BUN and creatinine clearances, were normal. Pulmonary function and chest x-ray are shown. A nasal mucosal biopsy and lung biopsy showed changes consistent with Wegener's granulomatosis. A renal biopsy was normal.

On prednisone the patient felt better and the chest x-ray improved. When an attempt was made to reduce the dose of prednisone the pulmonary lesions progressed to cavitation. The steroids were again increased and in January, 1965, Imuran, 450 mgm/day, was started. Again marked symptomatic and radiological improvement was noted. The patient's subsequent course was complicated by a pneumonia in March, 1965, and an infection in the left knee in January, 1966. The prednisone and Imuran were maintained, the latter at a dose of 150 mgm/day.

In July, 1966, the patient suffered a myocardial infarction, and the remainder of his life was punctuated by episodes of congestive failure and pyogenic infections involving the skin. Chest x-rays and pulmonary function were followed. Renal function remained normal.

The final admission was in April, 1967, for symptoms of cardiac failure. On the third day of hospitalization he developed left chest pain, hypotension, and oliguria and three days later died suddenly.

Radiology. A posteroanterior roentgenogram (*A*) in December, 1964, shows multiple well-defined nodules throughout both lungs, at least one of which had undergone cavitation.

In January, 1965, an anteroposterior tomogram (*B*) shows multiple thick-walled cavities scattered throughout both lungs but predominantly in the upper zones. The lesions range from 1.5 to 3 cm and are rather thick-walled. At least three lesions show no evidence of cavitation.

Corticosteroid and Imuran therapy resulted in gradual disappearance of these shadows over the subsequent months to a point at which only a small scar was identifiable in the right lung (*C*).

Final Admission. This 71-year-old male, with a three-year-old diagnosis of Wegener's granuloma, was admitted with dyspnea and ankle swelling. He had been on Imuran, prednisone, digoxin, and thiomerin. On the evening of admission he complained of chest pain and became hypotensive. He then developed anuria, cyanosis, and marked hyperventilation. His blood gases showed markedly reduced bicarbonates and P_{CO_2}. He was thought to be dehydrated. He continued to have episodes of dyspnea. He was found to have marked systemic lactic acidosis and died.

(Case report continued on page 312.)

	VC	FRC	RV	TLC	ME %	MMFR	$FEV_{0.75}$ ×40	pH^+	P_{CO_2}	HCO_3	P_{O_2}	O_2Hb %	$D_{Lco}SS_2$	CO Ext %
Predicted	3.8	3.7	2.4	6.2	47	2.8	88						11.1	36
Aug. 1964	3.3	3.7	2.7	6.0	49	3.0	98						17.0	38
Jan. 1966	3.1	3.4	2.2	5.3	37	3.1	91						11.3	30
Sept. 1967	3.1	3.9	2.7	5.8	34	3.2	103						9.1	27

In 1964 this patient showed normal function. Over the next three years there was a progressive fall in diffusing capacity, but other indices of function remained unchanged.

Wegener's Granulomatosis

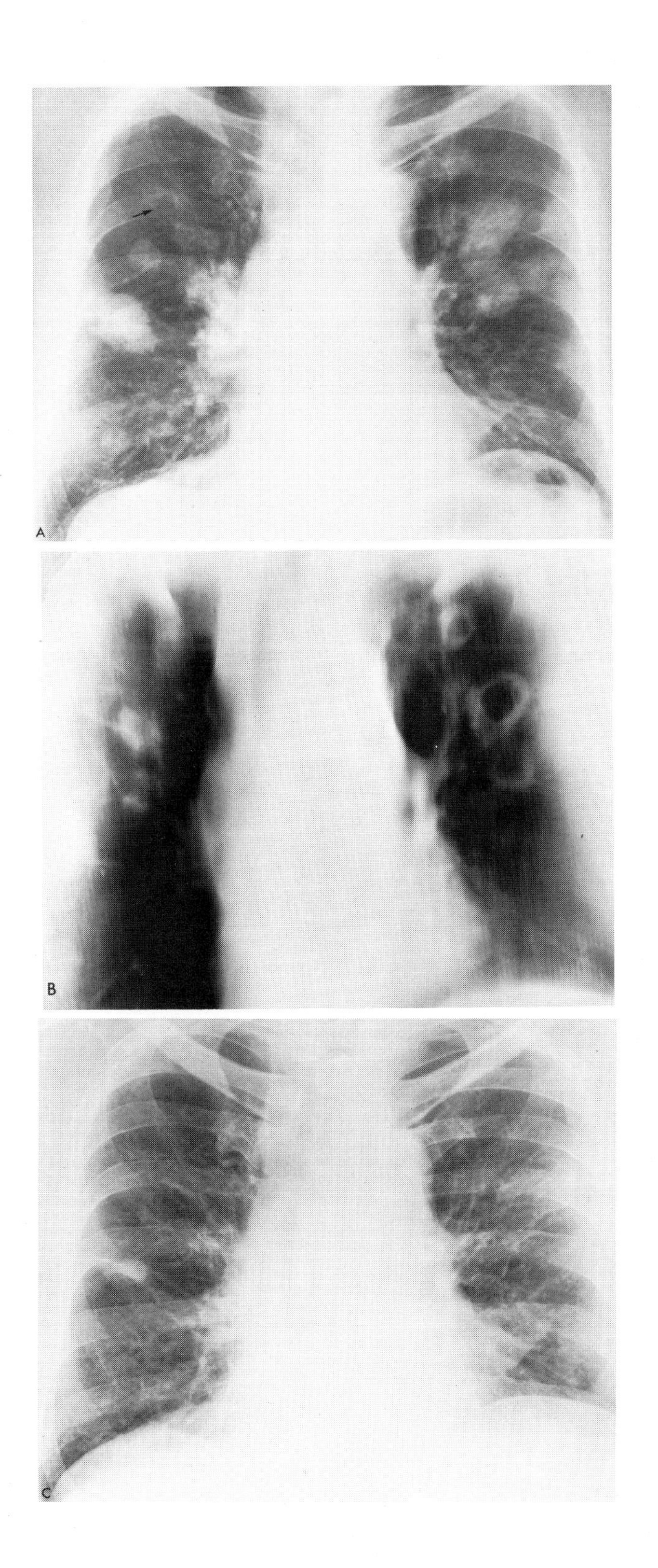

Case 30
Wegener's Granulomatosis (Continued)

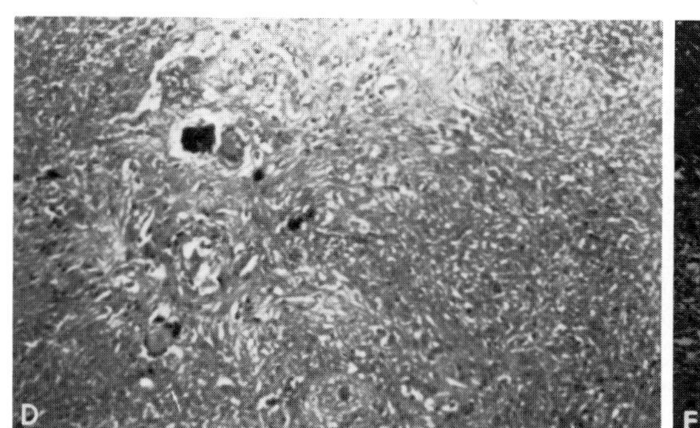

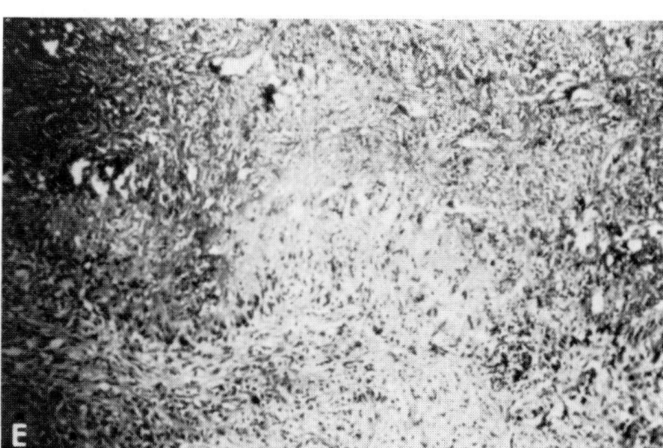

Autopsy showed a plethovic cyanotic male with multiple ecchymoses in the upper extremities. The main findings were in the thorax. The heart was enlarged, dilated, and hypertrophied. The main right coronary and the anterior descending arteries were occluded by old thrombi, corresponding areas of myocardial infarct were seen, and there was a recent subendocardial infarct. Both lungs were very heavy and together weighed 2000 gm. Sections showed focal scars, particularly in the left upper lobe, but no obvious active granulomas.

The liver showed central necrosis and chronic passive congestion, which correlates well with the patient's clinical history. Both adrenals were small and atrophied, representing after-effects of prolonged steroid therapy. There were focal superficial scars on the renal cortex. They may well represent healed focal arteritis, but are more likely just due to arteriosclerosis. However, there are no signs of active disease.

There was subacute inflammation of the nasal mucosa, with focal necrotizing angiitis of arterioles, together with fibroblastic proliferation and numerous bizarre multinucleate giant cells (Figure *D*). The lung biopsy showed nodules, about 0.75 mm in diameter, whose centers were necrotic and the margins of the viable tissue were serpiginous. Here there was palisading of fibroblasts with bizarre multinucleate giant cells similar to those in the nasal biopsy. The pulmonary vessels outside of the granulomas were free of vasculitis. At autopsy, there were multiple discrete linear and stellate scars throughout the lung but most commonly in the upper lobe. Many appeared around the bronchovascular bundles or were peripheral in the lobule. The lesions were inactive and there was striking intimal proliferation and narrowing of the pulmonary vessels in the scars with old destruction of the elastic tissue in their walls (Figure *E*).

There was severe coronary artery disease with old thrombosis and infarction and recent subendocardial infarction. Pulmonary emboli also contributed to death. The kidneys showed mild nephrosclerosis only.

Death was due to acute pneumonia and myocardial infarction in a patient with treated and currently inactive Wegener's granulomatosis.

Idiopathic pulmonary hemorrhage or pulmonary hemosiderosis

This is a comparatively rare disease, of unknown etiology, characterized by widespread pulmonary capillary hemorrhages. After a variable period of time, pulmonary hemosiderosis and fibrosis may develop.

Although the disease has been recognized in children for many years, in 1956 Florian could find only eight cases reported in adults.[1422] Four years later, in a thorough review of this interesting entity, Bronson found 34 such cases reported.[1423] He noted that the radiological changes might not appear until several years after onset of clinical symptoms, a circumstance suggesting that studies of disordered function might be of value and certainly of interest in this disease. One of the patients we have studied is shown in Case 33.

Some authorities consider idiopathic pulmonary hemosiderosis and Goodpasture's syndrome to be entirely distinct,[1558] but we have been impressed with the overlap between the two. The pulmonary lesions in idiopathic pulmonary hemorrhage are similar to those in Goodpasture's syndrome, and the gross appearance of the lungs is identical. The x-ray changes in the lung have been said to be more symmetrical than in Goodpasture's syndrome, and in hemosiderosis they are invariably bilateral.[3113] Macrophage-containing hemosiderin may be found in the sputum in this condition,[3114] and the history may extend over a period of years.[3115] Alveolitis, though uncommon, does occur.[1568, 1569] Inconspicuous glomerulonephritis or renal disease has been described,[1570–1573] as has necrotizing angiitis.[1574, 1575] In idiopathic pulmonary hemorrhage the pulmonary lesions are usually more chronic and hemosiderin induration of the lungs is more severe, and the appearance may resemble that in mitral stenosis. Soergel and Sommers stressed the frequent finding of hyperplasia, degeneration, and shedding of alveolar lining cells, with cytoplasmic inclusions, and dilatation and tortuosity of the alveolar capillaries.[2235] Peribronchial or perivascular chronic inflammatory-cell infiltrate also may be observed.[2236, 2237] Pulmonary fibrosis may be extensive in chronic cases of either disease. Deposition of iron and calcium on elastic fibers, often with fragmentation and giant-cell reaction, is also described, but this is not specific, occurring also in the lungs of patients with longstanding mitral stenosis. Cor pulmonale has been recorded in a few longstanding cases,[1576–1579] and we have seen severe emphysema develop in a young woman with this condition who died in respiratory failure. Fuleihan, Abboud, and Hubaytar[3116] have recently brought together published data on pulmonary function in this condition. They have reported that a reduced VC has been found in 8 of 14 patients; a reduced ventilatory ability in 5 of 7 patients; impairment of diffusing capacity in 3 out of 4 patients so studied; and a decreased arterial saturation in 3 of 7 patients.

Diffuse lupus erythematosus

The remarkable review of this condition published in 1954 by Harvey and his colleagues[1424] clearly established that pleural and, to a less extent, pulmonary involvement was a common feature. Subsequent data, particularly those of Myhre,[1425] indicate that bilateral involvement is the rule, with evanescent pleural effusions, ill-defined basal opacities, and areas of atelectasis that seem to have no real segmental distribution. Many who have written about this condition have recorded production of mucoid sputum,[1425, 1426] though to date there has been little pathological evidence that the bronchial tree is specially involved in patients with this syndrome. Indeed, the pathological findings are disappointingly nonspecific.[1580, 1581] Pleural effusions are commonly found, and mucinous edema of connective tissue,[1581] necrosis of pulmonary capillary walls[1582] and chronic interstitial pneumonitis[1583] have been described occasionally. One instance of pulmonary fibrosis has been reported.[1335] X-ray changes of one kind or another have been recorded in 50 of 78 patients with this condition,[3122] and it seems clear that the lungs are more commonly involved than has been generally imagined.[3055, 3123]

On the x-ray, focal areas of pneumonitis frequently are apparent; they may be associated with a variable degree of atelectasis and characteristically are more often in the lower portions of the lung fields. A common finding is that of bilateral pleural effusions with pericardial effusions, representing the manifestations of polyserositis. The combination

(Text continued on page 320.)

Case 31
Goodpasture's Syndrome

Summary of Clinical Findings. This 20-year-old man, a part-time bookkeeper for a bank, was referred for investigation of hemoptysis, anemia and renal disease. He gave a history of fatigue and dyspnea on exertion of two months' duration. For two weeks before admission he had coughed up small quantities of bright red blood. On physical examination he was a pale but well-developed white man in no apparent respiratory distress. Temperature was 101° F, pulse 120/min and regular, and blood pressure 145/80 mm Hg. Physical examination was otherwise normal and there were no cardiac murmurs or evidence of cardiac enlargement. The lungs were clear and the liver and spleen were not felt. Repeated urinalyses showed 2+ albuminuria, with 50 RBC per high-power field and granular and RBC casts. He was anemic, with a hemoglobin of 7.6 gm/100 ml, the red cells being hypochromic. There was a reticulocytosis of 3.8 per cent, and the platelet count was normal. Total and differential white-cell counts were within normal limits, with no eosinophilia. The serum bilirubin was not elevated. The patient ran a daily spiking fever to 100° F for three weeks. His anemia was corrected with blood transfusions and iron, and there was no further hemoptysis. A renal biopsy showed subacute glomerulonephritis.

When the function tests were repeated, at the end of November, 1958, the chest x-ray had been clear for six weeks and he had no dyspnea. Renal biopsy was repeated in January, 1959.

He has since been lost to follow-up.

Radiology. Innumerable indistinct patchy and nodular densities are scattered diffusely and evenly throughout both lung fields (*A*). The individual lesions measure between 5 and 10 mm in diameter and almost all are confluent over at least part of their circumference. The hila are not enlarged in either their vascular or nodal components. The left ventricle appears slightly enlarged. There is no pleural effusion.

A film of the chest made three days previously had shown no evidence of pulmonary disease. Intravenous pyelography had revealed rather poor function bilaterally but no structural deformity of the collecting systems of either kidney; the kidneys were normal in size and contour.

Four days later (*B*) the lungs had completely cleared and they remained normal in all subsequent films.

Pathology. The sputum showed very many macrophages containing brown pigment, which stained positively for iron.

The first renal biopsy showed an acute focal necrotizing glomerulonephritis (*C*), but no necrotizing angiitis was seen. The second biopsy showed subacute glomerulonephritis, with scarring and fibrosis of the glomeruli.

Summary. The combination of pulmonary and renal changes is characteristic of Goodpasture's syndrome. This patient showed normal ventilatory function but impaired diffusing capacity when the x-ray was grossly abnormal. Exercise diffusing capacity was still abnormal, however, after the x-ray had cleared and the hemoglobin had returned to normal, presumably indicating residual alveolar damage.

													EXERCISE					
	VC	FRC	RV	TLC	ME %	MMFR	$FEV_{0.75}$ ×40	pH	P_{CO_2}	HCO_3^-	O_2Hb %	$D_{LCO}SS_2$	MPH	GRADE	$\dot{V}O_2$	$\dot{V}_E$	$D_{LO}SS_3$
Predicted	5.3	3.7	1.7	7.0	70	4.7	155					25.2					35.0
Oct. 17, 1958	3.4	2.3	1.4	4.8	58	4.6	122					12.6	3	FLAT	1.1	36.5	16.7
Nov. 25, 1958													3	FLAT	1.1	29.2	18.4

The first set of function tests was done at the time of the first chest x-ray (*A*), when there was evidence of pulmonary infiltration and considerable anemia. Ventilatory function was normal, but the vital capacity and total lung capacity were reduced. There was a reduction in both rest and exercise diffusing capacity. By November 25, 1958, the chest x-ray had been clear for several weeks and the Hb was normal. There was still considerable impairment of the exercise diffusing capacity, however, indicative of definite residual abnormality despite the clear x-ray. Note the increased ventilation in relation to oxygen uptake, $\dot{V}O_2/\dot{V}_E$ being 3.5 on the first occasion and 3.8 on the second.

Goodpasture's Syndrome

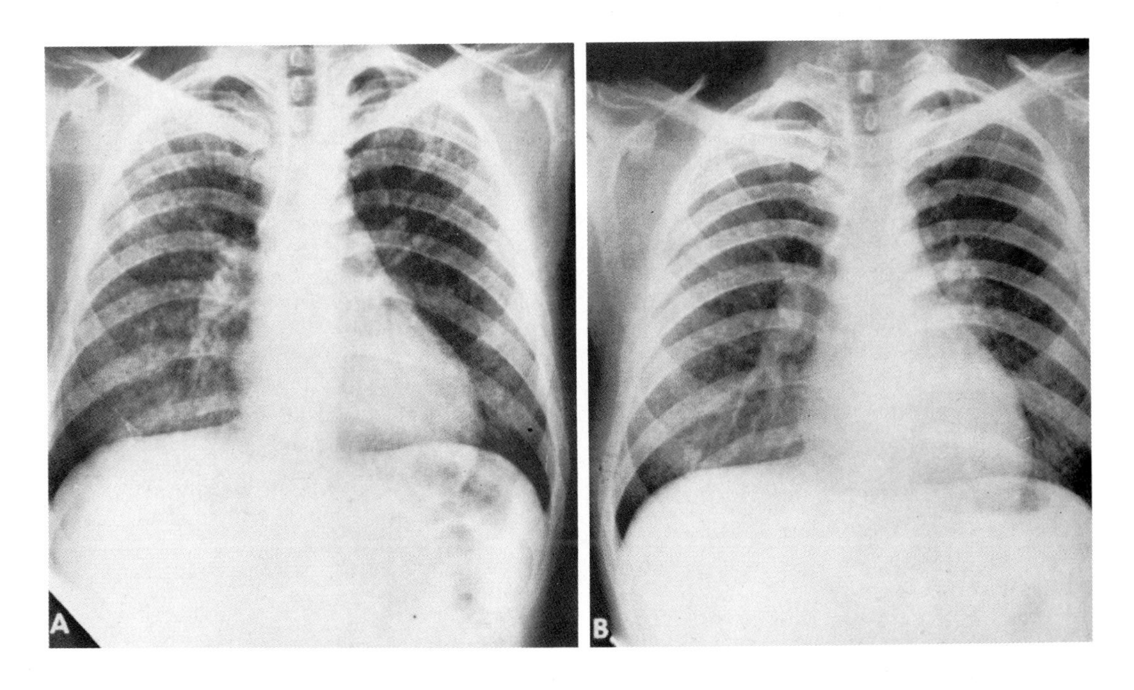

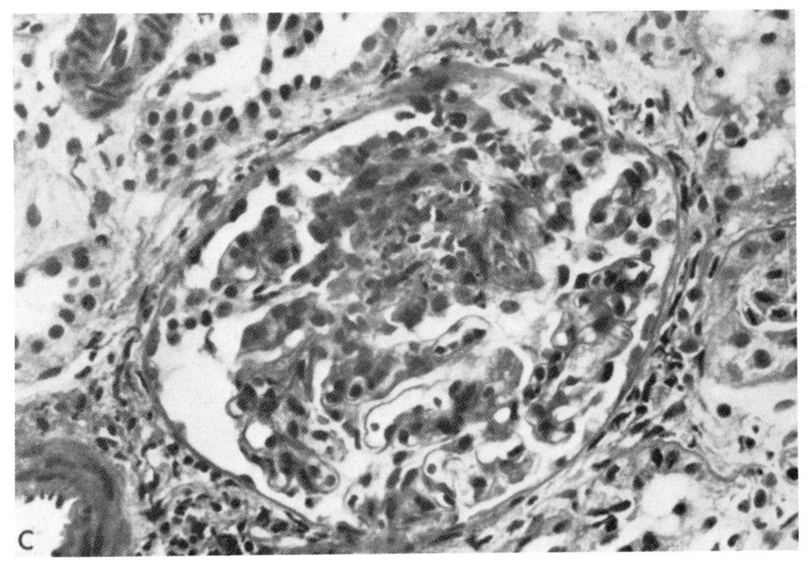

Case 32
Scleroderma

Summary of Clinical Findings. This 51-year-old unemployed construction worker was admitted to hospital in November 1960 complaining of a 22 lb weight loss (180 to 158) over the past eight months. His appetite was good and he had no symptoms of gastrointestinal upset. He had noticed gradually increasing shortness of breath over the previous five years and a nonproductive paroxysmal cough for one year. He was dyspneic after climbing one flight of stairs. During the previous two years, on exposure to cold, his hands had become purplish and sometimes white, but were not painful. One year previously, when seen at another hospital, he had been told he had chronic bronchitis.

Examination revealed a well-developed, well-nourished man. His blood pressure was 130/140 mm Hg; respiration rate was 20/min; pulse rate was 78/min. His hands and feet were cold, but no skin abnormalities were detected. The thorax moved well with respiration. Fine crepitations were audible over the entire chest. There were no other pertinent findings.

Routine urinalysis and hemogram were normal. A search for LE cells was negative. The level of $alpha_2$ globulin was increased. There was a moderate growth of *Diplococcus pneumoniae* from the sputum. On barium-swallow examination there were no primary or secondary peristaltic waves in the esophagus. Skin from the dorsum of a finger showed fibrosis consistent with scleroderma. Open lung biopsy was performed.

On steroids he improved symptomatically and was discharged from hospital. X-rays and function studies were repeated after two years on this medication, in November, 1962.

Radiology. A postero-anterior roentgenogram of the chest (*A*) reveals a generalized increase in density of the two lungs which is symmetrical and uniform. Although the density appears rather hazy and indistinct on this reproduction, close examination of the original film shows an extremely fine network of linear shadows in the form of a reticulation (difficult to reproduce photographically). The changes are somewhat more noticeable in the bases then elsewhere. This type of infiltration suggests a diffuse interstitial fibrosis and, in the absence of associated radiological abnormalities, must be regarded as of unknown etiology. Esophageal aperistalsis was observed in this patient fluoroscopically, and the diagnosis of scleroderma or diffuse systemic sclerosis could then be made with considerable conviction.

A magnified view of the lower portion of the left lung (*B*) reveals the nature of the reticulation to better advantage, although even with magnification the extremely fine network is difficult to visualize.

Pathology. The lung biopsy (*C*) showed great distortion of the lung tissue with formation of multiple microcysts. These contained a few desquamated cells and much mucoid material. The cysts were lined by cuboidal and columnar epithelium, the latter being often ciliated and occasionally mucus-secreting. The interstitial tissue showed mature collagen and much proliferated muscle and only minimal chronic inflammatory-cell infiltrate. The vessels showed striking medial thickening and intimal proliferation.

Summary. A case of scleroderma in a 51-year-old man. This case illustrates the importance of diffusing-capacity measurements, since a severe degree of lung involvement existed even though ventilatory ability was normal and the arterial blood showed no arterial desaturation at rest.

	VC	FRC	RV	TLC	ME %	MMFR	$FEV_{0.75}$ ×40	pH	P_{CO_2}	HCO_3^-	O_2Hb %	$D_{Lco}SS_2$	CO Ext %	EXERCISE MPH	GRADE	$\dot{V}O_2$	$\dot{V}_E$	$D_{Lco}SS_3$
Predicted	3.7	3.2	1.9	5.6	55	3.3	100	7.40	42	25	97	16.1	44					29.0
Oct. 1960	2.2	2.1	1.2	3.4	34	3.4	85					6.5	23	1.5	FLAT	1.0	26.2	12.1
Nov. 1962	2.2	1.8	1.3	3.5	36	3.8	83	7.33	46	23	99	6.9	21	2	FLAT	0.9	34.9	7.0

In October, 1960, the vital capacity and lung volumes were reduced. Mixing was slightly inefficient but the MMFR and FEV were normal. Diffusion was very low both at rest and exercise. Mechanics studies at this time showed a static compliance of 0.042 l/cm H_2O and an average airway resistance of 1.7 cm H_2O/l/sec. Two years later, after steroid therapy, there has been no change in vital capacity or total capacity. Although the resting D_{Lco} is the same as before, it now does not increase at all on exercise, whereas two years before it nearly doubled. The arterial blood at rest is still normal. It is of interest that the $\dot{V}O_2/\dot{V}E$ on exercise was 3.8 in October 1960 but had fallen to 2.58 two years later. In 1962, the arterial oxygen tension during maximal exercise was found to be 45 mm Hg.

Scleroderma

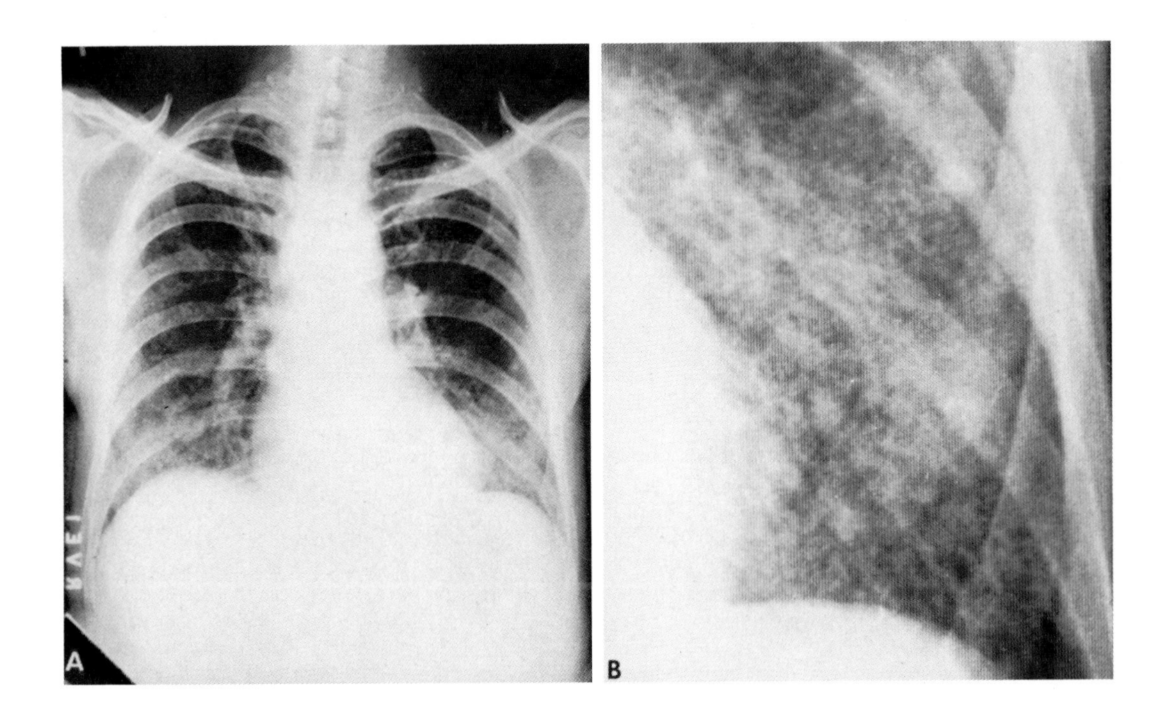

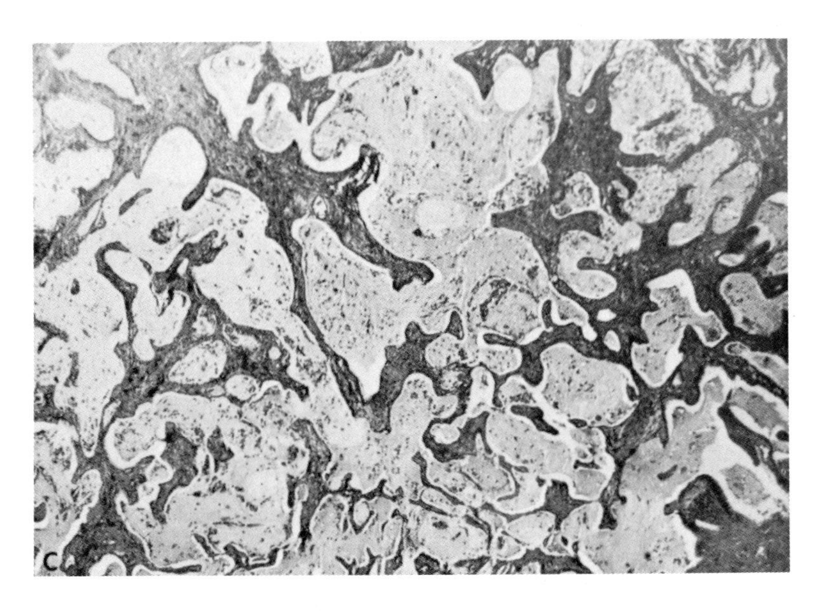

Case 33
Idiopathic Hemosiderosis

Summary of Clinical Findings. This 44-year-old taxi driver was admitted with hemoptysis on September 11, 1963. He had had several previous admissions to hospital for a bleeding duodenal ulcer and had undergone a hemigastrectomy and vagotomy in July, 1962. At the beginning of Septemper, 1963, he noticed the onset of an intermittent cough occasionally productive of small amounts of dark- or bright-red sputum. On the night of admission, he suddenly produced about half a cup of bright red blood and came to the Emergency Department. There an x-ray was taken and he was admitted. There was no prior history of cough, no chest pain and no orthopnea, although he had become alarmed by shortness of breath on the evening of admission. He smoked about 20 cigarettes per day.

On examination he was obese (250 lb) and pale but in no acute distress. Blood pressure was 165/85 mm Hg; pulse rate was 90/min and regular; respiratory rate was 25/min. The chest expanded equally. Breath sounds were harsh, and occasional high-pitched expiratory rhonchi were heard, especially over the left upper lobe. The heart did not appear enlarged but a grade II/IV systolic ejection murmur was heard best at the apex, radiating into the neck. There were no other findings of note.

Investigations included a normal urinalysis; hemoglobin was 7.8 gm/100 ml; reticulocytes 5.2 per cent; total white cells initially 17,300/cmm but dropping to 9800/cmm within five days, with an 8 per cent eosinophilia. Prothrombin activity was 25 per cent and did not rise after administration of vitamin K_1. Measurements of serum iron and iron-binding capacity were consistent with a state of iron deficiency, as was a bone-marrow examination. Sputum culture grew no pathogens, but a stain for iron showed macrophages loaded with iron pigment. No source of bleeding could be found in the nose or pharynx or on bronchoscopic examination. Kidney function was normal (ECC and PSP).

The patient was treated with sedation and codeine to suppress cough, and his symptoms rapidly subsided. He was started on iron sulfate, which was continued after his discharge.

He was readmitted one month later with similar symptoms of cough and hemoptysis. Routine examinations revealed anemia (Hb 9.4 gm/100 ml) and a slightly elevated white-cell count (10,200/cmm), with eosinophils varying between 1 and 4 per cent. Chest x-rays were similar to those obtained on his previous admission.

The patient has since been admitted on eleven occasions for similar episodes of hemoptysis, the last in May 1969. His course has also been complicated by a myocardial infarction in 1965. He continues to work as a taxi driver and denies shortness of breath between the episodes of hemoptysis. Follow-up pulmonary function studies are shown.

Radiology. The lungs are diffusely and evenly involved by patchy densities of varying size, which are so numerous that they are all at least partly confluent. There is no pleural effusion. The hila appear slightly enlarged and the heart is at the upper limit of normal in size. Subsequent films made at daily intervals showed gradual clearing over seven days, at which time the lungs had regained a normal appearance. A chest film had been normal in July 1962.

Such an appearance could easily be produced by pulmonary edema, but the slow rate of clearing and the history of gross hemoptysis suggest idiopathic hemosiderosis as a more likely diagnosis.

Summary. This case of idiopathic hemosiderosis in a 44-year-old man illustrates the preservation of ventilatory function but lowering of arterial saturation and diffusing capacity that one might expect to find in a condition diffusely involving alveolar walls.

	VC	FRC	RV	TLC	ME %	MMFR	$FEV_{0.75}$ ×40	pH	P_{CO_2}	HCO_3^-	O_2Hb %	$D_{Lco}SS_2$	CO Ext %	EXERCISE MPH	GRADE	$\dot{V}O_2$	$\dot{V}_E$	$D_{Lco}SS_3$
Predicted	3.7	3.0	1.6	5.3	60	3.6	111	7.40	42	25	97	18.6	48					32
Sept. 17, 1963	3.5	2.4	1.7	5.2	50	3.6	112	7.48	25	20	92	13.4	31	2	FLAT	1.9	42.8	21
Sept. 12, 1968	3.4	2.7	1.9	5.3	54	4.0	113					11.3	37					

The abnormalities seen are a reduction in the diffusing capacity both at rest and on exercise, and a hypoxemia in spite of hyperventilation (low P_{CO_2}). These tests were done a few days after x-ray had shown that clearing was still incomplete.

In the next five years, in spite of repeated episodes of hemoptysis, there has been remarkably little change in function.

Idiopathic Hemosiderosis

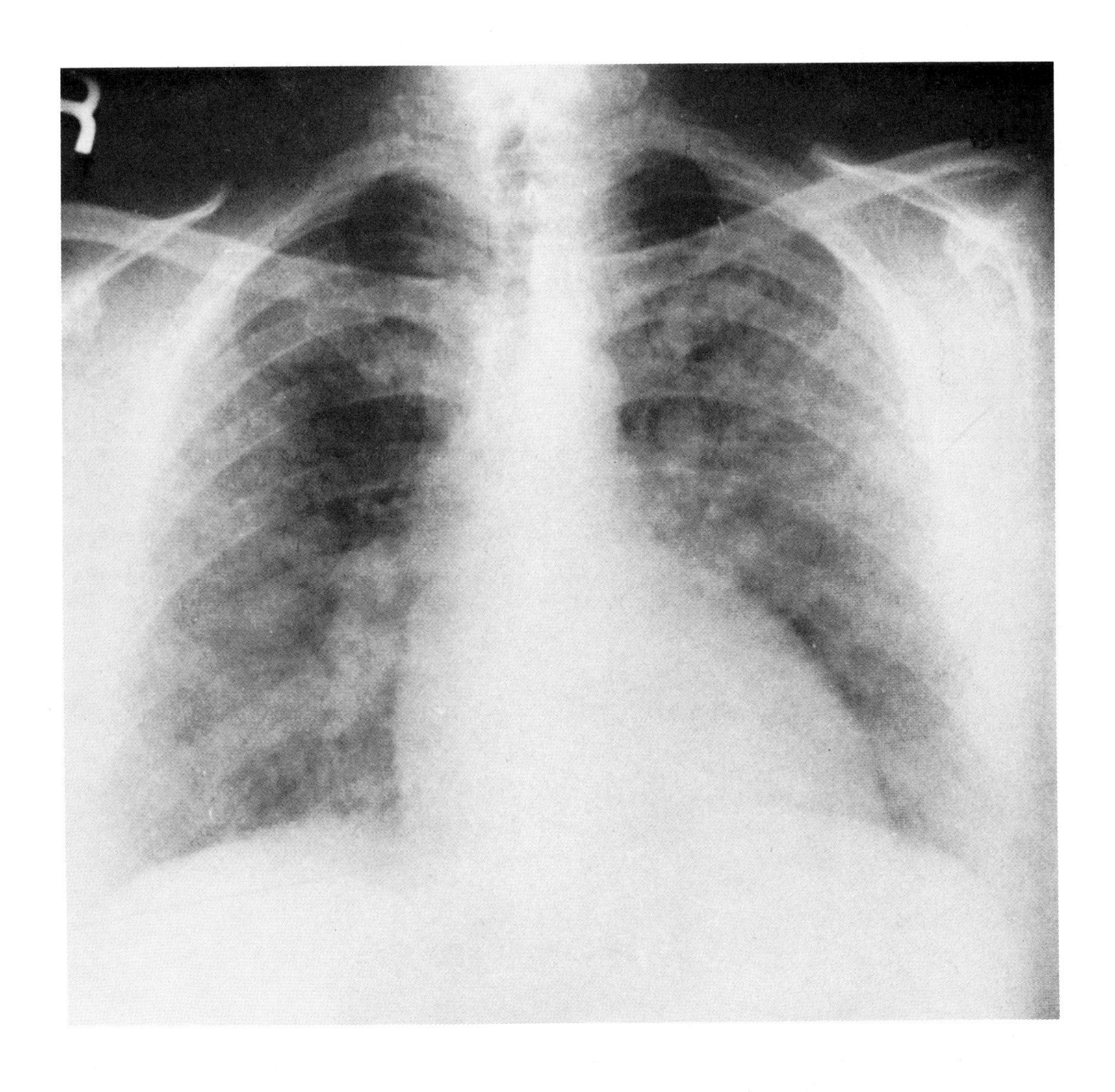

of focal areas of pneumonitis, generally in the bases, with a pleural or pericardial effusion should make one strongly suspect the possibility of this diagnosis.

In the first edition of this book we wrote, "As far as we are aware, no complete study of pulmonary function in a sufficient number of these patients has been published to enable an accurate picture to be drawn of the impairment of function usually present." This gap has been filled during the past four years, and nearly 100 patients have now been reported on. These studies have shown that pulmonary function is not infrequently abnormal in the presence of a normal chest x-ray (as in Case 31 in our first edition),[3057, 3117] that the vital capacity and lung volumes are commonly decreased,[3118, 3121] with a reduced pulmonary compliance;[3121] that some degree of airway obstruction occurs not uncommonly;[3120] and that the diffusing capacity[3057, 3119] and arterial oxygen saturation[3118, 3119] are commonly found to be reduced (*see* Case 29).

It may be concluded from this evidence that involvement of the pulmonary parenchyma in this disease is more common than might be judged from clinical or radiological criteria.[3055, 3123] Some degree of dyspnea or some history of sputum in a noncigarette smoker might be recorded more frequently if the physician carefully asks the patient about them; and this he is more likely to do if he is aware of the recent pulmonary function data on this condition.

PULMONARY FUNCTION IN HEART DISEASE AND IN PULMONARY HYPERTENSION

CHAPTER 15

Shall man into the mystery of breath
From his quick beating pulse a pathway spy?
GEORGE MEREDITH

INTRODUCTION

Although some of the earliest observations of abnormal pulmonary function were made in patients with heart failure and pulmonary congestion,[1] in general there has been little appreciation of the effect that heart disease may exert on the pulmonary parenchyma. These have now been well documented, however, and it is possible to state with some certainty the changes in pulmonary function that may occur in these patients. Yet, such is the effect of specialization, that, as Arnott has pointed out,[2061] many physicians and cardiologists are unaware of much of this important information. Even in a condition as common as mitral stenosis—in which the changes in pulmonary pathology have been known for 30 years, and in which pulmonary function has been studied in detail—clinical papers still appear in which no attention is paid to the state of the lungs in assessing operative results or long-term survival. It will be appreciated that the consequences of mitral-valve stenosis, in which the pulmonary capillary bed is placed between the stenosed orifice and the right ventricle, and in which pulmonary venous and arterial hypertension exist, are likely to be very different from the consequences of thrombotic obliteration of the arterial bed, in which situation there is no pulmonary venous elevation of pressure. Thus there is little sense in discussing the lung in "pulmonary hypertension" as if these two conditions could be equated.

THE LUNG IN MITRAL STENOSIS

Clinical features

In general terms, it is useful to recognize that some patients with mitral stenosis have the signs characteristic of the condition but have little or no disability; others, with relatively little cardiac enlargement, may have pulmonary hypertension and suffer mainly from recurrent episodes of pulmonary edema; in others, considerable cardiac enlargement, particularly of the left atrium, may have occurred, with some degree of dyspnea constantly present; and finally, a few may be seen who have suffered from the condition for many years, who have had several episodes of right ventricular failure, and in whom irreversible changes have taken place in the lungs. Any or most of these different types of patients may be included in a study of pulmonary function in mitral stenosis.

Dyspnea is the characteristic symptom of mitral stenosis, initially being noted on effort only, and often accompanied by orthopnea. A short unproductive cough is frequently present, and repeated attacks of bronchitis, often with considerable wheezing in the chest, may occur. Hemoptysis is an important symptom. These three complaints may continue unchanged for many years. The clinical picture may be dramatically changed by the complication of cerebral embolism or the onset of right ventricular failure. Rhonchi may be heard in the chest at any time, and rales are not infrequently audible, though it is equally common to note considerable dyspnea on exertion with no abnormal findings over the lungs.

In the later stages of the disease, and when it has been present for many years, considerable muscle wasting occurs, fatigue and weakness are commonly pronounced, and gross cardiac hypertrophy may be present.

Pathology

The classic description of the lungs in mitral stenosis written by Parker and Weiss[1436] in 1936 provided the first detailed discussion of the changes that might be encountered. Similar changes may occur as a consequence of any condition producing pulmonary venous hypertension—as, for example, mitral incompetence, ball-valve thrombus of the left atrium, left atrial myxoma, and rare congenital disorders such as cor triatriatum or mitral atresia. The lung changes are often described under the heading of "brown induration of the lung," and lesser grades of this may be seen also in patients who have had prolonged left ventricular failure or left atrial hypertension.

The term "brown induration" describes the two striking gross features of this condition, namely, deposition of iron pigment (hemosiderosis) and increased firmness of the lung parenchyma. The hemosiderosis results from intrapulmonary hemorrhage, probably venous in origin,[9, 1437] that may be seen in various degrees of organization. Hemosiderin from lysed red blood cells is phagocytosed by histiocytes (siderophages), which are found particularly in alveolar spaces, often forming visible nodules. They are present to a less striking degree in the interstitium of the lung, where, however, they may accumulate in the pleura or around respiratory bronchioles. Hemosiderosis is said to be most striking in the upper zones of the lung, and may be slight or even absent in the inferior lingular or basal part of the lower lobe even in advanced cases.[1438] Alveolar lining cells are swollen and cuboidal and the alveolar walls are thickened.[9, 1441, 1449] Schulz,[26] who attempted to measure this accurately by electron microscopy, concluded that in mitral stenosis the basement membrane varies from 2000 Å to 5000 Å in width, compared with a value of less than 1600 Å for this structure in the normal human lung. The alveolar capillaries may be tortuous and dilated initially, but in longstanding cases this change is often not readily apparent. In contrast to the appearance in the Hamman-Rich syndrome (*see* Chapter 12), the lung structure is generally intact and the increase in fibrous tissue is modest. In severe cases of long duration, iron may be deposited on elastic and reticulum fibers (siderofibrosis),[1439] which may fragment and elicit a foreign-body response. Very striking changes are present in the pulmonary lymphatics:[1440] they become tortuous and dilated, and their interlobular septa are thickened and edematous, giving rise to the appearance of "Kerley B lines."[715] Variable degrees of pulmonary edema may occur, the organization of which may result in fibrosis. There is recent evidence that the clinical horizontal Kerley lines can only be seen on radiographs when there is fibrosis of alveolar septae.[3132] Bone formation within alveolar spaces may occur[1441, 1442] and may be related to organization of fibrin in edema fluid.[1439]

Various changes occur in the pulmonary vessels.[9, 1443, 1444] The main and lobar arteries are dilated and may show severe atherosclerosis. The smaller elastic arteries are variable: in the upper zones of the lung they may be normal or slightly dilated; in the lower zones they are usually narrowed. Thickening of the media and intimal proliferation of the pulmonary arterioles and small muscular arteries may be striking, particularly in the lower zones, but changes beyond Grade 3[9, 1445] are rare, although fibrinoid necrosis has been observed. Several authors have noted that severe vascular changes may be present even when the pulmonary artery pressure is not greatly elevated.[3130] Pulmonary venules and small veins show intimal fibrosis[1443, 1444] and some medial thickening.[9] Pulmonary infarcts due to embolism or thrombosis commonly occur in patients with mitral stenosis. Varices of the bronchial arteries may be present,[1446, 1447] and in some patients these may be very prominent. It has been suggested that the bronchial artery anastomoses may be responsible for hemoptysis and, further, that they may be one of the causes of pulmonary hypertension in mitral stenosis.[1448]

Radiology

The radiological appearances in the thorax in mitral stenosis may vary from those of a chest that is almost normal to one in which there is severe cardiomegaly and advanced changes of pulmonary venous engorgement, pulmonary arterial hypertension, and pulmonary edema. The x-ray changes may be conveniently divided into cardiac and pulmonary, each of which generally present characteristics indicating the presence of left atrial hypertension. The changes to be described may occur in any abnormality producing left atrial hypertension, including mitral incompetence, left atrial myxoma, and cor triatriatum.

In the heart, the cardinal sign of mitral stenosis is enlargement of the left atrium, commonly of only slight to moderate degree. The main criteria for enlargement of the left atrium consist of a double density or contour on the right border of the heart, prominence of the left atrial appendage on the left heart border, and displacement of the esophagus backward and to the right. Enlargement of the right ventricular mass is common although not invariable, presumably on the basis of pulmonary arterial hypertension. It is surprising, however, how often fairly convincing evidence of right ventricular hypertrophy will be unassociated with clear-cut evidence of pulmonary arterial hypertension, an observation that lacks a satisfactory explanation. Other signs to be sought in the cardiovascular shadow in mitral stenosis are calcification of the mitral valve and smallness of the aortic shadow, the former being relatively uncommon in pure mitral stenosis and the latter a frequent finding.

Alteration in radiological appearance of the pulmonary vascular bed probably depends upon a combination of severity and duration of left atrial hypertension. There is a reasonably good correlation between the vascular changes in mitral stenosis, as assessed radiologically, and the measured pulmonary artery pressure.[3134] The earliest discernible changes are in the venous network of the lungs, the presence of venous hypertension giving rise to early "spasm" of the inferior pulmonary veins, and engorgement of the superior venous trunks. The discrepancy between upper- and lower-lobe pulmonary venous caliber is often striking and may be the only detectable abnormality in the pulmonary vasculature to indicate the presence of venous hypertension. With progressive elevation of venous pressure, the upper-lobe veins eventually return to relatively normal size; before this occurs, however, discernible changes of pulmonary arterial hypertension nearly always develop. The major criterion for arterial hypertension is a discrepancy between the relative sizes of hilar and peripheral arteries, commonly due to both increase in size of the former and decrease in size of the latter. Increased prominence of the main pulmonary artery along the left border of the heart is usually present. As with the pulmonary veins, peripheral arterial narrowing is generally more noticeable in the lower portions of the lungs than in the upper, at least in the early stages of arterial hypertension; with increasing severity and duration, however, peripheral arterial narrowing becomes generalized. It can readily be seen that patients with severe arterial and venous hypertension can have peripheral arteries and veins of almost normal caliber, although the increased size of the hilar artery complex should by this stage have reached striking proportions.

At any stage during the development of pulmonary venous hypertension, and generally in an unpredictable fashion, signs of pulmonary edema may appear. Being predominantly interstitial in location, pulmonary edema in mitral stenosis is usually readily distinguishable from the alveolar edema of acute left ventricular failure. It may show itself in one or both of two forms:

1. Since edema fluid accumulates in the perivascular interstitial tissues, the vascular markings of such lungs show a loss of sharp definition and the borders are hazy and indistinct. This change takes place throughout the substance of both lungs and in the hilar areas as well, so that the hila appear both enlarged and indistinct. Edema fluid tends to accumulate in the interlobular septa of the lung, particularly in the most dependent portions of the lower lobes. These engorged septa become visible radiologically as horizontal linear densities measuring up to 2 cm in length, with one end contiguous to the visceral pleura and generally most evident in the costophrenic sulci and in the lung immediately above. In most patients with mitral stenosis these lines appear and disappear at intervals, depending upon the level of pulmonary venous pressure, a figure of 16 to 25 mm Hg or more generally being regarded as necessary for their development. When the edema is chronic, however, deposition of hemosiderin occurs within the interlobular septa, with concomitant fibrosis, in which case the septal lines become permanent and do not disappear despite successful mitral commissurotomy.

2. The picture of the more severe varieties of pulmonary edema is fairly distinctive in mitral stenosis, but it is not always in the same form. The edema may be of the "bat's-wing" type; the localization of edema in the hilar and medullary areas of the lungs has generally been regarded as a characteristic of uremic edema, but we have seen typical examples in mitral stenosis. Perhaps a more usual distribution of edema in mitral stenosis is in the form of patchy indistinct densities, scattered diffusely throughout the lungs, but again more predominant in the medial and central lung zones. Being mainly interstitial in location, it may be fairly extensive in the absence of major physical signs.

As described in the section on pathology, certain of the pulmonary complications of chronic venous hypertension lead to chronic changes within the lungs, and these are frequently radiologically demonstrable.

Hemosiderosis

The accumulation of deposits of hemosiderin within the lung parenchyma may appear radiologically as a very fine granularity or stippling, generally more noticeable in the central lung zones. Hemosiderosis is seldom identifiable in the upper lung fields or bases.

Ossification

Well-defined ossific nodules measuring up to 4 or 5 mm in diameter are sometimes present in the lungs of patients with mitral stenosis. If they are large enough, bony trabeculae may be identified within them. They are generally not numerous and appear most often in the central lung zones. These nodules are considered to be pathognomonic of mitral stenosis.

Pulmonary fibrosis

Longstanding pulmonary edema may lead to the development of interstitial fibrosis; this may appear radiologically as an extremely fine reticulation, again more prominent usually in the central lung fields than elsewhere. It may be difficult to distinguish this reticulation from the fine mottling or stippling of hemosiderosis, but where one is present it is common to find the other.

THE CIRCULATION

With the advent of cardiac catheterization and the great advances in cardiac surgery, a tremendous volume of data on the hemodynamic consequences of mitral stenosis has accumulated. The principal changes that may follow significant stenosis may be summarized as follows:

There is elevation of the pulmonary artery pressure and of the pulmonary capillary wedge pressure,[2062] best measured during exercise.[9] Although the cardiac index may be normal at rest in some patients,[9, 1451, 1452, 2063] on exercise it usually does not rise to normal levels, and hence may be regarded as limited. This limitation of augmentation of cardiac output is a very important aspect of the condition.[628, 1453, 2064] The intrathoracic blood volume is increased, particularly in relation to the existing level of cardiac output.[1454–1456] As measured by the dye dilation method, the pulmonary blood volume is increased to about 420 ml/M^2 in moderately severe mitral stenosis, compared to a normal value of about 210 ml/M^2 found by the same technique.[3124] Finally, there are important adaptive responses in terms of differential blood flow to various organs in patients with mitral stenosis.[1457, 2065]

However, these generalizations, here summarized so briefly, may conceal the fact that some of the circulatory aspects of mitral stenosis are very puzzling. It has been suggested that the pulmonary hypertension found in this condition should be regarded as a protective mechanism,[1437] and administration of certain pharmacological agents will certainly reduce its degree.[9] It is a remarkable fact, however, that in mitral stenosis, obstruction of one pulmonary artery by a balloon catheter, with consequent diversion of the total cardiac output through one lung, may cause little change in pulmonary artery pressure–which indicates that, in this condition, "... despite very high initial resistance, increase in flow in the lung can occur with rapid reduction in resistance."[1458] Thus, the extent to which the pulmonary hypertension in mitral stenosis is structural or functional is very much open to question, and it seems likely that the abnormal perfusion distribution within the lung in mitral stenosis[341] must represent a balance between structural change and adaptive control.

A full discussion and documentation of these and other aspects of the circulation in mitral stenosis are beyond the scope of the present text.

PULMONARY FUNCTION

As was noted under Clinical Features, patients with mitral stenosis vary very greatly in their clinical condition. This must be remembered when one attempts to answer the question, for example, of whether ventilatory impairment is commonly present in this disease. Much depends upon the type of case or the clinical grade of severity. Thus, one sees some patients who have undoubted mitral stenosis but whose pulmonary function tests are normal; these appear in almost all series of cases that have been studied. In our view, however, there are now enough data on pulmonary function for the state of lung function to be broadly related to the stage of the disease, and this we have attempted under the following subheadings:

Subdivisions of lung volume

The observation that the vital capacity may be reduced in patients with heart disease was traced back by Peabody[1459] to as early as 1855. This reduction, though commonly if not invariably present,[1076, 1107, 1460] is not, in our experience, very closely related to the severity or stage of the disease (*see* Figure 15–1), although there may be no overlap between patients in the least-severe group and those who have congestive failure.[1461] It is evident that attacks of acute pulmonary edema will inevitably be accompanied by severe reductions in vital capacity. The inspiratory capacity is relatively more reduced than is the expiratory reserve volume. A small increase in residual volume, in absolute terms,[1460, 1462, 1463] occurs in some patients but not in others.[1107, 1464, 3127] As the inspiratory capacity is usually reduced, the total lung capacity is smaller than normal in many of these patients;[1076, 1107, 1465] consequently the ratio of residual volume to total capacity (RV/TLC) is not infrequently elevated in mitral stenosis. One group of authors has documented this increase,[1466, 1467] and in our view has accorded it much more functional significance than it possesses. Since the expiratory reserve volume is slightly decreased, the functional residual capacity is often normal. The cardiac enlargement present in some patients no doubt accounts for part of the fall in total lung capacity. The pathological changes in the lung, however, seem to provide perfectly valid reasons why both the vital capacity and the total lung capacity are likely to be reduced.

Inert-gas distribution

The patient with mitral stenosis has a reduced total lung capacity and often a resting ventilation higher than normal;[1452] it is not surprising, therefore, that gas distribution estimated from measurement of the alveolar nitrogen concentration after a set period of oxygen breathing does not reveal any significant abnormality in this aspect of function in mitral stenosis.[1465] By contrast, the closed-circuit helium-equilibration method, in which correction is applied for lung volume and minute volume, does reveal abnormal gas distribution in some of these patients.[1461, 1463] Using this method, we found the helium-mixing index normal in 20 of 35 patients with mitral stenosis and unequivocally abnormal in the remaining 15.[1107] Similar results with a similar circuit were reported by Englert and Denolin,[1462] who noted that, although the equilibration time was usually normal in this condition, the helium-mixing index was abnormal in about 11 of 28 such patients. In a recently published study of 20 cases, Raine and Bishop found the inert-gas distribution measured by the single-breath oxygen test to be uneven when the patients were at rest, and after exercise the degree of unevenness increased still further.[2063] As was noted earlier, the pathological changes in the lung in some of these patients may be so gross that it is difficult to conceive of normal gas distribution in them. It seems likely that this aspect of function in mitral stenosis has been underestimated in the past because of the inability of the seven-minute alveolar-nitrogen test to demonstrate the defect in patients with small lungs who are hyperventilating at rest.[1463]

In a recent study of pulmonary ventilation and perfusion distribution using radioactive ^{133}xenon, Dawson, Kaneko, and McGregor[3131] found that there was little abnormality in the regional distribution of a single inspiration in 15 patients with mitral-valve disease, but that the equilibration time during normal breathing was considerably delayed in the lower zones.

Ventilatory function

There is general agreement that ventilatory function as measured either by the maximal breathing capacity or by a single-breath test is not uncommonly impaired in patients with mitral stenosis. The maximal breathing capacity is reduced in most patients with any complaint of dyspnea,[1452, 1463–1465] and single-breath FEV measurements also are lower than predicted.[1460, 1461, 1469] Stock and Kennedy noted that values for this measurement were related to the stage of the disease, as indicated by clinical grading;[1469] our experience has been similar, particularly with the maximal midexpiratory flow rate, which showed no overlap between the least severe and most advanced groups[1461] (*see* Figure 15–1). It is possible, of course, that this and other single-breath measurements are unduly influenced by muscular weakness, though it is probably equally likely that fatigue influences the 15-second maximal breathing capacity tests. However, airway resistance is not infrequently elevated in mitral stenosis, and there is little reason not to attribute most of the fall in FEV to partial airway obstruction. Stock and Kennedy noted that, after exercise, the FEV was usually lower in patients with mitral stenosis than in normal subjects or in those with primary pulmonary conditions,[1469] which suggests that increasing pulmonary congestion may well determine airway diameter in this condition. In advanced stages, ventilatory function may be considerably reduced (*see* Case 34), and in these circumstances may present a considerable hazard to adequate ventilation postoperatively. Friedman and his colleagues noted that the maximal breathing capacity fell progressively with each advancing stage of the disease;[1464] we have found that the ventilatory defect parallels the pulmonary vascular resistance fairly closely (*see* Figure 15–1);

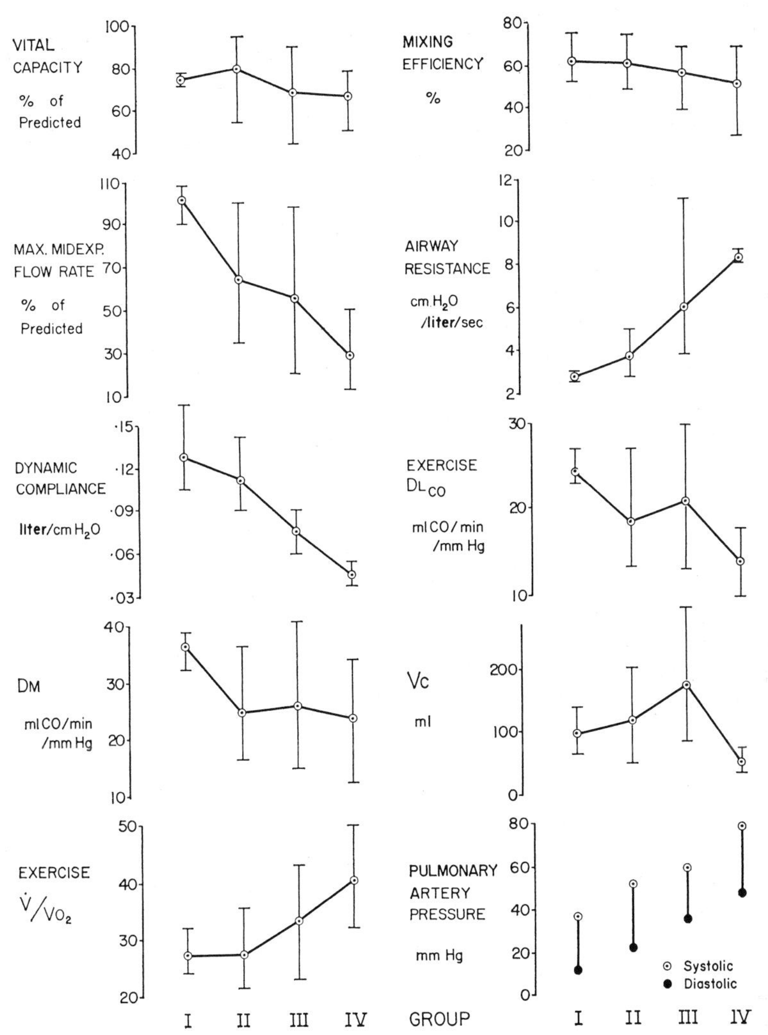

FIGURE 15–1. *Changes in Pulmonary Function in Mitral Stenosis.* The group grading corresponds to clinical severity. Note particularly the rising airway resistance and falling maximal midexpiratory flow rate as the disease becomes more severe. The high pulmonary capillary blood-volume values (V_c) in Group 3 probably represent a state of true pulmonary engorgement. The bars represent the extremes of observed values in each group. (Data from Palmer, Gee, Mills, and Bates.[1461])

these findings support the conclusion reached by Krautwald and his co-workers in their detailed studies of 153 patients with mitral stenosis,[1460] that ventilatory defect is related to pulmonary vascular resistance. The occasional occurrence of chronic bronchitis as a complication of mitral stenosis, particularly in smokers or in those living in heavily polluted areas, will interfere with this relationship. Thus, the finding of considerable impairment of ventilatory function and increased airway resistance in a patient with mitral stenosis whose hemodynamic changes are slight should suggest the possibility that chronic bronchitis is playing a predominant part in the production of dyspnea in that particular patient. It is erroneous, however, to regard the presence of bronchospasm as inevitably an independent phenomenon in mitral stenosis, as some physicians have done,[1470] since progressive ventilatory impairment is an important feature of the evolution of change in pulmonary function consequent upon mitral stenosis.

Pulmonary mechanics

It will be realized that, from the pulmonary point of view, the patient with mitral stenosis with associated severe pulmonary congestion is not very different from one whose pulmonary congestion, or edema, is consequent upon acute left ventricular failure. The mechanical effects of this clinical situation are considered in detail later (*see* page 338). Many patients with mitral stenosis who are not on the verge of pulmonary edema nevertheless experience severe dyspnea on exertion, and may have considerable abnormality of pulmonary compliance and airway resistance. The mechanical status of the "acutely congested lung" and the mechanism of orthopnea are discussed later (*see* page 338). The changes in these aspects of pulmonary function commonly found in less-severe cases of mitral stenosis may be regarded as earlier and milder examples of the picture seen in pulmonary edema, and the physician will realize that no hard and fast differentiation can be drawn, from the point of view of pulmonary function, between these different grades of severity.

Every observer has found that mitral stenosis is commonly accompanied by a fall in pulmonary compliance, usually demonstrable at rest but accentuated on exercise.[467, 498, 1076, 1461, 1471, 1472, 3127] This leads inevitably to a considerable increase in the work of breathing,[498, 1472] which on exercise at a level of ventilation of 25 liters/min may rise to 5.0 KgM/min, whereas in normal subjects at this ventilation it would not exceed 2.0 KgM/min. It is evident that this increase in work is caused also by the increase in airway resistance generally found in patients with mitral stenosis.[467, 1461] The administration of a bronchodilator aerosol not uncommonly leads to a reduction in respiratory work per liter of ventilation.[3127] The relative importance of the decreased compliance and increased air-flow resistance varies no doubt from patient to patient, but it should be noted here that there is some evidence that the air-flow change is at least as important as the decreased compliance in the genesis of orthopnea[496] (*see* page 338). Nisell and his colleagues noted that on exercise the compliance usually fell, but the airway resistance, rather than increasing, tended to decline;[467] so it may be supposed that the relative importance of these factors may be influenced by exercise. In a detailed study of 31 patients with mitral stenosis, Bühlmann, Behn, and Schuppli noted the commonly reduced compliance in mitral stenosis, but they found no close relationship between the severity of this reduction and the pulmonary capillary wedge pressure.[1471] This observation is of considerable interest and should caution one in assuming that these two aspects are inevitably closely interlinked—though such a relationship would certainly result from a correlation between normal subjects in whom wedge pressures are low and compliance high, and patients with mitral stenosis in whom pressures are high and compliance low.

Using a modified esophageal balloon technique, we have recently shown that this method was adequate for the estimation of the intrapleural pressure in patients with mitral stenosis.[2383] We confirmed that a decreased compliance and an increased total resistance with depression of the flow volume curve was characteristic of this condition. In addition, there were unique abnormalities of the static pressure volume curve of the lung; at low lung volumes, elastic recoil was diminished, and at high lung volumes it was increased. One may speculate that the decreased compliance at low lung volume was a consequence of the engorgement of the capillary bed, and that the increase in compliance at high lung volumes was occasioned by the pulmonary fibrosis secondary to chronic edema which occurs in this condition, but there is no direct evidence that this is the true explanation of the findings.

We have pointed out that the lowered compliance in mitral stenosis raises the respiratory frequency at which the most economical ventilation can be achieved;[495] and it is useful to regard the tachypnea as an adaptive mechanism. However, it has proved very difficult to understand how the respiratory rate can be so closely adjusted to a minimal work function. It seems very likely that pulmonary stretch-receptor activity may be modified by pulmonary congestion[1473, 2076] (in the same way as it may be changed by pulmonary fibrosis[1340]) to produce a level of alveolar ventilation that is excessive in relation to CO_2 production; but one cannot pretend that the physiological mechanism or the nervous paths by which these effects are exerted are well known or understood. There can be little doubt that the mechanical changes in the lungs of the patient with mitral stenosis play a major part in relation to his dyspnea. The integration of this defect with others that exist, in relation to his dyspnea, is more fully considered subsequently.

Blood-gas tensions

At rest, the arterial P_{CO_2} value is usually either normal or at the lower limit of normal in patients with mitral stenosis.[1452, 1471, 1474] The arterial oxygen tension is often normal or slightly reduced below the normal resting value, and Friedman and his colleagues noted that it fell from an average value of 78 mm Hg to an average of 68 mm Hg with increasing severity of the condition.[1464] Significant decreases in arterial oxygen saturation are rare, except when pulmonary edema has developed. Rinck and his co-workers found that patients with mitral stenosis had a greater than normal fall in arterial oxygen saturation, as measured by an oximeter, when the oxygen concentration of inspired air was progressively lowered; thus, when 10 per cent oxygen was being inspired, arterial saturation of the normal subjects was about 95 per cent and that of the patients with mitral stenosis was decreased to about 90 per cent.[424]

Blount, McCord, and Anderson, reporting from Denver, Colorado, which is at an altitude of one mile, found the resting arterial oxygen tension in patients with mitral stenosis to average 66.3 mm Hg, 8 mm Hg less than in normal subjects;[1475] exercise provoked no further decrease. Some workers have reported occasional significant reduction in arterial oxygen tension in patients with mitral stenosis, but this is the exception rather than the rule.[1452]

During exercise, the level of arterial $P\text{CO}_2$ may decrease, and De Coster and his co-workers noted that in 5 patients with mitral stenosis it averaged 36.4 mm Hg, compared with a mean value of 39.7 mm Hg in 11 normal subjects.[283]

Diffusing capacity

It is generally agreed that the diffusing capacity is commonly impaired in mitral stenosis, though there is some difference of opinion as to frequency of occurrence and importance of this finding. Analysis of the data shows that impairment has been found less frequently when the modified Krogh method has been used ($D_{L\text{co}}$SB) and when resting studies only have been performed.[362, 411, 1476–1478] Aber and Campbell,[3125] using this method in a study of 79 patients, have reported that the diffusing capacity is generally lowered, and the fall parallels the grade of functional incapacity and severity of pulmonary vascular changes; and others have also noted a correspondence between D_{co} and vascular changes.[3132] Carroll and his colleagues, using the oxygen-diffusing-capacity method, found the diffusing capacity impaired in 6 of 29 patients who had no concomitant distributional defects and in a further 10 patients in whom abnormal distribution patterns were demonstrable; thus, impairment of diffusing capacity was present in 16 of their 29 patients with mitral stenosis.[1468] Similar findings have been noted by others using this technique,[1464, 1479–1481] including Curti and his co-workers,[1452] who found a reduced $D_{L\text{O}_2}$ in 14 out of 16 patients with mitral stenosis. Riley and his colleagues restudied some of Carroll's patients after operation and noted that in most instances commissurotomy had had little effect on the $D_{L\text{O}_2}$ when this had been very low preoperatively.[419] Measurements of oxygen-diffusing capacity have been duplicated by steady-state measurement of CO uptake. At rest, there is a lowered fractional uptake of CO in some of these patients,[1107, 3129] and the end-tidal $D_{L\text{co}}$ ($D_{L\text{co}}SS_2$) is reduced;[1461] this reduction is sufficient to ensure no overlap between values in patients least affected and those in patients most severely affected. The Filley $D_{L\text{co}}$ ($D_{L\text{co}}SS_1$) is also commonly found to be low at rest in mitral stenosis.[3126] MacIntosh and his colleagues found the diffusing capacity lowered on exercise in almost all but those with the mildest grade of stenosis,[551] and they further commented that the degree of abnormality of diffusion measured by $D_{L\text{co}}SS_1$, using an arterial sample, was not closely correlated with the ratio of ventilation to oxygen uptake. In our experience, the level of diffusing capacity on exercise is significantly lower in the most severe grade of stenosis[1461] (*see* Figure 15–1). In detailed studies of hemodynamics and gas exchange in three patients with mitral stenosis, Linderholm noted that the striking feature was the failure of the diffusing capacity to increase normally during exercise.[628] In two patients, there was little defect at rest, but it rose only one or two units when oxygen uptake was trebled during exercise. In the third patient, a low resting value of 13.7 ml CO/min/mm Hg rose to only 14.8 on moderately severe effort.

Some of the puzzling features of the diffusing capacity in mitral stenosis may be explicable on the inference that, in early stages of the condition, there may be a reverse change in pulmonary capillary blood volume (V_c), which is elevated, and in membrane diffusing capacity (D_M), which may be lowered. This pattern of change, which we found in one patient,[399] leaves the total diffusing capacity (D_L) little changed. McNeill, Rankin, and Forster,[411] studying normal subjects and

Case 34
Mitral Stenosis

Summary of Clinical Findings. This 48-year-old invalid has had many admissions to hospital, the first in 1926 for "chorea." She subsequently developed mitral stenosis. Her course has been complicated by two episodes of cerebral embolism in 1942 and 1957, from both of which she recovered completely. In 1951 she was discovered to have slight bronchiectasis of the right middle lobe. Atrial fibrillation was present, although she had been in sinus rhythm in 1942, and therefore she was given digitalis. Until 1959, she had several admissions to hospital for episodes of apparent pulmonary edema and pneumonia.

She was admitted in November, 1959, for consideration of mitral commissurotomy. She had a chronic cough productive of white sputum, was short of breath on slight exertion and used three pillows at night, but did not complain of ankle swelling.

On examination she was thin and pale and appeared chronically ill. She was orthopneic, with an irregular pulse rate of 80/min. The jugular veins were distended two inches above the clavicle at 45°. The chest moved symmetrically. Breath sounds were poorly heard at both bases and a few moist rales were audible under the right breast. The heart was enlarged clinically. The first sound was loud and an opening snap was present. A grade III/VI mid-diastolic rumbling murmur could be heard at the apex. These findings were corroborated by phonocardiogram. There was no ankle edema.

Commissurotomy was performed on December 18, 1959. The mitral opening was extremely small and was opened to 2½ fingers-breadth. A lung biopsy was taken from the lingula at the time of surgery.

Four hours after operation, she was unresponsive and had a positive Babinski sign on one side. As there had been a considerable amount of blood clot in the left atrium, it was thought probable that she had had a cerebral embolus; however, the arterial P_{CO_2} was found to be 82 mm Hg, and following assisted ventilation for several hours she made a satisfactory recovery.

Two and a half years after operation her dyspnea had lessened slightly and she was no longer orthopneic. There has been no hospitalization since 1962.

Radiology. The heart is obviously enlarged (*A*), although its exact size is impossible to measure because of the obliteration of its right margin by chronic right middle-lobe disease. Other investigations had demonstrated atelectasis of the right middle lobe, the anterior basal segment of the right lower lobe and the anterior segment of the right upper lobe, all associated with bronchiectasis. Fluoroscopic examination revealed moderate enlargement of the left atrium and of the right ventricle, indicating a predominant mitral stenosis. The aortic shadow is small. Numerous horizontal lines of increased density measuring 1 to 2 cm in length are present in the axillary zone of both lung bases, extending inward from the pleural surfaces (*A*). These septal lines, or "Kerley" lines, represent lymphatic engorgement and edema of the interlobular septa. The upper-lobe pulmonary veins are engorged and the lower-lobe veins are narrowed. The hilar pulmonary arteries are enlarged and the lower-lung arteries are narrowed, so that these vessels taper more rapidly than normal. There is no evidence of generalized pulmonary edema, fibrosis or hemosiderosis.

Two years later (*B*) the heart is smaller, but an enlarged left atrium can still be identified through the right heart shadow. The septal lines on the left have completely disappeared, although a few thin lines remain on the right. Since all other signs of venous hypertension have cleared, it is probable that these residual lines represent interlobular septal fibrosis and hemosiderosis, the result of long-standing edema.

Pathology. Histological examination of the lingular biopsy showed greatly widespread and edematous interlobular septae, with dilated tortuous lymphatics (*C*). Siderophages in air spaces were widely distributed through the biopsy specimen. One small focus of recent intrapulmonary hemorrhage was present. The alveolar walls were moderately thickened, and the alveolar lining cells

														EXERCISE				
	VC	FRC	RV	TLC	ME %	MMFR	$FEV_{0.75}$ ×40	pH	P_{CO_2}	HCO_3^-	O_2Hb %	$D_{L_{CO}}SS_2$	MPH	GRADE	$\dot{V}_{O_2}$	$\dot{V}_E$	$D_{L_{CO}}SS_3$
Predicted	2.8	2.4	1.4	4.2	55	2.7	71	7.40	42	25	97	13.9					
Dec. 1959	1.8	2.4	1.6	3.4	67	1.5	51					9.1	1	FLAT	0.58	27.2	9.9
Aug. 1962	1.3	2.2	1.7	3.0	52	1.7	48					8.9					

Preoperatively in December, 1959, the vital capacity was reduced but the residual volume was normal, and therefore the total lung capacity was low. The gas distribution was normal but ventilatory ability was reduced significantly. The resting diffusing capacity was low and did not rise with exercise. She also required a very large minute volume to obtain an oxygen uptake of 0.58 liter/min ($\dot{V}_{O_2}/\dot{V}_E = 2.0$).

Two and a half years after mitral commissurotomy there has been no change in any of the indices of lung function.

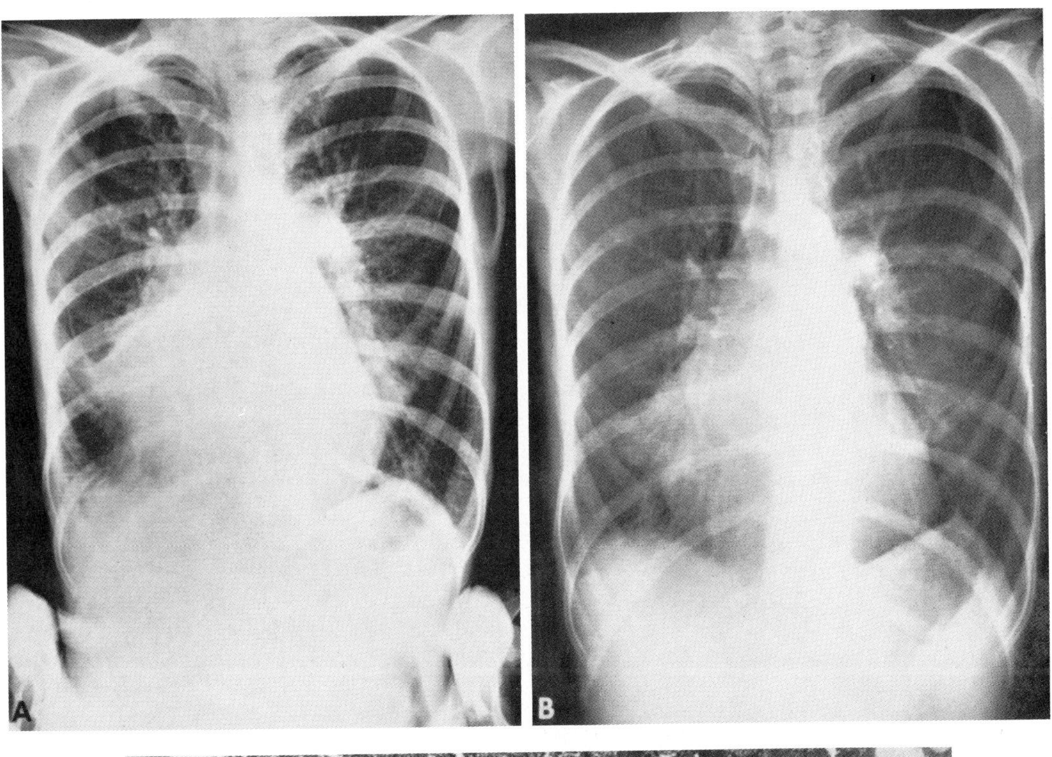

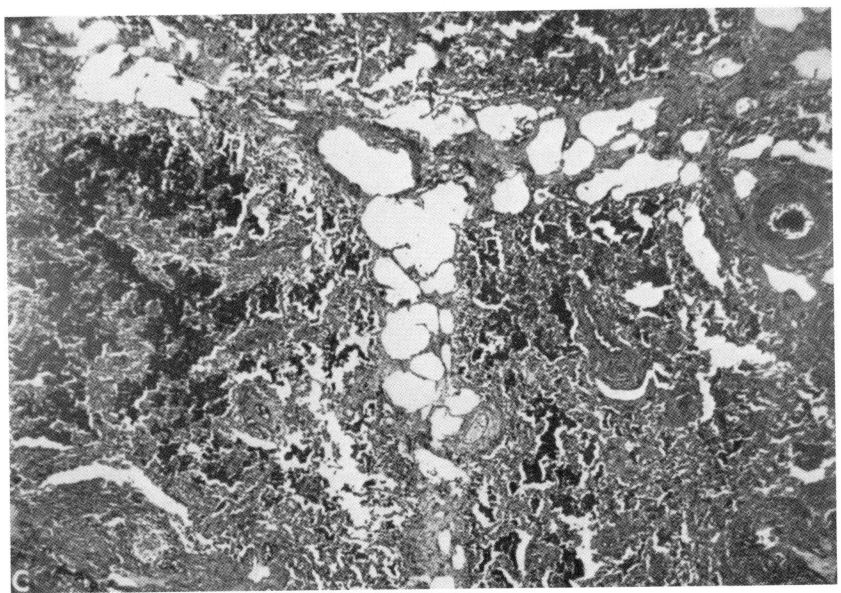

showed widespread cuboidal metaplasia. Striking medial thickening and slight intimal proliferation had occurred in the pulmonary arteries. Aggregates of chronic inflammatory cells were present focally around bronchioles, in interlobular septa, and in relation to nodular aggregates of siderophages. Mucus plugs were present in two large bronchioles.

Summary. Long-standing mitral stenosis with severe secondary lung changes and gross pulmonary function impairment. Spontaneous ventilation was inadequate during the postoperative period, presumably as a result of the state of the lung parenchyma. In spite of some subjective improvement postoperatively, pulmonary function status was unchanged.

patients with cardiopulmonary disorders, noted an abnormally high V_c value in their only patient with mitral stenosis. A recent attempt we have made to relate changes in V_c and D_M more closely to the various stages of the disease[1461] lends some support to the idea that the middle stages of the condition are characterized by elevation of V_c to a varying extent, with variable reduction in D_M. Flatley and his colleagues found an elevated V_c in some cases of mitral stenosis.[2288] In the most severe stage there is very considerable lowering of both V_c and D_M, and consequently of $D_{L_{CO}}$. McCredie,[3128] in a careful comparison between 18 controls and 18 patients with mitral stenosis, concluded that both D_M and V_c were usually lowered. This is the state of affairs represented by Case 34; in that patient irreversible changes were found to be present in the lung parenchyma.

It is obvious from much of the published pathological data on mitral stenosis that there are many reasons for expecting a fall in diffusing capacity in this condition. The explanation of the apparent discrepancy between results with different methods may be explained by two factors. First, the unusually high perfusion of the upper zones in this condition (*see* page 333) might increase the single-breath diffusing capacity disproportionately to the steady-state measurement. Second, and more important, the defect may become apparent and readily measurable only during exercise, when the cardiac output is trying to rise, the pulmonary compliance is falling, and the degree of pulmonary congestion may be approaching overt pulmonary edema. In a condition in which the state of the lung in relation to gas exchange is likely to be profoundly altered during exercise, it is unwise to infer, from data secured at rest, the factors that may limit gas exchange during exercise. The possible role of the lowered diffusing capacity in mitral stenosis, in relation to dyspnea and to limitation of physical exertion, is discussed later.

Effect of CO_2 administration

Observations on one patient with mitral stenosis by Meakins and Davies[1] apparently showed that in this condition there was an increased ventilatory response to inhaled CO_2. Recent and much more detailed evidence collected by Pauli, Noe, and Coates[1474] indicates clearly that, in the majority of these patients, there is a diminished response to inspired CO_2. Using an index based on the increase of ventilation in liters/min/sq m BSA in relation to the change in arterial P_{CO_2} in normal subjects, these workers found the ventilation so expressed altered by 1.12 liters/min/sq m BSA/1.0 mm Hg change in P_{CO_2}. In patients with mitral stenosis, breathing oxygen, the comparable figure was 0.73 liters/min/mm Hg change; in two, the value changed from 0.55 and 0.73 preoperatively to 1.61 and 1.79 postoperatively, respectively. The resting P_{CO_2} levels in these patients, as was noted under Blood-gas Tensions, usually were lower than normal. There does not appear to be any satisfactory explanation of these findings, which are, however, of particular relevance in discussion of the abnormal response of ventilation during physical exercise in patients with mitral stenosis.

Exercise studies

In mitral stenosis there is usually an inadequate or abnormally small increase in cardiac output on exercise, which results in very low values for the mixed venous oxygen saturation.[1482] As has been noted, there is a fall in compliance and there is an abnormally small increase in diffusing capacity in relation to oxygen uptake. Of more importance, however, is the fact that the level of total ventilation is excessive in relation to oxygen uptake. The interrelationship between these two variables has caused considerable confusion. Knipping and Moncrieff calculated a ventilation equivalent by dividing minute volume by oxygen uptake,[549] whereas others have preferred to calculate the reciprocal of this,[1482] since in fact it represents the oxygen extraction from respired air. This problem will be discussed here without reference to numerical values, in an effort to avoid further confusion.

Knipping and Moncrieff noted that there was excessive ventilation in relation to oxygen uptake in some patients with heart disease,[549] though when this measurement is made at rest there is very considerable overlap and scatter between values in normal and abnormal states. On exercise, however, the differences become more striking, and Donald and his colleagues carefully documented the lowered percentage oxygen extraction commonly encountered during exercise in patients with mitral stenosis.[1482] Similar observations have been recorded by others.[283, 551, 1461, 1483,

[1485] It seems quite clear that the lowered oxygen percentage extraction is closely related to the severity of the clinical grade of mitral stenosis;[551, 1461] or, in other words, the more severe the mitral stenosis, the higher the ventilation on exercise for a given oxygen uptake. MacIntosh and his colleagues were unable to demonstrate any very close relationship between the measured diffusing capacity and the extent of impairment of this aspect of function,[551] although insofar as both of these have a general relationship to severity[1461] they must in general be related. Cronin and MacIntosh also have observed that the patient with mitral stenosis takes up significantly less oxygen during steady-state exercise than does a normal subject of similar size performing the same work load.[2072] That the minute volume is excessive in relation to CO_2 production is shown by the lowered arterial P_{CO_2} found on exercise in this condition[283] and in the fact that no considerable increase in physiological dead space occurs. Furthermore, it is clear that the most striking respiratory consequence of successful relief of the mitral stenosis is diminution in ventilation by the patient in relation to oxygen uptake.[551, 1453]

It is far from certain what these observations mean in terms of changes in lung function and in control of minute ventilation in mitral stenosis. Discussion of this problem has been somewhat obscured by some authors, who have considered the lowered percentage oxygen extraction as indicative of more than the fractional oxygen removal.[1485] Of the possible mechanisms responsible for the relative hyperventilation in mitral stenosis, the reduced diffusing capacity seems unlikely to be important, since this is usually adequate for gas transfer. There is no reason to suppose that patients with mitral stenosis are abnormally sensitive to CO_2—indeed, the evidence available indicates the reverse. Four other possibilities exist:

1. That the increased pulmonary congestion on exercise stimulates receptors in the lung and overdrives ventilation, as happens occasionally in patients with pulmonary fibrosis.
2. That the increased ventilation is directly caused by pulmonary hypertension, perhaps via receptors in the pulmonary artery, a possibility supported by the occurrence of hyperventilation in patients with primary pulmonary hypertension (*see* page 347).
3. That ventilation is somehow stimulated by the very low mixed venous-oxygen tensions or raised CO_2 tensions that may exist on exercise in blood on the right side of the heart.
4. That the slowed circulation in some regions of the body consequent upon the restricted cardiac output may give rise to increased levels of cellular P_{CO_2} and decreased levels of tissue-oxygen tension, and that from these cells there may be a stimulus to increase ventilation.

We do not feel that it is possible to decide, on evidence presently available, which mechanism is most likely responsible. However, it is very important for the physician to realize that the increased ventilation in relation to oxygen uptake that occurs in these patients on exercise plays a major part in determining the level of their dyspnea.

Ventilation–perfusion distribution in the lung

Although there had been some evidence pathologically to indicate structural differences in the state of the pulmonary vessels in the upper and lower parts of the lung in mitral stenosis, definite evidence of abnormalities in perfusion distribution in this condition was not available until the demonstration by Dollery and West that such patients had an unusually increased perfusion of the upper zones of the lung when sitting upright.[341] It is now known that in this position, in normal subjects, there is relative overperfusion of the lower zones (*see* Chapter 2, page 48), whereas in those with mitral stenosis there is reversal or partial reversal of this distribution pattern.

Dawson, Kaneko, and McGregor[3131] have shown that the relative underperfusion of the lower zones was not affected by breathing 100 per cent oxygen; thus, although many experiments have illustrated the fact that the perfusion distribution in relation to ventilation in mitral stenosis is under vasomotor control,[9, 1486, 1487, 1489, 1490] it does not appear that raising the inspired oxygen tension affects the vasomotor tone of the lower lung vessels. The recent work by West and his colleagues[3135, 3173] suggests that, initially, blood flow through dependent parts of the lung is reduced by perivascular edema. Later this is replaced by fibrosis. In the final stages, when severe pulmonary hypertension is present, blood flow distribution may again be regionally more uniform,[3131] but severe parenchymal changes will have occurred in the lung.

Case 35
Arteriosclerotic Heart Disease; ?Cause of Dyspnea

Summary of Clinical Findings. In May, 1961, a request for studies of a 60-year-old man was sent to the Pulmonary Function Laboratory with the following note: "Marked dyspnoea but no orthopnoea for the past few years. He had coronary, but this does not seem to be L.V. failure. Chest film of no help. Has he lung disease? Mystery!" The patient was noted to have some degree of bronchospasm but no cough or expectoration.

He was in hospital at the time for investigation of chest pain and dyspnea. In 1954 and 1956 he had suffered two attacks of severe retrosternal chest pain associated with a drop in blood pressure. Although the ECG showed no change on either occasion, it was felt at the hospital at which he had been treated that he had suffered episodes of myocardial ischemia. He was treated with bed rest and anticoagulant therapy. After the second episode he began to experience frequent attacks of dyspnea, both exertional and nocturnal, associated with wheezing. The patient denied any cough or sputum. He had smoked 20 cigarettes per day for some years.

On physical examination blood pressure was 125/80 mm Hg, and pulse rate 78/min. The heart sounds were normal but distant. The chest was of normal contour with no increase in anteroposterior diameter; on percussion, it was possibly hyperresonant, and air entry seemed poor, but no rhonchi were audible. There was no clubbing or cyanosis and he had no signs of heart failure. The ECG showed right axis deviation and some ST changes compatible with a state of coronary insufficiency. During his stay in hospital he rarely coughed, and difficulty was experienced in obtaining a blob of sputum for bacteriological culture.

Radiology. Apart from moderate generalized overinflation of the lungs and the densely calcified scar in the right base, the appearance of the chest on plain films is unremarkable (*A* and *B*). A midsagittal tomogram (*C*) of both lungs reveals general reduction in caliber of the peripheral vasculature, with resultant discrepancy between hilar and peripheral artery size. This finding suggests diffuse emphysema.

Summary. This patient illustrates the occasional difficulty of deciding on clinical and on radiological evidence from plain films alone whether dyspnea is most likely to be a consequence of left ventricular failure or of primary lung disease. When the history of chronic bronchitis is unspectacular, and there are few signs of bronchospasm in the chest and sputum is negligible in volume, the diagnosis of emphysema may easily be overlooked.

	VC	FRC	RV	TLC	ME %	MMFR	$FEV_{0.75}$ ×40	pH	P_{CO_2}	HCO_3^-	O_2Hb %	$D_{L_{CO}}SS_2$
Predicted	4.1	3.7	2.3	6.4	50	3.10	94					14.1
May 1961	1.4	4.7	4.2	5.6	24	0.38	14					7.8

The vital capacity is grossly reduced. There are hyperinflation, impaired gas distribution and marked reduction in ventilatory flow rates. The diffusing capacity is half the predicted value. These findings are typical of moderately severe emphysema.

Arteriosclerotic Heart Disease; ?Cause of Dyspnea

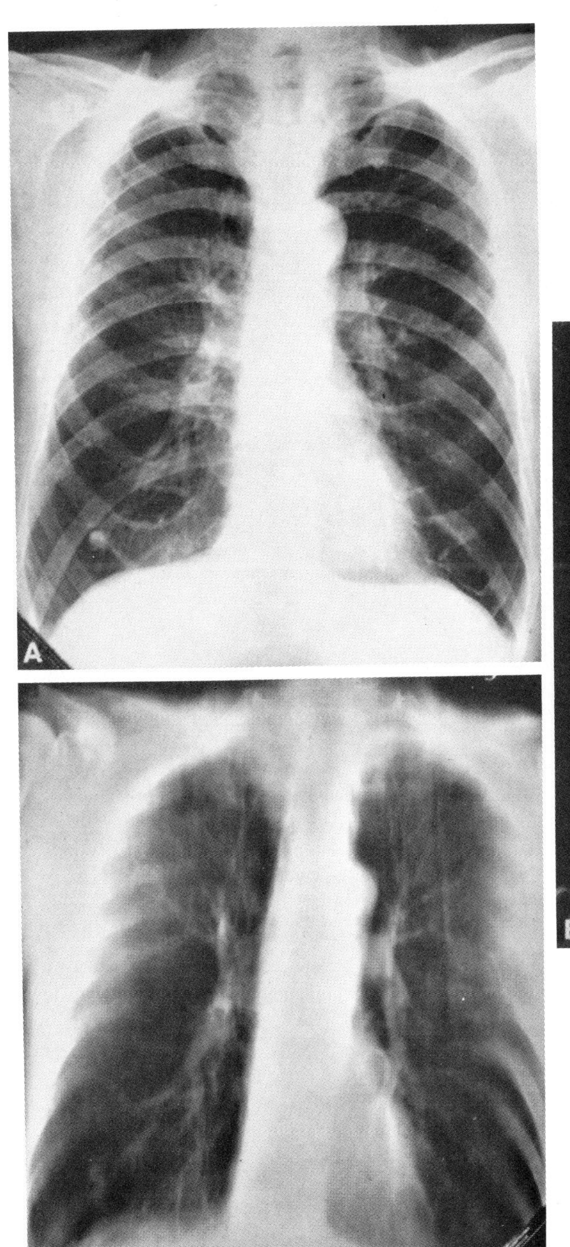

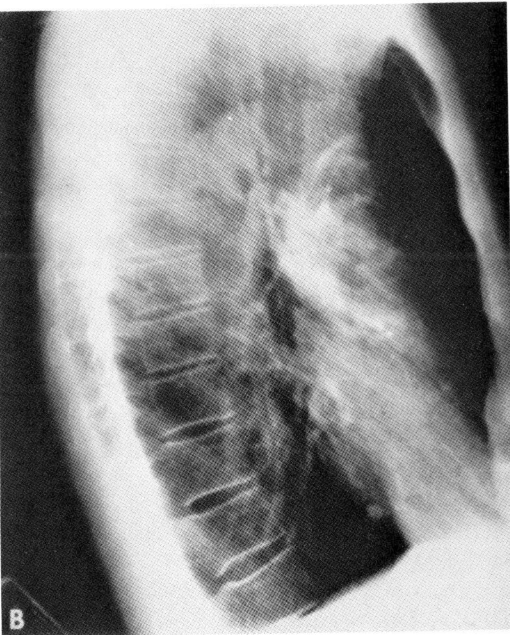

USE OF PULMONARY FUNCTION TESTS

In our experience there are three groups of patients with mitral stenosis in whom a careful assessment of pulmonary function may make a clear contribution to management. These are:

1. Patients with mitral stenosis who give a history of recurrent respiratory infections and in whom there may be evidence of chronic bronchitis. As has been noted (*see* page 327), the demonstration of ventilatory impairment out of proportion to the hemodynamic data indicates the presence of some factor additional to the stenosis that has an important bearing on the clinical situation. It is advisable, therefore, to test pulmonary function in any patient in whom the cardiologist feels there is a lack of correspondence between symptomatology and the probable state of the mitral valve.
2. Patients with the most severe grade of stenosis, in whom adequate ventilation can be difficult in the postoperative period after thoracic surgery. In some the impairment of ventilatory flow rates, diffusing capacity, and compliance may be severe enough to warrant performance of tracheostomy as an elective procedure to assist in ventilation during the postoperative period.
3. Patients in whom it is desirable to obtain an accurate estimate of the degree of dyspnea, necessitating study during exercise. In more than one case we have noted less dyspnea on exercise than the cardiologist had estimated from the patient's history; in others, we have found the reverse. There is real merit in watching such patients exercise, talking to them meanwhile, and measuring the ventilation and oxygen uptake at some level of effort they can manage comfortably. A purely clinical—or, as might be said more realistically, a solely dialectic—appraisal of effort dyspnea is inferior to this type of observation.

In view of the considerable documentation that now exists on the significant changes in pulmonary function that may result from mitral stenosis, it is remarkable that detailed, and in themselves wholly admirable, discussions of this condition and its natural history continue to be written without mention of this aspect of the disease.[1470] It seems clear that, in some patients with longstanding mitral stenosis, the secondary changes in the lung must play a dominant part in determining the degree of physical incapacity.

PULMONARY FUNCTION AND DYSPNEA

There is little doubt that the disorder in pulmonary mechanics, particularly on exercise, plays the major role in increasing respiratory work and in causing the sensation of dyspnea that these patients experience; and it is equally clear that an important secondary mechanism is their hyperventilation in relation to oxygen uptake, the cause of which is obscure. It is possible that the disturbances of ventilation–perfusion distribution and of diffusing capacity that are known to exist in many of these patients aggravate the situation further by necessitating a greater ventilation than would otherwise be needed. It is not clear to what extent the sensation of dyspnea may be accentuated by a feeling of fatigue or by the muscular weakness and wasting that may be very prominent in severe cases of mitral stenosis of long duration.

THE LUNG IN LEFT VENTRICULAR FAILURE

RADIOLOGY

In many respects the pulmonary changes of left ventricular failure are identical to those in mitral stenosis. In its milder forms, pulmonary venous hypertension leads to the development of mild pulmonary edema, which shows itself by the presence of septal lines in the costophrenic angles and by an increase in size and loss of definition of the pulmonary vasculature. In acute left ventricular failure, the development of acute pulmonary edema usually presents an x-ray picture that should not cause difficulty in diagnosis. Although the distribution of edema is variable, some lobes being more severely affected than others or one lung more severely involved than the other, the classic picture of a massive density occupying both lung fields, generally out to the periphery, is so distinctive as to require little description. Occasionally, distinctive peribronchial and perivascular "cuffing" may be visible.[3149] The heart may or may not appear much enlarged, although some left ventricular enlargement is common. Pleural effusions are uncommon.

In chronic or recurring left ventricular failure, there may be radiological evidence of left atrial enlargement of slight degree, and an alteration in size of the hilar pulmonary-artery complex and of the peripheral pulmonary arteries consistent with the presence of pulmonary arterial hypertension.

Pulmonary edema

The occurrence of frank pulmonary edema may be taken to represent the most severe and acute form of pulmonary congestion. Clinically this occurs most commonly as a result of acute left ventricular failure consequent upon coronary thrombosis or systemic hypertension, more rarely as a result of intracranial lesions,[2073] and only occasionally from other causes. It is not uncommon for episodic pulmonary edema to occur as a result of mitral stenosis, and it may be a complication of a variety of conditions, such as renal failure, cerebral injury and the inhalation of toxic substances. The classic clinical presentation is so familiar that no detailed description is needed; the shocked appearance of the patient, evident acute respiratory distress, copious moist sounds and wheezing in the lungs, and expectoration of a blood-tinged frothy fluid usually pinpoint the diagnosis. Less severe manifestations, however, may resemble an acute episode of spasmodic asthma, and in some clinical conditions, particularly uremia, there may be considerable radiological evidence of pulmonary edema without its giving rise to any very alarming symptoms.

Much has been written on various clinical aspects of pulmonary edema; this literature cannot be reviewed here, but it is important that the physician understand fully the state of lungs in which edema is occurring, whatever the cause of the edema may be. The observations made by Barcroft of the physiological changes that accompanied experimentally produced pulmonary edema are still relevant today: "The pathology of gas poisoning has to me been full of surprises, but never was I more surprised than when I discovered that it was possible for a goat to live with its arterial blood fully, or almost fully, oxygenated, but with its lung four times the ordinary weight.... The key to this situation lies in the fact that the blood almost ceases to circulate in the completely oedematous portions of the lung."[271]

It has become clear in recent years that pulmonary edema is best regarded as an "all or none" phenomenon. Parts of the lung are completely filled with fluid, and the circulation is reduced through these; the remainder functions fairly normally until it, too, closes as a result of fluid accumulation. Thus the arterial oxygen tension remains normal in experimental pulmonary edema until just before the occurrence of edema becomes grossly evident.[3142] In the acute stage there is gross reduction in vital capacity, and extremely low values for the pulmonary compliance have been reported, both in experimental animals[1488, 2094] and in patients.[495, 496, 1471, 1493, 1494] Working with animals, Cook and his colleagues concluded that the mechanical behavior of edematous lungs probably could be explained by "surface phenomena" rather than by congestion of pulmonary vessels or intrinsic tissue changes.[1488] There is some evidence to suggest that the fluid permeability of lung capillaries may be less in some capillary beds than in others.[2075] Widdicombe has shown that pulmonary edema in the cat increases the response of pulmonary stretch receptors to inflation.[2076]

Staub and his colleagues[3143] have recently thrown light on the sequence of events in the development of experimentally induced pulmonary edema. Their results show that the first observable phenomenon is the accumulation of fluid around the terminal bronchiole and accompanying arteriole just proximal to the terminal airway unit. Such an accumulation might have the effect of producing a concomitant reduction both of perfusion and of ventilation.

Sharp and his co-workers[1493, 1494] conducted very elegant observations of changes in pulmonary mechanics during treatment of pulmonary edema in humans and showed that positive-pressure breathing increased the compliance, as did the administration of intravenous aminophylline; conversely, morphine did not affect either compliance or airway resistance. The tachypnea of pulmonary edema presumably is explainable on the basis of the reduction in compliance that occurs.[495]

The terminal stage of pulmonary edema is one of ventilatory failure, with a considerable elevation of arterial P_{CO_2} and severe acidosis,[1481] and finally cardiac arrest. In some patients, prompt ventilation during this stage may be life-saving.[3147]

A discussion of the mechanism of pulmonary edema secondary to elevation of intracranial pressure is beyond the scope of the present volume. In a recent review, Luisada[3150] has suggested that inadequate left ventricular relaxation may be the determining factor in its production. Ducker[3151] has published a detailed review of 11 carefully observed patients with this interesting condition.

ORTHOPNEA

The increased respiratory discomfort when lying flat that is experienced by patients with cardiopulmonary disorders is a phenomenon that has attracted interest and speculation for hundreds of years.[1495] It has been recognized for 30 years[439] that sufferers from pulmonary congestion consequent upon mitral stenosis or left ventricular failure have decreased lung compliance when they are recumbent.[498] This change is accompanied by a considerable increase in the work of breathing, and a tachypnea that may be regarded as an adjustment to a respiratory rate at which minimal mechanical work will be required.[495] More recently it has become apparent that changes in airway resistance also play a major part in production of orthopnea. Cherniack and his colleagues, in a study of five patients with orthopnea, documented the increase in the work of breathing that occurred with transition from an upright to a supine position.[496] In one patient it increased from 123.7 Kg/cm/min to 186.3 Kg/cm/min with this change of position. They further noted that a major part of this increase was due to a considerable increase in viscous work, a result of interference with patency of the airways. It is to be presumed, therefore, that the total mechanical consequences of recumbency in the presence of pulmonary congestion of this type are a decrease in compliance and an increase in airway resistance. It is not difficult to understand, in these circumstances, why areas of atelectasis and bronchopneumonia are such common, if not invariable, accompaniments of bed rest or immobility of patients with marginal left ventricular inadequacy.

Mauck and his colleagues have recently shown[3141] that elevation of left atrial pressure is closely correlated with dyspnea in early left ventricular failure.

"PULMONARY CONGESTION"

Although physicians have for many years recognized a state of pulmonary congestion characterized by dyspnea and rales audible at the lung bases in patients known to have an inadequate left ventricle, it is far from clear what this condition is. Two useful reviews of contemporary knowledge of the congested lung have appeared,[1472, 1504] but relatively few studies have been published of pulmonary function before and after relief of such pulmonary congestion. Wilhelmsen and Varnauskas have recently shown that infusion of up to a liter of Rheomacrodex into normal subjects causes a shift to the right of static compliance curves and a decrease in maximal expiratory flow rate, without clinical pulmonary edema,[3139] and Giuntini and his colleagues noted a similar relationship.[3734]

It is now clear that the small airways in the dependent part of the lung are closed at residual volume in young normal subjects, and at FRC in older people (*see* page 47). It is to be assumed that pulmonary congestion with fluid accumulation around small vessels and bronchioles will lead to premature airway closure. In Table 15–1 are shown observations made on two men with essential hypertension. These cases illustrate the view that such pulmonary congestion essentially represents a subacute pulmonary edema and is not really distinguishable from it. Presumably, if the lung were abnormally congested with blood, a higher-than-normal diffusing capacity might be found, whereas in our experience it is usually lowered. It might be argued that the congestion of the lung with blood is offset by interstitial and alveolar edema, but if this is admitted, then it must be conceded that pulmonary congestion is unlikely to exist without concomitant edema. Such a reciprocal change in D_M and V_c does appear to occur in mitral stenosis (*see* page 329), but as far as we are aware this has not been demonstrated in left ventricular failure consequent upon aortic valve disease or systemic hypertension. The two cases shown in Table 15–1 illustrate the reduction in pulmonary compliance and increase in minute ventilation on exercise that together probably determine the exercise dyspnea. This is a sensitive early symptom of left ventricular failure, and it precedes the appearance of the physical signs of basal moist sounds in many of these patients. Rosenthal and Doyle[3137] have recently stressed the fact that the measurement of pulmonary compliance during exercise is a sensitive test of early left ventricular failure.

Saunders[3138] found that pulmonary con-

TABLE 15–1 EFFECT OF TREATMENT OF LEFT VENTRICULAR FAILURE ON PULMONARY FUNCTION IN TWO PATIENTS WITH ESSENTIAL HYPERTENSION

	A.T., AGED 51		R.S., AGED 51	
	10 March	*5 April*	*15 April*	*9 May*
Weight (lb)	195	187	181	174
Systemic BP (mm Hg)	210/150	140/90	220/150	150/100
TLC (liters)	3.5	4.6	3.9	4.7
VC (liters)	1.9	3.0	2.1	2.9
FRC (liters)	2.0	2.3	2.2	2.2
ME (%)	49	52	14	57
$D_{LCO}(SS_2)$(ml CO/min/mm Hg)	9.0	10.0	10.9	13.8
Compliance (l/cm H_2O)	0.113	0.186	0.067	0.185
Exercise: 1 mph flat:				
V_E (l/min)	26.0	18.1	34.2	27.5
V_{O_2} (l/min)	1.3	1.0	1.0	1.1
$D_{LCO}SS_3$ (ml CO/min/mm Hg)	18.0	28.0	11.9	15.8

Note that relief of pulmonary congestion was followed by improvement in vital capacity, increase in resting and exercise diffusing capacity, increased lung compliance, and reduction in exercise ventilation.

gestion resulted in a lowering of the physiological V_D/V_T ratio with the patient upright, an effect presumably caused by an increased perfusion of the lung apices.

CHEYNE-STOKES RESPIRATION*

Ever since Cheyne in 1818 accurately described the phenomenon of periodic breathing,[1496] physicians and physiologists have been intrigued by it. Haldane and Priestley,[2] who ascribed the first observation of it to John Hunter, conducted experiments on apnea and periodic breathing, and their observations played an important part in early research on the mechanisms controlling respiration. Meakins and Davies summarized their view as follows: "The combined effects of want of oxygen, diminished carbon dioxide, and the time required for the pulmonary blood to reach the respiratory centre, result in the well known manifestation of periodic or Cheyne-Stokes breathing."[1]

Clinically, periodic breathing consists of three elements: (1) hyperventilation, with progressive increase in tidal volume, followed by (2) diminution, followed by (3) periods of comparative or absolute apnea; usually each of these periods lasts 15 to 20 seconds. As can be seen from Figure 15–2, the ventilation during the hyperventilation phase may reach a level of 30 liters/min, and it may fall to only 5 liters/min during the apneic period. It is to be noted that this is a different phenomenon from Biot's respiration, in which there is no waxing and waning of the tidal volume when breathing occurs, and which is seen in severe respiratory depression.[1498]

Cheyne's patient not only had heart disease but also had suffered a cerebral seizure; and there is little doubt that the most severe forms of periodic respiration are seen in patients who have both cardiac and cerebral lesions. Pryor noted delayed circulation time to be a feature of the five patients he studied,[1499] but until recently there was considerable doubt as to whether the periodic breathing was caused by some cyclical change in the lungs—as a waxing and waning change of compliance, for example—or whether it reflected a periodic output from the respiratory center or centers. Mendel and McIlroy, studying esophageal pressure in this syndrome, were able to show conclusively that there was no cyclical change in pulmonary compliance, the increasing and decreasing ventilation being precisely paralleled by similar changes in intrapleural pressure.[1500] However, the reason for the oscillation became plain only when the new engineering understanding of the behavior of "controlled" systems began to extend into biology. Guyton, Crowell, and Moore showed that breathing of

*It seems very doubtful that Stokes' name should, in justice, be attached to this entity. He included a description of Cheyne's patient in his textbook written 36 years later,[1503] but added nothing to the description or understanding of the condition.

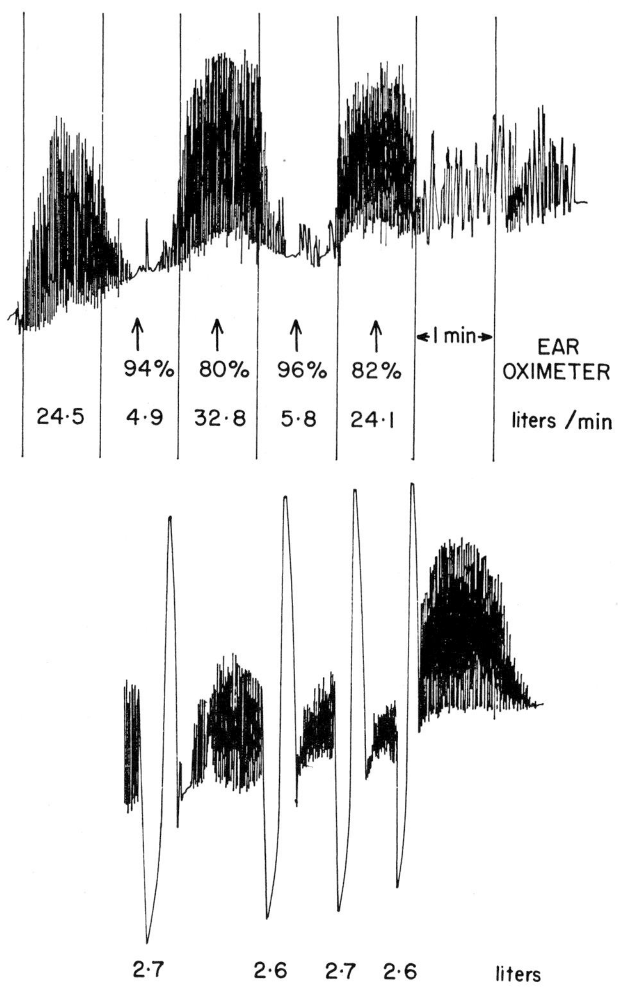

FIGURE 15–2. SEVERE CHEYNE-STOKES RESPIRATION IN A 72-YEAR-OLD MAN.

This man was known to have had a coronary thrombosis at the age of 55. There was considerable left ventricular enlargement and an abnormal electrocardiogram. He noticed his oscillatory breathing pattern, which interfered with his sleep. The top tracing shows the sequence of breathing pattern recorded on a closed circuit containing air. Note that in consecutive minute periods the ventilation is varying between about 28 and 5 liters/min. The oxygen saturation at the ear is high during the apneic periods and low during the hyperventilation. The lower tracing illustrates four vital-capacity maneuvers carried out during apneic and hyperventilation phases; their constancy illustrates the observation that there is no cyclical change in pulmonary compliance. The patient lived for two years after these tracings were made; at autopsy there was not only gross cardiomegaly but also severe obliterative arterial disease in both internal carotid arteries. There were no striking morphological changes in the region of the medulla. The lungs were normal.

the Cheyne-Stokes type could be produced by the insertion of plastic tubes between proximal carotid arteries and distal carotid or vertebral arteries in dogs.[1501] This preparation, therefore, had the effect of imposing a circulatory delay between the thorax and the respiratory centers, but did not cause any intrinsic abnormalities of lungs, heart or respiratory neurones. This concept has been supported by the observations reported by Lange and Hecht on nine patients with this condition.[1502] It seems quite clear, therefore, that the basic mechanism is the prolongation of lung-to-brain circulation time, a circumstance caused clinically by a combination of the following factors: left ventricular failure, low cardiac output, increased left atrial and left ventricular volume, and thrombosis or arteriosclerosis of cerebral vessels. Gross Cheyne-Stokes respiration of long duration, such as that illustrated in Figure 15–2, occurs only when all of these factors co-exist. It is noteworthy that the patient is able to take as large a deep breath during the period of apnea as during the hyperventilation, which indicates that there can be no significant cyclical change in compliance; furthermore, perhaps contrary to expectation, the arterial oxygen saturation as measured at the ear is normal during the period of apnea and low during the hyperpnea; that is, it is 90 degrees out of phase with the simultaneous blood saturation in the pulmonary vein. The level of P_{CO_2} is low during the apneic period and normal during the hyperventilation, though these determinations are more difficult to secure than those of the oxygen saturation. John Hunter in 1794 noted the rhythmical change in color of arterial blood during Cheyne-Stokes breathing.

Tanser,[3140] using an impedence pneumograph, has recently reported detailed studies of a 71-year-old man with essential hypertension and a slow circulation time with quite severe Cheyne-Stokes respiration during sleep, the end-tidal P_{CO_2} oscillating between 40 and 20 mm Hg. The sequence of events appeared to be: sleep; increased periodic breathing with increase of apneic interval from 5 to 30 seconds; right atrial pressure rise from 0 to 5 cm H_2O; wakes breathless; increased ventilation for 10 minutes; fall in right atrial pressure; sleep. Anoxia seems to be the cause of the right atrial pressure increase and of cardiac arrhythmias that have been noted.[3152]

It is of considerable interest to read the discussion by Meakins and Davies of this entity.[1] They possessed much of the relevant data, and they knew the correct conclusion, but they were uncertain about why a controlled system should oscillate.

Post myocardial infarction

Since 1966, several interesting observations have been made of the defect in gas exchange that may exist after myocardial infarction. McNicol and his colleagues[3157] studied the arterial oxygen tension during acute myocardial infarction and found values of about 53 mm Hg to be common if there was clinical evidence of pulmonary congestion or a lowered systemic blood pressure. In a later paper the same authors reported that six to twelve months after recovery from an infarct, 13 of 39 patients had a lowered arterial oxygen tension, and in 17 the alveolar–arterial oxygen difference was increased.[3158] These abnormalities were more common in those patients who had had evidence of cardiac failure at the time of the acute episode. Valentine and his co-workers have reported that the arterial P_{O_2} is often lowered for three to four weeks after infarction.[3730]

Similar findings during the acute stage have been reported by Pain and his colleagues in 33 patients,[3216] and by Higgs,[3154] who also observed a lower than normal arterial oxygen tension during 100 per cent oxygen breathing and suggested that airway closure as well as atelectasis and edema might have occurred. Pain noted that the arterial oxygen tension during air breathing was improved after the administration of diuretics.

Higgs, Clode, and Campbell studied 29 patients between 12 and 30 months after a myocardial infarction, and measured ventilation and gas exchange during exercise on a bicycle ergometer.[3155] In 10 patients, who could only manage 300 kpm/minute of exercise, the V_D/V_T ratio, the alveolar–arterial oxygen tension difference, and the venous admixture effect were all abnormal, and there was an abnormally high rise of blood lactate. The cardiac output, however, was within normal limits. There was no clinical evidence of left ventricular failure in any of these patients, and the ventilatory capability as measured by the FEV was not different in the more severely and less severely affected.

These findings indicate the importance of monitoring the arterial gas tensions in this condition and certainly suggest that 40 per cent oxygen might be administered with advantage to many patients with an acute infarct. If this is not done, respiratory depression as a consequence of morphine administration may lower the arterial P_{O_2} still further. Lal and his colleagues have recently suggested that pentazocine, which in contrast to morphine did not cause a widening of the alveolar–arterial oxygen difference, should be used in place of morphine.[3156]

The exact mechanism of these changes is not clear. It may be suggested that the situation after a severe myocardial infarction is similar to that seen after post-traumatic shock (*see* Chapter 22). Pulmonary edema, atelectasis, and airway closure probably all occur in varying degree, but it is not clear why complete recovery does not always follow restitution of the cardiac output.

Clinical differentiation between "cardiac asthma" and spasmodic asthma

It may be difficult sometimes to decide whether acute dyspnea of paroxysmal type is really due to acute pulmonary edema or whether it is primarily a manifestation of

Case 36 Pulmonary Embolism with Infarction

Summary of Clinical Findings. This 45-year-old housewife was transferred to the Cardiorespiratory Service of the Royal Victoria Hospital on October 21, 1965. She had undergone a radical vulvectomy with bilateral resection of inguinal and external iliac lymph nodes for a carcinoma of the vulva on September 29, 1965. On October 15 she developed symptoms and signs of a superficial phlebitis involving the right long saphenous vein, but by October 19 the redness and tenderness had disappeared and the patient was up and around. On the afternoon of October 20 the patient developed right lower anterior pleuritic chest pain which persisted, and during the night she coughed up a small amount of bright red blood. She was transferred on the following day.

At that time her temperature was 101° having previously been normal. Her blood pressure was 110/70; pulse rate was 40/min. She appeared pale and her respirations were grunting in character. There was no jugular vein distention. The percussion note was dull over the right base and in the right axilla inferiorly, and the breath sounds were distant. There was no pleural friction rub or other adventitial sounds. Induration was described over the right long saphenous vein from knee to groin but there was no tenderness.

The Hb was 12.0 gm, the white blood count was 12,000 on October 21, rising to 15,000 with 75 per cent neutrophils the next day. The sedimentation rate was 43 mm/hr. Serum glutamate oxaloacetate transaminase and lactic dehydrogenase were repeatedly normal. The blood gases on October 21, while the patient was on nasal O_2, are shown below. An ECG was normal on admission and showed no change following the chest pain.

Chest x-rays, radioactive macroaggregated albumin lung scan, and radioactive xenon studies are shown.

The patient was anticoagulated with heparin and the symptoms rapidly subsided. She was allowed to get up on October 29 and transferred back to the Gynecology Service on October 31 and placed on oral anticoagulants. The xenon study was repeated on November 9, 1965, and routine function studies were performed on November 12. She was discharged on November 13 in good health.

Radiology. An anteroposterior roentgenogram of the chest (*A*), exposed, with the patient in the supine position, demonstrates a uniform opacity over the right hemithorax, in all likelihood owing to a large accumulation of fluid in the pleural space. From this bedside examination, an area of parenchymal consolidation cannot be identified but its presence cannot be excluded. The descending branch of the right pulmonary artery appears enlarged. This combination of findings, particularly the enlargement of the pulmonary artery, is highly suggestive of pulmonary embolism with infarction. Two weeks later, an anteroposterior roentgenogram (*B*) reveals a moderate accumulation of fluid in the right pleural space some of which appears to be loculated posteriorly. The right hemidiaphragm is moderately elevated. A major area of parenchymal consolidation cannot be identified.

A radioactive macroaggregated albumin lung scan (*C*) performed on the same day as the roentgenogram (*A*) shows poor perfusion of the upper and lower zones of the right lung. This abnormality may be due, all or in part, to the large pleural effusion. Two weeks later the lung scan (*D*) had returned to normal.

Xenon Studies. The xenon studies performed 48 hours after embolization (Fig. E) showed normal values for perfusion ($\dot{Q}$), ventilation/perfusion ratio and ventilation ($T\frac{1}{2}$) throughout the left lung. In the right lung, perfusion was slightly decreased in the two apical regions, ventilation was normal, and ventilation/perfusion ratios were high. The mid-lung region showed normal values, while at the right base both perfusion and ventilation (long $T\frac{1}{2}$) were sharply curtailed and the ventilation/perfusion ratio was high. These findings were interpreted as indicating embolization without infarction at the apex and embolization with infarction and ventilation impairment at the base. It is worth noting that

														EXERCISE				
	VC	FRC	RV	TLC	ME %	MMFR	$FEV_{0.75}$ ×40	pH^+	P_{CO_2}	HCO_3	P_{O_2}	O_2Hb %	$D_{Lco}SS_2$	CO Ext%	GRADE	$\dot{V}O_2$	$\dot{V}_E$	$D_{Lco}SS_3$
Predicted	3.0	2.7	1.6	4.6		2.8	75	7.40	40	25	80	97	14.3	45				
Oct. 21, 1965								7.36	48	25		100						
Nov. 12, 1965	1.8	2.4	1.6	3.4		2.1	54						10.3	37				

Blood gases on the day following the pulmonary embolism, while the patient was receiving oxygen, revealed a normal oxygen saturation but slight carbon dioxide retention.

On November 12, studies of pulmonary function showed a reduction in vital capacity and a borderline diffusing capacity.

Pulmonary Embolism with Infarction

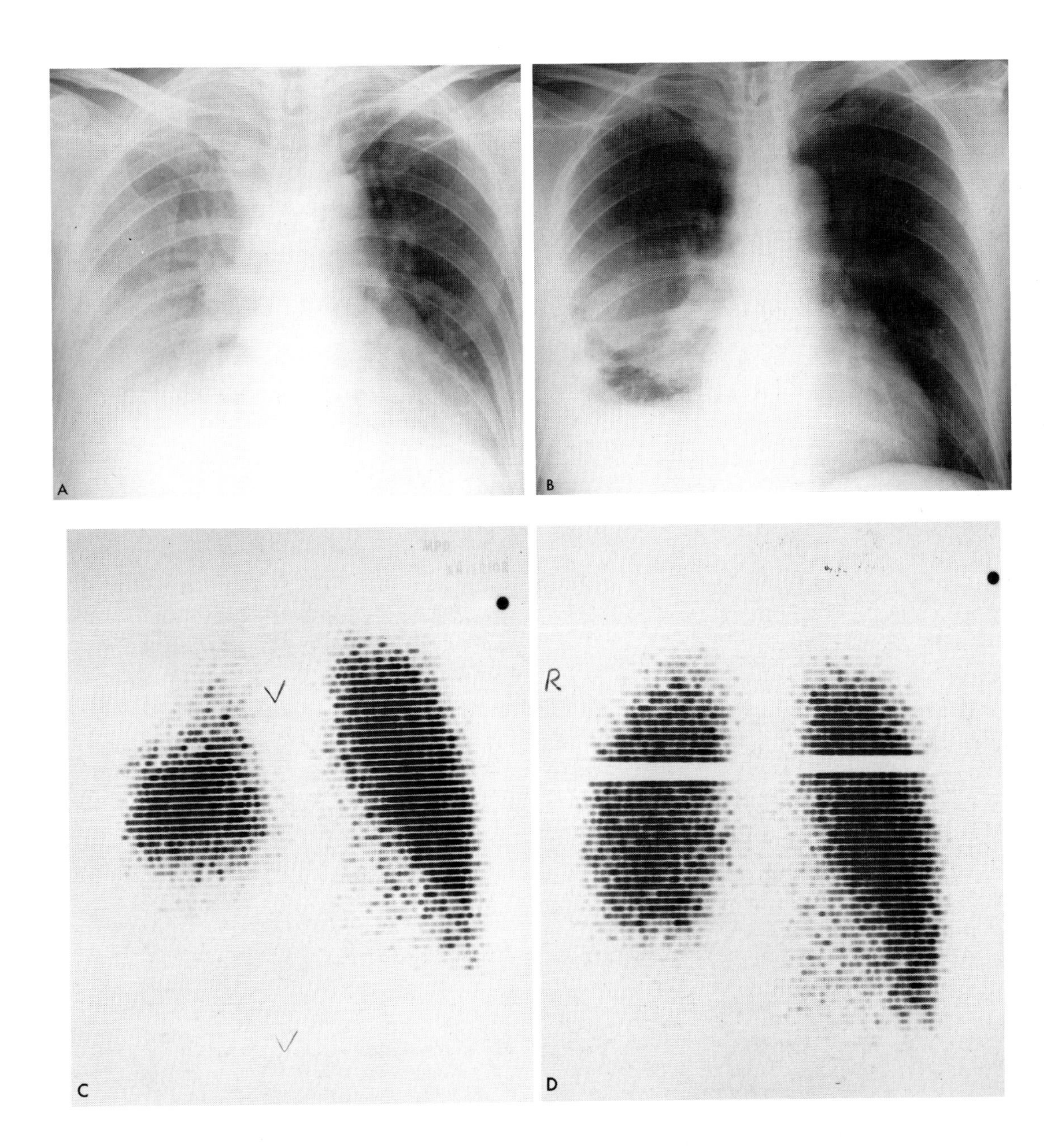

these studies are not affected by the presence or absence of pleural effusion.

Studies 20 days after embolization (Fig. F) showed again normal values on the left, decreased perfusion, decreased ventilation, and high ventilation/perfusion ratios at the right base. At the right apex, however, both perfusion and ventilation/perfusion ratios had returned to normal without any change in the ventilation of these regions.

Summary. This patient's clinical findings were typical of pulmonary embolism and infarction. Radioactive studies were useful in diagnosing and defining the pathologic process and course.

Pulmonary Embolism with Infarction (Continued)

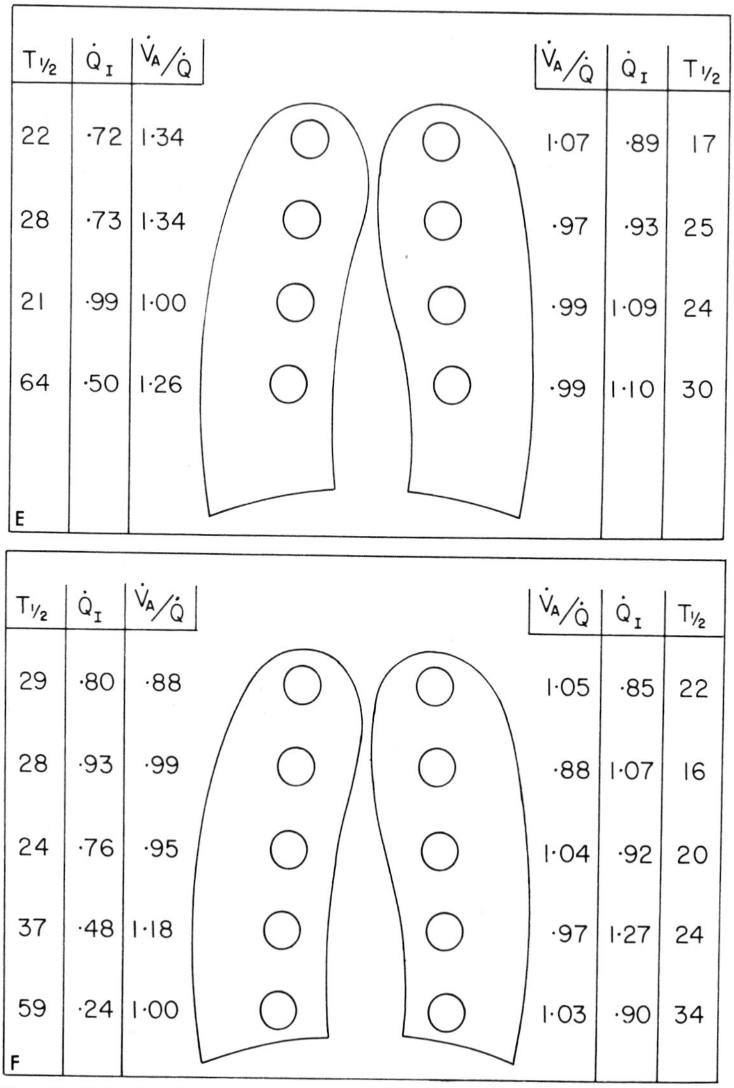

E

$T_{1/2}$	$\dot{Q}_I$	$\dot{V}_A/\dot{Q}$	$\dot{V}_A/\dot{Q}$	$\dot{Q}_I$	$T_{1/2}$
22	·72	1·34	1·07	·89	17
28	·73	1·34	·97	·93	25
21	·99	1·00	·99	1·09	24
64	·50	1·26	·99	1·10	30

F

$T_{1/2}$	$\dot{Q}_I$	$\dot{V}_A/\dot{Q}$	$\dot{V}_A/\dot{Q}$	$\dot{Q}_I$	$T_{1/2}$
29	·80	·88	1·05	·85	22
28	·93	·99	·88	1·07	16
24	·76	·95	1·04	·92	20
37	·48	1·18	·97	1·27	24
59	·24	1·00	1·03	·90	34

E, Results of Xe^{133} study 48 hours after embolization. Patient in supine position. There is a moderate reduction of perfusion to the right apex and upper zone, and severe reduction to the right lower zone. Ventilation is reduced, as shown by a prolonged $T_{1/2}$, only to the right lower zone; *F*, A similar study 20 days later. Perfusion is now normal to the right apical and upper zones, but is still reduced to the right lower zone.[3184]

---

acute bronchial obstruction. Since audible rhonchi over the chest and varying degrees of bronchial obstruction are common features of pulmonary edema, clinically such a differentiation can be difficult. Occasionally confusion between pulmonary edema and acute respiratory infection leads to the use of morphine and oxygen, with very deleterious effects, as exemplified in Case 58. In cases in which the clinical situation is confusing, an estimate of the level of arterial P_{CO_2} may be very valuable. If pulmonary congestion is present, this may be low; though, as noted previously (*see* page 337), it may rise in the terminal stages of pulmonary edema. When congestive failure is present, on a basis of longstanding emphysema, not only will the P_{CO_2} level usually be elevated, but the fact that this elevation is chronic may be revealed by the finding of an elevated level of serum bicarbonate when the arterial puncture is taken.

Since aminophylline is of considerable assistance in both conditions and is contraindicated in neither, we have found it useful to teach that emergency treatment should consist of the intravenous administration of this compound, until the clinical condition has been thoroughly evaluated.

CHRONIC BRONCHITIS AND EMPHYSEMA IN ASSOCIATION WITH CORONARY-ARTERY DISEASE OR ESSENTIAL HYPERTENSION

Physicians and pathologists stressed the interrelationship between chronic bronchitis and heart disease before the increasing prevalence of chronic bronchitis and its association with atmospheric pollution and cigarette-smoking were generally recognized. The fact that both chronic bronchitis and coronary artery disease are commoner in heavy cigarette-smokers indicates that an association between these two conditions is probably not fortuitous.

It not infrequently happens that chronic bronchitis is noted in a patient known to have had a coronary thrombosis or to suffer from systemic hypertension, and the physician is perplexed as to whether his dyspnea is primarily related to left ventricular failure and pulmonary congestion or to chronic bronchitis. It will be evident that the finding of relative preservation of ventilatory function and the normal residual capacity and diffusing capacity, together with a demonstrated decrease in pulmonary compliance – which are the common findings in a patient with early left ventricular failure – will readily assist one in forming a definite opinion in some cases. Sometimes, however, the distinction is less clear-cut, and it is to be assumed that some degree of left ventricular failure and chronic bronchitis may well co-exist. In interpreting the results of tests in patients known to have heart disease, therefore, the physician will sometimes find that no definite opinion as to which factor is mainly responsible for dyspnea is possible; however, if pulmonary function tests are repeated after appropriate treatment of the bronchitis or pulmonary congestion, the situation may become clearer, and one may be able to make a more precise estimate of the relative importance of these two factors.

PULMONARY HYPERTENSION (ARTERIAL)

PULMONARY SCHISTOSOMIASIS

It has been known for many years that the ova of schistosomiasis may be lodged in the pulmonary arterioles and may cause severe symptoms and death. Until 1952, clinical reports stressed the dyspnea, precordial pain, hemoptyses and cardiac enlargement that characterize this condition, occasionally mentioning the occurrence of pulmonary emphysema.[1505] More recently, published studies of hemodynamics and pulmonary function have outlined a clearer picture of the functional consequences of this disorder.[3159, 3160]

The formation of granulomata around the small pulmonary arterioles in which the ova lodge[1507, 3162] causes severe pulmonary hypertension – 58/31 mm Hg with a mean pressure of 41 mm Hg in the pulmonary artery of the patient reported by Cortes and Winters.[1506] Shunts may develop between the bronchial circulation and the pulmonary arterial tree.[1508] The maximal breathing capacity was 64 liters/min in Cortes and Winters' case[1506] and slightly decreased in the 15 patients studied in detail by Farid and his colleagues.[1509] In two patients reported by Wessel and his co-workers,[3161] the MBC was normal in one and reached 72 per cent of the predicted volume in the second. Frayser and De Alonso[3163] found moderate reductions of MBC and $FEV_{1.0}$ in 14 patients, however. Subdivisions of lung volume are little changed, and no abnormality of inert-gas distribution is demonstrable. Arterial saturation is usually normal at rest, though it may fall on exercise. The diffusing capacity is normal at rest, but increases significantly less on exercise than in normal subjects,[3161, 3163] and this may be an early sign of pulmonary involvement. Zaky and his colleagues[3159, 3160] have reported finding low values for pulmonary compliance in this condition. None of the case reports published contains function-test data to support a diagnosis of emphysema. Most authors mention a form of this disease that involves the pulmonary parenchyma and in which the changes are not confined to the pulmonary arterioles;

no function tests appear to have been reported in this variety of the condition. There is no doubt, however, that effort dyspnea is a prominent symptom of patients with pulmonary schistosomiasis when the lesions are arteriolar only, with no evidence of bronchial changes and no generalized alveolar-wall thickening.[1510, 3159] The dyspnea is probably attributable to a combination of lowered compliance and increased exercise ventilation.

EMBOLISM OF MAJOR PULMONARY VESSELS

Sudden death following a large acute pulmonary embolism in an otherwise healthy adult is a tragically familiar occurrence; yet, as Comroe has pointed out, its mechanism is far from obvious.[1511] Ever since Hanson showed that a right or left pulmonary artery could be completely blocked with a balloon catheter without any serious consequences,[308] it has been clear that the mechanism of these deaths is unlikely to be purely mechanical.

Patients who have just had a pulmonary infarct of any size are far too ill to undergo many physiological investigations. Arterial blood-gas studies are possible, however. Robin and his colleagues found significant arterial desaturation to be a feature of patients who had just suffered a major pulmonary infarction, and suggest that this finding may be of useful differential diagnostic value.[1515] In some of the patients they studied, a diminution of diffusing capacity appeared to have contributed to the anoxemia; in others it seemed clear that significant veno-arterial shunting must have been responsible for the anoxemia, since full saturation could not be achieved during oxygen breathing.

Until 1960 it was not known whether these patients, after recovery, suffered any residual abnormality of pulmonary function or of hemodynamics. Then Duner, Pernow, and Rigner[1512] demonstrated that, three months after recovery from a clinically severe pulmonary embolism, a patient may have normal pulmonary function, including exercise diffusing capacity, and normal values for cardiac output and pulmonary artery pressure, with a perfectly normal working capacity. (*See* Case 34 in reference 1512.) This case, together with some others they studied, illustrates that, with a normal cardiovascular system, complete recovery of such patients is possible. A few of those included in their careful follow-up survey of 113 patients who had suffered a pulmonary embolism had some worsening of symptoms from pre-existing heart disease or other clinical condition. Others have recently documented the complete recovery that may occur after embolization, and they have stressed that this is less common if there is pre-existing heart or lung disease.[3182] It has been demonstrated in dogs that obstruction of large branches of the pulmonary artery, caused by injected autologous blood clots, may disappear completely and spontaneously,[2070, 2071] and that reduction of $\dot{V}O_2$ and D_{LCO}, an early consequence of large pulmonary emboli in dogs, may show recovery to almost normal levels within two weeks.[2229]

The effects on pulmonary function of ligature of one pulmonary artery have been clearly documented by Roh and his colleagues.[1513] In their case, the left pulmonary artery had to be ligated during an operation on an aneurysmal communication between the aorta and pulmonary artery. The left bronchus was not tied, and the lung was left *in situ*. There was no disability postoperatively. The maximal breathing capacity, subdivisions of lung volume and nitrogen alveolar clearance were normal, as was the resting oxygen uptake. Bronchospirometry revealed absence of oxygen uptake from the left side, but there was a considerable output of CO_2, which the authors ascribed to the presence of a continuing bronchial circulation. These findings confirm that ligature of a major pulmonary artery does not have very serious functional consequences. In other case reports giving data of function tests there has usually been considerable chronic lung disease on the same side as the apparently absent pulmonary artery,[1514] and some of these cases might well be classified as examples of the type of unilateral lung emphysema described by Reid and Simon.[983]

MULTIPLE PULMONARY EMBOLI AND IDIOPATHIC PULMONARY HYPERTENSION

The use of cardiac catheterization has led to recognition of a well-defined syndrome of pulmonary hypertension not associated with chronic parenchymal lung disease or with intracardiac shunts. Since it is usually difficult, and occasionally impossible, to be sure whether or not the pulmonary arteriolar changes have been caused by recurrent embolism and thrombosis or whether there has been a progressive arteriolar sclerosis of unknown cause,[3189] both of these entities will be considered together.

There is a considerable volume of experimental work on the effects of embolism of small pulmonary vessels in animals. Such embolization causes tachypnea, an effect abolished by vagotomy but not by oxygen breathing;[2066] the pulmonary compliance falls,[1523, 2067] and recent work suggests that this is attributable to release of histamine and closure of terminal airway units.[1522] If occurring locally in the lung, this would have the effect of diverting ventilation away from the affected region.

From the clinical standpoint, such patients suffer from exercise dyspnea, which is a prominent and almost invariable symptom.[1521] There may be a complaint of precordial pain, and hemoptyses are not infrequent. Pregnancy often precedes its onset, in which case it is assumed that the emboli originated in ovarian or pelvic veins. Occasionally some other episode provides a possible antecedent history of thrombophlebitis. Clinically the lungs are normal on auscultation and radiologically clear, and the pulmonary vessels may appear either attenuated or small by contrast with the enlarged main pulmonary arteries. Selective angiography reveals filling defects and abnormal vessel cut-off.[3181] Clinical cardiac signs are those of right ventricular hypertrophy, and occasionally the murmur of pulmonary-valve incompetence may be heard. The patient is not cyanosed, and usually the fingers are not clubbed. There is respiratory distress at rest only in the terminal stages, though in severe cases there may be evident hyperventilation at rest. The introduction by Wagner and Sabiston[3165, 3166] of the micro-aggregate serum ^{131}I albumin technique with lung scanning represented a major diagnostic advance. Although this technique needs careful interpretation[3191] and does not replace selective angiography,[3178, 3179, 3181] it has led to a realization that pulmonary emboli are often missed clinically, and recurrent emboli are an important cause of unexplained dyspnea.[3170, 3175, 3183]

In such patients there is no significant change in the subdivisions of lung volume. In most cases the vital capacity is normal[2333] or slightly reduced,[3184] though it may be more reduced if the heart is greatly enlarged, in which case the total lung capacity also is lowered.[2074] The maximal breathing capacity may be slightly reduced,[2333] but usually is normal.[552, 1516, 1517, 2074] No striking changes are found in pulmonary compliance (*see* Case 16 in reference 1518) and airway resistance is usually normal or nearly so but the compliance has been reported to be low on exercise.[3171] The alveolar–arterial oxygen difference is usually increased, particularly if 15 per cent oxygen is breathed,[3728] and a major cause may be the diminished P_{O_2} of mixed venous blood. The level of arterial P_{CO_2} may be normal or sometimes subnormal,[552, 711] occasionally falling even further on exercise.[552] There is no defect in inert-gas distribution.[552, 1516, 1518, 2074, 2333, 3184] Arterial-oxygen-tension values may be low during air breathing,[552] but this is not an invariable finding, and the resting arterial saturation may be normal or nearly so.[2074, 3190] There is considerable variation in reported levels of pulmonary diffusing capacity. Ehrner and his colleagues found little reduction in steady-state $D_{L_{CO}}$ at rest, and in two of their three patients it rose further during exercise; in the third, however, it was lower during the performance of 300 kg/m/min of work than it had been at rest, presumably indicating a worsening of V/Q distribution on exercise.[552] In other cases diffusing capacity is slightly reduced,[1518, 3186, 3188, 3190] but values for single-breath $D_{L_{CO}}$ were normal or nearly so in the group of seven patients studied by Colp and Williams.[1516] Obrecht and his colleagues have recently found a significantly lowered $D_{L_{O_2}}$ in 10 women with primary pulmonary hypertension.[3728] Robin showed that, in this condition, the continued ventilation of significant volumes of lung that have little perfusion leads to decrease in the end-tidal CO_2 tension in relation to the arterial CO_2 tension.[1519] He and his colleagues have demonstrated that the same difference is present in dogs after occlusion of branches of the pulmonary artery,[1520, 2068] and that the percentage of lung volume involved in the occlusion may be calculated. The diagnostic value of a demonstration of discrepancy between end-tidal and arterial CO_2 values is unfortunately diminished by the common occurrence of this finding in pulmonary emphysema, as Robin himself has pointed out,[1519] and others have noted.[3177] We have had occasion to observe one patient in whom the diagnosis of infarct was suggested by the finding of a *normal* arterial P_{CO_2} in the presence of considerable and sustained elevation of the minute ventilation.

We have recently reported detailed studies of perfusion and ventilation distribution using

Case 37
Atrial Septal Defect

Summary of Clinical Findings. This patient was admitted in January, 1959, for assessment for open-heart surgery. He had a history of a cardiac murmur since birth and was said to be a "blue baby." He had had several admissions to hospital beginning in 1948 and slight cyanosis was noted on each examination. Cardiac catheterization in 1952 had revealed pulmonary hypertension and a large left-to-right shunt at the level of the atria. The brachial arterial saturation was 86 per cent. At that time his only complaints were undue fatigue and weakness. In 1956, however, he noticed increasing dyspnea on effort, with orthopnea and occasional episodes of paroxysmal nocturnal dyspnea, gradually increasing in severity since 1954.

On examination he showed slight peripheral cyanosis. The pulse rate was 100/min and irregular, blood pressure 118/80 mm Hg. There was a systolic pulse wave of the jugular veins and a precordial heave, a fixed split of the aortic and pulmonary closure sounds, and a grade III/VI ejection systolic murmur along the left sternal border. The chest moved symmetrically. There were diffuse inspiratory and expiratory high-pitched short rhonchi but no crepitations. The liver was enlarged three finger-breadths below the costal margin and was not tender. There was no peripheral edema.

Urinalysis and hemogram were normal. There was a BSP retention of 6.6 per cent. The electrocardiogram revealed atrial fibrillation and an incomplete right bundle branch block. Right heart catheterization was repeated and again revealed a left-to-right shunt at the atrial level. O_2 saturation of right and left atrial and brachial-artery samples were the same at 90 per cent. The pressure in the right ventricle was moderately elevated.

With extracorporeal cardiopulmonary bypass, repair of the defect was undertaken in February 1959. The size of the defect was estimated at 6 × 4 cm.

On the fifth postoperative day he died of pulmonary edema and cardiac arrest, the cause of which was obscure.

Radiology. The heart was markedly enlarged (*A*). On fluoroscopy a predominant enlargement of the right atrium and right ventricle was observed, and there was a considerable increase in the amplitude of pulsations in these two chambers and in the main hilar and peripheral pulmonary arteries. The pulmonary arteries were all increased in size to a considerable degree. The aortic shadow was small. The combination of pulmonary plethora, right atrial and right ventricular enlargement and an increase in the dynamic activity of these chambers and vessels is almost pathognomonic of interatrial septal defect.

Pathology. Autopsy disclosed severe acute congestion and edema of the lungs, and the main trunks of the pulmonary arteries were noted to be very dilated, but there were few atherosclerotic plaques. The interatrial defect had been surgically closed. The heart was greatly enlarged (640 grams), and both ventricles were hypertrophied, the right ventricle being particularly thick (10 mm).

Microscopical examination of the lungs showed acute congestion and edema. The pulmonary arteries and arterioles showed medial thickening only and the arteries appeared dilated. The pulmonary parenchyma was normal, showing no induration or fibrosis (*B*).

Summary. This case illustrates the fact that patients with an atrial septal defect may have an increased pulmonary blood flow for many years without its causing histological changes at the alveolar level, and consequently without causing impairment of pulmonary diffusing capacity.

													EXERCISE				
	VC	FRC	RV	TLC	ME %	MMFR	$FEV_{0.75}$ ×40	pH	P_{CO_2}	HCO_3^-	O_2Hb %	$D_{LCO}SS_2$	MPH	GRADE	$\dot{V}_{O_2}$	$\dot{V}_E$	$D_{LCO}SS_3$
Predicted	4.3	3.2	1.6	5.9	65	4.1	130	7.40	42	25	97	22					28
Jan. 1959	2.8	2.7	2.1	4.9	64	1.3	70	7.50	39	29	90	25	1.5	FLAT	0.60	21.6	31

The total lung capacity is reduced, probably a consequence of the space occupied by the greatly enlarged heart. Inert-gas distribution is normal, but there is some reduction in maximal midexpiratory flow rate and FEV. (Note: Rhonchi were audible over the lungs.) The arterial oxygen saturation is reduced and the bicarbonate slightly elevated. The diffusing capacity at rest and exercise is at the upper limits of normal. Measurement of the exercise diffusing capacity at two levels of oxygen tension showed that the pulmonary capillary blood volume was at the upper limit of normal, and the membrane components (D_M) were in the middle of the normal range. The ratio of $\dot{V}_{O_2}/\dot{V}_E$ on exercise is only 2.78 compared with a normal value of greater than 3.5 for this relationship.

Atrial Septal Defect

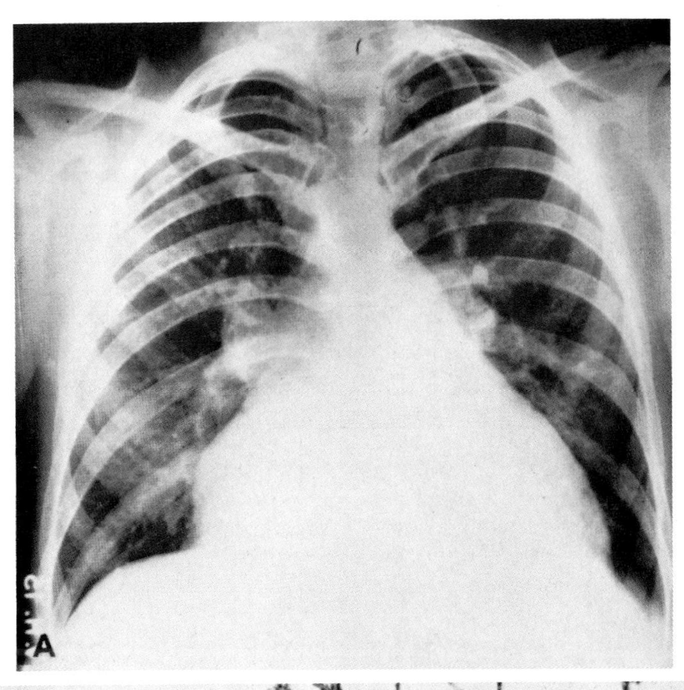

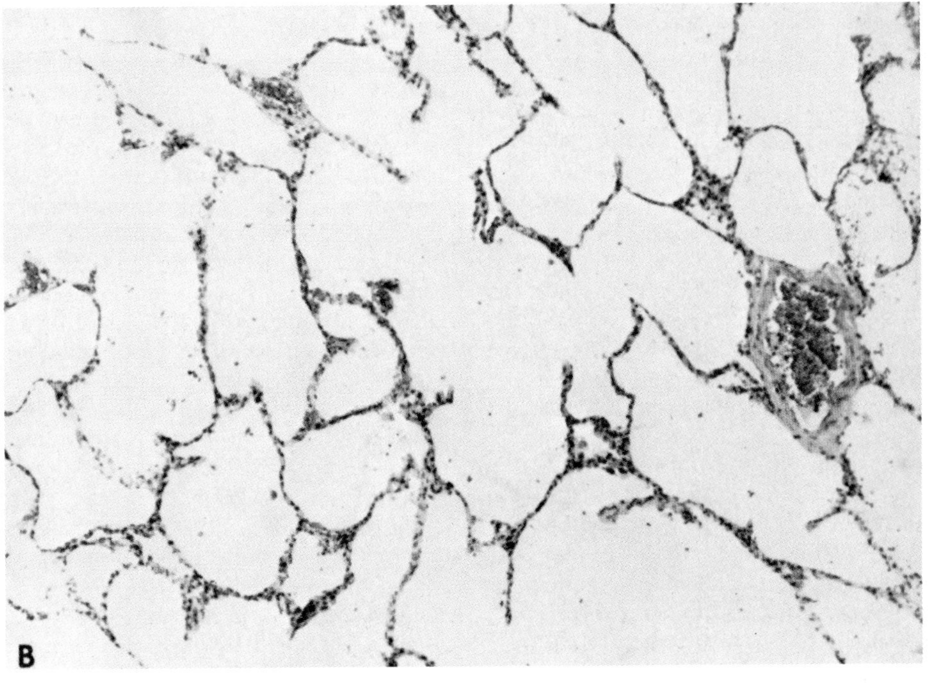

^{133}xenon in 7 patients, two or more days after pulmonary embolism had occurred.[3184] Regions with greatly reduced perfusion did not show evidence of reduced ventilation, and thus the $\dot{V}/\dot{Q}$ ratio in them was considerably elevated. It thus seems doubtful whether the shift of ventilation away from embolized zones noted in acute experimental studies in dogs[3172] continues to be operative in humans.

In marked distinction to the relatively minor changes in subdivisions of lung volume, pulmonary compliance, and pulmonary diffusing capacity that occur after recurrent pulmonary emboli is the very common and often very pronounced hyperventilation that occurs on exercise. This hyperpnea in relation to oxygen uptake was noted by McIlroy and Apthorp in one of their patients with idiopathic pulmonary hypertension who was exercised (*see* Case 16 in reference 1518), was present in most of the patients studied by others,[711, 1517, 1521, 3190] and was very pronounced in the three patients studied by Ehrner and his co-workers.[552] In these patients, the ratio $\dot{V}O_2/\dot{V}E$ on exercise was 2.04, 1.06, and 2.34, compared with average normal values of about 4.8 in this ratio in normal subjects exercising.[387] There can be little doubt that this exercise hyperpnea plays a major part in the effort dyspnea of which these patients complain[3169, 3171, 3180, 3186] Effort dyspnea was the commonest symptom in 54 cases of primary pulmonary hypertension collected by Yu, being present in all but one.[1521] It cannot be attributed to impairment of diffusing capacity or in pulmonary mechanics. It is understandable, in a general sense, since the physiological dead space is increased by many alveoli that are ventilated but that receive little perfusion. Its mechanism, however, is obscure. It may be that the restricted cardiac output bears some relation to the phenomenon, but it seems to us more probable that ventilation is being overdriven because of abnormal receptor impulses from the grossly hypertensive pulmonary circulation.[1536] As far as we know, no conclusive evidence for this exists; but disproportionate exercise hyperventilation is a feature of mitral stenosis and of arterial pulmonary hypertension, and is less prominent in patients who have other lesions, such as pulmonary-valve stenosis, that restrict cardiac output without giving rise to abnormal pressures in the lesser circulation.

In 1966, Nadel and his colleagues[3174] described three patients who had been referred for pulmonary function tests on account of dyspnea and were found to have a decrease in diffusing capacity and pulmonary capillary blood volume and an excess in exercise ventilation. Biopsy revealed unusual changes in pulmonary vessels. The serum gamma-A-globulin was increased, suggesting some immunological process. The origin of this condition could not be determined, but it seems possible that these patients either represent unusual cases of scleroderma, or are very early cases of pulmonary thromboembolic disease.

POST-TRAUMATIC FAT EMBOLISM AND LYMPHANGIOGRAPHY

Several recent papers have emphasized the disturbances in pulmonary function that may result from severe fat embolism after trauma. Clinically such patients have tachypnea, arterial unsaturation, and copious and occasionally blood-tinged sputum. The chest x-ray commonly shows a diffuse loss of pulmonary radiolucency and often some areas of diffuse and scattered pulmonary infiltration.[3207] The arterial–alveolar oxygen difference may be widened, and the diffusing capacity has been noted to be reduced.[3202] It has been pointed out that the diagnosis is probably often missed or confused with pulmonary edema,[3205] but occasionally the secretions are so copious and the arterial oxygen so low that tracheostomy and assisted ventilation with oxygen may be needed.[3201] Atypical recurrent cases have been recorded.[3203] Although the tachypnea seems to be a constant feature, it is not known whether the pulmonary compliance is lowered in this condition.

Experimental observations in dogs have revealed similar findings to the clinical situation,[2069] but arterial blood-gas changes are only produced if embolization is very gross and widespread.[3206] It has been suggested that fat emboli depress surfactant synthesis,[3200] and also that the normal lung, being directly concerned with fat metabolism,[3204] can usually dispose of small fat emboli.

Recently attention has been drawn to a pulmonary syndrome that may follow lymphangiography – essentially a specialized form of pulmonary embolization with oily radiopaque material. Clinically, there may be tachypnea and some transient radiological changes.[3185]

The clinical picture is rarely very severe, and although sputum may be produced, hemoptysis is rare.[3209, 3210, 3213, 3215] The arterial oxygen tension is most usually normal[3208] or only slightly reduced.[3213] In two studies, the diffusing capacity has been shown to be reduced,[3208, 3215] and, in one, a fall in pulmonary compliance was documented.[3208] Similar changes to these can be produced experimentally in dogs.[3212, 3214] Clinically, the changes might be of importance in compromising pulmonary function in patients with pre-existing heart or lung disease, but provided that the amount of material injected is limited to 15 ml, severe consequences appear to be unlikely.[3213]

Pulmonary veno-occlusive disease

Although from time to time it has been suggested that specific disease entities might be related to changes in the pulmonary veins,[3192] definitive case reports have only appeared within the past five years. One patient was described in 1965,[3195] another was described by Heath and his colleagues,[3193] who suggested the name of pulmonary veno-occlusive disease, since at autopsy the pulmonary veins were severely involved by cellular fibrous tissue. During life, the patient appeared to have primary pulmonary hypertension, and the laboratory findings appeared consistent with this diagnosis. In 1966, Brown and Harrison[3194] described a patient in whom the diagnosis had been made during life. All the pulmonary function tests were typical of those seen in severe obliterative pulmonary hypertension, but the nature of the lesion was revealed by lung biopsy. These authors collected eight similar cases from the literature and summarized the syndrome as consisting of a history resembling that of mitral stenosis; clinical and laboratory signs of pulmonary hypertension; radiological pulmonary edema without venous distention; and absence of structural heart disease. The etiology is not known.

THE LUNG IN CONGENITAL HEART DISEASE

Left-to-right shunt conditions

Several observations have been made of the pulmonary function status of patients with atrial or ventricular septal defects in whom there is a considerable increase in pulmonary in relation to systemic blood flow. There is customarily no alteration in subdivisions of lung volume,[1524] or slight reduction in TLC and VC with a relative increase in residual volume may be noted,[3198, 3199] no impairment of maximal breathing capacity,[1525] and no defect in inert-gas distribution[1525, 3198] (*see* Case 37). The arterial blood is usually normal, and there is no abnormality in pulmonary compliance.[1518] The level of resting diffusing capacity is higher than normal, particularly when estimated by the single-breath method ($D_{L_{CO}}SB$),[361, 362, 411, 1478, 2077, 3144] and on exercise it has been shown to increase normally:[1525] although this is the finding in a significant proportion of these patients, all reported series contain cases in which the resting diffusing capacity was within normal limits. Using a steady-state technique, we reported that on exercise the overall diffusing capacity in two patients with atrial septal defects was not significantly elevated, although values for pulmonary capillary blood volume were in the higher range of normal.[399] Flatley and his co-workers found higher values of V_c in cases of ventricular septal defect.[2288] In studies of children with atrial septal defects, Bucci and Cook found generally elevated values for resting $D_{L_{CO}}SB$; the pulmonary capillary blood volume (V_c) was elevated significantly in many of them, and the membrane component (D_M) was normal or at the upper limit of normal.[2077] Similar results have been reported by others.[3144] It has been shown by Dollery and his colleagues, using radioactive CO_2, that the increased pulmonary blood flow in these patients is accommodated preferentially in the upper zones of the lung,[339] and it is possible that this redistribution might cause a proportionately greater effect on the single-breath measurement than on the steady-state determinations of diffusing capacity. On exercise, there may be an excess ventilation in some patients with an increased pulmonary flow.[3145] Lees and his colleagues have shown that infants with left-to-right shunts and pulmonary hyperperfusion have a widened A–a O_2 difference which they attribute to an increased venous admixture rather than to $\dot{V}a/\dot{Q}$ disturbance.[3196]

Right-to-left shunt conditions

Auchincloss, Gilbert and Eich suggested that, when significant pulmonary hypertension occurs with shunt reversal in patients with atrial septal defects, a normal or low diffusing capacity may be found.[362] In long-standing congenital right-to-left shunt lesions, as in the tetralogy of Fallot, there is, in our experience, little if any disturbance of pulmonary function. Of considerable interest, however, is the fact that these patients adapt to their shunt hypoxia at the tissue level, since their blood lactate levels are not elevated;[1526] and they do not develop hyperventilation in response to hypoxemia, as occurs in normal subjects on exposure to the hypoxia of altitude. This latter distinction has been emphasized by Husson and Otis, who point out that, whereas hyperventilation is of assistance at altitude in raising the arterial P_{O_2}, it would be without effect in a patient with a right-to-left shunt.[696] In these patients there is a slight but significant tendency to metabolic acidosis, with a slightly decreased bicarbonate—a shift that is of assistance to the unloading of oxygen from blood to tissues. There appears to be no answer to the question of *how* the patient with a shunt lesion knows that hyperventilation would be ineffective. Husson and Otis found that "there is no significant difference between the oxygen consumption of patients with chronic hypoxia arising from circulatory anomalies and that of those who had circulatory anomalies but no hypoxia,"[696] and inferred that there was no depression of the resting oxygen requirement in the chronically hypoxic patients they studied, a conclusion at variance with some earlier data. Their experiments were so carefully conducted that it seems to us that this conclusion is more likely to be correct than that recorded in earlier investigations.

Occasionally, patients with right-to-left shunts of rare type, with central arterial unsaturation, constitute diagnostic puzzles of considerable complexity.[3735] In some of these, the demonstration of normal ventilation, gas distribution, and diffusing capacity is of much value in establishing the diagnosis. In a study of 14 patients, ranging in age from 8 to 37, who had palliative shunt operations for Fallot's tetralogy, Crawford, Simpson, and McIlroy[3197] found striking falls of oxygen saturation on exercise with a generally normal or low normal P_{aCO_2}. They concluded that the effect of high pulmonary blood flow and pulmonary venous congestion on lung volumes in this condition was essentially similar to that produced by pulmonary congestion in other diseases. It may lead to some fall in compliance.[3731] Mürtz[3732] has reported that patients with congenital cyanotic heart disease have a reduced ventilatory response to hypoxia.

SUMMARY

There are many points of interest in the interaction of changes in cardiac function and respiration. Some of these, such as the long-term pulmonary effects of mitral stenosis, have been recognized for many years, but less attention has been devoted to some of the other problems discussed in this chapter. In particular, the importance of mechanical changes in the lung and of an increase in airway resistance in the causation of orthopnea, the understanding of Cheyne-Stokes respiration (which we would prefer to see called "Cheyne's respiration") in terms of the oscillation of a controlled feedback circuit, and the mechanism for the exercise hyperventilation that seems to be closely associated with pulmonary hypertension of any genesis: these aspects of this subject have received less attention but contain many elements of great interest to the physiologist and to the physician.

In practical terms, there is little doubt that evaluation of pulmonary function may be helpful in the management of some patients with mitral stenosis and in the differentiation between chronic bronchitis and pulmonary congestion. The demonstration of normal pulmonary function in a patient with pulmonary hypertension, as far as maximal ventilation and diffusing capacity are concerned, may be valuable evidence in the elucidation of the etiology of his hypertension. More recently, the demonstrated abnormalities of arterial oxygen tension, both during an acute myocardial infarction and several months after recovery in some patients, have been of particular interest. Thus, the physician who has to understand the details of methods of measuring arterial blood-gas contents and tensions, and who is conversant with measurements of pulmonary function, should work in close conjunction with his colleagues in cardiology. Their collaboration at the bedside in cases of combined heart and lung disease can be, in our experience, very rewarding.

PRIMARY ALVEOLAR HYPOVENTILATION SYNDROME

CHAPTER 16

"For some of us are out of breath, And all of us are fat . . . ."

LEWIS CARROLL
("The Walrus and the Carpenter")

INTRODUCTION

It has become evident in recent years that an important defect in several clinical conditions is a hypoventilation limited to certain parts of the lung. Thus, the level of arterial $P\text{CO}_2$ may be elevated in patients with emphysema or thoracic deformity, even though total minute volume may appear adequate. Underventilation of all alveoli may follow severe respiratory depression or interference with ventilation such as that accompanying neuromuscular disorders. Only during the last few years, however, has the syndrome of primary alveolar hypoventilation been recognized, in which, by definition, maximal ventilatory ability may be normal and gas diffusion unimpaired, yet the level of resting (and particularly of sleeping) ventilation may be so low as to create arterial unsaturation and hypercapnia. In its commonest form this syndrome is seen in obese patients. It has been documented to occur also without obesity, but for descriptive purposes it is wise to discuss these two situations separately. The syndrome as a whole is of very considerable clinical importance and interest, and a complete understanding of it provides a valuable insight into a number of physiological processes and adaptations.

THE PICKWICKIAN SYNDROME

In 1955, Sieker,[1537] Auchincloss,[1538] and Ratto[1540] and their colleagues drew attention to a syndrome of obesity (usually of gross degree), somnolence, polycythemia, and arterial unsaturation. Other cases of this type began to be described in the literature,[588, 589,

[1539, 2079, 2080] and several systematic studies of pulmonary function in obese persons were reported (these were reviewed in Chapter 3). Burwell and his colleagues gave a full description of this syndrome in a 51-year-old businessman weighing 263 lb who had fallen asleep after being dealt a "full house" at poker—of which he consequently failed to take advantage.[587] They noted that a similar episodic somnolence had been described by Charles Dickens as occurring in the fat boy in *Pickwick Papers,* and they suggested that it be called the "Pickwickian syndrome."

The respiratory consequences of obesity have been fully discussed in Chapter 3, but it may be useful at this point to reiterate that, compared with one of similar height but normal weight, the very obese subject shows: (1) a higher resting absolute oxygen uptake; (2) a fall in expiratory reserve volume and a higher intra-abdominal pressure when lying flat; (3) an increased oxygen cost of breathing; (4) airway closure at FRC as a consequence of the reduced lung volume; (5) a resulting impairment of $\dot{V}/\dot{Q}$ ratios due to the presence of poorly ventilated alveoli in dependent parts of the lung; and (6) a consequent increase of A–a O_2 difference, but a normal diffusing capacity.

Lambertsen has pointed out that the normal population comprises people whose ventilatory response to CO_2 is high, average or, in about 5 per cent of the population, well below average.[1541] It seems to us that the primary alveolar hypoventilation syndrome in obese persons might be accounted for mainly by the occurrence of obesity in those with a low CO_2 response. Similar obesity in one who has a high or normal CO_2 response would not cause hypoventilation and, even if the obesity were gross, no CO_2 retention would occur. In those who do not respond to CO_2 with as great an increase in minute ventilation as the majority of the normal population, the development of obesity with its effects on pulmonary function would not be accompanied by the increased level of ventilation necessary to hold the arterial P_{CO_2} within normal limits. In such people, reduction in weight and active rehabilitation may well be expected to lead to improvement in arterial blood-gas values.

In order to understand the diagnostic criteria for the Pickwickian syndrome, the physician must realize, first, that polycythemia rubra vera does not produce any impairment of pulmonary function and that the arterial saturation in this condition is normal or nearly so.[1540, 1542] (*see* page 420), and second, that an obese patient may have concomitant bronchitis or even emphysema, so that in some it may be difficult to determine whether or not any degree of primary hypoventilation is present. In a typical and uncomplicated case of the Pickwickian syndrome, the following observations may be made:

1. It may be noted that the patient appears cyanosed during sleep or recumbency[3218] or during one of the many periods of somnolence during the day. Doll and his colleagues have documented the severe hypoxia and elevation of pulmonary artery pressure that occurs during sleep in this syndrome.[3727]
2. Arterial blood may be unsaturated and may have an elevated P_{CO_2} level with a normal pH. The bicarbonate level will be elevated: we have on occasion found this value to be a useful indicator of the average ventilatory function. The stimulus of an arterial puncture or of having to breathe through a mouthpiece may be sufficient, in some of these patients, to cause a period of adequate ventilation, with return to normal or near-normal of the arterial P_{CO_2} level. However, if in these circumstances the pH is elevated and the bicarbonate level is raised, it may be taken that their customary level of ventilation is considerably lower.
3. It may be demonstrated by use of an oximeter that hyperventilation on air produces prompt elevation in arterial saturation.
4. Ventilatory capacity should be normal or nearly so.
5. Inert-gas mixing should be normal, or nearly so, though with very low minute volumes it may be difficult to be sure of this.
6. The diffusing capacity should be normal or nearly so.
7. It may be possible to demonstrate that the resting oxygen uptake is high in relation to ventilation; this is usually the case, but, as was noted earlier, in our experience these patients tend to increase their ventilation when asked to breathe into any apparatus, and it may be difficult to obtain a satisfactorily representative record of their usual level of ventilation.

Recently, several additional cases of this syndrome have been described,[3219, 3220, 3233] many with unusual features. The condition has been reported in two children,[3232, 3726] in siblings,[3217] and in association with myxedema.[3229] The syndrome may be improved by treatment,[3226, 3725] and in one patient, eight weeks of assisted ventilation and a low-calorie diet resulted in marked improvement[3227] (*see* Case 38). Most authors recognize that a central failure of response to CO_2 is present,[3224] and there is doubt that the increased physical load of fat in the thorax plays any significant part in the syndrome.[3221] The airway closure that occurs no doubt predisposes these patients to bronchitis and some authors believe that bronchospasm plays a part in the symptomatology.[3223] Progesterone therapy has been reported to have a favorable effect.[3231] It is of interest that many distinguished physicians and acute observers, among whom one might mention Osler, failed to record a single case of hypoventilation in the many patients with polycythemia whom they saw and studied. It is exceedingly difficult to recognize hypoventilation on clinical grounds, as Mithoefer and his colleagues have recently clearly demonstrated.[3724] The exact delineation of the syndrome of primary alveolar hypoventilation inevitably depends upon the ability of the physician to demonstrate the presence of hypercapnia when ventilatory capacity, gas distribution, and diffusing capacity are normal. One of the most remarkable features of the syndrome as a whole is the fact that, without abnormality of these aspects of lung function and without intrinsic heart disease, a serious degree of congestive heart failure may follow the chronically altered levels of alveolar gas tension in this condition. This aspect of the disorder is discussed later (*see* page 358).

PRIMARY ALVEOLAR HYPOVENTILATION SYNDROME IN THE NONOBESE SUBJECT

In the nonobese subject there is no increased oxygen requirement at rest, no abnormality of pulmonary mechanics, and no increased mechanical disadvantage on lying flat; it is of particular significance, therefore, that this syndrome occurs also in patients of normal weight, in whom all of these aggravating factors are absent. It must be remembered that severe hypoventilation has been described in patients with neuromuscular disorders,[1286] and the finding of a significant degree of polycythemia in postparalytic poliomyelitis cases[1284] indicates that in these patients there is commonly some degree of chronic hypoventilation.

Several patients have been described who undoubtedly had primary alveolar hypoventilation and who were not obese. Of the four described by Rodman and his colleagues, one had chronic schizophrenia, another was thought to have some kind of diffuse organic brain disease, a third suffered from "spirochetal infection of the central nervous system," and the fourth had cervical syringomyelia.[1543] In the patient described by Pare and Lowenstein, some mental depression was apparent but there was no definite evidence of organic disorder of the central nervous system.[1544] Lawrence's patient was a 37-year-old man weighing 167 lb; at autopsy the lungs were normal and no brain lesions could be demonstrated.[1545] The 37-year-old man studied by Richter and his colleagues had no evidence initially of any systemic disorder but later developed an unexplained inflammation of the right fifth cervical nerve root.[1546] The patient studied by Garlind and Linderholm was known to have had encephalitis lethargica, had subsequently developed symptoms of Parkinsonism, and three years before he was first seen by these authors had suffered a minor head injury.[1547] The 44-year-old man weighing 145 lb, described by Fraser and his colleagues, undoubtedly had primary alveolar hypoventilation, although the clinical picture was somewhat confused.[2078] He was noted to have a tremor and nystagmus, and at necropsy it was considered that degenerative changes of unusual extent were demonstrable in the region of the medulla.

More recently, other patients with associated central nervous system disorders have been described.[3222, 3225, 3230, 3736, 3737] Of particular interest was the 33-year-old woman, studied by Mannhart and his colleagues,[3228] who had normal arterial blood-gas values at rest, but hypoventilated on exercise, with resultant hypoxemia. Hughes[3234] has described a patient with a glioblastoma multiforme involving the brain stem, the medulla, and the surface of the third, fourth, and lateral ventricles. He had no muscle paralysis, a normal $FEV_{1.0}$ and chest x-ray, and marked irregularity of respiratory rate and rhythm, described as "respiratory apraxia." The arterial P_{CO_2} was elevated, but returned to normal values after x-ray therapy to the brain.

The physician must be aware that chronic hypoxemia and hypercapnia as a consequence of alveolar hypoventilation may be responsible for such symptoms as headache, loss of memory, somnolence, and the like, and he

Case 38
Primary Alveolar Hypoventilation Syndrome

Summary of Clinical Findings. This 42-year-old woman was first seen in December, 1956, when she was admitted to hospital with shortness of breath and swelling of the legs of one year's duration. She was more comfortable in a sitting position while sleeping at night and had coughing spasms when she lay flat. It was not unusual for her to fall asleep during the day while sitting in a chair. Her weight at the time of onset of dyspnea had been 300 lb. On her marriage, some 15 years previously, she had weighed 180 lb.

On physical examination she was a plethoric, cyanotic and extremely obese woman weighing 310 lb. Blood pressure was 160/100 mm Hg; pulse rate, 76/min and regular. There was a faint ejection murmur over the pulmonary area, with an accentuated second sound. Pitting edema of the legs extended up to the groins.

Urinalysis showed 1+ albuminuria with normal sediment. The hemoglobin was 19 gm/100 ml, and the hematocrit 68 per cent. Blood-volume studies revealed a marked increase in red-cell mass. Urinary 17-ketosteroids and corticoids were within the normal range. An electrocardiogram was interpreted as showing right ventricular hypertrophy. The electroencephalographic pattern was that of narcolepsy, indicating "some disturbances in regulation of sleep mechanisms and structures located in the higher brain stem and adjacent diencephalon." She was placed on an 800-calorie diet and was treated for cardiac failure. During her one and a half months in hospital she lost 60 pounds. A diagnosis of primary alveolar hypoventilation was first made in January, 1957, as a result of pulmonary function studies.

During the next seven years this patient had several admissions to hospital for treatment of obesity and cardiac failure. Variations in arterial blood gases and pulmonary function are shown below. Cardiac catheterization was performed in October, 1960, when the patient weighed 213 pounds and did not show any signs of congestive heart failure.

In the recumbent position, the arterial saturation was 75 per cent, the P_{CO_2} was 62 mm Hg, the pulmonary arterial pressure was 55 mm Hg systolic and 16 mm Hg diastolic, the cardiac output was 4.7 l/min, and the pulmonary vascular resistance was 465 dynes/sec/sq cm. After a period of increased ventilation, the arterial oxygen saturation rose to 92 per cent and the P_{CO_2} fell to 40 mm Hg; at this time the pulmonary artery pressure was 30 mm Hg systolic and 16 mm Hg diastolic, and the cardiac output was virtually unchanged at 4.8 l/min.

In November, 1962, pulmonary function tests were repeated when she had an attack of bronchitis and a return of leg edema. Her weight at that time was 220 lb.

Over the next two years there was little further weight loss. She was admitted in July, 1964, with an incarcerated incisional hernia through an old appendectomy scar. Her weight on admission was 207 lbs. The symptoms associated with the hernia

													CO	EXERCISE				
	VC	FRC	RV	TLC	ME %	MMFR	$FEV_{0.75}$ ×40	pH	P_{CO_2}	HCO_3^-	O_2Hb %	$D_{Lco}SS_2$	Ext %	MPH	GRADE	$\dot{V}_{O_2}$	$\dot{V}_E$	$D_{Lco}SS_3$
Predicted	3.3	2.9	1.7	5.0	55	3.3	87	7.40	42	25	97	17.1	48					28.0
Jan. 1957	2.5	2.0	1.7	4.2	40			7.37	62	32	77	15.8	37					
April 1957	2.6	1.5	1.1	3.7	39	3.7	92	7.42	52	31	89	11.9	38					
March 1958	2.8	2.0	1.4	4.2	55	4.2	98	7.44	51	33	88	18.4	42	1¼	4%	0.97	17.5	29.0
Nov. 1962*	1.7	1.3	1.2	2.9	42	1.9	49	7.28	70	29.4	79	15.6	33					
Nov. 1962		ON HYPER-VENTILATION						7.46	44	29.5	100							
Dec. 1963	2.2	2.2	2.0	4.2	44	3.3	77	7.29	62	27	85	16.9	38					
Dec. 1963		ON HYPER-VENTILATION						7.44	40	25.8	98							
June 1968	2.6	3.0	2.0	4.6	63	3.3	90	7.32	35	17	94	8.1	37					

Apart from an occasion when she had bronchitis,* note the generally normal ventilatory ability and normal gas distribution. On exercise, ventilation increased to 17.5 l/min, but the ratio of $\dot{V}_{O_2}/\dot{V}_E$ (at 5.5) is high, indicating probable hypoventilation. Resting and exercise diffusing capacity are normal; the result in April 1957 was ascribed to a low tidal volume of only 300 ml. Voluntary hyperventilation results in a prompt fall in P_{CO_2} and rise of the arterial saturation to normal.

In June, 1968, lung volumes, including the expiratory reserve volume are normal. The diffusing capacity is low (predicted 12.1) but is probably due to a severe anemia. Blood gases show a mild metabolic acidosis felt to be due to malabsorption associated with the intestinal bypass.

Primary Alveolar Hypoventilation Syndrome

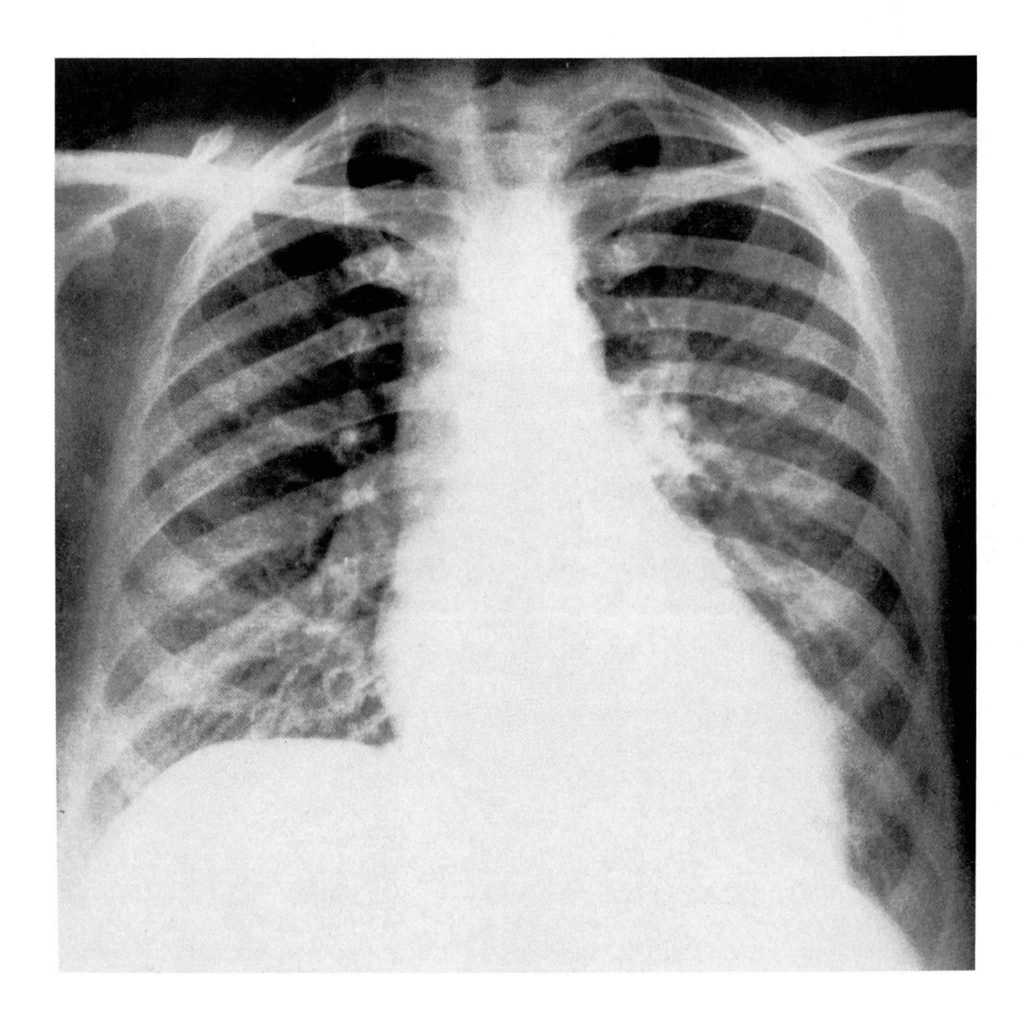

subsided on conservative treatment and a decision was made to perform a jejuno-coecal shunt in order to combat the intractable obesity. This was performed on September 1, 1964. Her postoperative course was complicated by two episodes of respiratory failure but by discharge on October 9 she was feeling well and had lost 37 lbs of weight.

Over the next four years her weight dropped to 101 lbs. She was having three to four loose bowel movements per day. The symptoms of congestive failure had cleared, but her course was complicated by a severe anemia (Hgb 7.0 gm%) and low serum albumin, potassium, and calcium. Pulmonary function studies are shown. On June 13, 1968, the intestinal bypass was closed, after which these deficiencies responded to treatment, and she was discharged on July 1.

Radiology. Apart from a slight degree of nonspecific cardiac enlargement and an increased prominence of the hila bilaterally, the chest x-ray is not very remarkable in appearance. The lungs are clear and there is no pleural effusion. Fluoroscopy revealed decreased diaphragmatic excursion bilaterally.

Summary. This obese woman shows most of the characteristic features of primary alveolar hypoventilation in obesity (Pickwickian syndrome). These disappeared when her weight was reduced to within normal limits.

must be on his guard against assuming that these necessarily indicate central nervous system damage.

These few clinical details concerning those nonobese patients in whom the phenomenon of alveolar hypoventilation has been carefully documented indicate the rarity of this syndrome without obesity or without evidence of considerable neurological abnormality. However, the difficulty of establishing the diagnosis, and the fact that—as most of the papers quoted make clear—the possibility of alveolar hypoventilation was not suspected in most of these patients for many years, may well indicate that the few instances reported reflect these difficulties rather than the rarity of the phenomenon.

Many of these patients have been shown to be virtually insensitive to CO_2. The P_{CO_2} value changed from 74 mm Hg to 94 mm Hg in one patient with no observable increase in minute volume;[1547] exercise in this patient did cause an increase in ventilation, however. In other patients, the level of arterial saturation has dropped still further on exercise.[1546] Although most of Rodman's patients showed a diminished response to CO_2, this was not invariable.[1543] Almost all of the patients showed a considerable degree of polycythemia, and in some this had been regarded for years as the primary diagnosis. In most of them, the maximal breathing capacity was normal, e.g., a value of 106 liters/min was recorded in one patient[1547] and 137 liters/min in another.[1544] Many other tests reported on these patients established the absence of any significant degree of chronic lung disease, although in the case described by Fraser and his coworkers the vital capacity was noted to be only 63 per cent of predicted.[2078]

PULMONARY HYPERTENSION SECONDARY TO ALVEOLAR HYPOVENTILATION

Many of the patients, both obese and nonobese, whose clinical course has been described in the papers referred to in the preceding sections had edema of the ankles when first seen. Right ventricular hypertrophy has been noted at necropsy;[1539, 1545] but there are relatively few recorded measurements of pulmonary artery pressure in those suffering from this syndrome. Hackney and his colleagues reported that, in four obese patients with hypoventilation whom they catheterized, they found "normal or increased cardiac output (mean, 8.1 L. per minute), and pulmonary hypertension (mean, 74/30 mm. Hg; range, 50/30 to 105/25 mm. Hg) . . ."[588] A patient with hypoventilation secondary to myotonic dystrophy had an elevated pulmonary arterial pressure.[1286] Garlind and Linderholm reported details of a cardiac catheterization study in their patient who had hypoventilation and was not obese.[1547] These very detailed hemodynamic studies clearly established that both the pulmonary hypertension and the increased pulmonary vascular resistance in this man were reduced by elevating the alveolar oxygen tension. This was done by inducing hyperventilation, in which case the P_{CO_2} level fell, and by administering oxygen, in which case there was no change in the P_{CO_2}; in both circumstances, as the arterial oxygen saturation rose the pulmonary vascular resistance fell. The authors concluded that the hypercapnia was playing no part in the genesis of the pulmonary hypertension in this particular patient. Similar observations were made by Gillam and Mymin in a 35-year-old man weighing 230 lb who had primary alveolar hypoventilation. The pulmonary arterial pressure fell from 80/30 mm Hg when the arterial saturation was 76 per cent to a value of 24/8 mm Hg after breathing oxygen for 10 minutes. This case report illustrates the actual pulmonary arterial-pressure tracings recorded.[2079] In support of these findings are the results of hemodynamic studies made in one of our obese patients with hypoventilation, shown in Case 38.

There are insufficient data on which to base a firm opinion, but at present it seems safe to conclude that the evidence available points to the lowered alveolar oxygen tension as the main, if not the only, determinant of the pulmonary hypertension that these patients have. The patient studied by Fraser and his colleagues did not show any change in pulmonary arterial pressure when breathing oxygen,[2078] so it may be premature to conclude that such a relationship is invariable. However, the finding of antemortem clot in his pulmonary vessels at necropsy might indicate that this patient's pulmonary hypertension was fixed and thus not capable of relief by elevation of the alveolar oxygen tension.

It is of interest to draw a parallel between the state of a patient suffering from alveolar hypoventilation who lives at sea level and that of a normal subject living at altitude. The normal subject resident at altitude (*see* page 103) has a lowered arterial oxygen tension, with consequent secondary polycythemia. In these respects he is no different from the patient with alveolar hypoventilation living at sea level. However, the resident at altitude has a *decreased* level of arterial P_{CO_2}, whereas the patient invariably has elevated levels of arterial P_{CO_2} and bicarbonate. The fact that at altitude everyone probably has some degree of pulmonary hypertension[700, 2245] – and it is likely that this constitutes an important part of the syndrome of chronic mountain sickness[704] – supports the conclusion that the pulmonary hypertension of the primary alveolar hypoventilation syndrome is mainly, if not entirely, attributable to the decreased alveolar oxygen tension of this condition. Although definite evidence of this is lacking, it may well be that the chronic hypercapnia in this condition aggravates the situation still further; such a possibility is suggested by the observation that cor pulmonale occurs in the hypoventilation syndrome at levels of arterial unsaturation that do not appear to cause this complication in normal subjects resident at altitude.

DIFFERENTIAL DIAGNOSIS AND DIAGNOSTIC CRITERIA

The first essential in establishing the diagnosis of primary alveolar hypoventilation is to show that chronic CO_2 retention exists; and, as has been noted, the finding of an elevated bicarbonate level in the arterial blood may sometimes be a more reliable indicator of this than a single value of the arterial P_{CO_2}. Second, the presence of any considerable degree of primary lung disease must be excluded. The demonstration of a normal maximal ventilatory ability excludes emphysema, and the finding of a normal diffusing capacity excludes a primary defect of gas transfer. By means of an ear oximeter, the demonstration of a rise in arterial saturation to normal values as soon as the patient takes a few deep breaths provides a valuable and simple indication of the essential normality of lung function in this condition. It may be more difficult to secure adequate spirometer tracings, since the patient will often increase his resting ventilation when breathing through a mouthpiece and noseclip.

Unexplained arterial desaturation, such as occurs in arteriovenous fistulae of the lung[1552] or in such rare entities as pulmonary telangiectasia,[1553] when not accompanied by retention of CO_2 can be wrongly attributed to hypoventilation, but a careful and complete arterial blood analysis usually enables one to make the differentiation without difficulty. It is important to exclude the presence of a primary musculoskeletal disorder in any patient with unexplained alveolar hypoventilation.

The physician is often called upon to establish whether or not hypoventilation is playing any part in the genesis of a polycythemia. Since in primary polycythemia there is no concomitant or consequential impairment of pulmonary function, nor of arterial CO_2 tension, it is easy to detect the presence or absence of significant hypoventilation in most patients. In our experience, difficult clinical differentiations arise mainly in three clinical situations:

1. In patients with polycythemia rubra vera and concomitant chronic bronchitis with some limitation of ventilatory function.
2. In patients with apparent clinical emphysema, as judged by pulmonary function impairment, with considerable secondary polycythemia and CO_2 retention that appears out of proportion to the severity of the pulmonary function loss. These patients, in whom a low responsiveness to CO_2 complicates the clinical picture, have been mentioned (*see* page 151).
3. In patients with probable previous pulmonary embolism and secondary cor pulmonale. In such instances, however, the arterial P_{CO_2} is usually reduced rather than increased, and the correct diagnosis can be made without difficulty.

SUMMARY

The syndrome of primary alveolar hypoventilation is of very considerable interest for many reasons, of which perhaps the following may be singled out for particular comment:

1. The part played by chronic hypoventilation in the genesis of polycythemia went undetected for very many years, in spite of careful clinical observation of such patients.
2. The demonstration that chronic hypoventilation of essentially normal lungs in patients with a normal cardiovascular system could cause pulmonary hypertension and even

congestive heart failure was of the greatest interest and importance.

3. The fact that some of these patients, who are very insensitive to CO_2 yet increase their ventilation on exercise, is relevant to an understanding of the control of ventilation on exercise.

4. Apart from these issues, the careful study of this syndrome has led to a wider appreciation of the importance of the possible role of alveolar hypoventilation – occurring not as a primary entity but as a consequence of kyphoscoliosis or emphysema, for example – in the genesis of pulmonary hypertension and of cor pulmonale.

5. Although the exact etiology of alveolar hypoventilation in the obese is not understood, it may be that in many clinical situations characterized by an increased work of breathing there is also a decreased CO_2 sensitivity. This may be true in obesity, in emphysema, or in chronic tracheal obstruction.

RESPONSE TO CHEMICAL AND PHYSICAL IRRITANTS

CHAPTER

17

"The time has come to give to the study of the responses that the living organism makes to its environment the same dignity and support which is being given at present to the study of the component parts of the organism. Exclusive emphasis on the individualist approach will otherwise lead biology and medicine into blind alleys. Unless a program of environmental research is vigorously prosecuted, medicine will remain a two-legged structure, unable to support the loads placed on it by the health problems arising from the new environmental forces created by modern life."

R. DUBOS[3361]

INTRODUCTION

In modern industrial society man is exposed to an increasing number of chemical and physical irritants. Although there has been a steady accumulation of knowledge regarding the pathological changes in the lung that these may cause,[33] much less is known about the variations in pattern of function to which they give rise. In some instances this has been due to the absence of any facilities for the testing of pulmonary function, in others to the fact

(*Text continued on page 367.*)

Case 39
Arc Welder's Lung (Siderosis)

Summary of Clinical Findings. This 52-year-old male was admitted to the hospital in April, 1965, for investigation of abdominal pain and hypertension. The abdominal pain was epigastric, not related to meals, but worse when lying down. It had been present for five years. He was known to have had hypertension since 1962. He had received no treatment. He described mild shortness of breath on exertion for seven or eight years but could walk three or four blocks on the level without difficulty. He had an occasional cough with small amounts of white sputum and had smoked one pack of cigarettes per day for many years.

He had worked for fifteen years as an arc welder until seven years prior to admission, but then worked in close proximity to arc welding till his admission. He had never worn a mask, although frequently was required to weld in poorly ventilated cylinders and boilers.

Physical examination revealed a blood pressure of 170/100 and pulse rate of 80/min and regular. He was not cyanosed; there was no clubbing. His chest moved well with good air entry throughout. There were no rales or rhonchi. There were no other specific findings.

Hemogram and urinalysis were normal. Chest x-rays and pulmonary function are shown. Investigations did not reveal a specific cause for the abdominal pain and were felt to exclude secondary hypertension. The patient was discharged on methyldopa and hydrochlorothiazide.

Radiology. A magnified view of the left lower lung zone shows a fine micronodular pattern. This was seen diffusely and evenly through both lungs.

Summary. This is a characteristic example of arc welder's lung or siderosis, in which widespread reticulation and nodulation in the lungs is often associated with no impairment of respiratory function.

	VC	FRC	RV	TLC	ME %	MMFR	$FEV_{0.75}$ ×40	pH^+	Pco_2	HCO_3	Po_2	O_2Hb %	$D_{L_{CO}}SS_2$	CO Ext %	EXERCISE: MPH	GRADE	$\dot{V}o_2$	$\dot{V}_E$	$D_{L_{CO}}SS_3$
Predicted	4.0	3.5	2.0	6.0	55	3.40	105						16.5	43					23.0
April 1965	3.3	3.0	2.3	5.6	41	1.95	87						13.0	45					24.7

Aside from mild reduction in flow, this patient showed normal function. In particular, both resting and exercise diffusing capacities were normal.

		Predicted	April 1965
	Resistance at FRC cm H_2O/l/sec	1–3	6
COMPLIANCE l/cm H_2O	STATIC	0.156	0.149
	DYNAMIC	0.156	0.143

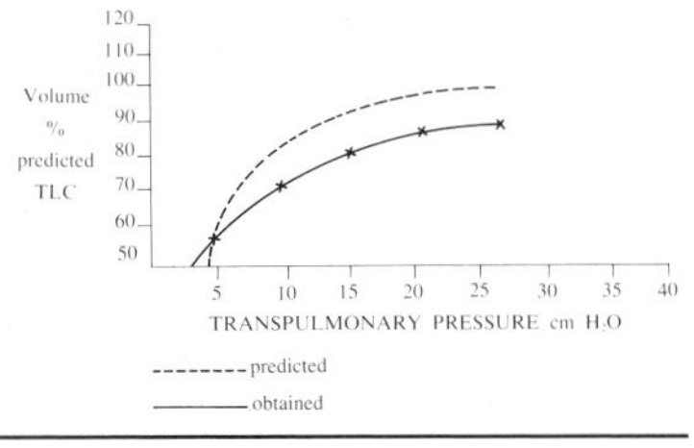

Volume % predicted TLC (50–120) vs. TRANSPULMONARY PRESSURE cm H_2O (5–40)

-------- predicted

——— obtained

Values were normal except for the increased resistance, which could have been due to glottis resistance.

Arc Welder's Lung (Siderosis)

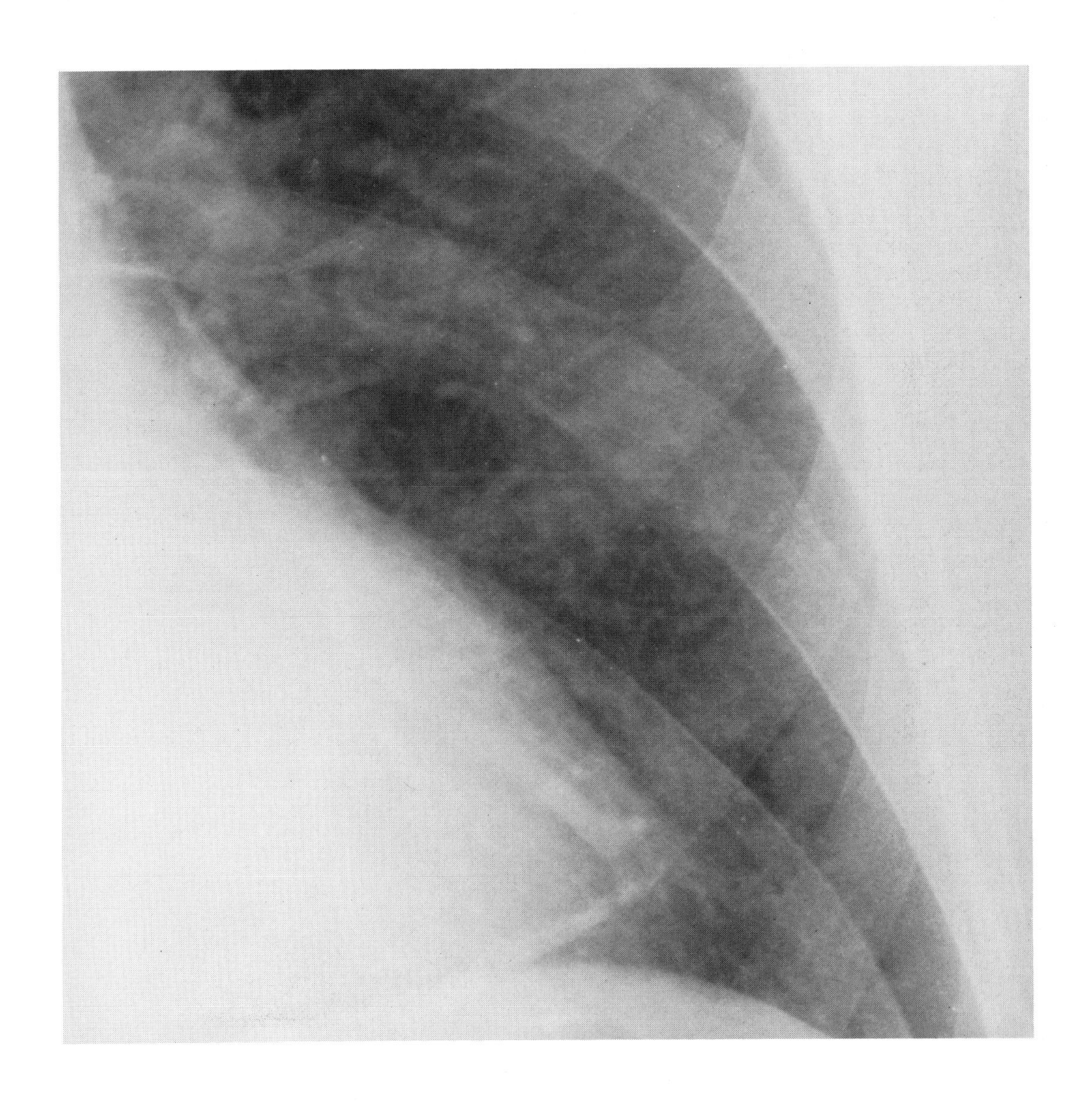

Cases 40 and 41
NO_2 Inhalation

Summary of Clinical Findings. On June 21, 1968, two male employees of a shipbuilding firm were admitted to the hospital, complaining of shortness of breath and cough. The patients, "JD," 40 years old, and "JF," 60 years old, had both been using oxyacetylene torches to free a shaft in the small rudder room of an icebreaker. Patient "JD" had worked for eight hours during the day on June 20, and "JF" for six hours that evening. After each had completed his shift, he noticed the onset of dyspnea and cough, accompanied by discomfort in the chest and headache. Patient "JD" was admitted the following morning with these symptoms. "JF" felt better in the morning but visited the infirmary and was referred to the Royal Victoria Hospital that evening.

On examination both had a tachycardia of 100 per min and a tachypnea of about 30 resp. per min. "JD" was cyanosed, but this was not noted in "JF." Diffuse fine inspiratory rales could be heard throughout the lung fields in both. There were no other pertinent physical findings.

Investigations showed a neutrophilic leukocytosis: 17,800 in "JD" and 12,000 in "JF." Other hematological and biochemical studies were normal. ECGs were normal, aside from the tachycardia. Chest x-rays and pulmonary function studies are shown.

Both patients required oxygen initially but responded quickly to treatment with steroids, antibiotics, and bronchodilators. "JF" was discharged on July 3 and "JD" six days later. "JD" continued to note mild dyspnea upon exertion and steroids were maintained for another month. At the end of that period his dyspnea was described as minimal. "JF" felt well when seen one week after discharge and steroids were discontinued.

Radiology. The postero-anterior roentgenogram (*A*) of patient "JD" reveals extensive involvement of both lungs by a process characteristic of air-space consolidation; the chest roentgenogram had returned to normal four days later, so that the process clearly was one of edema. The postero-anterior roentgenogram (*B*) of "JF" shows an identical pattern of diffuse bilateral air-space edema.

Summary. The pattern of illness presented by these patients consisted of pulmonary edema appearing soon after exposure. This is characteristic of exposure to oxides of nitrogen, which in this instance seems to have been the most likely cause of their illness.

CASE J. F.

	VC	FRC	RV	TLC	ME %	MMFR	$FEV_{0.75}$ ×40	pH^+	P_{CO_2}	HCO_3	P_{O_2}	O_2Hb %	$D_{Lco}SS_2$	CO Ext %	EXERCISE GRADE	$\dot{V}O_2$	$\dot{V}_E$	$D_{Lco}SS_3$
Predicted	3.7	3.5	2.2	5.9	50	2.9	92	7.40	40	25	80	97	12.1	40				
June 21, 1968								7.41	35	21	35	67						
June 25, 1968	3.1	3.3	2.3	5.4	61	4.7	98	7.42	39	25	75	95	21.0	40				
July 26, 1968	3.8	3.1	2.0	5.8	56	5.1	109	7.42	35	22	87	96	17.6	35				

A severe hypoxemia was present on the day of admission, which improved three days later. Function at that time was within normal limits. One month later P_{O_2} was normal.

CASE J. D.

	VC	FRC	RV	TLC	ME %	MMFR	$FEV_{0.75}$ ×40	pH^+	P_{CO_2}	HCO_3	P_{O_2}	O_2Hb %	$D_{Lco}SS_2$	CO Ext %	EXERCISE GRADE	$\dot{V}O_2$	$\dot{V}_E$	$D_{Lco}SS_3$
Predicted	4.3	3.5	1.9	6.2	60	3.8	124	7.40	40	25	80	97	17.0	46				
June 21, 1968								7.43	35	23	25	49						
June 25, 1968	2.1	1.2	0.8	2.9	77	1.7	58	7.44	41	27	72	93	13.3	46				
August 16, 1968	4.3	2.3	1.7	6.0	78	4.6	129						18.9	46				

On admission a severe hypoxemia was present, but three days later P_{O_2} was only slightly reduced (room air). At this time he showed marked reduction in all subdivisions of lung volume, a moderate degree of bronchial obstruction, and a slight reduction in diffusing capacity. The CO extraction percentage, however, was normal. Two months later, aside from a continued reduction in FRC, function had returned to normal. A blood gas in the interval had shown a P_{O_2} of 93.

Cases 40 and 41

NO_2 Inhalation

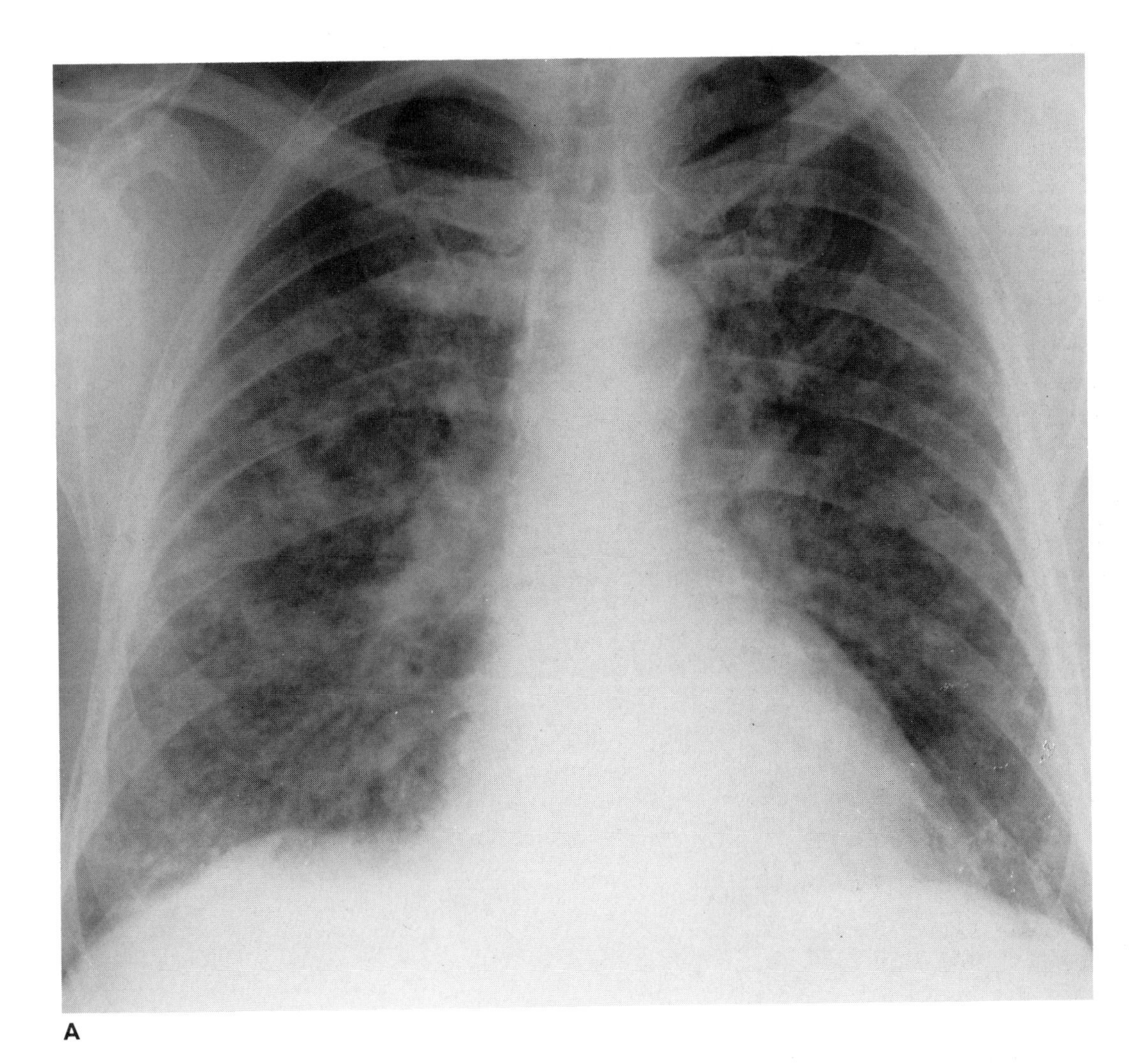

A

	July 2, 1968	Predicted	"JD"	"JF"
	Resistance at FRC cm H_2O/l/sec	1–2	3.5	1.7
COMPLIANCE l/cm H_2O	STATIC	0.160	0.182	0.147
	DYNAMIC	0.160	(f=3) 0.164 (f=50) 0.158	(f=16) 0.148 (f=50) 0.145

On July 2, "JD" showed a slight increase in airway resistance, but "JF" was normal. Both showed normal compliance. Both showed an increase in the maximum negative intrapleural pressure to about -50 cm H_2O. In addition, the slope of the flow volume curve in "JF" was significantly increased, which might indicate early fibrosis. These studies were repeated on July 26 and showed no change.

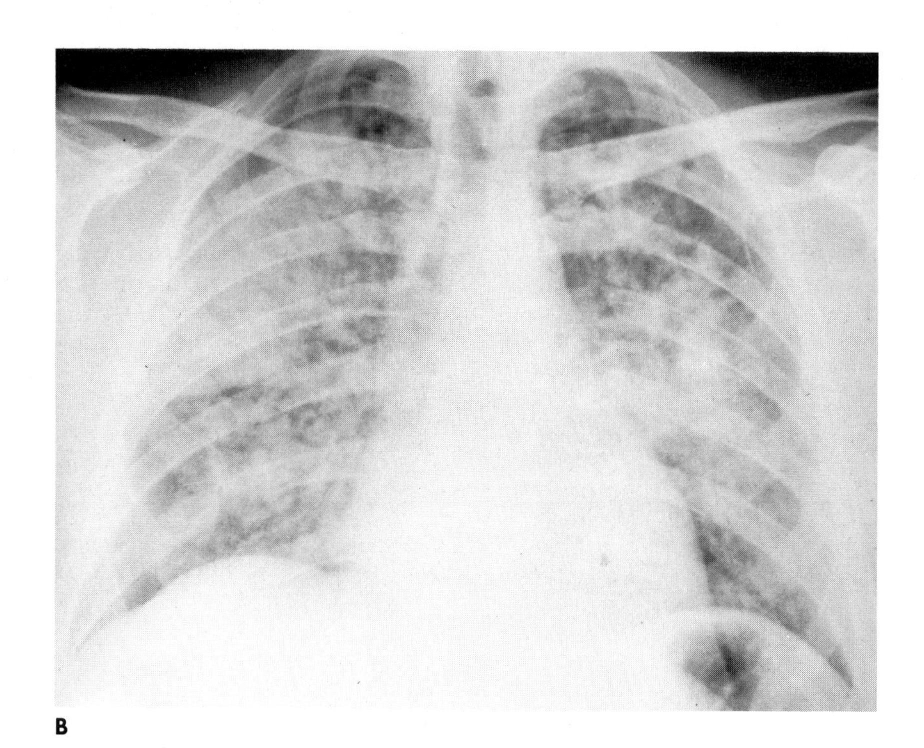

B

that only simple ventilatory tests have been employed in relation to a disease which, by its nature, would be expected to affect mainly other aspects of pulmonary function. Yet enough information has been secured to indicate that a careful assessment of pulmonary function is obligatory in relation to these disorders, not solely to assist in deciding legal problems of attributability but also to clarify the interrelationship between structural change and function.

The problems of radiological changes and pathological findings in the pneumoconioses embrace such an enormous field that no formal treatment of these aspects of the disease processes can be attempted in this volume. Brief mention will be made of these important aspects to enable the reader to integrate them with what is known of the changes in pulmonary function they cause.

The general term "pneumonokoniosis" was first suggested by Zenker[1601] to describe lung disease caused by inhalation of dust and is currently so used in its shortened form of "pneumoconiosis." The dust may be of mineral or organic origin, and it may be profoundly damaging to lung structures or may be almost inert. Consequently there are great differences in the effect on pulmonary function of different inhaled substances. There is also very considerable discrepancy between the degree of radiological abnormality these substances may produce and the severity of impairment of function that results.

Some consideration is given in the following sections to the functional consequences of the inhalation of various gases. Although some work has been done on the acute effects of breathing high concentrations of many of these chemicals, little is known of the consequences of human exposure over periods of years to very low concentrations of them—a general problem that underlies the difficulty of relating atmospheric pollution to chronic respiratory disease in any precise way.

So many areas of study impinge on the general field of industrial lung disease, that it is not easy to give the reader any general guide to the total bibliography. Problems of dust accumulation and aerosol retention have been dealt with in a number of review articles;[856, 1616, 2350] special consideration has been given to deposition and retention models of the respiratory tract;[3362] and problems of bulk flow in the respiratory tract have been discussed at a recent Ciba Symposium.[3363] To these references may be added general discussions of the place of respiratory function tests in industrial lung disease,[3250] and a special bibliography on asbestosis[3259] which was prepared for an international conference. The increase of interest and concern which Dr. Dubos has called for, has perhaps been reflected more by the proliferation of conferences than by a great increase in the amount of firm data or the number of new and definitive contributions that have been made to this field; at least now there are few who can doubt its importance.

PNEUMOCONIOSIS DUE TO MINERAL DUST

HIGH DUST CONTENT BUT LITTLE FIBROSIS (IRON, TIN, BARIUM, COALWORKER'S PNEUMOCONIOSIS [EARLY STAGE])

Iron

Oxides of iron are inhaled by men employed in three different occupations: welding, mining of iron ore, and silver-polishing. In general, iron oxide can accumulate in considerable amounts in lymphoid tissue and can cause considerable radiological change without producing any measurable impairment of pulmonary function, though it cannot be assumed that the pulmonary parenchyma is never involved as a result of its inhalation. In welders, the lung changes are generally described as "siderosis" or "arc-welder's lung." In a typical case, iron-oxide pigment is deposited in the lung in the perivascular and subpleural lymphatics, and this is not accompanied by any fibrotic change.[1602, 2303] With very heavy exposure, alveoli in some areas may be filled with macrophages containing black granules of iron oxide. The radiological appearances in this condition were first described by Doig and McLaughlin;[1603] they are relatively nonspecific, consisting of a generalized reticular and nodular pattern associated with considerable linear streaking. These radiological changes may be, and often are, associated with normal ventilatory function. In 1938, Enzer and Sander recorded normal values for vital capacity, exercise ventilation, and maximal ventilation in 15 welders who had lung changes radiologically,[1602] and others have since documented the finding of normal pulmonary function in this condition.[2303]

(Text continued on page 371.)

Case 42
Talcosis

Summary of Clinical Findings. This 30-year-old housewife was first admitted to this hospital in June, 1967, complaining of shortness of breath. She had been admitted to another hospital in December, 1966, with complaints of vague pain in the extremities and back and of shortness of breath on exertion of a few months' duration. She denied exposure to noxious dusts or fumes. Investigations included supraclavicular node biopsy and a diagnosis of sarcoidosis was made. Because of progression of her symptoms she was referred to the Royal Victoria Hospital six months later. On examination she appeared fatigued but in no acute distress. Blood pressure was 118/70; pulse rate was 96; temperature was 99°. The chest was clear; the air entry good and there were no rales or rhonchi. There were no palpable lymph nodes and no other significant findings. Investigations revealed a normal urinalysis and hemogram and a sedimentation rate of 39 mm per hour. LE cells were not found. Coombs' test and levels of BUN, creatinine, calcium, and phosphorus were normal. Serum electrophoresis showed an increased $alpha_2$ globulin and a marked elevation of gamma globulin. The OT skin test 1:1000 was negative but the histoplasmin skin test was positive. The slides of the lymph node were reviewed and showed granulomatous infiltration. Chest x-rays and pulmonary function are shown. Kweim antigen was injected and the patient was discharged. She was readmitted five weeks later for biopsy of the injection site. This showed vague granuloma formation but was felt to be a positive test. Investigations failed to further illuminate the problem and the patient was discharged and prednisone was prescribed.

She was readmitted three months later. Although her fatigue and extremity pain had improved the dyspnea had progressed until she could climb only 10 stairs without resting. Investigations again were not helpful. Pulmonary function tests are shown. An open-lung biopsy was performed. Because of the presence of the doubly refractile crystals (*see* figure) the patient was again closely questioned and this time admitted exposure to excessive amounts of talcum powder during her last pregnancy in 1964. Throughout the final three months of her pregnancy she would spread large amounts of a lavender-scented talcum powder over herself, her clothes, pillows, sheets and blankets. In addition she would frequently inhale it from her cupped hands. The obsession disappeared after her pregnancy.

Radiology. A postero-anterior roentgenogram (*A*) reveals extensive involvement of both lungs by a rather coarse reticular pattern. In the upper axillary zone on the right and in the left mid-lung are two areas of homogeneous consolidation possessing poorly defined margins B. Paratracheal lymph-node enlargement is present bilaterally, more markedly on the left.

Pathology. Sections of the lung and lymph nodes show similar granulomata (see Fig. C) some of the granulomata are fibrotic while others are hyalinized. The granulomata tend to be in close proximity to blood vessels. There is interstitial fibrosis. Special stains for A.F.B. and fungus are negative.

Diagnosis: Lung: Silicosis
Lymph node: Silicosis

Note: The doubly refractile crystals (see Fig. D) are extremely numerous and more closely resemble the silicates in talc. The histological reaction, however, is more like clinical silicosis than classic talcosis.

Summary. This diffuse fibrosis following the inhalation of talc (hydrated magnesium silicate) was associated with a loss of lung volume and a low diffusing capacity.

														EXERCISE				
	VC	FRC	RV	TLC	ME %	MMFR	$FEV_{0.75}$ ×40	pH^+	Pco_2	HCO_3	Po_2	O_2Hb %	$D_{Lco}SS_2$	CO Ext %	GRADE	$\dot{V}O_2$	$\dot{V}_E$	$D_{Lco}SS_3$
Predicted	3.0	2.3	1.3	4.3	65	3.2	87						16.3	52				
June, 1967	2.3	1.9	0.9	3.2	45	1.6	50						9.1	35				
December, 1967	1.9	1.7	1.0	2.9	65	2.4	66	7.42	37	24	78	94	7.1	32				

On admission in June, 1967, the patient showed loss of volume and a low diffusing capacity. Part of the flow rate reduction could be explained by the volume change. In December there had been little change except for a slight further reduction in diffusing capacity. Blood gases were normal.

Talcosis

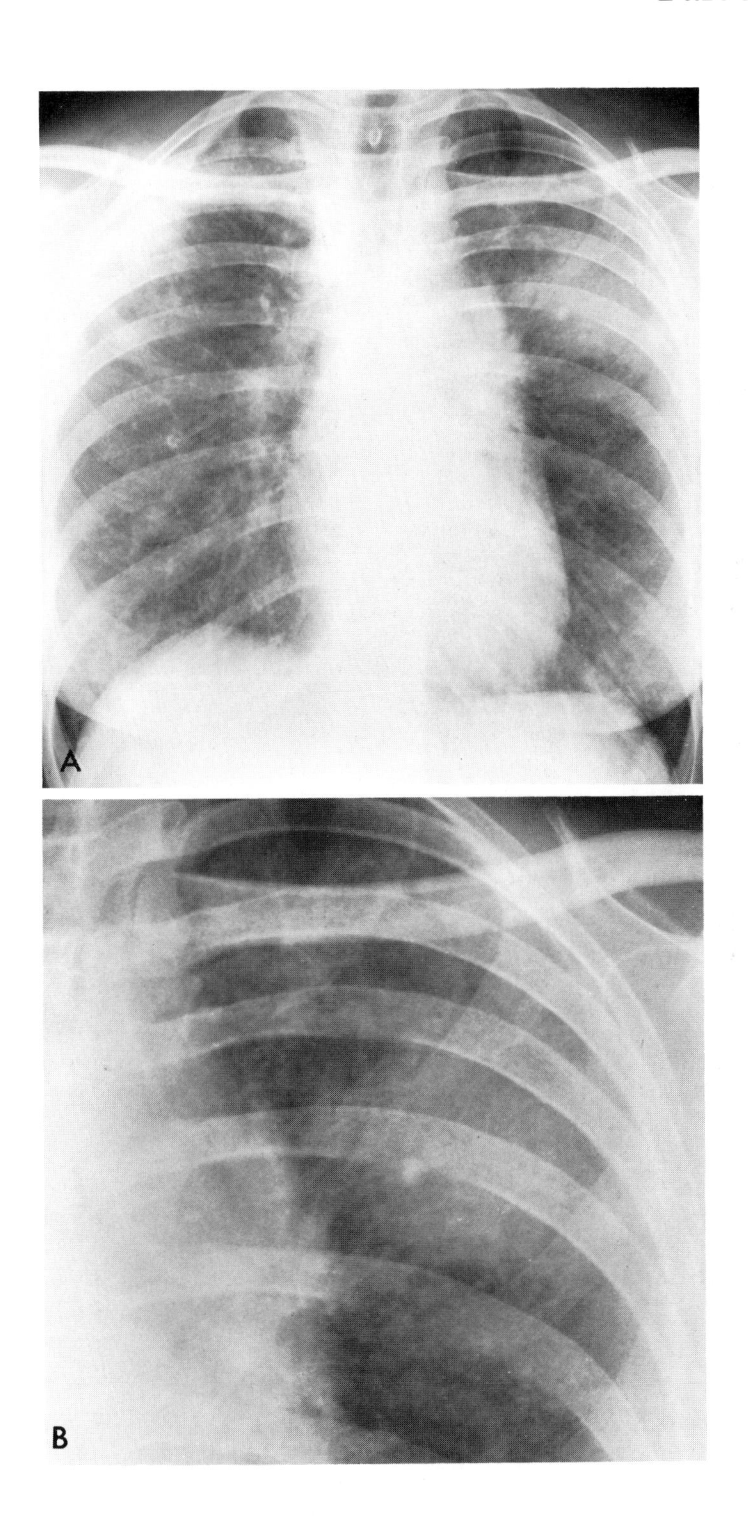

 Case 42
Talcosis (Continued)

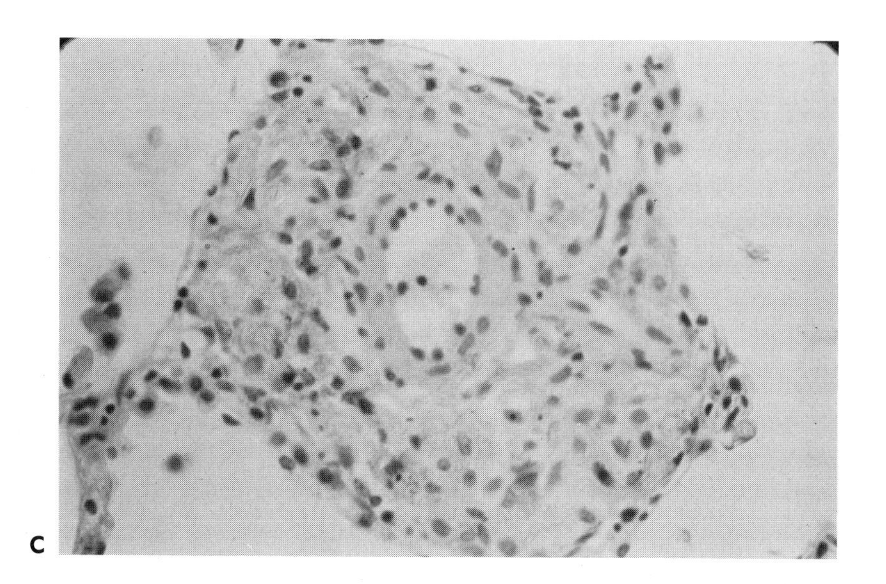

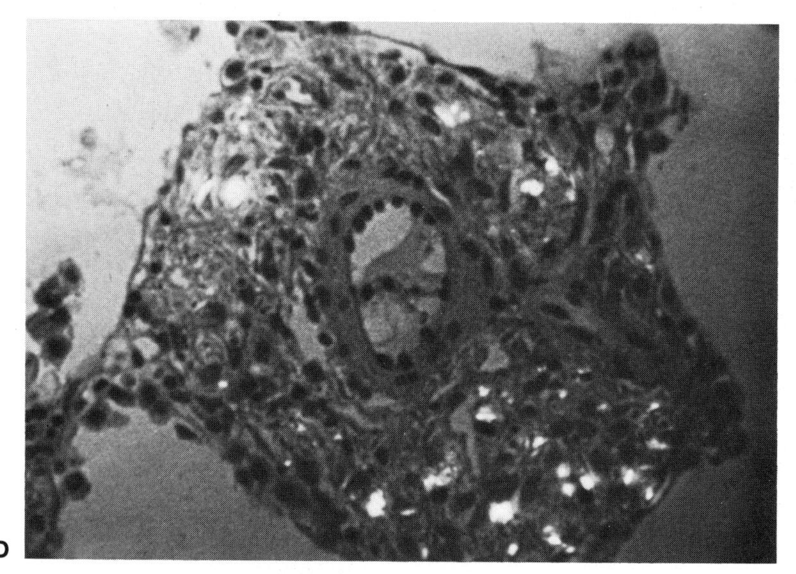

Doubly refractile crystals within a granuloma.

Marchand and Lefebvre[3358] found little evidence of ventilatory defect in a study of 402 arc welders, though Hunnicutt and his colleagues found a slight lowering of maximal midexpiratory flow rate.[3356] Single cases of pulmonary change in welders are reported,[3357] but this may be attributable to inhalation of metals or gases other than iron. Some reduction of pulmonary compliance has been reported by Stanescu and his co-workers in 7 out of 13 welders.[3359]

It must be emphasized, however, that men using the technique of argon-shielded welding are exposed to ozone; in addition, those engaged in cutting scrap metal may be exposed to a wide variety of metal fumes as well as to the relatively harmless oxide of iron. The problem of the effects of ozone is discussed later in this chapter.

Men employed in the mining of iron ore may develop a pneumoconiosis known as "hematite-miner's lung." This condition cannot be regarded as synonymous with siderosis, since the mine dust contains other minerals as well as iron. Pathologically it is described as taking three forms:[1605] diffuse, nodular, and massive fibrotic, very similar to that sometimes seen as a late development of anthracosis. The descriptions and illustrations of the pathological changes that may be seen in this condition[33] clearly indicate that some of these patients must experience considerable interference with pulmonary function, at least in the later stages of the disease process. Not only may considerable emphysema be present, but serious damage to many pulmonary arterioles has been noted to be present, and it seems clear that this change, if widespread, would give rise to impairment of diffusing capacity.

In many occupations, the inhalation of oxides of iron is accompanied inevitably by inhalation of other far more dangerous materials such as silica. In magnetite miners and sinterers, there is little evidence of pulmonary function disturbance,[3235] even though considerable radiological change may be noted.

Tin

Pneumoconiosis caused by inhalation of tin is often referred to as "stannosis" and is a relatively benign condition.[1597] Deposits of tin oxide are distributed around septa, beneath the pleura, and in relation to bronchioles and vessels, and there is no evidence that they excite fibrotic reactions.[33] It is not surprising, therefore, that in a study of 116 men engaged in processing tin, there was no difference in airway resistance or maximal breathing capacity between 26 with Grade 3 to Grade 4 radiological changes compared with the remainder, in whom no changes were visible.[1606] Similar and more recent studies have led to essentially the same conclusion.[3236]

Barium

The pneumoconiosis that develops from inhalation of barium sulfate dust during mining is known as barytosis. Although this produces relatively dense radiographic shadows, there appears to be little interference with pulmonary function.[1607] Although barium oxide is harmless,[3236] some workers exposed to barium sulfate in a factory environment did show ventilatory impairment,[3240] though the attributability of this is in some doubt. There is little doubt, however, that barium sulphate may cause granulomata in the lungs of rabbits,[3239] so it must be regarded as a potential hazard.

Coalworker's pneumoconiosis (Early stage)

Although it was initially considered that inhalation of coal dust unaccompanied by a significant silica content was not harmful (a view endorsed with authority by the Haldane Committee in the 1930's), this view has now been considerably modified. Accumulations of coal dust give rise to dilatation of the respiratory bronchioles, and these, surrounded by black dust, may be seen with the naked eye.[1608] Recent reviews of the fate of inhaled carbon particles[3247] and of the pathogenesis of coalworker's pneumoconiosis[3241] provide considerable insight into the processes that follow dust inhalation and removal. In the early stages, the x-ray is typically nodular in character, with a variable reticular element. It is believed that the nodules must be caused mainly by the tissue reaction, since the density of coal dust is only slightly greater than unity. There is a reasonably close correspondence between radiological category and lung pathology.[2244]

Initial studies of pulmonary function in this stage of coalworker's pneumoconiosis indicated that there was little gross interference.[152, 1611] Brasseur[2095] reported a widen-

Case 43
Coalworker's Pneumoconiosis

Summary of Clinical Findings. This 46-year-old Polish miner was admitted to this Service in October, 1960, complaining of increasing shortness of breath. He had had a previous admission to the Urological Service eight months earlier, when a papilloma of the bladder was resected. Chest x-rays at that time revealed the presence of a diffuse reticulation. He had worked underground in a Belgian coal mine for seven years from 1948 to 1955. While mining, he had been exposed to heavy concentrations of dust but had never worn a mask. On coming to Canada he obtained work with an iron-mine company, this time above ground and with no dust exposure.

He had had no respiratory symptoms until mid-September, 1960, when he developed a low-grade fever and a cough productive of white to yellow sputum. These symptoms persisted for only two weeks, but he said that then he began to note increasing shortness of breath with exertion. At the time of this admission, he said that he was short of breath after walking one hundred yards on the level or climbing seven to ten steps.

There were no remarkable physical findings. The chest moved well; a few scattered rhonchi were noted over both lung fields. Results of routine investigations were noncontributory.

Radiology. The normal pulmonary markings have superimposed upon them a rather coarse reticulonodular pattern composed of shadows which are of "low" density and therefore difficult to reproduce photographically (*A*). Involvement is diffuse, but the apices are relatively less affected. The hila are prominent and possess a nodular outline suggestive of lymph-node enlargement. There is no evidence of pleural effusion or thickening, and the cardiovascular silhouette is normal.

Although this radiological picture is not diagnostic, the character of the diffuse lung reticulation and nodularity combined with hilar lymph-node enlargement suggests a diagnosis of pneumoconiosis. A magnified view of the right lower lung field (*B*) shows the coarse reticulation but does not bring out the nodularity evident on the original film.

Summary. The normal values obtained on investigation, including exercise diffusing capacity and lung compliance, indicate that pulmonary function has not been interfered with by the dust accumulation in the lungs. No organic cause for the dyspnea could be found, and the patient was not short of breath after the exercise test, in spite of the clinical history obtained earlier.

													EXERCISE			
	VC	FRC	RV	TLC	ME %	MMFR	$FEV_{0.75}$ ×40	*pH*	P_{CO_2}	HCO_3^-	O_2Hb %	$D_{Lco}SS_2$	MPH GRADE	$\dot{V}_{O_2}$	$\dot{V}_E$	$D_{Lco}SS_3$
Predicted	4.1	3.5	2.0	6.1	55	3.4	105	7.40	42	25	97	16.5				35.0
Oct. 1960	4.2	2.6	1.4	5.6	54	2.8	121	7.41	38	23	97	17.7	ERGOMETER 400 kgm/min.	1.33	28.7	38.0

These results are within normal limits except for slight reduction in functional residual capacity. Additional studies of lung mechanics revealed normal compliance and airway resistance.

Coalworker's Pneumoconiosis

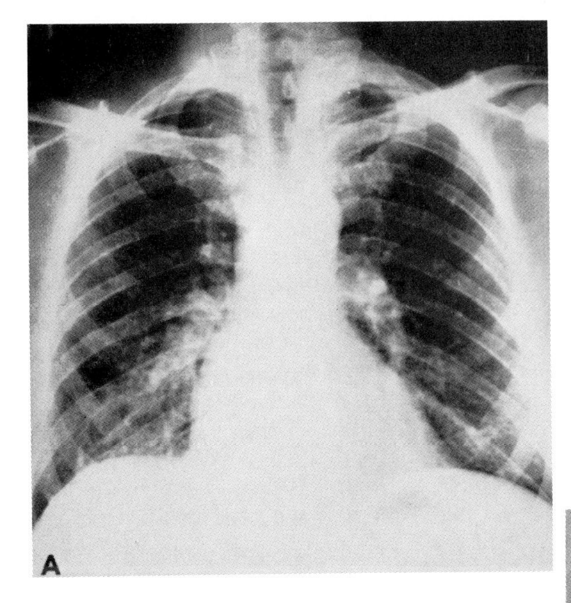

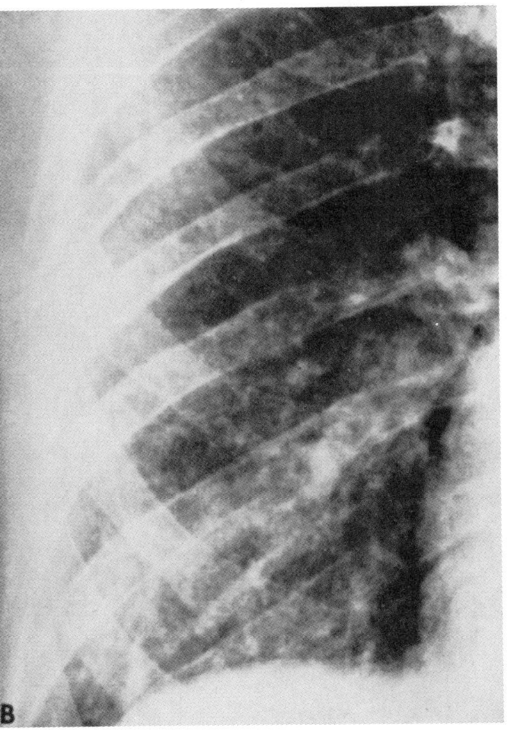

ing of the alveolar–arterial P_{O_2} difference, however, and this disturbance of $\dot{V}/\dot{Q}$ relationships has been confirmed by others.[3248]

A recent study by Ogilvie, Brown, and Kearns[3246] has shown that there is commonly a considerable increase in residual volume at an early stage of this condition, presumably to be explained by premature small airway closure rather than by the presence of significant alveolar destruction. In their group of 17 coalminers, the FEV was only slightly lowered and the single-breath $D_{L_{CO}}$ was normal in the presence of this elevation of residual volume, findings which lend support to this interpretation.

Lyons and his colleagues, however, have reported a lowered single-breath $D_{L_{CO}}$ in 10 of 16 men with simple pneumoconiosis attending a pneumoconiosis panel, confirming an earlier report of a lowered steady-state CO diffusing capacity at rest and on effort in such men.[3251] The pulmonary compliance may also be significantly lowered.[3243] These findings, taken together, indicate that coal-dust inhalation, when sufficient to produce radiological change, probably also produces changes in pulmonary function, though these are not of themselves severe. However, they may well be aggravated when increasing small airway closure occurs as a result of advancing age (*see* Chapter 3).

In general, therefore, it is unwise to dismiss this stage of pneumoconiosis as one that has not produced irreversible effects on pulmonary function, even though these are not severe enough to cause much effort limitation.

As the radiological category advances, ventilatory defect becomes greater.[883] However, it must be remembered that tests such as the FEV are very insensitive to quite large changes in resistance in small airways, and the FEV cannot now be regarded as a sensitive indicator of defect in a disease process that primarily involves the small airways. Changes in residual volume are likely to be more sensitive.

High dust content with massive localized fibrosis

This condition is also referred to as "progressive massive fibrosis of coalminers," and less often as "conglomerate pneumoconiosis." Earlier stages of coal-dust pneumoconiosis may progress to develop conglomerate lesions of dense massive fibrosis. These usually start in the midlung fields bilaterally, and eventually develop into large masses of fibrous tissue, replacing a significant volume of the normally air-filled lung. Often several centimeters in diameter, the fibrous-tissue tumor has well-defined edges, and may contain an irregular cavity. In 1000 autopsies on coalminers from South Wales, James found massive fibrosis with lesions more than 3 cm in diameter in the lungs of 245 cases.[1610] It is believed on both clinical and experimental grounds[33] that this lesion is due to a combination of coal-dust deposits and tuberculosis, and it is important to note that development from an earlier stage to progressive massive fibrosis may occur years after exposure to the dust has ceased. The radiological appearances at this stage of coalworker's pneumoconiosis are very characteristic, irregular masses of fibrous tissue visible usually in both lungs, the intervening lung tissue later appearing more translucent than in other areas, suggesting that significant secondary emphysema has developed in addition to the progressive massive fibrosis.

The onset of this stage of coalworker's pneumoconiosis usually, if not invariably, causes considerable disability. Attempting to correlate ventilatory defect with the extent of the radiological findings, Cochrane and Higgins concluded that the disability was not appreciable until the area of the shadows on the radiograph exceeded 20 sq cm.[2082] In a typical moderately advanced case, the vital capacity is decreased, leading to a reduction in total lung capacity.[152] If, as is often the case, the residual volume is little changed, the ratio of residual volume to total lung capacity is increased (RV/TLC). This increased ratio was initially misinterpreted as inevitably indicating the presence of secondary emphysema;[1612] but its rise in patients with progressive massive fibrosis, at least initially, is due to a reduction in total lung capacity, in contrast to the situation in emphysema, in which elevation of residual volume produces the same change in the ratio. Inert-gas distribution is more uneven than in simple pneumoconiosis[152] but less abnormal than that seen commonly in emphysema. A slight degree of arterial unsaturation on exercise has been noted,[1613] which has been attributed to poor ventilation of parts of the lung, since the alveolar–arterial gradient has been observed to diminish on positive-pressure breathing.[1614] Some reduction in diffusing capacity occurs, but this usually does not become severe until secondary emphysema is extensive. Brasseur has found that the alveolar–arterial Po_2 difference becomes progressively greater in coalminers as the radiological stage of the disease increases.[2095] This excellent study clearly indicates the probable future importance of gas-exchange studies in these patients if a comprehensive view of the nature of the pulmonary function defect is to be secured.

The mechanical function of the lung in progressive massive fibrosis is less seriously impaired than might be expected. Although the ventilatory ability of these patients is usually reduced,[152, 1594] often their flow resistance during quiet inspiration and expiration is normal.[1594] There is a decrease in dynamic compliance,[1594] and almost certainly a decrease in static compliance also, since the total lung volume is decreased.

Thus, the total pattern of function in a moderately severe case of progressive massive fibrosis is apparently explicable by the replacement of normally aerated lung by a space-occupying functionless mass of fibrous tissue.[1705] As the patient ages, and as recurrences of infection become more frequent, chronic bronchitis—and, later, severe emphysema—in relation to the fibrous masses may dominate the clinical and functional picture, leading to severe ventilatory defect, continuous bronchial obstruction, and ultimately arterial desaturation, CO_2 retention, and cor pulmonale. This stage, however, is not usually seen until advanced lung destruction is present. Lavenne has carefully studied and documented the prevalence of right ventricular hypertrophy and cor pulmonale in such patients.[1621]

It is important to recognize that the clinical and radiological picture of progressive massive fibrosis of the lung is not confined to coal-workers; severe cases have been described in others exposed to massive amounts of carbon dust. Recently this syndrome in a severe form has been recognized in carbon-electrode makers,[1615] and a milder degree, but causing impairment of function, has been observed in a man who inhaled synthetic graphite.[1682]

Relatively Little Dust but Generalized Nodular Fibrosis (Classic Silicosis)

Silica is an extremely widely distributed constituent of the earth's structure, and therefore it is not surprising that this element and its compounds occur very frequently in industry. Davies, in a valuable review of the physics and chemistry of dust, lists the occupations that involve inhalation of dusts containing silica and mentions more than a dozen in which there is a potential hazard, including hardrock-mining, rock-drilling, quarrying, working china clay, sand-blasting, and grinding.[1616]

Silica has an almost unique capacity to evoke a fibrous-tissue response in animal tissue of all kinds.[1617] Characteristically, a fibrous silicotic nodule consists of layers of whorled connective tissue arranged like those of an onion. Spencer[33] summarizes four contemporary theories of the mechanism underlying this reaction, which cannot be discussed in detail here. It is important to note, however, that high concentrations of silica dust in a very fine state of division are capable of producing a more diffuse type of fibrosis in the lung.[33, 1617–1619] Since exposure is much more often to mixed dusts than to pure, many mixed patterns of change within the lung are encountered in different industries. It is generally true, however, that the greater the free silica content of the dust and the smaller the particle size, the more severe the fibrosis. These differences are reflected in the variations in radiological appearances and are related also to the concomitant existence or the absence of tuberculosis.

The classic radiographic appearance of silicosis is of multiple nodular shadows varying from 1 to 10 millimeters in diameter. These tend to be well circumscribed and are generally of a uniform density. Since this appearance may be accompanied by or even preceded by a reticular pattern, there is often difficulty in establishing the diagnosis at its earliest stage, and such radiographs are often classified as "suspect" rather than either normal or clearly indicative of silicosis. Hilar lymph-node enlargement may be present, but the pleura is usually normal. Silicosis secondary to exposure to diatomaceous earth has a somewhat different pattern as compared to quartz silicosis. Nodularity is not conspicuous, and a linear and reticular pattern may progress directly to massive fibrosis and emphysema. Exposure to silicon dioxide has been suggested as the cause of the occasional occurrence of eggshell calcification of the lymph glands that may become a distinctive radiographic feature. Rarely, such calcification may involve lymph glands in the abdomen.

Case 44
Acute Silicosis

Summary of Clinical Findings. This 29-year-old man was first admitted to the hospital in June, 1963, with a six-month history of dyspnea, accompanied by a cough productive of thick yellow sputum for one week. On the day before admission he developed left chest pain aggravated by breathing.

The patient had worked since 1957 with a sandblasting company. For the first three years he had been exposed to the sand for only a few hours once weekly but for the last three years he had been engaged full time in sandblasting. The blasting was done inside huge nonventilated metal tanks. Loosely fitted masks were worn, supplied with a continuous flow of supposedly sand-free air. However, the air flow was not filtered and dust was sometimes blown into the mask. The men frequently worked without the air hose connected.

On examination the patient was flushed but not cyanosed, and there was pain with deep respirations. His temperature was 103.4° F, pulse rate 108/min, and rate of respiration 24/min. There were dullness, bronchial breathing, and occasional rales over the lower half of the left chest. There was conspicuous clubbing of the fingers. No signs of congestive failure were apparent.

The total white-cell count was 25,000/cmm, and differential count showed 90 per cent mature neutrophils. Sputum cultures grew no accepted pathogens, but chest x-ray revealed findings consistent with pneumonia of the left mid-lung zone in addition to a diffuse ground-glass appearance. The patient's acute symptoms and signs cleared rapidly with penicillin treatment. Numerous sputum and gastric washings were negative for tubercle bacilli on smear and on culture.

He was readmitted in October, 1963, complaining of a 25 lb weight loss and night sweats for two months. He continued to have mild dyspnea after walking two blocks on the level or climbing two flights of stairs.

Because of the possibility of tuberculous disease at the right apex he was started on PAS and INH. Function studies were repeated (*see* Table). Cardiac catherization showed no elevation of pulmonary artery pressure. A lung biopsy was performed on this admission, with findings as described under Pathology.

Ten days after discharge he required readmission for fever; this disappeared when administration of PAS was discontinued.

Over the next two years he deteriorated rapidly. Until his final admission in September, 1965, he was hospitalized on eleven further occasions, usually necessitated by exacerbations of his dyspnea and respiratory infections. In addition he suffered spontaneous pneumothoraces on the right in 1964 and on the left in early 1965. Since that time he had been completely bedridden requiring constant oxygen by nasal catheter.

(Case report continued on page 378.)

														EXERCISE				
	VC	FRC	RV	TLC	ME %	MMFR	$FEV_{0.75}$ ×40	pH	P_{CO_2}	HCO_3	P_{O_2}	O_2Hb %	$D_{Lco}SS_2$	MPH	GRADE	$\dot{V}O_2$	$\dot{V}_E$	$D_{Lco}SS_3$
Predicted	3.6	2.7	1.3	4.9	65	3.9	121	7.4	40	25		97	21.0					31.0
June 25, 1963	2.9	2.8	1.6	4.5	59	3.5	96						13.6					
Sept. 9, 1963	2.8	2.9	1.9	4.7	61	3.3	100	7.42	36	22		93	11.4	3	FLAT	0.90	24.9	12.5
Nov. 1964	1.1	1.7	1.2	2.3	50	0.9	30	7.32	44	21		92.5	8.5					
July 23, 1965								7.38	55	30	70	93.5						
Sept. 16, 1965								7.33	100	47		97						
Sept. 30, 1965								7.48	48	36	99	97						
Oct. 4, 1965								7.46	54	39	82	96						
Oct. 5, 1965								7.57	47	43	31	70						

Lung volumes, mixing efficiency, and flow rates were normal in June and September. Diffusing capacity at rest was low and did not rise with exercise. The ventilation during exercise was more than one would expect for the oxygen uptake achieved. Blood gases were normal; O_2 saturation was borderline. Mechanical properties of the lung were also studied and found to be within normal limits on the first occasion. Measurement of the pulmonary compliance in January, 1964, showed that this had fallen since June, 1963, to half its previous value.

In November, 1964, there has been marked worsening of function with very low volumes and flow rates and a drop in the diffusing capacity. Just prior to a tracheostomy on September 16, he showed marked CO_2 retention. The day following transplantation on September 29, 1965, his P_{CO_2} was almost normal. Five days after operation his P_{O_2} was beginning to fall and by the following day was severely decreased in spite of O_2 administration.

Acute Silicosis

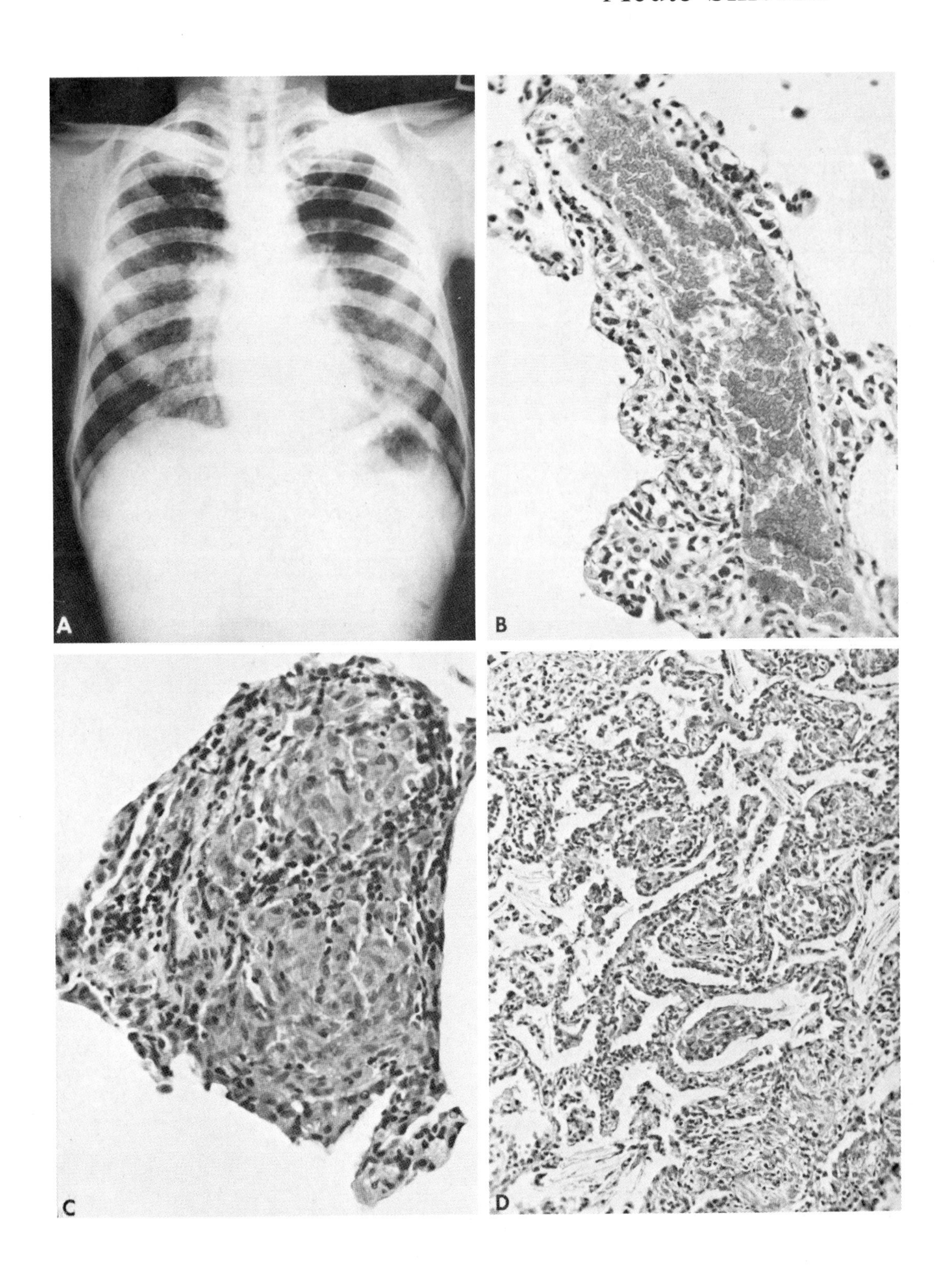

Case 44
Acute Silicosis (Continued)

He was admitted in what was felt to be a terminal state in September, 1965. A lung transplantation was proposed as an attempt to prolong his life.* A tracheostomy was performed in September and he was then maintained on a respirator until September 29, when a left lung transplantation was performed.

Although hypercapnia had persisted preoperatively on assisted ventilation, following operation his blood gases returned to normal and were easily maintained with respiratory assistance. He was treated pre- and postoperatively with steroids, Imuran, and a variety of antibiotics. After the fourth postoperative day, his condition began to deteriorate. His P_{O_2} began to fall in spite of 100 per cent oxygen administration and he died on the seventh postoperative day.

Radiology. Both lungs (*A*) show a diffuse haziness which is symmetrical and evenly distributed. Although it is difficult to reproduce photographically, the original films revealed a fine mottling throughout the lung fields, possessing both a reticular and a nodular component. There is minimal pleural thickening over the left diaphragmatic dome and in the right accessory fissure but no free pleural effusion. The hilar lymph nodes are slightly enlarged bilaterally.

The radiological appearance suggests either silicosis or sarcoidosis as the likeliest diagnostic possibility.

Pathology. Lung biopsy showed an unusual and varied histological picture. The dominant process was the formation of aggregates of epithelioid cells which were situated predominantly around small vessels, both arterial and venous (*B*). In other areas, these appeared interstitial and formed discrete granulomata (*C*), the epithelioid cells being arranged in whorls. Occasionally these granulomata were intra-alveolar. In addition, there was widespread thickening of the alveolar walls with a slight mononuclear infiltrate, and cuboidal metaplasia of the alveolar lining cells, usually associated with the changes noted above, but occasionally alone. In many of these areas cholesterol clefts were present in the alveolar spaces (*D*). Many of the epithelioid cells contained small, nonrefractile brown granules, staining for iron. Most of the pulmonary parenchyma was grossly disorganized, but about one quarter of the alveolar walls was normal. In these areas perivascular epithelioid cells were still present. A large muscular artery showed severe intimal proliferation with a slight inflammatory infiltrate, suggestive of microscopic "web" formation, resulting from organized thrombus.

Ashing of the lung biopsy specimen by the Department of Geology at McGill University showed that of the residuum 20 per cent was SiO_2. At autopsy the residual right lung was shrunken and fibrosed. The transplanted lung showed infarction of the mainstem bronchus distal to the anastomosis and an extensive lower lobe pneumonitis.

Summary. Inhalation of finely divided sand over a three-year period has led to severe changes within the lung. Initially only the exercise pulmonary diffusing capacity was clearly abnormal, but six months later the pulmonary compliance had fallen to 0.08 l/cm H_2O from an initially normal value of 0.15 l/cm H_2O.

This case illustrates the importance of detailed and thorough studies of pulmonary function in the clinical evaluation of such patients.

*See Reference 3018 for full clinical details.

It is not easy, with the presently available data, to present a complete and generally accurate picture of the pulmonary function disturbances that most frequently result from silicosis. It has been shown, however, that there may be little measurable impairment of function in a significant proportion of men who have radiologically typical nodular silicosis, this group totaling 15 per cent in one series[1585] and 18 per cent in another.[17] Conversely, it is clear that in some early cases the main defect may be in exercise diffusing capacity, which few investigators have measured; an example is illustrated in Case 44, a 29-year-old man who was a sand-blaster. Cases of longer duration show alterations in pulmonary function tests that reflect two pathological states with opposite effects on pulmonary function: on the one hand, there may be predominant fibrosis with reduction in functional residual capacity and residual capacity but with relative preservation of air flow,[1406, 1599, 1600] and, on the other, the development of secondary emphysema with its concomitant hyperinflation and decreased air flow.[2243]

Once the disease is clearly established, there is almost certain to be a fall in dynamic compliance and later in static compliance, too. Teculescu, Stanescu, and Pilat[3253] correlated these changes with careful radiological grading in 43 men who had been employed in rock-drilling and sand-blasting, and compared them to a normal group of 10 men. The mechanical changes were, in general, more severe than one might have inferred from the relatively small decline in FEV expressed as a percentage of vital capacity, which they also measured in their patients. Others have documented the fall in compliance in similar studies.[3243, 3252] There can also be little doubt that the diffusing capacity is usually found to be abnormal,[381, 761, 3245, 3251] though there is considerable variation in the degree of impairment found. There is also little correlation between the steady-state diffusing capacity and the measured arterial P_{O_2},[3251] and between the radiological appearance and the lowering of CO transfer.

It is important for the physician to recognize that the pattern of function disturbance may thus vary widely, depending upon the site of nodule formation and the extent of development of secondary emphysema. There is little doubt that when a high concentration of finely divided silica has been inhaled, the initial lesions develop predominantly in association with small pulmonary vessels.[33] In such patients, of whom the one shown in Case 44 is an example, there is little reason to anticipate interference with air flow or with the subdivisions of lung volume, and impairment of diffusing capacity may be the main defect.[1706] In early cases, arterial blood desaturation may not be present at rest[1585, 1620] or on exercise,[1585] though at a heavier exercise load a considerable proportion shows some degree of arterial desaturation.[1585] The alveolar–arterial CO_2 difference is only widened in advanced cases.[3254]

Classic silicosis, like coalminer's pneumoconiosis, may progress to conglomerate disease, probably usually on a basis of complicating tuberculous infection modified by the co-existent disease. There has been little detailed documentation of the effects on pulmonary function of this condition when it has followed classic silicosis, and no exact consecutive picture can yet be drawn of the pattern of function disorder that occurs in a man progressing from an early stage of diffuse nodular silicosis to this advanced degree of lung involvement and destruction. Severe disorders of ventilation–perfusion distribution must occur, however, and the terminal stages may be marked by CO_2 retention, chronic anoxia, and the development of cor pulmonale.

Pneumoconiosis Characterized by Diffuse Pulmonary Fibrosis (Asbestosis, Aluminosis, Berylliosis)

Asbestosis

Asbestosis was first recognized as a disease entity nearly 60 years ago,[1616] but it is only within the last few years that its effects on pulmonary function have been studied in detail. The world consumption of asbestos has increased about eightfold in the last 30 years, and increasing numbers of workers are exposed to secondary industrial products containing this substance.[2225]

A remarkable summary of the history of asbestos and of its effects on man has been published by Brodeur[3260]—a review which ought to be read by anyone interested in this mineral.

The initial report on the incidence of asbestos fibers in the lungs of random autopsies reported from Cape Town[2096] has been followed by similar reports from Tyneside in England,[3301] Milan,[3269] Montreal,[3305] Pittsburgh,[3263] and Israel.[3270] It seems clear that isolated bodies may be found in about half the adult population in these areas. The amount of asbestos seems too small to cause significant effects, but its general spread, possibly from wear of automobile brake linings, should clearly be a matter of general concern. An asbestos fiber has been captured from the air of London and identified by electron microscopy.[2720] A comprehensive bibliography on all aspects of asbestosis has been published in South Africa.[3259]

It has been postulated that the initial reaction to asbestos particles is a fluid exudation, recurrent with each fresh dust exposure.[1622] As the result of the inflammatory reaction, the particles become covered with a smooth protein film, which later becomes impregnated with iron, transforming the original particle into the characteristic golden-brown "asbestos body."[1623] Few of these seem to reach the lymphoid system or hilar lymph nodes, and they have not been found in the pleura[929, 1624]—a surprising finding, since the

Case 45 Asbestosis

Summary of Clinical Findings. This man had worked for nine years supervising the installation of asbestos as insulation for ceilings when he first became aware of dyspnea on exertion. This occupation was a dusty one and required a foil-and-cheesecloth face mask, which, as foreman, he frequently had to remove for the purpose of giving orders. He coughed a good deal while working and for half a day to a full day when he left this atmosphere during holidays. He had had pleural pain some seven years before admission but was unable to recollect on which side. The dyspnea, which developed on going up two flights of stairs or on walking half a mile on the flat, had not increased in severity over the four years since it had first been noted.

On physical examination he was a well developed man with conspicuous clubbing of the fingers and toes. Examination of the chest revealed good chest movement and breath sounds but many crepitations at the lung bases. In view of the radiographic findings it was decided that a bronchogenic carcinoma could not be excluded and thoracotomy was performed. Pulmonary function tests were done before operation and were repeated two weeks postoperatively. He has since been lost to follow-up.

Radiology. The lungs (*A*) are generally overinflated and large bullae are present in the left base. Irregular pleural thickening is present around both lungs, particularly at the bases. The right lower lung field, and to a much lesser extent the left, shows a fine reticular pattern which largely obscures the normal lung markings. In the left lung, behind the heart, there is rather poorly visualized an indistinctly defined mass measuring about 5 cm in diameter. In lateral projection (not reproduced here), this mass was seen to be roughly spherical and to be situated contiguous to the posterior pleural surface. The appearance of the chest suggested pulmonary fibrosis, predominantly basal in distribution, associated with bullous emphysema and with a left lower-lobe peripheral carcinoma.

A magnified view (*B*) of the right lower lung field shows the fine reticular pattern to better advantage.

Pathology. Two large pleural plaques and the left lower lobe were removed. On the lateral aspect of the lower lobe was a fibrous plaque $4 \times 3 \times 1$ cm, and focal localized pleural thickenings were seen on the diaphragmatic surface. The major portion of the lobe was greatly increased in consistency, grayish in color and relatively airless. Portions of the apical segment and posterior and medial basal segments were spared, but there was irregular emphysema here. Microscopical examination showed varying degrees of fibrosis, from dense, relatively acellular fibrous tissue obliterating lung structure to mild interstitial fibrosis (*C*), the general architecture of the lung being preserved. A small portion of the lung showed normal alveolar walls; in these areas fibrosis was centered around respiratory bronchioles. Many histiocytic cells were present in the alveolar spaces in the fibrotic areas and the alveolar lining cells were often swollen and cuboidal. Large numbers of asbestos bodies were seen both in alveolar spaces and in the interstitium (*D*). Scattered giant cells were seen engulfing the bodies. Elsewhere, giant cells were seen containing asteroid bodies (*D*). Moderate thickening of the pulmonary arteries was present. The pleural plaques were composed of dense acellular hyaline tissues. There was no evidence of malignancy.

Summary. The history of exposure, the lowered diffusing capacity and vital capacity with relatively good air flow in the bronchi, and the diffuse reticular pattern on the x-ray are characteristic findings in asbestosis. The slightly increased, rather than reduced, residual volume probably is explained by the presence of bullae at the left base.

The parenchymal shadow was interpreted as representing a carcinoma or mesothelioma, but fortunately it proved to be simply a pleural plaque.

	VC	FRC	RV	TLC	ME %	MMFR	$FEV_{0.75}$ ×40	pH	P_{CO_2}	HCO_3^-	O_2Hb %	$D_{Lco}SS_2$	EXERCISE MPH	GRADE	$\dot{V}_{O_2}$	$\dot{V}_E$	$D_{Lco}SS_3$
Predicted	4.0	3.2	1.7	5.7	60	3.7	115	7.40	42	25	97	18.9					24.5
Dec. 6, 1963	1.8	2.9	2.2	4.0	39	2.7	72	7.40	42	25	96	7.2	3	FLAT	0.9	31.8	13.5
Dec. 30, 1963	1.4	2.7	2.2	3.5	48	1.7	37					8.7					

Pulmonary function was studied one week before and seventeen days after thoracotomy.

Vital capacity was very low and decreased further after operation. The expiratory flow rates show proportionally less impairment preoperatively, and the postoperative values probably are influenced by the recent operative procedure. The diffusing capacity is grossly abnormal both at rest and on exercise.

Studies of lung mechanics showed a considerable increase in elastic recoil and a steep F–V slope.

Asbestosis

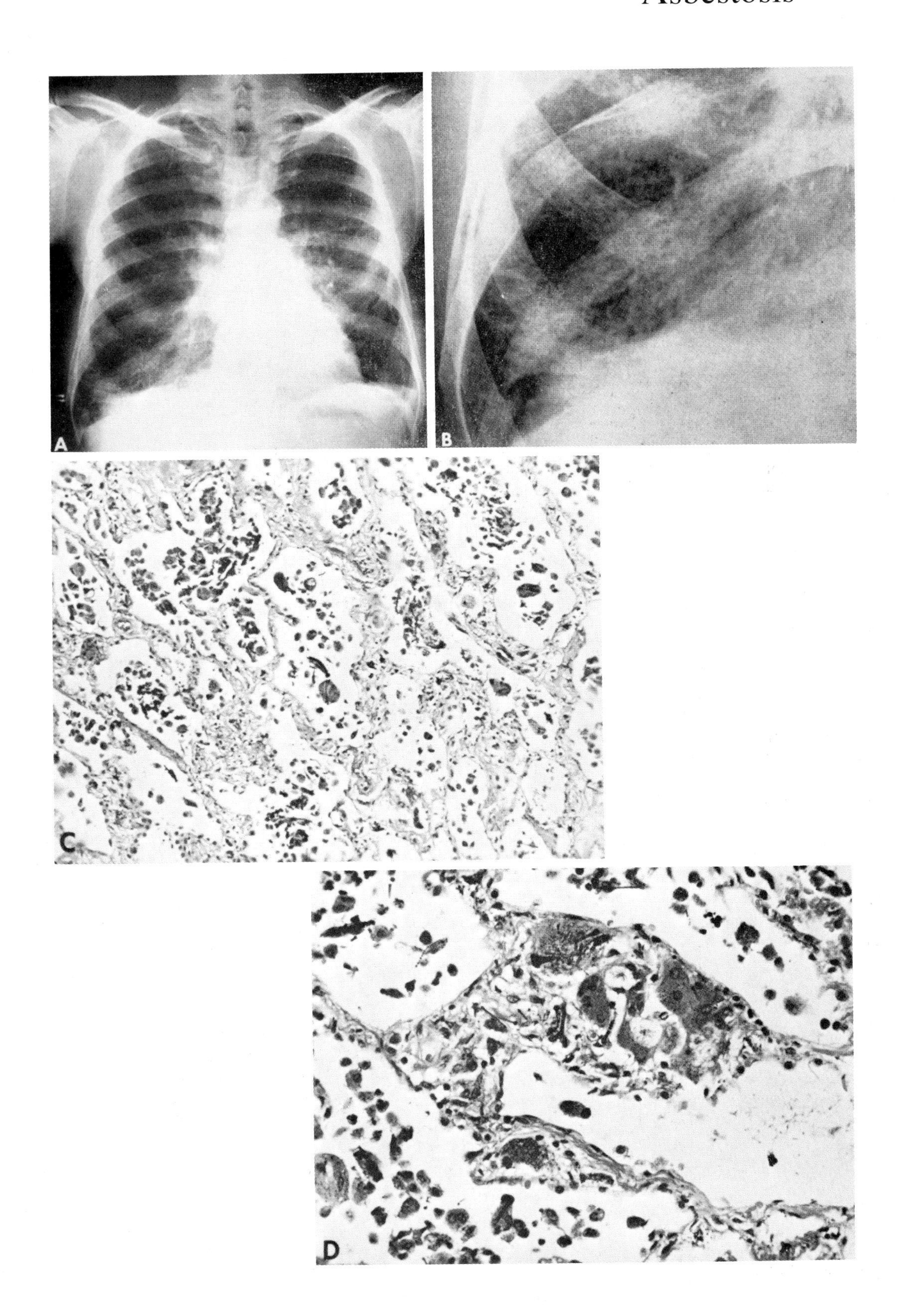

pleural involvement is often severe. In the course of time, a generalized reaction starts in lung tissue, beginning with a peribronchiolar fibrosis and subsequently spreading to obliterate many alveoli and produce general disorganization of the lung structure.

A recent electron-microscope study[3267] has given a more detailed description of the cellular events that apparently follow the deposition of an asbestos fiber in the lung.

Bronchiectasis may accompany the more advanced stages of the disease[929] and has been cited as the cause of two prominent clinical features in such patients: finger-clubbing and bilateral basal rales. In most cases the bases are more severely involved than the rest of the lungs throughout the course of the disease. Radiologically, it has been taught that the pattern of linear fibrosis with emphasis on the lung bases was characteristic, and even diagnostic, of asbestosis, but more recent studies[1625] have indicated very clearly that in many patients the radiological picture is far less specific.

Radiographically, asbestosis may be divided into three stages: (1) fine reticulation, predominantly in the lower zones; (2) a combination of more pronounced interstitial reticulation, often with evidence of chronic pleural change; and (3) a late stage, with considerable distortion and secondary bronchiectasis, often with obliteration of cardiac and diaphragmatic contours. In some groups of cases, pleural changes predominate, and in a significant number, pleural plaques may be the only evidence of disease. These are often bilateral. It seems clear that the frequency of pleural change and the incidence of pleural mesothelioma varies widely in different regions of the world, and this may be because of differences in the form of the mineral.

Changes in pulmonary function in asbestosis have been well documented. There is a generalized reduction in lung volume, in particular of the vital capacity, a change ascribed to the severe basal pleural reaction which undoubtedly may limit the range of lung expansion.[366, 960, 1595, 1626] Ventilatory capacity is relatively well preserved unless secondary emphysema develops. The most striking disorder of function, the decrease in pulmonary diffusing capacity, is one of the "hallmarks" of asbestosis. This change has been found by investigators using three different methods of measurement,[366, 960, 1584, 1595, 2225, 3261] and its importance is confirmed by the fact that the alveolar–arterial oxygen difference is consistently increased.[1626] The decrease in diffusing capacity may be present before there is definite radiological evidence of asbestosis, a finding in keeping with the pathologists' finding that the earliest lesion may be an alveolar exudate.[33] As the disease advances and radiological changes become evident, the diffusing capacity decreases further.[366] Measurements of the RQ in expired air have shown that considerable ventilation–perfusion inequality exists in patients with asbestosis.[1344] Thus, one cannot be sure how much of the decrease in diffusing capacity in this disease is ascribable to $\dot{V}/\dot{Q}$ abnormality, to decrease in lung volume, or to qualitative changes in the alveolar walls: no doubt all these processes play some part in most cases.[1705] However, this uncertainty does not lessen the importance of impairment in diffusing capacity as a *cardinal diagnostic sign* of early pulmonary involvement in men exposed to the inhalation of asbestos dust. The evidence for this view is so complete and unanimous that no survey of asbestos workers could be intelligently conducted that excluded some measurement of this aspect of pulmonary function.

Asbestosis is also associated with a marked reduction in pulmonary compliance,[1595] presumably the result of alteration by fibrosis of the mechanics of those lung units still functioning, and aggravated by a diminution in their total number.[434] Nonelastic work of breathing has been shown to be about twice normal at rest.[1595]

There is still some doubt concerning the correlation or lack of it between the amount of exposure, the extent of radiological change, and the sequence of impairment of pulmonary function in this condition. Williams and Hugh-Jones, in 1960,[366] drew attention to the disparity that might be found between function impairment and radiological change, and more recent studies[3261] have confirmed this view. It has been suggested that a significant fall in pulmonary compliance may occur before change is detectable on a chest film,[3266] and diminishing lung volume without much evidence of obstructive disease[3262, 3302] may occur as the disease progresses, and the radiological signs of worsening may be difficult to detect. The most extensive follow-up data on asbestos workers over several years is the important group studied by Hunt;[3265] it is evident from his data that the routine measurement of pulmonary function in workers exposed to asbestos may provide warning of pulmonary involvement before the routine chest film can do so, and removal from exposure at that stage may be a most important preventive measure.

A massive pulmonary fibrosis may develop after exposure to heavy concentrations of talc,[2083] and there are resemblances between this and the lesions of asbestosis.[1616] Kleinfeld and his colleagues[3257] found that the diffusing capacity in workers exposed to talc was significantly lowered once there were x-ray changes present.

In a survey of workers in a molten-glass plant, Wright[3238] found no evidence of any adverse lung effects.

Aluminosis

Aluminum dust is inert, as far as the lung is concerned, in many circumstances,[1629, 1630, 2084] but it is believed responsible, at least in part, for a diffuse pulmonary fibrosis that may develop in workers engaged in the processing of bauxite,[1631] particularly after exposure to fumes from fusion furnaces.[1632] These fumes consist of submicroscopic particles of aluminum and amorphous silica, and retention of such minute particles is high.[1633] The earliest pathological change is thought to be a septal edema, followed by infiltration with inflammatory cells in alveolar walls.[1634] Obliterative endarteritis is commonly found, and the end result is a diffuse interstitial fibrosis without nodules but with pleural thickening. Pulmonary function appears to have been studied in only five cases of this disease:[729, 1591] one patient who had minimal radiological change had normal lung volumes, ventilatory ability, and diffusing capacity; two had some impairment of these aspects of function; and the other two showed more severe volume restriction and airway obstruction.

Similar changes have been reported in workers exposed to fine aluminum dust in other processes,[729, 1591, 2351] but such cases appear to be rare. Recently, however, Freour and his colleagues have reported a carefully studied case of severe fibrosis leading to cor pulmonale that seems without doubt to have resulted from aluminum-dust exposure.[3271] A material used in aluminum-soldering flux, amino-ethyl ethanolamine, is believed to be responsible for causing severe bronchospasm in those exposed to these fumes. Sterling[2571] showed that in one man so exposed, the FEV_1 fell from 3.0 liters to 1.2 liters without any concomitant fall in steady-state D_{Lco}. It was of interest that the bronchospasm only began five hours after the episode of exposure and not immediately after it.

Chronic beryllium disease of the lung

This condition is more correctly classified as a manifestation of systemic poisoning by beryllium compounds than as a pneumoconiosis, though the toxin usually enters the body in the form of inhaled dust.[1635] In the chronic form of the disease, symptoms may start soon after exposure or may be delayed for as long as 10 years.[1635, 2085]

A recent review of this condition, based on experience with 174 cases, provides valuable information on the clinical course and manifestations,[3273] and long-term follow-up of cases has now been possible. The main incidence of this disease occurred in workers in electric incandescent-light plants between the years 1942 and 1950,[3273] but sporadic cases are not uncommon. Full recovery is possible,[3274] but, if exposure has been massive, early fatality has occurred.[3275]

The earliest pathological lesion in the affected tissue is a loose collection of cells surrounded by lymphocytes.[33, 1638] Giant cells appear as the lesion increases in size, forming noncaseating granulomata which are frequently indistinguishable microscopically from those of sarcoidosis.[1636, 1637] These may progress to hyalinization. In addition, in the lungs there is generalized cellular infiltration of alveolar walls,[1636] which may progress to form diffuse interstitial fibrosis. Many authors stress the difficulty of distinguishing chronic berylliosis from sarcoidosis in some cases.[1637, 1639] It is not surprising, therefore, to find that the pattern of pulmonary function change produced in these two diseases is very similar.

A study from one laboratory of the function-test changes found in patients with one or other of these diseases showed almost identical mean values and ranges in a wide selection of measurements.[1589] Both processes produce diminution in vital capacity and total capacity, with relative preservation of inert-gas distribution. Maximal ventilatory capacity is usually well maintained. A frequent though not invariable finding is a reduction in pulmonary diffusing capacity,[381, 1589] best demonstrated by exercise studies when the resting reduction is not gross in degree. This decrease in diffusing capacity cannot be taken as

Case 46
Farmer's Lung

Summary of Clinical Findings. This 56-year-old farmer was admitted for investigation in January, 1963. One year before admission he had developed a cough productive of about a quarter of a cup of white sputum per day, shortness of breath and episodic mild fever, which persisted throughout the winter months but gradually subsided in the spring except for a residual mild cough. In the fall the cough and shortness of breath recurred so severely that he was unable to carry on his farm work alone and had to hire an assistant. There had been no hemoptysis. He had stopped smoking three years previously. There had been exposure to moldy hay during the first episode of illness. The symptoms had improved during the two weeks before admission, when he avoided the barn.

On examination he appeared short of breath while talking and was frequently interrupted by coughing. His finger nails were beaked. There was no cyanosis, jugular vein distension, or ankle edema. The chest moved symmetrically but there was diminished air entry with scattered rales at both bases. The remainder of the examination was not contributory.

Investigations revealed a hemoglobin of 15.4 gm/100 ml; sedimentation rate 19 mm/hour; total WBC 9600/cmm, with a normal differential. Numerous sputum cultures were negative for acid-fast bacilli and bacterial and fungal pathogens. Tuberculin, blastomycin, and histoplasmin skin tests were negative. Chest x-rays and pulmonary function tests are reported here. Lung biopsy was performed and the description is reported under Pathology; the findings were consistent with a diagnosis of farmer's lung.

The patient was discharged with instructions to avoid contact with hay, and treatment with steroids was begun. Pulmonary function testing was repeated in April, 1963, but there has been no further follow-up.

Radiology. Fine reticulonodular densities are scattered diffusely throughout both lungs, more prominent in the bases than elsewhere (*A*). The hila are enlarged but possess a contour which suggests increased size of the pulmonary arteries rather than lymph-node enlargement. The heart is of normal size and there is no pleural effusion. The radiological appearance is not in any way diagnostic.

A magnified view of the lower portion of the right lung (*B*) demonstrates to better advantage the abnormality of pulmonary texture.

Pathology. Biopsy of the lung showed a patchy interstitial pneumonitis (*C*) involving about half of the alveolar parenchyma. The alveolar structure was intact, but an interstitial infiltrate of lymphocytes, mononuclear cells and occasional plasma cells thickened the involved alveolar walls. A few multinucleate giant cells were seen (*D*), containing doubly refractile particles. Epithelioid cells were scanty or absent, even in areas of giant-cell formation. Both large and small bronchioles showed a heavy infiltrate of mononuclear cells, and some of the large bronchioles contained much mucus. The histological appearance was typical of that seen in farmer's lung.

Summary. This case of farmer's lung illustrates the characteristic history of symptoms precipitated by exposure to moldy hay during the winter months. The lowered diffusing capacity, which is the chief defect of function, is related to the parenchymal changes described.

													EXERCISE				
	VC	FRC	RV	TLC	ME %	MMFR	$FEV_{0.75}$ ×40	pH	$P\text{CO}_2$	HCO_3^-	O_2Hb %	$D_{Lco}SS_2$	MPH	GRADE	$\dot{V}O_2$	$\dot{V}_E$	$D_{Lco}SS_3$
Predicted	3.7	3.5	2.2	5.9	50	3.0	90	7.40	42	25	97	13.7					14.5
Jan. 1963	2.3	3.3	2.6	4.9	34	1.5	59	7.47	38	26	98	9.2	1.5	FLAT	0.73	22.8	9.8
April 1963	2.2	3.1	2.5	4.7	40	1.0	45					9.9					

The vital capacity and flow rates are moderately reduced in this patient, but there is no evidence of hyperinflation. Diffusing capacity is reduced and does not rise with exercise. The $P\text{CO}_2$ and bicarbonate are within the normal range. Arterial blood is fully saturated. There has been essentially no change after a month on steroid therapy.

Farmer's Lung

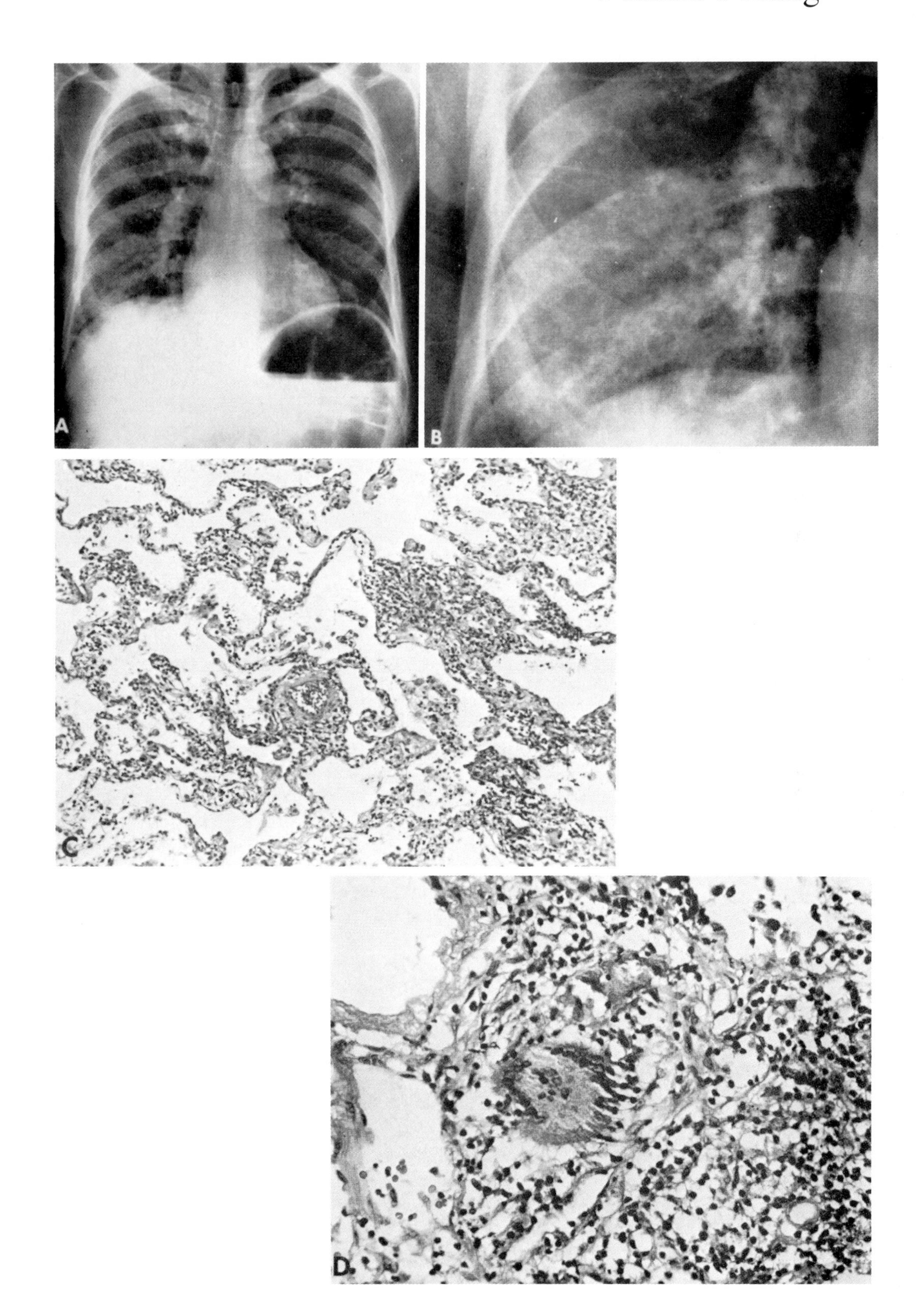

necessarily reflecting only the qualitative change in the alveolar membrane. In berylliosis, as in sarcoid, an important factor is the replacement of functioning alveoli by nodules of granulomata, with normal alveolar walls intervening. There is interference with vascularity, because of predilection of the granulomata for perivascular regions, and interference with normal $\dot{V}/\dot{Q}$ ratios in the lung. As noted in the discussion of asbestosis, uncertainty as to which of these mechanisms is responsible for the observed fall in diffusing capacity should not lead to the conclusion that it is not an important functional parameter to measure; indeed, no assessment of a suspected case of berylliosis can be considered complete without such a test. Some estimate of the relative importance of simple replacement of lung tissue in causing the lowered diffusing capacity can be obtained by relating this measurement to the observed lung volume,[1705] a technique first proposed in relation to sarcoidosis.[56] Only a small proportion of these patients shows the complicating features of emphysema as reflected by a reduced ventilatory capability and an increased residual volume. Patients with chronic beryllium disease studied between 1951 and 1955 showed a relatively high incidence of airway obstructive disease, with considerable ventilatory defect.[1589, 1640, 1641]

Redding, Hardy, and Gaensler[3272] have recently reported the detailed follow-up of a patient proven by lung biopsy to have berylliosis over a period of 16 years. Between 1954 and 1968, his maximal breathing capacity fell from 170 to 82 liters/min, his vital capacity from 3.5 to 1.9 liters, and his rest and exercise steady-state diffusing capacity from about 60 per cent of predicted values in 1954 to about 45 per cent of predicted values in 1968. The chest x-ray changed little over an eight-year period.

Although exposure to beryllium is now very rare, since the hazard is recognized, careful investigation and surveillance of those known to have been exposed to it are clearly important.

PNEUMOCONIOSIS DUE TO ORGANIC DUST

In contrast to the usually distinctive nature of the pathological changes caused in the lungs by inhalation of inorganic dust, those consequent upon inhalation of organic dust are much less specific. Some of these conditions are primarily, if not entirely, confined to changes in bronchial airways, and may represent an abnormal or conditioned response to the inhalation of a foreign protein or other molecule. Farmer's lung is an exception to this generalization, since the pulmonary parenchyma usually is involved in the pathological change.

Byssinosis

Schilling has reviewed the history of studies of respiratory disease in carding-room workers in factories where cotton is spun.[1598] It had been known for many years that these workers not only had a high incidence of chronic bronchitis, but in addition claimed that their symptoms were much more severe on Mondays; and this was such a distinctive feature that in some areas the symptoms were known as "Monday fever." It is of particular interest that McKerrow[1596] and Gilson[1590] and their colleagues, by careful use of serial ventilatory measurements, were able to show that carding-room workers with symptoms suffered a decline in ventilatory capacity throughout the Monday work-day after a weekend rest. In some groups of workers the changes were less marked during the rest of the week. Parallel changes in airway resistance occurred also. Saline extracts of mixed cotton dust are pharmacologically active in causing bronchial constriction,[1586] and it is believed[2086] that this substance may cause histamine release. However, hypersensitivity to histamine does not appear to be a feature,[3281] and the response to inhaled histamine seems similar to that of patients with chronic bronchitis without byssinosis.[3282]

Pathological changes have not been reported in any large number of such patients, and those that have been observed are mostly of chronic bronchitis with varying degrees of emphysema.[1598] Chronic inflammatory changes take place around the bronchi, but these do not appear to be particularly distinguishable from those seen in chronic bronchitis in the general population. Byssinosis bodies have been described,[1598] but there is no evidence of any generalized reaction occurring in the lung as with asbestos. Little appears to be known about the long-term effects of byssinosis on the lung or whether function changes appear to be in any way distinct from those commonly encountered in chronic bronchitis and pulmonary emphysema.

There is little doubt that the symptoms of byssinosis, at least in the early stages, are related to the fall in ventilatory capacity and an increase in airway resistance. It is of interest to note that such symptoms are apparently noticed by workers in whom the ventilatory capacity falls from an average of about 80 liters/min early on Monday morning to about 72 liters/min after eight hours' exposure, the airway resistance increasing over the same period.[1596] The fact that such small changes in ventilatory capacity can produce a distinctive clinical complaint of dyspnea is remarkable. Byssinosis is also of great interest as a classic example of the use of respiratory function tests to clarify a clinical entity, the accurate description of which was otherwise entirely dependent upon the subjective complaint of dyspnea, since usually the chest x-ray is normal.

There is now little doubt that byssinosis is a world-wide disease and not confined to any one country. Recently, cases have been reported from Sweden,[3279] Australia,[3280] Spain,[3276] and Belgium,[3283] where a relatively high incidence was found in workers in a flax-processing industry. Strict observance of preventive measures is needed.[3277]

Bouhuys and his colleagues have concluded[3276] that "a deleterious effect of long-term hemp dust exposure on pulmonary function is highly probable." It seems likely that the later consequences may be irreversible, but there is as yet little exact knowledge of the sequence of pathological changes in the lung that lead to this situation.

Bagassosis

Bagasse is the residue of cane from which the sugar has been extracted. Brief exposure to this dust may cause an acute febrile illness, with dyspnea and cough but with few residua, which is almost certainly an acute bronchiolitis.

It seems likely that continued exposure to this dust can cause a diffuse interstitial fibrosis,[33] and one patient had considerable bronchiectasis and emphysema on autopsy.[1643] In two patients in whom pulmonary function was studied, Buechner and his colleagues found impairment of vital capacity and a slightly lowered resting arterial oxygen saturation, though the maximal breathing capacities were reported as normal.[1588] No observations of diffusing capacity or of pulmonary compliance were made. More recently, Weill and his colleagues[3285] have reported on detailed function studies in 20 patients with this disease, finding a modest reduction in lung volumes and in gas transfer. Improvement in function followed clinical improvement and clearing of the radiographs. Pierce and his co-workers[3284] reported open-lung biopsies on 2 patients, which showed interstitial infiltrates, granulomata, and crystalline inclusions that rotated polarized light. Seven men had been involved in an epidemic of acute bagasse-worker's lung, and detailed pulmonary function studies were carried out initially and later, as the condition was subsiding. The authors concluded that the most sensitive measurement of impairment was the membrane diffusing capacity ($D_{M_{CO}}$). The total diffusing capacity remained significantly lower than normal after a year. During the initial acute phase, the arterial oxygen tension was considerably reduced, but no elevation of P_{CO_2} was observed. The administration of steroids seemed to have little effect on the course of the disease or its speed of resolution.

Sisal-worker's disease

An unusual type of apical fibrosis with bronchiectasis has been found in several workers in a Uganda factory for processing sisal.[1644] This may be another example of bronchial pathology following inhalation of organic dust, similar to the bronchiectasis noted in the worker with bagasse (*see* Bagassosis) and the apical fibrosis, cavitation and bronchiectasis reported in workers in the Hungarian pepper industry.[1645]

Operatives employed in sisal factories have more chest complaints and a lowered maximal ventilatory capacity in comparison with control subjects with no such exposure.[1644] It seems likely, therefore, that the main effect of the inhalation of this dust is to cause an increased prevalence of chronic bronchitis, and it is associated with occasional overt bronchiectasis.

Maple-bark-stripper's disease

In 1932 Towey and his colleagues described an acute respiratory disease occurring in a group of men engaged in stripping bark from maple logs. The syndrome is attributable to inhalation of the spores of *Coniosporum corticale.*[1646] The lung pathology has been described,[2113] and the spores have been demonstrated at lung biopsy.[3288] An agar-gel diffusion test is usually positive. Wenzel and Emanuel have recently reviewed the epidemiological and clinical features of this condition,[3287] which does not seem to cause anything very significant in the way of chronic clinical disability or impairment of pulmonary function,[3288] although the fibrotic change has been described as extensive.

Farmer's lung

Although the first description of this disease is often credited[1647] to Campbell in 1932,[1648] Spencer has pointed out[33] that Cadham, in Canada, described a similar entity eight years earlier.[1649]

The recent work of Pepys on the immunological aspects of this and related diseases has done much to clarify the nature of the pathological processes involved, and his recent summary of this information should be consulted by all those who treat clinical cases of this syndrome.[3364] Pepys and Jenkins in 1965 showed that 89 per cent of 205 farmers in Britain, regarded as having had this syndrome, had positive agar-gel precipitin tests to *Thermopolyspora polyspora.* The classic syndrome occurs most commonly after crops are harvested in rainy weather and stored in closed barns. When the moldy bales are forked out, the farmer may inhale a white irritant dust containing many fungus spores. Such inhalation in a previously sensitized person may lead to the swift onset of dyspnea, a dry irritant cough, fever, and, occasionally, hemoptysis.[2090] There is little evidence that bronchospasm occurs; moist sounds in the lung and cyanosis are common findings. Radiologically, in the acute stage there may be a "ground-glass" opacity extending to the periphery of both lung fields, and later a fine reticulation with granular mottling may be seen.[1654] Such an appearance may be misdiagnosed as miliary tuberculosis, though the granularity is finer in farmer's lung, the densities being 1 mm or less in diameter. The x-ray shows spontaneous resolution to occur usually over a period of weeks,[2090] but there is often considerable residual dyspnea. Recurrent exposure may result in chronic disability and even pulmonary fibrotic changes.

The differentiation from sarcoidosis may be difficult in some instances. The customary absence of significant lymph-gland enlargement in farmer's lung cannot be absolutely relied upon. We have encountered a patient in whom the diagnosis was proven by lung biopsy and by the presence of precipitating antibodies, and who showed clear-cut evidence of hilar lymph-node enlargement.

It is only in recent years that lung biopsies have been performed in this condition, yielding a better understanding of its pathology. Such biopsy material has shown focal granulomatous lesions said to be similar to those in sarcoidosis, diffuse interstitial inflammation involving alveoli and the walls of bronchioles, and resolution of the granulomatous lesions followed by interstitial fibrosis of variable degrees of severity.[1650, 1651] In fact, approximately two thirds of the cases have not shown these granulomata at the time of lung biopsy. In our experience of three cases, doubly refractile particles have been visible in the giant cells, and the granulomatous lesions have borne only a superficial resemblance to sarcoidosis (*see* Case 46). There is some evidence that the initial acute stage is essentially one of pulmonary edema,[33] though only one biopsy specimen appears to have been taken when the disease exists at this stage. It seems very likely that "farmer's lung" should be regarded as representing a granulomatous response to vegetable fiber to which some sensitization has occurred previously.[2091, 2092, 2315, 2349]

Recently, a number of authors have stressed that there exists both an acute and a chronic stage of this condition.[3295, 3298, 3299] Occasionally the acute stage may be very severe, and a fatal outcome in a 17-year-old patient has been described.[3300] The chronic stage is characterized by very considerable fibrosis,[3296] and the pathology described explains the considerable residual function impairment noted by a number of investigators.

Two annotations on "farmer's lung" three years apart in the same journal[1647, 1652] failed to make any mention of the impairment of pulmonary function this disease may cause. The later annotation was followed by correspondence in which the importance of this was stressed, the writers pointing out that significant abnormalities of function may continue after the radiograph has completely cleared.[1653] Dickie and Rankin and their colleagues documented the occurrence of arterial hypoxia, striking impairment in diffusing capacity, considerable reduction in vital capacity and moderate airway obstruction in the acute and early stage of the condition.[1650, 2354] The maximal breathing capacity was reduced in 6 of 10 patients studied by Bishop and his colleagues.[2349] Impairment of diffusing capacity persisting long after radiological clearing has been observed by several authors,[1650, 2093, 2298] and by us in 2 patients.

That residual function impairment must be common is indicated by Frank's observation that all of his 27 patients with this syndrome complained of exertional dyspnea at the time they were reviewed, several years after the acute episode;[1654] this paper should be consulted also for its excellent illustrations of the radiographic changes seen in this condition. Recently, Williams has carefully documented the changes in pulmonary function found in cases of farmer's lung.[2093] Ventilatory and total lung capacities are little affected, but there are significant reductions in pulmonary compliance and steady-state diffusing capacity in many of these patients months after the onset of symptoms. He found clear evidence of function impairment in several patients in whom the chest x-ray was normal, and drew attention to the importance of this defect by demonstrating low values of arterial P_{O_2} during exercise in these cases. Sanders and Martt[2298] and Bishop and his colleagues[2349] recently confirmed the importance of measurements of diffusing capacity and arterial P_{O_2} in the study of patients with this disease.

More recent work has fully confirmed these findings, particularly the low diffusing capacity.[3290, 3292, 3297] It is quite evident that chronic fibrotic change not uncommonly occurs, at least in areas where the disease is endemic. Barbee and his colleagues[3297] noted considerable functional impairment in 50 patients, followed for at least three years and for an average of six years. Diffuse fibrotic radiological changes and interference with CO transfer were commonly found in this series.

Bird-fancier's lung (pigeon-breeder's lung)

During the past four years, a considerable literature has been contributed to the study of a syndrome of pneumonitis caused by sensitivity to various avian antigens. Initially, the illness may be febrile, with patchy pneumonitis on the x-ray, and of moderately acute onset. Hargreave and his colleagues[3306] described 7 such cases among pigeon-breeders and 5 after contact with budgerigars. Dyspnea and cough were prominent features, and all had precipitins against avian antigens. In half the patients, there were crepitations in the lung and radiological changes. About the same number showed a lowered vital capacity and CO uptake, and one patient with fever and loss of weight had a lowered CO transfer with no other abnormal findings. These authors found that an attack could be precipitated by inhalation of the antigen. The pathology of this condition has been described,[3313] and lymph-gland enlargement has been reported.[3308] Although repetitive episodes of acute pneumonitis are characteristic,[3307] there may be a chronic afebrile stage,[3312] and acute airway obstruction has been noted.[3309] The relative rarity of this condition in Belgium, where many people are pigeon-fanciers, suggests that the syndrome must be relatively rare even among those in contact with these birds.[3311]

Miscellaneous syndromes

Hypersensitivity to inhaled pituitary snuff has been described, and in one instance the compliance was noted to be reduced, as were the single-breath $D_{L_{CO}}$ and the vital capacity.[3314] An allergic alveolitis has been described in a malt-worker, attributed to sensitivity to the spores of *Aspergillus clavatus*.[3316] Inhalation of these spores lowered the FEV and the vital capacity, and caused a febrile reaction. It has long been known that grain-handlers may suffer from a syndrome characterized by cough, dyspnea, and wheezing. A recent study of 55 men employed in this occupation showed generally normal values for vital capacity and FEV (though the cigarette smokers had generally worse function than the others).[3315]

ACUTE AND CHRONIC CHEMICAL IRRITANTS

Development of the chemical and allied industries has meant a great increase in the number of potentially dangerous fumes and gases to which man may be accidentally exposed. Knowledge of the effects of often-repeated inhalation of low concentrations of these has been gained very slowly, and even now this represents one of the most neglected

(Text continued on page 394.)

Case 47 Radiation Fibrosis

Summary of Clinical Findings. This 52-year-old housewife presented with a large lobulated and ulcerated mass of the right breast which she had watched grow from a small lump eight months previously. There were no palpable glands in the axillary region. A biopsy of the breast confirmed the diagnosis of carcinoma, and the patient was given 6000 roentgens of x-ray over a period of one month to the upper breast region, the mediastinum, the right axillary and supraclavicular areas, and to the tumor itself. A simple mastectomy was then performed, and the pathologist reported that the lymph nodes were uninvolved. Tumor tissue extended almost to the margins of the resection, however. Postoperative convalescence was uneventful.

Ten weeks later, on October 20, 1958, she developed a dry cough and noticed that she was increasingly dyspneic on exertion. A few days later she became febrile, anorexic and extremely weak and was immediately admitted to the hospital. Her temperature spiked daily to 102° F for the first week and then decreased to 101° F and 100° F over the next two weeks; it was unaffected by antibiotic therapy. Sputum cultures grew no accepted pathogens. Total white-cell count was 4400/cmm on admission, subsequently increasing to 13,000/cmm. She was treated with corticosteroids for one month. The dyspnea decreased in severity during her stay in the hospital. Subsequent follow-up examinations in 1959 and 1962 elicited shortness of breath on going upstairs or walking rapidly on the flat. The main physical signs were the contraction and the limitation of expansion of the right side of the chest and deviation of the trachea.

Over the next two years the carcinoma metastasized to cerebrum, bones, esophagus and lung. She developed a large metastatic mass in the left upper lobe, and coincident with this became increasingly dyspneic. On her final admission in May, 1964, the mass filled the upper left chest. The patient was severely short of breath and had great difficulty raising secretions. No extensive investigations or treatments were carried out and the patient died on May 10, 1964. Autopsy confirmed the presence of widespread metastases. The right lung was severely shrunken and fibrosed.

Radiology. On October 20, 1958, x-ray of the chest revealed subtle changes difficult to reproduce photographically (*A*). There was a slight but definite assymetry of radiolucency of the two lungs, a fine granularity and linear accentuation throughout the right lung creating an overall greater density on this side compared with the left. The right breast shadow is missing.

By November 13 (*B*), a remarkable change had occurred in the right lung. There was a severe degree of loss of volume manifested by elevation of the right diaphragmatic dome, shift of the mediastinum and approximation of ribs. A very fine, closely knit reticulation occupied the whole of the right lung so that little air-containing lung was visible. A tomogram made at this time demonstrated the bronchial tree to be air-containing out of the 6th- or 7th-stage divisions. The left lung showed a subtle change in texture similar to that present in the right lung on October 20.

	VC	FRC	RV	TLC	ME %	MMFR	$FEV_{0.75}$ ×40	pH	P_{CO_2}	HCO_3^-	O_2Hb %	$D_{Lco}SS_2$
Predicted	3.0	2.7	1.6	4.6	55	2.8	75	7.40	42	25	97	14.3
Nov. 13, 1958	1.2	1.8	1.3	2.5	44	1.1	39	7.53	35	28	85	5.4
Dec. 10, 1958	1.4	1.6	1.0	2.4	46	1.4	40					11.6
June 1959	1.6	1.8	1.2	2.8	46	1.3	44					11.0
April 1962	1.9	1.9	1.0	2.9	45	1.5	47					10.9

The first tests of function, on November 13, 1958, were made on the same day as the second chest film (*B*) was taken. The suspicion at this time of the *left* lung involvement is supported by the demonstration of a very low diffusing capacity and arterial unsaturation, which would have been unlikely had the left lung remained normal throughout. By December 1958, presumably the left lung has recovered from the pneumonitis, as pulmonary function is now about normal for someone with one lung destroyed and the other normal. Remarkable constancy of function is shown over the course of the next four years. There were no further studies before her death in 1964.

Radiation Fibrosis

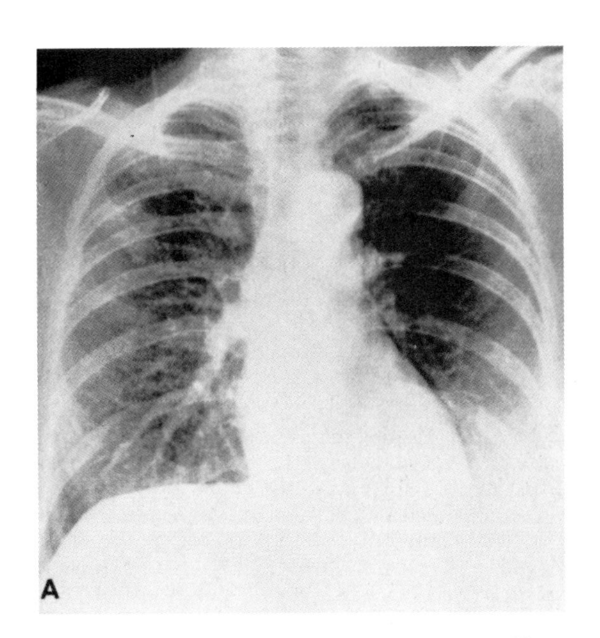

A

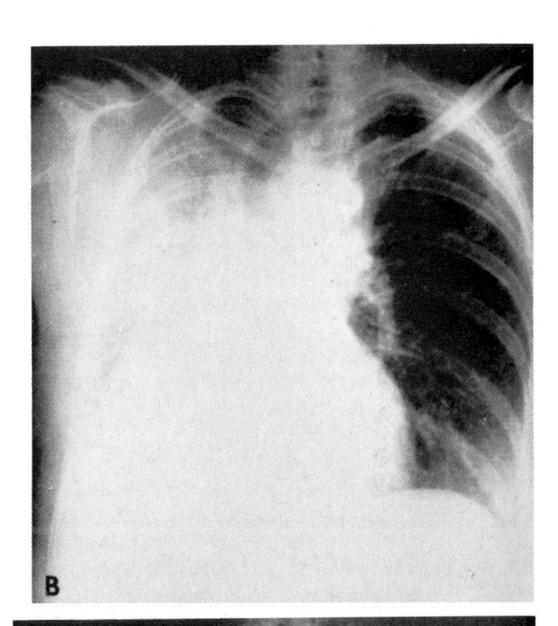

B

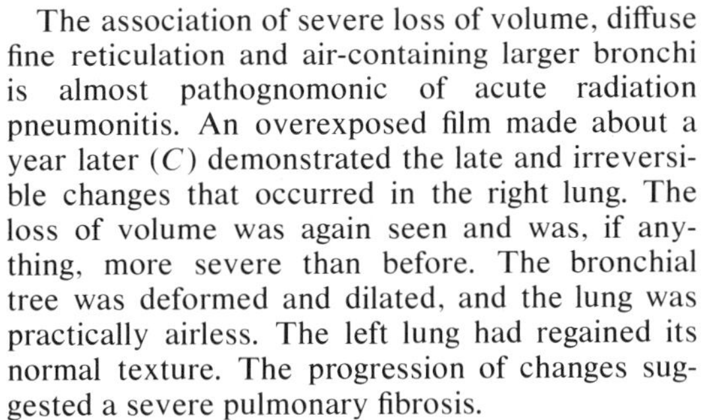

The association of severe loss of volume, diffuse fine reticulation and air-containing larger bronchi is almost pathognomonic of acute radiation pneumonitis. An overexposed film made about a year later (*C*) demonstrated the late and irreversible changes that occurred in the right lung. The loss of volume was again seen and was, if anything, more severe than before. The bronchial tree was deformed and dilated, and the lung was practically airless. The left lung had regained its normal texture. The progression of changes suggested a severe pulmonary fibrosis.

Summary. It seems clear that the radiation pneumonitis which progressed to a destructive fibrosis of the right lung involved the left lung also at the time of the first assessment of pulmonary function. The function of the left lung improved, so that the final pulmonary status, unchanged over four years, was similar to that of a patient who has had a pneumonectomy.

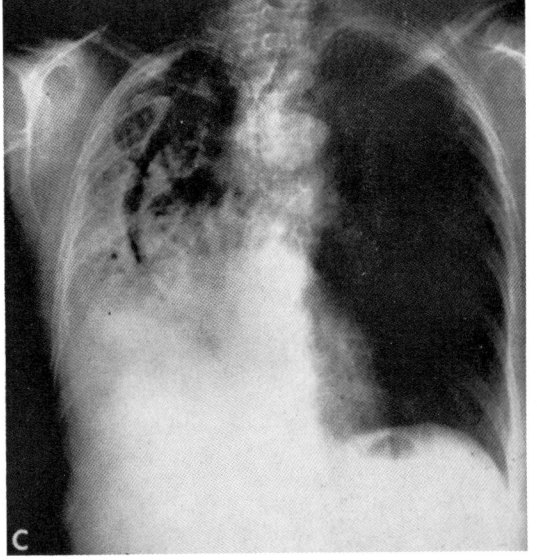

C

Case 48
"Chemical" Bronchiectasis; Acute Exposure to Oxides of Sulfur

Summary of Clinical Findings. This 33-year-old laborer working in a wood-pulp processing plant was accidentally exposed to fumes of SO_2 and SO_3 in November of 1958. This occurred when he was attempting to secure a metal plate on the top of a chemical tank. He immediately noticed a choking sensation and cough, and had difficulty in breathing. However, these symptoms cleared almost completely in a few minutes and he was able to return home three hours later at the end of his day's work. After he had been home for a few hours, his dyspnea became acutely worse and he was admitted urgently to the hospital, where he was treated with oxygen for three days. The x-ray revealed pulmonary edema, but this had cleared on his discharge three weeks later.

He was left with a productive cough and complained of dyspnea, however. In view of the normality of the x-ray, in February, 1959, he was referred for pulmonary function evaluation.

He stated on admission that he had been free of symptoms previously, but that since the episode he had coughed up half a cupful of sputum daily and had had severe dyspnea. He was orthopneic. The chest was symmetrical, but fine rales and rhonchi could be heard over most zones of both lungs. The quality of the breath sounds was not grossly abnormal. The cardiovascular system was normal. There was no finger-clubbing.

Re-examination two years later revealed the same findings, with the addition of definite finger-clubbing. The electrocardiogram was normal. He was admitted for reassessment in November, 1969. He had noticed gradually increasing dyspnea and now was short of breath when climbing stairs or walking quickly on the level. The cough was unchanged.

Radiology. A postero-anterior projection of the chest shows moderate symmetrical hyperinflation of both lungs (*A*), evidence for which was more convincing in the lateral view. The pulmonary markings and cardiovascular silhouette are essentially normal, and there are no localized or generalized parenchymal infiltrations. Films of the chest at the time of the acute episode three months previously were reported to show changes consistent with acute pulmonary edema, complete radiological clearing of which was said to have occurred within three or four days.

Midsagittal tomogram of the lungs shows normal peripheral vasculature (*B*). Situated along the distribution of the bronchovascular tree are several paired linear densities which run in parallel and which are seen predominantly in the middle third of the lung fields. These "tram lines" are thought to represent thickened bronchial walls. Tomographic sections made at different levels in the lungs showed these paired lines to be widely distributed through all lobes, but chiefly in the medial two-thirds of the lung fields.

Oblique films of the right (*C*) and left (*D*) bronchial trees following bronchography reveal a

(Case report continued on page 394.)

	VC	FRC	RV	TLC	ME %	MMFR	$FEV_{0.75}$ ×40	pH	P_{CO_2}	HCO_3^-	O_2Hb %	$D_{LCO}SS_2$	CO Ext %	EXERCISE MPH	GRADE	$\dot{V}_{O_2}$	$\dot{V}_E$	$D_{LCO}SS_3$
Predicted	4.3	3.2	1.6	5.9	65	4.1	130	7.40	42	25	97	21.7	52					24.0
Feb. 1959	2.5	3.2	2.4	4.9	21	0.5	32	7.46	45	30	94	8.7	30	1.5	FLAT	0.62	33	11.3
May 1961	3.1	3.4	2.4	5.5	18	0.3	16	7.38	35	20	94	9.1	31	1.5	FLAT	0.53	20	8.7
Nov. 1969	2.0	3.0	2.5	4.5	21	0.4	21					3.6	20	1.5	FLAT	0.48	19	5.4

In February, 1959, resting studies showed a diminution in vital capacity, a normal resting lung volume and considerable impairment of gas distribution. There is severe ventilatory disability as shown by the very low MMFR and low $FEV_{0.75} \times 40$. The resting diffusing capacity is decreased and this defect is confirmed by the low exercise figure. Mechanics studies showed a reduced compliance and a considerably increased airway resistance. Restudy two years later reveals that the vital capacity has improved, but inert-gas distribution is still grossly reduced. There has been a deterioration in ventilatory flow rates. Diffusion remains the same at rest, but is now even further reduced on exercise. These findings of severe derangement of function indicate that severe changes must be present not only in major bronchi but probably in bronchioles and in the lung parenchyma as well.

Eight years later there has been little further change in lung volumes and flow rates but the diffusing capacity has fallen markedly and rises very little with exercise. This again indicates severe parenchymal involvement. Pulmonary mechanics were restudied but unfortunately the condition of the patient precluded compliance measurements. The resistance was again quite high.

"Chemical" Bronchiectasis; Acute Exposure to Oxides of Sulfur

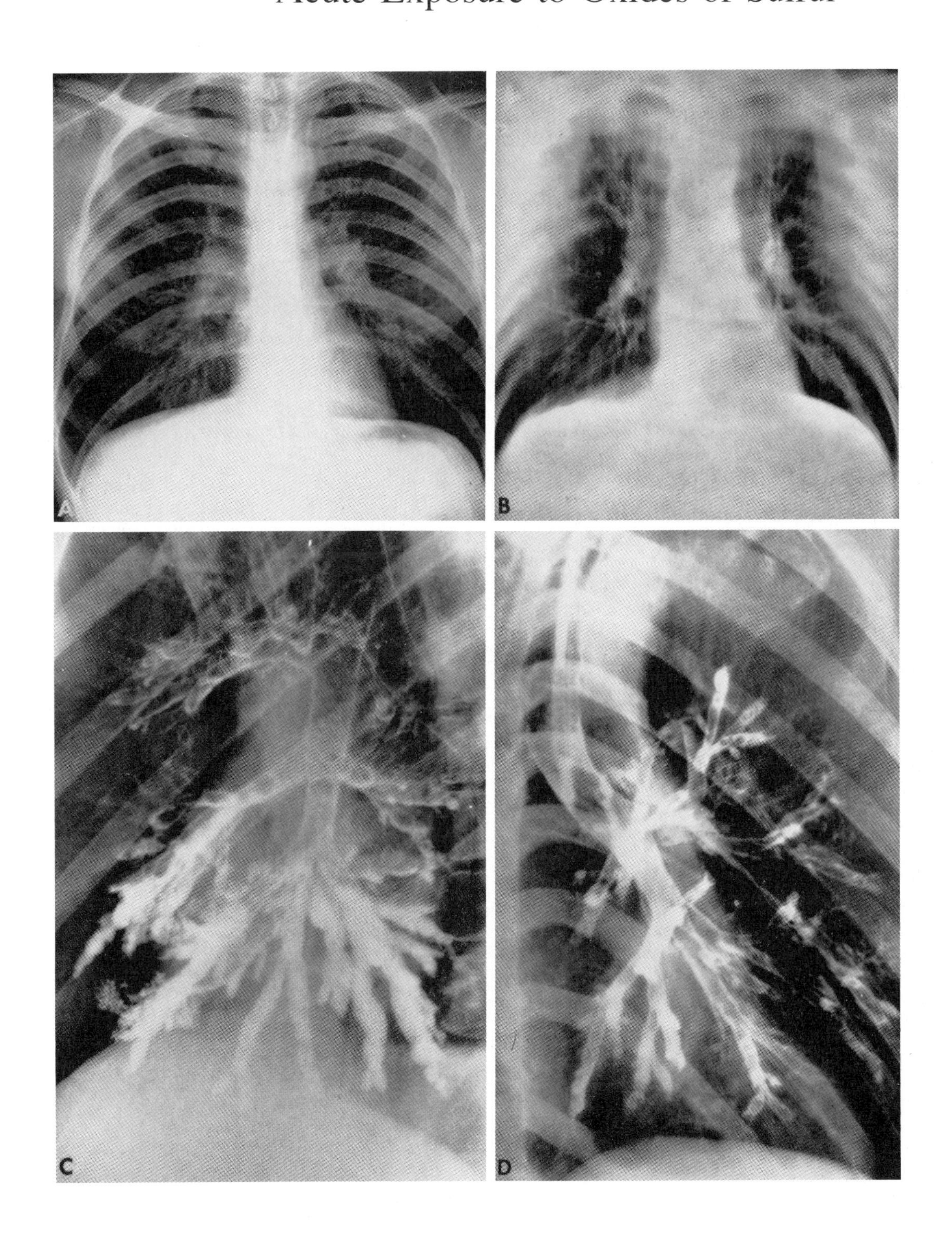

uniform dilatation and deformity of all segmental bronchi of both lungs. The bronchiectasis is varicose in type. The bronchi appear to end abruptly in rounded or bulbous extremities and there is little peripheral bronchiolar filling. In the absence of a history of pulmonary disease before the SO_2 exposure, it is to be presumed that this severe bronchial change has developed in the brief period of three months and that it is directly attributable to the toxic effects of the gas.

Summary. Severe lung destruction following accidental inhalation of oxides of sulphur. Pulmonary function defect was much more severe than was indicated on the plain x-ray, and bronchography revealed widespread and generalized bronchial damage. This case illustrates the importance of a careful assessment of function after exposure to corrosive gases.

---

areas in relation to lung disease. Even acute lung effects produced by inhalation of high concentrations of many of these gases are poorly documented and understood. Because no striking radiological changes, such as those that occur in silicosis, follow such episodes, general clinical recognition of permanent lung damage after inhalation of acute irritants has been long delayed. It is to be hoped that many of these deficiencies will be overcome as pulmonary function assessments become routine laboratory tools in most major hospital centers. The brevity of the following discussions does not indicate lack of importance of these entities, but reflects the paucity of relevant data.

Nitric acid, oxides of nitrogen, zinc chloride

In recent years it has been increasingly recognized that accidental exposure to oxides of nitrogen can occur in a wide variety of situations. Dangerous accumulations of NO and NO_2 can occur in agricultural silos, causing acute silage gassing,[1658] in enclosed mineshafts after detonation of explosives,[1659] in industrial processes requiring the handling of nitric acid,[1660] and in the slow combustion of nitrocellulose or plastics, as occurred in the Cleveland Clinic fire, in which x-ray films made of nitrocellulose burned slowly with little oxygen.[1661, 2097] Many observers have noted that there is often, perhaps invariably, a time interval of a few hours after exposure before symptoms develop.[1661]

Characteristically, after this interval, acute pulmonary edema, cyanosis, severe dyspnea, and radiological changes of widespread and patchy edema or bronchopneumonia develop, necessitating immediate oxygen administration and intravenous steroid therapy. When not immediately fatal, the acute episode may be followed by the development of bronchiolitis obliterans, which may cause death during the next few weeks[1658] or may lead to persistent abnormalities in air flow after the radiographic manifestations have completely cleared.[1659] Many of these patients will also be found to have a diffusion defect some weeks or months after the acute episode.[1662] It is of interest to note that Ogilvie and his colleagues, in their paper concerned with the development of the single-breath method of measuring diffusing capacity ($D_{L_{CO}}SB$), included two firemen (patients No. 14 and No. 15) who had been exposed to corrosive chemical fumes, one of whom showed very considerable diffusion impairment six weeks after the acute episode.[38] Tschumy has recorded a case of severe pulmonary change followed by recovery in a fireman who fought a fire in a fabrics and upholstery store.[1683] In addition to the papers quoted above, others have described typical cases or variations on the general pattern of clinical presentation.[1663–1667] It seems clear that, after a symptomless latent period of a few hours following inhalation, the clinical picture is one of acute pulmonary edema; the next stage, which may develop as the edema is subsiding, is one of intense bronchiolitis in which respiratory failure may necessitate respiratory care, and which often is fatal; and in the weeks following the episode either a progressive fibrosing obliterative bronchiolitis may develop[1666] as the main pathological change, or to this may be added a progressive interstitial pulmonary fibrosis.[1664] There seems little doubt that chronic pulmonary changes can occur in this condition,[1659,1662] though in some of the cases in which this has been claimed the evidence is incomplete and not wholly convincing.[1667] Cases 40 and 41 describe two patients we have seen with this condition.

A recent report of an episode involving 15 people, of whom 6 developed pulmonary edema, makes it clear that complete recovery with normal pulmonary function may occur.[3318]

The dangers of inhalation of smoke from smoke generators, usually zinc chloride, has been well documented; in one such case the smoke caused acute interstitial pulmonary fibrosis, the patient dying in respiratory failure 18 days after the acute episode.[2054]

Evaluation of pulmonary function in anyone known to have been exposed to any of these fumes is obviously an essential part of his clinical assessment, whether or not radiological appearances are normal. The pattern of function-test impairment varies from case to case, but it is clear from the literature that reduction of vital capacity, impaired air flow and increased airway resistance, abnormal inert-gas distribution, and a lowered diffusing capacity may all be encountered in variable degrees of severity. In some patients the arterial oxygen tension is lowered on exercise.[1662] Thus, a complete evaluation of such patients should include measurements of all of these parameters if a precise knowledge of the functional status of the lung is to be obtained.

There has recently been a series of studies on the effect of oxides of nitrogen, usually at concentrations of about 25 or 50 parts per million, on rats.[2733, 3317] These concentrations are very much higher than those occurring as a consequence of metropolitan automobile pollution, in episodes of which values of up to 0.80 parts per million have been recorded.[2704]

Ammonia, Oxides of Sulfur, Chlorine, Phosgene

All of these very corrosive gases will produce acute pulmonary edema if inhaled in a high enough concentration. When recovery occurs, there may be residual bronchial damage and considerable impairment of pulmonary function as a result, often with a deceptively normal-looking chest radiograph (a situation illustrated in Case 48). Lépine and Soucy have documented an example of considerable residual impairment of function in a patient who had inhaled ammonia and SO_3,[1662] and other similar cases have been described by Brille and her colleagues.[1668] There can be little doubt that inhalation of sublethal amounts of ammonia or SO_3 fumes can produce severe and irreversible lung damage involving the whole bronchial tree, and almost certainly resulting in alveolar damage. The inhalation of phosgene is characterized by a latent period of several hours before the development of pulmonary edema. It is not known definitely whether it causes residual lung damage. There is little doubt that residual chronic bronchitis appeared to be a sequel of inhalation of phosgene and chlorine during the 1914–1918 World War, though in many men this has appeared to run a benign course subsequently.[39]

The importance of sulfur dioxide as an air pollutant has led to considerable experimental work on the effects of this on the lung. It is mostly absorbed by the nose,[2718] but may be eliminated via the alveoli and so reach the lung parenchyma.[2717] In higher concentration (10 ppm) it stimulates the cough receptors[2569] and increases airway resistance via a reflex effect. If dust is present at the same time, the effect is potentiated.[2705] It can affect the surface activity of lung extracts.[3329] In episodes of air pollution, it may reach a concentration of 0.5 ppm,[2712] or exceptionally 1.0 ppm.[2726, 3325] Although respiratory symptoms can be correlated with levels of SO_2 in the general sense,[2710, 2715, 3365] it is far from established that the incidence of chronic respiratory disease is to be attributed to this particular chemical.

Kowitz and his colleagues[3330] have recently studied the effects of acute chlorine exposure on a group of 17 men accidentally exposed in 1961. On the basis of their findings, they conclude that initially, there was alveolar damage, followed by repair and by increasing airway resistance, finally with a decrease in lung volume and a persistently reduced diffusing capacity and pulmonary compliance. This paper contains an excellent review of all previous data on chlorine exposure.

Cadmium Oxide

It is not obvious whether this very irritant substance should be classified as a mineral dust or as an acutely irritant chemical vapor; several unusual features about its effects on the lung certainly justify its mention under a separate heading from other substances. Inhalation of the fumes of cadmium oxide may occur in a wide variety of industrial processes and, in addition, may be a danger to welders involved in cutting scrap metal that contains a high proportion of cadmium. Acutely, it causes severe pneumonitis with a mortality rate said to be at least 16 per cent.[33] Recovery from such an episode of acute bronchopneumonia may be very slow,[3333] but it seems likely that it may be complete, at least in some instances.[3334]

Chronically, inhalation of this substance seems not to cause chronic diffuse interstitial pneumonitis and fibrosis, but apparently it may give rise to parenchymal lung destruction or pulmonary emphysema. Lane and Campbell, who described the autopsy appearances in two cases, found a severe and unusual pattern of emphysema spreading out to the lung periphery; these lungs were found to contain 277 mg of cadmium/100 gm of fresh tissue.[1669] Experimental studies have demonstrated production of destructive lung lesions in guinea pigs after inhalation of cadmium.[1670] Bonnell described severe chronic lung disease and proteinuria in a group of cadmium workers,[1671] and one of his patients whom we saw had evidence of severe airway obstruction and moderate emphysema. Kazantzis has reported evidence of an increased incidence of emphysema, as judged by a ventilatory and gas-distribution index, in men exposed to alloys of cadmium.[2107] From this work and from Bonnell's careful survey of workers exposed to this substance, it seems clear that such occupations carry the risk of a high incidence of emphysema with associated bronchitis.[1671]

Ozone

Ozone is a very irritant and toxic gas, concentrations as low as 9 ppm (0.0009 per cent) producing acute pulmonary edema in animals and in human subjects. Exposure by inhalation or other surface contact occurs in industry in relation to argon-shielded welding; in acute smog episodes, in which ozone is formed by the effect of sunlight on hydrocarbons from automobile exhaust fumes, as in Los Angeles where the concentration may exceed 0.7 ppm for periods of an hour[1672, 3831]; and in certain closed-cabin environments, including high-altitude aircraft.[1673] Apart from its ability to cause pulmonary edema if breathed in high concentration, little is known of its effect on the lung.

Stokinger[2706] has reviewed the toxicology of ozone, and Jaffe[2703, 3337] has surveyed the literature up to 1968 on the adverse effects of ozone on men and animals.

Mendenhall and Stokinger suggested recently that ozone may interfere with the surface-active agent normally present in the lung,[2098] and they postulate that this inactivation may be the cause of atelectasis or even pulmonary edema consequent upon inhalation of ozone. We reported that a concentration of about 0.6 ppm breathed for two hours causes a 20 per cent fall in steady-state diffusing capacity in normal subjects, with very little associated fall in vital capacity or in air flow.[1679]

Kelly, Whiting, and Gill[3338] described an acute episode of poisoning with no sequelae in a 52-year-old man. Hallett[3336] found evidence of a fall in CO transfer and in FEV after 1.0 ppm of the gas had been inhaled for 30 minutes through a mouthpiece, and Goldsmith and Nadel reported that increases in airway resistance measured by body plethysmography were evident in some subjects after one hour's exposure to 0.4 ppm, and in all subjects after one hour of exposure to 1.0 ppm.[3339] In recent studies,[3830] we have found that a concentration of 0.7 ppm of ozone breathed for two hours while at rest without using a mouthpiece causes symptoms of upper respiratory tract irritation and just measurable changes in airway mechanics. The same concentration breathed during light exercise produces easily detectable changes. Experimental work on guinea pigs has shown that these animals have an increased sensitivity to histamine if they are pre-exposed to 0.5 ppm of ozone for two hours.

In Los Angeles, ozone levels have reached 0.8 parts per million over periods of half an hour in the middle of the day,[3831] and it is not clear why these concentrations have not been followed by overt symptoms that could be unequivocally attributed to the presence of the gas.[2731, 3366]

Much of the literature on lung changes in welders is confusing in that it is difficult to know what might be ascribable to ozone and what to the inhalation of the many oxidized dusts, including cadmium oxide, to which such men are exposed. Challen and his colleagues attributed to inhalation of ozone at a level of about 1.0 ppm the bronchitis suffered by workers in a tungsten-arc welding shop.[1678] In other studies, the clinical and pathological picture was less distinct.[1675–1677] We could find no evidence of pulmonary impairment in welders who were using the argon-shielded method in a shop where the ozone concentration appeared to be about 0.2 ppm.[1604] On the flight deck of modern jet airliners flying at 30,000 to 40,000 feet, the ozone concentration appears to be between 0.2 and 0.4 ppm.[1673, 1674]

GASOLINE VAPOR, KEROSENE, TURPENTINE, BENZENE, NAPHTHALENE

All of these compounds, when aspirated into the lungs, rapidly produce a severe degree of pulmonary edema, but there is considerable variation in the toxicity of their vapor. In particular, gasoline (petrol) vapor is very toxic,[2099] and it is claimed that symptoms may result from its inhalation in concentrations as low as 500 ppm.[1680] It is obvious that, with such substances, absorption across the lungs must be extremely rapid.

Kerosene, when inhaled, produces a pneumonitis; but it is far commoner for this substance to be accidentally drunk by children, and it is usually taught that it is relatively nontoxic in these circumstances, provided vomit is not aspirated. In spite of an extensive literature on clinical and experimental studies of kerosene toxicity,[2100–2105] there is still considerable doubt whether all of the pulmonary manifestations that occur after its ingestion into the stomach can be ascribed to aspiration into the lung. As a recent annotation has pointed out, pulmonary involvement seems to occur when neither vomiting nor gastric lavage has taken place.[2106]

The authors of a recent review of 200 cases of kerosene ingestion reported a mortality of 0.5 per cent, and they stress that gastric lavage is contraindicated.[3342] Experimentally, the administration of corticosteroids has no beneficial effect on this condition.[3343]

HAIR SPRAY

Pulmonary infiltration occurring in women who use large quantities of commercial hair spray was first reported from the USA in 1958.[2108] Apparently the ingredients of the sprays are secret, but it is known that they contain lanolin and many natural and synthetic resins, including dextran.

The first two cases, reported by Bergmann, Flance, and Blumenthal, were in women aged 27 and 22 years respectively; in one, chest x-rays showed bilateral hilar adenopathy and diffuse reticular infiltration, and a scalene-node biopsy revealed granulomatous change. The course of the disease was benign in both patients, with regression of the pulmonary process.[2108] A similar case of "thesaurosis" in a woman aged 26 was reported from England a year later; regression of the pulmonary lesions was slow.[2109] Pulmonary function tests were not reported in any of these three cases.

More recently, Bergmann and his colleagues have collected a further 12 cases, including three autopsies. Lung biopsy in three of their patients showed "interstitial fibrosis or pneumonia, with hyperplasia of alveolar lining cells and an accumulation of macrophages containing PAS-positive granules in their cytoplasm."[2110] Attempts to demonstrate polyvinylpyrolidone or related compounds in the lung tissue were unsuccessful. No cases were encountered in a survey of 505 hairdressers in England,[2352] suggesting that the condition is rare[2353] as judged by radiological criteria.

Discordant results continue to appear in the literature concerning this condition. Attempts to duplicate the syndrome in dogs were not successful.[3346] Individual sensitivity reactions have been reported in humans,[3347] and although in one study, low values for diffusing capacity were reported in 5 of 36 Italian hairdressers,[3345] Sharma and Williams[3344] studied 62 beauty parlor employees and 33 controls, and found no evidence of difference in lung volumes or single-breath diffusing capacity.

TOLUENE DI-ISOCYANATE

The toxicity of this irritant material, which is used in the manufacture of some plastics, has been recognized since 1955; Trenchard and Harris recently summarized its known pulmonary effects and reported 12 more cases of lung disease developing after its inhalation.[2111] They emphasize that the clinical manifestations are those of bronchitis and bronchospasm, and that the symptoms are likely to be ascribed to influenza or asthma. There seems little doubt that inhalation of this substance gives rise to a considerable degree of bronchial edema and bronchospasm.[3366] We have been unable to find detailed reports of pulmonary function tests in this syndrome; thus, the sensitivity of the bronchial tree to this chemical has yet to be accurately defined. There does not seem to be any evidence that this compound produces pulmonary fibrosis, but careful follow-up with pulmonary function evaluation of workers who have been exposed to it does not appear to have been undertaken.

Maxon has reviewed the literature on this condition,[3348] and studied 7 men exposed to toluene di-isocyanate. In most, the FEV_1 was reduced, and 5 of the men showed an improvement in this parameter at a second evaluation about three months later.

Aspiration pneumonia (Mendelson's syndrome)

Gardner has shown that minor degrees of food or liquid aspiration into the lungs postoperatively may be far commoner than is usually supposed.[1681] It has been known for many years that a small amount of water instilled into the lung disappears quickly without any after-effect; it is the rapid transfer of water into the blood, causing severe hemodilution, that accounts for the more rapid death of people drowned in fresh than in salt water. Aspiration of food into the trachea may cause death from foreign-body obstruction of a bronchus. The development of bronchiectasis in the presence of a pharyngeal esophageal pouch is often ascribed to repeated aspiration of small amounts of foreign material.

Much more common, however, is the aspiration of vomited stomach contents. This is much more serious, since the aspirated matter may be very acid, and inhalation of such fluid causes an intense chemical pneumonia very similar to that produced by other acid and corrosive substances. Such episodes may occur after severe trauma or burns, after spontaneous or induced convulsions, after intoxication with alcohol, during emergency anesthesia and during the postoperative period, in association with bulbar paralysis, and in other disease states.[3351] There is characteristically a latent period between such aspiration and the beginning of respiratory distress. An hour or so after aspiration, the respiratory rate increases, and a few—often deceptively few—rales may be heard over the lungs. X-ray examination reveals more extensive changes than the physical examination would suggest, involving both lungs and resembling patchy pulmonary edema. This edema is the response of the lung to the inhaled hydrochloric acid. In patients whose lungs are extensively involved, cyanosis develops, initially with a normal or low arterial CO_2 tension. However, as the patient becomes weaker, respiration begins to fail, the arterial P_{CO_2} rises, and death occurs in respiratory failure.

Management of these problems requires intravenous administration of steroids immediately the diagnosis is made;[3367] treatment with continuous oxygen by mask; careful observation of arterial P_{CO_2}; early tracheostomy in any patient with extensive lung involvement; and management as a case of respiratory failure, with assisted ventilation before secondary circulatory effects become clinically obvious. Saline lavage of the bronchial tree has been shown to be particularly effective in the treatment of animals into whose bronchial tree gastric contents have been introduced and of patients who have inhaled vomitus.[1713] Not all such patients require tracheostomy, and relatively few need respiratory assistance, but the physician must have the sequence of decisions clearly in his mind if he is to take the right steps early enough. Usually there is a latent period of two or three hours between aspiration and the development of symptoms. By that time it may be too late for bronchoscopy and lavage to be effective, and it should not be attempted then. When aspiration occurs under anesthesia, however, this procedure is obviously indicated at once, with removal of as much material as possible with the least possible delay; three hours later, such instrumentation may be too hazardous.

TRACE ELEMENTS IN THE LUNG

Although they normally occur in the lung only in minute quantities, measurable amounts of antimony, arsenic, cadmium, mercury, manganese, and zinc are found in human lungs. Molokhia and Smith[3360] and Tipton and Shafer[2716] have reported these values. The latter study made comparisons between lungs from nine U.S. cities and found, for example, a higher concentration of nickel in the lungs of residents of Seattle than of the other eight cities.

These studies are important in providing baselines for comparison between rural and urban populations and for providing an opportunity for lung analyses to be made in populations close to major industrial complexes dealing with these metals.

RADIATION PNEUMONITIS

Pathology and incidence

The reported incidence of pulmonary lesions developing after irradiation therapy shows a remarkably wide range,[1385] but it seems likely that a transient pneumonitis may commonly occur. For example, Warren and Spencer,[1386] in an autopsy study, found this condition in 12 per cent of 234 patients whose lungs had been thus exposed. In our experience, severe and irreversible pulmonary fibrosis after radiation therapy is seen infrequently; nevertheless, the syndrome deserves careful consideration.[1380]

In the acute phase after irradiation,[1387] the findings are those of severe pulmonary congestion, edema, lymphangiectasis,[1388] and hyaline membrane formation. It has been suggested that the first effect of radiation may be a consequence of interference with surface-active material in the lung, though this has yet to be established with certainty.[2112] There is desquamation of the alveolar lining cells, and necrosis of the bronchial and bronchiolar epithelium may occur.[3355] Thrombosis of the pulmonary vessels may be seen,[1389] and the picture may be confused by superimposed infection.

In the chronic phase,[1390] the overlying chest wall may show induration and the pulmonary changes may follow an identical geographical distribution without regard to lobar or segmental divisions. Pleural thickening and adhesions are often described, but may not be as common as is generally supposed.[1391] The affected lung becomes small and firm, and the mediastinum may be shifted to the involved side, with elevation of the diaphragm. The intercostal spaces may be narrowed and the spine curved toward the side of the lesion. Although the lung structure is often relatively intact, a dense interstitial fibrosis develops, clumps of elastic fibers being visible in the interstitial tissue. The alveolar lining cells undergo considerable change and appear cuboidal in form. Squamous metaplasia of the bronchi and bronchioles may be seen.[1392] The capillaries and pulmonary vessels are hyalinized and thickened, and the arterioles may be markedly narrowed.[1389, 3355]

Cor pulmonale occurs if the process is extensive enough;[2228] in some patients it may be difficult to determine whether this is the result of pulmonary parenchymal changes or whether it has been occasioned by involvement of the pulmonary veins in mediastinal fibrosis, which is a prominent feature in some cases.[1390, 1393] The factors controlling the occurrence, the extent, and particularly the resolution of radiation pneumonitis have not been satisfactorily delineated. In many instances it is presumed that the state of the lung before exposure to radiation may have been an important factor.[1394]

Acute irradiation pneumonitis is shown radiologically by consolidation of lung parenchyma and concomitant loss of volume. The appearances of an "air bronchogram" are characteristically seen at this stage. The subsequent course is one of progressive shrinkage of the lung, followed by distortion of adjacent structures. (*See* Case 47.)

Pulmonary function

The changes in pulmonary function that have been shown to result from radiation damage to the lung are those one would predict from the pathological changes described. Most observers have noted that pulmonary symptoms, usually an irritative cough and dyspnea,[1380] occur between 3 and 16 weeks after cessation of radiotherapy.[2340, 3353] Whitfield, Bond, and Arnott noted some reduction in maximal breathing capacity, vital capacity, and total lung capacity in all of the nine patients in whom the measurements were made, radiotherapy having been given for breast cancer in all cases. In one of their patients the arterial oxygen saturation was noted to fall to 83.3 per cent on exercise from a normal value at rest.[1380]

In an experimental study in dogs exposed to variable amounts of irradiation, Sweany and his co-workers showed that pulmonary compliance and diffusing capacity fell together in the period after exposure, the former from control values of 0.056 to 0.045 liter/cm H_2O, and the diffusing capacity from control values of about 4.5 to about 2.5 ml CO/min/mm Hg 130 days after irradiation.[1381] These observations were closely correlated with the finding of diffuse pulmonary fibrosis in the lungs of three of the animals examined more than 172 days after exposure.

Clinically the picture is often somewhat less clear-cut, since frequently there is preexistent intrathoracic disease or the radiation is applied unilaterally (*see* Case 47). However, Emirgil and Heinemann demonstrated a similar course of events in 15 patients they studied.[463] These patients sometimes develop arterial unsaturation on exercise,[1382] presumably attributable to a shunt of blood through almost totally destroyed lung. Some clinical reports have included no data on pulmonary function tests[1383] and in others the methods used were so indirect as to result in misleading conclusions, since, if only ventilatory function tests are employed, it is certain that only gross disturbances will be demonstrable.[1384] Measurements of compliance and diffusing capacity are clearly obligatory if minor changes in function are sought or if any complete evaluation of the cause of dyspnea is attempted.[2340] There is little doubt that a lowering of diffusing capacity is the most characteristic finding.[3377]

Hoffbrand, Gillam, and Heaf[3354] have studied the effect of pre-existent chronic bronchitis on the pattern of pulmonary function change after irradiation in a carefully controlled investigation. They concluded that there was no evidence that in patients with chronic bronchitis, irradiation is followed by deterioration of the bronchitis, nor do they show any greater tendency to develop functional changes of radiation fibrosis or pneumonitis. They observed a fall in steady-state $D_{L_{CO}}$ in most patients ten weeks after the end of irradiation treatment.

SUMMARY

This necessarily brief review of knowledge of the effects of inhaled substances on the lung leads, we feel, to the conclusion that the application of detailed studies of pulmonary function to the study of lung disease in industry will prove to be of major importance. The clarification of the symptomatology of byssinosis, employing only the simplest ventilatory tests, provides a remarkable, and almost a pioneer, application of such methods to the study of lung disease. There is an obvious need for much more general application of such methods to many industrial problems, and no one should feel any complacency about the present status of this field; all too often no use has been made of contemporary methods of study, involving gas tension, compliance, and diffusing-capacity measurement. It should be obvious that, *without* objective measurement of the extent to which lung function has been impaired, *no complete opinion can be given of the effects of any inhaled substance.* Illustrative case presentations in this chapter serve to document this viewpoint.

It is important to recognize also that we are still without any data on the effect on the lung of very low concentrations of known irritants over long periods of time. Such information is obviously needed, especially for cases of exposure to SO_3, ozone, cadmium oxide, and oxides of nitrogen.

It is perhaps worth pointing out that, once it has been shown—as we believe it has been—that asbestosis may seriously impair pulmonary function *without radiological change,* a fundamental alteration must occur in the *clinical* approach the physician should adopt to this condition. A similar statement may be made about farmer's lung, since it has been clearly shown that radiological clearing may occur even when considerable pulmonary damage persists.

The future application of pulmonary function tests to every kind of industrial pulmonary problem will of itself justify the considerable effort that has gone into a better understanding of these methods of study.

INVOLVEMENT OF THE LUNG IN PRIMARY AND SECONDARY MALIGNANT DISEASE

CHAPTER 18

INTRODUCTION

Pulmonary function tests can aid little in the diagnosis of primary bronchial carcinoma and are of importance in this disease only in relation to assessment of operative risk and probable postoperative function. It is therefore reasonable that this chapter should be brief.

When the lung is diffusely infiltrated by malignant disease, estimates of pulmonary function serve little practical purpose, although they may illustrate further the general relationship between structural change and functional disturbance.

PRIMARY BRONCHIAL CARCINOMA

EFFECT ON LUNG FUNCTION

It is obvious that a small carcinoma situated at the periphery of the lung will produce no impairment of function. Partial occlusion of a major bronchus causes a delay in inert-gas mixing as an early effect; thereafter the main consequences are a limitation of ventilatory capability, with progressive loss of diffusing capacity as the effective lung surface area that can be ventilated becomes reduced.

USE OF FUNCTION TESTS IN ESTIMATING OPERATIVE RISK AND PROBABLE RESIDUAL FUNCTION

In elderly patients, it is often of importance to assess pulmonary function before resectional surgery is undertaken to estimate the likely postoperative disability. It is often erroneously thought that tests of total function are of little value when the lesion is in one lung only and that bronchospirometry in such cases is the only type of study that can yield useful information. When one main bronchus is partially occluded by carcinoma, it is of little value to know that most of the resting oxygen uptake is from the uninvaded areas; in fact, the information usually required is whether the lung tissue that will be left behind is functioning normally or is significantly deranged by emphysematous changes. In our experience, which is similar to that recorded by Rossier,[2255] tests of total pulmonary function may be very useful in such a situation, provided that the physician reporting them has an accurate knowledge of the extent and situation of the carcinoma and of the extent of lobar collapse resulting from bronchial obstruction. Only then can he properly assess the significance of estimates of ventilatory capability and diffusing capacity on the basis of the volume of lung not affected by carcinoma. Not infrequently he will find that total function preoperatively in a patient with a bronchial carcinoma producing collapse of one lobe is worse than in a patient of similar age who has had a pneumonectomy. This finding may, we feel, be fairly confidently interpreted to indicate that the unaffected lung is almost certainly structurally abnormal. Bronchospirometry may reveal a lowered oxygen uptake on the affected side, even in the presence of a normal ventilation.[3375] In one recent series of 118 patients, a low FEV in 15 per cent of operable cases was considered to contraindicate surgical treatment.[3378] Alterations in mechanics of breathing appear to be independent of the site of the carcinoma.[3376] The results obtained must be discussed by the surgeon, the physician, and the radiologist. In some patients, after consideration in relation to radiological findings and bronchoscopic appearance, they will permit a confident statement to be made concerning the probable integrity of the lung tissue it is proposed to leave behind. Not infrequently, demonstrated impairment of function may indicate the advisability of attempting a lobectomy rather than a pneumonectomy. Occasionally function is so poor that any type of resectional surgery may appear too hazardous. In our opinion, there can be little doubt that methods of studying involving radioactive isotopes will play a major part in this kind of evaluation.[2317]

It is important to stress that the information the surgeon needs is knowledge of the structural integrity of the lung upon which the patient will be dependent postoperatively. An idea of this can sometimes be gained by a study of the effect of occlusion of the pulmonary artery to the affected side,[208] but too few data exist for an opinion to be given of the usefulness of such an evaluation. It seems very possible that studies of xenon clearance from the "normal" lung may provide a better indicator of its normality than any other method of investigation.[735, 1684, 2317]

SECONDARY CARCINOMA OF THE LUNG

Metastatic deposits of carcinoma in the lung produce only such changes in pulmonary function as are consequent upon replacement of alveolar tissue by solid tumors. Reduction in total capacity and vital capacity, little interference with inert-gas mixing or ventilatory capability, and a level of pulmonary diffusion that may be well preserved until lung involvement is gross have been features of the patients we have studied. This nearly normal condition should be contrasted with the considerable interference in pulmonary diffusion that is often an early feature of lymphangitic carcinoma of the lung or of the general involvement that develops consequent upon leukemic infiltration. As they contribute nothing to differential diagnosis, and as operative intervention is not usually undertaken, pulmonary function tests are of little importance in patients with secondary carcinoma in the lung.

In the few cases of tumor embolization studied with function tests, findings similar to those in primary pulmonary hypertension have been noted.[3380] In one patient with endometrial choriocarcinoma, a low D_{Lco} was observed.[3379]

LYMPHANGITIC CARCINOMA OF THE LUNG

Harold, in an excellent review of this condition, collected data on 178 reported cases in which the lungs had been involved by extensive spread of malignant cells through the lymphatic system.[1685] Common primary sites were stomach, breast, bronchus, pancreas and prostate. The pleural surface of the lung may reveal the network of lymphatics filled with neoplastic cells, and a reticular pattern on the chest radiograph may indicate the diagnosis. Both Harold[1685] and Hauser and Steer,[1686] who also reviewed this condition, stress that these patients may suffer a significant degree of dyspnea before the radiograph depicts abnormality; yet we have been unable to trace reports of pulmonary function in this condition in which diffusing capacity and, more particularly, pulmonary compliance have been measured. In one of our own patients a considerable loss of steady-state diffusing capacity was the only abnormal finding before radiographic appearances became abnormal, but no measurements of lung mechanics were made and postmortem examination was not permitted. Since the pulmonary compliance is affected early in mitral stenosis, in which pulmonary lymphatics are engorged by edema to produce the Kerley lines on the radiograph, it is likely that loss of pulmonary compliance is an early feature of lymphangitic carcinoma of the lung; and since all observers are agreed that severe dyspnea can antedate the radiological changes, it is possible that loss of pulmonary compliance with perhaps a reduction in diffusing capacity may account for this symptom. In any event, such a hypothesis may be tentatively advanced until evidence is produced that refutes it.

Since this condition is untreatable at the present time, the value of any test is somewhat limited. However, tests of function may be useful occasionally, as they were in one case we were asked to study. The patient complained of dyspnea but his chest x-ray was normal, and he was considered to be suffering from anxiety symptoms. The finding of a low diffusing capacity altered this outlook, however, and one month later the characteristic radiographic picture of lymphangitic carcinoma of the lung was present. In patients who have had radiation therapy after radical mastectomy for breast cancer, the measurement of pulmonary function may be of assistance occasionally to differentiate between lymphangitic carcinoma and interstitial pneumonitis due to irradiation.

ALVEOLAR-CELL CARCINOMA OF THE LUNG

Very few reports of this condition have included any estimate of pulmonary function, and none has been detailed. We have studied several patients who were later shown to be suffering from disseminated alveolar-cell carcinoma, and in general the degree of functional impairment reflected the extent of lung tissue replaced by carcinoma. In one patient, although most of one lobe was affected, pulmonary function was little disturbed. A second, in whom both lungs were involved, had loss of lung volume with remarkable preservation of ventilatory function until a late stage in the disease. In Case 50, at the time when the patient was first seen, there was considerable radiological change and a lowered arterial oxygen saturation.

One case of this condition associated with dermatomyositis has been reported.[3369]

LEUKEMIA AND HODGKIN'S DISEASE

It has been clearly established that there may be extensive infiltration by leukemic cells of the alveolar capillary surface in myelogenous[1687] and chronic lymphatic[1688] leukemia. Recent evidence has suggested that this may be rather more common than is often supposed,[3370] and Green and Nichols found leukemic infiltration of the lung in 27 per cent of 109 leukemia patients examined at autopsy;[1689] they concluded that this had been of clinical significance in about 7 per cent of the total. Resnick and his colleagues have clearly documented the diffusion defect to which this infiltration may give rise.[1687] Such evidence suggests that the complaint of dyspnea in a patient known to have leukemia should be an indication for performance of pulmonary function tests, although it must be admitted that, when extensive pulmonary infiltration has occurred, the prognosis is very poor.

Hodgkin's disease may cause partial bronchial obstruction by mediastinal lymphadenopathy but seldom, if ever, invades the alveoli. Rarely, large tumor masses may appear in the lung parenchyma in this condition; the extent of pulmonary function impairment

(Text continued on page 408.)

Case 49
Eosinophilic Granuloma

Summary of Clinical Findings. This 17-year-old high school student was first admitted to hospital on January 14, 1965, complaining of shortness of breath. This symptom had been present for two years, gradually increasing in severity until by admission he could walk no further than two city blocks or climb more than one flight of stairs without dyspnea. He developed a cough during the same period which was occasionally productive of small amounts of yellow sputum. He smoked about five cigarettes a day for a year before the onset of symptoms, but not since. There was no history of chest infections or tuberculosis. There had been no undue exposure to dusts or fumes. On enquiry he admitted that he urinated three or four times during the night and drank large quantities of fluid.

Examination revealed a well-developed, well-nourished boy in no distress. Vital signs were normal; there was no cyanosis. The head and neck were normal and visual fields full. The chest moved easily and symmetrically. Breath sounds were clear but fine inspiratory rales could be heard over both lung fields. There were no other significant findings.

Urinalysis revealed a specific gravity of 1.003, but was otherwise negative. Hemoglobin was 16.7 gm per 100 ml; hematocrit was 48; white blood count was 7700 with a normal differential. BUN was 8.5 mgm per 100 ml; AC and PC blood sugars were 79 and 73 mgm per 100 ml respectively. Electrophoresis showed an increase in the alpha globulins. Chest x-rays and pulmonary function studies are shown below. The patient was noted to have a daily urine output of 6000 cc with an average daily intake of 7000 cc. He did not concentrate his urine after a water-fast, but following the use of vasopressin nasal spray the urine osmolarity rose to twice that of the serum. A lung biopsy was performed. The patient was discharged and 60 mgm of prednisone daily was prescribed. This was gradually tapered at home and discontinued in May, 1965.

He was readmitted in September, 1965, for assessment. His symptoms had not progressed. Pulmonary function studies are shown.

Radiology. A postero-anterior roentgenogram (*A*) shows diffuse involvement of both lungs by a rather coarse reticular pattern affecting predominantly lower lung zones. There is no hilar involvement. The reticular pattern is seen to better advantage in a magnified view (*B*) of the lower portion of the left lung.

Pathology. The biopsy showed a massive cellular infiltration, particularly pronounced in the centrilobular regions. The infiltrate was pleomorphic, consisting dominantly of lymphocytes and large histiocytes with much eosinophilic cytoplasm. While not classic, the histological features are considered diagnostic of eosinophilic granuloma of the lung.

															EXERCISE			
	VC	FRC	RV	TLC	ME %	MMFR	$FEV_{0.75}$ ×40	pH^+	Pco_2	HCO_3	Po_2	O_2Hb %	$D_{Lco}SS_2$	CO Ext %	GRADE	$\dot{V}O_2$	$\dot{V}_E$	$D_{Lco}SS_3$
Predicted	4.6	3.2	1.4	6.0	70	4.5	145						24.5	55				37.6
Jan. 1965	2.1	2.9	2.3	4.4	30	0.87	37	43	41	22.5	59	90	6.5	23		1.1	28.8	11.1
Sept. 1965	2.1	2.6	2.0	4.1	32	0.84	46		37	23.5		93	7.5	27				

In January, 1965, although the vital capacity and TLC were reduced, the residual volume was high. Flow rates were low and the diffusing capacity was extremely reduced and rose very little with exercise. He was moderately hypoxemic. In September, although subjectively improved, there was little change in function. Po_2 was not measured on the second occasion but O_2 saturation had increased slightly.

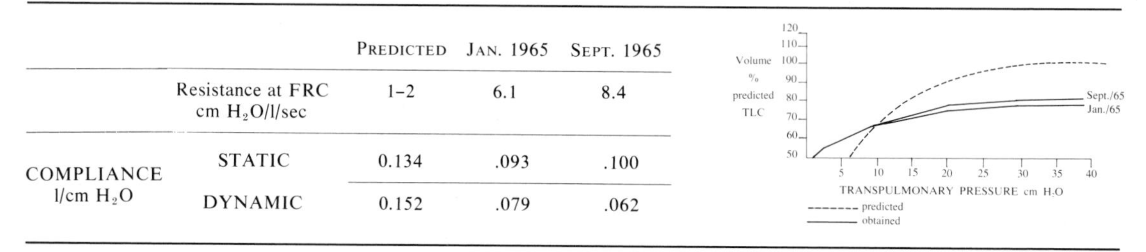

		Predicted	Jan. 1965	Sept. 1965
	Resistance at FRC cm H_2O/l/sec	1–2	6.1	8.4
COMPLIANCE l/cm H_2O	STATIC	0.134	.093	.100
	DYNAMIC	0.152	.079	.062

In January, 1965, studies of lung mechanics showed evidence of very stiff lungs and increased airway resistance. There had been very little change by September.

Eosinophilic Granuloma

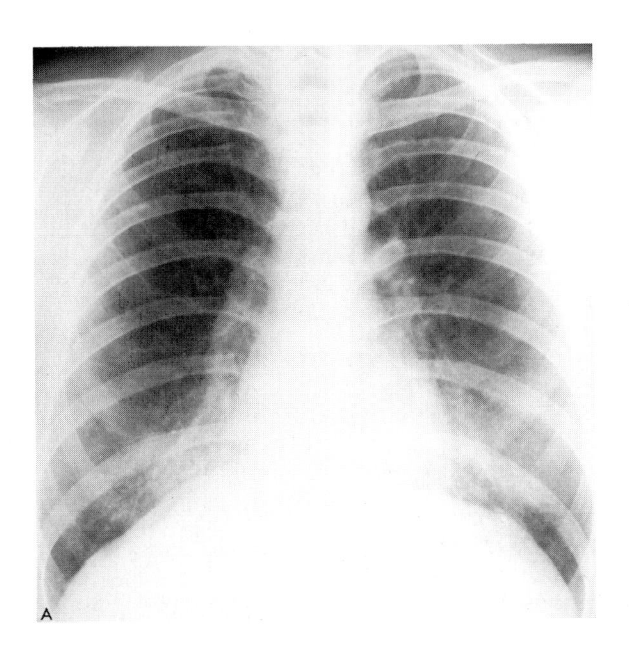

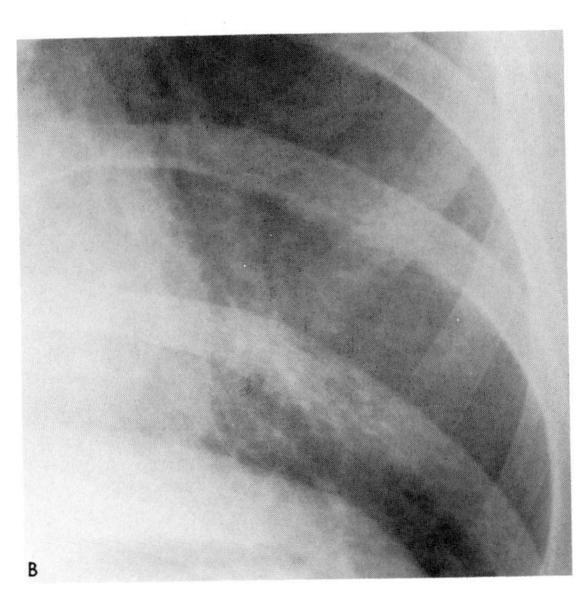

Summary. This young man had considerable disability and extensive pulmonary involvement as a result of eosinophilic granuloma. An unusual feature was the considerable increase in airway resistance that was measured, together with the evidence from the lung biopsy that there was extensive cellular infiltration around the bronchioles.

Case 50
Alveolar Cell Carcinoma

Summary of Clinical Findings. This 74-year-old retired accountant was admitted to hospital, complaining of shortness of breath in April, 1964. He had undergone a cholecystectomy in 1959 and at that time admitted to mild breathlessness upon brisk walking. A chest x-ray showed heavy linear markings at both bases. He had had a cough productive of small amounts of white sputum for many years and smoked 12 cigarettes a day. Following this hospitalization, his symptoms remained unchanged. In January, 1964, he noticed that the dyspnea was increasing and by admission in April he was breathless even with talking. In the two weeks prior to admission he became orthopneic, requiring two pillows to sleep. His sputum had increased slightly but there had never been hemoptysis. He had recently lost 10 lbs.

On examination he was a slightly cyanotic, thin, elderly male; his blood pressure was 110/60; pulse rate was 74/min and regular. There was no adenopathy. The chest moved poorly, but air entry was good. Medium rales could be heard throughout both lung fields. The liver was enlarged two finger-breadths below the costal margin. There were no other abnormal findings.

Urinalysis and hemogram were normal. Sputum grew normal flora on culture, and sputum cytology was repeatedly negative. Smears and cultures of sputum for tubercle bacilli and fungi were negative. The OT was 1:1000 and positive, but fungal skin tests were negative. Chest x-rays and pulmonary function studies are described.

The patient deteriorated rapidly in hospital. He became increasingly dyspneic and cyanotic even with O_2 administration. His sputum increased in quantity and was described as yellow and purulent. He died on May 23.

Radiology. The postero-anterior roentgenogram revealed widespread involvement of both lungs which consists of a mixed pattern of nodular shadows up to 3 mm in diameter, larger nodules 6 or 7 mm in diameter (representing acinar shadows), and coarse linear strands, seen particularly in the right upper zone (representing lymphangitic spread). Each of these patterns is common in diffuse broncho-alveolar carcinoma.

Pathology. Nodules of alveolar cell carcinoma, many with abscess formation, were scattered throughout both lungs. There were metastases in the pancreas. There was some emphysema, particularly in the upper lobes.

Summary. Widespread dissemination of alveolar cell carcinoma was associated with severe dyspnea and a low oxygen saturation and diffusing capacity. The vital capacity was reduced but the lung compliance could not be measured.

	VC	FRC	RV	TLC	ME %	MMFR	$FEV_{0.75}$ ×40	pH^+	P_{CO_2}	HCO_3	P_{O_2}	O_2Hb %	$D_{L_{CO}}SS_2$	CO Ext %
Predicted	3.8	3.7	2.5	6.3	45	2.7	79	7.40	40	25	80	97	11.3	36
April 15, 1964	2.3	3.0	2.0	4.3	38	2.2	62	7.47	38	26		77	6.9	20
May 11, 1964						1.7	63						8.4	33
May 22, 1964								7.39	41			46		

On admission in April, there was a decrease in vital capacity, but other subdivisions of lung volume were within normal limits. The diffusing capacity was low and oxygen saturation reduced. On the day prior to the patient's death, the oxygen saturation had fallen to an extremely low value although there was no hypercapnea.

Case 50

Alveolar Cell Carcinoma

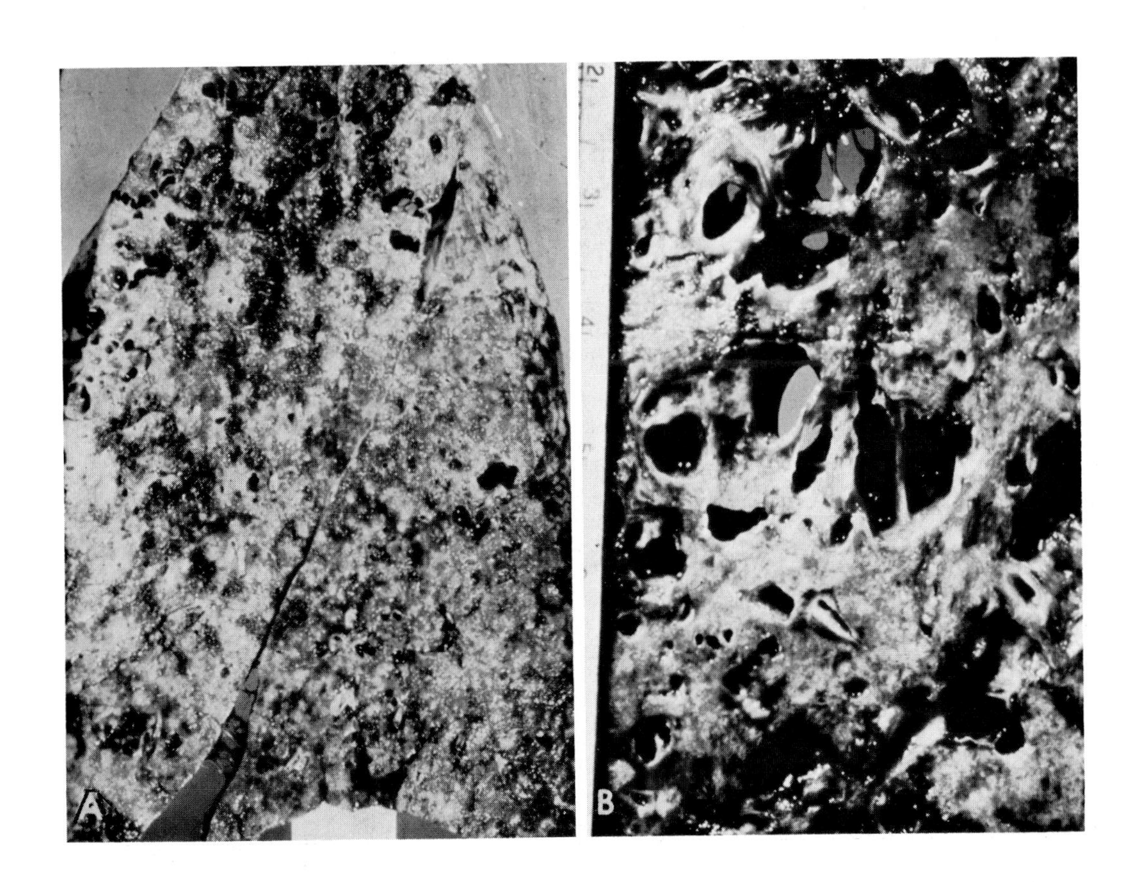

they cause depends upon the volume of lung tissue they replace.

EOSINOPHILIC GRANULOMA OF THE LUNG (HISTIOCYTOSIS X)

Eosinophilic granuloma may occur as a pulmonary manifestation[1692] of Hand-Schüller-Christian disease[1047, 1693–1695] or of Letterer-Siwe's disease,[1696] or may develop in association with eosinophilic granuloma of bone.[1047, 1695] More commonly, however, the disease is limited to the lungs, in which it often runs a relatively benign course.[1690, 1691, 1697] It is not clear whether it should be regarded as inflammatory or neoplastic, nor does it appear to be definitely classifiable as a "storage" disease. Knudson, Badger, and Gaensler have recently contributed a careful review of this condition, finding 75 cases in the literature to 1966.[3368]

Knowledge of the morphology of the lung changes is still incomplete, since most cases at an early stage of the disease have been studied on the basis of small biopsy specimens only. Gross examination of the lung shows widespread nodularity or granularity, and air-containing cysts may be visible. Nodules a few millimeters in diameter may be seen in the biopsy specimen. They consist of aggregates of cells with large vesicular nuclei, prominent nucleoli and abundant pale eosinophilic cytoplasm, which is occasionally finely vacuolated; these are the histiocytic components of eosinophilic granuloma, and they may form large multinucleate giant cells. Scattered through the histiocytes are variable numbers of eosinophils. Variable degrees of fibrosis are found at the margins. Later, fibrosis comes to dominate the picture, together with the development of numerous cysts of variable size, producing a pathological picture sometimes referred to as "honeycomb lung."[1046, 1047] Histiocytes are usually still visible in the walls of the spaces, but eosinophilic infiltration is often minimal or absent. The end stage may be entirely nonspecific. The exact mechanism of cyst formation is not understood, but evacuation of granulomata,[1692] bronchial obstruction[1696] and weakening of the bronchiolar walls[1046] have all been postulated as factors. Occasionally, involvement of blood vessels may occur early in the disease,[3372] and bronchiolar involvement may be an early feature in some patients. (*See* Case 49.)

The radiological picture may be indistinguishable from that in other types of diffuse interstitial fibrosis, though usually the opacities are more nodular than in the Hamman-Rich syndrome. Associated cystic change may suggest the presence of eosinophilic granuloma, but these changes are rarely definite enough for a firm diagnosis to be made on the radiological appearances.

Clinically, the diagnosis may be suggested by the finding of an associated bone lesion, or by the coexistence of pulmonary change and diabetes insipidus—a combination that should always suggest this diagnosis.[1047] The presence of cysts leads to an increased risk of spontaneous pneumothorax, which in these patients may be a dangerous complication. Several clinical reports on these cases have stressed the production of mucoid sputum as a notable symptom;[1698] and all of the patients we have seen have had this clinical feature, perhaps as a consequence of bronchial-wall involvement.

The reported results of pulmonary function studies in this condition fit well with the general pattern of pulmonary pathology just outlined. In the early stages, both maximal ventilatory ability and vital capacity may be normal,[3368] and there is no dyspnea.[1698] There is little interference initially with pulmonary compliance, and quite considerable radiological change may be visible before there is any alteration in pulmonary diffusion capacity.[1700] As more fibrosis develops, the lung volume becomes reduced[3368] though only rarely is this as conspicuous a feature as in the Hamman-Rich syndrome. Later, considerable defects in diffusing capacity are found, with an increase in the alveolar–arterial oxygen difference.[1700, 3368, 3371, 3373, 3374] If, at this stage, there is still little impairment of air flow, the arterial P_{CO_2} level may be reduced, and ventilation on exercise becomes excessive in relation to oxygen uptake. In addition to the references quoted above, others[1701–1703] attest the generally benign course of this disease, which may change little over the course of years, and often the patients continue with little dyspnea in spite of considerable change apparent radiologically.

In any patient in whom there is relatively good function despite obvious radiological change, the physician should suspect eosinophilic granuloma to be the diagnosis. This is not to suggest that pulmonary function may not become severely deranged, but it is generally true that relatively good function with considerable radiological change occurs more commonly in this condition than in the Hamman-Rich syndrome. The reason for this lies in the fact that generalized alveolar-wall change is not a feature of the pathology in eosinophilic granuloma, and authors have stressed the relative normality of the intervening walls in early cases.[1690]

Pulmonary function tests may be useful in following the progress of patients with this condition.[3368] If mucoid sputum is constantly present, the physician may be hesitant to advise long-term steroid therapy unless a progressive decline in pulmonary function has been documented. In one such case, steroids were shown to produce an objective improvement in function.[1700] Some other cases reach a static, "burnt-out" state in which no further deterioration of function occurs and therapy results in no improvement.

PULMONARY FUNCTION IN PULMONARY TUBERCULOSIS AND IN HISTOPLASMOSIS

CHAPTER
19

PULMONARY TUBERCULOSIS

INTRODUCTION

So much can be written on the epidemiology, pathology, radiology, diagnosis, and treatment of pulmonary tuberculosis that this subject occupies about one fifth of most volumes on lung disease. In most civilized countries the mortality rate from this disease has been decreasing since the end of the nineteenth century, and the introduction of effective chemotherapy hastened its decline as a major cause of death in all except primitive areas or in countries where control and supervision are difficult to maintain.

In regard to evaluation of pulmonary function, however, there is relatively little to be said. It is only in advanced cases in which surgery is considered that a careful assessment of pulmonary function is obligatory.[2217] Such problems, fortunately, are becoming progressively less common. In this section are summarized various aspects of pulmonary function in this disease, but no attempt has been made to deal with the many aspects of the pathogenesis or of the radiological changes of intrathoracic tuberculosis, which can be found in any standard text on the subject. Bromberg and Robin have contributed a useful review of pulmonary function in tuberculosis.[2215]

ACUTE PULMONARY TUBERCULOSIS

Acute miliary tuberculosis

McClement and his colleagues documented the sudden, severe fall in arterial oxygen tension and widening of the arterial–alveolar gradient that may be found in patients with acute miliary tuberculosis.[1704] Rossier and his co-workers reported detailed function tests in a 40-year-old man with subacute miliary tuberculosis, in whom an alveolar–arterial oxygen difference of 38 mm Hg was found[17] (normally in their laboratory this is 5 to 8 mm Hg). We have been able to study only one patient with acute miliary tuberculosis, a 17-year-old girl. The steady-state CO diffusing capacity was only 5.2 ml CO/min/mm Hg at rest when she was acutely ill; after one week's chemotherapy it was only 6.9 ml; and several months later, when radiological resolution was complete, it was still only one-half the normal value, being 8.5 ml at rest and 13.5 ml/CO/min mm Hg while the patient was walking at 3 mph. The rapid respiratory rate exhibited by these patients almost certainly indicates a considerable decrease in pulmonary compliance during the acute stage of the disease, but we are unaware of any measurements of this. Presumably the effect of acute miliary tuberculosis is to lower the lung volume, reduce compliance and interfere with gas diffusion.

Acute nonmiliary pulmonary tuberculosis

Very few studies have reported the effect on pulmonary function of the treatment of acute pulmonary tuberculosis. Williams and his colleagues, having devised a simplification of the single-breath ($D_{Lco}SB$) technique suitable for bedside use,[356] applied this very successfully to study the relationship between the radiological extent of infiltration and the vital capacity and diffusing capacity.[364] They were able to demonstrate, in 35 patients with acute tuberculosis, that there was a general relationship between the reduction of diffusing capacity and the extent of radiological involvement, though correlation with the vital-capacity change was less satisfactory.[364] Noting that pathological examination often reveals the presence of more extensive tuberculosis than was evident from the chest film, the authors concluded that their data might indicate "that the level of diffusing capacity is actually a more accurate index of the extent of pulmonary tuberculosis than is the chest roentgenogram." Whether this is substantiated by future work or not, the authors' data clearly demonstrate the significance of serial measurements of diffusing capacity in the evaluation of therapy in acute tuberculosis. It seems quite clear that future controlled trials of the effects of, for example, steroid therapy in treatment of tuberculosis[2223] should contain serial observations of pulmonary function.

Chronic pulmonary tuberculosis

Factors determining effect on function

The possible effect on function of chronic pulmonary tuberculosis is dependent upon the relative importance of three different factors in any individual patient: (1) the extent of parenchymal destruction of lung tissue; (2) the severity of involvement of pleura and diaphragm, where fibrotic thickening may produce considerable mechanical restriction of lung movement; and (3) the presence of complicating chronic bronchitis or actual chronic bronchial stenosis. The third factor may be responsible for considerable ventilatory defect despite very little parenchymal change. Martin, Cochran, and Katsura[3384] have recently analyzed the incidence of chronic bronchitis and morphological emphysema in 36 autopsied cases of pulmonary tuberculosis and compared them to 22 controls. They concluded that the incidence of emphysema and chronic bronchitis was no greater in the tuberculosis group than in the general population. The existence of these factors in different combinations in different patients with pulmonary tuberculosis makes any generalizations about their common effect on pulmonary function largely valueless. Rossier and his colleagues described in some detail seven patients who showed different patterns of lung-function impairment.[17] Uggla[623] and Söderholm,[1707] in their detailed monographs on this problem, provided many examples of restrictive and ventilatory defect in these patients, not a few of whom were found to have significant pulmonary hypertension. Other reviews of the problem have been published from Scandinavia,[1710] Switzerland,[1708] France,[1709] and Japan.[1711] The extensive literature on bronchospirometry also contains many illustrative case records. There is little doubt that simple tests of function, such as measurement of the FEV, the arterial blood gases, and the diffusing capacity may play a useful part in the evaluation of such patients; and the procedures essential to careful examination of differential lung function are necessary before resectional surgery is under-

Case 51
Post-thoracoplasty; Fibrothorax (Contralateral)

Summary of Clinical Findings. This 44-year-old male salesclerk had developed bilateral pulmonary tuberculosis in 1938. Over the next 10 years he received intermittent sanatorium care and numerous pneumothoraces. In 1948, a left upper-lobe cavity was demonstrated and a five-rib thoracoplasty was performed. In 1951, a left pleural-cutaneous fistula developed; a radical Schede operation was performed, with removal of the parietal pleura and two more ribs. After this he began to develop increasing shortness of breath with frequent disabling respiratory infections. Signs of right heart failure developed, for which he was given digitalis. By 1956, a permanent tracheostomy was found necessary as well as occasional assisted breathing on a respirator. In 1959 he required assisted respiration most of the time. He had been in the hospital for a year before being transferred to the Royal Victoria Hospital in 1960, when he could climb only three or four stairs without stopping, and slept sitting up. His blood pressure was 135/85 mm Hg and pulse rate 84/min; he had cyanosis of the nail beds. He had a severe scoliosis of the dorsal spine with convexity to the left. There was marked paradoxical movement of the extensive defect in the left chest wall, which moved inward as the diaphragm descended and outward during "expiration." The right chest was dull to percussion and breath sounds were distant. Fine rales were heard at the left apex and right base. The neck veins were engorged. The liver was three finger-breadths enlarged. The peripheral edema responded to diuretics.

Decortication of the right lung was performed in May, 1960, and a thick pleural peel was removed. He required four weeks of elective respirator care after operation.

Subsequently there was gradual clinical deterioration and in May, 1965, an Ivalon Prosthesis was inserted into the defect in the chest wall in an attempt to stabilize the chest. There was no apparent clinical improvement following this procedure. He has since required several admissions for treatment of respiratory infections. His exercise tolerance is extremely limited but he continues to do some clerical work in his home.

He was last admitted to the hospital in May, 1969, for an upper respiratory infection. His physical findings were unchanged and there were no signs of congestive failure.

Radiology. The postero-anterior roentgenogram of the chest in full inspiration reveals marked deformity of the thoracic cage. An eight-rib thoracoplasty has been performed on the left with the resultant development of a compensatory cervicothoracic scoliosis convex to the left. The right sixth rib has been resected. Because of the bony deformity, assessment of comparative volume of the two hemithoraces is impossible, but there has obviously been a considerable loss of volume of both lungs. On the right, this is shown by the high position of the diaphragmatic dome and by an approximation of ribs which is more than could be explained by the scoliosis *per se*. These latter changes are related to a marked generalized thickening of the pleura over the right lung, and as no change has occurred in this thickening for some years it is clear that this lung is encased in a thick envelope of fibrous tissue.

On the left, there is a deficiency of the axillary portion of the thoracic wall from the level of the 6th to the 9th ribs, through which a part of the left lung is protruding. This lung herniation was much more evident on direct fluoroscopic observation;

	VC	FRC	RV	TLC	ME %	MMFR	$FEV_{0.75}$ ×40	pH	P_{CO_2}	HCO_3^-	P_{O_2}	O_2Hb %	$D_{Lco}SS_2$	CO Ext %
Predicted	5.0	4.0	2.2	7.2	60	4.0	129	7.40	42	25		97	20.0	42
Feb. 1960	0.7	1.0	0.8	1.5	49			7.33	77	36		70	5.1	28
July 1960	1.0	1.7	1.4	2.4	22	0.9	29	7.42	50	30		87	7.2	22
Feb. 1965	1.1	1.6	1.2	2.3	36	0.8	29	7.31	59	27		76	6.6	23
Apr. 1966	1.0	1.6	1.3	2.3	41	0.8	29	7.46	53	34	56	85	8.4	36

In February, 1960, vital capacity and lung volumes were grossly reduced. There was severe chronic CO_2 retention and O_2 desaturation. One and a half months after decortication (which was performed in May, 1960), the vital capacity and lung volumes had shown a slight increase, but gas distribution had become less efficient, suggesting that part of the increased lung volume may have been very poorly ventilated. There was a marked improvement in the arterial blood-gas tensions, however, and a small increase in diffusing capacity after the operation. There was still slight retention of CO_2 and undersaturation. In February, 1965, prior to the insertion of the prosthesis there had been a further rise in the CO_2 tension and a drop in the O_2 saturation. One year after this operation blood gases had again improved.

Post-thoracoplasty; Fibrothorax (Contralateral)

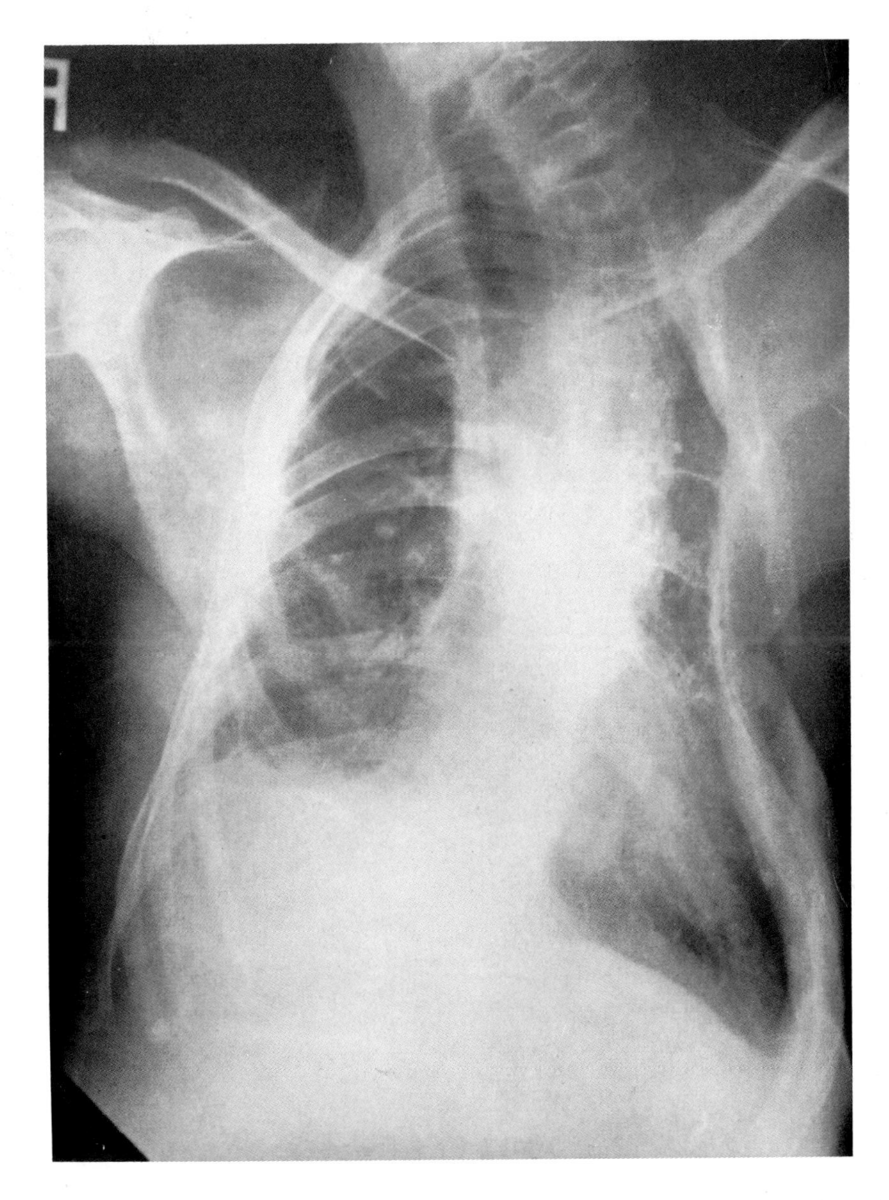

on inspiration, with descent of the left diaphragmatic dome, a sharp movement of the left chest wall occurred medially in the region of the defect; on expiration, as the left dome elevated, the axillary portion of the lung herniated through the defect to a remarkable degree so as to produce a prominent bulge in the axilla. With rapid respiration, the impression was gained of a double set of pistons moving in the left chest, the diaphragm moving upward and downward while at the same time the lateral chest wall in the region of the defect moved outward and inward through almost the same excursion. As a result, there was little total change in volume of the left chest from maximal inspiration through full expiration. On the right very little change in volume occurred even on deep inspiration, because of the marked pleural thickening.

Summary. A right-lung decortication in a man with a serious loss of function of the left lung has resulted in just sufficient improvement to permit him to hold an office job and prevent a return of right ventricular failure. Four weeks of elective respirator care were required to bring him through the postoperative period.

taken in advanced cases. As many authors have pointed out, facilities for such examinations are obligatory in any center in which resectional surgery for advanced pulmonary tuberculosis is undertaken. Blood gas changes occur only late in the disease,[3381] and obstructive impairment is commonly encountered,[3382] particularly in elderly patients.[3383]

Gregoire and his colleagues compared pulmonary function at rest and during exercise in patients with chronic pulmonary tuberculosis, fibrosis from other causes and pulmonary emphysema.[2216] They found that those with chronic tuberculosis commonly increased their ventilation considerably on exercise and usually there was no elevation of the arterial P_{CO_2} level.

Factors related to development of cor pulmonale in pulmonary tuberculosis

The monographs by Uggla[623] and Söderholm[1707] referred to in the preceding section contain studies of the hemodynamics of the pulmonary circulation in chronic pulmonary tuberculosis in relation to the extent of the pulmonary lesion and the impairment in ventilatory capacity and changes in arterial blood gases. Uggla concluded that there was a general correlation between ventilatory impairment, as measured by the MBC, and the level of pulmonary hypertension in these patients. Söderholm stressed the necessity for measurements during exercise and demonstrated a general relationship between pulmonary hypertension and lowering of the arterial oxygen saturation in his group of patients; he did not measure the arterial CO_2-tension levels. It is clear from the data of both these authors that significant pulmonary hypertension, likely eventually to produce overt cor pulmonale, can be found in these patients at a stage when ventilatory capacity is not grossly reduced and when arterial oxygen saturation is only slightly below normal values. In other patients, however, considerable arterial unsaturation and ventilatory defect can be demonstrated when the pulmonary arterial pressure is elevated. Neither author included any estimate of pulmonary mechanics or diffusing capacity. Uggla, who measured the arterial CO_2 tension, found it to be normal in some of his patients, although the arterial oxygen tension was significantly reduced;[623] Gregoire made similar observations.[2216] The importance of an exercise evaluation if this defect is to be uncovered is quite evident from all these studies.[623, 1707, 2216] It seems likely that estimates of exercise diffusing capacity might be useful in this group of patients, though no opinion can be formed from contemporary data of whether the lowered arterial oxygen tension in these patients is ascribable to parenchymal lung changes in themselves or to abnormalities of $\dot{V}/\dot{Q}$ distribution.

CHRONIC HISTOPLASMOSIS

Several excellent clinical reviews have been published of the many forms chronic histoplasmosis may assume,[1712] but we are unaware of any systematic study of the effect of this disease on pulmonary function. The pulmonary function pattern in one patient in whom the diagnosis was confirmed at autopsy* suggests that this disease may provide an example of loss of diffusion surface with minimal disturbance to air flow. It is likely that many cases of completely healed histoplasmosis infection, in which small calcified nodules are scattered throughout the lungs, will not show any defect in pulmonary function, since such lesions will not interfere to any considerable extent with air flow, mechanics, or diffusing capacity. Chronic histoplasmosis has been shown to cause a fibrosis mediastinitis in some patients, but too few of these cases have been reported as yet to permit an assessment to be made of the effect of this lesion on pulmonary function.[2218]

---

*Case 15 in first edition of this book.

ACUTE PULMONARY INFECTIONS

CHAPTER

20

The effect of different types of acute respiratory infection on pulmonary function has recently been reviewed.[3386, 3396]

ACUTE BACTERIAL PNEUMONIA

LOBAR PNEUMONIA

Meakins and Davies carried out a considerable number of arterial blood-gas studies in patients with acute lobar pneumonia, and the common pattern of change that was found was well established by the date when their textbook was written.[1] Most commonly, there was arterial oxygen desaturation, and the CO_2 content of the blood was reduced. They ascribed this to continued perfusion of affected lobes of the lung to which there was little ventilation, a conclusion supported by the experimental observations quoted that demonstrated a state of lobar "hyperaemia" during the acute or red-hepatization change, and "anaemia" during the stage of gray hepatization and resolution. Meakins and Davies also observed the close interrelationship between the state of delirium in acute lobar pneumonia and the level of arterial unsaturation. It is known not only that the CO_2 content of the blood is reduced in many of these patients, but also that often the arterial P_{CO_2} level is decreased, a consequence of the increased ventilation that follows reduction in arterial oxygen tension. Elevations of the P_{CO_2} level in these patients probably occur only terminally or in the presence of pre-existing—though often undiagnosed—pulmonary emphysema.

It has also been known for many years that the functional residual capacity is reduced in lobar pneumonia[1714] and that the vital capacity falls before it is further limited by the pain of concomitant pleurisy.

Little further work was reported on this disease until Marshall and Christie in 1954 measured the pulmonary compliance in patients with acute lobar pneumonia.[507] They found: "The rigidity of the lungs is increased considerably in the acute stage of the disease and this increase is more than can be accounted for by changes in the consolidated areas only." They were able to show also that the tachypnea which is a constant feature of these cases can be accounted for by the fact that, with a reduced pulmonary compliance, the most economical pattern of respiration in terms of work is one with a reduced tidal volume and an increased respiratory rate. Acute pneumonia, therefore, illustrates the remarkable ability of the human subject to breathe at the most economical rate and depth, and the dramatic fall in respiratory rate that occurs in this condition, as a result of treatment or spontaneously at the crisis of the disease, presumably is to be explained by a sudden reduction in lung rigidity. It should be realized, however, that although this hypothesis goes some way to explaining the necessity for the tachypnea of pneumonia, we are still a long way from understanding the mechanism whereby this adjustment to the most economical rate is accomplished.

Alexander and his colleagues have reported the results of bronchospirometric and hemodynamic studies in a group of patients with unilateral pneumococcal lobar pneumonia.[2219] Oxygen uptake was consistently reduced on the affected side in 10 patients studied by bronchospirometry, less decrease being observed in ventilation. Eight patients on whom right-heart catheterization was performed had an increased cardiac index but little change in pulmonary arterial pressure. Pulmonary arterial occlusion by balloon on the affected side did not result in a significant elevation of arterial oxygen tension in the three patients in whom this study was performed. Colp, Park, and Williams studied 12 patients with lobar pneumonia and found significantly low values of diffusing capacity in several.[2220]

Acute lobar pneumonia of classic type has become a relatively rare disease in hospital practice, and fortunately there are now few opportunities to observe the natural history of this condition. From the data on pulmonary compliance presented by Marshall and Christie[507] it may be inferred that much more of the lung is involved in this process than appears as consolidated lung on the chest x-ray. The stage of red hepatization is accompanied by considerable arterial unsaturation because of continued perfusion of congested and poorly ventilated lung, and it is to be presumed that in acute lobar pneumonia there is initially a failure to curtail perfusion through these affected areas. As organization and resolution occur, this adjustment takes place, with restoration of the arterial saturation to normal values.

Regional lung function studies in three children using ^{133}xenon after pneumonia have been reported by Kjellman.[3385] He found ventilation to be more affected than perfusion in the postacute stage and noted residual abnormal function in two cases in spite of a normal chest x-ray.

Bronchopneumonia

Diffuse bronchopneumonia, with patchy-consolidation often involving areas in both lungs, is associated with changes in respiratory function similar to those in lobar pneumonia. The severity of arterial desaturation, which may be much greater than in lobar pneumonia, is dependent upon the extent of lung involvement. Elevation of the arterial P_{CO_2} level is seen only in the terminal stages, in which essentially the clinical picture is one of respiratory failure.

Severe bronchopneumonia in small children is often accompanied by early circulatory failure, and the management of such cases may be very difficult.[3387]

ACUTE VARICELLA PNEUMONIA

This clinical entity has recently been reviewed in detail[3390] and may lead to death in respiratory failure. In such instances the lungs are the site of multiple nodular lesions, often peribronchial in location.[3389] After resolution there may be chronic impairment of gas transfer; this has been demonstrated both by oxygen diffusion measurement[3391] and steady-state $D_{L_{CO}}$ estimations.[3397] There is no residual ventilatory defect.

ACUTE VIRAL PNEUMONIA

As Spencer points out,[33] early descriptions of the pathology of acute viral pneumonia were confused by the presence of secondary bacterial infection in many patients. It is only since the clear recognition of the viral origin of this disorder and since bacterial invasion could be controlled by antibiotics that the pathological changes in the lungs have been clearly recognized. In fulminating cases the alveoli are filled with fibrin, fluid, red blood cells, and macrophages. Such patients have an intense cyanosis, often incompletely relieved by oxygen administration, and not infrequently require tracheostomy and ventilatory assistance.[1312] These patients are rare, however, and it is far more common to encounter cases in which patchy areas of viral pneumonitis, occurring during the course of an influenzal infection, are not extensive enough to cause severe arterial unsaturation. Indeed, the signs and symptoms of such episodes of pneumonitis may be less than the extent of involvement as seen radiologically might lead one to expect.

Berven's remarkable study[394] of pulmonary function after apparent clinical and radiological resolution of viral pneumonia should be consulted by any physician interested in this condition. He showed unequivocally that the steady-state diffusing capacity not infrequently was still impaired some months after the chest x-ray appearances had returned to normal; that this reduction was due to a lowered membrane-diffusion component (D_M); that this component was reduced not only in absolute terms but also in relation to the measured lung volume; and that, by contrast, after resolution following bacterial pneumonia no such residual abnormality could be demonstrated.

These findings are of the greatest interest and suggest that the changes in the alveolar lining cells and interstitial tissue may be slow to resolve even when there are no residual radiological abnormalities. Several of Berven's patients complained of some dyspnea, which he considered was related to the impairment of diffusing capacity.[394] He did not measure the pulmonary compliance, but it may be noted that if this, too, has not returned to normal some months after an acute episode, the combination of increased ventilation and reduced compliance might well be sufficient to account for the dyspnea. It seems clear that residual dyspnea in any patient who has had viral pneumonia should occasion a careful assessment of pulmonary function, whether or not the radiograph is clear.

Klocke and his colleagues[3395] could not confirm residual diffusion impairment after acute viral infections; they ascribe the difference between their findings and those of Berven to the lesser clinical severity of their cases of viral pneumonia.

It may be noted that Berven's findings are of particular interest in relation to the syndrome of "desquamative histiocytic pneumonitis" (*see* page 281). Perhaps the impact of viral infections in the lung should be viewed as possibly leading to an abnormal alveolar lining-cell response in some cases with development of this syndrome, to complete alveolar resolution in others, and to very slow or only partial restoration of normality in the rest, as shown to occur in Berven's study.

ACUTE BRONCHIOLITIS

Acute bronchiolitis is a feature of the lung damage caused by inhalation of irritant gases and, although difficult to diagnose, almost certainly plays a major part in the repetitive chest infections that are a feature of chronic bronchitis and emphysema. A case of bronchiolitis in an adult is described in Case 2, page 118. It is mainly in children, however, that this disease has a distinctive character, producing acute and occasionally fatal lower airway obstruction in patients between the ages of six months and three years. It seems clear that it is commonly due to an acute viral infection, sometimes occurring as an epidemic of infantile bronchiolitis.[2222] Little has been written on the pulmonary function changes that it produces, though the typical radiological appearance of overinflation of the lung in this disorder is familiar to most pediatricians. Reynolds found hypoxia, often severe, in 12 babies with bronchiolitis and bronchopneumonia, and in addition in 6 of them the $P\text{CO}_2$ level was elevated.[2221]

Simpson and Henley[3393] found that a $P\text{CO}_2$ of more than 65 mm Hg was of grave prognostic significance. The work of breathing is considerably increased in this condition,[3392] the dynamic compliance being reduced[3394] and the total gas volume increased. These parameters return to normal in about seven days after the onset of the illness.

Ventilatory tests of pulmonary function cannot be carried out on patients within this age group, but the study of the arterial blood is certainly of importance in relation to the management of acute bronchiolitis.

The reader should be reminded of the recent disquieting evidence that the incidence of acute lower chest infection in infants is related to air pollution level.[2724]

PULMONARY FUNCTION IN MISCELLANEOUS CONDITIONS

CHAPTER 21

BLOOD DISORDERS

Anemia

The level of arterial saturation is usually normal in patients with chronic anemia,[1] but the difference between alveolar and arterial oxygen tension is greater than normal. In a study of 10 patients with anemia, Ryan and Hickam found a mean A–a difference of 20.5 mm Hg, compared with 4.2 mm Hg in normal subjects. The arterial P_{O_2} tension averaged 82 mm Hg in air in the anemic patients compared with 94 mm Hg in the normal subjects; the arterial P_{CO_2} was on average 2 mm Hg lower in the patients.[1715] On exercise the differences may be greater.

In a more recent study,[3399] Housley found that recovery from severe chronic anemia was accompanied by a reduction in the $(A\text{–}a)D_{O_2}$ and attributed its previous widening to an increase in the anatomical shunt component. There is little evidence of a $\dot{V}/\dot{Q}$ defect in this condition.

Sproule and his colleagues studied four patients with sickle-cell anemia, two with pernicious anemia, and three with iron-deficiency anemia, during exercise at a level close to their maximal capability; their mean arterial oxygen tension was 73.2 mm Hg, compared with 86.0 mm Hg in normal subjects under the same conditions; and their $P\text{CO}_2$, at 34.5 mm Hg, was 5.5 mm Hg lower than in the normal subjects. Under the conditions of exercise they used, there was a significant difference in observed oxygen saturation between the two groups;[1716] Bishop, Donald and Wade noted decreased arterial oxygen saturation in 4 of the 11 anemic patients they studied during exercise.[1717] It is also of interest that in certain types of anemia (e.g., sickle-cell anemia) the oxyhemoglobin dissociation curve is shifted to the right, a factor that would contribute to arterial desaturation but would not affect arterial O_2 tension and, therefore, would not contribute to the (A–a) $P\text{O}_2$ difference.

The pulmonary diffusing capacity is the only other parameter of lung function that is deranged to any considerable extent in the anemic state. As the hematocrit level falls, the amount of hemoglobin around alveoli into which oxygen or carbon monoxide can pass (which might be termed the "effective" pulmonary capillary volume) will be reduced, although the total amount of blood in this location may be unchanged. Thus, the total diffusing capacity is reduced in anemia, though it is not clear whether this reduction is exactly proportional to the decrease in total hematocrit.[1718] Comparative data on a patient with pernicious anemia (*see* Table 21–1) show other aspects of pulmonary function to be normal during the anemic state; there is usually no change in pulmonary mechanics,[1719] in gas distribution, or in ventilatory capacity.

Studying the circulatory adjustment that occurs in chronic anemia, Bishop and his colleagues found that the cardiac output was usually elevated at rest and considerably higher at moderate grades of exercise than in normal subjects.[1717] Comparison of the findings in anemic patients with those in normal subjects studied by Sproule and his co-workers shows that, although the exercise level was apparently nearly maximal for all, the normal subjects had a mean absolute oxygen uptake of 3.2 liters/min, whereas in the patients this was only 1.84 liters/min.[1716] If both groups were in a steady state, presumably the anemic patients were capable of only a much lower exercise load. The measured average cardiac output was 23.6 liters/min in the patients and 23.4 liters/min in the normal subjects. One may conclude that in anemia the level of cardiac output during exercise is increased in relation to both oxygen uptake and the level of external work performed.

An outstanding feature of the anemic patient on exercise is his relative overventilation in relation to oxygen uptake, resulting in a decreased percentage extraction of oxygen from the expired air. This was particularly striking in the study by Bishop, Donald and

TABLE 21–1 PULMONARY FUNCTION TEST DATA BEFORE AND AFTER TREATMENT OF PERNICIOUS ANEMIA
(Male Aged 58, Height 167 cm, Weight 154 lb)

	BEFORE TREATMENT (JANUARY 1955)	AFTER TREATMENT (APRIL 1955)	PREDICTED VALUES
Hemoglobin percentage	48	95	95 to 100
Vital capacity (liters)	3.5	3.4	3.5
Functional residual capacity (liters)	2.6	3.2	3.2
Total lung capacity (liters)	5.4	5.7	5.5
Maximal breathing capacity (l/min)	75	88	90
Mixing efficiency	65	77	55
Resting $D_{Lco}SS_2$ (ml CO/min/mm Hg)	8.2	13.6	14.0
Exercise (2 mph, flat)			
Minute volume ($\dot{V}_E$) (l/min)	30.2	24.5	
Oxygen uptake ($\dot{V}O_2$) (l/min)	0.88	0.98	
$\dot{V}O_2/\dot{V}_E$	2.92	4.0	3.5 to 5.5
Diffusing capacity ($D_{Lco}SS_3$)	14.0	24.1	25.0

The chest x-ray was normal throughout in this patient. Note that restitution of the hematocrit to normal was followed by a considerable increase in diffusing capacity and a reduction in exercise ventilation.

Wade.[1717] It is this relative overventilation that accounts for the decrease in arterial P_{CO_2} on exercise in these patients.

Manfredi[3398] has suggested that the respiratory-center stimulation and arterial hypocapnia in anemia should be regarded as a defense mechanism to compensate for the expansion of the extracellular fluid that occurs in chronic anemia.

There have been few studies of the effect of acute blood loss on exercise capability. Balke and his co-workers used a progressive exercise test in which the subject reached exhaustion point before and one hour after donation of 500 ml of blood.[1720] One hour after blood loss the maximal oxygen uptake had fallen by 10 per cent, pulmonary ventilation had increased by about the same amount, the pulse rate had risen by about 6 beats/min, and the level of maximal work possible was reduced. All values had returned to normal levels by the second day.

It is not at all clear why the arterial oxygen tension should be reduced in these patients. Possible explanations are that the transit time through the lung is too fast for complete equilibration, that there is delay in equilibration in the alveolus because there is a wider layer of plasma between the red blood cell and the alveolar wall, and that there may be some change in the kinetics of combination of oxygen and hemoglobin in some types of chronic anemia. Another possibility is that the increased alveolar–arterial difference reflects some change in ventilation–perfusion relationships, though there is no direct evidence to support this theory. Freeman and Nunn, in studies of the effect of acute hemorrhage in dogs, found no evidence of abnormal shunting or of gross changes in $\dot{V}/\dot{Q}$ ratio. They concluded, however, that "The severe desaturation of mixed venous blood resulted in an alveolar-to-arterial P_{O_2} difference which was a significant factor in the oxygenation of the arterial blood."[2123] Studies of acute hemorrhage in animals have not as yet yielded a clear explanation of the mechanism of respiratory stimulation that occurs under these conditions.[1721] It has been shown recently by Bartlett and Tenney that, in the rat, the tissue oxygen tension is lowered as a consequence of acute anemia, the tension of CO_2 in the tissue gas pocket remaining unchanged.[2124]

The respiratory adaptation to anemia thus consists in increasing the alveolar oxygen tension both by hyperventilation and by tissue adaptation to anoxia,[1716] the hyperventilation possibly being related to the increase in extracellular fluid if the anemia is chronic. The circulatory adjustment consists in elevation of the cardiac output, in an effort to supply a normal quantity of oxygen to the tissues. Patients with moderately severe anemia are able to accomplish exercise without dyspnea at customary day-to-day levels, since they are acclimatized to the concomitant slight increase in ventilation. It seems clear, however, that chronic or severe anemia or acute blood loss inevitably entails a restricted maximal oxygen uptake and physical working capacity.

Polycythemia rubra vera

In most patients with polycythemia rubra vera, the subdivisions of lung volume, maximal ventilatory capacity, and inert-gas distribution are normal,[1540, 2125, 2126] and, in our experience, the resting steady-state diffusing capacity also is normal. Many authors have stressed that the demonstration of arterial desaturation in a patient believed to be suffering from polycythemia vera should immediately lead to the suspicion that he has some other condition, either as a cause of polycythemia or in addition to it.

Earlier studies indicated that the arterial saturation in primary polycythemia was normal,[1540, 1542] but Murray[3401] and Lertzmann and his colleagues[3400] have observed a lowered arterial oxygen tension in a few of their patients, in whom the presence of emphysema or alveolar hypoventilation has been carefully excluded. One such patient was noted by Calabresi and Meyer[1722] and another by Cassels and Morse.[1723] The latter authors confirmed the previous finding of a normal oxyhemoglobin dissociation curve in patients with polycythemia rubra vera. In 1927 Harrop and Heath,[352] using the original Krogh method for determining CO diffusing capacity, concluded that this parameter was often decreased in patients with this disease, but relied on the Krogh data for normal values. There is some uncertainty about the cases they studied, since they were at pains to point out the frequency with which emphysema and chronic bronchitis were found at autopsy in these patients. The studies of Harrop and Heath have been made obsolete by the investigation of 10 patients with polycythemia rubra vera, using the single-breath ($D_{Lco}SB$) modified Krogh method, published by Burgess and Bishop.[2125] These investigators found that, before treatment, the diffusing capacity was either normal or elevated. After treatment, with restoration of the hematocrit to normal, in five of their patients the $D_{Lco}SB$ was abnormally low. They concluded that the probable cause of this was the presence of thromboses in pulmonary vessels; and they illustrate such lesions in the lung of another patient with polycythemia, unfortunately not studied with pulmonary function tests. Similarly low diffusing-capacity values have been noted by Lertzmann and his co-authors[3400] using a steady-state technique. Bjure and his colleagues[3402] also found a lowered D_{Lco} when the hemoglobin content was restored to normal in some of their patients, and in addition reported a widening of the $(A–a)Do_2$ and some exercise hyperventilation. These important contributions raise the question of whether the pulmonary thromboses were in fact primary or secondary lesions—an important point not yet conclusively settled. It may be noted, however, that small pulmonary thrombi might well be responsible for most of these changes. The diffusing capacity may be normal in some patients with polycythemia and in pulmonary hypertension due to pulmonary embolism. In our own laboratory we have usually obtained normal values for the steady-state diffusing capacity in patients with polycythemia rubra vera referred from the Haematology Division. It is clear that the finding of a low value should lead to the suspicion of the presence of emphysema, of a right-to-left cardiac or pulmonary shunt, or possibly the occurrence of significant pulmonary infarction or thrombosis, which are thought to be common complications in some of these patients.

It is important to realize that the patient with polycythemia rubra vera may acquire chronic bronchitis, in which case the polycythemia may well be wrongly attributed by the physician to pulmonary emphysema. It has also been shown that significant alveolar hypoventilation may exist in patients who are not obese (*see* Chapter 16), and it may occur in those who have a neuromuscular disorder. On occasion it may be very difficult to decide whether the polycythemia is primary or secondary, and our experience leads us to suggest that this differentiation is usually most difficult when a patient with primary polycythemia has definite chronic bronchitis, or when a patient with emphysema and secondary polycythemia has splenomegaly as a result of recurrent splenic infarction. Particular attention should be paid to the bicarbonate level in the arterial blood as an indication of the presence of chronic hypoventilation in the differentiation between these syndromes.

ALVEOLAR PROTEINOSIS

This disease was first described in 1958 by Rosen, Castleman, and Liebow, who reported 27 cases with a clinical syndrome usually characterized by progressive dyspnea accompanied by a cough that was often productive of sputum.[1750] In half of their cases the onset followed a febrile illness that was considered at the time to be a pneumonia. Physical signs were few in relation to the extent of the radiological appearances, which were very similar in all of their patients. The changes visible on x-ray were described by the authors as follows: "There is a fine, diffuse, perihilar, radiating, feathery, or vaguely nodular, soft density, resembling in its 'butterfly' distribution the pattern seen in severe pulmonary edema." In some cases the shadows appeared to become denser with passage of time, but, in many, partial or complete resolution occurred. The appearances of the lung on biopsy or necropsy were equally characteristic, although the lesion was variable in extent and distribution. The bronchi and bronchioles appeared normal, and there was little evidence of alveolar-wall thickening or damage, but many alveoli were filled with dense eosinophilic material.

The microscopical appearance of alveolar proteinosis is immediately diagnostic, the alveoli and bronchioles being filled with eosinophilic material, which is often granular and flocculent, particularly when stained with PAS, which stains the material strongly. The material is rich in protein and lipid, and cholesterol crystals may be recognizable microscopically. It has been suggested that the material is secreted by the alveolar lining cells, which are swollen and increased in number and which may slough into the alveolar lumina, resulting finally in laminated bodies

(Text continued on page 425.)

Case 52 Pulmonary Myomatosis

Summary of Clinical Findings. This 37-year-old Chinese airline stewardess was admitted to the Royal Victoria Hospital in April, 1965. She had been well until four years previously when she began to notice mild shortness of breath on exertion. Yearly routine chest x-rays had revealed no abnormality, but nine months prior to admission the dyspnea began to progress in severity and two months later she noticed small amounts of blood in her sputum. At this time chest x-ray revealed an abnormality and she was admitted to the Vancouver General Hospital. Investigations included a lung biopsy interpreted as showing pulmonary myomatosis and the patient was discharged on steroids. In spite of this her symptoms progressed until she was completely incapacitated and short of breath at rest with five-pillow orthopnea. Pulmonary function studies were obtained one month prior to admission. Her symptoms showed a further exacerbation and she was admitted.

Her past history was uneventful and she had never smoked.

On examination she was extremely cyanosed and tachypneic. Her blood pressure was 130/80, pulse rate was 110/min and regular; respiration rate was 38/min. There was no clubbing. There were the signs of a small effusion at the right base. There was no jugular vein distention but a hepato-jugular reflux was present and the liver edge was two finger-breadths below the right costal margin. There was no ankle edema.

Investigations revealed a hemoglobin of 14.7 gm per 100 ml and a hematocrit of 46; white blood count was 11,000, with neutrophilia. Urinalysis, BUN, and creatinine levels were normal. A chest x-ray confirmed the presence of a right pleural effusion, and a thoracentesis on the day following admission yielded 1000 cc of creamy pink fluid. Shortly after this she developed a right pneumothorax. In spite of drainage this recurred and was difficult to control. The patient deteriorated rapidly and died eight days after admission.

Radiology. A magnified view of the lower portion of the left lung (*A*) reveals an extremely coarse reticular nodular pattern, in areas almost confluent. Generally these changes were much more marked in the lower than in the upper lung zones.

Pathology. At autopsy, both lungs were almost completely replaced by cysts 0.25 to 2 cm. in diameter (*B*), and many of the cysts were filled with hemorrhagic fluid. Microscopically there was interstitial proliferation of smooth muscle surrounding the greater portion of the cysts and elsewhere in the interstitium. The internal lining of the cysts was generally alveolar epithelium or alveoli and thus they were emphysematous spaces (*C*). In addition, proliferation of smooth muscle was found in cervical, hilar, abdominal, and psoas muscle lymph nodes. This case has been reported[3720] as an example of pulmonary and lymph node myomatosis, and the lesions are identical with those found in tuberous sclerosis.

Case report continues on page 424.

														EXERCISE				
	VC	FRC	RV	TLC	ME %	MMFR	$FEV_{0.75}$ ×40	pH^+	P_{CO_2}	HCO_3	P_{O_2}	O_2Hb %	$D_{Lco}SS_2$	CO Ext. %	GRADE	$\dot{V}_{O_2}$	$\dot{V}_E$	$D_{Lco}SS_3$
Predicted	3.5	2.9	1.6	5.1		3.3	87						17.2	48				
March, 1965	1.3	2.9	2.7	4.0		0.48	27	32	32	24		81.7	3.5	18				

There was a marked decrease in vital capacity but an increase in the residual volume and severe reduction in flow rates. The diffusing capacity was extremely low. She was hypoxic and hyperventilating. A part of the reduction in flow can be accounted for by the reduction in vital capacity.

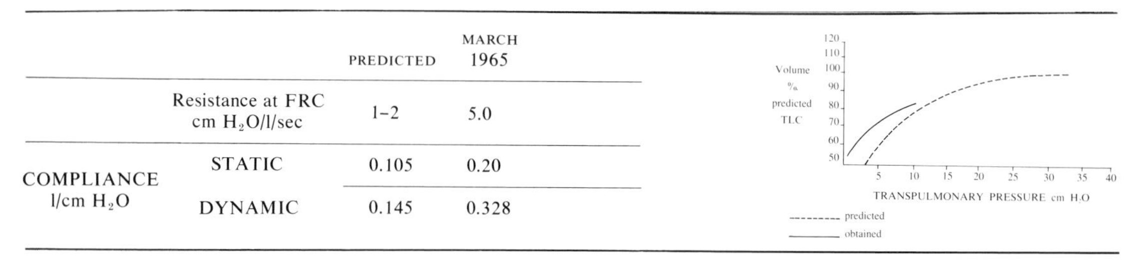

		PREDICTED	MARCH 1965
	Resistance at FRC cm H_2O/l/sec	1–2	5.0
COMPLIANCE l/cm H_2O	STATIC	0.105	0.20
	DYNAMIC	0.145	0.328

The increased compliance values suggested loss of elastic recoil. There is only moderately increased resistance.

Pulmonary Myomatosis

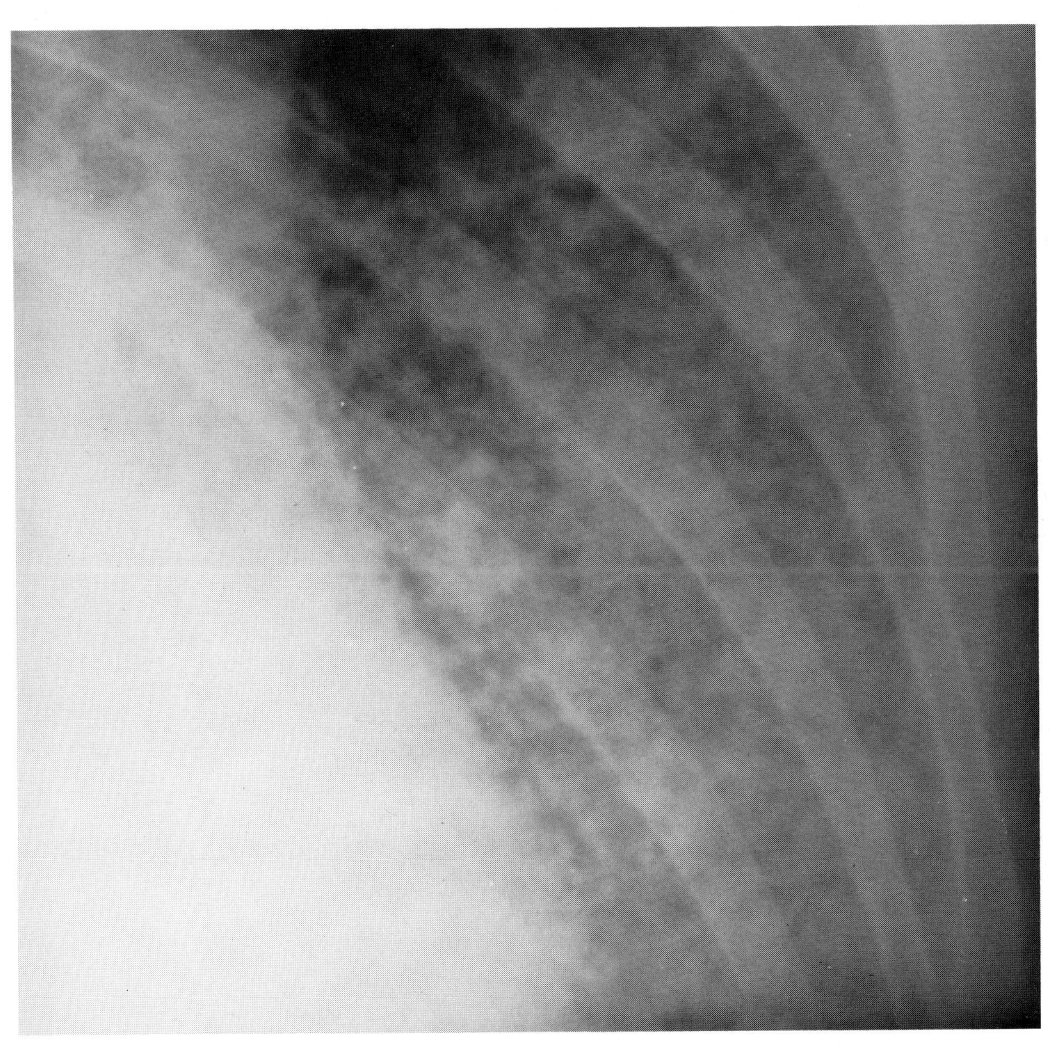

A

Case 52
Pulmonary Myomatosis (Continued)

Summary. This patient was an example of a rare condition leading to lung destruction and death about four years after the onset of symptoms. The function test data was of particular interest because although the vital capacity and total lung capacity were lowered, and the diffusing capacity grossly reduced, the compliance was increased and there was a moderate increase in airway resistance. The mechanics data were therefore unlike those found in restrictive lung disease of the Hamman-Rich type, or in scleroderma. Furthermore, the maximal negative intrapleural pressure in the patient was reduced, reaching only −9.5 cm H_2O compared to a predicted value of −31.0 cm H_2O, whereas in the purely fibrotic conditions, this pressure is most commonly more negative than the predicted value.

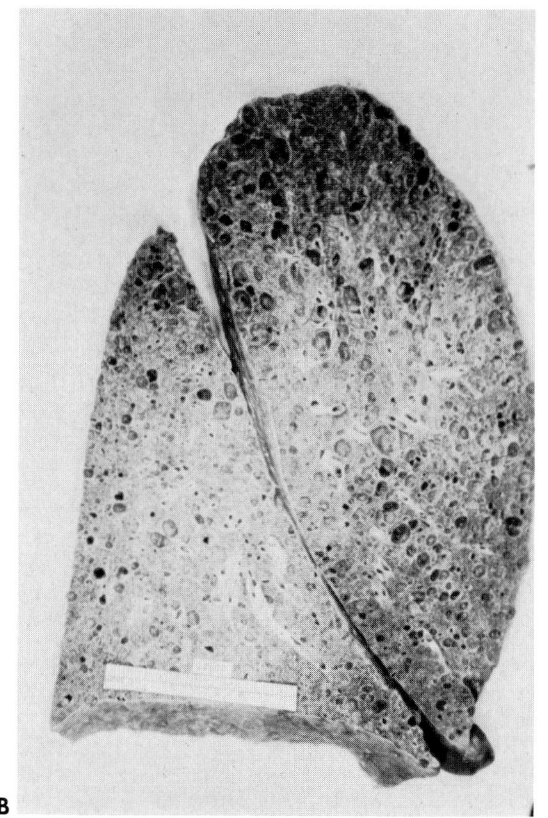

B

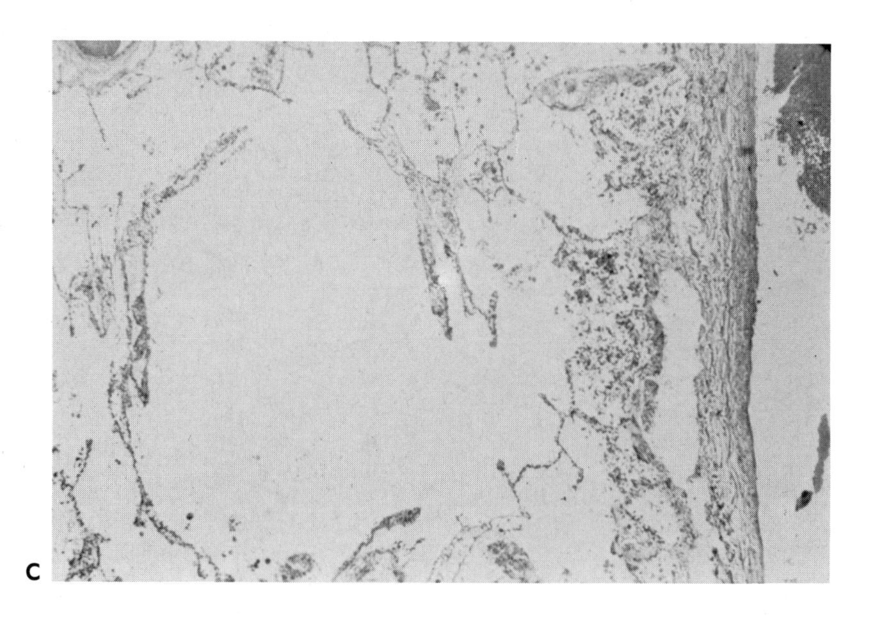

C

which are not infrequently seen in the alveoli in this condition. Larson and Gordinier in 1965[3403] found that 79 patients had been described and added a further 6 of their own. The electron microscopy study of this condition has not revealed much that was unexpected,[3406] and many recent papers have been concerned with the beneficial effects of pulmonary lavage in the treatment of this condition.[3404, 3407, 3408, 3409] One unusual case was considered to have been caused by adrenocorticosteroid.[3405]

Rosen and his colleagues described the pattern of pulmonary function in 10 of their patients. The maximal breathing capacity was generally normal, falling only six months before death in one patient. The arterial oxygen tension was commonly reduced, leading to a considerable increase in arterial–alveolar oxygen difference. In one patient (case 24 in reference 1750) the arterial oxygen tension on exercise was found to be as low as 39 mm Hg, resulting in an A–a difference of 89 mm Hg, and he had considerable pulmonary hypertension that was much reduced after he had breathed oxygen for 15 minutes.

Larson and Gordinier report serial studies over a period of 3½ years in one patient with progressive improvement being shown by increases in vital capacity, residual volume, and arterial oxygen tension to normal values. In only 5 of the 34 patients in the literature in whom the ventilatory ability has been measured has it been noted to be seriously impaired. These authors[3403] suggest that the syndrome is due to an overproduction of surfactant and note that half of the cases gave a history of virus infection and that electrical welding and metal work was given as the occupation in 12 of the reported cases.

Obviously the extent of impairment is directly dependent upon the extent of involvement of the lungs, with resultant variation in severity of the function defect in different patients. A low diffusing capacity, reduced functional residual capacity, and a normal maximal breathing capacity have been noted by several physicians.[1751–1754] In other recorded cases, every type of biochemical or bacteriological test has been described, but lung function has not been assessed.[1755–1757] Occasionally the clinical picture may become confused by complicating infection,[2128] and the disease may run a progressive and severe course.[2129] Case 53 describes a patient we have studied with this disorder.

HEXAMETHONIUM AND APRESOLINE LUNG; BUSULFAN LUNG

Hexamethonium, Apresoline (hydralazine) or busulfan may affect the lung when used therapeutically. The two former drugs are used in the treatment of hypertension, and busulfan (Myleran), although used in chronic myeloid leukemia, bears some similarity in molecular configuration to hexamethonium.[1593] "Hexamethonium lung" appears to be distinct from the other two entities; it is characterized by extensive intra-alveolar exudation of fibrin-rich material, with organization and resultant intra- and interalveolar fibrosis and granulation tissue.[1746, 1749] The gross appearance is of well-circumscribed nodular densities in the central and upper portions of lungs, consistent with the hypothesis that the lesion is due to organization and fibrosis of fibrin-rich pulmonary edema fluid.[1746] It has been pointed out also that the lesion is qualitatively similar to that of uremic pneumonitis.[2247] The same type of lesion may be seen in hypertensive patients treated with pentolinium tartrate.[1748] Interstitial pneumonitis and fibrosis, similar to that in Hamman-Rich disease, is the characteristic lesion resulting from administration of busulfan,[1194, 1593] hydralazine, and combined hydralazine and hexamethonium.[1745] Development of the pulmonary lesion in hydralazine-induced disease is rapid;[1745] it is more chronic with busulfan, and when due to this drug the changes may be reversible by administration of steroids[1593] or withdrawal of busulfan.[1194]

Heard and Cooke[3410] and Littler and his colleagues[3411] have recently contributed excellent analyses of busulfan lung, with light microscopy, electron microscopy, and clinical observations. This condition appears to start as a proliferation of granular pneumocytes[3411] and proceed to a fibrinous alveolar edema and fibrosis.[3410]

The x-rays show diffuse mottling, and dyspnea is a common feature of these and earlier cases.[1748, 1749] The patient described by Littler and his co-workers[3411] had a vital capacity only 45 per cent of that predicted and a total lung capacity of 64 per cent of predicted. The diffusing capacity was only 25 per cent of predicted, and the arterial P_{CO_2} was normal. Detailed studies of pulmonary mechanics do not seem to have been reported in these cases. Since busulfan is used in the treatment of chronic myelogenous leukemia, it may be difficult to distinguish the pulmonary infiltration that may occur spontaneously in that condition from pulmonary changes due to the drug.

MUSCULAR AND NEUROLOGICAL DISORDERS

Diaphragm paralysis

Paralysis of one dome of the diaphragm results in reduction, on that side, of ventilation to one quarter to one half the normal value, and of oxygen uptake to one half to three quarters the normal value.[1772] Söderholm and Widimsky studied three such patients and observed that the infusion of acetylcholine was followed by a measurable decrease in the arterial oxygen saturation.[1773]

Gould and his co-workers[3415] have recently studied the effect of experimentally produced hemidiaphragmatic paralysis in man, finding a diminution in lung volumes and in maximal ventilatory volume, particularly when the subject was supine.

McCredie and his colleagues have studied three patients with bilateral diaphragmatic paralysis.[2130] They have confirmed the earlier observation by Comroe and his co-workers[2131] of the prominence of orthopnea in such patients, and found considerable reductions in vital capacity, especially when the patient was supine. Expiratory flow rates were reduced, with, in two of the three patients, normal values for airway resistance. The diffusing capacity ($D_{L_{CO}}SB$) was normal in two and slightly reduced in one. In two of the patients there was a significant reduction in arterial oxygen saturation when they lay flat.

Parkinson's disease

Connolly and his co-workers have shown that alveolar ventilation is usually normal in this condition,[1775] which appears to affect respiration to a relatively small extent. Siegfried and Pitteloud[3416] found some evidence of impaired ventilatory ability and noted that this might be even more impaired after stereotoxic thalamotomy had been performed. It has been suggested that obstructive inspiratory dysfunction in patients with parkinsonism may be due to general parasympathetic overactivity.[3417]

Neuromuscular disorders

As is noted in Chapter 22, neuromuscular disorders are a relatively common cause of acute and chronic respiratory failure. Before this stage is reached, however, they may give rise to considerable diagnostic difficulty, since the complaint of dyspnea may lead to the performance of pulmonary function studies, and interpretation of these may be difficult in the circumstances. Miller and his colleagues have studied three such patients in detail, and emphasize that dyspnea may be noted before muscular atrophy or other signs become evident.[1777] In such cases, there is considerable impairment of maximal breathing capacity, though the shape of the expiratory tracing indicates that air flow is relatively satisfactory; the maximal midexpiratory flow rate may be relatively normal even though the vital capacity is reduced. Measurements of inert-gas distribution were not quite normal in two cases studied, but derangement was not severe.[1777] The diffusing capacity in these patients should be a useful indicator of normality, and one would predict that the diminution in expiratory force might be reflected in an inability to raise a mercury column on respiration. Gillam and his co-workers have recently published a valuable study of pulmonary function in patients with dystrophia myotonica.[2254] They stressed the sensitivity of these patients to respiratory depressants, but found normal values for arterial P_{CO_2} in some who had considerable respiratory-muscle weakness.

Keltz[3412] has also observed a lowered vital capacity and arterial P_{O_2} in one patient with myotonia dystrophia and in another with multiple sclerosis; Buchsbaum and his colleagues have recently documented the occurrence of alveolar hypoventilation in two patients with muscular dystrophy.[3418] The functional residual capacity is reduced in patients with chronic poliomyelitis,[2132] and the compliance is reduced roughly in proportion to the loss of vital capacity.[468]

The reader will find an elegant and comprehensive review of respiration in a variety of neurological disorders in a paper contributed by Plum to a Ciba Symposium.[3829]

Brain lesions

Cerebral tumors may lead to respiratory failure without concomitant respiratory muscle paralysis,[32, 34] though few such cases have been reported in detail. Davis[3413] has reported studies on patients with cerebellar disorders, finding no change in detection threshold of increased airway resistance in them in contrast to patients with upper spinal-cord lesions, who showed a diminution in detection capability.

Hemiplegia results in a 9 per cent reduction of chest movement over the upper chest but not over the lower chest during quiet breathing.[3414] Fluck, who reported this finding, noted that movements were symmetrical during deep breathing. Haas and his colleagues[3419] measured a considerably increased oxygen uptake during exercise in hemiplegic patients and believed that the mechanics of ventilation may have been impaired by the hemiplegia.

Trichinosis

Robin and his colleagues have drawn attention to an unusual syndrome caused by severe trichinosis.[1774] In their patient the vital capacity was reduced to 57 per cent of the predicted value, and x-ray revealed elevation of both sides of the diaphragm, but no other lesion. There was considerable dyspnea, and the pulmonary manifestations were entirely due to the severe muscular involvement consequent upon the heavy infection by *Trichinella spiralis*. Severe cases of this syndrome are occasionally reported.[3420]

CONGENITAL, FAMILIAL, AND DEVELOPMENTAL DISORDERS

Pulmonary alveolar microlithiasis

This remarkable condition was first described in detail by Sosman and his colleagues in 1957.[1769] As Gough has pointed out, the radiological appearances may give rise to confusion,[715] although once this rare condition has been encountered it is not difficult for the physician to recognize other cases. Conflicting claims of much earlier descriptions of this condition have been made,[3424, 3428] but we have not attempted to adjudicate between them. Its hereditary pattern has been studied in detail,[3427] and several reviews of it have appeared;[3427, 3429] about 110 cases have been described in the literature, including one of a 5-year-old boy[3423] and another in a 16-year-old patient.[3426] One case has been described in which it is thought that a similar lesion has been acquired.[3422] Fuleihan and his colleagues[3421] published pulmonary function data on 5 patients, confirming lowering of subdivisions of lung volume and increased $(A-a)O_2$ differences in all, with generally normal forced expiratory flow rates.

The pathology consists of "microliths" lying in individual alveoli.[1769] These bodies have a laminated appearance on section and are relatively constant in size. The alveolar walls may be normal or may show some evidence of thickening. In spite of exhaustive biochemical studies, no convincing explanation of the derangement responsible for this condition has yet been advanced. Reports of similar cases have appeared, and from these it is clear that on occasion the presence of microlithiasis can give rise to interstitial fibrosis which, in turn, can lead to considerable impairment of respiratory function.[1770, 1771, 2133, 3421, 3425] Other patients have very little permanent lung function impairment, however. (*See* Case 55.)

Telangiectasia and arteriovenous fistulae of the lung

It has been recognized for several years that arteriovenous fistulae, often multiple, are a feature of the lung pathology in patients with hereditary telangiectasia. In a remarkable survey of 231 members of a family suffering from hereditary telangiectasia, Hodgson and his colleagues found that 14 also had this associated condition.[1725] Several useful reviews of this entity have been published,[1552, 1726–1728, 3431, 3433, 3436] and many carefully documented individual cases have been reported.[1729–1734, 2134] Rossier and his colleagues recorded an arterial saturation value of 71 per cent on air-breathing and 77 per cent on oxygen in one such patient preoperatively; this rose to 94 per cent on air-breathing after removal of the lobe containing the fistula.[17] In the two patients studied by Armentrout and Underwood, the resting arterial saturation was 86.8 per cent in one and 84.4 per cent in the other in the presence of large arteriovenous fistulae that were easily demonstrable in the angiograms.[2135] In Hultgren and Gerbode's patient, removal of the lobe containing the fistula raised the arterial saturation from 80 per cent to 90 per cent, and the hemo-

Case 53
Alveolar Proteinosis

Summary of Clinical Findings. This 63-year-old clerical worker was admitted to the hospital in December, 1964, complaining of cough and shortness of breath. In August, 1964, he had suffered an episode of hematemesis and melena. The cause of this was undetermined, but was presumed to be and treated as an ulcer. A chest x-ray at that time was abnormal (*see* Radiology). He was a non-smoker and had no respiratory symptoms.

In October he began to notice a cough with occasional very slight mucus expectoration. In early December he found he was becoming short of breath on exertion and within two weeks he was unable to climb stairs. There was no orthopnea.

On admission he was not in acute distress nor cyanosed. Chest examination was entirely negative and there were no signs of congestive failure.

Urinalysis was normal. Hemoglobin was 14.8 gm per 100 ml and white blood count was 5900, with a normal differential. NPN, serum cholesterol, uric acid, alkaline phosphatase, and protein electrophoresis were all normal. Cultures of sputum were negative. The electrocardiogram was normal. OT was 1:1000 and histoplasmin skin tests were negative.

Pulmonary function studies are shown.

A lung biopsy was performed on January 20, 1965 (*see* figures).

The patient was placed on steroids and he slowly cleared clinically and radiologically.

Radiology.* A postero-anterior roentgenogram (*A*) in December, 1964, reveals involvement of the central and midzones of both lungs by patchy air-space consolidation which in many areas is confluent. The disease possesses a "butterfly" pattern of distribut on, the peripheral zones of the lungs being spared. An air bronchogram is visible. Cardiac size is normal. Five months later the x-ray was normal.

Pathology. Lung biopsy (*B*) shows the alveolar spaces to be filled with granular, eosinophilic material. The alveolar walls are normal.

Summary. This patient shows the characteristic clinical, radiological, and pathological features of alveolar proteinosis. The only significant abnormality of lung function was a diminution of diffusing capacity, which is also characteristic.

*X-rays courtesy of Dr. Adolph Glay, St. Mary's Hospital.

	VC	FRC	RV	TLC	ME %	MMFR	$FEV_{0.75}$ ×40	pH^+	Pco_2	HCO_3	Po_2	O_2Hb %	$D_{Lco}SS_2$	CO Ext. %	EXERCISE GRADE	$\dot{V}o_2$	$\dot{V}_E$	$D_{Lco}SS_3$
Predicted	4.0	3.8	2.5	6.5	48	2.9	92						11.5	37				
Jan. 5, 1965	4.4	3.7	2.1	6.5	41	2.3	102						7.8	27				
May 18, 1965	4.2	3.8	2.6	6.8	33	2.1	96						8.8	35				
Aug. 5, 1966	4.5	3.9	1.9	6.4	48	2.8	107						9.9	34				

In January, 1965, at the time of admission the only significant abnormality was a slight but definite reduction in diffusing capacity. Subsequent studies have shown gradual improvement in this measurement and in August, 1966, the result was within the range of normal.

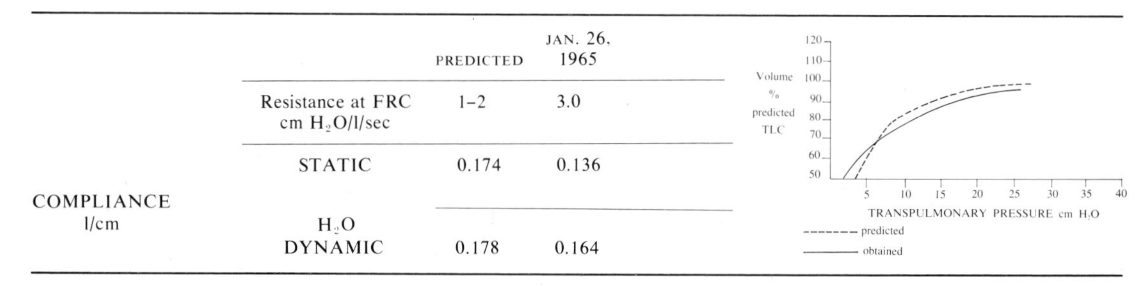

		PREDICTED	JAN. 26, 1965
	Resistance at FRC cm H_2O/l/sec	1–2	3.0
COMPLIANCE l/cm H_2O	STATIC	0.174	0.136
	DYNAMIC	0.178	0.164

The mechanical properties of the lung are within the range of normal.

Alveolar Proteinosis

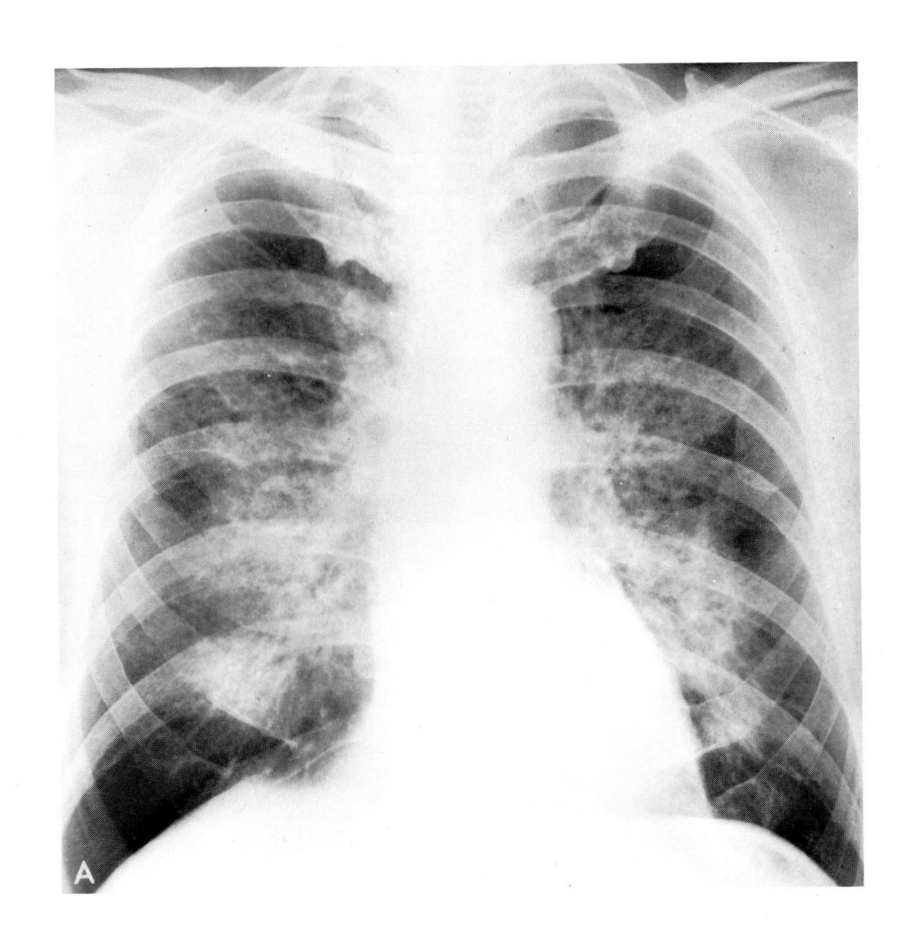

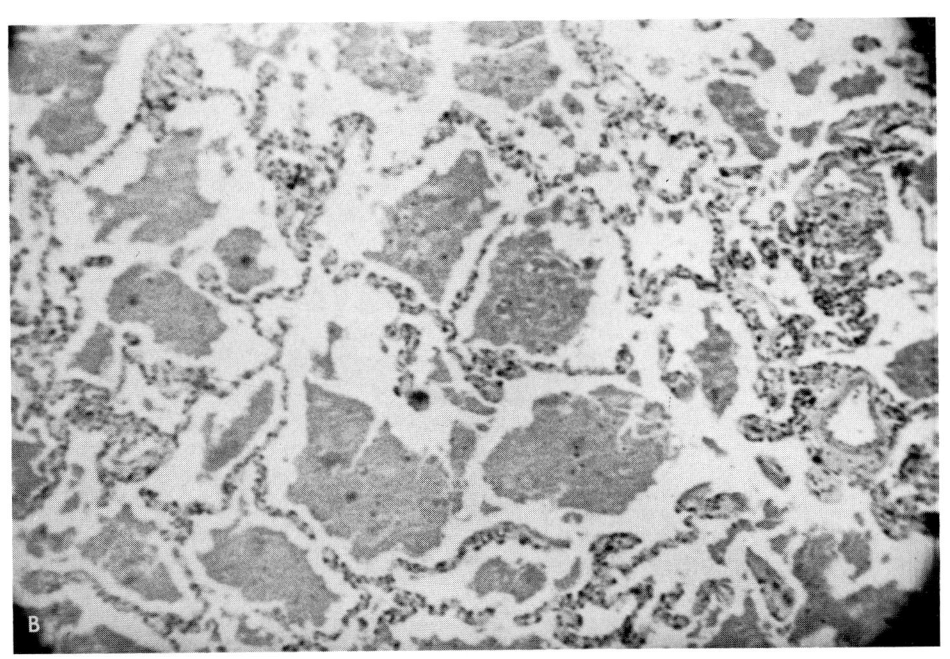

globin decreased from 26.5 to 15.8 gm/100 ml.[2136]

The diagnosis is apparent when arterial desaturation is found in a patient whose plain-chest or lateral radiograph reveals the presence of a lesion suggestive of a single fistula or multiple fistulae. In some patients, careful auscultation may reveal the presence of a murmur over the fistula, usually of maximal intensity during inspiration.[3432] Confirmation by angiocardiography is desirable, and a careful search for further lesions is mandatory before surgery is undertaken. Very few tests of pulmonary function in these patients have been reported, but the arterial P_{CO_2} is known to be normal,[17] and there was no abnormality of inert-gas distribution, diffusing capacity, or ventilatory ability in two cases we have studied. Presumably the lung mechanics are normal, and dyspnea is not a feature.

Less common, and much more difficult to diagnose, is the condition of pulmonary telangiectasia, in which normal alveoli are replaced by large capillary sinusoids. We have reported such a case diagnosed during life;[1553] this patient had considerable arterial unsaturation although there was no single arteriovenous fistula in the lungs. Similar cases, all associated with "juvenile" liver cirrhosis and telangiectasia, have been reported by others.[1735–1737]

In a recently reported case, the skin telangiectasia only appeared in later life.[3435] In one case there was an associated cerebral AV fistula,[3434] and the risk of brain abscess as a complication of pulmonary AV fistulae in children is stressed by a number of authors.[3437]

It is important to differentiate this entity; the clinical picture and pattern of function-test disorder is similar to that seen in patients with a single arteriovenous fistula, but no likely lesion is visible on the chest film and no shunt can be seen on angiography. A further point of confusion is that, in generalized pulmonary telangiectasia, as we noted in our patient,[1553] the arterial oxygen saturation may reach 100 per cent on oxygen-breathing, which does not occur in association with single large shunts. This observation was confirmed by Rydell and Hoffbauer in their similar patient, in whom arterial saturation increased from 73 per cent to 100 per cent on oxygen-breathing; the pathological findings, which were most carefully described, included multiple small shunts in the periphery of the lungs, with formation of capillary sinusoids.[1737]

ENDOCRINE DISORDERS

MYXEDEMA

The fact that serious hypercapnia may occur in myxedema coma, as noted in the section on respiratory failure (*see* page 462), was reported by Nordqvist and his associates.[1199] Of equal importance was the finding by Wilson and Bedell of significant elevation of arterial CO_2 tension in 5 obese patients with myxedema.[1765]

More recently, considerable hypoventilation has been reported in severe myxedema,[3439] with a suggestion of lowered CO_2 sensitivity possibly due to respiratory center involvement in addition to changes in thoracic muscles.[3438] As a result of the extensive studies in myxedema by these authors, a clear picture can be drawn of the pulmonary function defect in this condition. The vital capacity is reduced, probably as a result of interference with chest-muscle action; other subdivisions of lung volume, inert-gas mixing, and ventilatory capability are usually normal or nearly so. The pulmonary diffusing capacity, as measured by the single-breath technique ($D_{LCO}SB$) is often strikingly reduced. In 13 nonobese patients the $D_{LCO}SB$ before treatment averaged only 68 per cent of the predicted value, but increased to 93 per cent after treatment of the myxedema.[1765] The reader is referred to this excellent clinical study of myxedema for a discussion of the probable reasons for this decrease in diffusing capacity.

THYROTOXICOSIS

Although dyspnea on effort is the commonest symptom of thyrotoxicosis,[1766] there have been relatively few attempts to explain its origin in terms of alterations in function. Possibly it has been assumed that the alteration in metabolism is an explanation in itself, though the increment in resting basal oxygen uptake in this disease is quite insufficient to explain the hyperventilation commonly observed during exercise in thyrotoxic patients. In fact the oxygen uptake increment in relation to external work load is little different in thyrotoxicosis compared with the normal state.[1717, 3440] The high cardiac output on exercise in these patients has been well documented,[1717] the arterial–mixed-venous oxygen difference being narrower than normal. Bishop,

Donald, and Wade did not find definite evidence of hyperventilation in relation to oxygen uptake in their five patients with thyrotoxicosis;[1717] but Stein, Kimbel, and Johnson clearly documented a higher minute ventilation with a lower oxygen extraction ($\dot{V}O_2/\dot{V}E$) in hyperthyroid patients on exercise.[1767] This accords with our own experience of exercise studies in such patients.[3440] The hyperventilation on exercise cannot be explained by an abnormal sensitivity to CO_2 in thyrotoxicosis, since there is no evidence that this occurs and since Valtin and Tenney recorded no increase in CO_2 sensitivity in hyperthyroidism induced experimentally.[1768] Indeed, their data reveal that such a condition is, if anything, associated with a rise of a few millimeters in alveolar CO_2 tension.

Using the single-breath diffusing capacity ($D_{LCO}SB$), Stein and his co-workers observed that the resting levels in patients with thyrotoxicosis were low in relation to the considerably elevated resting cardiac output they had, but noted little change in this after therapy.[1767] Our own observations have indicated that the exercise diffusing capacity, measured by steady-state techniques, often is considerably lower than the predicted value in relation to oxygen uptake, in spite of the fact that the patient is hyperventilating and usually has a higher than normal cardiac output.[3440]

It has been known for many years that the vital capacity is lowered in thyrotoxicosis;[1] in the patients studied by Stein and his co-workers it increased from a mean value of 2.6 liters before, to 3.0 liters after treatment. This is partly due to muscle weakness, and these workers showed that both the maximal inspiratory and maximal expiratory pressures were reduced in thyrotoxicosis.[1767] They also found a considerable reduction in pulmonary compliance during the hyperthyroid state, in contradiction to the earlier report by McIlroy, Eldridge, and Stone that it was little altered in this condition.[1719] Airway resistance is normal.

All these findings taken together provide some basis for explaining the dyspnea noticed by these patients. For reasons not altogether clear, ventilation is higher than normal on exercise[3440] and there is some diminution in pulmonary compliance, so that the effort of breathing in relation to the level of external exercise undertaken will be significantly increased. Finally, there is weakness of the respiratory muscles, as part of the general muscle weakness that is characteristic of the condition, that may be reflected by a reduced vital capacity.[3440]

Werner's syndrome (Progeria of adults)

This remarkable syndrome of premature aging has been fully described, but it is difficult to know whether any unusual changes occur in the lungs. In a very completely documented case in a man aged 62, Boyd and Grant noted that death was due to lipoid pneumonia, and the autopsy report includes the statement that "the lungs were emphysematous."[1776] No pulmonary function tests were performed in this patient.

In view of the changes in pulmonary function that occur with age, it would be of great interest to know whether any of these bizarre endocrinological disorders are associated with any evidence of premature change in lung function.

Cushing's syndrome

Although some distinctive changes in the respiratory function in this condition have been claimed by Russian authors,[3441] it seems likely that these may be mostly attributed to obesity.

METABOLIC DISORDERS AND FEVER

Metabolic acidosis

Although it has been known for many years[1] that metabolic acidosis results in hyperventilation, lowering the arterial P_{CO_2} with a resultant partial restoration of the arterial pH to a more normal level, few studies have been made of the actual level of ventilation that occurs in acidotic patients. The carefully collected observations of Pauli and Reubi indicate that although in uremia there is undoubted hyperventilation, the level of this is less than would be predicted for control subjects with a similar reduction in pH, suggesting that the respiratory center adapts to the acidosis, at least in patients with chronic renal failure.[2138] There is no doubt that, in normal subjects, an acidosis due to ammonium chloride causes a

Case 54
(1) Chronic Myelogenous Leukemia; (2) Arteriosclerotic Heart Disease with Cardiac Failure; (3) Busulfan Lung

Summary of Clinical Findings. This 62-year-old charwoman was admitted to the hospital in September, 1959, complaining of fatigue, loss of weight, and a dragging feeling on the left side of the abdomen. On physical examination she was pale, the liver was palpable just below the costal margin, and the spleen extended to the level of the umbilicus. Examination of the blood revealed findings indicative of myelogenous leukemia and mild anemia. Myleran (busulfan) therapy produced a satisfactory remission in her leukemia; this treatment was continued for three years. In December, 1962, the patient was readmitted, complaining of shortness of breath, dry cough, anginal pain, loss of 50 pounds in weight and increasing weakness. Examination revealed moderate hepatomegaly and splenomegaly and a diffuse brown pigmentation of the skin. She had anemia and leukopenia, and marrow biopsy showed early myelofibrosis. A chest x-ray (*see* Figure *A*) showed clear lung fields. It was felt that the myelofibrosis and skin pigmentation represented overtreatment with Myleran, which was discontinued (Dec., 1962). She was transfused and the anemia was corrected, but she continued to complain of a dry cough and of dyspnea on exertion. A chest x-ray in April, 1963, showed a diffuse infiltration which increased considerably in degree over the next two months (*see* Figure *B*). In early April she was also found to be in mild cardiac failure, which was quickly controlled by treatment with digitalis and diuretics.

This patient has continued to show anemia necessitating transfusions. The leukemia relapses from time to time and has responded to various drugs and irradiation therapy. Myleran treatment has not been reinstituted, and corticosteroids have not been given. Dyspnea on exertion is less and the chest x-ray has shown considerable clearing (*see* Figure *C*). A summary of relevant function tests, hematological findings, and chest x-ray is shown in the table.

Radiology. In December, 1962, (*A*), the chest x-ray was normal in all respects. By May, 1963, (*B*), there had appeared moderate-sized nodular densities scattered diffusely and evenly throughout both lungs. The hila were slightly enlarged but cardiac size was unchanged. By February, 1964, (*C*), much clearing had occurred, although a few indistinct nodular densities and some fine reticulation could still be identified. The heart had undergone considerable enlargement in this relatively brief interval, suggesting the development of cor pulmonale and right heart failure.

Summary. This case illustrates the difficulty in interpreting changes in diffusing capacity in the presence of a varying degree of anemia. The diffuse pulmonary infiltration, the myelofibrosis and the skin pigmentation suggest overtreatment with Myleran. It is of interest that the x-ray changes became apparent after the development of dyspnea and the cessation of Myleran therapy.

Addendum. This patient died in May, 1964. The pathological findings in the lungs were typical of the changes reported to occur in "busulfan lung."

	VC	FRC	RV	TLC	ME%	MMFR	$FEV_{0.75}$ ×40	$D_{LCO}SS_2$	HEMOGLOBIN	HEMATOCRIT	RADIOLOGICAL PULMONARY INFILTRATION
Predicted	2.6	2.4	1.5	4.1	50	2.35	63	11.4	12–16 gm/100 ml	37–47%	
Jan. 7, 1963	2.0	2.5	2.0	4.0	35	1.88	52	7.9	6.8	21	None (Fig. *A*) (Dec. 27, 1962)
Jan. 16, 1963								10.0	9.5	30	
Jan. 22, 1963								15.0	10.4	35	
May 10, 1963								5.3	7.2	24	Marked (Fig. *B*) (May 16, 1963)
Feb. 25, 1964	1.4	3.1	2.7	4.1	32	0.86	30	6.8	7.2	22	Slight (Fig. *C*) (Feb. 24, 1964)
March 11, 1964								9.1	10.8	34	

There are minor changes in ventilatory function in keeping with slight bronchial obstruction and hyperinflation. The reduction in vital capacity may well reflect a diffuse fibrosis. The changes in the diffusion are more difficult to interpret. It would appear that the anemia is the major cause for a lowering of the diffusing capacity, since there was a return to normal with restoration of the hemoglobin by whole-blood transfusion. However, with the appearance of a diffuse infiltration as seen on x-ray there is a further decrease which is not corrected by further transfusion.

Case 54
(1) Chronic Myelogenous Leukemia; (2) Arteriosclerotic Heart Disease with Cardiac Failure; (3) Busulfan Lung

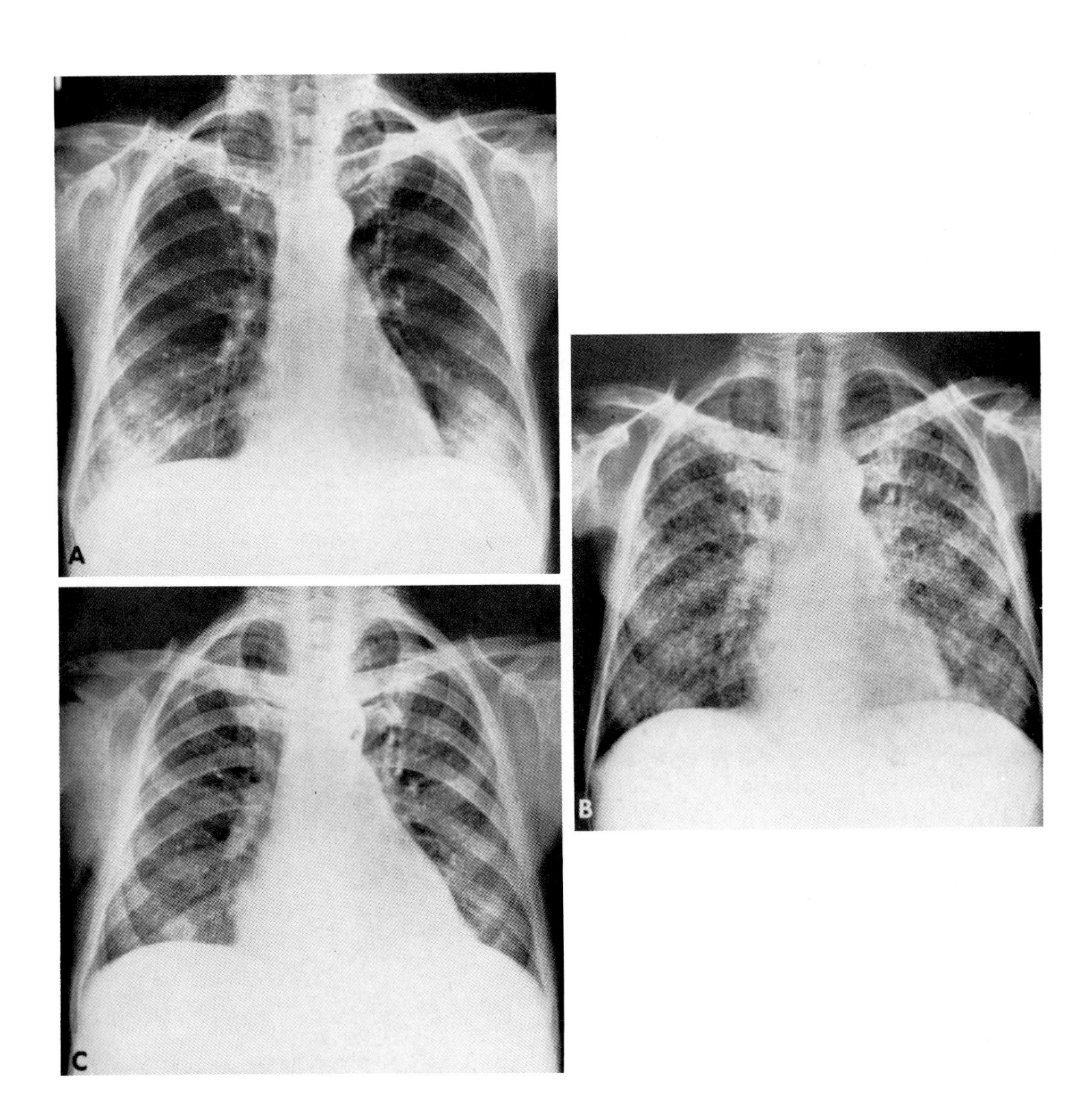

Case 55
Alveolar Microlithiasis

Clinical History and Physical Examination. This 42-year-old businessman was referred for assessment of pulmonary function in 1959. Twenty years previously he had been rejected by the armed services because of an abnormal chest x-ray. He subsequently noticed that he was slightly more dyspneic than his companions on particularly strenuous hunting trips, but he denied any increase in the severity of this symptom over the interval of 20 years. A slight dry cough was present occasionally first thing in the morning. He had never expectorated any stony material. His general health remained excellent, and he could not remember having missed a day from his work since 1937.

On physical examination, he was observed to be a slightly obese man with a florid complexion. There were no abnormal physical signs over the lungs, and no finger-clubbing was present. The cardiovascular system was similarly normal, as was the electrocardiogram.

He was seen again in 1966 and 1969. He had no respiratory symptoms and was working full-time.

In 1963, studies were made on the brother of this patient, who was also symptomless but whose x-ray was identical. The function tests on the brother were similar in all respects to those found in this patient.

Radiology. The postero-anterior view (*A*) of the chest reveals a generalized increase in the density of both lung fields, more obvious in the lower than in the upper regions. The vascular markings, although partly obscured, do not appear to be enlarged. The heart is normal in size, and no hilar or mediastinal lymph-node enlargement is present. There is no pleural effusion. The nature of the diffuse increase in density becomes apparent only when the lung pattern is examined with a magnifying glass.

The magnified view of a small area of the right upper lung (*B*) reveals multiple tiny nodular densities of uniform size, diffusely scattered throughout the lung substance. These nodules measure less than 1 mm in diameter and, in order to be seen so clearly and discretely at this magnification, must be of calcific density. Since such microliths are intra-alveolar and histologically measure only up to 1.0 mm in diameter, their radiological visibility must be due to the superimposition of many nodules. A roentgenogram in 1969 revealed the same pattern.

Analysis of Function Tests. The only significant findings are the lowered values for the FRC, RV, and TLC. Although the diffusing capacity at rest is slightly below that predicted, the normal CO extraction and exercise values indicate that this aspect of function is not disturbed. Studies of static and dynamic compliance were normal. Presumably the lowered lung volume is to be explained by the presence of microliths occupying space in the alveoli, but their presence in this patient has not resulted in any interference with air flow, gas distribution, or diffusing capacity. Repeat studies in 1966 and 1969 were essentially unchanged.

																EXERCISE				
	VC	FRC	RV	TLC	ME %	MMFR	$FEV_{0.75}$ ×40	pH	P_{CO_2}	HCO_3^-	pO_2	O_2Hb %	$D_{LCO}SS_2$	CO Ext. %	MPH	GRADE	$\dot{V}_{O_2}$	$\dot{V}_E$	$D_{LCO}SS_3$
Predicted	4.6	3.7	2.0	6.6	60	3.9	124	7.40	42	24	42	80	19.6	42					26.0
Feb. 1959	4.0	1.7	1.1	5.1	61	4.3	134	7.43	42	26			14.4	42	3	FLAT	1.2	27.7	24.3
July 1966	4.2	2.8	1.2	5.4	75	3.9	125	7.39	40	22	97	97	21.1	52					
April 1969	4.5	2.3	1.5	6.0									16.6	49					

Alveolar Microlithiasis

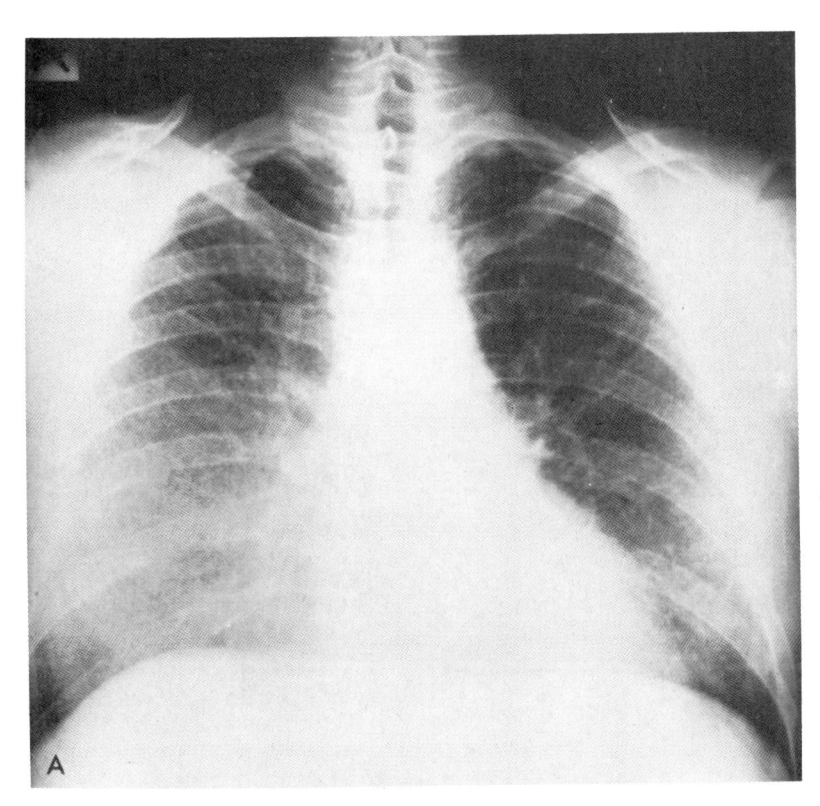

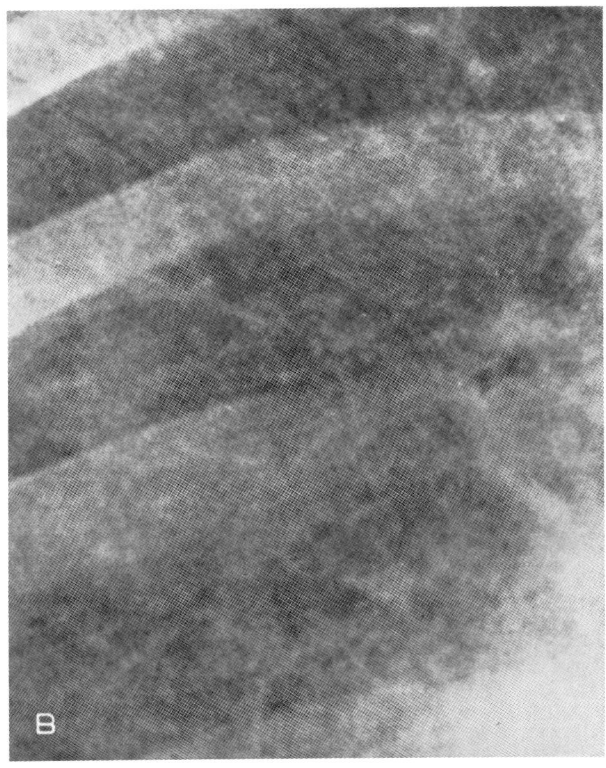

very considerable increase in ventilation during exercise.[2139] It has been demonstrated recently in dogs that sustained hypocapnia caused by mechanical hyperventilation is followed by a decrease in the bicarbonate level, but the mechanism of this secondary metabolic acidosis has not yet been elucidated. Eichenholz and his colleagues, who have reported some recent experiments of this type, point out that one can regard the metabolic acidosis with fall in bicarbonate and elevation of lactic- and pyruvic-acid levels as essentially compensatory in nature,[2141] but it is not clear how this adaptation occurs. Clinically, many complex patterns of interaction between respiratory and metabolic effects are observed. Common examples are seen in salicylate poisoning, in the respiratory failure that may occur terminally in uremia, and in the renal failure that is a not uncommon accompaniment of terminal respiratory failure.[2140]

The importance of metabolic acidosis in respiratory failure is discussed in Chapter 22.

Metabolic alkalosis

There is some conflict of evidence in relation to respiratory or ventilation changes as a result of an induced metabolic alkalosis in experimental animals. Some investigators have concluded that no depression of ventilation occurs, the arterial $P\text{CO}_2$ remaining at normal levels,[2144] whereas others find evidence for such an effect and consider that some degree of respiratory inhibition is demonstrable.[2142, 2143] There seems little doubt that, in normal man, when a metabolic alkalosis has been induced by oral administration of sodium bicarbonate, the ventilation response to breathing CO_2 mixtures is reduced.[2145] Very few data seem to exist to indicate whether this kind of change occurs normally; the arterial $P\text{CO}_2$ level was normal the only time we have had an opportunity to measure it in the presence of a severe metabolic alkalosis, when the pH was 7.58. Goldring and Heinemann have reported data suggesting that total-body hydrogen ion has to be depleted before any effect on ventilation can be observed.[2253]

Fever

Fever causes significant elevations in oxygen uptake and cardiac output, with considerable increases in alveolar ventilation,[2147] but Cander and Hanowell found that the single-breath diffusing capacity ($D_{L\text{CO}}SB$) was not increased during induced fever in man, and that the pulmonary compliance also was unaffected.[2146]

LIVER DISEASE

Cirrhosis hepatis

It has been known for many years that patients with cirrhosis of the liver may have arterial unsaturation, but it is only since the introduction of gas-tension measurements that this has been clearly attributable to a shunt between the right and left sides of the circulation. Of 28 consecutive patients with the diagnosis of liver cirrhosis investigated by Georg and his colleagues, the arterial saturation was less than 93 per cent in 14.[1738] Although few respiratory data—apart from arterial-blood studies—have been published, it is our experience that there is no abnormality of ventilation or of diffusing capacity in these patients. It is very far from clear, however, where the shunt occurs into the left side of the heart. As noted earlier (*see* page 427), in "juvenile" cirrhosis and in telangiectasia the shunt may exist at the level of the pulmonary arterioles. Careful histological studies of the lung in several cases of "adult" cirrhosis with known arterial desaturation failed to reveal any similar lesion;[1738, 1739] in other cases this was thought to be the site of the shunt.[1740] There seems little doubt that shunting may occur from the portal vein via peri-esophageal and mediastinal veins into bronchial and pulmonary veins,[1741, 1742] and in some patients this may represent the sole shunt. As Williams has observed, determination of the exact site of the shunt in these patients does not seem possible by analysis of arterial blood-gas tensions;[1743] and Rodman and his colleagues were unable to determine the site at autopsy in one patient.[1744]

However, recent studies have thrown some additional light on this problem. The elegant studies of Karlish and Berthelot[3445] and their colleagues have shown the existence of "spider naevi" in the lung, and in advanced cases these no doubt contributed significantly to the lower arterial oxygen tension. Very recently we have reported studies on patients with liver cirrhosis and lowered serum albumin[3443] which indicate that alterations in both ventilation and perfusion occur, presumably as a consequence of fluid transudation at the level of the terminal bronchiole causing airway closure. The $\dot{V}/\dot{Q}$ imbalance contributes further to lowering the P_{O_2} and it seems likely that in some patients it is the most important factor lowering the oxygen tension. There is increased CO_2 sensitivity in some of these patients,[3446] and the increased ventilation has also been linked to the hyponatremia.[3447]

Cotes and his co-workers[3444] found impairment of pulmonary function after portacaval anastomosis, attributing this to precapillary pulmonary vasodilation.

Ascites

As would be expected, the presence of ascites causes a reduction in total lung capacity and a slight decrease in functional residual capacity, with a slight to moderate decrease in maximal breathing capacity.[2148] These changes are similar to those that occur in pregnancy, although usually at full term there is a more significant change in total lung capacity than is commonly encountered as a result of ascites. It must be assumed that ascites will produce impairment of ventilation to dependent lung zones as does obesity, with resulting airway closure and significant $\dot{V}/\dot{Q}$ abnormality, particularly at low tidal volumes.

Hepatic coma

Vanamee and his co-workers have pointed out that in hepatic coma the arterial P_{CO_2} is not uncommonly lower than normal and that the pH may be elevated.[1778] They have suggested that ammonium compounds may stimulate respiration, resulting in production of a respiratory alkalosis in these patients. Renzetti, Harris, and Bowen, however, studied the effect of intravenous administration of 2 M glycine in nine patients, and concluded that "elevating the concentration of ammonia in the blood to as high as 500 μg/100 ml does not stimulate respiration and may depress it perhaps by changing the pH within chemosensitive cells toward alkalinity."[2149] It seems clear that the reduced arterial P_{CO_2} level in hepatic coma cannot be attributed to the effects of ammonia, and its mechanism of production is obscure. As noted earlier, the increased CO_2 sensitivity in his condition has been documented.[3446]

TRACHEAL STENOSIS

Several authors have commented on the functional consequences of tracheal obstruction, but the largest series of cases of tracheal stenosis is that of 20 patients observed by Castillon du Perron and his colleagues.[2150] Administration of bronchodilators to their patients did not reduce the degree of obstruction, but the authors conclude that the abnormality is indistinguishable on spirographic evidence from more common forms of airway obstruction. We have seen only two patients who in adult life had a severe degree of tracheal stenosis; in one of these, who is described in Case 56, there were several features that indicated the site of the obstruction and the absence of pulmonary emphysema, although chronic hypercapnia was present. Simonsson and Malmberg[3449] have noted that a low $FEV_{1.0}$ with a *normal* single-breath alveolar nitrogen test were features of two cases of tracheal stenosis, one due to aortic aneurysm and the other to a thymoma, that they studied. Jordanoglou and Pride[3448] were able to distinguish a case of tracheal stenosis from emphysema and asthma on the basis of analysis of inspiratory and expiratory flow curves.

One distinct form of tracheal obstruction is that due to an abnormal vascular ring round the trachea,[3450] and several cases of this anomaly have been described in which there was considerable effort dyspnea.[2151] It is of interest that in none of these does morphological emphysema seem to have developed as a consequence of many years of major tracheal obstruction.

FUNCTIONAL DISORDERS

Respiration in anxiety disorders; chronic hyperventilation syndrome

In 1935 one of us reported on the different patterns of breathing commonly encountered in patients with different types of anxiety

(Text continued on page 440.)

Case 56
Tracheal Stenosis

Summary of Clinical Findings. This 38-year-old man was admitted to another hospital in 1961 for hypertension, when he was noted to have a hoarse voice and gave a history of an injury to his larynx at the age of 9 years, caused by falling over the handle of a wheelbarrow. He complained of shortness of breath. He stated that his exercise ability had always been limited compared with that of others of similar age, and that his throat was frequently dry, stimulating an unproductive cough. There was no history of respiratory infection. Examination then revealed a slightly obese (85 kg) hypertensive (BP 160/120 mm Hg) male with a hoarse voice and with audible stridor over his trachea. The breath sounds were slightly diminished at the apices, but elsewhere air entry was good. There were no other physical findings and there was no finger-clubbing. An otolaryngologist described the vocal cords as paralyzed in abduction so that there was a small airway. During this admission the hemoglobin was found to be 18.2 gm/100 ml and the hematocrit 52 per cent.

This patient was first seen here in May, 1961, when he was referred to the Royal Victoria Hospital as an outpatient for one day of respiratory investigation, on the basis of which it was felt that there was minimal, if any, parenchymal lung disease. The elevated P_{CO_2} was felt to be due to hypoventilation consequent upon the longstanding laryngeal obstruction. A tracheal reconstruction operation was advised. In June, 1961, a tracheostomy was performed elsewhere. He improved symptomatically, although the FEV measured through the tracheostomy tube had not increased. We have not seen him since.

Radiology. The chest is unremarkable in appearance (*A*). The lungs do not appear to be particularly overinflated. There is slight fullness in the region of the pulmonary conus.

An AP tomogram of the trachea taken in full inspiration (*B*) in the region of the thoracic inlet reveals a sharp indentation in its left lateral wall with an outpouching of similar magnitude directly opposite on the right lateral wall. This "kink" is quite localized and on this view would not appear to reduce the caliber of the trachea to any gross degree. Cinefluorographic studies of the airway were not performed.

Summary. Tracheal obstruction consequent upon a laryngeal injury at the age of 9 appeared to have resulted in chronic hypoventilation but not in changes characteristic of pulmonary emphysema. The considerable increase in ventilatory ability while breathing 80 per cent helium in oxygen is characteristic of large-airway (turbulent flow) obstruction, and helped to confirm the probable site of the increased airway resistance.

	VC	FRC	RV	TLC	ME %	MMFR	$FEV_{0.75}$ ×40	pH	P_{CO_2}	HCO_3^-	O_2Hb %	$D_{Lco}SS_2$	CO Ext. %	EXERCISE MPH	GRADE	$\dot{V}_{O_2}$	$\dot{V}_E$	$D_{Lco}SS_3$
Predicted	5.0	4.0	2.2	7.2	60	4.0	129	7.40	42	25	97	20.0	46					26.2
May 1961	3.3	4.3	2.8	6.1	45	1.2	46	7.34	57	28	91	15.1	41	1	FLAT	1.02	19.5	24.2

	BREATHING AIR	BREATHING 80% HELIUM, 20% OXYGEN	
Compliance: Static	0.150		
Dynamic	0.094	0.107	l/cm H_2O
$FEV_{0.75}$ × 40	46	66	l/min
MMFR	1.18	1.78	l/sec
Airway resistance	16.6	12.5	cm H_2O/l/sec
Vital capacity	3.3	3.3	liters

Radioactive xenon studies showed a normal distribution of ventilation and perfusion in this man except for a slight reduction in ventilation to the right lower zone. Quiet ventilation at rest showed an oxygen uptake of 0.4 l/min and a minute volume of 6.7 l/min. The ratio of the $O_2/\dot{V}_E$ was 6.02, and this high figure confirms the presence of resting hypoventilation. The normal exercise diffusing capacity and xenon studies exclude the presence of significant morphological emphysema. The improvement in ventilatory ability on 80 per cent helium indicates that the tracheal "kink" is very likely to be the site of the airway obstruction.

Case 56
Tracheal Stenosis

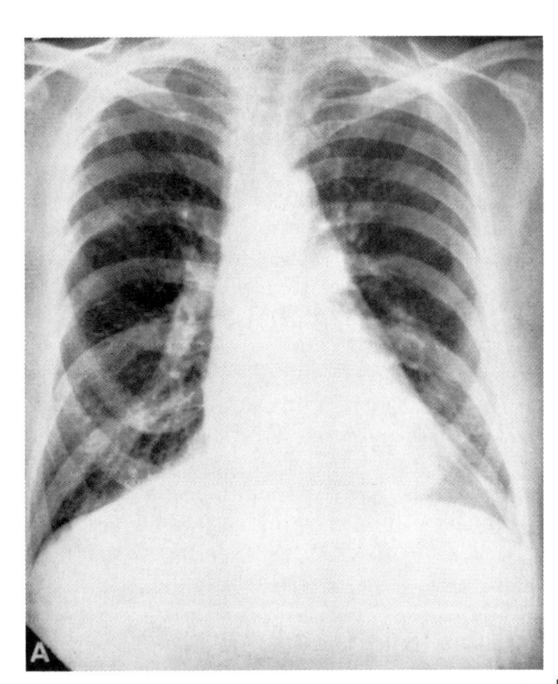

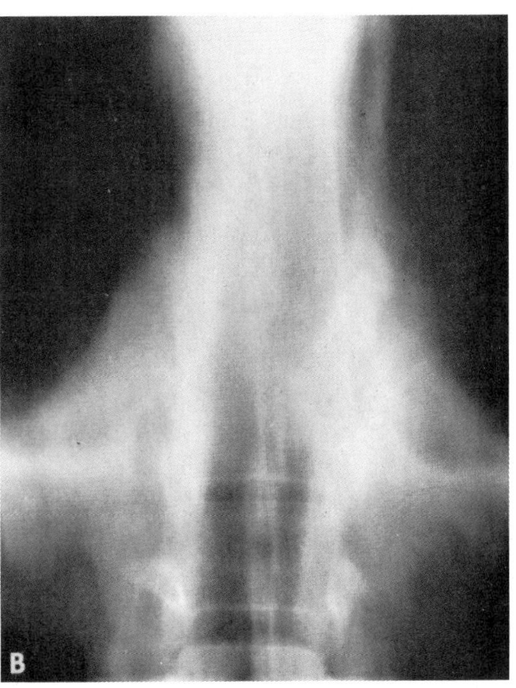

neuroses.[1758] Such patients tend to breathe with an irregular pattern, frequent changes in baseline level, intermittent deep sighing respirations, and occasionally definite resting hyperventilation. To these observations, Bülow has added the interesting note that such patients may record an impaired maximal breathing capacity when this is measured over a 15- to 20-second period, whereas the ventilatory capacity measured from a single expiration may be normal.[1759] In such patients, all measurements of respiratory function that are independent of their voluntary effort, such as compliance, inert-gas distribution, and diffusing capacity, are found to be normal. Several recent reviews of this condition have appeared,[3451, 3456] and it has been stated that these patients are abnormally sensitive to CO_2.[3452]

The clinical features of patients suffering from chronic hyperventilation have been reviewed by Lewis, although he makes no mention of the usefulness of a measurement of the arterial blood gases in this condition.[1760] We have studied one patient in whom the demonstration of a low bicarbonate level in arterial blood, in the absence of any cause for a metabolic acidosis, pointed toward such a diagnosis, and others in whom the normality of this figure suggested that the episodes of hyperventilation were only transient. There is considerable uncertainty about the extent to which the symptomatology of chronic hyperventilation can be accounted for by the lowered arterial CO_2 tension. As a result of experiments on normal subjects, Saltzman and his colleagues concluded that lowering of the arterial-CO_2 tension to 22 mm Hg was not accompanied by symptoms, but no tests of psychomotor or motor performance were included.[1627] It should be remembered, however, that acute attacks of hysterical hyperventilation, leading to a similar fall in the level of alveolar P_{CO_2}, may be associated with a severe respiratory alkalosis and all of the physical signs of tetany.[1758]

Vasoregulatory asthenia

The findings during detailed studies of circulation in this condition, reported by Holmgren and his colleagues,[1761, 1762] justify its consideration as a separate entity from that of chronic hyperventilation. They found that during physical work patients with this condition had an unusually high cardiac output, resulting in a much narrower difference between mixed-venous and arterial oxygen content than is found in normal subjects. Thus the tachycardia constantly noted in these patients represents an actual increase in cardiac output disproportionate to the exercise work load. At the same time there was a tendency for these patients to show an increased ventilation in relation to oxygen uptake, although not all of them were found to have a significant decrease in arterial CO_2 tension. Of particular interest was the demonstration that, after the patients had received physical training, all of these values returned toward normal.[1762–1764]

The mechanism involved in this syndrome seems quite obscure. The authors attribute their findings to "an inadequate regulation of peripheral blood flow at rest and during work (apparent as an abnormally low arterio-venous oxygen difference),"[1763] but it is not clear precisely why or how this occurs.

RESPIRATORY FAILURE

CHAPTER

22

INTRODUCTION AND DEFINITIONS

It is not an exaggeration to claim that the advances made in the last six years in the treatment of respiratory failure are much greater than those that have occurred in relation to cardiac or renal failure. In 1964, when the first edition of this book was published, relatively few centers had equipment or trained staff for the special care of those with respiratory failure, the rational basis of controlled oxygen therapy was not understood, and little attention had been focused on the respiratory failure that is now known to occur in patients with shock or who are severely burned. Furthermore, the occurrence of atelectasis not visible on an x-ray, although known to occur, had not been studied in detail and its mechanism was unknown. Although obesity, mild chronic bronchitis, and abdominal distention, particularly in the elderly patient, were known to be particular hazards, the precise reasons for this were not known.

Much of the chapter on respiratory failure in the first edition was therefore taken up with emphasis on the importance of early diagnosis and of active treatment once a dangerous degree of hypercapnia had occurred. A very important re-orientation in this field was pioneered in 1967 by Campbell,[3791] who pointed out that the extreme hypercapnia reported by many was a consequence of uncontrolled oxygen administration. If the patient is breathing air, it is not possible for the P_{CO_2} to be much above 80 mm Hg in order for the P_{O_2} to be compatible with life. He developed the Venturi mask, which permits 28 or 35 per cent oxygen to be delivered, and showed that, for many patients, careful management of the inspired oxygen tension permitted the respiratory failure to be successfully treated without recourse to mechanical ventilation and tracheostomy. A second area of advance has been the recognition that the main—and an important— manifestation of respiratory failure may be a lowered arterial oxygen tension without significant hypercapnia. This has been shown to be the case in asthma (*see* Chapter 5), but it also occurs in patients in shock. In some patients this hypoxia is followed by systemic hypotension before hypercapnia has developed.

For purposes of definition, it may be convenient to regard as cases of respiratory failure all those in whom the arterial P_{O_2} is below 60 mm Hg, *or* the arterial P_{CO_2} is above 49 mm Hg, at rest at sea level, as a consequence of impaired respiratory function. Campbell, who first suggested this definition, has referred to a Type-I category in which there is hypoxemia but a normal or even lowered arterial P_{CO_2}, and a Type-II group in which the arterial P_{CO_2} is elevated and the P_{O_2} is lowered as well.

PHYSIOLOGICAL CONSIDERATIONS OF IMPORTANCE IN THE MANAGEMENT OF RESPIRATORY FAILURE

ALVEOLAR VENTILATION

It is of the utmost importance that the physician recognize two important facts concerning alveolar ventilation: First, that it is very difficult to assess clinically—and he may too often rely on his clinical impression of this when he should not do so; and second, that a slow and insidious reduction of alveolar ventilation, from whatever cause, produces a significant fall in arterial oxygen tension before the CO_2 tension has risen greatly. This point is discussed in Chapter 2. Mithoefer and his colleagues[3724] have elegantly demonstrated the impossibility of guessing the alveolar ventilation from a clinical examination. Many clinical situations are so complex, that only the arterial P_{CO_2} can be relied upon as an indicator of alveolar ventilation, and the physician should be taught that, whenever possible, the arterial oxygen tension should be simultaneously measured, since this may be dangerously reduced in the absence of hypercapnia.

Once the baseline has been determined, serial measurements of ventilation on the ward at regular intervals may be very helpful in management. This is particularly the case in such disorders as myasthenia gravis, in which the lungs may be normal and the ventilatory capability may fluctuate over a relatively short period of time; but it is also of value in following the course of the asthmatic.

In many intensive care units, the routine measurement of minute volume and even vital capacity by the nursing staff every hour has become a common practice; elsewhere it will no doubt take many years before these measurements take their place alongside the time-honored "temperature, pulse, and respiration" measurements that used to delimit the nurses' jurisdiction. The depressive effect of many compounds such as fentanyl and meperidine is to cause a larger reduction in tidal volume than in frequency;[3767] as noted later, small-airway patency in the elderly is critically dependent on the magnitude of the tidal volume, and simple observation of frequency of respiration is far from adequate.

EFFECTS OF ANOXIA

The immediate effect of anoxia is stimulation of respiration, with an increase in the cardiac output[1434, 1435] and in renal blood flow,[1433] together with various effects on the central nervous system, which are well documented in textbooks of physiology. The adaptations to living at altitude that occur have been described in Chapter 3; these enable men to live at altitudes of 15,000 feet. Yet there can be little doubt that residence at high altitude invariably results in the development of pulmonary hypertension. If there is time for adaptation, the effects of anoxia are usually not serious, but, for reasons which are not properly understood, the rapid onset of anoxia may be followed by cardiovascular and neurological changes, with considerable elevation of circulating lactic acid. A severe and dangerous degree of acidosis may result. The complexity of the changes that occur in respiratory failure is evident. For example, Greene and Phillips have produced evidence that the metabolic consequences of hypoxia at the tissue level are made worse by the presence of epinephrine,[2159] both of which are released in response to hypercapnia. In newborn piglets, Glauser, McCance, and Widdowson found a greater reduction in glycogen in the diaphragm than in other muscles after a period of "respiratory embarrassment" induced by an atmosphere of 8 per cent O_2 and 10 per cent CO_2 for 24 hours.[2185] Another effect, of particular importance in emphysema, is the rise in pulmonary artery pressure that follows reduction of the alveolar Po_2 level.[1210]

Cross and his colleagues have recently measured the total body exchangeable-oxygen stores in both men and dogs.[3771] They found a value of about 11.0 ml per kilogram of body weight in both groups. For an average man this means a volume of only about 840 ml of oxygen is stored—enough to last about 4 minutes. In 8 patients with severe anemia, the total oxygen stores were only half that of normal subjects. The shape of the oxygen dissociation curve is such that an elevation of arterial Po_2 from 25 mm Hg to 40 mm Hg increases the O_2Hb percentage from 40 to 70 per cent, and the oxygen delivery from 200 to 500 ml/minute; thus, as Campbell points out,[3791] in terms of function such an elevation of tension, although small numerically, has a tremendous effect on tissue oxygen tension. Luft and Finkelstein have developed an excellent classification of hypoxia, which we have found very valuable for teaching purposes.[3762]

The importance of hypoxia in leading to systemic hypotension in the postoperative period has been stressed by Bendixen and his co-workers.[3788] They have documented the frequent occurrence of systemic hypotension as a result of undiagnosed hypoxia; that the reverse may occur, namely, a lowered arterial oxygen tension as a result of hypotension and shock, is noted later (*see* page 461).

EFFECTS OF CO_2

The recognition of the toxic effects of CO_2 has been partly responsible for the recent progress in the treatment of respiratory failure, and we should not forget that this is a development that stems from the laboratory rather than the bedside.

We know remarkably little of the effect of hypercapnia occurring independently of hypoxia on the cortical behavior of the normal human. Agitation, euphoria, and a loss of judgment are known features of hypoxia, and CO_2 in high enough concentration is known to be narcotic. On the single occasion when we were able to elevate the Pco_2 level from 35 mm Hg to 75 mm Hg over a period of five days in a mentally normal patient breathing 40 per cent oxygen, the main phenomena were drowsiness and inability to concentrate, together with irritability and dissatisfaction with nursing care, food, and other environmental features; inability to sleep at night; slight headache and anorexia; and a slight elevation of systemic blood pressure. The patient did not complain of dyspnea at any time, which is contrary to the experience of Patterson and his colleagues in another patient with respiratory-muscle paralysis.[2155] A dramatic change in our patient occurred when the Pco_2 level was restored to normal over a three-hour period, the patient remarking that she had felt on the preceding days as if she had had influenza. Neither the patient nor the nurses were aware of the elevation of Pco_2 level that had been allowed to occur.

These observations closely parallel those of Chapin, Otis, and Rahn, who in 1955 reported the consequences in two normal subjects of a 78-hour stay in an atmosphere of 3 per cent CO_2.[2211] Mental cloudiness and apathy, dull headache, anorexia, and inability to do mathematical computations were noted; dyspnea was absent. Each subject apparently noted the irritability of the other. It seems quite clear, therefore, that one cannot think of the cerebral effects of CO_2 in terms of narcosis only. Schaefer and his colleagues recently documented the course of adaptation to 1.5 per cent CO_2 over a period of 42 days.[2283]

Elevation of the arterial Pco_2 level leads to an increase in cerebrospinal-fluid pressure, probably caused by the increase in cerebral blood flow that develops during hypercapnia.[1211] This can be severe enough to cause papilledema,[951, 1328] which may result in the misdiagnosis of cerebrovascular accident. In the dog, both hypoxia and elevation of the arterial Pco_2 tension cause elevation of intracranial pressure independently of each other.[1212] The combined effect of hypoxia and hypercapnia is no doubt considerable. Changes in electrical activity over the brain occur in dogs when they are exposed to low concentrations of CO_2, and apparently are first evident over the frontal regions.[2328]

Of equal importance to these effects is that on the kidneys. Stone and his colleagues have shown in experimental work with dogs that inhalation of 30 per cent CO_2 in oxygen is followed by a prompt decrease in renal blood flow and severe oliguria.[1432] It seems that this, too, is more dependent upon the pH change

Case 57
Acute Respiratory Failure; ?Asthma

Summary of Clinical Findings. This 54-year-old Jewish housewife gave a three-year history of cough and expectoration and a one-year history of periodic attacks of dyspnea. She had never smoked cigarettes nor had she suffered from any allergic condition. In August, 1960, in an emergency admission because of severe bronchospasm, she required corticosteroids for relief of symptoms. The blood smear revealed a 10 per cent eosinophilia.

Three months later, one month after she had been weaned off steroids, she was readmitted in a severe asthmatic attack. For the first four days after admission she appeared to show a satisfactory response to bronchodilators. Urinalysis revealed glycosuria, albuminuria, and red and white blood cells as well as casts. Blood-sugar levels were high and the patient was started on insulin. Her peripheral blood continued to show a eosinophilia of from 9 to 20 per cent. Early on the morning of the fifth hospital day she was found unconscious, cyanosed, and barely breathing. A hypoglycemic reaction was suspected but she failed to respond to the intravenous administration of glucose. There were no localizing signs indicative of a cerebrovascular accident. Arterial blood gas analysis at 11:00 A.M. on the morning of November 25 revealed severe hypercapnia. A tracheostomy was performed and she was ventilated on a triggered respirator. Corticosteroids were given intravenously. Within 24 hours the patient was fully conscious and within 48 hours artificial respiration was discontinued. A subsequent renal biopsy showed focal glomerulonephritis. The patient was discharged on continued treatment with insulin and corticosteroids.

Between 1960 and 1964 she was admitted on five occasions for exacerbations of symptoms and in 1962 again suffered an episode of respiratory failure. On this occasion she was treated successfully without resorting to tracheostomy or endotracheal tube. There was no deterioration of renal function. She was last admitted in 1969 for a Colles fracture of the left wrist. She was still on corticosteroids but suffered one or two attacks of asthma per week. She was active although short of breath on moderate exertion. A urinalysis was normal. Pulmonary function was not studied.

Radiology. A postero-anterior roentgenogram of the chest, taken on November 24, 1960, (*A*), reveals numerous patchy and linear densities scattered throughout both lungs, more numerous on the right. The densities are generally along the vascular distribution. Neither this view nor the lateral suggested the presence of much hyperinflation. Since a chest film made a few days previously had shown clear lung fields, the changes seen here suggested an acute diffuse bronchopneumonia. A postero-anterior film made 10 days later (*B*) shows complete resolution of the diffuse pneumonia. The lungs are now clear.

A midsagittal tomogram (*C*) of both lungs shows a normal caliber of the pulmonary arterial tree. There is no peripheral vascular deficiency to suggest the presence of emphysema.

Summary. The initial clinical diagnosis was difficult in this patient, as there were several possible causes for the coma. Although the course of her illness suggested the possibility of periarteritis nodosa, this diagnosis could not be substantiated. In the absence of evidence for any other condition, this might be classified as a case of "chronic infective asthma" with acute respiratory failure.

	VC	FRC	RV	TLC	ME %	MMFR	$FEV_{0.75} \times 40$	pH	P_{CO_2}	HCO_3^-	O_2Hb %	$D_{L_{CO}}SS_2$
Predicted	2.5	2.2	1.3	3.8	55	2.6	67	7.40	42	25	97	13.5
Aug. 1960	1.4	2.7	2.4	3.8	28	0.3	19					9.9
11 A.M., Nov. 25, 1960								7.02	130	29		
8 P.M., Nov. 25, 1960								7.22	69	26		
Nov. 28, 1960								7.48	37	27	86	
Dec. 1, 1960								7.42	34	22	95	
Dec. 11, 1960												9.9

The resting studies in August revealed a severe ventilatory defect that persisted unchanged after bronchodilator therapy. The resting diffusing capacity was reduced, but the significance of this is hard to assess when ventilatory function is so limited. The severe respiratory failure in November was controlled by respirator treatment within three days. A repeat estimate of diffusing capacity after this episode showed the same result as had been obtained four months earlier.

Acute Respiratory Failure; ?Asthma

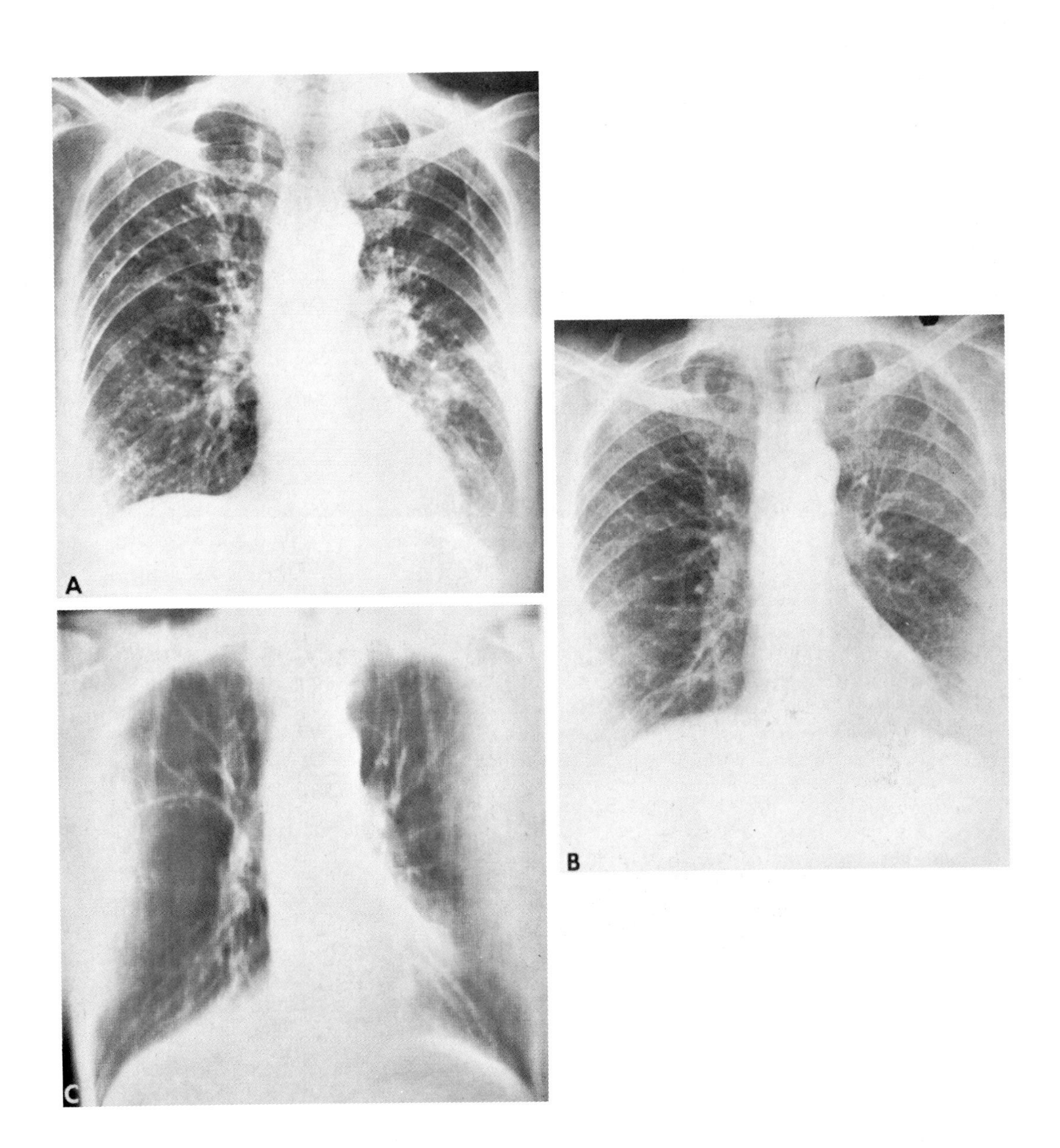

than the $P\text{CO}_2$ elevation, since Nahas found that THAM administration under these conditions leads to a prompt re-establishment of renal function, even when the $P\text{CO}_2$ level is very high.[31]

EFFECTS OF OXYGEN ADMINISTRATION

In this section, no extensive review of the literature on oxygen toxicity can be attempted.[2161] Nevertheless, it is essential that the physician be familiar with the effects of "overdose" of oxygen in exactly the same way as he is made aware of consequences of overdose of chemical compounds.

The first observable effects of oxygen on the lung, when administered as pure gas at ambient pressure, is damage to the capillary endothelium.[3797] The air–blood barrier next becomes thickened due to edema,[3757] and an increase in alveolar cells, especially the granular pneumocytes, is next observed.[3756] A decrease in surface area of alveolar capillary exposed to the air space occurs as a consequence of widening of the septum, and an increase in the number of septal (or nonalveolar) capillaries has been noted.[3756] Later stages consist in atelectasis and formation of hyaline membranes.[2166]

Normal dogs die after about 70 hours' exposure to 100 per cent oxygen at ambient pressure,[2165] the cause of death being neither hypoxia nor circulatory failure. A normal man shows a drop in diffusing capacity after varying amounts of time. These amounts were found by some observers to be three hours,[1245] by others to be nine hours,[2213] and most recently to be 30 hours of oxygen breathing.[3758] The vital capacity falls after 24 to 60 hours of oxygen breathing.[2163, 2164, 2168, 3759]

At 2 atmospheres of pressure, exposure for 6 to 11 hours causes symptoms of pulmonary irritation and significant changes in vital capacity, pulmonary compliance, and lung volumes, with no observable effect on the appearance of the chest x-ray.[3759] The safe upper limit for oxygen inhalation appears to be a pressure of about 280 mm Hg (40 per cent oxygen at average ambient pressure). Clinical cases are reported in which this limit has been exceeded, usually because the respirator delivered a far higher oxygen percentage than that indicated on the regulator dial. One such patient being treated for status epilepticus received approximately 90 per cent oxygen for 20 days. The resulting alveolar damage regressed satisfactorily as a result of slow withdrawal of oxygen over a nine-day period.[3764]

The problem of safe oxygen administration to those in danger of hypercapnia is discussed later in this chapter.

CIRCULATORY FAILURE SECONDARY TO RESPIRATORY FAILURE

Type-I respiratory failure in which hypoxemia occurs without hypercapnia may lead to a falling systemic blood pressure and also to a lowering of cardiac output. As noted earlier, this phenomenon has been observed by Bendixen and his colleagues.[3788] There is, however, relatively little information on the mechanism of this relationship, and the factors that influence it are not well understood. It seems very clear that there is the same variation in response to and tolerance of arterial hypoxemia in relation to the systemic circulation, that exists in the pulmonary response to alveolar hypoxia. A more common clinical situation is in the Type-II respiratory failure in which $P\text{O}_2$ is lowered and $P\text{CO}_2$ is elevated.

In 1915 Patterson clearly documented the effects on the heart of an elevation of CO_2 tension, the first sentence of the summary of his paper being "Carbon dioxide alone depresses all the functions of the isolated heart. . . ."[1427] He noted also that this effect was partially counteracted by epinephrine. This interaction has been carefully studied more recently by Tenney, who found that in the cat CO_2 acted as a specific stimulus to increase the circulating catecholamines.[1428] He further pointed out that the higher levels of circulating pressor substances caused by elevation of the CO_2 level might be responsible for an apparent inhibition of response to administered epinephrine.

Millar showed that a similar release occurred in dogs during artificially produced diffusion respiration or apneic oxygenation, and he concluded that, during the first 30 minutes of increase in the level of $P\text{CO}_2$, the rise was predominantly in norepinephrine. Subsequently the plasma epinephrine increased further, reaching levels of up to 30 μg/liter after 60 minutes of apnea.[1431] The extent to which these and other effects are caused by CO_2 itself, or by the fall in pH that occurs in such experiments, is not wholly settled. Nahas and his colleagues, using THAM to prevent a fall in pH, concluded that catecholamine release did not occur even at very high levels of P_{CO_2} in these circumstances.[1429, 1430] There seems little doubt, however, that the direct depressant effect on the myocardium of an elevated P_{CO_2} level is at least partly attributable to the concomitant fall in pH.[1201]

It can thus be appreciated that acute respiratory acidosis due to hypercapnia causes a depression of cardiac output. When this results in circulatory collapse and inadequate tissue perfusion, a metabolic acidosis is superimposed on the respiratory acidosis, driving the hydrogen-ion concentration still higher. It is this vicious circle of events that has to be broken if the treatment of respiratory failure is to be successful.

In patients in whom we have been unable to relieve alveolar hypoventilation, a period of severe CO_2 narcosis has been followed by a secondary fall in systemic blood pressure, and finally, and often quite quickly, by cardiac arrest. There is little information in the literature as to what constitutes a dangerous level of arterial P_{CO_2} or pH from the circulatory point of view. In our experience, however, an arterial P_{CO_2} value greater than 80 mm Hg or a pH of less than 7.2 must be considered dangerous, and means of immediate resuscitation must be available at a moment's notice for patients in whom such values have been recorded.

Other effects

Rapid changes in ventilation may be followed by shifts in electrolytes of sufficient magnitude to endanger the circulatory system. Hyperventilation of normal subjects causes an increase in serum potassium,[1213, 1231] and this increase may be considerable if a patient with marked elevation of the arterial P_{CO_2} and of bicarbonate is rapidly hyperventilated to reduce the P_{CO_2} value to normal. This maneuver can result in cardiac arrest; for this reason, when the P_{CO_2} value is very high (more than 100 mm Hg), it is safer to reduce the P_{CO_2} level to about 60 mm Hg and not to lower it further until bicarbonate has been excreted. In this way sudden marked shifts in serum potassium can be avoided.

Although it has been reported that serious convulsions may occur after therapy for alveolar hypoventilation in a few patients,[3779] we have not encountered this problem. Addington, Kettel, and Cugell observed alkalosis due to mechanical hyperventilation in 3 patients but noted that the symptoms were very easily reversed and not of a serious nature.[3789] Addis has stressed the importance of adequate bicarbonate therapy in acute exacerbations of respiratory failure,[3790] and Mithoefer and his colleagues[2621] have sucessfully managed cases of intractable asthma by giving intravenous sodium bicarbonate. They advise a single dose of 1.5 mEq/kg intravenously, and noted a dramatic recovery in a 12-year-old girl with a pH of 6.6 and a normal serum-lactic acid, using this therapy together with an endotracheal tube and assisted ventilation.

There is little doubt that prompt treatment of severe base deficit is important in all cases of respiratory failure. It is because therapy must be planned with knowledge of the blood-gas tensions and the hydrogen-ion concentration in the more severely ill patients that we feel that the physician should be taught that optimal management of such patients requires an initial analysis of a sample of arterial blood.

Noble, Trenchard, and Guz[3782] have pointed out the value of diuretics in some cases of respiratory failure. There is little doubt that these are indicated if there is any evidence of congestive heart failure, but these workers point out that the pulmonary compliance is lowered in respiratory failure and that a diuretic may break a vicious cycle of fluid retention in the lung, reduced compliance, lowered alveolar ventilation, and worsening failure.

LABORATORY AND CLINICAL DIAGNOSIS

Physicians who are unaware of the fact that accurate knowledge of respiratory failure has been attendant upon arterial blood-gas measurements and who have not made available to themselves the facilities for such determinations not uncommonly question the necessity for these in practice. An expression of such an opinion in 1962 is illustrative of some contemporary thought that we believe to be wholly misleading: "From the point of view of clinical assessment of the patient, however, arterial blood is probably not actually necessary and it is certain that multiple arterial punctures are not one hundred per cent safe. Such methods of assessment are in fact only required in cases where there is gross disorder of lung function. Where the lungs are substantially normal and there is no electrolyte upset, the determination of the carbon dioxide combining power of the venous blood in a patient, whose limb distal to the site of vein puncture is warm, will be sufficient."[1197]

Davenport has pointed out that dependence upon the measurement of CO_2 combining power as a diagnostic aid is dangerous in cases of acute respiratory failure.[29] In many departments, including our own, many hundreds of arterial punctures are performed every year without complications. The clinical signs of respiratory failure are so nonspecific that errors in diagnosis are almost certain unless arterial or mixed-venous blood-gas tensions are known. One need only consider the wide variety of conditions in which respiratory failure is known to play an important part, including thoracic injuries,[1198] myxedema coma,[1199] septicemia,[1200] and many others discussed in the last major section of this chapter, to recognize the obvious fact that facilities for precise diagnosis—which cannot depend solely upon clinical criteria—are essential in any major medical center.

In his 1967 Burns Amberson Lecture, Moran Campbell discussed the relative merits of different procedures to measure the blood-gas status of the patient. At that time he complained that "instrumentation in this field has recently run ahead of education," and he stressed that the physician must understand the basis and interpretation of whatever methods he is using. He recommended that full arterial blood analysis should be available in a teaching center and advised the use of the rebreathing P_{CO_2} as a simpler method of control. In the cases he described he noted that the measurement of blood P_{O_2} was not particularly valuable.

Recent evidence that in a variety of conditions, particularly in asthma, after myocardial infarction, and in states of shock, there may be serious depression of arterial oxygen tension without elevation of P_{CO_2} should be taken to indicate that, in a major teaching center at least, full facilities for arterial blood-gas analysis are obligatory if Type-I cases of respiratory failure are to be intelligently managed and promptly diagnosed. The recognition of cyanosis is clinically extremely unreliable;[1779] guessing the arterial oxygen tension is impossible. Fortunately the recent advances in electrode design and stability have made the routine measurement of blood-gas tensions and pH much simpler to maintain and provide on a routine basis.

Having stressed that the diagnosis of respiratory failure is primarily dependent on the laboratory and that the physician should be trained to suspect his clinical ability to diagnose respiratory failure, mention may be made of the clinical evidence of hypercapnia. Gross and Hamilton[3820] noted (in order of frequency) peripheral vasodilation and a bounding pulse, small pupils, engorged veins in the fundus, confusion and drowsiness, depressed tendon reflexes and muscular twitching, extensor plantar responses, headache, and coma in a series of 23 patients. However, the presence of any one of these signs was very poorly correlated with the level of mixed-venous P_{CO_2} that was found. Probably much depends on the rapidity with which the P_{CO_2} has risen and whether or not the patient had chronic hypercapnia for a period before the acute episode.

The clinical suspicion of Type-I respiratory failure is much less easy to describe. By the time the arterial blood pressure has fallen, serious hypoxemia has probably usually been present for some hours. Anxiety, restlessness, and fatigue may be ascribed to pain rather than hypoxemia, and these slight evidences of hypoxemia may easily be masked by the effects of a narcotic given to control the discomfort. The lowering of tidal volume by the narcotic further lowers the oxygen tension; many patients have moved quietly down this slope to a nearly irreversible situation until their condition was recognized and properly treated.

METHODS OF TREATMENT OF RESPIRATORY FAILURE

Oxygen administration

There are many papers and review articles dealing with different methods of oxygen administration. One of the most recent is a monograph published by the Scottish Health Services Council[3753] which contains an excellent and up-to-date analysis of the advantages and disadvantages of different methods of oxygen administration in a wide variety of clinical situations.

When a maximally high tension of oxygen is required, as in a patient being treated for cardiac arrest or unconscious from carbon monoxide, a face mask should invariably be used until such time as endotracheal intubation has been performed. Most of these masks effectively deliver about 60 per cent oxygen to the patient if the oxygen flow into them is at a rate of 6 liters/min. Some of these masks have an unacceptably high dead space,[3753] though it is not clear whether they lead to an elevation of P_{CO_2} as normally used.[3760] The introduction of the Venturi mask by Campbell represented a major step forward in the treatment of respiratory failure in patients with chronic lung disease.[3791] The masks commonly in use deliver 28 or 35 per cent oxygen with great reliability, using a fixed flow of oxygen.

The Venti-mask may be used in conjunction with a head tent, the oxygen entering the dome of this through a Venturi jet. Campbell and Gebbie[3792] have found this device useful for controlled oxygen therapy in patients who are intolerant of a mask.

Nasal catheters continue to be used for oxygen administration. At a flow of 1 liter of oxygen/min., these generally produce an inspired oxygen percentage of between 25 and 30 per cent; at 3 liters/min. flow, the inspired percentage approximates 36 per cent. Bethune and Collis[3781] have recently restudied this method of oxygen administration and they point out that the amount of oxygen that the patient receives is dependent on whether he is breathing through his nose or his mouth. The Venti-mask is generally preferable to the nasal catheter if enriched oxygen is indicated.

Oxygen tents provide concentrations varying between 25 and 50 per cent, depending on how recently the tent was opened. In our opinion they suffer from the major disadvantage that the patient is too removed from close, minute-to-minute observation, and for this reason they have little place in an intensive-care ward.

Tracheostomy and Endotracheal Intubation

The introduction by Campbell of controlled oxygen therapy has greatly reduced the number of tracheostomies performed on patients with chronic respiratory disease and acute respiratory failure. Since these patients constitute a large fraction of those being treated in intensive-care units, the introduction of more conservative management procedures has reduced significantly the number of tracheostomies considered necessary. In our own respiratory intensive-care unit, 143 tracheostomies were performed in treating 149 episodes of respiratory failure up to 1964, whereas in 1967 and 1968, only 19 tracheostomies were required in treating 60 episodes of failure in a comparable group of patients. The total mortality over the two periods for all cases was 44 per cent up until 1964 and 40 per cent since 1968.

There is still much discussion of the indications for endotracheal intubation versus tracheostomy.[3763] In our opinion, the prime indication for tracheostomy is for the sake of tracheal toilet and in cases in which assisted ventilation is clearly indicated after failure to respond to controlled oxygen administration. Endotracheal intubation is ideal in the unconscious patient and may be tolerated for several days in the conscious patient. Secretions are, however, less easily removed by this method than through a tracheostomy,[3763] and, in our experience, restlessness and movement by the patient not uncommonly necessitate removal of an endotracheal tube. Particular attention must be given to possible collapse of the left lung induced by a malpositioned endotracheal tube.[3786]

There have been several advances in the design of tracheostomy tubes fitted with inflatable cuffs.[3795] Divergent figures continue to be published on the complications of tracheostomy. McLelland analyzed 389 tracheostomies in 1965[3761] and reported that 252 of these had complications of one sort or another, and 13 deaths (3.4 per cent) were considered to be directly ascribable to the tracheostomy. The mechanical complications of tracheostomy have been excellently analyzed by Clarke,[3794] and Grillo[3801] has recently reported the successful treatment by resection of 10 out of 13 patients with tracheal stenosis consequent upon tracheostomy. This, the most serious long-term complication, is caused by pressure erosion and repair by cicatrization. It is evident that the indications for tracheostomy in particular patients must be clear to the physician and surgeon; when these indications are present,

Case 58
Clinical Emphysema; Acute Respiratory Failure

Summary of Clinical Findings. This 65-year-old man was first admitted to hospital on October 20, 1960, complaining of severe shortness of breath. He had had a chronic cough for 15 years, with frequent episodes of nocturnal dyspnea for the last two years. These symptoms had been treated with bronchodilators and with digitalis. Two days before admission his shortness of breath had increased greatly, and on admission he was orthopneic and cyanotic. He also complained of left-sided chest pain. His temperature was 102° F, his pulse rate 120 per minute, and respiration rate 28 per minute. There was jugular vein distention and pitting edema of his ankles. The chest was increased in the AP diameter and was hyperresonant. Breath sounds were reduced at both bases and diffuse rhonchi and moist rales were heard.

In the Emergency Department he was thought to be in acute pulmonary edema and was given oxygen and morphine. On admission to the ward, he was noted to be drowsy. Five hours after admission, a second injection of morphine was given to relieve the severe left-sided pain. Four hours later, he was unconscious, and the first arterial blood sample was drawn. This revealed a pH of 7.09 and a P_{CO_2} of 100 mm Hg (*see* Figure D). Tracheostomy was performed, and thick purulent sputum was aspirated from the trachea. The patient was placed on an Engström respirator and penicillin therapy was started. Although the P_{CO_2} decreased to about 70 mm Hg over the next two days, the patient's general condition deteriorated, with persistent high fever and tachycardia. Two days later he was started on chloramphenicol and intravenous cortisone and began to improve.

On discharge he was not orthopneic and could walk without marked dyspnea. The arterial blood was normal. Pulmonary function tests indicated chronic ventilatory impairment and a lowered diffusing capacity.

He was readmitted in August, 1961, with an exacerbation of his chronic symptoms. On this occasion, he responded quickly to antibiotics and bronchodilators, and respiratory assistance was not required.

Over the next two years the patient gradually deteriorated. He was readmitted on several occasions for exacerbations of symptoms. His dyspnea became more severe and the congestive failure more difficult to control. He had difficulty adhering to a medical regime and continued to smoke heavily.

His final admission was in August, 1963. He was in severe congestive failure and did not respond to treatment. He died suddenly on August 17th. Autopsy was not performed.

Radiology. An anteroposterior projection of the chest made at the bedside with the patient supine (*A*) reveals numerous ill-defined patchy densities scattered widely throughout both lung fields. There is little evidence of hyperinflation. A tracheostomy tube has been inserted. The lung changes are consistent with, but not diagnostic of, acute diffuse bronchopneumonia.

Postero-anterior and lateral views of the chest made a few weeks later (*B* and *C*), after recovery from the acute episode, show clearing of the diffuse disease seen originally. Hyperinflation is present but is not severe. The hila are clearly enlarged, and although the peripheral vessels of the lungs are not obviously reduced in number or caliber, the discrepancy between hilar and peripheral arterial size suggests the presence of moderately severe pulmonary arterial hypertension. The heart is only slightly enlarged.

Summary. In this patient, an acute respiratory infection with a left-sided pleurisy was misdiagnosed as acute pulmonary edema. Treatment with oxygen and morphine precipitated him into acute respiratory failure from which he was rescued with difficulty after several days of respirator care.

Clinical Emphysema; Acute Respiratory Failure

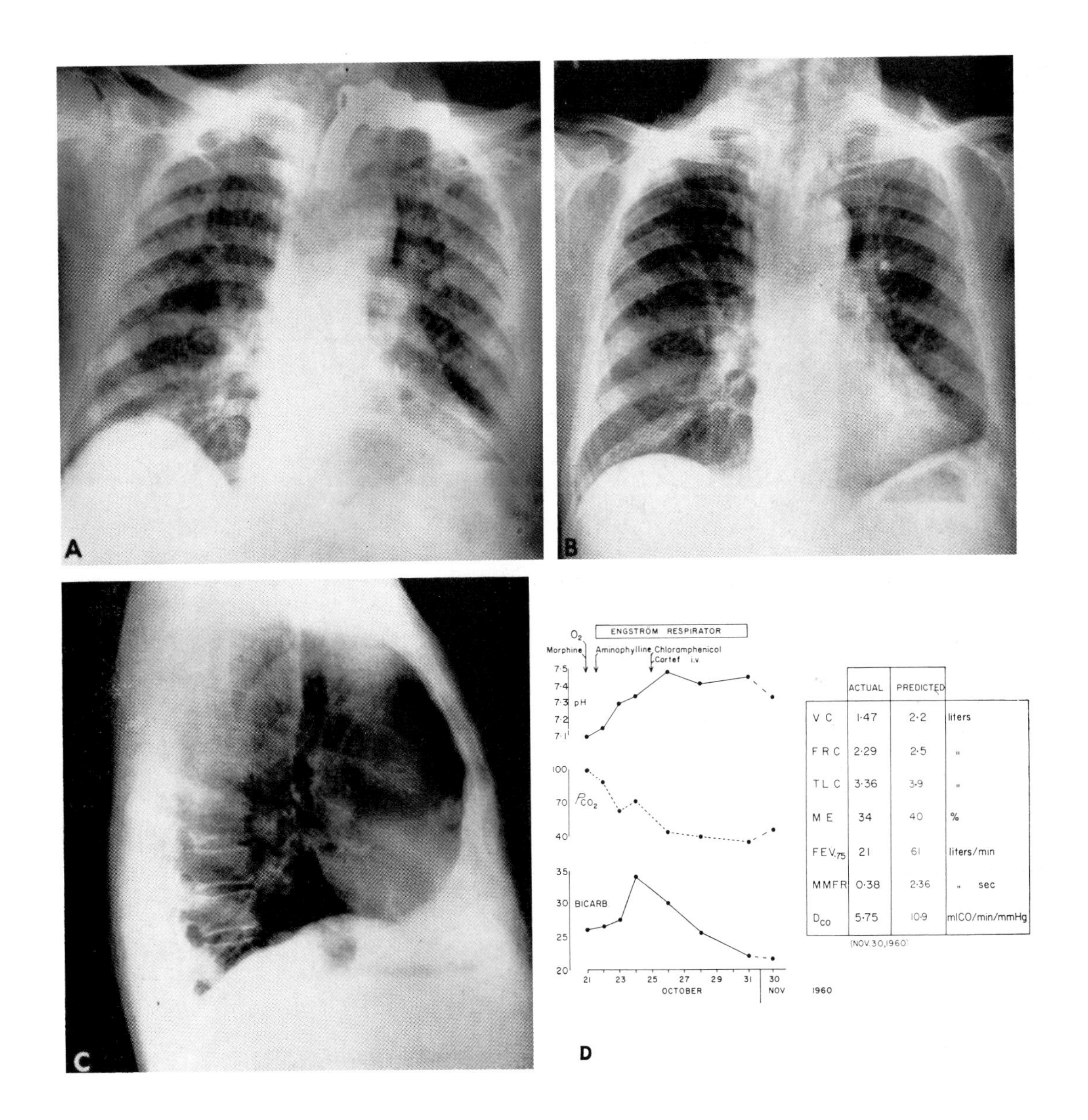

	ACTUAL	PREDICTED	
V C	1·47	2·2	liters
F R C	2·29	2·5	"
T L C	3·36	3·9	"
M E	34	40	%
$FEV_{.75}$	21	61	liters/min
MMFR	0·38	2·36	" sec
D_{CO}	5·75	10·9	mlCO/min/mmHg

(NOV. 30, 1960)

however, the possibility of complications should not, in our opinion, deter them from advising tracheostomy. The reduction in the number of tracheostomies required is a direct reflection of a better understanding by physicians of the physiological basis of treatment of respiratory failure—an advance that can be dated from Moran Campbell's paper in 1967.[3791] The indications for tracheostomy in patients with chronic respiratory disease are discussed in the next section (*see* page 453).

Assisted ventilation

A complete review of respirator equipment is beyond the scope of this volume; nevertheless, some changes in outlook in this field have occurred since 1964 and these may be noted. Many patients can be successfully managed on either a volume-cycled or a pressure-cycled respirator, and most intensive-care units have both types of equipment available. The design and cost of volume-cycled respirators have changed considerably over the past few years, and these respirators are now simpler to use, easier to maintain, and much less costly than was formerly the case. The pressure-cycled respirator can be successfully used in many clinical situations, but the unconscious patient and the patient more or less completely paralyzed may be more comfortably and safely managed on a volume respirator. The physician and anesthetic staff usually have little difficulty selecting which types of respirator they propose to use, and in most instances it is wise to choose one of each type.

With well-trained nursing supervision, patients may be managed successfully for many days on these machines. Whitehouse and Petty have recently described a patient with paralysis for 266 days, who eventually recovered following successful maintenance in a modern intensive-care unit.[3800]

Use of bicarbonate buffer

As noted earlier, the prompt administration of bicarbonate in some clinical situations of extreme acidemia may be life-saving. The staff of an intensive-care unit must be trained in the technique of administration and the necessary materials must always be available.

Respiratory stimulants

Over the past five years, there has been a steady decrease in enthusiasm for the use of respiratory stimulants in the treatment of respiratory failure. Cherniack and Young[3793] reported that ethamivan was of value in the treatment of barbiturate poisoning but not useful in emphysema and obesity, the increase in ventilation being negated by the associated increase in metabolism and CO_2 production attributable to the drug. Edwards and Leszczynski[3785] reported a double-blind trial of five respiratory stimulants and concluded that doxapram was the most effective and nikethamide the least useful in lowering the P_{CO_2}.

MANAGEMENT OF RESPIRATORY FAILURE

General principles

The management of respiratory failure consists of decisions made consecutively as the progress of the patient is closely observed. Moran Campbell[3791] has described the sequence of decisions commonly followed when controlled oxygen therapy is employed in the treatment of a patient with chronic respiratory disease. These may be broadened to cover other conditions, and in our experience the course of events may be usefully divided into the following stages:

1. *Establishing the diagnosis and status of the patient.* A first necessity is accurate diagnosis and a clear knowledge of whether the main problem is hypoxia or hypercapnia or both. An arterial-blood analysis for the degree of saturation, P_{O_2}, P_{CO_2}, and pH is essential at this stage. Careful clinical examination and a chest x-ray also are obligatory, together with information on the electrolyte balance and other biochemical data. Recent medication must be reviewed carefully; not infrequently the administration of a respiratory depressant may have precipitated the failure. If conscious, the patient should be encouraged to expectorate and cough. In many cases, medication with digitalis and diuretics will be indicated. Patients with chronic lung disease should usually start treatment with antibiotics, on the assumption that the respiratory failure was precipitated by an episode of

infection. Careful assessment of the situation as a whole should include evaluation of prognosis, and a tentative decision should be made as to the lengths to which therapy should be extended to assure adequate ventilation; for instance, if there is any contraindication to assisted ventilation, it should be decided at this stage not to proceed to tracheostomy and assisted ventilation, regardless of the P_{CO_2} level.

2. *Controlled oxygen administration.* If practical, the patient should be encouraged to cough and clear as much secretion from the chest as possible. The vital capacity and resting ventilation should be carefully recorded at this stage, and controlled oxygen administration may be started with a Venti-mask. A careful reassessment of the patient at least every hour is required so that the inspired oxygen may be adjusted and, if necessary, increased, and the effect on the P_{CO_2} may be observed.

3. *Assisted ventilation.* If controlled oxygen is not maintaining an adequate level of oxygenation, or the level of total ventilation is observed to be declining with a rising P_{CO_2}, assistance to ventilation may be given with a triggered respirator and mask. The effect of this must be most closely observed, since ventilation may, on occasion, decrease as a result of initiation of this treatment. If deterioration continues, it will be necessary to consider the following stage.

4. *Endotracheal intubation or tracheostomy.* In some cases of status asthmaticus, full ventilatory control may be necessary to achieve an adequate ventilation, and full control may be evidently necessary in cases of barbiturate or CO poisoning from the first moment that the patient is seen. If thick secretions are present, it is usually wiser to advise tracheostomy than endotracheal intubation; if the lungs are clear and the patient unconscious (as in barbiturate poisoning), an endotracheal tube will be the preferred method of treatment.

In general terms there are, we believe, two absolute indications for assisted ventilation in cases of respiratory failure. These are (1) when the condition from which the patient is suffering is known to be potentially completely reversible—as, for example, bronchial asthma, chest injuries, etc., and (2), when the respiratory failure, of whatever origin, has been precipitated by the administration of respiratory depressants. In general, all patients seen for the first time when they are in severe respiratory failure (as often happens) should be actively treated. Exceptions to this are the very old and, usually, those patients known to have advanced emphysema and who have been disabled for years. The only invariable contraindication to assisted ventilation for respiratory failure is the presence of advanced incurable disease. Thus, it is, we feel, obviously an error of judgment to assist ventilation when respiratory failure occurs as a result of cerebral metastases. In spite of these considerations, assisted ventilation will be begun in some such cases, and only later may it become evident that there is no prospect of recovery of cortical activity.

SPECIAL PROBLEMS

Chronic lung disease

As we noted in 1965, the general mortality for the treatment of respiratory failure in patients with chronic bronchitis and emphysema with an acute exacerbation is approximately 50 per cent. This figure does not seem to have varied much over the past few years, though it may have fallen slightly. In our own ward, the mortality in these patients was 46 per cent between 1958 and 1964 and 47 per cent in 1967 and 1968. Cullen and Kaemmerlen[3802] have reported a 30-day mortality of 36 per cent in these patients, with most of the deaths occurring in the first four days, half of them from causes other than ventilatory failure. A number of authors have reported their experiences with controlled oxygen therapy. Most recently, Bedon, Block, and Ball[3755] confirmed the usefulness of this technique in two groups of patients. In 21 ambulatory patients, the 28 per cent mask elevated the arterial P_{O_2} from a mean of 62 mm Hg to a mean of 74 mm Hg. In 23 more severely ill patients, the arterial P_{O_2} before treatment was 32 mm Hg and rose to 45 mm Hg with use of the Venturi mask. They note that this mask may not achieve an adequate level of oxygenation in some patients in their most severely ill group, and higher inspired-oxygen tensions are required. The arterial P_{CO_2} rose from a pretreatment mean of 63 mm Hg to 66 mm Hg after about an hour of treatment. These authors state however, "If P_{aO_2} of 40 mm Hg and a saturation of 70 per cent are necessary to prevent hypoxic tissue dam-

Case 59
?Pulmonary Edema—?Cor Pulmonale

Summary of Clinical Findings. This 64-year-old man was admitted to hospital in severe respiratory distress. He gave a history of persistent chronic cough with expectoration of one to two ounces of mucoid material per day for many years. Slight dyspnea on exertion had been present for three years, but this symptom had become much more noticeable during the three-week period before admission. Physical examination revealed an orthopneic, apparently cyanosed man with diffuse wheezing over both lungs and some basal rales. The jugular venous pressure was increased and there was slight pitting edema of the ankles. The heart sounds were faint and there was a gallop rhythm. The ECG showed a pattern of left bundle branch block. The attending physician felt that the clinical picture was compatible with a diagnosis of emphysema and cor pulmonale consequent upon an acute respiratory infection. An arterial blood-gas analysis was requested one hour after admission. Treatment with digitalis and diuretics resulted in satisfactory inprovement in his clinical condition.

Radiology. *A* and *B*, The pulmonary vessels are larger and less distinct than normal and the hila are hazy and ill defined. Short horizontal lines of increased density, extending to the pleural surface, are present in the right costophrenic region, representing septal edema and lymphatic engorgement (not well seen in illustration). There are small bilateral pleural effusions. A moderate degree of cardiomegaly is due to predominant left ventricular enlargement.

The picture suggests left heart failure, with pulmonary venous engorgement, interstitial edema and pleural effusion.

Summary. In certain circumstances, an arterial blood-gas analysis may be useful in excluding congestive failure due to lung disease.

	VC	FRC	RV	TLC	ME %	MMFR	$FEV_{0.75}$ ×40	pH	P_{CO_2}	HCO_3^-	O_2Hb %	$D_{Lco}SS_2$	CO Ext. %
Predicted	3.0	3.0	1.9	4.9	48	2.57	73	7.40	42	25	97	11.6	41
Feb. 3, 1961								7.43	38	24	92.8		
Feb. 11, 1961	3.0	3.7	2.6	5.6	43	1.5	64					9.2	38

At the time of his admission, on the afternoon of February 3, 1961, the patient was acutely ill and in severe respiratory distress. The absence of hypercapnia makes a diagnosis of congestive heart failure secondary to lung disease unlikely. The lowered arterial saturation and normal P_{CO_2} suggest the probability of bronchopneumonia or pulmonary edema.

When he was fit enough to co-operate in resting function tests, the results indicated slight hyperinflation, minimal impairment of inert-gas distribution, and slight reduction in ventilation ability and resting diffusing capacity. Any significant degree of morphological emphysema seems unlikely.

?Pulmonary Edema – ?Cor Pulmonale

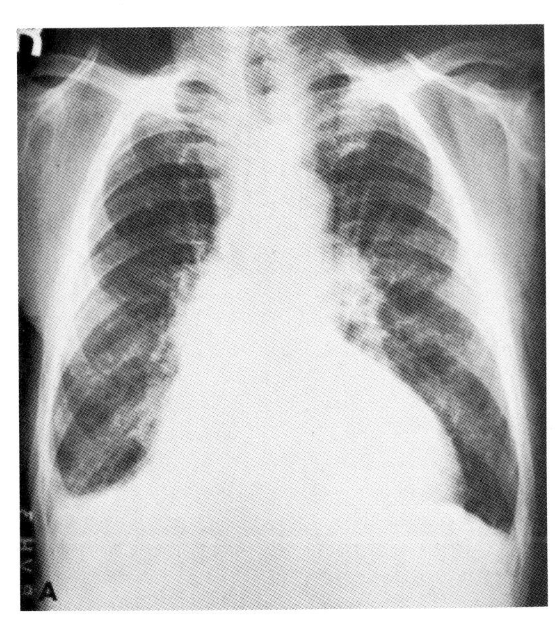

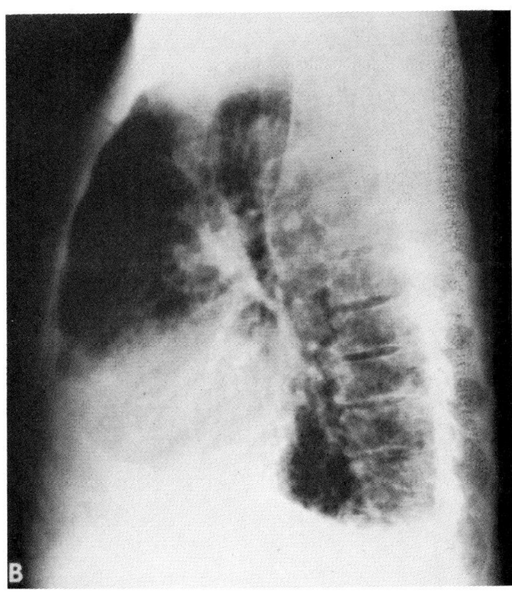

age, as claimed by Campbell, then only 14 of our 23 acutely ill patients achieved adequate oxygenation." This emphasizes the need for constant surveillance of these patients until adequate oxygenation and ventilation have been reached.

The problem of the long-term prognosis of patients with chronic respiratory disease after hospital treatment for an episode of acute respiratory failure has been discussed in two papers since the first edition of this book. Sukumalchantra and his co-workers[3783] followed 43 such patients, finding that 23 (54 per cent) were alive three years later. The mean age of these men was 62, with a range from 42 to 79. Seventy-four per cent were alive one year after the hospitalization. Jessen, Kristensen, and Rasmussen reported on a group of 111 patients treated mostly with tracheostomy and assisted ventilation. In the chronically disabled group, none was alive three years later. By contrast, in the group who had been working before their episode of failure, 58 per cent were alive three years after discharge and 20 per cent were alive seven years after discharge.

These figures reflect the common occurrence that some of these patients are thrown into respiratory failure when an acute infection compromises the function of a region of the lung on which they are dependent—and resolution is accompanied by reasonable pulmonary function. As all physicians who deal every day with these problems know, it is far from easy to decide initially which patients are in this category. It is certainly valuable to have available pulmonary function data recorded during a previous hospital visit when the patient was not acutely ill.

Neuromuscular disorders

The occurrence of widespread outbreaks of acute poliomyelitis in modern times has resulted in the development of methods for providing assisted ventilation in the treatment of this and other diseases; in particular, it was after the 1952 poliomyelitis epidemic in Copenhagen[1266] that the use of tracheostomy and positive-pressure ventilation was generally accepted.

The vast literature on the management of acute paralytic poliomyelitis cannot be reviewed here, but it may be pertinent to point out that after partial recovery from the acute stage, when a vital capacity of several hundred milliliters may enable the patient to dispense with mechanical aids, it is not uncommon to find that the lungs have an abnormally low compliance;[468, 1285] increasing lung stiffness also occurs in patients on continuous tank-respirator care, presumably because of chronic atelectatic changes in the lungs. The development of a significant degree of polycythemia in patients who have recovered partially from paralytic poliomyelitis[1284] indicates that many of these patients are suffering from chronic hypoventilation. It is convenient to use the level of bicarbonate in the arterial blood as an indicator of the generally adequate or inadequate ventilation that may exist in such cases.

Assisted ventilation is often required in patients suffering from the Guillain-Barré syndrome, and we have already noted the remarkable case of this syndrome in a 56-year-old woman who required respirator support for 266 days before making a complete recovery.[3800] Assisted ventilation may also be indicated in myotonic dystrophy,[1286] polymyositis,[1287] and other chronic disorders, particularly when an intercurrent respiratory infection occurs.[1288] Patients suffering an acute exacerbation during the course of myasthenia gravis not infrequently require respirator care, and a dangerous degree of respiratory failure can occur in the postoperative period after thymectomy. In severe cases it is often wise to establish tracheostomy a week or two before thymectomy is performed, since the simultaneous midline sternal incision and tracheostomy may give rise to difficulties in management and risk of infection.

Several papers have dealt with the successful treatment by paralyzing drugs and artificial respiration of tetanus in adults[1289, 1290] and in infants.[1291] There is little doubt that this technique should invariably be adopted in severe cases of this infection.

Reporting from South Africa, Adams and his colleagues[3766] state that the use of IPPB halved the mortality of patients with this condition, as compared to that of a control group treated conservatively.

Carbon-monoxide poisoning

Although a patient with chronic anemia and a hemoglobin value of only 40 per cent may be almost normally active, one with 60 per cent carboxyhemoglobin and 40 per cent normal hemoglobin is severely incapacitated. Haldane's elucidation of this phenomenon was one of his major contributions.[2] He showed that, with a carboxyhemoglobin content of 60 per cent, the oxyhemoglobin dissociation curve of the residual hemoglobin is markedly shifted to the left, and its shape is altered. These changes profoundly reduce the efficiency of the remaining blood as an oxygen carrier, with the result that, in Haldane's words, "An enormous fall in oxygen pressure is needed to make the bulk of the oxygen in the oxyhaemoglobin dissociate. . . ." For this reason the tissue oxygen tension is much higher in the man with anemia than in the one with 60 per cent carboxyhemoglobin. The extensive literature on carbon monoxide was excellently summarized by Lilienthal in 1950.[376] The rate of uptake and of dissociation of carbon monoxide with hemoglobin is determined by the oxygen tension. Thus, admixture of 100 per cent oxygen slows the rate of uptake of CO and increases its rate of elimination. CO poisoning, when acute, usually presents little difficulty in diagnosis once it has been suspected. The alveolar-gas equilibration method described by Henderson and Apthorp may be very useful in measuring the COHb level without venepuncture, and is very precise even at low levels of COHb.[2198]

The first requirement in the treatment of CO poisoning, therefore, is to ensure adequate ventilation of the patient by administration of 100 per cent oxygen. The tissue oxygen tension may be further raised, with resultant faster elimination and quicker recovery, if the subject is placed in oxygen under pressure.[30, 1306] It seems doubtful that it is ever advisable to add 5 per cent CO_2 to the inspired oxygen, as some have advocated, since there is evidence that inhalation of carbon monoxide may be attended by a considerable metabolic acidosis and even hyperventilation in some instances.[1308] If, in a severely poisoned patient, ventilation is poor, it would be much safer to pass an endotracheal tube and artificially ventilate the patient with 100 per cent O_2 than it would be to administer 5 per cent CO_2. Carbon-monoxide poisoning is notoriously insidious and, even during exercise, a saturation of 40 per cent COHb may be reached without any change in oxygen uptake or ventilation and with no sensation of dyspnea.[1307]

Although there has recently been much interest in the experience of treating CO poisoning by the use of hyperbaric oxygen—and there are sound theoretical reasons for expecting this treatment to be valuable in this condition—as far as we are aware there has been no controlled comparison between this method of treatment and modern assisted ventilation with 100 per cent oxygen at ambient pressure.[3753] It is not possible, therefore, to be sure that it offers any decisive advantage.

After cardiac arrest

The fact that cardiac arrest is swiftly followed by the development of severe metabolic acidosis due to lactic-acid accumulation has now been well documented.[2200, 2201, 2204–2206] The provision of ventilation immediately to prevent an additional respiratory acidosis, and the prompt intravenous administration of bicarbonate or THAM, must be supplemented by complete respiratory control. The severe acidosis develops so quickly after circulatory arrest that it may well play a part in causing some of the residual cerebral damage that is conventionally ascribed to anoxia.

Acute left ventricular failure and pulmonary edema

In an earlier section (*see* Chapter 15) we noted that severe hypercapnia may occur as a terminal event in patients with pulmonary edema due to acute left ventricular failure. Some of these patients may be saved by prompt assisted ventilation with 100 per cent oxygen.[3147] Gibson,[3777] in catheter studies of 7 patients with extensive radiological pulmonary edema in renal failure, found that pulmonary vascular pressures were normal in 2 cases and lower in the remaining 5 than those commonly recorded in mitral stenosis or left ventricular failure. The pulmonary edema due to this extensive capillary damage is very difficult to treat; the most that can be done is to maintain the blood gases at values as near physiological values as possible until resolution has had a chance to occur.

After cardiac or thoracic surgery

The early experience of Björk and Engström in the use of assisted ventilation in the postoperative period has been duplicated by others,[1195, 1305, 1309] and most thoracic centers have now had some experience in elective or emergency respirator care of such patients. Norlander and his colleagues have reported a series of 522 patients, many of them in the

Case 60
Hyaline Membrane Disease

Summary of Clinical Findings. This 28-week gestation, 1840 gm premature male infant was delivered spontaneously on June 20th, 1966, at 12:32 P.M. Pregnancy had been normal to that point. Delivery was easy with spontaneous rupture of membranes, but there was a placenta praevia with premature separation. At birth the infant was pink, active but showed some respiratory difficulty. At 4 hours of age he became cyanosed and had a short apneic spell. This led to his transfer to the Montreal Children's Hospital where he was admitted at 9 hours of age.

On arrival he was observed to be cyanosed even while receiving 100 per cent oxygen. His respiratory rate was 70 per minute with expiratory grunting, subcostal and substernal retraction, and decreased air entry on auscultation. He was flaccid with depressed neurological responses.

The first acid–base and blood gas assessment of arterial blood obtained from an umbilical artery catheter was performed at 11 hours of age. The arterial Po_2 was 25 mm Hg while the child was breathing 100 per cent oxygen. The Pco_2 was 75 mm Hg and the $[H^+]$ was 120 μEq/l. Within 15 minutes of this evaluation, the child was placed in a negative pressure respirator. As the base excess was −20 mEq/l, 14 ml of a solution of sodium bicarbonate containing 0.9 mEq/ml was infused over a 10-minute period and 10 ml of the same solution was added to the infusion of 10 per cent glucose and water to run in the next eight hours. Repeat evaluation of blood gases and acid–base status was done one and a half hours later and at regular intervals thereafter, as indicated in the accompanying table.

The immediate response in oxygenation and ventilation was dramatic as illustrated by the Po_2 and Pco_2 values obtained on repeat examination. The course of the disease was typical in that after an immediate improvement after initiating assisted ventilation, there was radiological and clinical worsening in the disease process and a gradual deterioration in ventilation and oxygenation over the next three days in spite of consistently high ventilator pressures. He began to improve on the fourth day of life and on the sixth day was able to maintain satisfactory Po_2 and Pco_2 blood level without respirator assistance. Because of hyperbilirubinemia an exchange transfusion was performed on the fifth day while the patient was in the respirator.

He continued to require 100 per cent oxygen for an extra day to maintain normal blood oxygen levels, but it was possible to reduce this to 40 per

Case report continues on page 459

RESPIRATORY CHART

TIME OF BIRTH June 20/66 @ 12:32

DATE June	20	21	21	22	24	25	25	26
TIME	2320	0120*	2240	2200	1115	1600	2335**	2130
AGE IN HOURS	10¾	12¾	34	57¼	94½	123½	130¾	152¾
TYPE OF BLOOD	Arterial	Arterial	Arterial	Arterial	Arterial	Arterial	Arterial	Arterialized Capillary
RESPIRATORY AIDS	None	Negative Pressure Resp.	Negative Pressure Resp.	Negative Pressure Resp.	Negative Pressure Resp.	Negative Pressure Resp.	None	None
AMBIENT O_2 %	100	100	100	100	100	100	100	95
Po_2	25	138	136	41	75	103	63	
O_2 SATURATION	28	98	98	69	93	96	84	
$[H^+]$	120	58	47	56	47	54	66	59
Pco_2	73	44	50	61	46		66	65
BASE EXCESS	−19.9	−8.6	−0.1	−1.9	−2.6		−5.8	0.5
STANDARD BICARBONATE	10.5	17.5	23.9	22.4	22.0		19.5	24.5

*After 1 hour 50 minutes on respirator.
**After being off respirator for 3 hours and 45 minutes.

Hyaline Membrane Disease

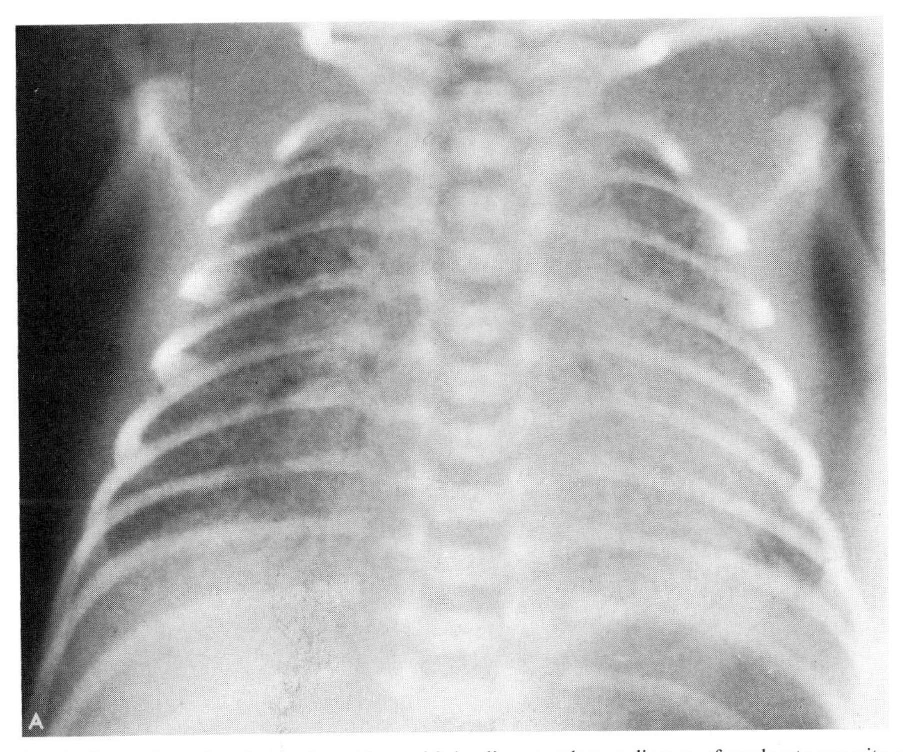

FIGURE A. Radiograph of the chest of a patient with hyaline membrane disease of moderate severity at age eight hours. There is a diffuse reticulo-granular pattern of increased density throughout both lungs, evenly distributed. The air content of the bronchi is abnormally visible—the "air bronchogram." (Courtesy of Dr. J. S. Dunbar.)

cent by the eleventh day of life, and to room air by the fifteenth day. He was discharged without obvious sequellae at 6 weeks of age weighing 2900 gm. At 4 months of age he successfully underwent a herniorrhaphy at which time the chest x-ray was normal and he was otherwise well. When seen at 2 years of age, he was considered to be in normal health.

Summary. This premature infant with severe hyaline membrane disease required ventilatory assistance with 100 per cent ambient O_2 for a period of six days in order to prevent dangerous hypoxemia or excessive hypercarbia. Early development of severe respiratory failure is usually accompanied by a fatal outcome. Rapid intervention to support respiration and correct metabolic disturbances in this child might very well be responsible for the favorable outcome.

Hyaline Membrane Disease (Continued)

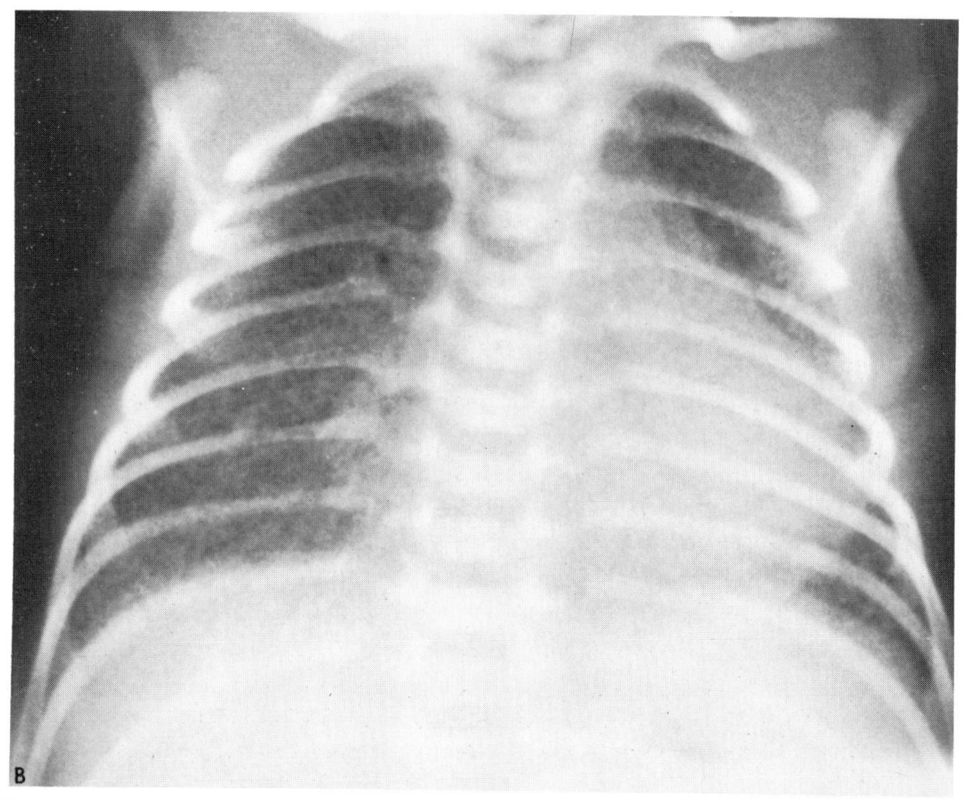

FIGURE B. The same patient as in Figure A at age eight days. Clinical recovery is accompanied by radiographic improvement. The reticulo-granular pattern and the increased visibility of bronchial airways are still evident but less marked. (Courtesy of Dr. J. S. Dunbar.)

---

postoperative state, who were treated with controlled ventilation during a five-year period.[1297] This valuable experience clearly documents the importance of the availability of a well-trained, competent team to handle such problems, and shows that the commonest reason for failure of such treatment is irreversible damage or disease in some other organ, usually the heart, brain, or kidney. These authors stress the occasional necessity for ventilatory assistance during the postoperative period after cardiac surgery, often with a midsternal incision, *before* derangement of the blood gases has occurred. Ventilation is just sufficient in such patients, but one can observe them becoming progressively more exhausted and fatigued, and effective pain relief cannot be given because respiratory depression is feared. Adequate sedation with full ventilatory control enables them to enjoy necessary rest and sleep and may result in obvious improvement in circulation. We have encountered this clinical situation, which deserves mention since it is important to stress that, on occasion, it may be wise to assist ventilation or to assume full control of it before gross hypercapnia has occurred.

Elective respirator care with a planned tracheostomy and ventilatory control has revolutionized the management of many patients who require thoracic surgery but in whom this would otherwise be attended by a major operative and postoperative mortality rate (*see* Case 51, page 412). It is very striking that such patients, being able to receive adequate medication for complete pain control, undoubtedly often have a more comfortable recovery from an operation such as a pneumonectomy than do those whose remaining lung is normal and whose ventilation does not require assistance.

Of particular interest and importance have been the recent observations of the state of the lung after prolonged cardiopulmonary bypass procedures. There is now a formidable amount of evidence that patients in whom this technique has been used may develop atelectasis and may suffer reduction of lung compliance, probably because of inactivation of the surface-active material in the lung upon which its integrity depends. The mechanism of this inactivation is not known. This syndrome, often called "generalized congestive atelectasis,"[26] occurs in dogs under experimental conditions,[2194–2197] and widespread atelectasis[2192] and a decreased diffusing capacity[2173, 2190, 2191, 2193] have been observed in human subjects by many investigators.

After operation, therefore, the cardiac case represents a major problem for four reasons. The lungs may be abnormal as a consequence of heart disease, the thorax is entered often through a midline incision, cardiac output may be poor postoperatively, and patchy atelectasis may occur as a consequence of the bypass procedure. Very careful management of many of these patients, with monitoring of blood gases, may make the difference between their dying and their survival.[2246]

Acute chest injury

Although some thoracic surgeons have realized that respirator treatment is often indicated in the management of thoracic injuries[1198] and that adequate lung inflation is the best method of chest-wall fixation, such an approach has only slowly gained general acceptance. Norlander and his co-workers noted: "Trauma to the chest with mechanical instability of the thoracic cage and pulmonary contusion is a very important indication for primary tracheostomy and respirator treatment."[1297]

It has been our experience that such patients not infrequently pass through the following stages: at first, there is considerable blood flow through unventilated parts of the lung; this leads to a low oxygen saturation (and a low level of $P\text{O}_2$[2289]) but no hypercapnia. This hypoxia may so stimulate ventilation that the arterial $P\text{CO}_2$ level may be subnormal.[2270] The tremendous effort of ventilation, usually evident from the bedside, induces considerable fatigue, and pain may be severe, so that, although the $P\text{O}_2$ level can be maintained by administration of oxygen, finally ventilation begins to fail, and the arterial $P\text{CO}_2$ level rises. Management of such patients, often complicated by the presence of severe injuries elsewhere, requires very close observation and assessment.[2275] In our experience, it is often helpful, after deciding whether assisted ventilation is indicated or not, to record this decision on the chart every hour, thus ensuring that this re-evaluation is made frequently enough to enable ventilatory assistance to be given before respiratory failure has occurred.

Ambiavagar and his co-workers have recently summarized published experience in treating acute chest injuries with ventilators up to 1966.[3772] Of 123 so treated there were 91 survivors. They also have documented the tremendous alveolar–arterial oxygen differences that may be observed in these patients. In 6 patients breathing 100 per cent oxygen with assisted ventilation, the arterial $P\text{O}_2$ was measured at values between 65 and 187 mm Hg, indicating A–a differences of 500 mg Hg or so. The arterial $P\text{CO}_2$ was normal or low in these patients.

Respiratory failure in shock and burns (Post-traumatic pulmonary insufficiency)

A considerable amount of attention has recently been focused on a syndrome of progressive Type-I respiratory failure with deficient oxygen exchange occurring in patients who have extensive body injuries and are in shock and also in patients who have been burned. The now considerable literature on this phenomenon has been summarized by Collins in a recent review article,[3751] and the reader will also find valuable information in the monograph published by Moore and his colleagues,[3774] and in other publications.[3750, 3776, 3788, 3806] The observations indicate that there is a progressive decline in arterial oxygen tension, which finally cannot be maintained even with assisted ventilation, and at autopsy there are areas of atelectasis and hemorrhage in the lung. In patients who have been burned, this pulmonary complication carries a very serious prognosis, and Shook, MacMillan, and Altemeier[3804] report only one survivor of 13 such patients, all of whom required continuous positive-pressure ventilation for more than 48 hours. A Russian author has reported on 32 cases in burned patients, and notes that atelectasis seems to be the dominant feature.[3805]

It is evident that much basic work lies ahead to clarify the origin of this syndrome. It is perhaps useful to recall that widened $(A\text{–}a)O_2$ differences occur in patients with myocardial infarction (*see* Chapter 15), and thus hypoperfusion may be an important element in its genesis. We have recently been able to simulate this syndrome in the pig; it may be that it occurs more easily in the well-lobulated pig and human lung than in the dog lung, in which there is a tremendous capability of collateral ventilation. It seems clear that some biochemical process on which endothelial integrity depends has been deranged. It is hard to believe that the syndrome can be primarily attributed to loss of surfactant, since it occurs rapidly; nevertheless, destruction of surfactant may be a part of the complex changes that are occurring.

From the point of view of clinical management, there is no alternative to maintaining the patient on a combination of ventilation and inspired oxygen that will keep his blood gases in the physiological range. This may necessitate higher oxygen concentrations for longer than is normally desirable, but usually the physician or surgeon has no alternative but to adopt this approach.

Miscellaneous conditions

We have had experience of successful resuscitation and treatment of a patient with postabortion septicemia who had an arterial $P\text{CO}_2$ level of 82 mm Hg and severe pulmonary edema before respirator treatment was started. The successful use of a respirator in a similar case was reported by Thomeret and his colleagues.[1200] Nordqvist and his associates described two patients in myxedema coma in whom the arterial $P\text{CO}_2$ levels were 109 and 86 mm Hg, respectively.[1199] No doubt there are other conditions in which a fatal outcome can be prevented by the prompt recognition of respiratory failure. For some patients with barbiturate poisoning, treatment by respiratory stimulants is all that is required,[1315, 1316] but others will need respirator care, in which case ventilatory assistance may be satisfactorily given through a cuffed endotracheal tube until consciousness begins to return, thereby avoiding the need for tracheostomy. As discussed in Chapter 5, if the arterial $P\text{CO}_2$ level is dangerously elevated in a patient in status asthmaticus, a decision may have to be made to assist ventilation. Such patients, in whom restoration of normal function after the acute episode is the rule, cannot be allowed to pass into the stage of circulatory failure as a consequence of hypercapnia; when this danger is present, treatment should be vigorous.

Slapak, Lee, and Hume[3778] have documented the occurrence of Type-I respiratory failure in patients who have undergone renal transplant operations. They characterize this as "transplant lung"—a somewhat confusing name in view of the interest in lung transplantation. They note that lung infiltrates occur and the arterial $P\text{O}_2$ falls, and they state, "The fact is stressed that in two of the patients the diagnosis was made on a characteristic pulmonary function abnormality which was detected by arterial gas studies before there were any clinical or radiological manfestations."

IDIOPATHIC RESPIRATORY DISTRESS SYNDROME OF INFANTS (HYALINE-MEMBRANE DISEASE)

There are a number of causes of respiratory distress on the first day of life, but of these this condition is by far the most common. It is believed to account for the death of about 3.8 per cent of live premature births.[3807] The condition has to be differentiated from pneumonia, lobar emphysema, aspiration of amniotic fluid, pulmonary hemorrhage, pneumothorax, tracheo-esophageal atresia, diaphragmatic eventration or hernia, and the rare Wilson-Mikity syndrome, all of which may be responsible for respiratory distress in newborn infants.

The lungs of an infant dying from the respiratory-distress syndrome are airless and liver-like at autopsy. Eosinophilic hyaline membranes can be seen uniformly lining the terminal bronchioles and alveolar ducts in all cases except those dying in the first few hours after birth. By electron microscopy, the membrane is found to be composed of a matrix with the periodicity of fibrin and cellular fragments. It has been shown to be derived from blood.

Infants at risk are mainly those born prematurely and those born of diabetic mothers. Whether cesarean section itself or the factors leading to it predispose to the occurrence of this syndrome has not yet been definitely determined.[3808, 3809] Symptoms always occur before six to eight hours of life in children who have had some respiratory difficulty at birth. It is believed that reports of a longer delay in the onset of symptoms are probably attributable to inadequate earlier observation.[3807] The most prominent features are increased respiratory rate, grunting, retraction of the soft tissues of the chest during inspiration, a "seesaw" pattern of respiration with the abdomen protruding during inspiration, harsh breath sounds, and, occasionally, fine rales. Systemic hypotension and poor peripheral circulation are commonly seen, and cyanosis is evident in the more severely affected infants. In uncomplicated but untreated cases, death occurs within 72 hours as a rule, and if it occurs later it is usually associated with either pulmonary or intracranial hemorrhage, or pneumonia. Radiographic examination is essential to exclude other causes of respiratory distress and confirm the presence of hyaline-membrane syndrome. It shows characteristic diffuse reticulogranular infiltrates throughout both lung fields, usually about equally distributed, with an air bronchogram.

Whether the primary factor in the initiation of the full-blown syndrome be asphyxia,[707] hypoperfusion of the pulmonary vasculature,[3810, 3811] or a fibrinolytic-enzyme defect,[3812] there is little doubt that a loss or inactivation of surfactant plays an important and possibly primary role in the syndrome.[537, 3803, 3813]

The pulmonary function derangements in this syndrome have been extensively studied. Tidal volume is decreased and minute volume normal or increased. Compliance is reduced to one fourth or one fifth of the predicted value. The functional residual capacity is decreased and the crying vital capacity is diminished. Airway resistance is essentially unchanged.[1911, 3814] There is a significant alveolar–arterial CO_2 difference,[2285] indicating the presence of significant $\dot{V}/\dot{Q}$ imbalance. There is often, but not invariably, an increased P_{CO_2}, indicating alveolar hypoventilation. The P_{O_2} is usually moderately or severely decreased; the presence of a widened alveolar–arterial O_2 difference during oxygen breathing indicates a significant shunt component, which is probably mostly intrapulmonary but may also be due to actual shunting through the foramen ovale or the still patent ductus arteriosus. It is the frequently profound hypoxemia that is the main threat to the survival of the infant.

Initial treatment is supportive, and such measures as maintenance of body temperature, correction of metabolic acidosis using infusion of bicarbonate or THAM, alleviation of hypoglycemia and hyperkalemia with glucose and insulin, and treatment of shock with a blood transfusion are often indicated. The hypoxemia is relieved with oxygen in sufficient concentration to keep the arterial P_{O_2} between 60 and 70 mm Hg. The presence of an elevated P_{CO_2} or a failure to maintain the P_{O_2} above 50 mm Hg necessitates the use of assisted or controlled ventilation. When the arterial P_{O_2} falls below 50 mm Hg, survival is low, being only about 5 per cent.[3815] Considerable work has been reported recently on the use of positive-pressure[3796, 3816, 3817] and negative-pressure ventilators,[3752, 3818] following the pioneering (but commonly unrecognized) work of Alexander Graham Bell in 1882,[3819] and that of Donald in 1955.[22] The immediate benefits of such measures are not easy to assess, though there seems little doubt that they are of benefit in severe cases. There is some evidence to indicate that there may be some long-term lung effects in survivors,[3768, 3769] but in many the lungs appear normal a year or so later.

PULMONARY FUNCTION AND ANESTHESIA

There are many ways in which the relationship between these two fields may be viewed. Some of the interesting problems concerning gas exchange that are directly relevant to anesthesia[433, 1214–1216, 2174] are beyond the scope of this volume. Others must be considered in some detail if the physician is to view the problem from the anesthetist's standpoint. Nunn[3825] has recently published a useful review of respiratory physiology in relation to anesthesia.

After a period in which there was some conflict of evidence concerning the effect of anesthesia on pulmonary mechanics,[1217–1222] it was shown by Safar and Bachman that, whereas succinylcholine had no effect on pulmonary compliance, tubocurarine reduced it significantly, probably by releasing histamine.[464] The conclusions of some of the early workers on this problem were faulty because they did not take into account the development of pulmonary atelectasis after anesthesia, which would cause a change in the compliance, as has been clearly demonstrated in dog lungs by Mead and Collier.[1410] The important practical implication of their study, however, is the demonstration that a single deep breath can reverse the progressive fall in compliance which, they showed, occurred with time in anesthetized dogs receiving assisted ventilation. Thus, this is the physiological basis for the excellent anesthetic practice of giving a forceful breath at intervals during prolonged anesthesia, to open up the lung units that tend to close off in these circumstances. That areas of atelectasis not visible on radiographs do occur as a result of general anesthesia was demonstrated by Gordh and his colleagues by their finding of an arterial oxygen tension that was reduced, compared with the value preoperatively, during administration of 100 per cent oxygen in the immediate postoperative period.[422] Such areas of atelectasis are presumed to result from immobility during surgery, combined with the effects of oxygen breathing. Bendixen and his co-workers recently confirmed Gordh's work and showed that during anesthesia the level of P_{CO_2} may be held constant but that of the arterial P_{O_2} falls steadily.[2056]

These and more recent observations on the occurrence of atelectasis before and during anesthesia[3770, 3773] are easier to explain now than they were five years ago. As noted in Chapter 3 (*see* pages 96–99), it is now evident that airway closure occurs in dependent lung regions even at FRC in older normal subjects. Anything that reduces lung volume, such as obesity or ascites, or lowers tidal volume, such as respiratory depression or an upper abdominal incision, or causes "subclinical" lung edema with fluid collection around the terminal bronchiole, will lead to airway closure. As the lung loses elasticity with age, the phenomenon occurs at higher lung volumes. Anything that may jeopardize the terminal bronchiole, such as cigarette smoking, will aggravate the situation. Inspiration of a high-oxygen mixture will also favor the development of atelectasis, as shown by the experiments of Burger and Macklem.[2969] Such a concept is supported by the experiments of Georg, Hornum, and Mellemgaard[3669] who concluded that the main cause of postoperative hypoxemia after a laparotomy is an uneven $\dot{V}/\dot{Q}$ ratio distribution in the lungs and not a veno-arterial shunt through completely atelectatic areas. Palmer and Diament[3798] have also noted that arterial P_{O_2} values were lower after upper abdominal surgery than after lower abdominal incisions (a fall from preoperative values of 18.0 mm Hg in the former and 9.5 mm Hg in the latter case).

In the section on the effects of age on the lung it was pointed out that airway closure occurs at progressively higher lung volumes as the lung loses elastic recoil with advancing age. Nunn[3765] studied 169 patients, 120 analyzed from the literature and 49 directly observed by himself, and noted a highly significant correlation between the arterial P_{O_2} in the postoperative period and the age of the patient. The explanation of this important phenomenon is almost certainly the phenomenon of airway closure, since this probably explains the lower resting arterial P_{O_2} in elderly subjects even without anes-

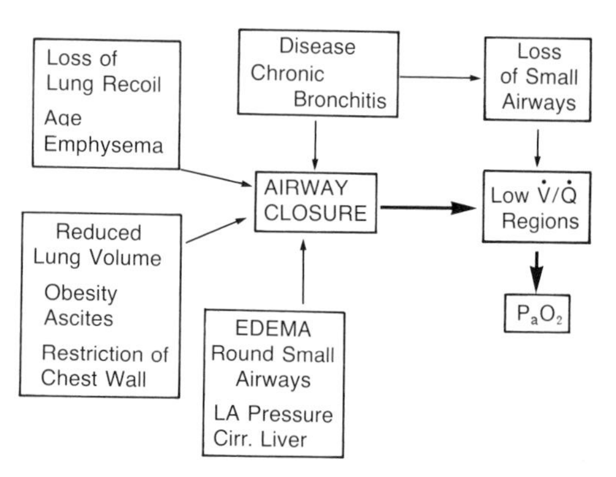

FIGURE 22–1. Diagram of processes believed to be related to airway closure in the lung. This occurs, in the absence of disease, at progressively higher lung volumes as a consequence of the loss of lung recoil that accompanies age; this phenomenon is enhanced by the presence of any of the other factors. In such circumstances, the arterial oxygen tension will be dependent on the depth of the tidal volume and on the functional residual capacity.

thesia, in the presence of the same P_{CO_2} as is found in young subjects. It is of interest that some anesthesiologists are using a positive end expiratory pressure during controlled ventilation; this may be beneficial in some cases because it prevents airway closure from occurring.

Although very high arterial P_{CO_2} and low pH values during anesthesia have been reported by some authors,[1223, 2172] and lesser but still significant changes noted by others,[2358] in general the anesthetist has little difficulty in ventilating the patient, and dangerous CO_2 retention is now a very rare event in normal circumstances. Special problems, such as the maintenance of ventilation during bronchoscopy, have been discussed.[2153] It is important that adequate attention be devoted to the design and care of the anesthetic apparatus,[1224, 1225] but there should be as much concern for the maintenance of adequate ventilation in the postoperative period as when strict control is possible during the operation itself.

The factors involved in CO_2 elimination during anesthesia may be complex.[2174] Although dependent upon the metabolic production of CO_2,[1227] the blood levels may be modified by shifts in ventilation-perfusion ratios consequent upon adoption of unusual body positions during surgery, or other maneuvers,[1226] and may also be influenced by sudden changes in nitrous-oxide uptake or elimination.[1215] The physiological dead space is found to increase slightly during anesthesia, even under controlled assisted respiration,[2171] although artificial ventilation and anesthesia of themselves have little or no effect on the uniformity of inert-gas distribution.[2269] The necessity for assisted ventilation is generally recognized,[2169] and many anesthetists have come to appreciate the value of being able to measure the arterial P_{CO_2} of the patient routinely in the recovery room.

Hypothermia does not appear to alter pulmonary mechanics significantly,[1228] but may give rise to some degree of metabolic acidosis. Several observers have noted that, under anesthesia, elevation of the arterial P_{CO_2} level is usually accompanied by a simultaneous metabolic acidosis.[1229] It is not known whether this commonly observed bicarbonate deficit is secondary to inadequate circulation, such as that which occurs during cardiorespiratory bypass with an inadequate flow,[1230] or to changes in regional circulation during anesthesia.

PREOPERATIVE EVALUATION AND POSTOPERATIVE CARE

However effective the treatment of respiratory failure, it is clearly better to anticipate and, if possible, prevent its development. In the case of intrathoracic disease, the preoperative assessment of patients may present a complex problem of evaluation and study before one can forecast residual function and its adequacy. The provision of adequate ventilation and oxygenation while the patient is under anesthesia in these and other types of cases does not present a major problem, since ventilation is easily maintained by way of an endotracheal tube in a fully relaxed patient. It is the postoperative period that represents the danger to the patient's life. The physician, surgeon, and anesthetist can often be assisted in their management of individual cases by a knowledge of the preoperative function status.

When thoracic surgery is scheduled, careful preoperative evaluation of ventilatory function is essential; if it is seriously disordered, an arterial blood-gas analysis should be performed. Swenson and his colleagues have found that the degree of postoperative elevation of CO_2 tension occurring in patients who have undergone pulmonary resection correlates with the preoperative ventilatory status.[1317] They also found that "Postoperative difficulties with atelectasis and poor expansion (resulting in significant hypoxemia) were, paradoxically, more common in the group of patients with better preoperative ventilatory function. The factors thought to be responsible for the good results in the ventilatory dysfunction cases include the preoperative training, intraoperative procedures aimed at minimizing function loss, and unflagging postoperative care concentrated upon them."

Careful preoperative preparation of any patient with chronic lung disease includes attempts to reduce the amount of sputum and to clear up residual infection, adequate use of bronchodilators, and training in breathing exercises and coughing. We have found, as did Swenson, that monitoring of minute ventilation and arterial blood gases before and after surgical procedures is an essential part of proper preparation and postoperative care of these patients. Their finding of fewer postoperative complications in those with initially more impairment of function provides striking confirmation of the efficacy of these methods

Case 61 Respiratory Failure; Pulmonary Emphysema; Severe $\dot{V}/\dot{Q}$ Disturbance

Summary of Clinical Findings. This 38-year-old taxi driver was admitted to hospital on February 26, 1962. He had a long history of productive cough and of dyspnea on effort. These symptoms had become severe over the last three years, accompanied by definite cyanosis for the last six months. Two weeks before admission he had developed an upper respiratory infection, which had engendered episodes of cough syncope. At that time his family had noticed a change in his behavior with a tendency to somnolence and confusion. There had been no evidence of heart failure.

On the day of admission he drove his taxi to the hospital and walked into the emergency room. He was severely dyspneic and deeply cyanosed and had generalized muscle twitching. His blood pressure was 140/90 mm Hg and his pulse rate 112/min. His fundal veins were engorged and the pharynx injected. The chest was increased in the AP diameter, with indrawing of the costal margins on inspiration and hyperresonance over the upper lobes. There were high-pitched rhonchi scattered throughout and a few fine rales at the left base. There were no signs of heart failure. An arterial blood sample revealed: $P\text{CO}_2$, 87 mm Hg; bicarbonate, 38 mM/l; pH 7.30; O_2 saturation, 70 per cent.

On investigation, the hemoglobin was 18.8 gm/100 ml, the ESR was 1 mm/hr, and the total white-cell count was 8500 per cmm. *Haemophilus influenzae* grew on sputum culture.

The patient was treated with penicillin, tetracycline, bronchodilators, and intermittent positive-pressure breathing with the Bird respirator, using 40 per cent O_2. The accompanying chart illustrates the course of his illness. The $P\text{CO}_2$ level fell during the first two days, with a rise in pH and a gradual increase in O_2 saturation. The improvement was only temporary, and on March 18 it was felt necessary to establish a tracheostomy and to maintain continuous artificial ventilation. Again the improvement was short-lived, and on March 27 he was switched to the Engström respirator in an attempt to increase ventilation, since he became breathless and deeply cyanosed when off the respirator for even short periods. His course had been complicated by a phlebitis of the right foot and an episode of melena, both of which cleared quickly. A barium meal revealed no abnormality. Respiratory infections were another complicating factor despite continued administration of a variety of antibiotics. The chest x-ray shown in *B* illustrates one such episode of infection. At no time did the $P\text{CO}_2$ drop to a normal level. Another trial on the Bird respirator was unsuccessful. It was during this period that he had an episode of severe anoxia due to some displacement of the tracheostomy tube and the next day noticed that his vision was hazy. This progressed to complete blindness within a week. He became severely depressed and completely dependent upon the Engström respirator. His condition gradually deteriorated and he died on May 19 after nearly three months of respirator therapy.

Radiology. On admission (*A*), the lungs were clear, although there was slight hyperinflation which was more evident in lateral projection through deepening of the retrosternal air space. The peripheral vasculature did not appear deficient but there was obvious prominence of the main pulmonary artery and enlargement of the hilar arteries. There was thus a discrepancy between hilar and peripheral arterial caliber which indicated the presence of pulmonary arterial hypertension.

An anteroposterior film made with the patient in bed (*B*) one month later reveals ill-defined densities in both lower lung fields consistent with bilateral lower-lobe pneumonia. Enlargement of the hilar pulmonary arteries is even more striking. A tracheostomy tube is in position.

A tomogram of both lungs (*C*) through the midsagittal plane showed a general reduction in the caliber and number of peripheral arterial radicals, the upper lung fields being more deficient than the lower. This arterial deficiency was not suspected from the plain film (*A*). Hilar enlargement is clearly evident. This combination of findings is highly suggestive of diffuse emphysema with pulmonary arterial hypertension.

Case report continues on page 468

	VC	FRC	RV	TLC	ME %	MMFR	$FEV_{0.75}$ ×40	pH	$P\text{CO}_2$	HCO_3^-	O_2Hb %	$D_{L_{CO}}SS_2$	CO Ext %
Predicted	4.0	3.2	1.7	5.7	60	3.7	115	7.40	42	25	97	18.9	48
March 1, 1963	1.9	6.0	5.4	7.3	25	0.15	11	7.33	70	30	79	7.3	20

The above measurements were made three days after admission. They show a severe impairment of ventilatory function with much air-trapping and gross overinflation. Diffusion is low. The patient is still acidotic because of CO_2 retention and is undersaturated with oxygen. See the figure for details of the course of this patient's illness.

Respiratory Failure; Pulmonary Emphysema; Severe $\dot{V}/\dot{Q}$ Disturbance

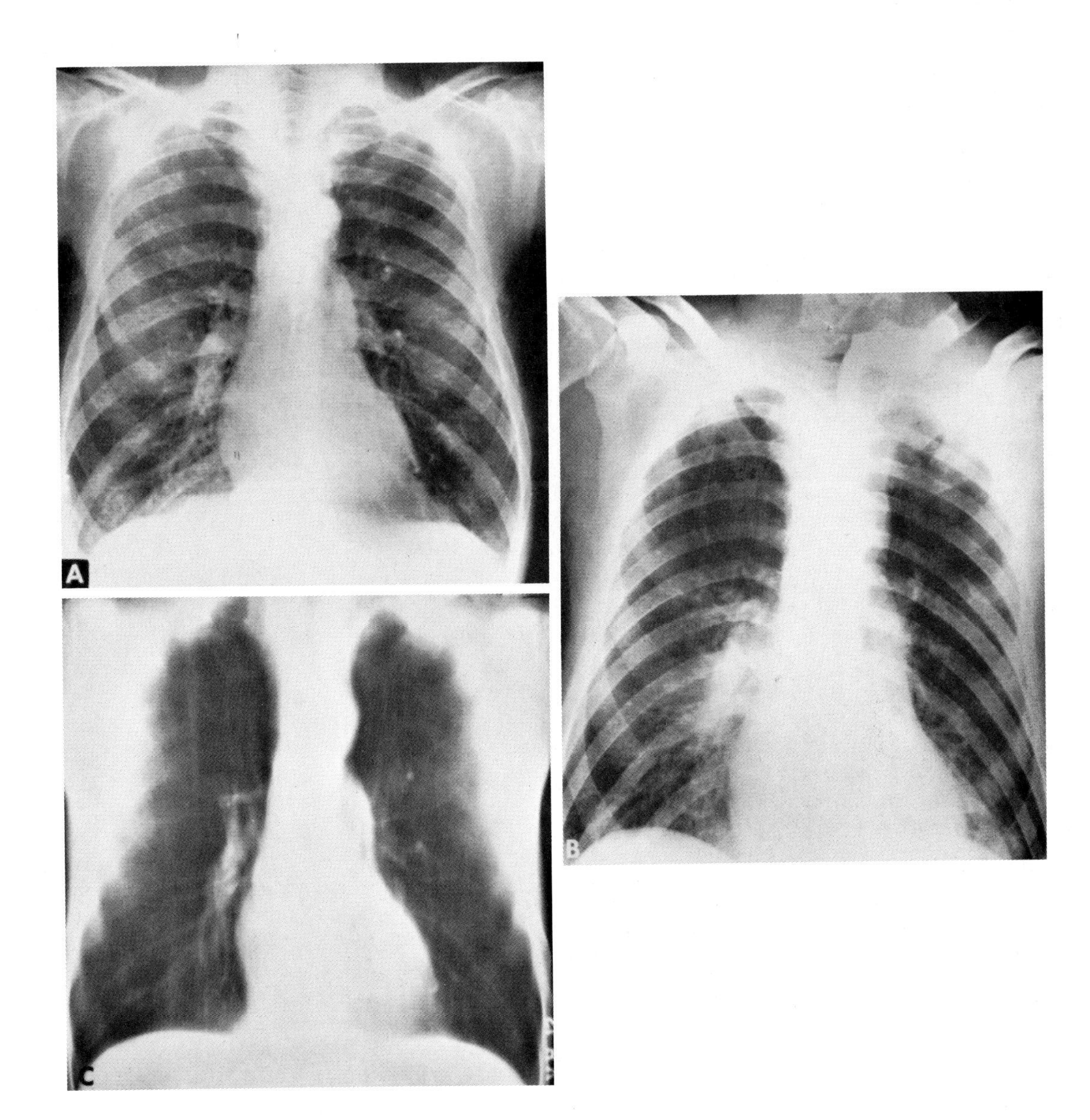

Case 61
Respiratory Failure; Pulmonary Emphysema; Severe $\dot{V}/Q$ Disturbance (Continued)

Pathology. Both upper lobes were involved by emphysema which had destroyed and distorted much of the pulmonary parenchyma (*D*). In some areas this could be categorized as centrilobular emphysema, but in the majority of instances the type could not be accurately determined, being apparently mixed centrilobular, paraseptal, and irregular, and associated with much fibrosis. Similar but milder and less widespread emphysema was present in the apical segments and anterior basal segments of both lower lobes, and along the superior and anterior margins of the lingula and middle lobe. The parenchyma of most of the lower, middle, and lingular lobes was congested but intact. Patchy hemorrhagic bronchopneumonia was present in both upper lobes, the middle and lingular lobes, and both apical lower lobes. There was widespread plugging of bronchi and bronchioles by mucopurulent secretions. Active chronic bronchiolitis of gross degree was apparent in areas uninvolved by emphysema. Focal squamous metaplasia was present in some affected bronchioles. The bronchioles were narrowed by granulation tissue situated between epithelium and muscle walls (*E*). Small scattered foci of organizing pneumonia were present throughout both lungs. The pulmonary vessels showed mild medial thickening. The bronchial mucous glands were hypertrophied; the Reid index was 0.52. The right ventricle of the heart showed considerable hypertrophy.

(*See next page*)

Summary. In retrospect, it is clear that the severe $\dot{V}/\dot{Q}$ discrepancy was due to ventilation of the upper destroyed zones and perfusion of the structurally intact lower zones to which ventilation was prevented by severe bronchiolitis. Assisted or controlled total ventilation of 13 l/min failed to restore the level of arterial P_{CO_2} to normal.

---

in preventing the development of "the postoperative chest."

Of equal importance are older patients, often suffering from chronic bronchitis, who undergo abdominal surgery, usually with little respiratory preparation. It has been shown that upper (as opposed to lower) abdominal incisions produce considerable impairment of vital capacity[1318] and of peak expiratory flow rate.[1319] The arterial P_{O_2} has been shown to be lower after upper abdominal surgery than after lower abdominal incisions.[3798] Ross and his colleagues demonstrated changes in inert-gas distribution and lung volumes in such patients after herniorrhaphy.[2322] These reductions may prove critical in a patient with chronic bronchitis and some degree of emphysema. It is a valuable preoperative practice routinely to estimate the ventilatory capacity of these patients and to estimate the arterial P_{CO_2} level in those with any considerable impairment. In this way, special attention can be directed at those patients who represent a potential postoperative hazard. With an increasing volume of major surgery being performed on older patients, this service makes a valuable contribution to the management of this kind of patient.[1320] In this context, the paragraph written by McCann, Lovejoy, and Yu nearly 20 years ago is relevant: "For some reason or other, most doctors tend to ignore the presence of emphysema and to remain oblivious to its insidious way of bringing a patient to disaster. Its physical signs are so unobtrusive, its appearance in chest x-rays so inconspicuous or so easily obscured by more spectacular lesions that we forget it until some intervening situation precipitates pulmonary failure."[1321]

Throughout the postoperative period, supervision of drugs that depress respiration and a careful watch for the development of atelectasis and retention of secretions are very important in the total care of the patient.[2307] Routine checks of arterial blood are required when the P_{CO_2} level was elevated before operation or when the patient appears less alert than he should be. Measurements of arterial P_{O_2} are also important, as Bendixen[3788] has documented. Measurements of total ventilation and of vital capacity may be valuable, though absolute reliance cannot be placed on these.

Now that much more is known of the mechanisms that cause respiratory failure, this kind of meticulous postoperative care

Respiratory Failure; Pulmonary Emphysema; Severe V/Q Disturbance

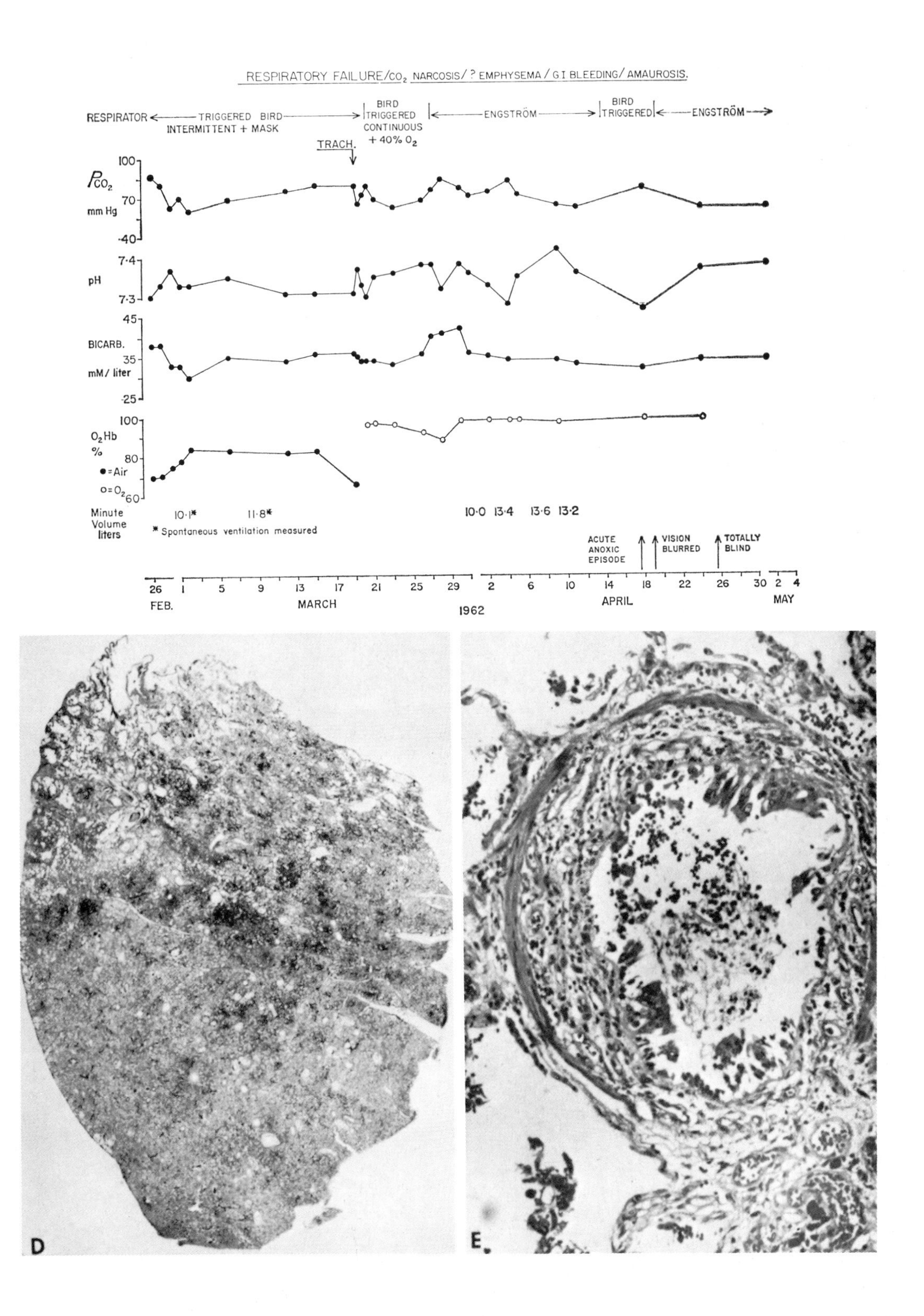

should obviate the need for an emergency tracheostomy in the early hours of the morning, followed by an attempt to reverse the circulatory or renal complications of a period of progressive respiratory failure. Decisions on intervention with ventilatory assistance must be taken at the right moment, and not postponed until emergency resuscitation is required.

SUMMARY

It is indicative of the great progress that has been made in the recognition and skilled treatment of respiratory failure that it does not seem necessary to conclude this chapter, as was done in the first edition, with a section on the organization of an intensive-care unit. There are now so many excellently organized and staffed centers that most physicians would be better advised to visit one or two of these than to read a description of their operation.

It seems clear that the next major advance should come in understanding the mechanisms that underlie respiratory failure secondary to trauma and shock; it may be suspected, however, that our knowledge of lung biochemistry is too deficient at the present time for quick results to be expected in this field.

This chapter may be fittingly concluded by drawing the reader's attention to a paper by Mithoefer and his co-workers,[3799] entitled "A method of distinguishing death due to cardiac arrest from asphyxia"—a technique that one hopes will rarely have to be used under normal circumstances.

DYSPNEA, DISABILITY, AND PULMONARY FUNCTION

CHAPTER

23

PULMONARY FUNCTION AND DYSPNEA

Until 20 years ago, when the measurable aspects of pulmonary function were few, the problem of the interrelationship between function defect and dyspnea could not be discussed intelligently on a scientific basis. Then, with the rapid development of new laboratory techniques and tests, resulting in improved methods of measurement, so much attention was focused on defining the exact mechanism of production of the sensation of dyspnea that now the general tendency is to overlook the fact that many more definite and reliable answers can be given to specific questions than was possible even 10 years ago.

Dyspnea is usually related to an awareness of respiratory effort, and it is now known that in most disease states there is a measurable abnormality that increases the muscular effort required to ventilate the lungs. It is known also that, in most diseases, the degree of dyspnea is related to the degree of function disturbance—a correlation that can be measured, particularly if measurements are made during exercise as well as at rest.

No attempt is made in this chapter to review the vast literature on dyspnea in health and disease, since this would have to be a monograph in itself. Instead, the problem is approached by attempting to answer three primary questions.

1. What is the relationship between normal lung function and the complaint of dyspnea?

If normal values are obtained for lung volume, ventilatory capacity, inert-gas mixing, pulmonary compliance, and arterial gas tensions, and for exercise ventilation, oxygen uptake, and diffusing capacity, the physician can state with confidence that the normality of pulmonary function has been demonstrated beyond doubt. He may go one step further and note that there is no derangement that would, in a normal person, give rise to a sensation of dyspnea, which symptom, therefore, must be caused by some such mechanism as muscular weakness, anxiety, or an abnormal receptor sensitivity. When all of these measurements are normal, there can be no pathological process extensive enough to interfere with total function; but, of course, a localized process, such as a small carcinoma, can exist without having any effect on total function.

2. What is the relationship between disturbance of function and the complaint of dyspnea?

The first important point in attempting to answer this question is to understand that, whereas the disturbance of function can be approximately quantitated numerically, the sensation of dyspnea inevitably remains subjective, and therefore its evaluation is as difficult as that of other similar sensations, such as hunger, thirst, pain, appreciation of cold, etc. There has perhaps been a tendency to pay too much respect to the physician's grading of dyspnea—especially when this is assessed in accordance with some published classification that appears to give it a stamp of accuracy it clearly does not possess—and too little endeavor directed toward studying particularly those patients who seem to show a marked discrepancy between the degree of effort dyspnea they have noticed and the severity of function derangement recorded. It seems to us that, in addition, there has been a tendency to assume that all sensations of dyspnea are similar—to assume, for example, that the effort dyspnea noted by a normal subject attempting to exercise with his chest wall strapped (which does produce a most disagreeable sensation of suffocation) is similar to that noted by the patient with bronchial obstruction. In general, it seems likely that the sensation of dyspnea may be caused by any one or a combination of three mechanisms: increased respiratory work, reduced ventilatory capacity, and increased subjective sensitivity. A fourth mechanism—increased stimulation of receptors—may have to be added to explain, for example, the dyspnea of pulmonary hypertension, but the nature or even existence of reflexes of this kind is largely speculative. No one knows whether these mechanisms give rise to the same or different sensations, though all such effects are noted as "dyspnea."

With these points in mind, an attempt can now be made to answer the second question. In general, the relationship between disturbance of function and sensation of dyspnea is a close one *within any one distinct disease entity*. Thus, in emphysema, there is in general a satisfactory correlation between ventilatory dysfunction and the increase in respiratory effort it entails, and the severity of dyspnea. In diffuse interstitial fibrosis there is a similar correlation between the degree of dyspnea and the increase in mechanical work that results from the increased exercise ventilation and decreased pulmonary compliance. In mitral stenosis, in the later stages, to these defects is added an increase in airway resistance that increases still further the work of breathing in relation to a given external task. In kyphoscoliosis, the severity of dyspnea is similarly broadly related to the degree of thoracic deformity and interference with ventilation. Thus, as a generality, within any one clearly defined disease group, the relationship between pulmonary function defect and dyspnea is reasonably close. It is very important to note, however, that the influence of individual defects of function is not the same in different types of disease, and that no one measurement of function could possibly be taken as accurately defining the general pattern of dysfunction.[2329]

Dyspnea also appears to be a prominent symptom in some conditions in which the disorder of function in the lung is much less clearly defined or in which pulmonary function is demonstrably normal. These conditions include the following.

NEUROMUSCULAR WEAKNESS. There is little doubt that, in progressive or remittent neuromuscular disorders, dyspnea may be noted by the patient even though lung structure may be normal. It is to be presumed that the patient's awareness of being unable to increase ventilation normally or to take a full deep breath is noted as dyspnea, and it seems likely that muscular weakness involving the intercostal muscles may give rise to a sensation not easily distinguishable from that of other types of dyspnea. Many more studies on such patients will be required before this aspect of dyspnea is understood.

MUSCULAR WEAKNESS IN ADDITION TO LUNG CHANGES. In sarcoidosis there may be pulmonary infiltration together with considerable skeletal-muscle weakness, which may result in a subnormal level of sustainable maximal ventilation even though the single expiration may be of normal velocity. In thyrotoxicosis, dyspnea is one of the commonest symptoms, although interference with pulmonary function is not gross; however, the combination of increased exercise ventilation, decreased pulmonary compliance and muscular weakness, all of which have been noted in this condition (*see* page 430), probably accounts for the prominence of the sensation. Also there is a possibility that the hyperthyroid state may produce a heightened awareness of the proprioceptive impulses, which may be an additional factor of importance.

ANEMIA. As is well known, the patient with megaloblastic anemia may be unaware of dyspnea even when the hemoglobin level is much decreased. However, when the oxygen-carrying capacity falls precipitately in acute conditions, the increased ventilation usually found in these patients may be noticed as dyspnea. The mechanism of this hyperpnea is obscure. It is of interest that acute carbon-monoxide poisoning is not accompanied by dyspnea. In this state, the arterial oxygen tension is normal though the capacity is much reduced; there is no hyperventilation in relation to oxygen uptake; and the lungs are mechanically normal. Thus, there is no reason why dyspnea should be noticed in this condition.

ANXIETY STATES. In anxiety states, the patient's feeling of being unable to take a deep breath—although he is demonstrably capable of this—is often interpreted as dyspnea. Such patients, particularly those with the syndrome of neurocirculatory asthenia (*see* page 440), often overventilate on exercise in relation to oxygen uptake, and this may be noted as dyspnea. There is little doubt that there is an increased perception of breathing effort in some of these patients, just as in others the complaint of palpitations may indicate a preoccupation with the heart. Yet it is easy to be misled, and the physician should be aware that, in the absence of some measurements of function, he may be in danger of dismissing as "functional" a complaint of dyspnea in a patient with organic lung changes. In our experience this is particularly likely to happen when the chest x-ray is clear although function is clearly impaired, as occurs in sarcoidosis, asbestosis, and scleroderma, for example; in emphysema unaccompanied by chronic bronchitis; and in cases in which complaints of dyspnea seem to the physician disproportionate to the clinical or radiological findings and in which it is easy to unearth reasons why the patient may be anxious about his or her condition.

3. What is the mechanism whereby dyspnea is signaled?

Much effort has been expended in trying to develop a unified, comprehensive theory of the perception of dyspnea, and many ingenious and stimulating explanations have been formulated. Campbell has suggested that there may be a neurophysiological basis for an awareness of disproportion between muscular effort of respiratory muscles and the level of ventilation produced.[26, 2214]

It is not possible to undertake a full discussion of this important area in this volume. Many interesting ideas will be found in a recent symposium on breathlessness,[2372] and some recent advances appear to be of particular interest. A valuable discussion of the whole problem of afferent signals from the lung and of reflexes that may be involved in modifying respiration will be found in a recent Ciba Symposium devoted to this topic.[3829] Widdicombe and his colleagues have documented the existence of "lung irritant receptors" in rabbits. He notes that: "The receptors are stimulated by strong inflations and deflations of the lungs, pneumothorax, asphyxial hyperpnea, pulmonary congestion, the inhalation of ammonia vapor or cigarette smoke, pulmonary microembolism, anaphylactic reactions, and bronchostriction induced by injections of histamine and phenyl diguanide. It is concluded that the reflex action of the receptors is to cause hyperpnea and probably bronchoconstriction, and that these receptors may contribute to unpleasant respiratory sensation in human subjects and patients."[3829] Guz and his colleagues[3821] have shown that vagal block does not have any effect on quiet respiration in man, but that bilateral ninth- and tenth-nerve block[3822] result in man in a prolongation of the maximal breath-holding time, with alleviation of the associated distress. Campbell in 1967 showed that muscular paralysis induced by tubocurarine enabled a resting subject to hold his breath for 240 seconds with no accompanying distressing sensation,[3823] supporting the concept that the sensation of distress arises by contraction of respiratory muscles and does not originate in the lungs. Eisele and his co-workers found that spinal anesthesia to the level of T1 did not affect the subject's ability to detect added elastic loads,[3824] and the response to 7 per cent CO_2 was unchanged, as was the sensation and duration of breath-holding.

It is not yet possible to weld these and other observations into a coherent whole. They are certainly relevant to an understanding of the basic mechanism of dyspnea, but they leave much unexplained.

PULMONARY FUNCTION AND DISABILITY

Questions concerning defects of lung function in relation to occupation and disability usually are not open to simple answers. Any physician responsible for giving an opinion on patients in such situations must be fully aware of the clinical history, radiological appearances, and resting and exercise pulmonary function data as a necessary preliminary to his consideration.

We have found it useful to approach such problems by attempting to answer three questions: (1) To what extent has function been impaired and what degree of this impairment can be confidently attributed to one particular pathological process? (2) To what extent is physical ability limited by dyspnea, and is the degree of dyspnea less or more severe than one would predict from the defect in function? (3) To what extent has prognosis been limited by the lung disease? Although such an attempt to assess the salient features is an aid to the overall evaluation, it cannot be pretended that precise answers can be given to these questions. It is equally clear that no intelligent answer can be framed without knowledge of objective measurements of pulmonary function in such persons (*see* Cases 43–48).

Thus, as stressed in Chapter 17, careful appraisal of function, including exercise tests, *must* be available to any panel of physicians charged with responsibility for decisions concerning the effect of a particular disease entity on physical capability.

It is obvious that the degree of disability in relation to dyspnea can be evaluated only when the nature of the patient's work is taken into consideration. No disability, in the industrial sense, may be present in someone with moderately severe emphysema whose job is clerical, though his spare-time athletic pursuits may be curtailed. On the other hand, a similar loss of effort tolerance may result in unemployment for a man trained only in hard physical work.[2249]

Annotated Guide to the Bibliography

Under 41 General Headings

All references between the numbers 1 and 2358 date from before 1964; almost all those between 2359 and 3833 date from 1964.

This index is not extensively cross-referenced. For example, "blood-gas tensions in emphysema" will be found under "emphysema" and not under "blood-gas tensions." Most of the references under the heading "blood-gas tensions" are concerned with methodology or normal values.

Occupational Lung Diseases (including Pigeon Breeder's Lung)

152, 366, 727, 728, 729, 878, 881, 882, 883, 921, 929, 960, 961, 1532–1534, 1584–1614, 1615–1683, 1705, 2082–2093, 2095–2098, 2107–2111, 2225, 2243, 2244, 2298, 2303, 2315, 2349–2354, 2531, 2723, 3235–3323, 3330–3338, 3348–3352, 3356–3360, 3362, 3715.

Pneumonectomy (including Lung Transplantation)

242, 307, 313, 363, 388, 1151–1195, 2044–2047, 2234, 2226, 2252, 2277, 2278, 2977–3031, 3719, 3827.

Pneumonia

394, 507, 1049, 1416–1418, 1714, 2219, 2220, 3385–3397.

Pneumothorax (including Hemothorax)

304, 1130–1150, 2241, 2970, 2971–2976.

Pulmonary Circulation

1827, 1829, 1833, 1920, 1921, 1947–1995, 2023, 2230, 2267, 2284, 2323, 2442, 2451, 2461, 2466–2473, 2475–2484, 3173, 3542, 3543.

Pulmonary Edema (including Left Ventricular Failure and Myocardial Infarction)

271, 1488, 1492–1494, 2073, 2075, 2076, 2094, 2481, 3137–3143, 3145–3158, 3173, 3216, 3629–3631, 3730, 3734, 3750, 3751, 3777.

Pulmonary Emboli (including Primary Pulmonary Hypertension)

552, 711, 1505–1523, 2066–2071, 2074, 2229, 2333, 3159–3191, 3200–3215, 3380, 3728.

Radiation Pneumonitis and Fibrosis

463, 1380–1394, 2112, 2340, 3353–3355, 3377.

Regional Lung Function

119, 127, 171–176, 266, 290–300, 303–306, 308–319, 326–345, 574–577, 579, 735, 1790–1792, 1810, 1812, 2302, 2304, 2318, 2431, 2432, 2436–2438, 2440, 2442, 2444–2447, 2450, 2452, 2455–2460, 2464, 2465, 2466, 2473, 2479, 2484, 2532, 2811, 2812, 2815, 2831, 2873, 2880, 2894, 2945, 3131, 3165, 3166, 3178, 3385, 3443, 3652, 3717, 3826, 3834.

Respiratory Failure (including Shock and Trauma)

43, 280, 678, 1012, 1195–1213, 1243, 1244, 1249–1265, 1267–1281, 1297–1328, 1364, 1367, 1427–1434, 2123, 2138, 2140, 2152, 2154–2159, 2161, 2175–2182, 2186–2189, 2192, 2198–2201, 2207, 2209–2213, 2233, 2240, 2259, 2261, 2270, 2275, 2289, 2291, 2305, 2307, 2313, 2332, 2355, 2356, 2366, 2609, 2610, 2612, 2844, 2864, 2877, 2886, 2914, 3234, 3724, 3732, 3750, 3751, 3752–3820, 3834.

Sarcoidosis

56, 393, 418, 528, 1395–1405, 2060, 3076–3092.

Ventilation Distribution (see also Regional Lung Function)

94, 95–97, 100 101, 112–114, 130–134, 142–145, 147–151, 153–170, 233, 236–240, 249, 250, 315, 320–322, 325, 578, 593, 653, 1283, 1946, 2269, 2276, 2341, 2374, 2375, 2423, 2425, 2426, 2430–2433, 2745, 2772, 2848, 2850, 2859, 2870, 2871, 2881, 3522, 3652, 3653, 3718.

$\dot{V}$ / $\dot{Q}$ Distribution

231, 233, 234, 249, 261–264, 272, 289, 315, 336–345, 412–416, 423, 653, 1811, 2123, 2268, 2377, 2439, 2442, 2488, 2489–2491, 2872, 2873, 2875, 2894, 3523, 3539, 3554, 3581, 3633, 3639, 3640, 3652, 3654–3657, 3661.

Books and Monographs

1–4, 6–20, 23, 25, 27–29, 31–35, 88, 189, 222, 231, 542, 561, 663, 671, 810, 822, 823, 824, 856, 857, 2224, 2227, 2434, 2456, 2470, 2487, 2488, 2489, 2878, 3455, 3670, 3688, 3807, 3825, 3826, 3828.

Symposia

5, 21, 22, 24, 26, 30, 171, 181, 203, 563, 662, 670, 672, 815, 842, 886, 894, 910, 915, 2319, 2360, 2372, 2437, 2644, 2701, 3363, 3454, 3516, 3829.

References

1. Meakins, J. C., and Davies, H. W.: *Respiratory Function in Disease.* Edinburgh, Oliver & Boyd, 1925.
2. Haldane, J. S., and Priestley, J. G.: *Respiration.* 2nd ed. Oxford, Clarendon Press, 1935.
3. Comroe, J. H., Jr., Forster, R. E., II, DuBois, A. B., Briscoe, W. A., and Carlsen, E.: *The Lung: Clinical Physiology and Pulmonary Function Tests.* 2nd ed. Chicago, Year Book Medical Publishers, 1962.
4. Campbell, E. J. M., Agostoni, E., and Davis, J. N.: *The Respiratory Muscles: Mechanics and Neural Control.* Philadelphia & London, W. B. Saunders Company, 1970, p. 348.
5. Harbord, R. P., and Woolmer, R. (eds.): *Symposium on Pulmonary Ventilation, Leeds, 1958.* Altrincham, England, John Sherratt & Son, 1959.
6. Stuart-Harris, C. H., and Hanley, T.: *Chronic Bronchitis, Emphysema and Cor Pulmonale.* Bristol, John Wright & Sons, 1957.
7. Oswald, N. C.: *Recent Trends in Chronic Bronchitis.* London, Lloyd-Luke, 1958.
8. Campbell, E. J. M., and Dickinson, C. J. (eds.): *Clinical Physiology.* Oxford, Blackwell Scientific Publications, 1960.
9. Harris, P., and Heath, D.: *The Human Pulmonary Circulation; Its Form and Function in Health and Disease.* Edinburgh, E. & S. Livingstone, 1962.
10. Feather, N.: *Mass, Length and Time.* Edinburgh, University Press, 1959; Harmondsworth, Penguin Books, 1961 (Pelican Book No. A532).
11. Barach, A. L., and Bickerman, H. A. (eds.); *Pulmonary Emphysema.* Baltimore, Williams & Wilkins, 1956.
12. Rubin, E. H.: *The Lung as a Mirror of Systemic Disease.* Springfield, Ill., Charles C Thomas, 1956.
13. Comroe, J. H., Jr. (ed.): Pulmonary function tests. In: *Methods in Medical Research,* vol. 2. Chicago, Year Book Medical Publishers, 1950, p. 74 (part II).
14. Karpovich, P. V.: *Physiology of Muscular Activity.* 5th ed. Philadelphia, W. B. Saunders Co., 1959.
15. Hinshaw, H. C., and Garland, L. H.: *Diseases of the Chest.* 2nd ed. Philadelphia, W. B. Saunders Co., 1963.
16. Cherniack, R. M., and Cherniack, L.: *Respiration in Health and Disease.* Philadelphia, W. B. Saunders Co., 1961.
17. Rossier, P. H., Bühlmann, A. A., and Wiesinger, K. (P. C. Luchsinger and K. M. Moser, editors and translators): *Respiration: Physiologic Principles and Their Clinical Applications.* St. Louis, C. V. Mosby Co., 1960.
18. Knowles, J. H.: *Respiratory Physiology and Its Clinical Application.* Cambridge, Mass., Harvard University Press, 1959.
19. Mushin, W. W., Rendell-Baker, L., and Thompson, P. W.: *Automatic Ventilation of the Lungs.* Oxford, Blackwell Scientific Publications; Springfield, Ill., Charles C Thomas, 1959.
20. Ryle, G.: *Dilemmas* (The Tarner Lectures, 1953). London, Cambridge University Press, 1954.
21. Wolstenholme, G. E. W., and Cameron, M. P. (eds.): *Ciba Foundation Colloquia on Ageing.* Vol. I: *General Aspects.* London, J. & A. Churchill, 1955.
22. *Symposium on Pulmonary Circulation and Respiratory Function, Dundee, 1955.* Edinburgh, E. & S. Livingstone (for University of St Andrews), 1956.
23. von Hayek, H. (V. E. Krahl, translator): *The Human Lung.* New York, Hafner Publishing Co., 1960.
24. *Symposium on Emphysema and the "Chronic Bronchitis" Syndrome, Aspen, Colorado, 1958.* Am. Rev. Resp. Dis., *80*:1, 1959.
25. *Summary of a Report of The Royal College of Physicians of London on Smoking in Relation to Cancer of the Lung and Other Diseases.* London, Pitman Medical Publishing Co., 1962.
26. de Reuck, A. V. S., and O'Connor, M. (eds.): *Ciba Foundation Symposium on Pulmonary Structure and Function.* London, J. & A. Churchill, 1962.
27. Simon, G.: *Principles of Chest X-Ray Diagnosis.* London, Butterworth & Co., 1956.
28. Barcroft, J.: *The Respiratory Function of the Blood.* London, Cambridge University Press, 1914.
29. Davenport, H. W.: *The A B C of Acid-Base Chemistry.* 4th ed. Chicago, University of Chicago Press, 1958.
30. Cunningham, D. J. C., and Lloyd, B. B. (eds.): *The Regulation of Human Respiration:* Proceedings of the J. S. Haldame Centenary Symposium, Oxford, 1961. Oxford, Blackwell Scientific Publications, 1963.
31. Nahas, G. G. (ed.): *In vitro* and *in vivo* effects of amine buffers. Ann. N.Y. Acad. Sci., *92*:333–812, 1961.
32. Boothby, W. M. (ed.): *Handbook of Respiratory Physiology: Respiratory Physiology in Aviation* (Project No. 21-2301-0003). Randolph Field, Texas, USAF School of Aviation Medicine, 1954.
33. Spencer, H.: *Pathology of the Lung (Excluding Pulmonary Tuberculosis).* New York, The Macmillan Company; Galt, Canada, Brett-Macmillan; London, Pergamon Press; 1962, p. 850.
34. Wade, O. L., and Bishop, J. M.: *Cardiac Output and Regional Blood Flow.* Oxford, Blackwell Scientific Publications, 1962.
35. Ministry of Health Report on Public Health, No. 95. *Mortality and Morbidity during the London Fog of December 1952.* London, HMSO, 1954.
36. Perkins, J. F., Jr.: Plastic Douglas bags. J. Appl. Physiol., *6*:445, 1954.
37. Donald, K. W., and Christie, R. V.: A new method of clinical spirometry. Clin. Sci., *8*:21, 1949.
38. Ogilvie, C. M., Forster, R. E., Blakemore, W. S., and Morton, J. W.: A standardized breath holding technique for the clinical measurement of the diffusing capacity of the lung for carbon monoxide. J. Clin. Invest., *36*:1, 1957.
39. Bates, D. V., Woolf, C. R., and Paul, G. I.: Chronic bronchitis. A report on the first two stages of the co-ordinated study of chronic bronchitis in the Department of Veterans Affairs, Canada. Med. Serv. J. Canada, *18*:211, 1962.
40. Shepard, R. J., Carey, G. C. R., and Phair, J. J.: Evaluation of a portable box-bag for field testing of pulmonary diffusion. J. Appl. Physiol., *12*:79, 1958.
41. Gandevia, B., and Hugh-Jones, P.: Terminology for measurements of ventilatory capacity. Thorax, *12*:290, 1957.
42. Hermannsen, J.: Untersuchungen über die maximale Venti-

lationgrösse (Atemgrenzwert). Z. Ges. Exper. Med., *90*:130, 1933.

43. Baldwin, E. de F., Cournand, A., and Richards, D. W., Jr.: Pulmonary insufficiency. I. Physiological classification, clinical methods of analysis, standard values in normal subjects. Medicine, *27*:243, 1948.
44. Bernstein, L., and Mendel, A.: The accuracy of spirographic recording at high respiratory rates. Thorax, *6*:297, 1951.
45. Matheson, H. W., Spies, S. N., Gray, J. S., and Barnum, D. R.: Ventilatory function tests. II. Factors affecting the voluntary ventilation capacity. J. Clin. Invest., *29*:682, 1950.
46. Gray, J. S., Barnum, D. R., Matheson, H. W., and Spies, S. N.: Ventilatory function tests. I. Voluntary ventilation capacity. J. Clin. Invest., *29*:677, 1950.
47. Stead, W. W., Wells, H. S., Gault, N. L., and Ognanovich, J.: Inaccuracy of the conventional water-filled spirometer for recording rapid breathing. J. Appl. Physiol., *14*:448, 1959.
48. Wells, H. S., Stead, W. W., Rossing, T. D., and Ognanovich, J.: Accuracy of an improved spirometer for recording of fast breathing. J. Appl. Physiol., *14*:451, 1959.
49. Wright, G. W., and Gilford, S. R.: A method for the simultaneous measurement of maximum breathing capacity, pulmonary volumina, and effective lung ventilation. J. Thorac. Cardiov. Surg., *38*:643, 1959.
50. Bartlett, R. G., Jr., and Specht, H. S.: Maximum breathing capacity with various expiratory and inspiratory resistances (single and combined) at various breathing rates. J. Appl. Physiol., *11*:79, 1957.
51. Zwi, S., Theron, J. C., McGregor, M., and Becklake, M. R.: The influence of instrumental resistance on the maximum breathing capacity. Dis. Chest, *36*:361, 1959.
52. Shephard, R. J.: Some factors affecting the open-circuit determination of maximum breathing capacity. J. Physiol. (London), *135*:98, 1957.
53. Theron, J. C., Zwi, S., and McGregor, M.: A low-resistance respiratory valve. Lancet, *1*:415, 1958.
54. McKerrow, C. B., and Otis, A. B.: Low resistance valve for hyperventilation. J. Appl. Physiol., *9*:497, 1956.
55. Bartlett, R. G., Jr., Brubach, H., and Specht, H.: Some factors determining the maximum breathing capacity. J. Appl. Physiol., *12*:247, 1958.
56. Marshall, R., Smellie, H., Baylis, J. H., Hoyle, C., and Bates, D. V.: Pulmonary function in sarcoidosis. Thorax, *13*:48, 1958.
57. Gaensler, E. A.: Evaluation of pulmonary function: Methods. Ann. Rev. Med. *12*:385, 1961.
58. Anderson, W. H.: A comparison of various segments of the forced expirogram with the maximum breathing capacity. Dis. Chest, *38*:370, 1960.
59. Brille, D., and Hatzfeld, C.: Critique de l'aspect rectiligne de la premiére portion de la courbe d'expiration forcée de l'épreuve de Tiffeneau. Path. Biol. Semaine Hop., *6*:591, 1958.
60. Shephard, R. J.: The direct interpretation of the fast vital capacity record. Thorax, *11*:223, 1956.
61. Drutel, P., and Dechoux, J.: Un test spirographique de la perméabilité bronchique: Le rapport de la capacité pulmonaire utilisable a l'effort avec la capacité vitale. J. Franc. Med. Chir. Thorac., *6*:517, 1952.
62. Kennedy, M. C. S.: Practical measure of the maximum ventilatory capacity in health and disease. Thorax, *8*:73, 1953.
63. Bernstein, L., and Kazantzis, G.: The relation between the fast vital capacity curves and the maximum breathing capacity. Thorax, *9*:326, 1954.
64. Bernstein, L.: A critical discussion of the recorded form of the fast vital capacity record. Thorax, *9*:63, 1954.
65. Gillis, S., and Butterworth, B. A.: Modifications of a spirometer for timed capacity and mid-expiratory flow measurements. Lancet, *1*:723, 1958.
66. McKerrow, C. B., McDermott, M., and Gilson, J. C.: A spirometer for measuring the forced expiratory volume with a simple calibrating device. Lancet, *1*:149, 1960.
67. Miller, W. F., Johnson, R. L., Jr., and Wu, N.: Relationships between fast vital capacity and various timed expiratory capacities. J. Appl. Physiol., *14*:157, 1959.
68. Hyatt, R. E., Schilder, D. P., and Fry, D. L.: Relationship between maximum expiratory flow and degree of lung inflation. J. Appl. Physiol., *13*:331, 1958.
69. Fry, D. L.: Theoretical considerations of the bronchial pressure-flow-volume relationships with particular reference to the maximum expiratory flow volume curve. Phys. Med. Biol., *3*:174, 1958.
70. Fry, D. L., and Hyatt, R. E.: Pulmonary mechanics. A unified analysis of the relationship between pressure, volume and gasflow in the lungs of normal and diseased human subjects. Am. J. Med., *29*:672, 1960.
71. Gilson, J. C.: Lung function tests: An assessment of their usefulness. Lectures Sci. Basis Med., *6*:58, 1956.
72. Horton, G. E., and Phillips, S.: The expiratory ventilagram. Application of total and timed vital capacities and maximal expiratory flow rate, as obtained by a bellows apparatus, for bedside and office use. Am. Rev. Resp. Dis., *80*:724, 1959.
73. McKerrow, C. B.: The McKesson Vitalor. J.A.M.A., *177*:865, 1961.
74. Leuallen, E. C., and Fowler, W. S.: Maximal mid-expiratory flow. Am. Rev. Tuberc., *72*:783, 1955.
75. Fairbairn, A. S., Fletcher, C. M., Tinker, C. M., and Wood, C. H.: A comparison of spirometric and peak expiratory flow measurements in men with and without chronic bronchitis. Thorax, *17*:168, 1962.
76. Kory, R. C., Callahan, R., Boren, H. G., and Syner, J. C.: The Veterans Administration–Army Cooperative Study of Pulmonary Function, I. Clinical spirometry in normal men. Am. J. Med., *30*:243, 1961.
77. Bouhuys, A.: The clinical use of pneumotachography. Acta Med. Scand., *159*:91, 1957.
78. Wright, B. M., and McKerrow, C. B.: Maximum forced expiratory flow rate as a measure of ventilatory capacity. Brit. Med. J., *2*:1041, 1959.
79. Heaf, P. J. D., and Gillam, P. M. S.: Peak flow rates in normal and asthmatic children. Brit. Med. J., *1*:1595, 1962.
80. Jackson, J. M.: Peak expiratory flow rates. Brit. Med. J., *1*:1760, 1961.
81. Tinker, C. M.: Peak expiratory flow rates. Brit. Med. J., *2*:177, 1961.
82. Ritchie, B.: A comparison of forced expiratory volume and peak flow in clinical practice. Lancet, *2*:271, 1962.
83. Shephard, R. J.: Some observations on peak expiratory flow. Thorax, *17*:39, 1962.
84. Tinker, C. M.: Peak expiratory flow measured by the Wright peak flow meter: Distribution of values in men aged 30–50 who denied respiratory symptoms. Brit. Med. J., *1*:1365, 1961.
85. Nairn, J. R., Bennet, A. J., Andrew, J. D., and Macarthur, P.: A study of respiratory function in normal school children. The peak flow rate. Arch. Dis. Child., *36*:253, 1961.
86. Cherniack, R. M.: Ventilatory function in normal children. Canad. M. A. J., *87*:80, 1962.
87. Federation of American Societies for Experimental Biology: Standardization of definitions and symbols in respiratory physiology. Fed. Proc., *9*:602, 1950.
88. Davy, H. (J. Davy, ed.): *Collected Papers.* Vol. 3: *Researches, Chiefly Concerning Nitrous Oxide.* London, Smith Elder, 1939, p. 242.
89. Hutchinson, J.: On the capacity of the lungs, and on the respiratory functions, with a view of establishing a precise and easy method of detecting disease by the spirometer. Med.-Chir. Trans. (London), *29*:137, 1846.
90. Van Slyke, D. D., and Binger, C. A. L.: The determination of lung volume without forced breathing. J. Exper. Med., *37*:457, 1923.
91. Christie, R. V.: The lung volume and its subdivisions. I. Methods of measurement. J. Clin. Invest., *11*:1099, 1932.
92. Hurtado, A., and Fray, W. W.: Studies of total pulmonary capacity and its subdivisions. II. Correlation with physical and radiological measurements. J. Clin. Invest., *12*:807, 1933.
93. Lassen, H. C. A., Cournand, A., and Richards, D. W., Jr.: Distribution of respiratory gases in closed breathing circuits. I. In normal subjects. J. Clin. Invest., *16*:1, 1937.
94. Darling, R. C., Cournand, A., Mansfield, J. S., and Richards, D. W., Jr.: Studies on the intrapulmonary mixture of gases. I. Nitrogen elimination from blood and body tissues during high oxygen breathing. J. Clin. Invest., *19*:591, 1940.
95. Darling, R. C., Cournand, A., and Richards, D. W., Jr.:

Studies on the intrapulmonary mixture of gases. III. An open circuit method for measuring residual air. J. Clin. Invest., *19:*609, 1940.

96. Cournand, A., Baldwin, E. D., Darling, R. C., and Richards, D. W., Jr.: Studies on the intrapulmonary mixture of gases. IV. Significance of pulmonary emptying rate and simplified open circuit measurement of residual air. J. Clin. Invest., *20:*681, 1941.
97. Bateman, J. B., Boothby, W. M., and Helmholz, H. F., Jr.: Studies of lung volumes and intrapulmonary mixing: Notes on open-circuit methods, including use of a new pivoted type gasometer for lung clearance studies. J. Clin. Invest., *28:*679, 1949.
98. Gilson, J. C., and Hugh-Jones, P.: The measurement of the total lung volume and breathing capacity. Clin. Sci., *7:*185, 1949.
99. Curtis, J. K., Emanuel, D., and Rasmussen, H. K.: Improved apparatus for determining the functional residual capacity of the lung by the open circuit method. Am. J. Med., *18:*531, 1955.
100. Luft, U. C., Roorbach, E. H., and MacQuigg, R. E.: Pulmonary nitrogen clearance as a criterion of ventilatory efficiency. Am. Rev. Tuberc., *72:*465, 1955.
101. Hickam, J. B., Blair, E., and Frayser, R.: An open-circuit helium method for measuring functional residual capacity and defective intrapulmonary gas mixing. J. Clin. Invest., *33:*1277, 1954.
102. Emmanuel, G., Briscoe, W. A., and Cournand, A.: A method for the determination of the volume of air in the lungs: Measurements in chronic pulmonary emphysema. J. Clin. Invest., *40:*329, 1961.
103. McMichael, J.: A rapid method of determining lung capacity. Clin. Sci., *4:*167, 1939.
104. Herrald, F. J. C., and McMichael, J.: Determination of lung volume: A simple constant volume modification of Christie's method. Proc. Roy. Soc. (London), *s.B, 126:*491, 1939.
105. Aslett, E. A., Hart, P. D., and McMichael, J.: Lung volume and its subdivisions in normal males. Proc. Roy. Soc. (London), *s.B, 126:*502, 1939.
106. Birath, G.: Lung volume and ventilation efficiency. Changes in collapse-treated and non-collapse-treated pulmonary tuberculosis and in pulmonectomy and lobectomy. Acta Med. Scand., Suppl. 154, 1945.
107. Meneely, G. R., and Kaltreider, N. L.: The volume of the lung determined by helium dilution. Description of the method and comparison with other procedures. J. Clin. Invest., *28:*129, 1949.
108. Cara, M., and Economides, E.: Spectre de fréquence de l'air courant et de la ventilation lors de l'épreuve de la ventilation maxima, rélation avec la courbe d'expiration forcée. Compt. Rend. Soc. Biol. (Paris), *146:*709, 1952.
109. Whitfield, A. G. W., Waterhouse, J. A. H., and Arnott, W. M.: The total lung volume and its subdivisions. A study in physiological norms. I. Basic data. Brit. J. Social Med., *4:*1, 1950.
110. Weiner, R. S., and Cooper, P.: Measurement of functional residual capacity. A comparision of two closed-circuit helium-dilution methods. Am. Rev. Tuberc., *74:*729, 1956.
111. Birath, G., and Swenson, E. W.: A nomographic solution for lung volume determinations in the closed system helium dilution method. Scand. J. Clin. Lab. Invest., *8:*329, 1956.
112. Nye, R. E., Jr.: Closed circuit method for measuring uneven ventilation. J. Appl. Physiol., *16:*1109, 1961.
113. Visser, B. F.: *Clinical Gas Analysis Based on Thermal Conductivity.* Thesis for the degree of Ph.D., University of Utrecht, 1957. Utrecht, Kemink & Zoon, 1957.
114. Bates, D. V., and Christie, R. V.: Intrapulmonary mixing of helium in health and in emphysema. Clin. Sci., *9:*17, 1950.
115. Björklund, O., and Dahlström, H.: On the accuracy of determinations of the functional residual air. Scand. J. Clin. Lab. Invest., *4:*345, 1952.
116. Birath, G., and Swenson, E. W.: A correction factor for helium absorption in lung volume determinations. Scand. J. Clin. Lab. Invest., *8:*155, 1956.
117. Meneely, G. R., Ball, C. O. T., Kory, R. C., Callaway, J. J., Merrill, J. M., Mabe, R. E., Roehm, D. C., and Kaltreider, N. L.: A simplified closed circuit helium dilution method for the determination of the residual volume of the lungs. Am. J. Med., *28:*824, 1960.
118. Goldman, H. I., and Becklake, M. R.: Respiratory function tests: Normal values of median altitudes and the prediction of normal results. Am. Rev. Tuberc, *79:*457, 1959.
119. Fleming, H. A., and West, L. R.: An appreciation of bronchospirometry as a method of investigation based on 125 cases. Thorax, *9:*273, 1954.
120. Comroe, J. H., Jr., Botelho, S. Y., and DuBois, A. B.: Design of a body plethysmograph for studying cardiopulmonary physiology. J. Appl. Physiol., *14:*439, 1959.
121. Bedell, G. N., Marshall, R., DuBois, A. B., and Comroe, J. H., Jr.: Plethysmographic determination of the volume of gas trapped in the lungs. J. Clin. Invest., *35:*664, 1956.
122. DuBois, A. B.: New concepts in cardio-pulmonary physiology, developed by the use of the body plethysmograph. (Third Bowditch Lecture.) Physiologist, *2:*8, 1959.
123. Schmidt, A. M., and Cohn, J. E.: Modified body plethysmograph for study of cardiopulmonary physiology. J. Appl. Physiol., *16:*935, 1961.
124. Mead, J.: Volume displacement body plethysmograph for respiratory measurements in human subjects. J. Appl. Physiol., *15:*736, 1960.
125. Wade, O. L., and Gilson, J. C.: The effect of posture on diaphragmatic movement and vital capacity in normal subjects, with a note on spirometry as an aid in determining radiological chest volumes. Thorax, *6:*103, 1951.
126. Cobb, S., Blodgett, D. J., Olson, K. B., and Stranahan, A.: Determination of total lung capacity in disease from routine chest roentgenograms. Am. J. Med., *16:*39, 1954.
127. Autio, V.: Bronchospirometric studies relating to a radiographic method for determining differential vital capacity. Acta Med. Scand., *158:*Suppl. 329, 1957.
128. Anthony, A. J.: Untersuchungen über Lungenvolumina und Lungenventilation. Deutsch. Arch. klin. Med., *167:*129, 1930.
129. Lanphier, E. H.: Determination of residual volume and residual volume/total capacity ratio by single breath technics. J. Appl. Physiol., *5:*361, 1953.
130. Siebeck, R.: Über den Gasaustausch zwischen der Aufsenluft und den Alveolen. Z. Biol., *55:*267, 1911.
131. Lundsgaard, C., and Schierbeck, K.: Studies on the mixture of air in the lungs with various gases. II. The quantitative influence of certain factors in producing a full mixture of hydrogen with air in the lungs. Am. J. Physiol., *64:*231, 1923.
132. Sonne, C.: Inequality of ventilation of different parts of the lung as a source of error in respiratory-physiological experiments. Skand. Arch. Physiol., *75:*127, 1936.
133. Sonne, C.: Modern views of the mechanism of the lung function and its significance to physiology and clinical medicine. Acta Med. Scand., *90:*315, 1936.
134. Roelsen, E.: The composition of the alveolar air investigated by fractional sampling. Comparative investigations on normal persons and patients with bronchial asthma and pulmonary emphysema. Acta Med. Scand., *98:*141, 1939.
135. Roelsen, E.: Fractional analysis of alveolar air after inspiration of hydrogen as a method for the determination of the distribution of inspired air in the lungs. Examination of normal persons and of patients suffering from bronchial asthma and pulmonary emphysema. Acta Med. Scand., *95:*452, 1938.
136. McGregor, M.: The value of an index of maximal expiratory force in the interpretation of tests of maximal ventilatory capacity. Am. Rev. Tuberc., *78:*692, 1958.
137. McKerrow, C. B.: The assessment of respiratory function. Proc. Roy. Soc. Med. (London), *46:*532, 1953.
138. Gad, U.: Fractionated analysis of the alveolar air in pulmonary tuberculosis. I. Examinations after inhalation of pure hydrogen at various degrees of the disease and during collapse-treatment. Acta Tuberc. Scand., *17:*88, 1943.
139. Gad, U.: Fractionated analysis of the alveolar air in pulmonary tuberculosis. II. Examinations after inhalation of atmospheric air at various degrees of the disease and during collapse-treatment. Acta Tuberc. Scand., *17:*116, 1943.
140. Mundt, E., Schoedel, W., and Schwarz, H.: Über den effektiven Schädlichen Raum der Atmung. Arch. ges. Physiol., *244:*107, 1940.

141. Mundt, E., Schoedel, W., and Schwarz, H.: Über die Gleichmässigkeit der Lungenbelüftung. Arch. ges. Physiol., *244*:99, 1940.
142. Comroe, J. H., Jr., and Fowler, W. S.: Lung function studies. VI. Detection of uneven alveolar ventilation during a single breath of oxygen; a new test of pulmonary disease. Am. J. Med., *10*:408, 1951.
143. Greifenstein, F. E., King, R. M., Latch, S. S., and Comroe, J. H., Jr.: Pulmonary function studies in healthy men and women 50 years and older. J. Appl. Physiol., *4*:641, 1952.
144. Fowler, W. S.: Lung function studies. III. Uneven pulmonary ventilation in normal subjects and in patients with pulmonary disease. J. Appl. Physiol., *2*:283, 1949.
145. Fowler, W. S.: Intrapulmonary distribution of inspired gas. Physiol. Rev., *32*:1, 1952.
146. Briscoe, W. A.: Comparison between alveolo-arterial gradient predicted from mixing studies and the observed gradient. J. Appl. Physiol., *14*:299, 1959.
147. Otis, A. B., McKerrow, C. B., Bartlett, R. A., Mead, J., McIlroy, M. B., Selverstone, N. J., and Radford, E. P., Jr.: Mechanical factors in distribution of pulmonary ventilation. J. Appl. Physiol., *8*:427, 1956.
148. Shephard, R. J.: Assessment of ventilatory efficiency by the single-breath technique. J. Physiol. (London), *134*:630, 1956.
149. Kjellmer, I., Sandqvist, L., and Berglund, E.: Alveolar plateau' of the single breath nitrogen elimination curve in normal subjects. J. Appl. Physiol., *14*:105, 1959.
150. Sandqvist, L., and Kjellmer, I.: Normal values for the single breath nitrogen elimination test in different age groups. Scand. J. Clin. Lab. Invest., *12*:131, 1960.
151. Lundin, G.: Nitrogen meter in respiratory research. Scand. J. Clin. Lab. Invest., *4*:71, 1952.
152. Gilson, J. C., and Hugh-Jones, P.: *Lung Function in Coalworkers' Pneumoconiosis* (M.R.C. Spec. Rep. Ser. No. 290). London, H.M.S.O., 1955.
153. Robertson, J. S., Siri, W. E., and Jones, H. B.: Lung ventilation patterns determined by analysis of nitrogen elimination rates; use of the mass spectrometer as a continuous gas analyzer. J. Clin. Invest., *29*:577, 1950.
154. Fowler, W. S., Cornish, E. R., Jr., and Kety, S.: Lung function studies. VIII. Analysis of alveolar ventilation by pulmonary N_2 clearance curves. J. Clin. Invest., *31*:40, 1952.
155. Blair, E., and Hickam, J. B.: Quantitative study of intrapulmonary gas mixing in emphysema. Am. J. Med., *18*:519, 1955.
156. Blair, E., and Hickam, J. B.: The effect of change in body position on lung volume and intra-pulmonary gas mixing in normal subjects. J. Clin. Invest., *34*:383, 1955.
157. Cohen, A. A., Hemingway, A., and Hemingway, C.: Standardization of the pulmonary nitrogen clearance test using older normal men. J. Lab. Clin. Med., *54*:603, 1959.
158. Bouhuys, A.: Jönsson, R., and Lundin, G.: Nonuniformity of pulmonary ventilation in chronic diffuse obstructive emphysema. Acta Med. Scand., *162*:29, 1958.
159. Briscoe, W. A.: Further studies on the intrapulmonary mixing of helium in normal and emphysematous subjects. Clin. Sci., *11*:45, 1952.
160. Briscoe, W. A., and Cournand, A.: Uneven ventilation of normal and diseased lungs studied by an open-circuit method. J. Appl. Physiol., *14*:284, 1959.
161. Nye, R. E., Jr.: Theoretical limits to measurement of uneven ventilation. J. Appl. Physiol., *16*:1115, 1961.
162. Bouhuys, A., and Lundin, G.: Distribution of inspired gas in lungs. Physiol. Rev., *39*:731, 1959.
163. Becklake, M. R.: A new index of the intrapulmonary mixture of inspired air. Thorax, *7*:111, 1952.
164. Englert, M., Denolin, H., and De Coster, A.: Étude de la ventilation pulmonaire par la méthode a l'hélium. J. Franc. Med. Chir. Thorac., *9*:14, 1955.
165. Needham, C. D., Rogan, M. C., and McDonald, I.: Normal standards for lung volumes, intrapulmonary gas-mixing, and maximum breathing capacity. Thorax, *9*:313, 1954.
166. Kanagami, H., Shiroishi, K., Katsura, T., and Aonuma, K.: Studies on the new method of the intrapulmonary gas distribution by the helium closed circuit method. Resp. Circ., *8*:99, 1960.
167. Briscoe, W. A., Becklake, M. R., and Rose, T. F.: Intrapulmonary mixing of helium in normal and emphysematous subjects. Clin. Sci., *10*:37, 1951.
168. Orinius, E., and Ståhle, I.: The helium-dilution method in determination of ventilatory disturbances: A new method for data treatment. Am. Rev. Resp. Dis., *79*:450, 1959.
169. Buxton, R. S. J., and D'Silva, J. L.: Use of the helium-dilution method to assess the mixing of gases in the lungs. Tubercle, *37*:264, 1956.
170. Becklake, M. R., and Goldman, H. I.: The influence of pulmonary dead space on lung mixing indices. S. African J. Med. Sci. *19*:21, 1954.
171. Venrath, H.: The test of lung function with the help of isotopes. In: *Bad Oeynhausener Gespräche*, 1956. Berlin: Springer, 1957, p. 144.
172. Knipping, H. W., Bolt, W., Valentin, H., Venrath, H., and Endler, P.: Technik und Möglichkeiten der regionalen Ventilationsanalyse mittels des radioktiven Edelgases $Xenon^{133}$ (Isotopenthorakographie). Z. Tuberk., *117*:51, 1961.
173. Dyson, N. A., Hugh-Jones, P., Newbery, G. R., Sinclair, J. D., and West, J. B.: Studies of regional lung function using radioactive oxygen. Brit. Med. J., *1*:231, 1960.
174. Ball, W. C., Jr., Stewart, P. B., Newsham, L. G. S., and Bates, D. V.: Regional pulmonary function studied with $xenon^{133}$. J. Clin. Invest., *41*:519, 1962.
175. Dollery, C. T., Hugh-Jones, P., and Matthews, C. M. E.: Use of radioactive xenon for studies of regional lung function. Brit. Med. J., *2*:1006, 1962.
176. Steiner, R. E., Laws, J. W., Gilbert, J., and McDonnell, M. J.: Radiological lung-function studies. Lancet, *2*:1051, 1960.
177. Campbell, E. J. M.: R I pH. Lancet, *1*:681, 1962.
178. Nahas, G. G.: Spectrophotometric determination of hemoglobin and oxyhemoglobin in whole hemolyzed blood. Science, *113*:723, 1951.
179. Nahas, G. G.: A simplified Lucite cuvette for the spectrophotometric measurement of hemoglobin and oxyhemoglobin. J. Appl. Physiol., *13*:147, 1958.
180. Verel, D., Saynor, R., and Kesteven, A. B.: A spectrophotometric method of estimating blood oxygen using the Unicam SP 600. J. Clin. Pathol., *13*:361, 1960.
181. Sendroy, J.: Problems in measurement of pH of blood and other biological fluids. In: *Symposium on pH Measurements*, Spec. Tech. Publ. No. 190. Philadelphia, American Society for Testing Materials, 1956, pp. 55–64.
182. Semple, S. J. G., Mattock, G., and Uncles, R.: A buffer standard for blood pH measurements. J. Biol. Chem., *237*:963, 1962.
183. Astrup, P., and Schrøder, S.: Apparatus for anaërobic determination of the pH of blood at 38° Centigrade. Scand. J. Clin. Lab. Invest., *8*:30, 1956.
184. Astrup, P.: A simple electrometric technique for the determination of carbon dioxide tension in blood and plasma, total content of carbon dioxide in plasma, and bicarbonate content in "separated" plasma at a fixed carbon dioxide tension (40 mm Hg). Scand. J. Clin. Lab. Invest., *8*:33, 1956.
185. Astrup, P.: Ultra-micro-methods for determining pH, $P\text{co}_2$ and standard bicarbonate in capillary blood. Lecture delivered at the Ciba Foundation Research Forum on "Acid Base Balance," London, December, 1958.
186. Astrup, P.: Erkennung der Störungen des Säure/Base-Stoffwechsels und ihre klinische Bedeutung. Klin. Wchnschr., *35*:749, 1957.
187. Astrup, P.: On the recognition of disturbances in the acid-base metabolism. Danish Med. Bull., *2*:136, 1955.
188. Astrup, P., Jørgensen, K., Siggaard Andersen, O., and Engel, K.: Acid-base metabolism. A new approach. Lancet, *1*:1035, 1960.
189. Weisberg, H. F.: *Water, Electrolyte, and Acid-Base Balance: Normal and Pathological Physiology as a Basis for Therapy*. 2nd ed. Baltimore, Williams & Wilkins, 1962.
190. Paine, E. G., Boutwell, J. H., and Soloff, L. A.: The reliability of "arterialized" venous blood for measuring arterial pH and $P\text{co}_2$. Am. J. Med. Sci., *242*:431, 1961.
191. Maas, A. H. J., and van Heijst, A. N. P.: The accuracy of the micro-determination of the $P\text{co}_2$ blood from the earlobe. Clin. Chim. Acta, *6*:34, 1961.
192. Riley, R. L., Proemmel, D. D., and Franke, R. E.: A direct

method for determination of oxygen and carbon dioxide tensions in blood. J. Biol. Chem., *161*:621, 1945.
193. Riley, R. L., Campbell, E. J. M., and Shepard, R. H.: A bubble method for estimation of P_{CO_2} and P_{O_2} in whole blood. J. Appl. Physiol., *11*:245, 1957.
194. Filley, G. F., Gay, E., and Wright, G. W.: The accuracy of direct determinations of oxygen and carbon dioxide tensions in human blood *in vitro*. J. Clin. Invest., *33*:510, 1954.
195. Cotes, J. E., and Oldham, P. D.: Calibration of a modified Riley bubble method for estimation of P_{CO_2} and P_{O_2} in whole blood. J. Appl. Physiol., *14*:467, 1959.
196. Asmussen, E., and Nielsen, M.: A bubble method for determination of P_{CO_2} and P_{O_2} in blood. Scand. J. Clin. Lab. Invest., *10*:267, 1958.
197. Björk, V. O., and Hilty, H. J.: Microvolumetric determination of CO_2 and O_2 tensions in arterial blood. J. Appl. Physiol., *6*:800, 1954.
198. Shepard, R. H., and Meier, P.: Analysis of the errors of a bubble method for estimation of P_{CO_2} and P_{O_2} in whole blood. J. Appl. Physiol., *11*:250, 1957.
199. Bates, D. V., and Harkness, E. V.: Notes on the application of the Hersch galvanic oxygen cell to measurement of blood oxygen content and tension. Canad. J. Biochem., *39*:991, 1961.
200. Strang, L. B.: Blood gas tension measurement using a mass spectrometer. J. Appl. Physiol., *16*:562, 1961.
201. Bartels, H., Beer, R., Koepchen, H. P., Wenner, J., and Witt, I.: Messung der alveolär-arteriellen O_2-Druckdifferenz mit verschiedenen Methoden am Menschen bei Ruhe und Arbeit. Arch. ges. Physiol., *261*:133, 1955.
202. Bartels, H., Beer, R., Fleischer, E., Hoffheinz, H. J., Krall, J., Rodewald, G., Wenner, J., and Witt, I.: Bestimmung von Kurzschlussdurchblutung und Diffusionskapazität der Lunge bei Gesunden und Lungenkranken. Arch. ges. Physiol., *261*:99, 1955.
203. Connelly, C. M.: Methods for measuring tissue oxygen tension; theory and evaluation: The oxygen electrode. In: *Symposium on Tissue Oxygen Tension*, Am. Physiol. Soc., Chicago, 1957. Fed. Proc., *16*:681, 1957.
204. Kreuzer, F., Watson, T. R., Jr., and Ball, J. M.: Comparative measurements with a new procedure for measuring the blood oxygen tension *in vitro*. J. Appl. Physiol., *12*:65, 1958.
205. Sproule, B. J., Miller, W. F., Cushing, I. E., and Chapman, C. B.: An improved polarographic method for measuring oxygen tension in whole blood. J. Appl. Physiol., *11*:365, 1957.
206. Rooth, G., Sjöstedt, S., and Caligara, F.: Oxygen tension measurements in whole blood with the Clark cell. Clin. Sci., *18*:379, 1959.
207. Drenckhahn, F. O.: Über eine Methode zur Messung des Sauerstoffdruckes im Blut mit der Platin-Kathode. Arch. ges. Physiol., *262*:169, 1956.
208. Bishop, J. M.: The measurement of blood gas tensions: Measurement of blood oxygen tension. Proc. Roy. Soc. Med. (London), *53*:177, 1960.
209. Bishop, J. M., and Pinock, A. C.: A method of measuring oxygen tension in blood and gas using a covered platinum electrode. J. Physiol. (London), *145*:20*P*, 1959.
210. Polgar, G., and Forster, R. E.: Measurement of oxygen tension in unstirred blood with a platinum electrode. J. Appl. Physiol., *15*:706, 1960.
211. Severinghaus, J. W., and Bradley, A. F.: Electrodes for blood P_{O_2} and P_{CO_2} determination. J. Appl. Physiol., *13*:515, 1958.
212. Said, S. I., Davis, R. K., and Crosier, J. L.: Continuous recording in vivo of arterial blood P_{O_2} in dogs and man. J. Appl. Physiol., *16*:1129, 1961.
213. Meyer, J. S., Gotoh, F., and Tazaki, Y.: Continuous recording of arterial P_{O_2}, P_{CO_2}, pH, and O_2 saturation in vivo. J. Appl. Physiol., *16*:896, 1961.
214. Lukas, D. S., and Ayres, S. M.: Determination of blood oxygen content by gas chromatography. J. Appl. Physiol., *16*:371, 1961.
215. Wilson, R. H., Jay, B., Doty, V., Pingree, H., and Higgins, E.: Analysis of blood gases with gas adsorption chromatographic technique. J. Appl. Physiol., *16*:374, 1961.
216. Lawther, P. J., and Apthorp, G. H.: A method for the determination of carbon monoxide in blood. Brit. J. Indust. Med., *12*:326, 1955.
217. Gaensler, E. A., Cadigan, J. B., Jr., Ellicott, M. F., Jones, R. H., and Marks, A.: A new method for rapid precise determination of carbon monoxide in blood. J. Lab. Clin. Med., *49*:945, 1957.
218. Lawther, P. J., and Bates, D. V.: A method for the determination of nitrous oxide in blood. Clin. Sci., *12*:91, 1953.
219. Fowler, W. S., and Comroe, J. H., Jr.: Lung function studies. I. The rate of increase of arterial oxygen saturation during the inhalation of 100 per cent O_2. J. Clin. Invest., *27*:327, 1948.
220. Perkins, J. F., Jr., Adams, W. E., and Flores, A.: Arterial oxygen saturation vs. alveolar oxygen tension as a measure of venous admixture and diffusion difficulty in the lung. J. Appl. Physiol., *8*:455, 1956.
221. Comroe, J. H., Jr., and Walker, P.: Normal human arterial oxygen saturation determined by equilibration with 100 per cent O_2 in vivo and by the oximeter. Am. J. Physiol., *152*:365, 1948.
222. Zijlstra, W. G.: *Fundamentals and Applications of Clinical Oximetry* (Van Gorcum's Medical Library, No. 117). 2nd ed. Assen, Holland, Van Gorcum, 1953.
223. Woolf, C. R., Gunton, R. W., and Paul, W.: Simple tests of respiratory function using a direct-writing ear oximeter. Am. Rev. Tuberc., *74*:511, 1956.
224. Enson, Y., Briscoe, W. A., Polanyi, M. L., and Cournand, A.: In vivo studies with an intravascular and intracardiac reflection oximeter. J. Appl. Physiol., *17*:552, 1962.
225. Collier, C. R.: Determination of mixed venous CO_2 tensions by rebreathing. J. Appl. Physiol., *9*:25, 1956.
226. Hackney, J. D., Sears, C. H., and Collier, C. R.: Estimation of arterial CO_2 tension by rebreathing technique. J. Appl. Physiol., *12*:425, 1958.
227. Campbell, E. J. M., and Howell, J. B. L.: Simple rapid methods of estimating arterial and mixed venous P_{CO_2}. Brit. Med. J., *1*:458, 1960.
228. Campbell, E. J. M., and Howell, J. B. L.: Rebreathing method for measurement of mixed venous P_{CO_2}. Brit. Med. J., *2*:630, 1962.
229. Scholander, P. F.: Analyzer for accurate estimation of respiratory gases in one-half cubic centimeter samples. J. Biol. Chem., *167*:235, 1947.
230. Krogh, A., and Lindhard, J.: The volume of the "dead space" in breathing. J. Physiol. (London), *47*:30, 1913.
231. Rahn, H., and Fenn, W. O.: *A Graphical Analysis of the Respiratory Gas Exchange. The O_2–CO_2 Diagram.* Washington, D.C., American Physiological Society, 1955.
232. Fenn, W. O., Rahn, H., and Otis, A. B.: A theoretical study of the composition of the alveolar air at altitude. Am. J. Physiol., *146*:637, 1946.
233. Rahn, H.: Inhomogeneity of alveolar air. Am. J. Physiol., *155*:462, 1948.
234. Rahn, H.: A concept of mean alveolar air and the ventilation-bloodflow relationships during pulmonary gas exchange. Am. J. Physiol., *158*:21, 1949.
235. Fowler, W. S.: Lung function studies. II. The respiratory dead space. Am. J. Physiol., *154*:405, 1948.
236. Bartels, J., Severinghaus, J. W., Forster, R. E., Briscoe, W. A., and Bates, D. V.: The respiratory dead space measured by single breath analysis of oxygen, carbon dioxide, nitrogen or helium. J. Clin. Invest., *33*:41, 1954.
237. Birath, G.: Respiratory dead space measurements in a model lung and healthy human subjects according to the single breath method. J. Appl. Physiol., *14*:517, 1959.
238. Roos, A., Dahlstrom, H., and Murphy, J. P.: Distribution of inspired air in the lungs. J. Appl. Physiol., *7*:645, 1955.
239. Shepard, R. H., Campbell, E. J. M., Martin, H. B., and Enns, T.: Factors affecting the pulmonary dead space as determined by single breath analysis. J. Appl. Physiol., *11*:241, 1957.
240. Nunn, J. F., Campbell, E. J. M., and Peckett, B. W.: Anatomical subdivisions of the volume of respiratory dead space and effect of position of the jaw. J. Appl. Physiol., *14*:174, 1959.
241. Fowler, W. S.: Lung function studies. V. Respiratory dead space in old age and in pulmonary emphysema. J. Clin. Invest., *29*:1439, 1950.

242. Fowler, W. S., and Blakemore, W. S.: Lung function studies. VII. The effect of pneumonectomy on respiratory dead space. J. Thoracic Surg., *21*:433, 1951.
243. Fowler, W. S.: Lung function studies. IV. Postural changes in respiratory dead space and functional residual capacity. J. Clin. Invest., *29*:1437, 1950.
244. Tenney, S. M., and Miller, R. M.: Dead space ventilation in old age. J. Appl. Physiol., *9*:321, 1956.
245. Birath, G., Malmberg, R., Beck, M., and Bergh, N. P.: The airway dead space in tracheotomized patients. Acta Chir. Scand., suppl. 245, p. 51, 1959.
246. Severinghaus, J. W., and Stupfel, M.: Alveolar dead space as an index of distribution of blood flow in pulmonary capillaries. J. Appl. Physiol., *10*:335, 1957.
247. Barcroft, H.: A source of error in measurement of the circulation rate by Henderson and Haggard's method. J. Physiol. (London), *63*:162, 1927.
248. Krogh, A., and Lindhard, J.: On the average composition of the alveolar air and its variations during the respiratory cycle. J. Physiol. (London), *47*:431, 1914.
249. Rauwerda, P. E.: Unequal ventilation of different parts of the lung and the determination of cardiac output. Thesis for the degree of Doctor of Medicine, in Rijks-Universiteit, Groningen, Holland, 1946.
250. Forssander, C. A., and White, C.: Mixing of alveolar air with dead space air during expiration. J. Appl. Physiol., *2*:110, 1949.
251. Suskind, M., Bruce, R. A., McDowell, M. E., Yu, P. N. G., Lovejoy, F. W., Jr., and Vernarelli, S. J.: Normal variations in end-tidal air and arterial blood carbon dioxide and oxygen tensions during moderate exercise. J. Appl. Physiol., *3*:282, 1950.
252. Lambertsen, C. J., and Benjamin, J. M., Jr.: Breath-by-breath sampling of end-expiratory gas. J. Appl. Physiol., *14*:711, 1959.
253. DuBois, A. B., Britt, A. G., and Fenn, W. O.: Alveolar CO_2 during the respiratory cycle. J. Appl. Physiol., *4*:535, 1952.
254. DuBois, A. B.: Alveolar CO_2 during breath holding, expiration, and inspiration. J. Appl. Physiol., *5*:1, 1952.
255. Collier, C. R., Affeldt, J. E., and Farr, A. F.: Continuous rapid infrared CO_2 analysis. Fractional sampling and accuracy in determining alveolar CO_2. J. Lab. Clin. Med., *45*:526, 1955.
256. Berengo, A., and Cutillo, A.: Single-breath analysis of carbon dioxide concentration records. J. Appl. Physiol., *16*:522, 1961.
257. Sivertson, S. E., and Fowler, W. S.: Expired alveolar carbon dioxide tension in health and in pulmonary emphysema. J. Lab. Clin. Med., *47*:869, 1956.
258. Göpfert, H., and Henneberg, W.: Der Anstieg der CO_2-konzentration in der Exspirationsluft im Verlauf einzelner Atemzüge. Arch. ges. Physiol., *263*:1, 1956.
259. Aitken, R. S., and Clark-Kennedy, A. E.: On the fluctuation in the composition of the alveolar air during the respiratory cycle in muscular exercise. J. Physiol. (London), *65*:389, 1928.
260. Asmussen, E., and Nielsen, M.: Physiological dead space and alveolar gas pressures at rest and during muscular exercise. Acta Physiol. Scand., *38*:1, 1956.
261. Marshall, R., Bates, D. V., and Christie, R. V.: Fractional analysis of the alveolar air in emphysema. Clin. Sci., *11*:297, 1952.
262. West, J. B., Fowler, K. T., Hugh-Jones, P., and O'Donnell, T. V.: Measurement of the ventilation-perfusion ratio inequality in the lung by the analysis of a single expirate. Clin. Sci., *16*:529, 1957.
263. West, J. B., Fowler, K. T., Hugh-Jones, P., and O'Donnell, T. V.: The measurement of the inequality of ventilation and of perfusion in the lung by the analysis of single expirates. Clin. Sci., *16*:549, 1957.
264. West, J. B., and Hugh-Jones, P.: Experimental verification of the single breath tests of ventilatory and ventilation–perfusion ratio inequality. Clin. Sci., *18*:553, 1959.
265. Read, J.: Pulmonary ventilation and perfusion in normal subjects and in patients with emphysema. Clin. Sci., *18*:465, 1959.
266. Martin, C. J., and Young, A. C.: Lobar ventilation in man. Am. Rev. Tuberc, *73*:330, 1956.
267. Radford, E. P., Jr.: Ventilation standards for use in artificial respiration. J. Appl. Physiol., *7*:451, 1955.
268. Briscoe, W. A., Forster, R. E., and Comroe, J. H., Jr.: Alveolar ventilation at very low tidal volumes. J. Appl. Physiol., *7*:27, 1954.
269. Robin, E. D., Corson, J. M., and Dammin, G. J.: The respiratory dead space of the giraffe. Nature, *186*:24, 1960.
270. Visser, B. F.: Pulmonary diffusion of carbon dioxide. Phys. Med. Biol., *5*:155, 1960.
271. Barcroft, J.: Some problems of the circulation during gas poisoning. J. Roy. Army Med. Corps, *34*:155, 1920.
272. Briscoe, W. A., and Gurtner, H. P.: The alveolo urinary N_2 partial pressure difference compared to other measures of the distribution of ventilation and perfusion within the lung. Fed. Proc., *19*:381, 1960.
273. Gray, J. S., Grodins, F. S., and Carter, E. T.: Alveolar and total ventilation and the dead space problem. J. Appl. Physiol., *9*:307, 1956.
274. Pappenheimer, J. R., Fishman, A. P., and Borrero, L. M.: New experimental methods for determination of effective alveolar gas composition and respiratory dead space, in the anesthetized dog and in man. J. Appl. Physiol., *4*:855, 1952.
275. Folkow, B., and Pappenheimer, J. R.: Components of the respiratory dead space and their variation with pressure breathing and with bronchoactive drugs. J. Appl. Physiol., *8*:102, 1955.
276. Asmussen, E., and Nielsen, M.: Alveolo-arterial gas exchange at rest and during work at different O_2 tensions. Acta Physiol. Scand., *50*:153, 1960.
277. Fishman, A. P.: Studies in man of the volume of the respiratory dead space and the composition of the alveolar gas. J. Clin. Invest., *33*:469, 1954.
278. Filley, G. F., Gregoire, F., and Wright, G. W.: Alveolar and arterial oxygen tensions and the significance of the alveolar-arterial oxygen tension difference in normal men. J. Clin Invest., *33*:517, 1954.
279. Hatch, T., Cook, K. M., and Palm, P. E.: Respiratory dead space. J. Appl. Physiol., *5*:341, 1953.
280. Rossier, P. H., and Wiesinger, K.: Pulmonary failure, its pathophysiology and its treatment. J. Internat. Chir. Thorax, *1*:35, 1949.
281. Rossier, P. H., Bühlmann, A., and Müller, H. R.: Espace mort respiratoire et clearance alvéolaire. Schweiz. Med. Wchnschr., *83*:577, 604, 1953.
282. Rossier, P. H., and Bühlmann, A.: The respiratory dead space. Physiol. Rev., *35*:860, 1955.
283. De Coster, A., Denolin, H., and Englert, M.: Étude de la ventilation alvéolaire et de l'espace mort physiologique au repos et à l'effort chez les sujets normaux et pathologiques. Acta Med. Scand., *163*:47, 1958.
284. De Coster, A., and Denolin, H.: Détermination de la ventilation alvéolaire et de l'espace mort physiologique chez les sujets normaux et les emphysémateux. Rev. Med. Nancy, *82*:732, 1957.
285. Wilson, R. H., Jay, B. E., Meador, R. S., and Evans, R.: The pulmonary physiologic dead space as an index of effective alveolar perfusion. Am. J. Med. Sci., *234*:547, 1957.
286. Riley, R. L., Permutt, S., Said, S., Godfrey, M., Cheng, T. O., Howell, J. B. L., and Shepard, R. H.: Effect of posture on pulmonary dead space in man. J. Appl. Physiol., *14*:339, 1959.
287. Larson, C. P., Jr., and Severinghaus, J. W.: Postural variations in dead space and CO_2 gradients breathing air and O_2. J. Appl. Physiol., *17*:417, 1962.
288. Strang, L. B.: Alveolar gas and anatomical deadspace measurements in normal newborn infants. Clin. Sci., *21*:107, 1961.
289. Briscoe, W. A., Cree, E. M., Filler, J., Houssay, H. E. J., and Cournand, A.: Lung volume, alveolar ventilation and perfusion interrelationships in chronic pulmonary emphysema. J. Appl. Physiol., *15*:785, 1960.
290. Björkman, S.: Bronchospirometrie. Eine Klinische Methode, die Funktion der menschlichen Lungen getrennt und

gleichzeitig zu Untersuchen. Acta Med. Scand., Supply. 56, 1934.
291. Carlens, E.: A new flexible double-lumen catheter for bronchospirometry. J. Thoracic Surg., *18*:742, 1949.
292. Gaensler, E. A.: Some problems of bronchospirometry. Analysis of 1,000 procedures. Dis. Chest, *24*:390, 1953.
293. Gaensler, E. A., and Cugell, D. W.: Bronchospirometry. V. Differential residual volume determination. J. Lab. Clin. Med., *40*:558, 1952.
294. Birath, G., Ställberg-Stenhagen, S., and Swenson, E. W.: Significance of bronchospirometric values. Am. Rev. Tuberc., *75*:699, 1957.
295. Brille, D., Hatzfeld, C., and Kourilsky, R.: Valeur des techniques endobronchiques pour l'exploration fonctionelle des poumons séparés. Bronches, *5*:381, 1955.
296. Sadoul, P., Grilliat, J. P., and Braun, P.: La bronchospirométrie ou séparation des airs. Poumon Coeur, *11*:939, 1955.
297. Wright, G. W., and Woodruff, W.: Bronchospirography: Ventilation and oxygen absorption of normal and diseased lungs during nitrogen respiration in the opposite lung. J. Thoracic Surg., *11*:278, 1942.
298. Rothstein, E., Landis, F. B., and Narodick, B. G.: Bronchospirometry in the lateral decubitus position. J. Thoracic Surg., *19*:821, 1950.
299. Carlens, E., and Dahlström, G.: The clinical evaluation of bronchospirometry: with special reference to posture and exercise. Am. Rev. Resp. Dis., *83*:202, 1961.
300. Siebens, A. A., Newman, M. M., Smith, R. E., and Vaughan, L. H.: Measurements of the unilateral residual volume. J. Thoracic Surg., *31*:569, 1956.
301. Savage, T., and Fleming, H. A.: Decortication of the lung in tuberculous disease: A study in 43 cases. Thorax, *10*:293, 1955.
302. Siebens, A. A., Storey, C. F., Newman, M. M., Kent, D. C., and Standard, J. E.: The physiological effects of fibrothorax and the functional results of surgical treatment. J. Thoracic Surg., *32*:53, 1956.
303. Birath, G., Swenson, E. W., Andér, L., and Bergh, N. P.: The definitive functional results after partial pulmonary resection. Bronchospirometric investigation. Am. Rev. Tuberc., *76*:983, 1957.
304. Fleming, H. A.: Pulmonary function before and after segmental resection and after "ideal" pneumothorax treatment. Brit. Med. J., *1*:485, 1957.
305. Birath, G., Bergh, N. P., and Swenson, E. W.: Bronchospirometric investigations before and after segmental resection and lobectomy for pulmonary tuberculosis. Am. Rev. Tuberc., *75*:710, 1957.
306. Birath, G., and Söderholm, B.: Bronchospirometric investigations before and after a small thoracoplasty. Am. Rev. Tuberc., *75*:724, 1957.
307. Semb, C., Erikson, H., Bergan, F., and Müller, C.: Cardiorespiratory function in pulmonary surgery. Acta Chir. Scand., *109*:235, 1955.
308. Hanson, H. E.: Temporary unilateral occlusion of the pulmonary artery in man. A method for preoperative determination of the function of each lung. Acta Chir. Scand., Suppl. 187, 1954.
309. Kanagami, H., Suzuki, K., Katsura, T., Shiroishi, K., Baba, K., and Mori, A.: On measurement of the CO pulmonary capacity in each lung by a modified endtidal sampling method. Resp. Circ., *9*:169, 1961.
310. Samet, P., Fierer, E. M., and Bernstein, W. H.: Anomalous pulmonary venous drainage. Diagnostic value of bronchospirometry. Am. J. Med., *25*:654, 1958.
311. Birath, G.: Simultaneous samples of alveolar air from each lung and parts thereof. A preliminary report of a method using bronchial catheterization. Am. Rev. Tuberc., *55*:444, 1947.
312. Martin, C. J., Cline, F., Jr., and Marshall, H.: Lobar alveolar gas concentrations: Effect of body position. J. Clin. Invest., *32*:617, 1953.
313. Martin, C. J., Cline, F., Jr., and Marshall, H.: Lobar alveolar gas concentration after pneumonectomy. J. Clin. Invest., *34*:875, 1955.
314. Mattson, S. B., and Carlens, E.: Lobar ventilation and oxygen uptake in man: Influence of body position. J. Thoracic Surg., *30*:676, 1955.
315. Martin, C. J., and Young, A. C.: Ventilation-perfusion variations within the lung. J. Appl. Physiol., *11*:371, 1957.
316. Vaccarezza, R. F., Bence, A., Lanari, A., Labourt, F., and Gonzalez Segura, R.: The study of the two lungs separately in practical and research work. Dis. Chest, *9*:95, 1943.
317. Armitage, G. H., and Taylor, A. B.: Non-bronchospirometric measurement of differential lung function. Thorax, *11*:281, 1956.
318. West, J. B.: A bronchial flow meter. Lancet, *2*:908, 1960.
319. Hugh-Jones, P., and West, J. B.: Detection of bronchial and arterial obstruction by continuous gas analysis from individual lobes and segments of the lung. Thorax, *15*:154, 1960.
320. West, J. B.: Observations on gas flow in the human bronchial tree. In: Davies, C. N. (ed.): *Inhaled Particles and Vapours.* New York, Pergamon Press, 1961, p. 3.
321. West, J. B., and Hugh-Jones, P.: Patterns of gas flow in the upper bronchial tree. J. Appl. Physiol., *14*:753, 1959.
322. West, J. B.: Measurement of bronchial air flow. J. Appl. Physiol., *15*:976, 1960.
323. West, J. B., and Hugh-Jones, P.: Effect of bronchial and arterial constriction on alveolar gas concentrations in a lobe of the dog's lung. J. Appl. Physiol., *14*:743, 1959.
324. West, J. B., and Hugh-Jones, P.: Rate of fall of O_2 tension in a lobe of dog lung after bronchial occlusion. J. Appl. Physiol., *14*:897, 1959.
325. West, J. B., and Hugh-Jones, P.: Pulsatile gas flow in bronchi caused by the heart beat. J. Appl. Physiol., *16*:697, 1961.
326. Marchal, M., and Marchal, M. T.: Perfectionnement en stati-densigraphie. Compt. Rend. Acad. Sci. (Paris), *238*:2560, 1954.
327. Marchal, M., Marchal, M. T., and Kourilsky, R.: Enregistrement photo-électrique de la ventilation des poumons séparés dans les sténoses bronchiques par la statidensigraphie. Bronches, *11*:102, 1961.
328. Kourilsky, R., and Marchal, M.: Étude cinédensigraphique de la circulation artérielle du poumon dans différentes affections pathologiques du poumon, des bronches et du médiastin. J. Franc. Med. Chir. Thorac., *7*:113, 1953.
329. Kourilsky, R.: Une nouvelle méthode électronique d'exploration de la circulation pulmonaire: La cinédensigraphie (de Maurice Marchal): Résultats obtenus dans les cancers du poumon et les tumeurs du médiastin. Un. Med. Canada, *82*:1, 1953.
330. Knipping, H. W., Bolt, W., Venrath, H., Valentin, H., Ludes, H., and Endler, P.: Eine neue Methode zur Prüfung der Herz- und Lungenfunktion. Die regionale Funktionsanalyse in der Lungen- und Herzklinik mit Hilfe des radioaktiven Edelgases Xenon^{133} (Isotopen Thorakographie). Deutsch. Med. Wchnschr., *80*:1146, 1955.
331. Knipping, H. W., Bolt, W., Valentin, H., Venrath, H., and Endler, P.: Technik und Möglichkeiten der regionalen Ventilationsanalyse mittels des radioktiven Edelgases Xenon^{133} (Isotopen Thorakographie). Z. Tuberk., *111*:259, 1958.
332. Knipping, H. W., Bolt, W., Valentin, H., Venrath, H., and Endler, P.: Regionale Funktionsanalyse in der Kreislauf- und Lungen-Klinik mit Hilfe der Isotopenthorakographie und der selektiven Angiographie der Lungengefässe. Beitrag zur präoperativen Funktionsanalyse in der Thoraxchirurgie. Muench. Med. Wchnschr., *99*:1, 46, 1957.
333. Bolt, W., and Rink, H.: Studien zur regionalen Analyse der Lungenventilation und Lungenzirkulation (mittels der Isotopenthorakographie und der selektiven Lungenangiographie). Thoraxchirurgie, *5*:379, 1958.
334. Fucks, W., and Knipping, H. W.: Bildiche Darstellung der Verteilung und der Bewegung von radioaktiven Substanzen in Raum ("Röntgen ohne Röntgenröhre") unter Berücksightigung einiger Probleme der Herzund Lingenklinik. Atomkernenergie, *3*:209, 1958.
335. Trippe, H.: Zur Diagnose regionaler Ventilations-störungen der Lunge mit Hilfe von Xenon^{133}. Thesis for the degree of Doctor of Medicine, University of Cologne, 1959.
336. West, J. B., Holland, R. A. B., Dollery, C. T., and Matthews, C. M. E.: Interpretation of radioactive gas clearance rates in lung. J. Appl. Physiol., *17*:14, 1962.

337. Dollery, C. T., Heimburg, P., and Hugh-Jones, P.: The relationship between blood flow and clearance rate of radioactive carbon dioxide and oxygen in normal and oedematous lungs. J. Physiol. (London), *162*:93, 1962.
338. West, J. B., and Dollery, C. T.: Distribution of blood flow and ventilation-perfusion ratio in the lung, measured with radioactive CO_2. J. Appl. Physiol., *15*:405, 1960.
339. Dollery, C. T., West, J. B., Wilcken, D. E. L., Goodwin, J. F., and Hugh-Jones, P.: Regional pulmonary blood flow in patients with circulatory shunts. Brit. Heart J., *23*:225, 1961.
340. Dollery, C. T., West, J. B., Wilcken, D. E. L., and Hugh-Jones, P.: A comparison of the pulmonary blood flow between left and right lungs in normal subjects and patients with congenital heart disease. Circulation, *24*:617, 1961.
341. Dollery, C. T., and West, J. B.: Regional uptake of radioactive oxygen, carbon monoxide and carbon dioxide in the lungs of patients with mitral stenosis. Circ. Res., *8*:765, 1960.
342. West, J. B., Dollery, C. T., and Hugh-Jones, P.: The use of radioactive carbon dioxide to measure regional blood flow in the lungs of patients with pulmonary disease. J. Clin. Invest., *40*:1, 1961.
343. West, J. B.: Distribution of gas and blood in the normal lungs. Brit. Med. Bull., *19*:53, 1963.
344. West, J. B.: Regional differences in gas exchange in the lung of erect man. J. Appl. Physiol., *17*:893, 1962.
345. Dollery, C. T., and Hugh-Jones, P.: Distribution of gas and blood in the lungs in disease. Brit. Med. Bull., *19*:59, 1963.
346. Forster, R. E.: Exchange of gases between alveolar air and pulmonary capillary blood: pulmonary diffusing capacity. Physiol. Rev., *37*:391, 1957.
347. Krogh, A., and Krogh, M.: On the rate of diffusion of carbonic oxide into the lungs of man. Skand. Arch. Physiol., *23*:236, 1910.
348. Krogh, M.: The diffusion of gases through the lungs of man. J. Physiol. (London), *49*:271, 1915.
349. Forster, R. E., Fowler, W. S., and Bates, D. V.: Considerations on the uptake of carbon monoxide by the lungs. J. Clin. Invest., *33*:1128, 1954.
350. Forster, R. E., Fowler, W. S., Bates, D. V., and van Lingen, B.: The absorption of carbon monoxide by the lungs during breathholding. J. Clin. Invest., *33*:1135, 1954.
351. Constantine, H. P., and Perkins, P. T.: Correction for carbon dioxide in the measurement of lung diffusing capacities by carbon monoxide single breath techniques. J. Appl. Physiol., *14*:668, 1959.
352. Harrop, G. A., Jr., and Heath, E. H.: Pulmonary gas diffusion in polycythemia vera. J. Clin. Invest., *4*:53, 1927.
353. Bøje, O.: Über die Grösse der Lungendiffusion des Menschen während Rube under körperlicher Arbeit. Arbeitsphysiol., *7*:157, 1934.
354. Cadigan, J. B., Marks, A., Ellicott, M. F., Jones, R. H., and Gaensler, E. A.: An analysis of factors affecting the measurement of pulmonary diffusing capacity by the single breath method. J. Clin. Invest., *40*:1495, 1961.
355. McGrath, M. W., and Thomson, M. J.: The effect of age, body size and lung volume change on alveolar-capillary permeability and diffusing capacity in man. J. Physiol. (London), *146*:572, 1959.
356. Williams, M. H., Jr., and Zohman, L.: A simplified method for estimation of the diffusing capacity of the lung in subjects without airway obstruction. Am. Rev. Tuberc., *78*:173, 1958.
357. Mittman, C., and Burrows, B.: Uniformity of pulmonary diffusion: Effect of lung volume. J. Appl. Physiol., *14*:496, 1959.
358. Shephard, R. J.: "Breath-holding" measurement of carbon monoxide diffusing capacity. Comparision of a field test with steady-state and other methods of measurement. J. Physiol. (London), *141*:408, 1958.
359. Jones, R. S., and Meade, F.: Pulmonary diffusing capacity: An improved single-breath method. Lancet, *1*:94, 1960.
360. Jones, R. S., and Meade, F.: A theoretical and experimental analysis of anomalies in the estimation of pulmonary diffusing capacity by the single breath method. Quart. J. Exper. Physiol., *46*:131, 1961.
361. Bedell, G. N., and Adams, R. W.: Pulmonary diffusing capacity during rest and exercise. A study of normal persons and persons with atrial septal defect, pregnancy, and pulmonary disease. J. Clin. Invest., *41*:1908, 1962.
362. Auchincloss, J. H., Jr., Gilbert, R., and Eich, R. H.: The pulmonary diffusing capacity in congenital and rheumatic heart disease. Circulation, *19*:232, 1959.
363. Burrows, B., Harrison, R. W., Adams, W. E., Humphreys, E. M., Long, E. T., and Reimann, A. F.: The postpneumonectomy state. Clinical and physiologic observations in thirty-six cases. Am. J. Med., *28*:281, 1960.
364. Williams, M. H., Jr., Seriff, N. S., Akyol, T., and Yoo, O. H.: The diffusing capacity of the lung in acute pulmonary tuberculosis. Am. Rev. Resp. Dis., *84*:814, 1961.
365. Rankin, J., McNeill, R. S., and Forster, R. E.: The effect of anemia on the alveolar-capillary exchange of carbon monoxide in man. J. Clin. Invest., *40*:1323, 1961.
366. Williams, R., and Hugh-Jones, P.: The significance of lung function changes in asbestosis. Thorax, *15*:109, 1960.
367. Apthorp, G. H., and Marshall, R.: Pulmonary diffusing capacity: A comparison of breath-holding and steady state methods using carbon monoxide. J. Clin. Invest., *40*:1775, 1961.
368. Rosenberg, E., and Forster, R. E.: Changes in diffusing capacity of isolated cat lungs with blood pressure and flow. J. Appl. Physiol., *15*:883, 1960.
369. Forster, R. E.: The determination and significance of the diffusing capacity of the lungs and its clinical applications. Progr. Cardiov. Dis., *1*:268, 1959.
370. Bates, D. V.: The measurement of the pulmonary diffusing capacity in the presence of lung disease. J. Clin. Invest., *37*:591, 1958.
371. Bates, D. V., Boucot, N. G., and Dormer, A. E.: The pulmonary diffusing capacity in normal subjects. J. Physiol. (London), *129*:237, 1955.
372. Pace, N., Consolazio, W. V., White, W. A., Jr., and Behnke, A. R.: Formulation of the principal factors affecting the rate of uptake of carbon monoxide by man. Am. J. Physiol., *147*:352, 1946.
373. Hatch, T. F.: Carbon monoxide uptake in relation to pulmonary performance. A.M.A. Arch. Indust. Hyg., *6*:1, 1952.
374. Forbes, W. H., Sargent, F., and Roughton, F. J. W.: The rate of carbon monoxide uptake by normal men. Am. J. Physiol., *143*:594, 1945.
375. Lilienthal, J. L., Jr., and Pine, M. B.: The effect of oxygen pressure on the uptake of carbon monoxide by man at sea level and at altitude. Am. J. Physiol., *145*:346, 1946.
376. Lilienthal, J. L., Jr.: Carbon monoxide. Pharmacol. Rev., *2*:324, 1950.
377. Roughton, F. J. W.: The average time spent by the blood in the human lung capillary and its relation to the rates of CO uptake and elimination in man. Am. J. Physiol., *143*:621, 1945.
378. Filley, G. F., MacIntosh, D. J., and Wright, G. W.: Carbon monoxide uptake and pulmonary diffusing capacity in normal subjects at rest and during exercise. J. Clin. Invest., *33*:530, 1954.
379. Ross, J. C., Frayser, R., and Hickam, J. B.: A study of the mechanism by which exercise increases the pulmonary diffusing capacity for carbon monoxide. J. Clin. Invest., *38*:916, 1959.
380. Turino, G. M., Brandfonbrener, M., and Fishman, A. P.: The effect of changes in ventilation and pulmonary blood flow on the diffusing capacity of the lung. J. Clin. Invest., *38*:1186, 1959.
381. Cugell, D. W., Marks, A., Ellicott, M. F., Badger, T. L., and Gaensler, E. A.: Carbon monoxide diffusing capacity during steady exercise. Am. Rev. Tuberc., *74*:317, 1956.
382. Marks, A., Cugell, D. W., Cadigan, J. B., and Gaensler, E. A.: Clinical determination of the diffusion capacity of the lungs: Comparison of methods in normal subjects and patients with "alveolar-capillary block" syndrome. Am. J. Med., *22*:51, 1957.
383. Linderholm, H.: On the significance of CO tension in pulmonary capillary blood for determination of pulmonary diffusing capacity with the steady state CO method. Acta Med. Scand., *156*:413, 1957.
384. Williams, M. H., Jr., and Zohman, L. R.: Cardiopulmonary

function in bronchial asthma: A comparison with chronic pulmonary emphysema. Am. Rev. Resp. Dis., *81*:173, 1960.

385. Williams, M. H., Jr., and Zohman, L. R.: Cardiopulmonary function in chronic obstructive emphysema. Am. Rev. Resp. Dis., *80*:689, 1959.
386. Stahlman, M. T.: Pulmonary ventilation and diffusion in the human newborn infant. J. Clin. Invest., *36*:1081, 1957.
387. Donevan, R. E., Palmer, W. H., Varvis, C. J., and Bates, D. V.: Influence of age on pulmonary diffusing capacity. J. Appl. Physiol., *14*:483, 1959.
388. McIlroy, M. B., and Bates, D. V.: Respiratory function after pneumonectomy. Thorax, *11*:303, 1956.
389. Bates, D. V., Pare, J. A. P., and Meakins, J. F.: The clinical usefulness of routine tests of pulmonary function. Canad. M. A. J., *83*:192, 1960.
390. MacNamara, J., Prime, F. J., and Sinclair, J. D.: An assessment of the steady-state carbon monoxide method of estimating pulmonary diffusing capacity. Thorax, *14*:166, 1959.
391. Marshall, R.: Methods of measuring pulmonary diffusing capacity and their significance. Proc. Roy. Soc. Med. (London), *51*:101, 1958.
392. Bates, D. V., Knott, J. M. S., and Christie, R. V.: Respiratory function in emphysema in relation to prognosis. Quart. J. Med., *(n.s.)25*:137, 1956.
393. Svanborg, N. (ed.): Studies on the cardiopulmonary function in sarcoidosis. Acta Med. Scand., Suppl. 366, 1961; and Stockholm, Tryckeriaktiebolaget, 1961.
394. Berven, H.: Studies on the cardiopulmonary function in the post-infectious phase of "atypical" pneumonia. Acta Med. Scand., *172*. Suppl. 382, 1962.
395. Marshall, R.: A comparison of methods of measuring the diffusing capacity of lungs for carbon monoxide. Investigation by fractional analysis of the alveolar air. J. Clin. Invest., *37*:394, 1958.
396. Lewis, B. M., Lin, T. H., Noe, F. E., and Hayford-Welsing, E. J.: The measurement of pulmonary diffusing capacity for carbon monoxide by a rebreathing method. J. Clin. Invest., *38*:2073, 1959.
397. Bates, D. V.: The uptake of carbon monoxide in health and in emphysema. Clin. Sci., *11*:21, 1952.
398. West, J. B.: Diffusing capacity of the lung for carbon monoxide at high altitude. J. Appl. Physiol., *17*:421, 1962.
399. Bates, D. V., Varvis, C. J., Donevan, R. E., and Christie, R. V.: Variations in the pulmonary capillary blood volume and membrane diffusion component in health and disease. J. Clin. Invest., *39*:1401, 1960.
400. Roughton, F. J. W., and Forster, R. E.: Relative importance of diffusion and chemical reaction rates in determining rate of exchange of gases in the human lung, with special reference to true diffusing capacity of pulmonary membrane and volume of blood in the lung capillaries. J. Appl. Physiol., *11*:290, 1957.
401. Forster, R. E., Roughton, F. J. W., Cander, L., Briscoe, W. A., and Kreuzer, F.: Apparent pulmonary diffusing capacity for CO at varying alveolar O_2 tensions. J. Appl. Physiol., *11*:277, 1957.
402. Roughton, F. J. W., Forster, R. E., and Cander, L.: Rate at which carbon monoxide replaces oxygen from combination with human hemoglobin in solution and in the red cell. J. Appl. Physiol., *11*:269, 1957.
403. Staub, N. C., Bishop, J. M., and Forster, R. E.: Importance of diffusion and chemical reaction rates in O_2 uptake in the lung. J. Appl. Physiol., *17*:21, 1962.
404. Staub, N. C., Bishop, J. M., and Forster, R. E.: Velocity of O_2 uptake by human red blood cells. J. Appl. Physiol., *16*:511, 1961.
405. Gibson, Q. H.: The direct determination of the velocity constant of the reaction $Hb_4(CO)_3 + CO \rightarrow Hb_4(CO)_4$. J. Physiol. (London), *134*:123, 1956.
406. Gibson, Q. H., Kreuzer, F., Meda, E., and Roughton, F. J. W.: The kinetics of human haemoglobin in solution and in the red cell at 37°C. J. Physiol. (London), *129*:65, 1955.
407. Gibson, Q. H., and Roughton, F. J. W.: The velocity constant, k_4, of the reaction $Hb_4O_8 \rightarrow Hb_4O_6 + O_2$ in dilute sheep haemoglobin solutions. J. Physiol. (London), *145*:32*P*, 1959.
408. Bishop, J. M., Forster, R. E., Johnson, R. L., and Spicer, W. S.: The relationship between pulmonary capillary blood flow, pulmonary capillary blood volume and diffusing capacity during rest and exercise. J. Physiol. (London), *146*:5*P*, 1959.
409. Johnson, R. L., Jr., Spicer, W. S., Bishop, J. M., and Forster, R. E.: Pulmonary capillary blood volume, flow and diffusing capacity during exercise. J. Appl. Physiol., *15*:893, 1960.
410. Lewis, B. M., Lin, T. H., Noe, F. E., and Komisaruk, R.: The measurement of pulmonary capillary blood volume and pulmonary membrane diffusing capacity in normal subjects; the effects of exercise and position. J. Clin. Invest., *37*:1061, 1958.
411. McNeill, R. S., Rankin, J., and Forster, R. E.: The diffusing capacity of the pulmonary membrane and the pulmonary capillary blood volume in cardiopulmonary disease. Clin. Sci., *17*:465, 1958.
412. Lilienthal, J. L., Jr., Riley, R. L., Proemmel, D. D., and Franke, R. E.: An experimental analysis in man of the oxygen pressure gradient from alveolar air to arterial blood during rest and exercise at sea level and at altitude. Am. J. Physiol., *147*:199, 1946.
413. Riley, R. L., and Cournand, A.: "Ideal" alveolar air and the analysis of ventilation-perfusion relationships in the lungs. J. Appl. Physiol., *1*:825, 1949.
414. Riley, R. L., and Cournand, A.: Analysis of factors affecting partial pressures of oxygen and carbon dioxide in gas and blood of lungs: Theory. J. Appl. Physiol., *4*:77, 1951.
415. Riley, R. L., Cournand, A., and Donald, K. W.: Analysis of factors affecting partial pressures of oxygen and carbon dioxide in gas and blood of lungs: Methods. J. Appl. Physiol., *4*:102, 1951.
416. Donald, K. W., Renzetti, A., Riley, R. L., and Cournand, A.: Analysis of factors affecting concentrations of oxygen and carbon dioxide in gas and blood of lungs: Results. J. Appl. Physiol., *4*:497, 1952.
417. Riley, R. L., Shepard, R. H., Cohn, J. E., Carroll, D. G., and Armstrong, B. W.: Maximal diffusing capacity of the lungs. J. Appl. Physiol., *6*:573, 1954.
418. Riley, R. L., Riley, M. C., and Hill, H. M.: Diffuse pulmonary sarcoidosis: Diffusing capacity during exercise and other lung function studies in relation to ACTH therapy. Bull. Johns Hopkins Hosp., *91*:345, 1952.
419. Riley, R. L., Johns, C. J., Cohen, G., Cohn, J. E., Carroll, D. G., and Shepard, R. H.: The diffusing capacity of the lungs in patients with miral stenosis studied post-operatively. J. Clin. Invest., *35*:1008, 1956.
420. Shepard, R. H., Cohn, J. E., Cohen, G., Armstrong, B. W., Carroll, D. G., Donoso, H., and Riley, R. L.: The maximal diffusing capacity of the lung in chronic obstructive disease of the airways. Am. Rev. Tuberc., *71*:249, 1955.
421. Cohn, J. E., Carroll, D. G., Armstrong, B. W., Shepard, R. H., and Riley, R. L.: Maximal diffusing capacity of the lung in normal male subjects of different ages. J. Appl. Physiol., *6*:588, 1954.
422. Gordh, T., Linderholm, H., and Norlander, O.: Pulmonary function in relation to anesthesia and surgery evaluated by analysis of oxygen tension of arterial blood. Acta Anaesthesiol. Scand., *2*:15, 1958.
423. Fritts, H. W., Jr., Hardewig, A., Rochester, D. F., Durand, J., and Cournand, A.: Estimation of pulmonary arteriovenous shunt-flow using intravenous injections of T-1824 dye and Kr^{85}. J. Clin. Invest., *39*:1841, 1960.
424. Rinck, H., Venrath, H., Valentin, H., and Schmitz, T.: Diffusionsstörungen in den Lungen bei alten Insuffizienzen des linken Herzens und bei der Mitralstenose nebst einigen Bemerkungen zur Operation der Mitralfehler. Thoraxchirurgie, *1*:403, 1954.
425. Shepard, R. H.: Effect of pulmonary diffusing capacity on exercise tolerance. J. Appl. Physiol., *12*:487, 1958.
426. Finley, T. N., Swenson, E. W., and Comroe, J. H., Jr.: The cause of arterial hypoxemia at rest in patients with "alveolar-capillary block syndrome." J. Clin. Invest., *41*:618, 1962.
427. West, J. B., Lahiri, S., Gill, M. B., Milledge, J. S., Pugh, L. G. C. E., and Ward, M. P.: Arterial oxygen saturation during exercise at high altitude. J. Appl. Physiol., *17*:617, 1962.
428. Austrian, R., McClement, J. H., Renzetti, A. D., Jr., Don-

ald, K. W., Riley, R. L., and Cournand, A.: Clinical and physiologic features of some types of pulmonary diseases with impairment of alveolar-capillary diffusion. The syndrome of "alveolar-capillary block." Am. J. Med., *11*:667, 1951.

429. Burrows, B., Kasik, J. E., Niden, A. H., and Barclay, W. R.: Clinical usefulness of the single-breath pulmonary diffusing capacity test. Am. Rev. Resp. Dis., *84*:789, 1961.
430. Becklake, M. R., Varvis, C. J., Pengelly, L. D., Kenning, S., McGregor, M., and Bates, D. V.: Measurement of pulmonary blood flow during exercise using nitrous oxide. J. Appl. Physiol., *17*:579, 1962.
431. Krogh, A., and Lindhard, J.: Measurements of the blood flow through the lungs of man. Skand. Arch. Physiol., *27*:100, 1912.
432. Jacobs, M. H.: Diffusion processes. In: Ruhland, W. (ed.): *Ergebnisse der Biologie*. Berlin, Springer-Verlag, 1935, vol. 11.
433. Kety, S. S.: The theory and applications of the exchange of inert gas at the lungs and tissues. Pharmacol. Rev., *3*:1, 1951.
434. Mead, J.: Mechanical properties of lungs. Physiol. Rev., *41*:281, 1961.
435. Rohrer, F.: Der Strömungswiderstand in den menschlichen Atemwegen und der Einfluss der unregelmässigen Vertzweigung des Bronchialsystems auf den Atmungsverlauf in verschiedenen Lungenbezirken. Arch. ges. Physiol., *162*:225, 1915.
436. von Neergaard, K., and Wirz, K.: Die Messung der Strömungswiderstände in den Atemwegen des Menschen, insbesondere bei Asthma und Emphysem. Z. klin. Med., *105*:51, 1927.
437. Christie, R. V., and McIntosh, C. A.: The measurement of the intrapleural pressure in man and its significance. J. Clin. Invest., *13*:279, 1934.
438. Christie, R. V.: The elastic properties of the emphysematous lung and their clinical significance. J. Clin. Invest., *13*:295, 1934.
439. Christie, R. V., and Meakins, J. C.: The intrapleural pressure in congestive heart failure and its clinical significance. J. Clin. Invest., *13*:323, 1934.
440. Buytendijk, H. J.: Oesophagusdruck en longelasticiteit. Thesis, University of Groningen, 1949. Groningen, Oppenheim, 1949.
441. Lim, T. P. K., and Luft, U. C.: Alterations in lung compliance and functional residual capacity with posture. J. Appl. Physiol., *14*:164, 1959.
442. Fenn, W. O.: Mechanics of respiration. Am. J. Med., *10*:77, 1951.
443. Otis, A. B.: The work of breathing. Physiol. Rev., *34*:449, 1954.
444. Daly, W. J., and Bondurant, S.: A comparison of esophageal pressure (balloon technique) and direct interpleural pressure in the estimation of lung compliance. [Abstr.] Fed. Proc., *21*:447, 1962.
445. Fry, D. L., Stead, W. W., Ebert, R. V., Lubin, R. I., and Wells, H. S.: The measurement of intraesophageal pressure and its relationship to intrathoracic pressure. J. Lab. Clin. Med., *40*:664, 1952.
446. Schilder, D. P., Hyatt, R. E., and Fry, D. L.: An improved balloon system for measuring intraesophageal pressure. J. Appl. Physiol., *14*:1057, 1959.
447. Mead, J., and Gaensler, E. A.: Esophageal and pleural pressures in man, upright and supine. J. Appl. Physiol., *14*:81, 1959.
448. Petit, J. M., and Milic-Emili, G.: Measurement of endoesophageal pressure. J. Appl. Physiol., *13*:481, 1958.
449. Farhi, L., Otis, A. B., and Proctor, D. F.: Measurement of intrapleural pressure at different points in the chest of the dog. J. Appl. Physiol., *10*:15, 1957.
450. Knowles, J. H., Hong, S. K., and Rahn, H.: Possible errors using esophageal balloon in determination of pressure-volume characteristics of the lung and thoracic cage. J. Appl. Physiol., *14*:525, 1959.
451. Cherniack, R. M., Farhi, L. E., Armstrong, B. W., and Proctor, D. F.: A comparison of esophageal and intrapleural pressure in man. J. Appl. Physiol., *8*:203, 1955.
452. Milic-Emili, G., and Petit, J. M.: Relationship between endoesophageal and intrathoracic pressure variations in dog. J. Appl. Physiol., *14*:535, 1959.
453. Petit, J. M., and Milic-Emili, G.: Mesure simultanée des variations respiratoires de la pression pleurale et de la pression oesophagienne. Arch. Int. Physiol. Biochim., *67*:341, 1959.
454. Bondurant, S., Carlson, M., Hawley, R., and Klatte, E.: Respiratory compression of the esophagus by mediastinal structures. Physiologist, *3*/3:26, 1960.
455. Milic-Emili, G., and Melon, J.: Le modificazioni delle proprieta' meccaniche dell'esofago in pazienti pneumectomizzati, quale cause di errore nella misura della variazioni di pressione endotoracica per via endoesofagea. Boll. Soc. Ital. Biol. Sper., *36*:1268, 1960.
456. Bondurant, S., Mead, J., and Cook, C. D.: A reevaluation of effects of acute central congestion on pulmonary compliance in normal subjects. J. Appl. Physiol., *15*:875, 1960.
457. Fry, D. L., Hyatt, R. E., McCall, C. B., and Mallos, A. J.: Evaluation of three types of respiratory flowmeters. J. Appl. Physiol., *10*:210, 1957.
458. Fry, D. L.: Physiologic recording by modern instruments with particular reference to pressure recording. Physiol. Rev., *40*:753, 1960.
459. Nisell, O., and Ehrher, L.: The resistance to breathing determined from time-marked respiratory pressure volume loops. Acta Med. Scand., *161*:427, 1958.
460. Marshall, R.: The physical properties of the lungs in relation to the subdivisions of lung volume. Clin. Sci., *16*:507, 1957.
461. Cook, C. D., Helliesen, P. J., and Agathon, S.: Relation between mechanics of respiration, lung size and body size from birth to young adulthood. J. Appl. Physiol., *13*:349, 1958.
462. Crosfill, M. L., and Widdicombe, J. G.: Physical characteristics of the chest and lungs and the work of breathing in different mammalian species. J. Physiol. (London), *158*:1, 1961.
463. Emirgil, G., and Heinemann, H. O.: Effects of irradiation of chest on pulmonary function in man. J. Appl. Physiol., *16*:331, 1961.
464. Safar, P., and Bachman, L.: Compliance of the lungs and thorax in dogs under the influence of muscle relaxants. Anesthesiology, *17*:334, 1956.
465. Frank, N. R., Mead, J., and Ferris, B. G., Jr.: The mechanical behavior of the lungs in healthy elderly persons. J. Clin. Invest., *36*:1680, 1957.
466. West, J. R., and Alexander, J. K.: Studies on respiratory mechanics and the work of breathing in pulmonary fibrosis. Am. J. Med., *27*:529, 1959.
467. Nisell, O., Carlberger, G., and Bevegård, S.: The mechanics of respiration in patients with mitral heart disease. Acta Med. Scand., *162*:277, 1958.
468. Cherniack, R. M., Adamson, J. D., and Hildes, J. A.: Compliance of the lungs and thorax in poliomyelitis. J. Appl. Physiol., *7*:375, 1955.
469. Ehrner, L.: Lung compliance and respiratory resistance, determined from time-marked esophageal pressure-tidal volume curves, and their relation to some other tests of lung function: A clinical and pathophysiological study of 148 cases with various chest diseases. Acta Med. Scand., *167*: suppl. 353, 1960.
470. Kreuger, J. J., Bain, T., and Patterson, J. L., Jr.: Elevation gradient of intrathoracic pressure. J. Appl. Physiol., *16*:465, 1961.
471. Mead, J., and Whittenberger, J. L.: Physical properties of human lungs measured during spontaneous respiration. J. Appl. Physiol., *5*:779, 1953.
472. Otis, A. B., and Proctor, D. F.: Measurement of alveolar pressure in human subjects. Am. J. Physiol., *152*:106, 1948.
473. Jeker, K., and Wyss, F.: Vergleichende Bronchialwiderstandsmessungen mit der Verschlussdruck und Oesophagusdruckmethode. Helv. Med. Acta, *19*:383, 1952.
474. Mead, J., and Whittenberger, J. L.: Evaluation of airway interruption technique as a method for measuring pulmonary air-flow resistance. J. Appl. Physiol., *6*:408, 1954.

475. Clements, J. A., Sharp, J. T., Johnson, R. P., and Elam, J. O.: Estimation of pulmonary resistance by repetitive interruption of airflow. J. Clin. Invest., *38*:1262, 1959.
476. Cheng, T. O., Godfrey, M. P., and Shepard, R. H.: Pulmonary resistance and state of inflation of lungs in normal subjects and in patients with airway obstruction. J. Appl. Physiol., *14*:727, 1959.
477. Jaeger, M.: Zur Messung des Bronchialwiderstandes. Schweiz. Med. Wchnschr., *90*:648, 1960.
478. Petit, J. M., Melon, J., and Milic-Emili, G.: Application pratique de la technique de l'interruption du courant aérien dans les tests de provocation. Intern. Arch. Allergy Appl. Immunol., *16*:141, 1960.
479. DuBois, A. B., Botelho, S. Y., and Comroe, J. H., Jr.: A new method for measuring airway resistance in man using a body plethysmograph: Values in normal subjects and in patients with respiratory disease. J. Clin. Invest., *35*:327, 1956.
480. Marshall, R., and Dubois, A. B.: The viscous resistance of lung tissue in patients with pulmonary disease. Clin. Sci., *15*:473, 1956.
481. Briscoe, W. A., and DuBois, A. B.: The relationship between airway resistance, airway conductance and lung volume in subjects of different age and body size. J. Clin. Invest., *37*:1279, 1958.
482. DuBois, A. B., and Dautrebande, L.: Acute effects of breathing inert dust particles and of carbachol aerosol in the mechanical characteristics of the lungs in man. Changes in response after inhaling sympathomimetic aerosols. J. Clin. Invest., *37*:1746, 1958.
483. Nadel, J. A., and Comroe, J. H., Jr.: Acute effects of inhalation of cigarette smoke on airway conductance. J. Appl. Physiol., *16*:713, 1961.
484. Nadel, J. A., and Tierney, D. F.: Effect of a previous deep inspiration on airway resistance in man. J. Appl. Physiol., *16*:717, 1961.
485. Hyatt, R. E.: The interrelationships of pressure, flow, and volume during various respiratory maneuvers in normal and emphysematous subjects. Am. Rev. Resp. Dis., *83*:676, 1961.
486. McIlroy, M. B., Marshall, R., and Christie, R. V.: The work of breathing in normal subjects. Clin. Sci., *13*:127, 1954.
487. Cooper, E. A.: The work of ventilating the lungs on exertion. Quart. J. Exper. Physiol., *46*:13, 1961.
488. Margaria, R., Milic-Emili, G., Petit, J. M., and Cavagna, G.: Mechanical work of breathing during muscular exercise. J. Appl. Physiol., *15*:354, 1960.
489. Milic-Emili, G., and Petit, J. M.: Mechanical efficiency of breathing. J. Appl. Physiol., *15*:359, 1960.
490. Milic-Emili, G., Petit, J. M., and Delhez, L.: Les relations entre le travail mécanique ventilatoire pendant l'exercice musculaire et la capacité pulmonaire totale chez l'individu sain. Arch. Int. Physiol. Biochim., *67*:417, 1959.
491. Milic-Emili, G., Petit, J. M., and Deroanne, R.: Effect of respiration rate on mechanical work of breathing during muscular exercise. Int. Z. Angew. Physiol., *18*:330, 1960.
492. Milic-Emili, G., and Petit, J. M.: Il lavoro meccanico della respirazione a varia frequenza respiratoria. Arch. Sci. Biol. (Bologna), *43*:326, 1959.
493. Milic-Emili, G., Petit, J. M., and Deroanne, R.: Mechanical work of breathing during exercise in trained and untrained subjects. J. Appl. Physiol., *17*:43, 1962.
494. Petit, J. M., Milic-Emili, G., and Sadoul, P.: L'influence de la position corporelle sur le travail ventilatoire dynamique pendant l'exercice musculaire chez l'individu sain. Arch. Int. Physiol. Biochim., *68*:437, 1960.
495. Christie, R. V.: Dyspnoea in relation to the viscoelastic properties of the lung. Proc. Roy. Soc. Med. (London), *46*:381, 1953.
496. Cherniack, R. M., Cuddy, T. E., and Armstrong, J. B.: Significance of pulmonary elastic and viscous resistance in orthopnea. Circulation, *15*:859, 1957.
497. McIlroy, M. B., and Christie, R. V.: The work of breathing in emphysema. Clin. Sci., *13*:147, 1954.
498. Marshall, R., McIlroy, M. B., and Christie, R. V.: The work of breathing in mitral stenosis. Clin. Sci., *13*:137, 1954.
499. Marshall, R., Stone, R. W., and Christie, R. V.: The relationship of dyspnoea to respiratory effort in normal subjects, mitral stenosis and emphysema. Clin. Sci., *13*:625, 1954.
500. Bühlmann, A., and Behn, H.: Klinische Ergebnisse atemmechanischer Untersuchungen. Schweiz. Med. Wchnschr., *87*:1500, 1957.
501. Rossier, P. H., and Bühlmann, A.: Dyspnoe und Atemarbeit. Atemmachanische Untersuchungen während Hyperventilation und grosser körperlicher Arbeit. Schweiz. Med. Wchnschr., *89*:543, 1959.
502. Gilbert, R., Sipple, J. H., and Auchincloss, J. H., Jr.: Respiratory control and work of breathing in obese subjects. J. Appl. Physiol., *16*:21, 1961.
503. Cherniack, R. M., and Guenter, C. A.: The efficiency of the respiratory muscles in obesity. Canad. J. Biochem. Physiol., *39*:1215, 1961.
504. Fritts, H. W., Jr., Filler, J., Fishman, A. P., and Cournand, A.: The efficiency of ventilation during voluntary hyperpnea: Studies in normal subjects and in dyspneic patients with either chronic pulmonary emphysema or obesity. J. Clin. Invest., *38*:1339, 1959.
505. Nisell, O.: The respiratory work and pressure during exercise, and their relation to dyspnea. Acta Med. Scand., *166*:113, 1960.
506. Agostoni, E., Thimm, F. F., and Fenn, W. O.: Comparative features of the mechanics of breathing. J. Appl. Physiol., *14*:679, 1959.
507. Marshall, R., and Christie, R. V.: The visco-elastic properties of the lungs in acute pneumonia. Clin. Sci., *13*:403, 1954.
508. Milic-Emili, G., and Petit, J. M.: Il lavoro meccanico respiratorio durante la massima ventilazione polmonare volontaria. Boll. Soc. Ital. Biol. Sper., *35*:431, 1959.
509. McKerrow, C. B., and Otis, A. B.: Oxygen cost of hyperventilation. J. Appl. Physiol., *9*:375, 1956.
510. Cournand, A., Richards, D. W., Jr., Bader, R. A., Bader, M. E., and Fishman, A. P.: The oxygen cost of breathing. Tr. A. Am. Physicians, *67*:162, 1954.
511. Campbell, E. J. M., Westlake, E. K., and Cherniack, R. M.: Simple methods of estimating oxygen consumption and efficiency of the muscles of breathing. J. Appl. Physiol., *11*:303, 1957.
512. Bartlett, R. G., Jr., and Specht, H.: Energy cost of breathing determined with a simplified technique. J. Appl. Physiol., *11*:84, 1957.
513. Bartlett, R. G., Jr., Brubach, H. F., and Specht, H.: Oxygen cost of breathing. J. Appl. Physiol., *12*:413, 1958.
514. Millahn, H. P., and Eckermann, P.: Der Sauerstoffverbrauch der Atmungsmuskulatur bei hohen Ventilation. Int. Z. Angew. Physiol., *19*:120, 1961.
515. Campbell, E. J. M., Westlake, E. K., and Cherniack, R. M.: The oxygen consumption and efficiency of the respiratory muscles of young male subjects. Clin. Sci., *18*:55, 1959.
516. Bader, R. A., Mortimer, E., and Rose, D. J.: The oxygen cost of breathing in dyspneic subjects as studied in normal pregnant women. Clin. Res. Proc., *5*:226, 1957.
517. Cherniack, R. M.: The oxygen consumption and efficiency of the respiratory muscles in health and emphysema. J. Clin. Invest., *38*:494, 1959.
518. Murray, J. F.: Oxygen cost of voluntary hyperventilation. J. Appl. Physiol., *14*:187, 1959.
519. Bartlett, R. G., Jr., Brubach, H. F., and Specht, H.: Oxygen cost of forced breathing in submerged resting subjects. J. Appl. Physiol., *11*:377, 1957.
520. McGregor, M., and Becklake, M. R.: The relationship of oxygen cost of breathing to respiratory mechanical work and respiratory force. J. Clin. Invest., *40*:971, 1961.
521. von Neergaard, K.: Neue Auffassungen über einem Grundbegriff der Atemmechanik. Die Retraktionskraft der Lunge, abhängig von der Oberflächenspannung in den Alveolen. Z. Ges. Exper. Med., *66*:373, 1929.
522. Macklin, C. C.: The pulmonary alveolar mucoid film and the pneumonocytes. Lancet, *1*:1099, 1954.
523. Macklin, C. C.: Pulmonary sumps, dust accumulations, alveolar fluid and lymph vessels. Acta Anat. (Basel), *23*:1, 1955.
524. Radford, E. P.: Recent studies of mechanical properties of

mammalian lungs. In: Remington, J. W. (ed.): *Tissue Elasticity*. Washington, D. C.: American Physiological Society, 1957.

525. Pattle, R. E.: Properties, function and origin of the alveolar lining layer. Nature, *175*:1125, 1955.
526. Clements, J. A., Hustead, R. F., Johnson, R. P., and Gribetz, I.: Pulmonary surface tension and alveolar stability. J. Appl. Physiol., *16*:444, 1961.
527. Clements, J. A.: Surface tension in the lungs. Sci. Am., *207*:120, 1962.
528. Mallory, T. B.: Pathology of pulmonary fibrosis, including chronic pulmonary sarcoidosis. Radiology, *51*:468, 1948.
529. Pattle, R. E.: The lining layer of the lung alveoli. Brit. Med. Bull., *19*:41, 1963.
530. Mead, J., Whittenberger, J. L., and Radford, E. P., Jr.: Surface tension as a factor in pulmonary volume-pressure hysteresis. J. Appl. Physiol., *10*:191, 1957.
531. Clements, J. A.: Surface tension of lung extracts. Proc. Soc. Exper. Biol. Med., *95*:170, 1957.
532. Brown, E. S.: Lung area from surface tension effects. Proc. Soc. Exper. Biol. Med., *95*:168, 1957.
533. Clements, J. A., Brown, E. S., and Johnson, R. P.: Pulmonary surface tension and the mucus lining of the lungs: Some theoretical considerations. J. Appl. Physiol., *12*:262, 1958.
534. Pattle, R. E.: Properties, function, and origin of the alveolar lining layer. Proc. Roy. Soc. (London), *s.B, 148*:217, 1958.
535. Brown, E. S., Johnson, R. P., and Clements, J. A.: Pulmonary surface tension. J. Appl. Physiol., *14*:717, 1959.
536. Miller, D. A., and Bondurant, S.: Surface characteristics of vertebrate lung extracts. J. Appl. Physiol., *16*:1075, 1961.
537. Avery, M. E., and Mead, J.: Surface properties in relation to atelectasis and hyaline membrane disease. A.M.A. J. Dis. Child., *97*:517, 1959.
538. Pattle, R. E., Claireaux, A. E., Davies, P. A., and Cameron, A. H.: Inability to form a lung-lining film as a cause of the respiratory-distress syndrome in the newborn. Lancet, *2*:469, 1962.
539. McIlroy, M. B., and Christie, R. V.: A post-mortem study of the visco-elastic properties of normal lungs. Thorax, *7*:291, 1952.
540. McIlroy, M. B., and Christie, R. V.: A post-mortem study of the visco-elastic properties of the lungs in emphysema. Thorax, *7*:295, 1952.
541. Hugh-Jones, P.: A simple standard exercise test and its use for measuring exertion dyspnoea. Brit. Med. J., *1*:65, 1952.
542. Morehouse, L. E., and Miller, A. T., Jr.: *Physiology of Exercise* (Harvard University Monograph No. 11). St. Louis, C. V. Mosby Co., 1948.
543. Mitchell, J. H., Sproule, B. J., and Chapman, C. B.: The physiological meaning of the maximal oxygen intake test. J. Clin. Invest., *37*:538, 1958.
544. Reeves, J. T., Grover, R. F., Blount, S. G., Jr., and Filley, G. F.: Cardiac output response to standing and treadmill walking. J. Appl. Physiol., *16*:283, 1961.
545. Linroth, K.: Physical working capacity in conscripts during military service: Its relation to some anthropometric data; methods to assess individual physical capabilities. Acta Med. Scand., *157*: suppl. 324, 1957.
546. Holmgren, A., Jonsson, B., and Sjöstrand, T.: Circulatory data in normal subjects at rest and during exercise in recumbent position, with special reference to the stroke volume at different work intensities. Acta Physiol. Scand., *49*:343, 1960.
547. Åstrand, P. O., and Saltin, B.: Oxygen uptake during the first minutes of heavy muscular exercise. J. Appl. Physiol., *16*:971, 1961.
548. Wyndham, C. H., Strydom, N. B., Maritz, J. S., Morrison, J. F., Peter, J., and Potgieter, Z. U.: Maximum oxygen intake and maximum heart rate during strenuous work. J. Appl. Physiol., *14*:927, 1959.
549. Knipping, H. W., and Moncrieff, A.: The ventilation equivalent for oxygen. Quart. J. Med., *(n.s.) 1*:17, 1932.
550. Denolin, H., Lequime, J., De Coster, A., and Lewillie, L.: Evolution du coefficient d'utilisation d'oxygène lors de l'effort, au cours du récécissement mitral. Arch. Mal. Coeur, *46*:423, 1953.
551. MacIntosh, D. J., Sinnott, J. C., Milne, I. G., and Reid, E. A. S.: Some aspects of disordered pulmonary function in mitral stenosis. Ann. Int. Med., *49*:1294, 1958.
552. Ehrner, L., Garlind, T., and Linderholm, H.: Chronic cor pulmonale following thromboembolism. A clinical and pathophysiological study of three cases. Acta Med. Scand., *164*:279, 1959.
553. Åstrand, I.: The physical work capacity of workers 50–64 years old. Acta Physiol. Scand., *42*:73, 1958.
554. Robinson, S.: Experimental studies of physical fitness in relation to age. Arb. Physiol., *10*:251, 1958.
555. Bühlmann, A., Scherrer, M., and Herzog, H.: Vorschläge zur einheitlichen Beurteilung der Arbeitsfähigkeit durch die Lungenfunktionsprüfung. Schweiz. Med. Wchnschr., *91*:105, 1961.
556. Negus, V.: Protection of the respiratory tract. Brit. Med. J., *2*:723, 1961.
557. Christie, R. V., and Loomis, A. L.: The pressure of aqueous vapour in the alveolar air. J. Physiol. (London), *77*:35, 1932.
558. Bruck, E.: Water in expired air; Physiology and measurement. J. Pediat., *60*:869, 1962.
559. Hartroft, W. S., and Macklin, C. C.: The size of human lung alveoli expressed as diameter of selected alveolar outlines as seen in specially prepared 25μ microsections. Tr. Roy. Soc. Canad., Sect. V., *38*:63, 1944.
560. Weibel, E. R., and Gomez, D. M.: Architecture of the human lung. Science, *137*:577, 1962.
561. Miller, W. S.: *The Lung*. Springfield, Ill., Charles C Thomas, 1937.
562. Boren, H. G.: Alveolar fenestrae. Relationship to the pathology and pathogenesis of pulmonary emphysema. Am. Rev. Resp. Dis., *85*:328, 1962.
563. Bates, D. V., and Christie, R. V.: Effects of ageing on respiratory function in man. In Wolstenholme, G. E. W., and Cameron, M. P. (eds.): *Ciba Foundation Colloquia on Ageing*, vol. 1. London, J. & A. Churchill, 1955, p. 58.
564. Whitfield, A. G. W., Waterhouse, J. A. H., and Arnott, W. M.: The total lung volume and its subdivisions. A study in physiological norms. II. The effect of posture. Brit. J. Social Med., *4*:86, 1950.
565. Stewart, C. A.: The vital capacity of the lungs of children in health and disease. Am. J. Dis. Child., *24*:451, 1922.
566. Stephen, C. R.: The influence of posture on mechanics of respiration and vital capacity. Anesthesiology, *9*:134, 1948.
567. Mills, J. N.: The influence upon the vital capacity of procedures calculated to alter the volume of blood in the lungs. J. Physiol. (London), *110*:207, 1949.
568. Osher, W. J.: Change of vital capacity with the assumption of the supine position. Am. J. Physiol., *161*:352, 1950.
569. Lagneau, D., Namur, M., and Petit, J. M.: Influence de la position corporelle sur les volumes pulmonaires de l'homme normal. Arch. Int. Physiol., *68*:596, 1960.
570. Moreno, F., and Lyons, H. A.: Effect of body posture on lung volumes. J. Appl. Physiol., *16*:27, 1961.
571. Sjöstrand, T.: The significance of the pulmonary blood volume in the regulation of the blood circulation under normal and pathological conditions. Acta Med. Scand., *145*:155, 1953.
572. Sjöstrand, T.: Determination of changes in the intrathoracic blood volume in man. Acta Physiol. Scand., *22*:114, 1951.
573. Dock, W.: Effect of posture on alveolar gas tension in tuberculosis. Explanation for favored sites of chronic pulmonary lesions. A.M.A. Arch. Int. Med., *94*:700, 1954.
574. Bates, D. V.: Measurements of regional distribution. In: *Handbook of Physiology*, Respiration Sect., vol. I, ch. 57. Washington, D.C., American Physiological Society, 1964.
575. Bergan, F.: The relative function of the lungs in supine, left and right lateral position. J. Oslo City Hosp., *2*:185, 1952.
576. Svanberg, L.: Influence of posture on the lung volumes, ventilation and circulation in normals. A spirometric-bronchospirometric investigation. Scand. J. Clin. Lab. Invest., *9*: suppl. 25, 1957.
577. Autio, V.: Normal distribution of pulmonary function between the lungs. A bronchospirometric study. Ann. Med. Intern. Fenn., *48*:9, 1959.

578. Lillington, G. A., Fowler, W. S., Miller, R. D., and Helmholz, H. F., Jr.: Nitrogen clearance rates of right and left lungs in different positions. J. Clin. Invest., *38*:2026, 1959.
579. Miller, R. D., Fowler, W. S., and Helmholz, H. F., Jr.: Relative volume and ventilation of the two lungs with change to the lateral decubitus position. J. Lab. Clin. Med., *47*:297, 1956.
580. Granath, A., Horie, E., and Linderholm, H.: Compliance and resistance of the lungs in the sitting and supine positions at rest and during work. Scand. J. Clin. Lab., Invest., *11*:226, 1959.
581. Ehrner, L., and Nisell, O.: Variability of some characteristics of respiratory mechanics in normal adults. Acta Med. Scand., *164*:95, 1959.
582. Frank, N. R., Mead, J., Siebens, A. A., and Storey, C. F.: Measurements of pulmonary compliance in seventy healthy young adults. J. Appl. Physiol., *9*:38, 1956.
583. Macklem, P. T., and Becklake, M. R.: The relationship between the mechanical and diffusing properties of the lung in health and disease. Am. Rev. Resp. Dis., *87*:47, 1963.
584. Butler, J., White, H. C., and Arnott, W. M.: The pulmonary compliance in normal subjects. Clin. Sci., *16*:709, 1957.
585. Bates, D. V., and Pearce, J. F.: The pulmonary diffusing capacity; a comparison of methods of measurement and a study of the effect of body position. J. Physiol. (London), *132*:232, 1956.
586. Newman, F., and Thomson, M. L.: The effect of the inverted position on alveolar-capillary diffusion and volumes of the human lung. J. Physiol. (London), *153*:71 *P*, 1960.
587. Burwell, C. S., Robin, E. D., Whaley, R. D., and Bickelmann, A. G.: Extreme obesity associated with alveolar hypoventilation—A Pickwickian syndrome. Am. J. Med., *21*:811, 1956.
588. Hackney, J. D., Crane, M. G., Collier, C. C., Rokaw, S., and Griggs, D. E.: Syndrome of extreme obesity and hypoventilation: Studies of etiology. Ann. Int. Med., *51*:541, 1959.
589. Kaufman, B. J., Ferguson, M. H., and Cherniack, R. M.: Hypoventilation in obesity. J. Clin. Invest., *38*:500, 1959.
590. Lillington, G. A., Anderson, M. W., and Brandenburg, R. O.: Cardiorespiratory dysfunction and polycythemia in patients with extreme obesity. Proc. Staff Meet., Mayo Clin., *32*:585, 1957.
591. Naimark, A., and Cherniack, R. M.: Compliance of the respiratory system and its components in health and obesity. J. Appl. Physiol., *15*:377, 1960.
592. Said, S. I.: Abnormalities of pulmonary gas exchange in obesity. Ann. Int. Med., *53*:1121, 1960.
593. Tucker, D. H., and Sieker, H. O.: The effect of change in body position on lung volumes and intrapulmonary gas mixing in patients with obesity, heart failure, and emphysema. Am. Rev. Resp. Dis., *82*:787, 1960.
594. Cullen, J. H., and Formel, P. F.: The respiratory defects in extreme obesity. Am. J. Med., *32*:525, 1962.
595. Cherniack, R. M.: Respiratory effects of obesity. Canad. M. A. J., *80*:613, 1959.
596. Alexander, J. K., Amad, K. H., and Cole, V. W.: Observations on some clinical features of extreme obesity, with particular reference to cardiorespiratory effects. Am. J. Med., *32*:512, 1962.
597. Berlyne, G. M.: The cardiorespiratory syndrome of extreme obesity. Lancet, *2*:939, 1958.
598. Bedell, G. N., Wilson, W. R., and Seebohm, P. M.: Pulmonary function in obese persons. J. Clin. Invest., *37*:1049, 1958.
599. Siggaard-Andersen, O., Engel, K., Jørgensen, K., and Astrup, P.: A micro method for determination of pH, carbon dioxide tension, base excess and standard bicarbonate in capillary blood. Scand. J. Clin. Lab. Invest., *12*:172, 1960.
600. Siggaard-Andersen, O., and Engel, K.: A new acid-base nomogram. An improved method for the calculation of the relevant blood acid-base data. Scand. J. Clin. Lab. Invest., *12*:177, 1960.
601. Cunningham, D. J. C.: Some quantitative aspects of the regulation of human respiration in exercise. Brit. Med. Bull., *19*:25, 1963.
602. Asmussen, E., and Nielsen, M.: Studies on the regulation of respiration in heavy work. Acta Physiol. Scand., *12*:171, 1946.
603. Burton, A. C.: The control of pulmonary ventilation. [Letter to the Editor.] Canad. M. A. J., *84*:1027, 1961.
604. Dejours, P.: La régulation de la ventilation au cours de l'exercice musculaire chez l'homme. J. Physiol. (Paris), *51*:163, 1959.
605. Dejours, P., Labrousse, Y., Raynaud, J., Girard, F., and Teillac, A.: Stimulus oxygène de la ventilation au repos et au cours de l'exercice musculaire, à basse altitude (50m), chez l'homme. Rev. Franc Etud. Clin. Biol., *3*:105, 1958.
606. Dejours, P., Labrousse, Y., Raynaud, J., and Teillac, A.: Stimulus oxygène chémoréflexe de la ventilation à basse altitude (50m) chez l'homme. I. Au repos. J. Physiol. (Paris), *49*:115, 1957.
607. Asmussen, E., and Nielsen, M.: Pulmonary ventilation and effect of oxygen breathing in heavy exercise. Acta Physiol. Scand., *43*:365, 1958.
608. May, P.: L'action immédiate de l'oxygène sur la ventilation chez l'homme normal. Helv. Physiol. Pharmacol. Acta, *15*:230, 1957.
609. Kao, F. F., Schlig, B. B., and Brooks, C. M.: Regulation of respiration during induced muscular work in decerebrate dogs. J. Appl. Physiol., *7*:379, 1955.
610. Kao, F. F.: Regulation of respiration during muscular activity. Am. J. Physiol., *185*:145, 1956.
611. Asmussen, E., and Nielsen, M.: Studies on the initial changes in respiration at the transition from rest to work and from work to rest. Acta Physiol. Scand., *16*:270, 1948.
612. Torelli, G., and Brandi, G.: Regulation of the ventilation at the beginning of muscular exercise. Int. Z. Angew. Physiol., *19*:134, 1961.
613. Donevan, R. E., Anderson, N. M., Sekelj, P., Papp, O., and McGregor, M.: Influence of voluntary hyperventilation on cardiac output. J. Appl. Physiol., *17*:487, 1962.
614. Holmgren, A., and Linderholm, H.: Oxygen and carbon dioxide tensions of arterial blood during heavy and exhaustive exercise. Acta Physiol. Scand., *44*:203, 1958.
615. Rushmer, R. F., and Smith, O. A., Jr.: Cardiac control. Physiol. Rev., *39*:41, 1959.
616. Brandfonbrener, M., Landowne, M., and Shock, N. W.: Changes in cardiac output with age. Circulation, *12*:557, 1955.
617. Holmgren, A.: Circulatory changes during muscular work in man, with special reference to arterial and central venous pressures in systemic circulation. Scand. J. Clin. Lab. Invest., *8*: suppl. 24, 1956.
618. Christensen, E. H.: Beiträge zur Physiologie schwerer körperlicher Arbeit. VII. Über die Brauchbarkeit der Acetylenmethode zur Bestimmung des Herzminutenvolumens während körperlicher Arbeit. Arb. Physiol., *5*:479, 1932.
619. Christensen, E. H.: Beiträge zur Physiologie schwerer körperlicher Arbeit. III. Gasanalytische Methoden zur Bestimmung des Herzminutenvolumens in Rube und während körperlicher Arbeit. Arb. Physiol., *4*:175, 1931.
620. Barratt-Boyes, B. G., and Wood, E. H.: Cardiac output and related measurements and pressure values in the right heart and associated vessels, together with an analysis of the hemodynamic response to the inhalation of high oxygen mixtures in healthy subjects. J. Lab. Clin. Med., *51*:72, 1958.
621. Donald, K. W., Bishop, J. M., Cumming, G., and Wade, O. L.: The effect of exercise on the cardiac output and circulatory dynamics of normal subjects. Clin. Sci., *14*:37, 1955.
622. McGregor, M., Adam, W., and Sekelj, P.: Influence of posture on cardiac output and minute ventilation during exercise. Circ. Res., *9*:1089, 1961.
623. Uggla, L. G.: Pulmonary hypertension in tuberculosis of the lungs: A clinical study in advanced cases examined with cardiac catheterization and temporary unilateral occlusion of the pulmonary artery. Acta Tuberc. Scand., suppl. *41*:1, 1957.
624. Yu, P. N. G., Lovejoy, F. W., Jr., Joos, H. A., Nye, R. E., Jr., and McCann, W. S.: Studies of pulmonary hypertension. I. Pulmonary circulatory dynamics in patients with pulmonary emphysema at rest. J. Clin. Invest., *32*:130, 1953.
625. MacNamara, J., Prime, F. J., and Sinclair, J. D.: The in-

crease in diffusing capacity of the lungs on exercise: Experimental and clinical study. Lancet, *1*:404, 1960.
626. Hanson, J. S., and Tabakin, B. S.: Steady state carbon monoxide diffusing capacity in normal females. J. Appl. Physiol., *16*:839, 1961.
627. Hanson, J. S., and Tabakin, B. S.: Carbon monoxide diffusing capacity in normal male subjects, age 20–60, during exercise. J. Appl. Physiol., *15*:402, 1960.
628. Linderholm, H.: Diffusing capacity of the lungs as a limiting factor for physical working capacity. Acta Med. Scand., *163*:61, 1959.
629. Newman, F., Smalley, B. F., and Thomson, M. L.: Effect of exercise, body and lung size on CO diffusion in athletes and nonathletes. J. Appl. Physiol., *17*:649, 1962.
630. Astrand, P. O.: Human physical fitness with special reference to sex and age. Physiol. Rev., *36*:307, 1956.
631. Holmgren, A., Mossfeldt, F., Sjöstrand, T., and Ström, G.: Effect of training on work capacity, total hemoglobin, blood volume, heart volume and pulse rate in recumbent and upright positions. Acta Physiol. Scand., *50*:72, 1960.
632. Sloan, A. W., and Keen, E. N.: Physical fitness of oarsmen and rugby players before and after training. J. Appl. Physiol., *14*:635, 1959.
633. Stuart, D. G., and Collings, W. D.: Comparison of vital capacity and maximum breathing capacity of athletes and nonathletes. J. Appl. Physiol., *14*:507, 1959.
634. Margaria, R., Cerretelli, P., Marchi, S., and Rossi, L.: Maximum exercise in oxygen. Int. Z. Angew. Physiol., *18*:465, 1961.
635. Robinson, S., Robinson, D. L., Mountjoy, R. J., and Bullard, R. W.: Influence of fatigue on the efficiency of men during exhausting runs. J. Appl. Physiol., *12*:197, 1958.
636. Verzár, F.: The regulation of the lung volume and its disturbances. Schweiz. Med. Wchnschr., *76*:932, 1946.
637. Asmussen, E., and Christensen, E. H.: Die Mittelkapazität der Lungen bei erhöhtem O_2-Bedarf. Skand. Arch. Physiol., *82*:201, 1939.
638. Alleröder, H., and Landen, H.: Das Verhalten der Komplementärluft, der Reserveluft und der Sauerstoffaufnahme im Arbeitsversuch. Z. Ges. Exper. Med., *108*:406, 1940.
639. Petit, J. M., Milic-Emili, G., and Koch, R.: Le volume de réserve expiratoire pendant l'exercise musculaire chez l'homme sain. Arch. Int. Physiol. Biochim., *67*:350, 1959.
640. Hanson, J. S., Tabakin, B. S., and Caldwell, E. J.: Response of lung volumes and ventilation to posture change and upright exercise. J. Appl. Physiol., *17*:783, 1962.
641. Norris, A. H., Shock, N. W., Landowne, M., and Falzone, J. A., Jr.: Pulmonary function studies: Age differences in lung volumes and bellows action. J. Gerontol, *11*:379, 1956.
642. Bower, G.: Respiratory symptoms and ventilatory function in 172 adults employed in a bank. Am. Rev. Resp. Dis., *83*:684, 1961.
643. Bink, B.: The physical working capacity in relation to working time and age. Ergonomics, *5*:25, 1962.
644. Woodruff, W.: Thoracic surgery after the age of fifty. New York J. Med., *52*:1990, 1952.
645. Thurlbeck, W. M.: The incidence of pulmonary emphysema: With observations on the relative incidence and spatial distribution of various types of emphysema. Am. Rev. Resp. Dis., *87*:206, 1963.
646. Comfort, A.: The biology of ageing. Lancet, *2*:772, 1956.
647. Richards, D. W.: The aging lung. Bull. N.Y. Acad. Med., *32*:407, 1956.
648. Pierce, J. A., and Hocott, J. B.: Studies on the collagen and elastin content of the human lung. J. Clin. Invest., *39*:8, 1960.
649. Pierce, J. A., and Ebert, R. V.: The elastic properties of the lung collagen and elastin. Am. Rev. Resp. Dis., *80*:45, 1959.
650. Pierce, J. A., Hocott, J. B., and Ebert, R. V.: Studies of lung collagen and elastin. Am. Rev. Resp. Dis., *80*:45, 1959.
651. Pierce, J. A., and Ebert, R. V.: The barrel deformity of the chest, the senile lung and obstructive pulmonary emphysema. Am. J. Med., *25*:13, 1958.
652. Briscoe, A. M., and Loring, W. E.: Elastin content of the human lung. Proc. Soc. Exper. Biol. Med., *99*:162, 1958.
653. Briscoe, W. A.: A method for dealing with data concerning uneven ventilation of the lung and its effects on blood gas transfer. J. Appl. Physiol., *14*:291, 1959.
654. Heard, B. E.: A pathological study of emphysema of the lungs with chronic bronchitis. Thorax, *13*:136, 1958.
655. Heppleston, A. G., and Leopold, J. G.: Chronic pulmonary emphysema: Anatomy and pathogenesis. Am. J. Med., *31*:279, 1961.
656. Wright, R. R.: Elastic tissue of normal and emphysematous lungs. A tridimensional histologic study. Am. J. Pathol., *39*:355, 1961.
657. Weibel, E. R., and Gomez, D. M.: A principle for counting tissue structures on random sections. J. Appl. Physiol., *17*:343, 1962.
658. Spriggs, A. I., and Sladden, R. A.: The influence of age on red cell diameter. J. Clin. Pathol., *11*:53, 1958.
659. Galdston, M., Wolfe, W. B., and Steele, J. M.: Derangements of pulmonary function in individuals without clinical evidence of disease of heart or lungs. J. Appl. Physiol., *5*:17, 1952.
660. Norris, A. H., Shock, N. W., and Wiengst, M. J.: Age differences in ventilatory and gas exchange responses to graded exercise in males. J. Gerontol., *10*:145, 1955.
661. Joos, H., Rossier, P. H., and Bühlmann, A.: Die Lungenfunktion im Alter. Schweiz. Med. Wchnschr., *87*:806, 1957.
662. *Colloquium on Exercise and Fitness, Monticello, Illinois, 1959.* Chicago, Athletic Institute and University of Illinois, 1960.
663. Jokl, E.: *The Clinical Physiology of Physical Fitness and Rehabilitation.* Springfield, Ill., Charles C Thomas, 1958, p. 194.
664. Hettinger, T., Birkhead, N. C., Horvath, S. M., Issekutz, B., and Rodahl, K.: Assessment of physical work capacity. J. Appl. Physiol., *16*:153, 1961.
665. Cureton, T. K.: Relationship of physical fitness to athletic performance and sports. J.A.M.A., *162*:1139, 1956.
666. Berglund, G., and Karlberg, P.: Determination of the functional residual capacity in newborn infants. Preliminary report. Acta Paediat., *45*:541, 1956.
667. Polgar, G.: Airway resistance in the newborn infant. J. Pediat., *59*:915, 1961.
668. Cook, C. D., Sutherland, J. M., Segal, S., Cherry, R. B., Mead, J., McIlroy, M. B., and Smith, C. A.: Studies of respiratory physiology in the newborn infant. III. Measurements of mechanics of respiration. J. Clin. Invest., *36*:440, 1957.
669. Cook, C. D., Cherry, R. B., O'Brien, D., Karlberg, P., and Smith, C. A.: Studies of respiratory physiology in the newborn infant. I. Observations on normal premature and full-term infants. J. Clin. Invest., *34*:975, 1955.
670. Wolstenholme, G. E. W., and O'Connor, M. (eds.): *Ciba Foundation Symposium on Somatic Stability in the Newly Born.* London, J. & A. Churchill, 1961.
671. Smith, C. A.: *The Physiology of the Newborn Infant.* 3rd ed. Oxford: Blackwell Scientific Publications; Springfield, Ill., Charles C Thomas, 1959.
672. *Symposium on Normal and Abnormal Respiration in Children, Kansas City, 1960;* Report of the 37th Ross Conference on Pediatric Research. Columbus, Ohio, Ross Laboratories, 1961.
673. Agostoni, E., Taglietti, A., Agostoni, A. F., and Setnikar, I.: Mechanical aspects of the first breath. J. Appl. Physiol., *13*:344, 1958.
674. Cooperman, N. R., Rubovits, F. E., and Hesser, F.: Oxygen saturation in the newborn infant. Am. J. Obst. & Gynec., *81*:385, 1961.
675. McIlroy, M. B., and Tomlinson, E. S.: The mechanics of breathing in newly born babies. Thorax, *10*:58, 1955.
676. Weisbrot, I. M., James, L. S., Prince, C. E., Holaday, D. A., and Apgar, V.: Acid-base homeostasis of the newborn infant during the first 24 hours of life. J. Pediat., *52*:395, 1958.
677. Reardon, H. S., Baumann, M. L., and Haddad, E. J.: Respiratory alkalosis – a frequent phenomenon observed in newborn infants. A.M.A. Am. J. Dis. Child., *88*:371, 1954.
678. Miller, H. C., Behrle, F. C., Smull, N. W., and Blim, R. D.: Studies of respiratory insufficiency in newborn infants. II. Correlation of hydrogen-ion concentration, carbon dioxide

tension, carbon dioxide content, and oxygen saturation of blood with trend of respiratory rates. Pediatrics, *19*:387, 1957.
679. Wulf, H.: Blutgaswerte und Neugeborenenatmung. Klin. Wchnschr., *36*:234, 1958.
680. Roberts, H., and Please, N.: The respiratory minute volume in the newborn infant. J. Obst. Gynaec. Brit. Emp., *65*:33, 1958.
681. McCance, R. A., and Hatemi, N.: Control of acid-base stability in the newly born. Lancet, *1*:293, 1961.
682. Engström, I., Karlberg, P., and Swarts, C. L.: Respiratory studies in children. IX. Relationships between mechanical properties of the lungs, lung volumes and ventilatory capacity in healthy children 7-15 years of age. Acta Paediat., *51*:68, 1962.
683. Helliesen, P. J., Cook, C. D., Friedlander, L., and Agathon, S.: Studies of respiratory physiology in children. I. Mechanics of respiration and lung volumes in 85 normal children 5 to 17 years of age. Pediatrics, *22*:80, 1958.
684. Bucci, G., Cook, C. D., and Barrie, H.: Studies of respiratory physiology in children. V. Total lung diffusion, diffusing capacity of pulmonary membrane, and pulmonary capillary blood volume in normal subjects from 7 to 40 years of age. J. Pediat., *58*:820, 1961.
685. Cassels, D. E., and Morse, M.: Arterial blood gases and acid-base balance in normal children. J. Clin. Invest., *32*:824, 1953.
686. Bengtsson, E.: The working capacity in normal children, evaluated by submaximal exercise on the bicycle ergometer and compared with adults. Acta Med. Scand., *154*:91, 1956.
687. Hurtado, A., and Aste-Salazar, H.: Arterial blood gases and acid-base balance at sea level and at high altitudes. J. Appl. Physiol., *1*:304, 1948.
688. Chiodi, H.: Respiratory adaptations to chronic high altitude hypoxia. J. Appl. Physiol., *10*:81, 1957.
689. Kellogg, R. H., Pace, N., Archibald, E. R., and Vaughan, B. E.: Respiratory response to inspired CO_2 during acclimatization to an altitude of 12,470 feet. J. Appl. Physiol., *11*:65, 1957.
690. Reed, D. J., and Kellogg, R. H.: Changes in respiratory response to carbon dioxide during natural sleep at sea level and at altitude. J. Appl. Physiol., *13*:325, 1958.
691. Hock, R. J.: Effect of altitude on endurance running of *Peromyscus maniculatus*. J. Appl. Physiol., *16*:435, 1961.
692. Hultgren, H. N., Spickard, W. B., Hellriegel, K., and Houston, C. S.: High altitude pulmonary edema. Medicine, *40*:289, 1961.
693. Tenney, S. M., Rahn, H., Stroud, R. C., and Mithoefer, J. C.: Adaption to high altitude: Changes in lung volumes during the first 7 days at Mt. Evans, Colorado. J. Appl. Physiol., *5*:607, 1953.
694. Anderson, L. L., Wilcox, M. L., Silliman, J., and Blount, S. G., Jr.: The pulmonary physiology of normal individuals living at an altitude of one mile. J. Clin. Invest., *32*:490, 1953.
695. Rahn, H., and Hammond, D.: Vital capacity of reduced barometric pressure. J. Appl. Physiol., *4*:715, 1952.
696. Husson, G., and Otis, A. B.: Adaptive value of respiratory adjustments to shunt hypoxia and to altitude hypoxia. J. Clin. Invest., *36*:270, 1957.
697. Cerretelli, P., and Margaria, R.: Maximum oxygen consumption at altitude. Int. Z. Angew. Physiol., *18*:460, 1961.
698. Cerretelli, P.: Some aspects of the respiratory function in man acclimatized to high altitudes (the Himalayas). Int. Z. Angew. Physiol., *18*:386, 1961.
699. Schilling, J. A., Harvey, R. B., Becker, E. L., Velasquez, T., Wells, G., and Balke, B.: Work performance at altitude after adaptation in man and dog. J. Appl. Physiol., *8*:381, 1956.
700. Rótta, A., Cánepa, A., Hurtado, A., Velásquez, T., and Chávez, R.: Pulmonary circulation at sea level and at high altitudes. J. Appl. Physiol., *9*:328, 1956.
701. Rótta, A.: Peso del corazon en el hombre normal de la altura. Rev. Peru. Cardiol., *4*/1:71, 1955.
702. Pugh, L. G. C., and Ward, M. P.: Some effects of high altitude on man. Lancet, *2*:1115, 1956.
703. Pugh, L. G. C. E.: Resting ventilation and alveolar air on Mount Everest: With remarks on the relation of barometric pressure to altitude in mountains. J. Physiol. (London), *135*:590, 1957.
704. Hecht, H. H., and McClement, J. H.: A case of "chronic mountain sickness" in the United States: Clinical, physiologic and electrocardiographic observations. Am. J. Med., *25*:470, 1958.
705. Monge, C. C., Cazorla, T. A., Whittembury, M. G., Sakata, B. Y., and Rizo-Patrón, C.: A description of the circulatory dynamics in the heart and lungs of people at sea level and at high altitude by means of the dye dilution technique. Acta Physiol. Lat. Amer., *5*:198, 1955.
706. Comroe, J. H.: *The Functions of the Lung*. Harvey Lectures, series 48. New York, Academic Press, 1952, p. 110.
707. James, L. S.: Physiology of respiration in newborn infants and in the respiratory distress syndrome. Pediatrics, *24*:1069, 1959.
708. Robertson, A. J., and Coope, R.: Râles, rhonchi, and Laennec. Lancet, *2*:417, 1957.
709. Fletcher, C. M.: The clinical diagnosis of pulmonary emphysema—an experimental study. *In:* Discussion on the diagnosis of pulmonary emphysema. Proc. Roy. Soc. Med. (London), *45*:577, 1952.
710. Fraser, R. G., and Bates, D. V.: Body section Roentgenography in the evaluation and differentiation of chronic hypertrophic emphysema and asthma. Am. J. Roentgenol., *82*:39, 1959.
711. Heilman, R. S., Tabakin, B. S., Hanson, J. S., and Naeye, R. L.: Alterations of circulatory and ventilatory dynamics in pulmonary vascular obstruction secondary to recurrent pulmonary emboli. Case report, with studies of pulmonary physiology. Am. J. Med., *32*:298, 1962.
712. Gilson, J. C., and Oldham, P. D.: Lung function tests in the diagnosis of pulmonary emphysema: The use of discriminant analysis. *In:* Discussion on the diagnosis of pulmonary emphysema. Proc. Roy. Soc. Med. (London), *45*:584, 1952.
713. Shephard, R. J., and Turner, M. E.: On the probability of correct diagnosis by pulmonary function tests. Thorax, *14*:300, 1959.
714. Widdicombe, J. G.: Regulation of tracheobronchial smooth muscle. Physiol. Rev., *43*:1, 1963.
715. Gough, J.: Correlation of radiological and pathological changes in some diseases of the lung. Lancet, *1*:161, 1955.
716. Ganz, P., and Vetter, W.: Über die operative Behandlung des Asthma bronchiale. Ein vorläufiger Bericht über die Exstirpation des Paraganglion caroticum bei 20 Asthmakranken. Med. Klin. Munich, *54*:779, 1959.
717. Dimitrov-Szokodi, D., Husvéti, A., and Balogh, G.: Lung denervation in the therapy of intractable bronchial asthma. J. Thorac. Surg., *33*:166, 1957.
718. Overholt, R. H.: Pulmonary denervation and resection in asthmatic patients. Ann. Allergy, *17*:534, 1959.
719. Il'inskiĭ, P. I., and Rukhimovich, G. S.: Rentgenoterapüia bronchial'noĭ astmy u deteĭ. (Predvaritel'noe soobshchenie.) [Roentgen therapy of bronchial asthma in children. (Preliminary communication.)] Vestn. Rentgen. Radiol., *33*/3:71, 1958. [Excerpta Med. (XV), *12*:537, 1959.]
720. Roget, J., Beaudoing, A., and Mathieu, G.: Enquête sur l'action de la cuve climatique d'altitude dans l'asthme infantile. J. Med. Lyon, *41*:91, 1960.
721. Baker, A. G.: Treatment of chronic bronchial asthma. Aerosol of staphylococcus bacteriophage lysate as an adjunct to systemic hyposensitization. Am. Practitioner, *9*:591, 1959.
722. Edwards, G.: Hypnotic treatment of asthma: Real and illusory results. Brit. Med. J., *2*:492, 1960.
723. Sinclair-Gieben, A. H. C.: Treatment of status asthmaticus by hypnosis. Brit. Med. J., *2*:1651, 1960.
724. Gandevia, B., Hume, K. M., and Prime, F. J.: Outpatient bronchodilator therapy. Lancet, *1*:956, 1957.
725. Pestalozzi, C., and Schnyder, U. W.: Zur Frage der Bäckerrhinitis und des Bäckerasthmas. Schweiz. Med. Wchnschr., *85*:496, 1955.
726. Kux, E., and Kurrek, H.: Die thorakoskopischvegetative Denervation als Therapie des Asthma bronchiale. Muench. Med. Wchnschr., *100*:1049, 1958.
727. McKerrow, C. B., Roach, S. A., Gilson, J. C., and Schilling, R. S. F.: The size of cotton dust particles causing

byssinosis: An environmental and physiological study. Brit. J. Indust. Med., *19*:1, 1962.

728. Bruusgaard, A.: Astmalignende sykdom blant Norske aluminiumsarbeidere. Tidsskr. Norske Laegeforen, *80*:796, 1960.
729. Mitchell, J., Manning, G. B., Molyneux, M., and Lane, R. E.: Pulmonary fibrosis in workers exposed to finely powdered aluminum. Brit. J. Indust. Med., *18*:10, 1961.
730. Widdicombe, J. G.: Respiratory reflexes in man and other mammalian species. Clin. Sci., *21*:163, 1961.
731. Widdicombe, J. G., Kent, D. C., and Nadel, J. A.: Mechanism of bronchoconstriction during inhalation of dust. J. Appl. Physiol., *17*:613, 1962.
732. Tiffeneau, R.: L'hyperexcitabilité des terminaisons sensitives pulmonaires de l'asthmatique. Mesure; caractères; causes. Son rôle en tant que facteur asthmogène réflexe. Presse Med., *66*:1250, 1958.
733. Tiffeneau, R.: Hypersensibilité cholinergo-histaminique pulmonaire de l'asthmatique: Relation avec l'hypersensibilité allergénique pulmonaire. Acta Allergol., *12*: suppl. 5, p. 187, 1958.
734. Arborelius, M., Ekwall, B., Jernérus, R., Lundin, G., and Svanberg, L.: Unilateral provoked bronchial asthma in man. J. Clin. Invest., *41*:1236, 1962.
735. Bentivoglio, L. G., Beerel, F., Bryan, A. C., Stewart, P. B., Rose, B., and Bates, D. V.: Regional pulmonary function studied with xenon[133] in patients with bronchial asthma. J. Clin. Invest., *42*:1193, 1963.
736. Kennedy, M. C. S., and Thursby-Pelham, D. C.: Cortisone in treatment of children with chronic asthma. Brit. Med. J., *1*:1511, 1956.
737. Beaudry, P. H., and Becklake, M. R.: A trial of SA-97 in the treatment of asthma in children. J. Allergy, *33*:210, 1962.
738. Phelps, H. W., Sobel, G. W., and Fisher, N. E.: Air pollution asthma among military personnel in Japan. Some of the clinical characteristics of this disease and therapeutic measures that seem to give patients most relief. J.A.M.A., *175*:990, 1961.
739. Hume, K. M., and Jones, E. R.: Bronchodilators and corticosteroids in asthma: Forced expiratory volume as an aid to diagnosis and treatment. Lancet, *2*:1319, 1960.
740. Herschfus, J. A., Bresnick, E., and Segal, M. S.: Pulmonary function studies in bronchial asthma. I. In the control state. Am. J. Med., *14*:23, 1953.
741. Herschfus, J. A., Bresnick, E., and Segal, M. S.: Pulmonary function studies in bronchial asthma. II. After treatment. Am. J. Med., *14*:34, 1953.
742. Beale, H. D., Fowler, W. S., and Comroe, J. H., Jr.: Pulmonary function studies in 20 asthmatic patients in the symptom-free interval. J. Allergy, *23*:1, 1952.
743. McNeill, R. S., and McKenzie, J. M.: An assessment of the value of breathing exercises in chronic bronchitis and asthma. Thorax, *10*:250, 1955.
744. Thursby-Pelham, D. C., and Kennedy, M. C. S.: Prednisolone compared with cortisone in treatment of children with chronic asthma. Brit. Med. J., *1*: 243, 1958.
745. Engström, I., Escardó, F. E., Karlberg, P., and Kræpelien, S.: Respiratory studies in children. VI. Timed vital capacity in healthy children and in symptom-free asthmatic children. Acta Pediat, *48*:114, 1959.
746. Heese, H. de V.: The forced expiratory volume and forced vital capacity test in asthmatic children. S. African J. Lab. Clin. Med., *7*:53, 1961.
747. Lowell, F. C., Schiller, I. W., and Lynch, M. T.: Estimation of daily changes in the severity of bronchial asthma. J. Allergy, *26*:113, 1955.
748. Bates. D. V.: Impairment of respiratory function in bronchial asthma. Clin. Sci., *11*:203, 1952.
749. Sonne, L. M., and Georg, J.: The respiratory changes during attacks of bronchial asthma. Acta Med. Scand., *138*: suppl. 239, p. 333, 1950.
750. Briscoe, W. A., and McLemore, G. A., Jr.: Ventilatory function in bronchial asthma. Thorax, *7*:66, 1952.
751. Campbell, E. J. M.: Mechanisms of airway obstruction in emphysema and asthma. Proc. Roy. Soc. Med. (London), *51*:108, 1958.
752. Wells, R. E., Jr.: Mechanics of respiration in bronchial asthma. Am. J. Med., *26*:384, 1959.
753. Ruth, W. E., and Andrews, C. E.: Airway resistance studies in bronchial asthma. J. Lab. Clin. Med., *54*:889, 1959.
754. McIlroy, M. B., and Marshall, R.: The mechanical properties of the lungs in asthma. Clin. Sci., *15*:345, 1956.
755. Fraser, R. G.: Measurements of the calibre of human bronchi in three phases of respiration by cinebronchography. J. Canad. Radiol., *12*:102, 1961.
756. Campbell, E. J. M., Martin, H. B., and Riley, R. L.: Mechanisms of airway obstruction. Bull. Johns Hopkins Hosp., *101*:329, 1957.
757. Dominjon-Monnier, F., Carton, J., Buffe, D., Burtin, P., Brille, D., and Kourilsky, R.: Étude comparative des seuils de réactions cutanées et ventilatoires à la poussière de maison et de leur intérêt diagnostique. Rev. Franc. Allerg., *1*:161, 1961.
758. Dekker, E., and Groen, J.: Asthmatic wheezing: Compression of the trachea and major bronchi as a cause. Lancet, *1*:1064, 1957.
759. Gaensler, E. A.: Evaluation of pulmonary function: Results in chronic obstructive lung disease. Ann. Rev. Med., *13*:319, 1962.
760. Lorriman, G.: The effects of bronchodilators on pulmonary ventilation and diffusion in asthma and emphysema. Thorax, *14*:146, 1959.
761. Kanagami, H., Katsura, T., Shiroishi, K., Baba, K., and Ebina, T.: Studies on the pulmonary diffusing capacity by the carbon monoxide breath holding technique. II. Patients with various pulmonary diseases. Acta Med. Scand., *169*:595, 1961.
762. Lewis, B. M., Hayford-Welsing, E. J., Furusho, A., and Reed, L. C., Jr.: Effect of uneven ventilation on pulmonary diffusing capacity. J. Appl. Physiol., *16*:679, 1961.
763. Bates, D. V.: Unusual forms of emphysema. Am. Rev. Resp. Dis., *80*:172, 1959.
764. Bouhuys, A., Georg, J., Jönsson, R., Lundin, G., and Lindell, S. E.: The influence of histamine inhalation on the pulmonary diffusing capacity in man. J. Physiol. (London), *152*:176, 1960.
765. Simon, G., and Galbraith, H. J. B.: Radiology of chronic bronchitis. Lancet, *2*:850, 1953.
766. Simon, G.: The lateral position in chest tomography. J. Fac. Radiologists, *4*:77, 1952.
767. Newell, R. R., and Garneau, R.: The threshold visibility of pulmonary shadows. Radiology, *56*:409, 1951.
768. Christoforidis, A. J., Nelson, S. W., and Tomashefski, J. F.: Effects of bronchography on pulmonary function. Am. Rev. Resp. Dis., *85*:127, 1962.
769. Reid, L. M.: Reduction in bronchial subdivision in bronchiectasis. Thorax, *5*:233, 1950.
770. Reid, L., and Simon, G.: The peripheral pattern in the normal bronchogram and its relation to peripheral pulmonary anatomy. Thorax, *13*:103, 1958.
771. Reid, L. M.: Correlation of certain bronchographic abnormalities seen in chronic bronchitis with the pathological changes. Thorax, *10*:199, 1955.
772. Macklem, P. T., Fraser, R. G., and Bates, D. V.: Bronchial pressures and dimensions in health and obstructive airway disease. J. Appl. Physiol., *18*:699, 1963.
773. Fraser, R. G., and Brown, W.: Unpublished observations on bronchial dynamics in bronchiectasis studied cinefluorographically.
774. Sicard, J. A., and Forestier, J.: Méthode générale d'exploration radiologique par l'huile iodée (lipiodol). Bull. Mem. Soc. Med. Hop. Paris, *46*:463, 1922.
775. Reid, L.: Measurement of the bronchial mucous gland layer; a diagnostic yardstick in chronic bronchitis. Thorax, *15*:132, 1960.
776. Schiller, I. W., Beale, H. D., Franklin, W., Lowell, F. C., and Halperin, M. H.: The potential danger of oxygen therapy in severe bronchial asthma. J. Allergy, *22*:423, 1951.
777. Fein, B. T., Cox, E. P., and Green, L. H.: Respiratory and physical exercise in the treatment of bronchial asthma. Ann. Allergy, *11*:275, 1953.
778. Strang, L. B., and Knox, E. G.: Choline theophyllinate in

children with asthma: A controlled trial. Lancet, *1*:260, 1960.

779. Bickerman, H. A., Beck, G. J., Itkin, S., and Drimmer, F.: The evaluation of oral bronchodilator agents in patients with bronchial asthma and pulmonary emphysema. Ann. Allergy, *11*:301, 1953.
780. Braun, K., Samueloff, M., and Cohen, A. M.: Effects of intravenously administered ACTH on the pulmonary function in bronchial asthma and emphysema. Dis. Chest, *24*:76, 1953.
781. Toogood, J. H.: Betamethasone in the treatment of bronchial asthma. Canad. M. A. J., *86*:273, 1962.
782. Hume, K. M., and Gandevia, B.: Forced expiratory volume before and after isoprenaline. Thorax, *12*:276, 1957.
783. Roy, E. C., Seabury, J. H., and Johns, L. E.: Spirometric evaluation of Orthoxine in bronchial asthma. J. Allergy, *20*:364, 1949.
784. Dunnill, M. S.: The pathology of asthma, with special reference to changes in the bronchial mucosa. J. Clin. Pathol., *13*:27, 1960.
785. Houston, J. C., de Nevasquez, S., and Trounce, J. R.: A clinical and pathological study of fatal cases of status asthmaticus. Thorax, *8*:207, 1953.
786. Thomson, J. G.: Fatal bronchial asthma showing the asthmatic reaction in an ovarian teratoma. J. Path. Bact., *57*:213, 1945.
787. Williams, D. A., and Leopold, J. G.: Death from bronchial asthma. Acta Allergol., *14*:83, 1959.
788. Gough, J.: Post mortem differences in "asthma" and in chronic bronchitis. Acta Allergol., *16*:391, 1961.
789. Thieme, E. T., and Sheldon, J. M.: A correlation of the clinical and pathologic findings in bronchial asthma. J. Allergy, *9*:246, 1938.
790. Thurlbeck, W. M.: A clinico-pathological study of emphysema in an American hospital. Thorax, *18*:59, 1963.
791. Colebatch, H. J. H., Olsen, C. R., and Nadel, J. A.: Effects of intravenous histamine and 48/80 on lung mechanics. [Abstr.] Fed. Proc., *21*:445, 1962.
792. Holmes, E. L.: Pulmonary function in the normal male. J. Appl. Physiol., *14*:493, 1959.
793. Jouasset, D.: Normalisation des épreuves fonctionnelles respiratoires dans les pays de la communauté européenne du charbon et de l'acier. Poumon Coeur, *16*:1145, 1960.
794. Massachusetts General Hospital Case Records. Presentation of Case 36041. New Engl. J. Med., *242*:149, 1950.
795. Anderson, D. O., and Ferris, B. G., Jr.: Role of tobacco smoking in the causation of chronic respiratory disease. New Engl. J. Med., *267*:787, 1962.
796. Ferris, B. G., Jr., and Anderson, D. O.: The prevalence of chronic respiratory disease in a New Hampshire town. Am. Rev. Resp. Dis., *86*:165, 1962.
797. Heard, B. E.: Pathology of pulmonary emphysema: Methods of study. Am. Rev. Resp. Dis., *82*:792, 1960.
798. Gough, J.: The pathological diagnosis of emphysema. *In:* Discussion on the diagnosis of pulmonary emphysema. Proc. Roy. Soc. Med. (London), *45*:576, 1952.
799. Leopold, J. G., and Gough, J.: The centrilobular form of hypertrophic emphysema and its relation to chronic bronchitis. Thorax, *12*:219, 1957.
800. Hartroft, W. S., and Macklin, C. C.: Intrabronchial fixation of human lung for purposes of alveolar measurement using 25 μ microsections made therefrom. Tr. Roy. Soc. Can., Sect. V, *37*:75, 1943.
801. Hartung, W.: Gefrier-Grossschnite von ganzen Organen, speziell der Lunge. Zbl. Allg. Path., *100*:408, 1960.
802. Weibel, E. R., and Gomez, D.: Geometry and dimensions of the human airways. Fed. Proc., *21*:439, 1962.
803. Jones, E.: Study of lung specimens prepared by fume fixation. Am. Rev. Resp. Dis., *82*:704, 1960.
804. Weibel, E. R., and Vidone, R. A.: Fixation of the lung by formalin steam in a controlled state of air inflation. Am. Rev. Resp. Dis., *84*:856, 1961.
805. Sweet, H. C., Wyatt, J. P., Fritsch, A. J., and Kinsella, P. W.: Panlobular and centrilobular emphysema. Correlation of clinical findings with pathologic patterns. Ann. Int. Med., *55*:565, 1961.
806. Gough, J., and Wentworth, J. E.: Thin sections of entire organs mounted on paper. Harvey Lect., 1957-58, *ser.53*:182, 1959.
807. Schlesinger, M. J.: New radiopaque mass for vascular injection. Lab. Invest., *6*:1, 1957.
808. Wyatt, J. P., Fischer, V. W., and Sweet, H. C.: Panlobular emphysema: Anatomy and pathodynamics. Dis. Chest, *41*:239, 1962.
809. Liebow, A. A., Hales, M. R., Lindskog, G. E., and Bloomer, W. E.: Plastic demonstrations of pulmonary pathology. Bull. Int. A. Med. Museums, *27*:116, 1947.
810. Tompsett, D. H.: *Anatomical Techniques.* Edinburgh, E. & S. Livingstone, 1956, p. 240.
811. McIlroy, M. B.: The physical properties of normal lungs removed after death. Thorax, *7*:285, 1952.
812. Pratt, P. C., and Klugh, G. A.: A technique for the study of ventilatory capacity, compliance, and residual volume of excised lungs and for fixation, drying, and serial sectioning in the inflated state. Am. Rev. Resp. Dis., *83*:690, 1961.
813. Heppleston, A. G.: Cinephotography of serial sections: Technic for demonstration of microanatomy in depth. Lab. Invest., *4*:374, 1955.
814. Cowdrey, C. R., Kleinerman, J., and Wright, G. W.: Photographic reconstruction of a three-dimensional model of the lung, with special reference to centrilobular emphysema. Am. Rev. Resp. Dis., *87*:239, 1963.
815. Fletcher, C. M. (ed.): *Ciba Guest Symposium Report:* Terminology, definitions, and classification of chronic pulmonary emphysema and related conditions; Symposium, Sept., 1958. Thorax, *14*:286, 1959.
816. Cromie, J. B.: Correlation of anatomic pulmonary emphysema and right ventricular hypertrophy. Am. Rev. Resp. Dis., *84*:657, 1961.
817. Sweet, H. C., Wyatt, J. P., and Kinsella, P. W.: Correlation of lung macrosections with pulmonary function in emphysema. Am. J. Med., *29*:277, 1960.
818. Dunnill, M. S.: Quantitative methods in the study of pulmonary pathology. Thorax, *17*:320, 1962.
819. Dunnill, M. S.: Postnatal growth of the lung. Thorax, *17*:329, 1962.
820. Moolten, S. E.: A simple apparatus for fixation of lungs in the inflated state. Arch. Pathol., *20*:77, 1935.
821. McLean, K. H.: The macroscopic anatomy of pulmonary emphysema. Aust. Ann. Med., *5*:73, 1956.
822. Laennec, R. T. H.: *A Treatise on the Diseases of the Chest and on Mediate Auscultation,* translated from the 3rd rev. London ed., with additional notes, by J. Forbes, New York, Wood, 1830.
823. Louis, P. C. A.: *Researches on Emphysema of the Lungs* (translated by T. Stewardson, Jr.). Philadelphia, Dunglison's American Medical Library, 1838.
824. Waters, A. T. H.: *Researches on the Nature, Pathology and Treatment of Emphysema of the Lungs, and Its Relations with Other Diseases of the Chest.* London, J. & A. Churchill, 1862.
825. Tobin, C. E.: Methods of preparing and studying human lungs expanded and dried with compressed air. Anat. Rec., *114*:453, 1952.
826. Blumenthal, B. J., and Boren, H. G.: Lung structure in three dimensions after inhalation and fume fixation. Am. Rev. Tuberc., *79*:764, 1959.
827. Hentel, W., and Longfield, A. N.: Stereoscopic study of the inflated lung. Dis. Chest, *38*:357, 1960.
828. Cureton, R. J. R., and Trapnell, D. H.: Postmortem radiography and gaseous fixation of the lung. Thorax, *16*:138, 1961.
829. Martin, H.: *Cited in ref. No. 804.* Am. Rev. Resp. Dis., *84*:860, 1961.
830. Rackemann, F. M.: A working classification of asthma. Am. J. Med., *3*:601, 1947.
831. Johnston, R. N., Lockhart, W., Ritchie, R. T., and Smith, D. H.: Haemoptysis. Brit. Med. J., *1*:592, 1960.
832. Reid, D. D.: General epidemiology of chronic bronchitis. In: *Symposium on chronic bronchitis.* Proc. Roy. Soc. Med. (London), *49*:767, 1956.
833. Gorham, E.: Bronchitis and the acidity of urban precipitation. Lancet, *2*:691, 1958.
834. Stocks, P.: Cancer and bronchitis mortality in relation to atmospheric deposit and smoke. Brit. Med. J., *1*:74, 1959.

835. Olsen, H. C., and Gilson, J. C.: Respiratory symptoms, bronchitis and ventilatory capacity in men: An Anglo-Danish comparison, with special reference to differences in smoking habits. Brit. Med. J., *1*:450, 1960.
836. Christensen, O. W., and Wood, C. H.: Bronchitis mortality rates in England and Wales and in Denmark. Brit. Med. J., *1*:620, 1958.
837. Mork, T.: A comparative study of respiratory disease in England and Wales and Norway. Acta Med. Scand., *172*: suppl. 384, 1962.
838. Roberts, L., and Batey, J. W.: Atmospheric pollution, temperature inversion, and deaths from bronchitis. Lancet, *1*:579, 1957.
839. Goldmith, J. R.: Epidemiologic studies of obstructive ventilatory disease of the lung. I. A review of concepts and nomenclature. Am. Rev. Resp. Dis., *82*:485, 1960.
840. McGregor, D.: Sickness absence among forestry workers in the North of Scotland, 1958. Brit. J. Indust. Med., *17*:310, 1960.
841. Cornwall, C. J., and Raffle, P. A. B.: Bronchitis–Sickness absence in London Transport. Brit. J. Indust. Med., *18*:24, 1961.
842. Joules, H.: In: *Symposium on Chronic Bronchitis*, London, 1956. Proc. Roy. Soc. Med. (London), *49*:779, 1956.
843. Fletcher, C. M., Elmes, P. C., Fairbairn, A. S., and Wood, C. H.: The significance of respiratory symptoms and the diagnosis of chronic bronchitis in a working population. Brit. Med. J., *2*:257, 1959.
844. Fairbairn, A. S., Wood, C. H., and Fletcher, C. M.: Variability in answers to a questionnaire on respiratory symptoms. Brit. J. Prev. Soc. Med., *13*:175, 1959.
845. Schilling, R. S. F., Hughes, J. P. W., and Dingwall-Fordyce, I.: Disagreement between observers in an epidemiological study of respiratory disease. Brit. Med. J., *1*:65, 1955.
846. Phillips, A. M., Phillips, R. W., and Thompson, J. L.: Chronic cough: Analysis of etiologic factors in a survey of 1,274 men. Ann. Int. Med., *45*:216, 1956.
847. Greene, B. A., and Berkowitz, S.: Tobacco bronchitis: An anesthesiologic study. Ann. Int. Med., *40*:729, 1954.
848. Brown, R. G., McKeown, T., and Whitfield, A. G. W.: Observations on the medical condition of men in the seventh decade. Brit. Med. J., *1*:555, 1958.
849. Flick, A. L., and Paton, R. R.: Obstructive emphysema in cigarette smokers. A.M.A. Arch. Int. Med., *104*:518, 1959.
850. Franklin, W., and Lowell, F. C.: Unrecognized airway obstruction associated with smoking: A probable forerunner of obstructive pulmonary emphysema. Ann. Int. Med., *54*:379, 1961.
851. Higgins, I. T. T.: Tobacco smoking, respiratory symptoms, and ventilatory capacity. Studies in random samples of the population. Brit. Med. J., *1*:325, 1959.
852. Lawther, P. J.: Climate, air pollution and chronic bronchitis. In: *Symposium on Weather and Disease*. Proc. Roy. Soc. Med. (London), *51*:262, 1958.
853. Flint, F. J.: Cor pulmonale: Incidence and aetiology in an industrial city. Lancet, *2*:51, 1954.
854. Williams, D. A.: Deaths from asthma in England and Wales. Thorax, *8*:137, 1953.
855. Higgins, I. T. T.: Respiratory symptoms, bronchitis, and ventilatory capacity in random sample of an agricultural population. Brit. Med. J., *2*:1198, 1957.
856. Pilcher, J. M. (ed.): *Monograph on the Behaviour of Aerosols*. Ann. N.Y. Acad. Sci., *105*(art. 2): 25, 1963.
857. *Air Pollution* (Monograph ser. No. 46). Geneva and New York, World Health Organization, 1961.
858. Fletcher, C. M.: Disability and mortality from chronic bronchitis in relation to dust exposure. A.M.A. Arch. Indust. Health, *18*:368, 1958.
859. Kuenssberg, E. V.: Are duodenal ulcer and chronic bronchitis family diseases? In *Discussion: Do Diseases Run in Families?* A study of methods of recording morbidity in family groups and its results. Proc. Roy. Soc. Med. (London), *55*:299, 1962.
860. Sklaroff, S. A.: Suitability of housing estate general practice for family studies of chronic disease. In: *Discussion: Do Diseases Run in Families?* A study of methods of recording morbidity in family groups and its results. Proc. Roy. Soc. Med. (London), *55*:295, 1962.
861. Marshall, A. G., Hutchinson, E. O., and Honisett, J.: Heredity in common diseases: A retrospective survey of twins in a hospital population. Brit. Med. J., *1*:1, 1962.
862. Polgar, G., and Denton, R.: Cystic fibrosis in adults. Studies of pulmonary function and some physical properties of bronchial mucus. Am. Rev. Resp. Dis., *85*:319, 1962.
863. Marks, B. L., and Anderson, C. M.: Fibrocystic disease of the pancreas in a man aged 46. Lancet, *1*:365, 1960.
864. Karlish, A. J., and Tárnoky, A. L.: Mucoviscidosis as a factor in chronic lung disease in adults. Lancet, *2*:514, 1960.
865. Wood, J. A., Fishman, A. P., Reemtsma, K., Barker, H. G., and di Sant' Agnese, P. A.: A comparison of sweat chlorides and intestinal fat absorption in chronic obstructive pulmonary emphysema and fibrocystic disease of the pancreas. New Engl. J. Med., *260*:951, 1959.
866. Muir, D., Batten, J., and Simon, G.: Mucoviscidosis and adult chronic bronchitis: Their possible relationship. Lancet, *1*:181, 1962.
867. Fletcher, C. M.: Chronic bronchitis. Its prevalence, nature, and pathogenesis. Am. Rev. Resp. Dis., *80*:483, 1959.
868. Fletcher, C. M.: Chronic disabling respiratory disease. Ends and means of study. California Med., *88*:1, 1958.
869. Fletcher, C. M., and Tinker, C. M.: Chronic bronchitis. A further study of simple diagnostic methods in a working population. Brit. Med. J., *1*:1491, 1961.
870. Medvei, V. C.: Diagnosis of chronic bronchitis. Brit. Med. J., *2*:503, 1959.
871. Christie, R.: Chronic bronchitis and emphysema. Tr. Coll. Physicians Phila., *27*:12, 1959.
872. Holland, W. W., Tanner, E. I., Pereira, M. S., and Taylor, C. E. D.: A study of the aetiology of respiratory disease in a general hospital. Brit. Med. J., *1*:1917, 1960.
873. Leese, W. L. B.: An investigation into bronchitis. Lancet, *2*:762, 1956.
874. Medvei, V. C.: The natural history of chronic bronchitis. Lancet, *1*:1227, 1958.
875. Goodman, N., Lane, R. E., and Rampling, S. B.: Chronic bronchitis: An introductory examination of existing data. Brit. Med. J., *2*:237, 1953.
876. Bower, G.: Deaths and illness from bronchitis, emphysema, and asthma. Am. Rev. Resp. Dis., *83*:894, 1961.
877. Lowell, F. C., Franklin, W., Michelson, A. L., and Schiller, I. W.: Chronic obstructive pulmonary emphysema: A disease of smokers. Ann. Int. Med., *45*:268, 1956.
878. Higgins, I. T. T., Cochrane, A. L., Gilson, J. C., and Wood, C. H.: Population studies of chronic respiratory disease: A comparision of miners, foundryworkers, and others in Staveley, Derbyshire. Brit. J. Indust. Med., *16*:255, 1959.
879. Higgins, I. T. T., and Cochrane, A. L.: Chronic respiratory disease in a random sample of men and women in the Rhondda Fach in 1958. Brit. J. Indust. Med., *18*:93, 1961.
880. Higgins, I. T. T., Oldham, P. D., Cochrane, A. L., and Gilson, J. C.: Respiratory symptoms and pulmonary disability in an industrial town. Survey of a random sample of the population. Brit. Med. J., *2*:904, 1956.
881. Pemberton, J.: Chronic bronchitis, emphysema, and bronchial spasm in bituminous coal workers: An epidemiological study. A.M.A. Arch. Indust. Health, *13*:529, 1956.
882. Ashford, J. R., Forwell, G. D., and Routledge, R.: A study of the repeatability of ventilatory tests, anthropometric measurements, and answers to a respiratory symptoms questionnaire in working coal-miners. Brit. J. Indust. Med., *17*:114, 1960.
883. Rogan, J. M., Ashford, J. R., Chapman, P. J., Duffield, D. P., Fay, J. W. J., and Rae, S.: Pneumoconiosis and respiratory symptoms in miners at eight collieries. Brit. Med. J., *1*:1337, 1961.
884. Lawther, P. J.: Chronic bronchitis and air pollution. Roy. Soc. Health J., *79*:4, 1959.
885. Katz, M.: Some toxic effects of air pollution on public health. Med. Serv. J. Canada, *16*:504, 1960.
886. Lawther, P. J.: *Some Clinical Aspects of the Atmospheric Pollution Problem in London:* Proc. Third National Air Pollution Symposium. Pasadena, Calif., Stanford Research Institute, 1955, p. 160.
887. Pemberton, J., and Goldberg, C.: Air pollution and bronchitis. Brit. Med. J., *2*:567, 1954.
888. Holland, W. W., Spicer, C. C., and Wilson, J. M. G.:

Influence of the weather on respiratory and heart disease. Lancet, *2*:338, 1961.
889. Reid, D. D.: Environmental factors in respiratory disease. Lancet, *1*:1289, 1958.
890. Reid, D. D.: Environmental factors in respiratory disease. Lancet, *1*:1237, 1958.
891. Reid, D. D., and Fairbairn, A. S.: The natural history of chronic bronchitis. Lancet, *1*:1147, 1958.
892. Stuart-Harris, C. H., Twidle, R. S. H., and Clifton, M.: A hospital study of congestive heart failure with special reference to cor pulmonale. Brit. Med. J., *2*:201, 1959.
893. Stuart-Harris, C. H., Pownall, M., Scothorne, C. M., and Franks, Z.: The factor of infection in chronic bronchitis. Quart. J. Med., (*n.s.*)*22*:121, 1953.
894. Stuart-Harris, C. H.: Field studies in relation to chronic bronchitis. In: *Symposium on Chronic Bronchitis*. Proc. Roy. Soc. Med. (London), *49*:776, 1956.
895. Stuart-Harris, C. H.: The epidemiology and evolution of chronic bronchitis. Brit. J. Tuberc. Dis. Chest, *48*:169, 1954.
896. Anderson, A. E., Jr., and Foraker, A. G.: Pathogenic implications of alveolitis in pulmonary emphysema. Arch. Pathol., *72*:520, 1961.
897. Thurlbeck, W. M., Angus, G. E., and Paré, J. A. P.: Mucous gland hypertrophy in chronic bronchitis and its occurrence in smokers. Brit. J. Dis. Chest, *57*:73, 1963.
898. Reid, L., and Simon, G.: Part III: Pathological findings and radiological changes in chronic bronchitis and in emphysema. In: *Chronic Bronchitis and Emphysema: A Symposium;* Ann. Congr., Brit. Inst. Radiol., 1958. Brit. J. Radiol., *32*:291, 292, 294, 303, 1959.
899. Reid, L. M.: Pathology of chronic bronchitis. Lancet, *1*:275, 1954.
900. Cardon, L., Lemberg, L., and Greenebaum, R. S.: Acute suppurative bronchitis and bronchiolitis in chronic pulmonary disease: Diagnosis and management. Ann. Int. Med., *34*:559, 1951.
901. Prior, J. A.: Chronic bronchitis and acute bronchiolitis in adults. Ohio Med. J., *48*:310, 1952.
902. Morgan, E. H., Pearsall, H. R., Tolan, J. F., and Wilson, H. L.: Acute obstructing bronchiolitis: A medical emergency. Ann. Otol., *67*:1180, 1958.
903. Hentel, W., Longfield, A. N., Vincent, T. N., Filley, G. F., and Mitchell, R. S.: Fatal chronic bronchitis. Am. Rev. Resp. Dis., *87*:216, 1963.
904. Ebert, R. V., and Pierce, J. A.: Pathogenesis of pulmonary emphysema. Arch. Int. Med., *111*:34, 1963.
905. Thurlbeck, W. M., and Angus, G. E.: The relationship between emphysema and chronic bronchitis, as assessed morphologically. Am. Rev. Resp. Dis., *87*:815, 1963.
906. McLean, K. H.: The pathogenesis of pulmonary emphysema. Am. J. Med., *25*:62, 1958.
907. Kourilsky, R., and Hinglais, J. C.: Étude histopathologique de la muqueuse des grosses bronches dans les bronchorrhées muco-purulentes chroniques. J. Franc. Med. Chir. Thorac., *15*:1, 1961.
908. Kourilsky, R., Decroix, G., Verley, J. M., Matossy, Y., Hinglais, J. C., Pieron, R., and Brille, D.: Histologie de la muqueuse bronchique au cours des inflammations chroniques non tuberculeuses des bronches (étude sur prélèvements biopsiques). Bronches, *10*:76, 1960.
909. Laurenzi, G., Guarneri, J., Carey, J., and Endriga, R.: Bacterial clearance from the lungs of mice. Fed. Proc., *22*:255, 1963.
910. *Symposium on Chronic Bronchitis*, London, 1956. 3rd ed. London, The Chest & Heart Association, 1959.
911. Palmer, K. N. V.: Reduction of sputum viscosity by a water aerosol in chronic bronchitis. Lancet, *1*:91, 1960.
912. Palmer, K. N. V.: A new mucolytic agent by aerosol for inhalation in chronic bronchitis. Lancet, *2*:802, 1961.
913. Forbes, J., and Wise, L.: Expectorants and sputum viscosity. Lancet, *2*:767, 1957.
914. Krueger, A. P., and Smith, R. F.: Effects of gaseous ions on tracheal ciliary rate. Proc. Soc. Exper. Biol. Med., *98*:412, 1958.
915. Mulder, J.: Bacteriology of bronchitis: I. Chronic bronchitis. In: *Symposium on Chronic Bronchitis*. Proc. Roy. Soc. Med. (London), *49*:773, 1956.
916. Elmes, P. C., Dutton, A. A. C., and Fletcher, C. M.: Sputum examination and the investigation of "chronic bronchitis." Lancet, *1*:1241, 1959.
917. Brumfitt, W., Willoughby, M. L. N., and Bromley, L. L.: An evaluation of sputum examination in chronic bronchitis. Lancet, *2*:1306, 1957.
918. Brumfitt, W., and Willoughby, M. L. N.: Laboratory differentiation of chronic bronchial disease: An investigation of 117 cases. Lancet, *1*:132, 1958.
919. Laurent, R.: *Le Role de l'Atteinte Bronchiolaire dans l'Emphyseme Pulmonaire Chronique*. Paris, Amédée Legrand, 1955.
920. Passey, R. D.: Some problems of lung cancer. Lancet, *2*:107, 1962.
921. DuBois, A. B.: Industrial bronchitis and the function of the lungs. Arch. Environ. Health, *4*:128, 1962.
922. Karrel, I., and Place, R.: Pulmonary volumina and ventilation studies in chronic bronchitis. Canad. M.A.J., *67*:458, 1952.
923. Sadoul, P., and Saunier, C.: Aspects spirographiques des bronchites chroniques. Presse Med., *67*:1741, 1959.
924. Fox, R. E., Dowling, H. F., Saxton, G. A., Jr., and Mellody, M.: Treatment of chronic bronchitis and bronchiectasis with intravenous tetracycline. Results, as judged by studies of the sputum and tests of pulmonary function. A.M.A. Arch. Int. Med., *100*:11, 1957.
925. Clifton, M., and Stuart-Harris, C. H.: Steroid therapy in chronic bronchitis. Lancet, *1*:1311, 1962.
926. Hume, K. M., and Gandevia, B.: Ventilatory capacity in chronic bronchitis after oral ephedrine. Tubercle, *38*:199, 1957.
927. Christie, R. V.: Emphysema of the lungs. Brit. Med. J., *1*:105, 1944.
928. Best, E. W. R.: Lung cancer mortality trends in Canada, 1931–1960. Canad. M.A.J., *88*:133, 1963.
929. Heard, B. E., and Williams, R.: The pathology of asbestosis with reference to lung function. Thorax, *16*:264, 1961.
930. Hodson, C. J., and Trickey, S. E.: Bronchial wall thickening in asthma. Clin. Radiol., *11*:183, 1960.
931. Overholt, R. H.: Trigger mechanisms in asthma. Dis. Chest., *35*:587, 1959.
932. Felson, B., and Felson, H.: Acute diffuse pneumonia of asthmatics. Am. J. Roentgenol., *74*:235, 1955.
933. Friend, J.: The variability of ventilatory function in emphysema. Clin. Sci., *13*:491, 1954.
934. Baldwin, E. de F., Cournand, A., and Richards, D. W., Jr.: Pulmonary insufficiency. III. A study of 122 cases of chronic pulmonary emphysema. Medicine, *28*:201, 1949.
935. Hurtado, A., Kaltreider, N. L., Fray, W. W., Brooks, W. D. W., and McCann, W. S.: Studies of total pulmonary capacity and its subdivisions. VI. Observations on cases of obstructive pulmonary emphysema. J. Clin. Invest., *13*:1027, 1934.
936. Schultz, J.: The vital capacity difference. Acta Med. Scand., *160*:497, 1958.
937(a). Attinger, E. O., Monroe, R. G., and Segal, M. S.: The mechanics of breathing in different body positions. I. In normal subjects. J. Clin. Invest., *35*:904, 1956.
937(b). Attinger, E. O., Herschfus, J. A., and Segal, M. S.: The mechanics of breathing in different body positions. II. In cardiopulmonary disease. J. Clin. Invest., *35*:912, 1956.
938. Steady, W. W., Fry, D. L., and Ebert, R. V.: The elastic properties of the lung in normal men and in patients with chronic pulmonary emphysema. J. Lab. Clin. Med., *40*:674, 1952.
939. Dayman, H.: Mechanics of airflow in health and in emphysema. J. Clin. Invest., *30*:1175, 1951.
940. Hammond, J. D. S.: The physical properties of the lungs in chronic cor pulmonale. Clin. Sci., *16*:481, 1957.
941. Cherniack, R. M.: The physical properties of the lung in chronic obstructive pulmonary emphysema. J. Clin. Invest., *35*:394, 1956.
942. Ting, E. Y., and Lyons, H. A.: Pressure-volume relations of the lung and thoracic cage in pulmonary emphysema. J. Appl. Physiol., *16*:517, 1961.
943. Rau, G., Behn, H., Gebhardt, W., Rossier, P. H., and Bühlmann, A.: Atemmechanische Untersuchungen am Lungenmodell, bei Lungengesunden und bei Patienten mit obstruktiven Emphysem. Schweiz. Med. Wchnschr., *87*:374, 1957.

944. Riley, R. L.: The work of breathing and its relation to respiratory acidosis [Editorial]. Ann. Int. Med., *41*:172, 1954.
945. Prime, F. J., and Westlake, E. K.: The respiratory response to CO_2 in emphysema. Clin. Sci., *13*:321, 1954.
946. Sadoul, P., and Saunier, C.: L'équilibre acidobasique en pathologie respiratoire. Rev. Med. Nancy, *84*:557, 1959.
947. Platts, M. M., and Greaves, M. S.: Arterial blood gas measurements in the management of patients with chronic bronchitis and emphysema. Thorax, *12*:236, 1957.
948. Miller, R. D., Fowler, W. S., and Helmholz, H. F., Jr.: The relationship of arterial hypoxemia to disability and to cor pulmonale with congestive failure in patients with chronic pulmonary emphysema. Proc. Staff Meet., Mayo Clin., *28*:737, 1953.
949. Goggio, A. F.: The abnormal physiology of chronic pulmonary emphysema: Three contrasting illustrative cases. New Engl. J. Med., *231*:672, 1944.
950. Platts, M. M., and Greaves, M. S.: The composition of the blood in respiratory acidosis. Clin. Sci., *16*:695, 1957.
951. Westlake, E. K., Simpson, T., and Kaye, M.: Carbon dioxide narcosis in emphysema. Quart. J. Med., *(n.s.)24*:155, 1955.
952. Moltke, E., and Worning, H.: Studies on the hydrogen ion concentration, oxygen saturation, and carbon dioxide tension of the arterial blood in patients with cardiac dyspnoea. Acta Med. Scand., *160*:397, 1958.
953. Campbell, E. J. M., and Short, D. S.: The cause of oedema in "cor pulmonale." Lancet, *1*:1184, 1960.
954. Holland, R. A. B., and Blacket, R. B.: Pulmonary diffusing capacity in chronic obstructive lung disease: Studies at rest and on exercise by the steady state, physiological dead space method. Aust. Ann. Med., *10*:38, 1961.
955. West, J. R., Baldwin, E. de F., Cournand, A., and Richards, D. W., Jr.: Physiopathologic aspects of chronic pulmonary emphysema. Am. J. Med., *10*:481, 1951.
956. Holland, R. A. B., and Blacket, R. B.: The carbon monoxide diffusing capacity of the lung in normal subjects. Aust. Ann. Med., *7*:192, 1958.
957. Yokoyama, T., Ii, G., Matsumura, H., Tamura, F., and Sasamoto, H.: Studies on the pulmonary diffusing capacity of carbon monoxide in cases with chronic pulmonary emphysema. Resp. Circ., *9*:197, 1961.
958. Ogilvie, C.: Patterns of disturbed lung function in patients with chronic obstructive vesicular emphysema. Thorax, *14*:113, 1959.
959. Campbell, E. J. M.: Disordered pulmonary function in emphysema. Postgrad. Med. J., *34*:30, 1958.
960. Thomson, M. L., McGrath, M. W., Smither, W. J., and Shepherd, J. M.: Some anomalies in the measurement of pulmonary diffusion in asbestosis and chronic bronchitis with emphysema. Clin. Sci., *21*:1, 1961.
961. McGrath, M. W., and Thomson, M. L.: Pulmonary diffusion at small lung volumes in asbestosis and chronic bronchitis with emphysema. Clin. Sci., *21*:15, 1961.
962. Cherniack, R. M., and Snidal, D. P.: The effect of obstruction to breathing on the ventilatory response to CO_2. J. Clin. Invest., *35*:1286, 1956.
963. Donald, K. W., and Christie, R. V.: The respiratory response to carbon dioxide and anoxia in emphysema. Clin. Sci., *8*:33, 1949.
964. Tenney, S. M.: Ventilatory response to carbon dioxide in pulmonary emphysema. J. Appl. Physiol., *6*:477, 1954.
965. Tuttle, M. J., and Jenkins, E. K.: The respiratory response to inhaled carbon dioxide (7%)—an indication of pulmonary emphysema. Med. Serv. J. Canada, *16*:98, 1960.
966. Tenney, S. M.: Respiratory control in chronic pulmonary emphysema: A compromise adaptation. J. Maine Med. A., *48*:375, 1957.
967. Harvey, R. M., Ferrer, M. I., Richards, D. W., Jr., and Cournand, A.: Influence of chronic pulmonary disease on the heart and circulation. Am. J. Med., *10*:719, 1951.
968. Ebert, R. V.: Pulmonary emphysema. Ann. Rev. Med., *7*:123, 1956.
969. Mounsey, J. P. D., Ritzmann, L. W., Selverstone, N. J., Briscoe, W. A., and McLemore, G. A.: Circulatory changes in severe pulmonary emphysema. Brit. Heart J., *14*:153, 1952.
970. Whitaker, W.: Pulmonary hypertension in congestive heart failure complicating chronic lung disease. Quart. J. Med., *(n.s.)23*:57, 1954.
971. Orie, N. G. M., van Buchem, F. S. P., and Homan, B. P. A. A.: Heart failure in chronic pulmonary disease. Acta Med. Scand., *148*:123, 1954.
972. Denolin, H.: Contribution à l'étude de la circulation pulmonaire en clinique. Acta Cardiol., suppl. 10, 1961.
973. Wilson, V. H., and Gilroy, J. C.: The effects of oxygen administration upon pulmonary hypertension in patients with chronic widespread respiratory disease and cor pulmonale. S. African J. Med. Sci., *17*:47, 1952.
974. Tourniaire, A., Tartulier, M., Deyrieux, F., and Faucon, M.: L'inhalation d'oxygène chez les emphysémateux au stade du cœur pulmonaire chronique. Son effet sur la pression artérielle pulmonaire. Arch. Mal. Cœur, *51*:650, 1958.
975. Taquini, A. C., and González Fernández, J. M.: The cardiac output in different stages of chronic cor pulmonale. Acta. Physiol. Lat. Amer., *1*:200, 1951.
976. Mounsey, J. P. D.: Emphysema heart disease. Brit. J. Tuberc., *48*:63, 1954.
977. Harvey, R. M., and Ferrer, M. I.: A clinical consideration of cor pulmonale. Circulation, *21*:236, 1960.
978. Filley, G. F.: Pulmonary ventilation and the oxygen cost of exercise in emphysema. Trans. Am. Clin. Climat. A., *70*:193, 1958.
979. Woolf, C. R., Gunton, R. W., and Paul, W.: Cardiac output and blood volume in chronic cor pulmonale. Canad. M.A.J., *85*:1271, 1961.
980. Panchenko, I. A.: Carbon dioxide sensitivity of the respiratory centre in chronic hypercapnia. Bull. Exper. Biol. Med., *49*:444, 1960.
981. Swyer, P. R., and James, G. C. W.: A case of unilateral pulmonary emphysema. Thorax, *8*:133, 1953.
982. Macleod, W. M.: Abnormal transradiancy of one lung. Thorax, *9*:147, 1954.
983. Reid, L., and Simon, G.: Unilateral lung transradiancy. Thorax, *17*:230, 1962.
984. Darke, C. S., Chrispin, A. R., and Snowden, B. S.: Unilateral lung transradiancy: A physiological study. Thorax, *15*:74, 1960.
985. Margolin, H. N., Rosenberg, L. S., Felson, B., and Baum, G.: Idiopathic unilateral hyperlucent lung: A roentgenelogic syndrome. Am. J. Roentgenol., *82*:63, 1959.
986. Fouché, R. F., Spears, J. R., and Ogilvie, C.: Unilateral emphysema. Brit. Med. J., *1*:1312, 1960.
987. Dornhorst, A. C., Heaf, P. J., and Semple, S. J. G.: Unilateral "emphysema." Lancet, *2*:873, 1957.
988. Belcher, J. R., Capel, L., Pattison, J. N., and Smart, J.: Hypoplasia of the pulmonary arteries. Brit. J. Dis. Chest, *53*:253, 1959.
989. Smith, R. A., and Bech, A. O.: Agenesis of lung. Thorax, *13*:28, 1958.
990. Lull, G. F., Jr., and Taylor, R. R.: Agenesis in the pulmonary arterial circulation. Report of two cases. Am. Rev. Tuberc., *79*:641, 1959.
991. Simon, G., and Medvei, V. C.: Chronic bronchitis: Radiological aspects of a five-year follow-up. Thorax, *17*:5, 1962.
992. Ogilvie, C., and Catterall, M.: Patterns of disturbed lung function in patients with emphysematous bullae. Thorax, *14*:216, 1959.
993. Siebens, A. A., Grant, A. R., Kent, D. C., Klopstock, R., and Cincotti, J. J.: Pulmonary cystic disease: Physiologic studies and results of resection. J. Thoracic Surg., *33*:185, 1957.
994. Capel, L. H., and Belcher, J. R.: Surgical treatment of large air cysts of the lung. Lancet, *1*:759, 1957.
995. Baldwin, E. de F., Harden, K. A., Greene, D. G., Cournand, A., and Richards, D. W., Jr.: Pulmonary insufficiency: IV. A study of 16 cases of large pulmonary air cysts or bullae. Medicine, *29*:169, 1950.
996. Richards, D. W.: Pulmonary emphysema: Etiologic factors and clinical forms. Ann. Int. Med., *53*:1105, 1960.
997. Laurenzi, G. A., Turino, G. M., and Fishman, A. P.: Bullous disease of the lung. Am. J. Med., *32*:361, 1962.
998. Postgraduate Medical School of London, Clinicopatholog-

ical Conference: A case of bronchiectasis. Brit. Med. J., *2*:1417, 1961.
999. Goodwin, J. F., Harrison, C. V., and Wilcken, D. E. L.: Obliterative pulmonary hypertension and thrombo-embolism. Brit. Med. J., *1*:701, 777, 1963.
1000. McAdams, G. B.: Bronchiolar emphysema: Report of a case. Arch. Int. Med., *108*:279, 1961.
1001. Donohue, W. L., Laski, B., Uchida, I., and Munn, J. D.: Familial fibrocystic pulmonary dysplasia and its relation to the Hamman-Rich syndrome. Pediatrics, *24*:786, 1959.
1002. Burman, S. O., and Kent, E. M.: Bronchiolar emphysema (cirrhosis of the lung). J. Thorac. Cardiov. Surg. *43*:253, 1962.
1003. McKusick, V. A., and Fisher, A. M.: Congenital cystic disease of the lung with progressive pulmonary fibrosis and carcinomatosis. Ann. Int. Med., *48*:774, 1958.
1004. Meador, R. S., and Shields, D. O.: Pulmonary cysts. Five cases with preoperative and postoperative pulmonary function studies. Am. Rev. Tuberc., *75*:53, 1957.
1005. Kröker, P.: Zur Frage der sogenannten progressiven Lungendystrophie. Fortschr. Geb. Roentgenstr., *93*:1, 1960.
1006. Alarcón, D. G.: Regressive giant bullous emphysema in tuberculosis of adults. Dis. Chest, *27*:31, 1955.
1007. Burke, R. M.: Vanishing lungs: A case report of bullous emphysema. Radiology, *28*:367, 1937.
1008. Stanford, W. R., and Nalle, B. C., Jr.: Some notes on cystic disease of the lungs, with a report of one case. Ann. Int. Med., *17*:65, 1942.
1009. Tauber, K., Keyssler, H., and Parhofer, R.: Über die Blutverteilung in der Lung bei mangelhafter Sauerstoffversorgung eines Lappens. Muench. Med. Wchnschr., *100*:1106, 1958.
1010. Lister, W. A.: The check-valve mechanism and the meaning of emphysema. Lancet, *1*:66, 1958.
1011. Fry, J.: Fate of 424 patients with pneumonia and bronchitis. Brit. Med. J., *2*:1483, 1960.
1012. Sieker, H. O., and Hickam, J. B.: Carbon dioxide intoxication: The clinical syndrome, its etiology and management with particular reference to the use of mechanical respirators. Medicine, *35*:389, 1956.
1013. Simpson, T.: Anoxia in emphysema: its relief by oxygen. Lancet, *2*:105, 1957.
1014. Cornet, E., Kerneis, J. P., Dupon, H., and Coiffard, P.: Trois cas d'emphysème lobaires géants. Poumon Coeur, *15*:613, 1959.
1015. Eiken, M.: Congenital obstructive emphysema in infants. Acta Paediat., *50*:17, 1961.
1016. Fournier, H.: Deux cas d'emphysème lobaire géant du nourrisson opérés et guéris. Mem. Acad. Chir., *84*:383, 1958.
1017. Santy, P., Jeune, M., Galy, P., Jaubert de Beaujeu, M., Bethenod, M., and Bailly, E.: L'emphysème malformatif lobaire géant du petit enfant. A propos de 4 observations avec guérison par exérèse. J. Franc. Med. Chir. Thorac., *11*:457, 1957.
1018. Venturini, A.: Congenital lobar emphysema. Arch. Chir. Torace, *11*:209, 1957.
1019. Joseph, R., Nezelof, C., Ribierre, M., and Plainfosse, B.: Le rôle des anomalies des cartilages bronchiques dans la pathogénie de l'emphysème lobaire géant. Sem. Hop. Paris, *34*/2:536, 1958.
1020. Cottom, D. G., and Myers, N. A.: Congenital lobar emphysema. Brit. Med. J., *1*:1394, 1957.
1021. Stovin, P. G. I.: Congenital lobar emphysema. Thorax, *14*:254, 1959.
1022. Nanson, E. M.: Pulmonary resection in infancy and childhood. Canad. M. A. J., *87*:275, 1962.
1023. Ehrenhaft, J. L., and Taber, R. E.: Progressive infantile emphysema: A surgical emergency. Surgery, *34*:412, 1953.
1024. Minnis, J. F., Jr.: Congenital cystic disease of the lung in infancy. Successful lobectomy in a one-day-old infant. J. Thorac. Cardiov. Surg., *43*:262, 1962.
1025. Klosk, E., Bernstein, A., and Parsonnet, A. E.: Cystic disease of the lung. Ann. Int. Med., *24*:217, 1946.
1026. Mannix, E. P., Jr., and Haight, C.: Anomalous pulmonary arteries and cystic disease of the lung. Medicine, *34*:193, 1955.
1027. Myers, N. A.: Congenital lobar emphysema. Aust. New Zeal. J. Surg., *30*:32, 1961.
1028. Campbell, D., Bauer, A. J., and Hewlett, T. H.: Congenital localized emphysema. J. Thorac. Cardiov. Surg., *41*:575, 1961.
1029. Kountz, W. B., and Alexander, H. L.: Emphysema. Medicine, *13*:251, 1934.
1030. Wimpfheimer, F., and Schneider, L.: Familial emphysema. Am. Rev. Resp. Dis., *83*:697, 1961.
1031. Wilson, R. H., Borden, C. W., Ebert, R. V., and Johnson, J. J.: Hematologic adaptation to anoxemia in chronic pulmonary emphysema. J. Lab. Clin. Med., *36*:1004, 1950.
1032. Verel, D., and Kerridge, D. F.: Mean corpuscular hemoglobin concentration in anoxic lung disease. J. Appl. Physiol., *16*:847, 1961.
1033. Lerzman, M., Israels, L. G., and Cherniack, R. M.: Erythropoiesis and ferrokinetics in chronic respiratory disease. Ann. Int. Med., *56*:821, 1962.
1034. Grant, J. L., Macdonald, A., Edwards, J. R., Stacy, R. R., and Stueck, G. H., Jr.: Red cell changes in chronic pulmonary insufficiency. J. Clin. Invest., *37*:1166, 1958.
1035. Tabakin, B. S., Adhikari, P. K., and Miller, D. B.: Objective long-term evaluation of the surgical treatment of diffuse obstructive emphysema. A physiologic study. Am. Rev. Resp. Dis., *80*:825, 1959.
1036. McKeown, F.: The pathology of pulmonary heart disease. Brit. Heart J., *14*:25, 1952.
1037. Carasso, B., Maheux, P., and Gregoire, F.: Progressive bilateral bullous emphysema: With special reference to pulmonary function tests. Am. Rev. Tuberc., *71*:867, 1955.
1038. Brodovsky, D., Macdonell, J. A., and Cherniack, R. M.: The respiratory response to carbon dioxide in health and in emphysema. J. Clin. Invest., *39*:724, 1960.
1039. Zocche, G. P., Fritts, H. W., Jr., and Cournand, A.: Fraction of maximum breathing capacity available for prolonged hyperventilation. J. Appl. Physiol., *15*:1073, 1960.
1040. Alexander, J. M.: Cystic disease of the lungs in childhood. Med. J. Aust., *2*:676, 1957.
1041. Shek, J. L., Cope, J. A., and Myers, G. D.: Giant air cyst(s) as a sequela of pulmonary tuberculosis. J. Thoracic Surg., *32*:96, 1956.
1042. Berthrong, M.: Pulmonary "cyst" formation following treatment of tuberculosis with antibiotics[Editorial]. Am. J. Clin. Pathol., *26*:396, 1956.
1043. Warring, F. C., Jr., and Lindskog, G. E.: Surgical management of giant air cysts of the lungs. Physiologic improvement after resection. Am. Rev. Tuberc., *63*:579, 1951.
1044. Abbott, O. A., Hopkins, W. A., Van Fleit, W. E., and Robinson, J. S.: A new approach to pulmonary emphysema. Thorax, *8*:116, 1953.
1045. Von Bramann, C., Plenge, K., and Zadek, I.: Intrathorakale Zysten. Deutsch. Med. J., *8*:149, 1957.
1046. Heppleston, A. G.: The pathology of honeycomb lung. Thorax, *11*:77, 1956.
1047. Oswald, N., and Parkinson, T.: Honeycomb lungs. Quart, J. Med., *(n.s.)18*:1, 1949.
1048. Opie, E. L.: The pathologic anatomy of influenza: Based chiefly on American and British sources. Arch. Pathol., *5*:285, 1928.
1049. McNeil, C., Macgregor, A. R., and Alexander, W. A.: Studies of pneumonia in childhood. IV. Bronchiectasis and fibrosis of the lung. Arch. Dis. Child., *4*:170, 1929.
1050. Bachman, A. L., Hewitt, W. R., and Beekley, H. C.: Bronchiectasis. A bronchographic study of sixty cases of pneumonia. A.M.A. Arch. Int. Med., *91*:78, 1953.
1051. Perry, K.M.A., and King, D. S.: Bronchiectasis: A study of prognosis based on follow-up of 400 patients. Am. Rev. Tuberc., *41*:531, 1940.
1052. Whitwell, F.: A study of the pathology and pathogenesis of bronchiectasis. Thorax, *7*:213, 1952.
1053. Corbett, E. U.: The visceral lesions in measles; with a report of Koplik spots in the colon. Am. J. Pathol., *21*:905, 1945.
1054. Wiglesworth, F. W.: Bronchiectasis: An evaluation of present concepts. McGill Med. J., *24*:189, 1955.
1055. Diamond, S., and Van Loon, E. L.: Bronchiectasis in childhood. J.A.M.A., *118*:771, 1942.

1056. Ogilvie, A. G.: The natural history of bronchiectasis. A clinical, roentgenologic and pathologic study. Arch. Int. Med., *68*:395, 1941.
1057. Roles, F. C., and Todd, G. S.: Bronchiectasis: Diagnosis and prognosis in relation to treatment. Brit. Med. J., *2*:639, 1933.
1058. Amdur, M. O.: The effect of aerosols on the response to irritant gases. In: Davies, C. N. (ed.): *Inhaled Particles and Vapours*. New York, Pergamon Press, 1961, p. 281.
1059. Moore, J. R., Koberick, S. D., and Wiglesworth, F. W.: Bronchiectasis. A study of the segmental distribution of the pathologic lesions. Surg. Gynec. Obstet., *89*:145, 1949.
1060. Mallory, T. B.: The pathogenesis of bronchiectasis. New Engl. J. Med., *237*:795, 1947.
1061. Liebow, A. A., Hales, M. R., and Lindskog, G. E.: Enlargement of the bronchial arteries, and their anastomoses with the pulmonary arteries in bronchiectasis. Am. J. Pathol., *25*:211, 1949.
1062. Conway, D. J.: A congenital factor in bronchiectasis. Arch. Dis. Child., *26*:253, 1951.
1063. Kartagener, M.: Zur Pathogenese der Bronchiektasien; über Lungencysten. Beitr. Klin. Tuberk., *85*:45, 1934.
1064. Vaughan, B. F.: Syndromes associated with hypoplasia or aplasia of one pulmonary artery. J. Fac. Radiologists, *9*:161, 1958.
1065. Pryce, D. M.: Lower accessory pulmonary artery with intralobar sequestration of lung. A report of seven cases. J. Path. Bact., *58*:457, 1946.
1066. Wyman, S. M., and Eyler, W. R.: Anomalous pulmonary artery from the aorta associated with intrapulmonary cysts (intralobar sequestration of lung): Its roentgenologic recognition and clinical significance. Radiology, *59*:658, 1952.
1067. Smith, R. A.: A theory of the origin of intralobar sequestration of the lung. Thorax, *11*:10, 1956.
1068. Smith, R. A.: Intralobar sequestration of the lung. Thorax, *10*:142, 1955.
1069. Roosenburg, J. G., and Deenstra, H.: Bronchialpulmonary vascular shunts in chronic pulmonary affections. Dis. Chest., *26*:664, 1954.
1070. Cherniack, N., Vosti, K. L., Saxton, G. A., Lepper, M. H., and Dowling, H. F.: Pulmonary function tests in fifty patients with bronchiectasis. J. Lab. Clin. Med., *53*:693, 1959.
1071. Cook, C. D., and Bucci, G.: Studies of respiratory physiology in children. IV. The late effects of lobectomy on pulmonary function. Pediatrics, *28*:234, 1961.
1072. Kamener, R., Becklake, M. R., Goldman, H., and McGregor, M.: Respiratory function following segmental resection of the lung for bronchiectasis. Am. Rev. Tuberc., *77*:209, 1958.
1073. Brown, C. C., Jr., Fry, D. L., and Ebert, R. V.: The mechanics of pulmonary ventilation in patients with heart disease. Am. J. Med., *17*:438, 1954.
1074. Verstraeten, J. M.: Klinische en experimentele onderzoekingen over de "elastance" van de longen. Thesis, Ghent, 1956.
1075. Permutt, S., and Martin, H. B.: Static pressure-volume characteristics of lungs in normal males. J. Appl. Physiol., *15*:819, 1960.
1076. Frank, N. R., Lyons, H. A., Siebens, A. A., and Nealon, T. F.: Pulmonary compliance in patients with cardiac disease. Am. J. Med., *22*:516, 1957.
1077. Proctor, D. F., Hardy, T. B., and McLean, R.: Studies of respiratory air flow. II. Observations on patients with pulmonary disease. Bull. Johns Hopkins Hosp., *87*:255, 1950.
1078. Fry, D. L., Ebert, R. V., Stead, W. W., and Brown, C. C.: The mechanics of pulmonary ventilation in normal subjects and in patients with emphysema. Am. J. Med., *16*:80, 1954.
1079. Mead, J., Lindgren, I., and Gaensler, E. A.: The mechanical properties of the lungs in emphysema. J. Clin. Invest., *34*:1005, 1955.
1080. Marshall, R., and Dubois, A. B.: The measurement of the viscous resistance of the lung tissues in normal man. Clin. Sci., *15*:161, 1956.
1081. Attinger, E. O., Goldstein, M. M., and Segal, M. S.: The mechanics of breathing in normal subjects and in patients with cardiopulmonary disease. Ann. Int. Med., *48*:1269, 1958.
1082. Butler, J., Caro, C. G., Alcala, R., and DuBois, A. B.: Physiological factors affecting airway resistance in normal subjects and in patients with obstructive respiratory disease. J. Clin. Invest., *39*:584, 1960.
1083. Otis, A. B., Fenn, W. O., and Rahn, H.: Mechanics of breathing in man. J. Appl. Physiol., *2*:592, 1950.
1084. Newhouse, M. T., Becklake, M. R., Macklem, P. T., and McGregor, M.: Effect of alterations in end-tidal CO_2 tension on flow resistance. J. Appl. Physiol., *19*:745, 1964.
1085. Jeker, K.: Die Bestimmung des Strömungswiderstandes im Bronchialsystem des Menschen. Helv. Med. Acta, *20*:459, 1953.
1086. Smith, G. A., Siebens, A. A., and Storey, C. F.: Preoperative and postoperative cardiopulmonary function studies in patients with bronchiectasis. Am. Rev. Tuberc., *69*:869, 1954.
1087. Bergofsky, E. H., Turino, G. M., and Fishman, A. P.: Cardiorespiratory failure in kyphoscoliosis. Medicine, *38*:263, 1959.
1088. Liebow, A. A.: Pulmonary emphysema with special reference to vascular changes. In: *Symposium on Emphysema and The "Chronic Bronchitis" Syndrome,* Aspen, Colorado, 1958. Am. Rev. Resp. Dis., *80*/1: Part II, 1959.
1089. Gray, F. D., Jr.: Kyphoscoliosis and heart disease. J. Chron. Dis., *4*:499, 1956.
1090. Abrahamson, M. L.: Pulmonocardiac failure associated with deformity of the chest. Lancet, *1*:449, 1959.
1091. Naeye, R. L.: Kyphoscoliosis and cor pulmonale. A study of the pulmonary vascular bed. Am. J. Path., *38*:561, 1961.
1092. Zorab, P. A.: The lungs in ankylosing spondylitis. Quart. J. Med., *(n.s.)31*:267, 1962.
1093. Hanley, T., Platts, M. M., Clifton, M., and Morris, T. L.: Heart failure of the hunchback. Quart. J. Med., *(n.s.)27*:155, 1958.
1094. James, J. I. P.: Idiopathic scoliosis: The prognosis, diagnosis, and operative indications related to curve patterns and the age at onset. J. Bone Joint Surg. (Brit.), *36B*:36, 1954.
1095. Gucker, T., III. Changes in vital capacity in scoliosis: Preliminary report on effects of treatment. J. Bone Joint Surg. (Amer.), *44A*:469, 1962.
1096. Coombs, C. F.: Fatal cardiac failure occurring in persons with angular deformity of the spine. Brit. J. Surg., *18*:326, 1930.
1097. Chapman, E. M., Dill, D. B., and Graybiel, A.: The decrease in functional capacity of the lungs and heart resulting from deformities of the chest: Pulmonocardiac failure. Medicine, *18*:167, 1939.
1098. Kerwin, A. J.: Pulmonocardiac failure as a result of spinal deformity. Report of five cases. Arch. Int. Med., *69*:560, 1942.
1099. Samuelsson, S.: Cor pulmonale resulting from deformities of the chest. Acta Med. Scand., *142*:399, 1952.
1100. Daley, R.: Morphine hypersensitivity in kyphoscoliosis. Brit. Heart J., *7*:101, 1945.
1101. Martins de Oliveira, J., Sambhi, M. P., and Zimmerman, H. A.: The electrocardiogram in pectus excavatum. Brit. Heart J., *20*:495, 1958.
1102. Reusch, C. S.: Hemodynamic studies in pectus excavatum. Circulation, *24*:1143, 1961.
1103. Caro, C. G., Butler, J., and DuBois, A. B.: Some effects of restriction of chest cage expansion on pulmonary function in man: An experimental study. J. Clin. Invest., *39*:573, 1960.
1104. McIlroy, M. B., Butler, J., and Finley, T. N.: Effects of chest compression on reflex ventilatory drive and pulmonary function. J. Appl. Physiol., *17*:701, 1962.
1105. Price, F. W. (ed.): *A Textbook of The Practice of Medicine*. 5th ed. London, Oxford University Press, 1937.

1106. Caro, C. G., and DuBois, A. B.: Pulmonary function in kyphoscoliosis. Thorax, *16*:282, 1961.
1107. Bates, D. V.: The assessment of pulmonary function. Thesis for the degree of M.D., Cambridge, England, May 1954.
1108. Bruderman, I., and Stein, M.: Physiologic evaluation and treatment of kyphoscoliotic patients. Ann. Int. Med., *55*:94, 1961.
1109. Shaw, D. B., and Read, J.: Hypoxia and thoracic scoliosis. Brit. Med. J., *2*:1486, 1960.
1110. Iticovici, H. N., and Lyons, H. A.: Ventilatory and lung volume determinations in patients with chest deformities. Am. J. Med. Sci., *232*:265, 1956.
1111. The lungs in kyphoscoliosis [Annotation]. Lancet, *1*:205, 1963.
1112. Hart, F. D., Robinson, K. C., Allchin, F. M., and Maclagan, N. F.: Ankylosing spondylitis. Quart. J. Med., *(n.s.)18*:217, 1949.
1113. D'Silva, J. L., Freeland, D. E., and Kazantzis, G.: The performance of patients with ankylosing spondylitis in the maximum ventilatory capacity test. Thorax, *8*:303, 1953.
1114. Rogan, M. C., Needham, C. D., and McDonald, I.: Effect of ankylosing spondylitis on ventilatory function. Clin. Sci., *14*:91, 1955.
1115. Travis, D. M., Cook, C. D., Julian, D. G., Crump, C. H., Helliesen, P., Robin, E. D., Bayles, T. B., and Burwell, C. S.: The lungs in rheumatoid spondylitis: Gas exchange and lung mechanics in a form of restrictive pulmonary disease. Am. J. Med., *29*:623, 1960.
1116. Carr, J. G.: The cardiac complications of trichterbrust. Ann. Int. Med., *6*:885, 1933.
1117. Bär, C. G., Zeilhofer, R., and Heckel, K.: Über die Beeinflussung des Herzens und der Atmung durch die Trichterbrust. Deut. Med. Wchnschr., *83*:282, 1958.
1118. Fink, A., Rivin, A., and Murray, J. F.: Pectus excavatum. An analysis of twenty-seven cases. Arch. Int. Med., *108*:427, 1961.
1119. Brown, A. L., and Cook, O.: Cardio-respiratory studies and pre- and post-operative funnel chest (pectus excavatum). Dis. Chest., *20*:378, 1951.
1120. Koop, C. E.: The management of pectus excavatum. Surg. Clin. North Am., *36*:1627, 1956.
1121. Lam, C. R., and Brinkman, G. L.: Indications and results in the surgical treatment of pectus excavatum. A.M.A. Arch. Surg., *78*:322, 1959.
1122. Schaub, F., Bühlmann, A., Kälin, R., and Wegmann, T.: Zur Klinik und Pathogenese des sogenannten Kyphoskilioseherzens. Schweiz. Med. Wchnschr., *84*:1147, 1954.
1123. Halmagyi, D. F. J.: Dorsal kyphosis in chronic obstructive lung disease. Lancet, *1*:446, 1959.
1124. Finley, F. G.: Spinal deformity as a cause of cardiac hypertrophy and dilatation. Canad. M. A. J., *11*:719, 1921.
1125. Geelen, E. E. M., Orie, N. G. M., and Eerland, L. D.: Resection in bronchiectasis. Acta Med. Scand., *155*:171, 1956.
1126. James, U., Brimblecombe, F. S. W., and Wells, J. W.: The natural history of pulmonary collapse in childhood. Quart. J. Med., *(n.s.)25*:121, 1956.
1127. Dale, W. A., and Rahn, H.: Experimental pulmonary atelectasis. Changes in chest mechanics following block of one lung. J. Appl. Physiol., *9*:359, 1956.
1128. Dale, W. A., and Rahn, H.: Ventilation of the open lung during unilateral experimental atelectasis. In: Rahn, H., and Fenn, W. O. (eds.): *Studies in Respiratory Physiology*, 2nd Ser. Wright Air Development Center, WADC T-R 55-357, 1955, p. 115.
1129. Pump, K. K.: The effect on respiration of the occlusion of a bronchus in man during bronchospirometry. J. Clin. Invest., *33*:611, 1954.
1130. Berglund, E., Simonsson, B., and Birath, G.: Effect of induced pneumothorax on the pulmonary shunt and the ventilation in a patient with atelectasis of the lung. Am. J. Med., *31*:959, 1961.
1131. Christie, R. V., and McIntosh, C. A.: The lung volume and respiratory exchange after pneumothorax. Quart. J. Med., *(n.s.)5*:445, 1936.
1132. Christie, R. V.: Pulmonary congestion following artificial pneumothorax: Its clinical significance. Quart. J. Med., *(n.s.)5*:327, 1936.
1133. Stewart, H. J., and Bailey, R. L., Jr.: The effect of unilateral spontaneous pneumothorax on the circulation in man. J. Clin. Invest., *19*:321, 1940.
1134. Richards, D. W., Jr., Riley, C. B., and Hiscock, M.: Cardiac output following artificial pneumothorax in man. Arch. Int. Med., *49*:994, 1932.
1135. Riska, N.: The reticulocyte reaction as an indicator of respiratory insufficiency. Acta Med. Scand., suppl. 237, 1950.
1136. Simmons, D. H., and Hemingway, A.: Acute respiratory effects of pneumothorax in normal and vagotomized dogs. Am. Rev. Tuberc., *76*:195, 1957.
1137. Gaensler, E. A., Watson, T. R., Jr., and Patton, W. E.: Bronchospirometry. VI. Results of 1,089 examinations. J. Lab. Clin. Med., *41*:436, 1953.
1138. Osinska, K., Koziorowski, A., and Bednarski, Z.: Zaburzenia oddychania w przebiegu odmy opulcnej. III. Fibrothorax poodmowy. [Respiratory disturbances during pneumothorax therapy. III. Fibrothorax as a sequel of pneumothorax therapy.] Gruzlica, *24*:269, 1956. [Excerpta Med. (XV), *10*:206, 1957.]
1139. Autio, V.: The reduction of respiratory function by parenchymal and pleural lesions. A bronchospirometric study of patients with unilateral involvement. Acta Tuberc. Scand., *37*:112, 1959.
1140. Pätiälä, J., and Karvonen, M. J.: Studies on pulmonary function after pneumothorax therapy. Acta Tuberc. Scand., *29*:193, 1954.
1141. Sartorelli, E., Grieco, A., and Mancosu, M.: Ventilatory insufficiency as a consequence of intrapleural pneumothorax. Acta Gerontol., *10*:116, 1960.
1142. Gaensler, E. A.: Parietal pleurectomy for recurrent spontaneous pneumothorax. Surg. Gynec. Obstet., *102*:293, 1956.
1143. Guliaev, G. V.: Narusheniia vneshnego dykhaniia pri toraka'nykh operatsiiakh. II. Izmeneniia dykhaniia pri khirurgicheskom pnevmotorakse. [Disturbances of respiration during chest operations II. Respiratory changes associated with surgical pneumothorax.] Eksperim. Khirurg., 5/1:14, 1960. [Excerpta Med. (XV), *14*:76, 1961.]
1144. Uglov, F. G., and Martynchev, A. N.: O davlenii v sosudakh malogo kruga krovoobraschcheniia pri otkrytom pnevmotorakse. [Blood pressure in vessels of the pulmonary circulation system in open pneumothorax.] Klin. Med. (Moskva), 35/7:75, 1957.
1145. Petty, T. L., Filley, G. F., and Mitchell, R. S.: Objective functional improvement by decortication after twenty years of artificial pneumothorax for pulmonary tuberculosis: Report of a case and review of the literature. Am. Rev. Resp. Dis., *84*:572, 1961.
1146. Hertz, C. W.: Pleuraschwarte und Lungenfunktion. Folgezustände nach Pneumothorax mit Röntgenologisch nachweisbarer Pleuraschwarte. Beitr. Klin. Tuberk., *112*:503, 1954.
1147. Dark, J., and Chatterjee, S. S.: Pulmonary decortication. Lancet, *2*:950, 1959.
1148. Patton, W. E., Watson, T. R., Jr., and Gaensler, E. A.: Pulmonary function before and at intervals after surgical decortication of the lung. Surg. Gynec. Obstet., *95*:477, 1952.
1149. Carroll, D., McClement, J., Himmelstein, A., and Cournand, A.: Pulmonary function following decortication of the lung. Am. Rev. Tuberc., *63*:231, 1951.
1150. Falk, A., Pearson, R. T., and Martin, F. E.: A bronchospirometric study of pulmonary function after decortication in pulmonary tuberculosis. Am. Rev. Tuberc., *66*:509, 1952.
1151. Longacre, J. J., and Johansmann, R.: An experimental study of the fate of the remaining lung following total pneumonectomy. J. Thoracic Surg., *10*:131, 1940.
1152. Birkun, A. A.: Vnutrilegochnye kompensatornye protsessy pri obshirnykh operachiiakh na legkikh. K voprosy o kompensatornoĭ gipertrofii legkikh. (Eksperimental'noe issledovanie.) [Intrapulmonary compensatory processes dur-

ing major pulmonary surgery. Compensatory hypertrophy of the lungs. (Experimental study.)] Arkh. Patol., *20*/12:41, 1958. [Excerpta Med. (XV), *13*:241, 1960.]
1153. Romanova, L. K.: Regenerative hypertrophy of the lungs in rats after one-stage removal of the entire left lung and the diaphragmatic lobe of the right lung. I. Changes in the number and dimensions of the alveoli and in the thickness of the interalveolar septa. Bull. Exper. Biol. Med., *50*:1192, 1961.
1154. Fiornovelli, F.: Rilievi isto-funzionali sul polmone residuo a pneumonectomia nell'animale. Gazz. Int. Med. Chir., *62*:1421, 1957.
1155. Harrison, R. W., Adams, W. E., Beuhler, W., and Long, E. T.: Effects of acute and chronic reduction of lung volumes on cardiopulmonary reserve. A.M.A. Arch. Surg., *75*:546, 1957.
1156. Rudolph, A. M., Neuhauser, E. B. D., Golinko, R. J., and Auld, P. A. M.: Effects of pneumonectomy on pulmonary circulation in adult and young animals. Circ. Res., *9*:856, 1961.
1157. Williams, M. H., Jr., Canney, P. C., and Rayford, C. R.: The acute effects of resection of pulmonary tissue on some pulmonary functions in the dog. J. Thoracic Surg., *31*:643, 1956.
1158. Schilling, J. A., Harvey, R. B., Balke, B., and Rattunde, H. F.: Extensive pulmonary resection in dogs: Altitude tolerance, work capacity, and pathologic-physiologic changes. Ann. Surg., *144*:635, 1956.
1159. Keszler, P.: Compensatory phenomena in the residual lung following resection. Acta Med. Acad. Sci. Hung., *9*:181, 1956.
1160. Gorlin, R., Knowles, J. H., and Storey, C. F.: Effects of thoracotomy on pulmonary function. Patients with localized pulmonary disease. J. Thoracic Surg., *34*:242, 1957.
1161. Shephard, R. J.: The surgical treatment of pulmonary tuberculosis in flying personnel. A.M.A. Arch. Indust. Health, *15*:516, 1957.
1162. Miller, R. D., Bridge, E. V., Fowler, W. S., Helmholz, H. F., Jr., Ellis, F. H., Jr., and Allen, G. T.: Pulmonary function before and after pulmonary resection in tuberculous patients. J. Thoracic Surg., *35*:651, 1958.
1163. Kibrik, B. S., and Nefedov, V. B.: Izmenenie vneshnego dykhaniia posle operatsii udaleniia doli legkogo u bol'nykh tuberkulezom. [Changes in external respiration after removal of a pulmonary lobe in tuberculous patients.] Probl. Tuberk., *39*/6:87, 1961. [Excerpta Med. (XV), *15*:583, 1962.]
1164. Denk, W., and Helmer, F.: Spätergebnisse der Lungenresektion im Kindesalter. Wien. Klin. Wchnschr., *72*:704, 1960.
1165. Donno, L., Scalfi, G. F., and Rossi, B.: Il valore energetico del resecato polmonare. Ann. Villag. Sanat. Sondalo, *1*:15, 1953.
1166. Nikly, J., and Villemin, J.: Capacité vitale et volume expiratoire maximal/seconde avant et après exérèse pour tuberculose pulmonaire. Bull. Soc. Med. Passy, *26*:31, 1960.
1167. Wu, S. C., and Li, H. T.: The effects of pulmonary resection and extraperiosteal plombage on pulmonary function. Chinese Med. J., *77*:310, 1958.
1168. Cournand, A., and Berry, F. B.: The effect of pneumonectomy upon cardiopulmonary function in adult patients. Ann. Surg., *116*:532, 1942.
1169. Lester, C. W., Cournand, A., and Riley, R. L.: Pulmonary function after pneumonectomy in children. J. Thoracic Surg., *11*:529, 1942.
1170. Cournand, A., Himmelstein, A., Riley, R. L., and Lester, C. W.: A follow-up study of the cardiopulmonary function in four young individuals after pneumonectomy. J. Thoracic Surg., *16*:30, 1947.
1171. Cournand, A., Riley, R. L., Himmelstein, A., and Austrian, R.: Pulmonary circulation and alveolar ventilation-perfusion relationships after pneumonectomy. J. Thoracic Surg., *19*:80, 1950.
1172. Friend, J.: Respiratory insufficiency after pneumonectomy. Lancet, *2*:260, 1954.
1173. Frank, N. R., Siebens, A. A., and Newman, M. M.: The effect of pulmonary resection on the compliance of human lungs. J. Thorac. Cardiov. Surg., *38*:215, 1959.
1174. Dayman, H.: The expiratory spirogram. Am. Rev. Resp. Dis., *83*:842, 1961.
1175. Sadoul, P., Héran, J., and Lacoste, J.: Limites de la spirographie pour l'étude de la fonction respiratoire après pneumonectomie. J. Franc. Med. Chir. Thorac., *16*:427, 1962.
1176. Kunz, H., Muhar, F., and Wenzl, M.: Untersuchungen über die Funktion der Restlunge nach jahrelang zurückliegender Pneumonektomie. Chirurg., *32*:166, 1961.
1177. Larmi, T. K. I., Turunen, M., and Heinonen, A. O.: The loss of pulmonary function, especially of pulmonary diffusing capacity, following some thoracic operations. Scand. J. Clin. Lab. Invest., *11*:20, 1959.
1178. Dietiker, F., Lester, W., and Burrows, B.: The effects of thoracic surgery on the pulmonary diffusing capacity. Am. Rev. Resp. Dis., *81*:830, 1960.
1179. Bruck, A., Löhr, B., and Ulmer, W.: Untersuchungen über die Wirksamkeit der Ventilation nach thoraxchirurgischen Eingriffen (Pleuraeröffnung, Lobektomie, Pneumonektomie). Z. Ges. Exper. Med., *127*:605, 1956.
1180. Adams, W. E., Perkins, J. F., Harrison, R. W., Buhler, W., and Long, E. T.: The significance of cardiopulmonary reserve in the late results of pneumonectomy for carcinoma of the lung. Dis. Chest, *32*:280, 1957.
1181. Adams, W. E., and Perkins, J. F.: Physiologic effects of collapse and excisional surgery. In: Gordon, B. L. (ed.): *Clinical Cardiopulmonary Physiology*. 2nd rev. ed. New York, Grune & Stratton, 1960, p. 689.
1182. Harrison, R. W., Adams, W. E., Long, E. T., Burrows, B., and Reimann, A.: The clinical significance of cor pulmonale in the reduction of cardiopulmonary reserve following extensive pulmonary resection. J. Thoracic Surg., *36*:352, 1958.
1183. Witz, J. P., Schmidt, C., Zimmermann, C., Reys, P., and Miech, G.: Le cœur des pneumonectomisés. Arch. Mal. Cœur, *54*:780, 1961.
1184. Warembourg, H., Pauchant, M., and Sergeant, Y.: Le cœur des pneumonectomisés. Arch. Mal. Cœur, *52*:301, 1959.
1185. Peters, R. M., Roos, A., Black, H., Burford, T. H., and Graham, E. A.: Respiratory and circulatory studies after pneumonectomy in childhood. J. Thoracic Surg., *20*:484, 1950.
1186. Görgényi-Göttche, O., and Szöts, I.: Was wird aus unseren pneumonektomierten Kindern? Tuberkulosearzt, *14*:757, 1960.
1187. Gaensler, E. A., and Watson, T. R., Jr.: Bronchospirometry. III. Complications, contraindications, technique, and interpretation. J. Lab. Clin. Med., *40*:223, 1952.
1188. Harden, K. A., Johnson, J. B., McKnight, H. V., Washington, W., and Carr, C.: An evaluation of tests of pulmonary and cardiac function in relation to chest surgery. Med. Ann. D. C., *26*:451, 1957.
1189. Tammeling, G. J., and Laros, C. D.: An analysis of the pulmonary function of ninety patients following pneumonectomy for pulmonary tuberculosis. J. Thoracic Surg., *37*:148, 1959.
1190. Hurt, R. L.: Respiratory function before and after plombage. Tubercle, *37*:341, 1956.
1191. Källqvist, I.: Pulmonary resection in middle-aged and elderly patients. Am. Rev. Tuberc., *73*:40, 1956.
1192. Zohman, L. R., and Williams, M. H., Jr.: The clinical usefulness of measurement of the diffusing capacity of the lung. New York J. Med., *59*:453, 1959.
1193. Björkman, S., Bruce, N. E. T., Carlens, C. E. S., Hanson, H. E., and Uggla, L. G.: Function tests in pulmonary surgery. Am. J. Surg., *89*:30, 1955.
1194. Leake, E., Smith, W. G., and Woodliff, H. J.: Diffuse interstitial pulmonary fibrosis after busulphan therapy. Lancet, *2*:432, 1963.
1195. Le Brigand, H., Bastin, R., Pocidalo, J. J., Ranson-Bitker, B., Liot, F., Goulon, M., and Rapin, M.: Insuffisance

respiratoire grave après pneumonectomie; traitement par trachéotomie et respiration artificielle. J. Franc. Med. Chir. Thorac, *10*:562, 1956.
1196. Björk, V. O., and Engström, C. G.: The treatment of ventilatory insufficiency after pulmonary resection with tracheostomy and prolonged artificial ventilation. J. Thoracic Surg., *30*:356, 1955.
1197. Hunter, A. R.: Essentials of artificial ventilation of the lungs. London, J. & A. Churchill, 1962, pp. 43-44.
1198. Barrett, N. R.: Early treatment of stove-in chest. Lancet, *1*:293, 1960.
1199. Nordqvist, P., Dhunér, K. G., Steinberg, K., and Örndahl, G.: Myxoedema coma and CO_2-retention. Acta Med. Scand., *166*:189, 1960.
1200. Thomeret, G., Dubost, C., Duranteau, A., and Cara, M.: Nouvelle possibilité de la réanimation respiratoire. A propos d'un cas de coma asphyxique au cours d'une péritonite post-abortum. Mem. Acad. Chir., *83*:844, 1957.
1201. Nahas, G. G., and Cavert, H. M.: Cardiac depressant effect of CO_2 and its reversal. Am. J. Physiol., *190*:483, 1957.
1202. Barach, A. L.: Physiological methods in the diagnosis and treatment of asthma and emphysema. Ann. Int. Med., *12*:454, 1938.
1203. Godfrey, L., Pond, H. S., and Wood, F. C.: The Millikan oximeter in the recognition and treatment of anoxemia in clinical medicine. Am. J. Med. Sci., *126*:605, 1948.
1204. Davies, C. E., and Mackinnon, J.: Neurological effects of oxygen in chronic cor pulmonale. Lancet, *2*:883, 1949.
1205. Donald, K.: Neurological effects of oxygen [Letter to the Editor]. Lancet, *2*:1056, 1949.
1206. Comroe, J. H., Jr., Bahnson, E. R., and Coates, E. O., Jr.: Mental changes occurring in chronically anoxemic patients during oxygen therapy. J.A.M.A., *143*:1044, 1950.
1207. Penman, R. W. B.: The hypoxic drive in respiratory failure. Clin. Sci., *22*:155, 1962.
1208. Penman, R. W. B.: Blood lactate levels and some blood acid-base changes in respiratory failure and their significance in oxygen induced respiratory depression. Clin. Sci., *23*:5, 1962.
1209. Campbell, E. J. M.: A method of controlled oxygen administration which reduces the risk of carbon-dioxide retention. Lancet, *2*:12, 1960.
1210. Fishman, A. P.: Respiratory gases in the regulation of the pulmonary circulation. Physiol. Rev., *41*:214, 1961.
1211. Patterson, J. L., Jr., Hayman, A., and Duke, T. W.: Cerebral circulation and metabolism in chronic pulmonary emphysema. With observations on the effects of inhalation of oxygen. Am. J. Med., *12*:382, 1952.
1212. Small, H. S., Weitzner, S. W., and Nahas, G. G.: Cerebrospinal fluid pressures during hypercapnia and hypoxia in dogs. Am. J. Physiol., *198*:704, 1960.
1213. Hickam, J. B., Wilson, W. P., and Frayser, R.: Observations on the early elevation of serum potassium during respiratory alkalosis. J. Clin. Invest., *35*:601, 1956.
1214. Severinghaus, J. W.: The rate of uptake of nitrous oxide in man. J. Clin. Invest., *33*:1183, 1954.
1215. Rackow, H., Salanitre, E., and Frumin, M. J.: Dilution of alveolar gases during nitrous oxide excretion in man. J. Appl. Physiol., *16*:723, 1961.
1216. Frumin, M. J., Salanitre, E., and Rackow, H.: Excretion of nitrous oxide in anesthetized man. J. Appl. Physiol., *16*:720, 1961.
1217. Nims, R. G., Conner, E. H., and Comroe, J. H., Jr.: The compliance of the human thorax in anesthetized patients. J. Clin. Invest., *34*:744, 1955.
1218. Brownlee, W. E., and Allbritten, F. F., Jr.: The significance of the lung-thorax compliance in ventilation during thoracic surgery. J. Thoracic Surg., *32*:454, 1956.
1219. Foster, C. A., Heaf, P. J. D., and Semple, S. J. G.: Compliance of the lung in anesthetized paralyzed subjects. J. Appl. Physiol., *11*:383, 1957.
1220. Howell, J. B. L., and Peckett, B. W.: Studies of the elastic properties of the thorax of supine anaesthetized paralysed human subjects. J. Physiol. (London), *136*:1, 1957.
1221. Bromage, P. R.: Total respiratory compliance on anæsthetized subjects and modifications produced by noxious stimuli. Clin. Sci., *17*:217, 1958.
1222. Butler, J., and Smith, B. H.: Pressure-volume relationships of the chest in completely relaxed anaesthetised patients. Clin. Sci., *16*:125, 1957.
1223. Lucas, B. G. B., and Milne, E. H.: Acid base balance and anaesthesia. Thorax, *10*:354, 1955.
1224. Elam, J. O., and Brown, E. S.: Carbon dioxide homeostasis during anesthesia. III. Ventilation and carbon dioxide elimination. IV. An evaluation of the partial rebreathing system. Anesthesiology, *17*:116, 128, 1956.
1225. Nealon, T. F., Jr., Haupt, G. J., Chase, H. F., Price, J. E., and Gibbon, J. H., Jr.: Inefficient carbon dioxide absorption requiring increased pulmonary ventilation during operations. J. Thoracic Surg., *32*:464, 1956.
1226. Beecher, H. K., Quinn, T. J., Jr., Bunker, J. P., and D'Alessandro, G. L.: Effect of position and artificial ventilation on the excretion of carbon dioxide during thoracic surgery. J. Thoracic Surg., *22*:135, 1951.
1227. Theye, R. A., and Fowler, W. S.: Carbon dioxide balance during thoracic surgery. J. Appl. Physiol., *14*:552, 1959.
1228. Sechzer, P. H.: Effect of hypothermia on compliance and resistance of the lung-thorax system of anesthetized man. J. Appl. Physiol., *13*:53, 1958.
1229. Holaday, D. A., Ma, D., and Papper, E. M.: The immediate effects of respiratory depression on acid-base balance in anesthetized man. J. Clin. Invest., *36*:1121, 1957.
1230. Paneth, M., Sellers, R., Gott, V. L., Weirich, W. L., Allen, P., Read, R. C., and Lillehei, C. W.: Physiologic studies upon prolonged cardiopulmonary bypass with the pump-oxygenator with particular reference to (1) acid-base balance, (2) siphon caval drainage. J. Thoracic Surg., *34*:570, 1957.
1231. Scribner, B. H., Fremont-Smith, K., and Burnell, J. M.: The effect of acute respiratory acidosis on the internal equilibrium of potassium. J. Clin. Invest., *34*:1276, 1955.
1232. Knott, J. M. S., and Christie, R. V.: Radiological diagnosis of emphysema. Lancet, *1*:881, 1951.
1233. Schoenmackers, J., and Vieten, H.: Das Verhalten der Lungengefässe bei verändertem Luftgehalt der Lunge. (Untersuchungen am postmortalen Gefässbild.) Fortschr. Geb. Roentgenstr., *76*:24, 1952.
1234. Barden, R. P.: The interpretation of some radiologic signs of abnormal pulmonary function. Radiology, *59*:481, 1952.
1235. Hornykiewytsch, T., and Stender, H. S.: Normale und pathologisch veränderte Lungengefässe im Schichtbild. [I-X] Fortschr. Geb. Roentgenstr., *79*:44, 639, 704, 1953; *80*:458, 1954; *81*:36, 134, 455, 642, 1954; *82*:228, 331, 1955.
1236. Goldenthal, S., Armstrong, B. W., and Lowman, R. M.: Roentgen studies of ventilatory dysfunction: An analysis of diaphragmatic movement in obstructive emphysema. Am. J. Roentgenol., *79*:279, 1958.
1237. Andrews, A. H., Jr., Jensik, R., and Pfisterer, W. H.: Fluoroscopic pulmonary densiography. Dis. Chest, *35*:117, 1959.
1238. Bates, D. V., and Fraser, R. G.: Unpublished observations on the use of tomography in differentiation of emphysema and asthma; Observer-error experiment.
1239. Stone, D. J., Schwartz, A., and Feltman, J. A.: Bullous emphysema. A long-term study of the natural history and the effects of therapy. Am. Rev. Resp. Dis., *82*:493, 1960.
1240. Leopold, J. G., and Seal, R. M.: The bronchographic appearance of "peripheral pooling" attributed to the filling of centrilobular emphysematous spaces. Thorax, *16*:70, 1961.
1241. Parsons, W. D., de Villiers, A. J., Bartlett, L. S., and Becklake, M. R.: Lung cancer in a fluospar mining community. II. Prevalence of respiratory symptoms and disability. Brit. J. Indust. Med., *21*:110, 1964.
1242. Rainer, W. G., Mitchell, R. S., Filley, G. F., and Eiseman, B.: Significance of tracheal collapse in pulmonary emphysema—cinefluorographic observations. Surg. Forum, *12*:70, 1961.
1243. Campbell, E. J. M.: Respiratory failure. The relation be-

tween oxygen concentrations of inspired air and arterial blood. Lancet, *2*:10, 1960.
1244. Massaro, D. J., Katz, S., and Luchsinger, P. C.: Effect of various modes of oxygen administration on the arterial gas values in patients with respiratory acidosis. Brit. Med. J., *2*:627, 1962.
1245. Ernsting, J.: The effect of breathing high concentrations of oxygen upon the diffusing capacity of the lung in man. J. Physiol. (London), *155*:51*P*, 1960.
1246. Pratt, P. C.: Pulmonary capillary proliferation induced by oxygen inhalation. Am. J. Pathol., *34*:1033, 1958.
1247. Burton, J. D. K.: Effects of dry anaesthetic gases on the respiratory mucous membrane. Lancet, *1*:235, 1962.
1248. Cotes, J. E.: Respiratory function and portable oxygen therapy in chronic non-specific lung disease in relation to prognosis. Thorax, *15*:244, 1960.
1249. Westlake, E. K., and Campbell, E. J. M.: Effects of aminophylline, nikethamide, and sodium salicylate in respiratory failure. Brit. Med. J., *1*:274, 1959.
1250. Naimark, A., Brodovsky, D. M., and Cherniak, R. M.: The effect of a new carbonic anhydrase inhibitor (dichlorphenamide) in respiratory insufficiency. Am. J. Med., *28*:368, 1960.
1251. Simpson, T.: Dichlorphenamide for respiratory insufficiency [Letter to the Editor]. Lancet, *1*:54, 1961.
1252. Little, G. M.: Use of amiphenazole in respiratory failure. Brit. Med. J., *1*:223, 1962.
1253. Sadoul, P., Robert, J., Saunier, C., Pham, Q. T., and Lacoste, J.: Action du dichlorphénamide chez les insuffisants respiratoires. Rev. Med. Nancy, *87*:151, 1962.
1254. Christensen, P. J.: The carbonic anhydrase inhibitor dichlorphenamide in chronic pulmonary emphysema. Lancet, *1*:881, 1962.
1255. Harris, L. H.: Dichlorphenamide for respiratory insufficiency [Letter to the Editor]. Lancet, *1*:398, 1961.
1256. Hugh-Jones, P.: Oligopnoea [Abridged]. Proc. Roy. Soc. Med. (London), *51*:104, 1958.
1257. Davidson, L. A. G.: Tracheotomy in acute respiratory disease. Lancet, *1*:597, 1959.
1258. Harris, L. H., and Houston, J.: Tracheotomy for acute respiratory infections in emphysema. Lancet, *2*:1170, 1961.
1259. Lee, G. J.: The circulatory effects of acute respiratory failure: with special reference to acute cor pulmonale. Postgrad. Med. J., *37*:31, 1961.
1260. Friedman, R. L.: Atelectasis in upper respiratory infections in post-traumatic paralyzed patients. Ann. Int. Med., *40*:924, 1954.
1261. Björk, V. O., and Engström, C. G.: The treatment of ventilatory insufficiency by tracheostomy and artificial ventilation. A study of 61 thoracic surgical cases. J. Thoracic Surg., *34*:228, 1957.
1262. Pryer, D. L., Pryer, R. R. L., and Williams, A. F.: Fatal respiratory obstruction due to faulty endotracheal tube. Lancet, *2*:742, 1960.
1263. Pearce, D. J., and Walsh, R. S.: Respiratory obstruction due to tracheal granuloma after tracheostomy. Lancet, *2*:135, 1961.
1264. Blossom, R. A., and Affeldt, J. E.: Chronic poliomyelitic respiratory deaths. Am. J. Med., *20*:77, 1956.
1265. Boutourline-Young, H. J., and Whittenberger, J. L.: The use of artificial respiration in pulmonary emphysema accompanied by high carbon dioxide levels. J. Clin. Invest., *30*:838, 1951.
1266. Lassen, H. C. A.: A preliminary report on the 1952 epidemic of poliomyelitis in Copenhagen with special reference to the treatment of acute respiratory insufficiency. Lancet, *1*:37, 1953.
1267. Emerson, P. A., Torres, G. E., and Lyons, H. A.: The effect of intermittent positive pressure breathing on the lung compliance and intrapulmonary mixing of gases. Thorax, *15*:124, 1960.
1268. Burris, O. F., Brownlee, W. E., and Allbritten, F. F., Jr.: The efficiency of ventilation with various methods of controlled ventilation. A study of total ventilation, alveolar ventilation, and effieiency of ventilation in anesthetized dogs. J. Thorac. Cardiov. Surg., *42*:12, 1961.
1269. Watson, W. E.: Observations on physiological deadspace during intermittent positive pressure respiration. Brit. J. Anaesth., *34*:502, 1962.
1270. Campbell, E. J. M., Nunn, J. F., and Peckett, B. W.: A comparison of artificial ventilation and spontaneous respiration with particular reference to ventilation-bloodflow relationships. Brit. J. Anesth., *30*:166, 1958.
1271. Scherrer, M., and Hodler, J.: Gasaustauch und Hämodynamik bei künstlicher Beatmung. Schweiz. Med. Wchnschr., *87*:1509, 1957.
1272. Maloney, J. V., Jr., Elam, J. O., Handford, S. W., Balla, G. A., Eastwood, D. W., Brown, E. S., and Ten Pas, R. H.: Importance of negative pressure phase in mechanical respirators. J.A.M.A., *152*:212, 1953.
1273. Watson, W. E., Smith, A. C., and Spalding, J. M. K.: Transmural central venous pressure during intermittent positive pressure respiration. Brit. J. Anaesth, *34*:278, 1962.
1274. Opie, L. H., Spalding, J. M. K., and Smith, A. C.: Intrathoracic pressure during intermittent positive-pressure respiration. Lancet, *1*:911, 1961.
1275. Bernéus, B., and Carlsten, A.: Effect of intermittent positive-pressure ventilation on cardiac output in poliomyelitis. Acta Med. Scand., *152*:19, 1955.
1276. Bernéus, B., Gordh, T., Linderholm, H., Ström, G., and Werneman, H.: On the effect of head-low position during intermittent positive-pressure ventilation. Acta Med. Scand., *152*:31, 1955.
1277. Marshall, J.: Alterations in the diurnal excretion of electrolytes during intermittent positive-pressure respiration. Brit. Med. J., *2*:85, 1959.
1278. Currie, J. C. M., and Ullmann, E.: Polyuria during experimental modifications of breathing. J. Physiol. (London), *155*:438, 1961.
1279. Gauer, O. H., and Henry, J. P.: Circulatory basis of fluid volume control. Physiol. Rev., *43*:423, 1963.
1280. Hickam, J. B., Sieker, H. O., Pryor, W. W., and Frayser, R.: The use of mechanical respirators in patients with a high airway resistance. Ann. N.Y. Acad. Sci., *66*:866, 1957.
1281. Jones, R. H., Macnamara, J., and Gaensler, E. A.: The effects of intermittent positive pressure breathing in simulated pulmonary obstruction. Am. Rev. Resp. Dis., *82*:164, 1960.
1282. Cherniack, R. M., and Hodson, A.: Compliance of the chest wall in chronic bronchitis and emphysema. J. Appl. Physiol., *18*:707, 1963.
1283. Cournand, A., Lassen, H. C. A., and Richards, D. W., Jr.: Distribution of respiratory gases in a closed breathing circuit. II. Pulmonary fibrosis and emphysema. J. Clin. Invest., *16*:9, 1937.
1284. Cherniack, R. M., Ewart, W. B., and Hildes, J. A.: Polycythemia secondary to respiratory disturbances in poliomyelitis. Ann. Int. Med., *46*:720, 1957.
1285. Ferris, B. G., Jr., Mead, J., Whittenberger, J. L., and Saxton, G. A., Jr.: Pulmonary function in convalescent poliomyelitic patients. III. Compliance of the lungs and thorax. New Engl. J. Med., *247*:390, 1952.
1286. Kilburn, K. H., Eagen, J. T., and Heyman, A.: Cardiopulmonary insufficiency associated with myotonic dystrophy. Am. J. Med., *26*:929, 1959.
1287. James, J. L., and Park, H. W. J.: Respiratory failure due to polymyositis treated by intermittent positive-pressure respiration. Lancet, *2*:1281, 1961.
1288. Brain, R.: Discussion on the acquired myopathies: Clinical aspects. Proc. Roy. Soc. Med. (London), *53*:821, 1960.
1289. Foye, L. V., Jr.: Neuromuscular blockade and artificial respiration in severe tetanus. A.M.A. Arch. Int. Med., *99*:298, 1957.
1290. Smith, A. C.: The treatment of severe tetanus by paralysing drugs and intermittent pressure respiration. Proc. Roy. Soc. Med. (London), *51*:1006, 1958.
1291. Wright, R., Sykes, M. K., Jackson, B. G., Mann, N. M., and Adams, E. B.: Intermittent positive-pressure respiration in tetanus neonatorum. Lancet, *2*:678, 1961.
1292. Strang, L. B.: Respiratory distress in new-born infants. Brit. Med. Bull., *19*:45, 1963.
1293. Strang, L. B., and MacLeish, M. H.: Ventilatory failure

and right-to-left shunt in newborn infants with respiratory distress. Pediatrics, *28*:17, 1961.

1294. Swensson, S. A., and Feychting, H.: Viewpoints on the technique in respirator treatment of the newborn and infants. Acta Anaesthesiol. Scand., suppl. 6, p. 17, 1960.
1295. Benson, F., Celander, O., Haglund, G., Nilsson, L., Paulsen, L., and Renck, L.: Positive-pressure respirator treatment of severe pulmonary insufficiency in the newborn infant; a clinical report. Acta Anaesthesiol. Scand., *2*:37, 1958.
1296. Usher, R.: The respiratory distress syndrome of prematurity. Pediat. Clin. N. Am., *8*:525, 1961.
1297. Norlander, O. P., Björk, V. O., Crafoord, C., Friberg, O., Holmdahl, M., Swensson, A., and Widman, B.: Controlled ventilation in clinical practice. Anaesthesia, *16*:285, 1961.
1298. Noehren, T. H.: Relief of carbon dioxide narcosis by simple intermittent positive pressure therapy. Dis. Chest., *28*:515, 1955.
1299. Sadoul, P., Lacoste, J., and Saunier, C.: Les gestes essentiels de la réanimation respiratoire chez les pulmonaires chroniques. J. Franc. Med. Chir. Thorac., *15*:747, 1961.
1300. Lovejoy, F. W., Jr., Yu, P. N. G., Nye, R. E., Jr., Joos, H. A., and Simpson, J. H.: Pulmonary hypertension. III. Physiologic studies in three cases of carbon dioxide narcosis treated by artificial respiration. Am. J. Med., *16*:4, 1954.
1301. Munck, O., Kristensen, H. S., and Lassen, H. C. A.: Mechanical ventilation for acute respiratory failure in diffuse chronic lung disease. Lancet, *1*:66, 1961.
1302. Bühlmann, A., Schaub, F., and Rossier, P. H.: Zur Ätiologie und Therapie des Cor pulmonale. Schweiz. Med. Wchnschr., *84*:587, 1954.
1303. Westlake, E. K.: Emergencies in general practice: Dangerous bronchitis. Brit. Med. J., *2*:960, 1955.
1304. Stone, D. J., Schwartz, A., Newman, W., Feltman, J. A., and Lovelock, F. J.: Precipitation by pulmonary infection of acute anoxia, cardiac failure and respiratory acidosis in chronic pulmonary disease. Pathogenesis and treatment. Am. J. Med., *14*:14, 1953.
1305. Cara, M., Rudler, J. C., Angles, C., and Fourcade, R.: Notre expérience de la respiration artificielle avec l'appareil d'Engstroem en chirurgie thoracique. J. Franc. Med. Chir. Thorac., *11*:82, 1957.
1306. Lawson, D. D., McAllister, R. A., and Smith, G.: Treatment of acute experimental carbon-monoxide poisoning with oxygen under pressure. Lancet, *1*:800, 1961.
1307. Apthorp, G. H., Bates, D. V., Marshall, R., and Mendel, D.: Effect of acute carbon monoxide poisoning on work capacity. Influence of 5% CO_2 on rate of recovery. Brit. Med. J., *2*:476, 1958.
1308. Leathart, G. L.: Hyperventilation in carbon-monoxide poisoning. Brit. Med. J., *2*:511, 1962.
1309. Gaensler, E. A.: Respiratory acidosis as seen following surgery. Am. J. Surg., *103*:289, 1962.
1310. Erlanson, P., Lindholm, T., Lindqvist, B., and Swenson, A.: Artificial respiration in severe renal failure with pulmonary insufficiency. Acta Med. Scand., *166*:81, 1960.
1311. Beck, M., Berglund, E., and Simonsson, B.: Treatment of respiratory failure in two patients with pneumonia and with restricted pulmonary function. Acta Med. Scand., *163*:467, 1959.
1312. Herzog, H., Staub, H., and Richterich, R.: Gas-analytical studies in severe pneumonia. Observations during the 1957 influenza epidemic. Lancet, *1*:593, 1959.
1313. Walker, W. C., Douglas, A. C., Leckie, W. J. H., Pines, A., and Grant, I. W. B.: Respiratory complications of influenza. Lancet, *1*:449, 1958.
1314. Carlens, E., Widman, B., and Norlander, O.: Respirator treatment in cases of acute laryngotracheobronchitis. Acta. Otolaryngol., *52*:331, 1961.
1315. Wheeldon, P. J., and Perry, A. W.: The use of Ethamivan in the treatment of barbiturate poisoning. Canad. M. A. J., *89*:20, 1963.
1316. Cole, G. W., Marks, A., and Baum, G. L.: Barbiturate poisoning. Management with a new respiratory stimulant. J.A.M.A., *174*:156, 1960.
1317. Swenson, E. W., Ställberg-Stenhagen, S., and Beck, M.: Arterial oxygen, carbon dioxide, and pH levels in patients undergoing pulmonary resection. Intra-operative and early post-operative observations. J. Thorac. Cardiov. Surg., *42*:179, 1961.
1318. Anscombe, A. R., and Buxton, R. S. J.: Effect of abdominal operations on total lung capacity and its subdivisions. Brit. Med. J., *2*:84, 1958.
1319. Palmer, J. N. V.: Changes in ventilatory function after abdominal operations. Lancet, *1*:191, 1961.
1320. Miller, W. F., Wu, N., and Johnson, R. L., Jr.: Convenient method of evaluating pulmonary ventilatory function with a single breath test. Anesthesiology, *17*:480, 1956.
1321. McCann, W. S., Lovejoy, F. W., Jr., and Yu, P. N. G.: The failing lung. In: *Symposium on Pulmonary Problems in The Older Age Group*. New York J. Med., *52*:1983, 1952.
1322. Klassen, G. A., Broadhurst, C., Peretz, D. I., and Johnson, A. L.: Cardiac resuscitation in 126 medical patients using external cardiac massage. Lancet, *1*:1290, 1963.
1323. Woolf, C. R.: The respiratory unit at the Toronto General Hospital. Canad. M. A. J., *84*:466, 1961.
1324. Aronovitch, M., Kahana, L. M., Meakins, J. F., Place, R. E. G., and Laing, R.: Vanillic diethylamide in the management of acute respiratory insufficiency. A preliminary report. Canad. M. A. J., *85*:875, 1961.
1325. Silipo, S., Hagedorn, C., Rosenstein, I. N., and Baum, G. L.: Experiences with Ethamivan, a new respiratory stimulant and analeptic agent. A preliminary report. J.A.M.A., *177*:378, 1961.
1326. Said, S. I., and Banerjee, C. M.: Effects of a newer respiratory stimulant (vanillic diethylamide) in respiratory acidosis due to obstructive pulmonary emphysema or obesity. Am. J. Med., *33*:845, 1962.
1327. Miller, W. F., Archer, R. K., Taylor, H. F., and Ossenfort, W. F.: Severe respiratory depression. Role of a respiratory stimulant, Ethamivan, in the treatment. J.A.M.A., *180*:905, 1962.
1328. Simpson, T.: Papilloedema in emphysema. Brit. Med. J., *2*:639, 1948.
1329. Catterall, M., and Rowell, N. R.: Respiratory function in progressive systemic sclerosis. Thorax, *18*:10, 1963.
1330. Hamman, L., and Rich, A. R.: Acute diffuse interstitial fibrosis of the lungs. Bull. Johns Hopkins Hosp., *74*:177, 1944.
1331. Scadding, J. G.: Chronic diffuse interstitial fibrosis of the lungs. Brit. Med. J., *1*:443, 1960.
1332. Broch, O. J., Moe, T., and Wehn, M.: Pulmonary fibrosis. Acta Med. Scand., *148*:189, 1954.
1333. Grant, I. W. B., Hillis, B. R., and Davidson, J.: Diffuse interstitial fibrosis of the lungs (Hamman-Rich syndrome). A review with a report of three additional cases. Am. Rev. Tuberc., *74*:485, 1956.
1334. Hoff, H. R.: The Hamman-Rich syndrome. Review of the literature and report of a case treated with prednisone. New Engl. J. Med., *259*:81, 1958.
1335. Rubin, E. H., and Lubliner, R.: The Hamman-Rich syndrome: Review of the literature and analysis of 15 cases. Medicine, *36*:397, 1957.
1336. Bates, D. V.: Respiratory disorders associated with impairment of gas diffusion. (Alveolo-capillary block syndrome.) Ann. Rev. Med., *13*:301, 1962.
1337. Knipping, H. W.: Die Pneumonose. Ergebn. Inn. Med. Kinderheilk., *48*:249, 1935.
1338. Dickie, H. A., and Rankin, J.: Interstitial diseases of the lung. The alveolar-capillary block syndrome. In: Gordon, B. L. (ed.): *Clinical Cardiopulmonary Physiology*. 2nd rev. ed. New York, Grune & Stratton, 1960, sect. 9, chapt. 51, p. 810.
1339. Said, S. I., Thompson, W. T., Jr., Patterson, J. L., Jr., and Brummer, D. L.: Shunting effect of extreme impairment of pulmonary diffusion. Bull. Johns Hopkins Hosp., *107*:255, 1960.
1340. Turino, G. M., Lourenso, R. V., Davidson, L. A. G., and Fishman, A. P.: The control of ventilation in patients with reduced pulmonary distensibility. In: Nahas, G. G. (ed.): *Regulation of Respiration*, part V. Ann. N.Y. Acad. Sci., *109*:932, 1963.
1341. Tabakin, B. S., Hanson, J. S., Adhikari, P. K., and Naeye, R. L.: Circulatory and ventilatory dynamics in alveolar-

capillary membrane block. Am. Rev. Resp. Dis., *83*:194, 1961.
1342. Perret, C.: La mécanique respiratoire dans la fibrose pulmonaire. Schweiz. Med. Wchnschr., *90*:1129, 1960.
1343. Holland, R. A. B.: Physiologic dead space in the Hamman-Rich syndrome. Physiologic and clinical implications. Am. J. Med., *28*:61, 1960.
1344. Read, J., and Williams, R. S.: Pulmonary ventilation. Blood flow relationships in interstitial disease of the lungs. Am. J. Med., *27*:545, 1959.
1345. Finley, T. N.: The determination of uneven pulmonary blood flow from the arterial oxygen tension during nitrogen washout. J. Clin. Invest., *40*:1727, 1961.
1346. Staub, N. C.: Alveolar-arterial oxygen tension gradient due to diffusion. J. Appl. Physiol., *18*:673, 1963.
1347. Miller, R. D., Fowler, W. S., and Helmholz, F. H., Jr.: Scleroderma of the lungs. Proc. Staff Meet., Mayo Clin., *34*:66, 1959.
1348. Adhikari, P. K., Bianchi, F. A., Boushy, S. F., Sakamoto, A., and Lewis, B. M.: Pulmonary function in scleroderma. Its relation in the chest roentgenogram and in the skin of the thorax. Am. Rev. Resp. Dis., *86*:823, 1962.
1349. Hughes, D. T. D., and Lee, F. I.: Lung function in patients with systemic sclerosis. Thorax, *18*:16, 1963.
1350. Mahrer, P. R., Evans, J. A., and Steinberg, I.: Scleroderma: Relation of pulmonary changes to esophageal disease. Ann. Int. Med., *40*:92, 1954.
1351. Piper, W. N., and Helwig, E. B.: Progressive systemic sclerosis. Visceral manifestations in generalized scleroderma. A.M.A. Arch. Derm., *72*:535, 1955.
1352. Opie, L. H.: The pulmonary manifestations of generalised scleroderma (progressive systemic sclerosis). Dis. Chest, *28*:665, 1955.
1353. West, J. R., McClement, J. H., Carroll, D., Bliss, H. A., Kuschner, M., Richards, D. W., Jr., and Cournand, A.: Effects of cortisone and ACTH in cases of chronic pulmonary disease with impairment of alveolar-capillary diffusion. Am. J. Med., *10*:156, 1951.
1354. Andrews, E. C., Jr.: Five cases of an undescribed form of pulmonary interstitial fibrosis caused by obstruction of the pulmonary veins. Bull. Johns Hopkins Hosp., *100*:28, 1957.
1355. Bindelglass, I. L., and Trubowitz, S.: Pulmonary vein obstruction: An uncommon sequel to chronic fibrous mediastinitis. Ann. Int. Med., *48*:876, 1958.
1356. Ellman, P., Weber, F. P., and Goddier, T. E. W.: A contribution to the pathology of Sjögren's disease. Quart. J. Med., *20*:33, 1951.
1357. Hatch, H. B., and Boese, H. L.: Sjögren's syndrome associated with obstructive collapse of the middle lobe of lung. Ochsner Clin. Rep., *1*:42, 1955.
1358. Bucher, U. G., and Reid, L.: Sjögren's syndrome. Report of a fatal case with pulmonary and renal lesions. Brit. J. Dis. Chest, *53*:237, 1959.
1359. Doctor, L., and Snider, G. L.: Diffuse interstitial pulmonary fibrosis associated with arthritis. With comments on the definition of rheumatoid lung disease. Am. Rev. Resp. Dis., *85*:413, 1962.
1360. Gross, P.: The concept of the Hamman-Rich syndrome. A critique. Am. Rev. Resp. Dis., *85*:828, 1962.
1361. Solomon, M.: Interstitial pulmonary fibrosis secondary to pulmonary venous hypertension. Report of a case due to myxoma of the left atrium. J.A.M.A., *174*:464, 1960.
1362. Williams, W. J.: The pathology of the lungs in five nickel workers. Brit. J. Indust. Med., *15*:235, 1958.
1363. Cruickshank, B.: Interstitial pneumonia and its consequences in rheumatoid disease. Brit. J. Dis. Chest, *53*:226, 1959.
1364. Cawthorne, T., Hewlett, A. B., and Ranger, D.: Tracheostomy in a respiratory unit at a neurological hospital. In: *Discussion: Tracheostomy Today*. Proc. Roy. Soc. Med. (London), *52*:403, 1959.
1365. McIlroy, M. B., Mead, J., Selverstone, N. J., and Radford, E. P.: Measurement of lung tissue viscous resistance using gases of equal kinematic viscosity. J. Appl. Physiol., *7*:485, 1955.
1366. Simpson, T.: Carbonic anhydrase inhibitor [Letter to the Editor]. Lancet, *1*:920, 1955.
1367. Hugh-Jones, P.: Management of tracheostomies. In: *Discussion: Tracheostomy Today*. Proc. Roy. Soc. Med. (London), *52*:412, 1959.
1368. Caplan, H.: Honeycomb lungs and malignant pulmonary adenomatosis in scleroderma. Thorax, *14*:89, 1959.
1369. Cudkowicz, L., Madoff, I. M., and Abelmann, W. H.: Rheumatoid lung disease. A case report which includes respiratory function studies and a lung biopsy. Brit. J. Dis. Chest., *55*:35, 1961.
1370. Edge, J. R., and Rickards, A. G.: Rheumatoid arthritis with lung lesions. Thorax, *12*:352, 1957.
1371. Golden, A., and Bronk, T. T.: Diffuse interstitial fibrosis of lungs. A form of diffuse interstitial angiosis and reticulosis of the lungs. A.M.A. Arch. Int. Med., *92*:606, 1953.
1372. Gray, F. D., Jr., and Field, A. S., Jr.: Muscular hyperplasia of the lung: A physiopathologic analysis. Ann. Int. Med., *53*:683, 1960.
1373. Rubinstein, L., Gutstein, W. H., and Lepow, H.: Pulmonary muscular hyperplasia (muscular cirrhosis of the lungs). Ann. Int. Med., *42*:36, 1955.
1374. Inkley, S. R., and Abbott, G. R.: Unilateral pulmonary arteriosclerosis. Unusual fibrous connective tissue growth associated: Review of literature and discussion of possible physiological mechanisms involved in these changes. Arch. Int. Med., *108*:903, 1961.
1375. Ogilvie, A. G., and Hulse, E. V.: Some observations on a case of diffuse interstitial fibrosis of the lungs. Brit. J. Tuberc., *48*:200, 1954.
1376. Silverman, J. J., and Talbot, T. J.: Diffuse interstitial pulmonary fibrosis camouflaged by hypermetabolism and cardiac failure: Antemortem diagnosis with biopsy and catheterization studies. Ann. Int. Med., *38*:1326, 1953.
1377. Hall, Z. M., and Wilson, R. R.: A new syndrome? Brit. Med. J., *2*:820, 1961.
1378. Langfeld, S. B., Hopkins, F. T., and Theurkauf, E. A., Jr.: Chronic cor pulmonale due to multiple pulmonary emboli and accompanied by diffuse interstitial fibrosis. Am. J. Med., *27*:494, 1959.
1379. Moore, F. H., Hamlin, J. W., and Lindsay, S.: Progressive diffuse interstitial fibrosis of the lungs (Hamman-Rich syndrome). Report of a case of seven years' duration. Arch. Int. Med., *100*:651, 1957.
1380. Whitfield, A. G. W., Bond, W. H., and Arnott, W. M.: Radiation reactions in the lung. Quart. J. Med., (*n.s.*)*25*:67, 1956.
1381. Sweany, S. K., Moss, W. T., and Haddy, F. J.: The effects of chest irradiation on pulmonary function. J. Clin. Invest., *38*:587, 1959.
1382. Stone, D. J., Schwartz, M. J., and Green, R. A.: Fatal pulmonary insufficiency due to radiation effect upon the lung. Am. J. Med., *21*:211, 1956.
1383. Ross, W. M.: The radiotherapeutic and radiological aspects of radiation fibrosis of the lungs. Thorax, *11*:241, 1956.
1384. Sutton, M.: The functional effect of pulmonary irradiation. Brit. Med. J., *2*:838, 1960.
1385. Smith, J. C.: Radiation pneumonitis. A review. Am. Rev. Resp. Dis., *87*:647, 1963.
1386. Warren, S., and Spencer, J.: Radiation reaction in the lung. Am. J. Roentgenol., *43*:682, 1940.
1387. McIntosh, H. C., and Spitz, S.: A study of radiation pneumonitis. Am. J. Roentgenol., *41*:605, 1939.
1388. Warren, S.: Effects of radiation on normal tissues. V. Effects on the respiratory system. Arch. Path., *34*:917, 1942.
1389. Jacobsen, V. C.: The deleterious effects of deep roentgen irradiation on lung structure and function. Am. J. Roentgenol., *44*:235, 1940.
1390. Freid, J. R., and Goldberg, H.: Post-irradiation changes in the lungs and thorax. Clinical, roentgenological and pathological study, with emphasis on the late and terminal stages. Am. J. Roentgenol., *43*:877, 1940.
1391. Chu, F. C. H., Phillips, R., Nickson, J. J., and McPhee, J. G.: Pneumonitis following radiation therapy of cancer of the breast by tangential technic. Radiology, *64*:642, 1955.
1392. Hutchison, H. E.: Irradiation pneumonitis: Report of a case with description of histological findings. Glasgow Med. J., *152*:299, 1953.

1393. Leach, J. E., Farrow, J. H., Foote, F. W., Jr., and Wawro, N. W.: Fibrosis of the lung following roentgen irradiation for cancer of the breast. A clinical study. Am. J. Roentgenol., *47*:740, 1942.
1394. Widmann, B. P.: Irradiation pulmonary fibrosis. Am. J. Roentgenol., *47*:24, 1942.
1395. *Proceedings of the International Conference on Sarcoidosis*, Washington, D. C., June 1960. Am. Rev. Resp. Dis., *84*/5: part 2, 1961.
1396. Smellie, H., and Hoyle, C.: The natural history of pulmonary sarcoidosis. Quart. J. Med., *(n.s.)29*:539, 1960.
1397. Scadding, J. G.: Prognosis of intrathoracic sarcoidosis in England. A review of 136 cases after five years' observation. Brit. Med., J., *2*:1165, 1961.
1398. James, D. G., and Thomson, A. D.: The course of sarcoidosis and its modification by treatment. Lancet, *1*:1057, 1959.
1399. Longcope, W. T., and Freiman, D. G.: A study of sarcoidosis. Based on a combined investigation of 160 cases including 30 autopsies from the Johns Hopkins Hospital and Massachusetts General Hospital. Medicine, *31*:1, 1952.
1400. Hoyle, C.: Prognosis of pulmonary sarcoidosis. Lancet, *2*:611, 1961.
1401. Coates, E. O., and Comroe, J. H., Jr.: Pulmonary function studies in sarcoidosis. J. Clin. Invest., *30*:848, 1951.
1402. McClement, J. H., Renzetti, A. D., Himmelstein, A., and Cournand, A.: Cardiopulmonary function in the pulmonary form of Boeck's sarcoid and its modification by cortisone therapy. Am. Rev. Tuberc., *67*:154, 1953.
1403. Lyons, H. A.: Pulmonary compliance in granulomatous disease of the lung. Am. J. Med., *25*:23, 1958.
1404. Stone, D. J., Schwartz, A., Feltman, J. A., and Lovelock, F. J.: Pulmonary function in sarcoidosis. Results with cortisone therapy. Am. J. Med., *15*:468, 1953.
1405. Williams, M. H., Jr.: Pulmonary function in Boeck's sarcoid. J. Clin. Invest., *32*:909, 1953.
1406. Baldwin, E. de F., Cournand, A., and Richards, D. W., Jr.: Pulmonary insufficiency. II. A study of thirty-nine cases of pulmonary fibrosis. Medicine, *28*:1, 1949.
1407. Smellie, H., Apthorp, G. H., and Marshall, R.: The effect of corticosteroid treatment on pulmonary function in sarcoidosis. Thorax, *16*:87, 1961.
1408. Wigderson, A., Williams, M. H., Jr., Zohman, L. R., and Childress, W. G.: Impaired diffusion in pulmonary sarcoidosis. New York J. Med., *59*:2420, 1959.
1409. Cournand, A.: The syndrome of "alveolar-capillary block." Clinical, physiologic, pathologic and therapeutic considerations. Report of Annual Meeting and Proceedings, Royal College Physicians and Surgeons of Canada, October 1952, p. 34.
1410. Mead, J., and Collier, C.: Relation of volume history of lungs to respiratory mechanics in anesthetized dogs. J. Appl. Physiol., *14*:669, 1959.
1411. Arnott, W. M., Butler, J., and Pincock, A. C.: A pressure-volume diagram recorder for respiration in man. J. Physiol. (London), *124*:*6P*, 1954.
1412. Rose, G. A.: The natural history of polyarteritis. Brit. Med. J., *2*:1148, 1957.
1413. Löffler, W.: Zur Differential-Diagnose der Lungeninfiltrierungen. I. Frühinfiltrate unter besonderer Berücksichtigung der Rückbildungszeiten. II. Über flüchtige Succedan-Infiltrate (mit Eosinophilie). Beitr. Klin. Tuberk., *79*:338, 368, 1932.
1414. Eldridge, F.: Pulmonary infiltration with eosinophilia and the alveolar-capillary block syndrome. Am. J. Med., *25*:796, 1958.
1415. Reeder, W. H., and Goodrich, B. E.: Pulmonary infiltration with eosinophilia (PIE) syndrome. Ann. Int. Med., *36*:1217, 1952.
1416. Goodpasture, E. W.: The significance of certain pulmonary lesions in relation to the etiology of influenza. Am. J. Med. Sci., *158*:863, 1919.
1417. Cruickshank, J. G., and Parker, R. A.: Pulmonary haemosiderosis with severe renal lesions (Goodpasture's syndrome). Thorax, *16*:22, 1961.
1418. Parkin, T. W., Rusted, I. E., Burchell, H. B., and Edwards, J. E.: Hemorrhagic and interstitial pneumonitis with nephritis. Am. J. Med., *18*:220, 1955.
1419. Walton, E. W.: Giant-cell granuloma of the respiratory tract (Wegener's granulomatosis). Brit. Med. J., *2*:265, 1958.
1420. Gordon, G. B., Gechman, E., Rosengarten, R., and Neptune, A. P.: Wegener's granulomatosis. Ann. Int. Med., *47*:1260, 1957.
1421. Reeves, E. H., DeGroat, A., and Chapman, P. T.: Wegener's syndrome. Case with unusual features. Am. Rev. Resp. Dis., *82*:394, 1960.
1422. Florian, J.: Zur Klinik der idiopathischen Lungenhämosiderose der Erwachsenen. Muench. Med. Wchnschr., *98*:1597, 1956.
1423. Bronson, S. M.: Idiopathic pulmonary hemosiderosis in adults. Report of a case and review of the literature. Am. J. Roentgenol., *83*:260, 1960.
1424. Harvey, A. M., Shulman, L. E., Tumulty, P. A., Conley, C. L., and Schoenrich, E. H.: Systemic lupus erythematosus: Review of the literature and clinical analysis of 138 cases. Medicine, *33*:291, 1954.
1425. Myhre, J. R.: Pleuropulmonary manifestations in lupus erythematosus disseminatus. Acta Med. Scand., *165*:55, 1959.
1426. Matthews, H. L., and Meynell, M. J.: Acute diffuse lupus erythematosus. Report of a case with predominant pulmonary manifestations. Brit. Med. J., *2*:1140, 1954.
1427. Patterson, S. W.: The antagonistic action of carbon dioxide and adrenalin on the heart. Proc. Roy. Soc. (London) *s.B, 88*:371, 1915.
1428. Tenney, S. M.: Sympatho-adrenal stimulation by carbon dioxide and the inhibitory effect of carbonic acid on epinephrine response. Am. J. Physiol., *187*:341, 1956.
1429. Nahas, G. G., Jordan, E. C., and Ligou, J. C.: Effects of a "CO_2 buffer" on hypercapnia of apneic oxygenation. Am. J. Physiol., *197*:1308, 1959.
1430. Nahas, G. G., Ligou, J. C., and Mehlman, B.: Effects of pH changes on O_2 uptake and plasma catecholamine levels in the dog. Am. J. Physiol., *198*:60, 1960.
1431. Millar, R. A.: Plasma adrenalin and noradrenalin during diffusion respiration. J. Physiol. (London), *150*:79, 1960.
1432. Stone, J. E., Wells, J., Draper, W. B., and Whitehead, R. W.: Changes in renal blood flow in dogs during inhalation of 30% carbon dioxide. Am. J. Physiol., *194*:115, 1958.
1433. Berger, E. Y., Galdston, M., and Horwitz, S. A.: The effect of anoxic anoxia on the human kidney. J. Clin. Invest., *28*:648, 1949.
1434. Asmussen, E., and Nielsen, M.: The cardiac output in rest and work at low and high oxygen pressures. Acta Physiol. Scand., *35*:73, 1955.
1435. Doyle, J. T., Wilson, J. S., and Warren, J. V.: The pulmonary vascular responses to short-term hypoxia in human subjects. Circulation, *5*:263, 1952.
1436. Parker, F., Jr., and Weiss, S.: The nature and significance of the structural changes in the lungs in mitral stenosis. Am. J. Path., *12*:573, 1936.
1437. Wood, P.: An appreciation of mitral stenosis. I. Clinical features. Brit. Med. J., *1*:1051, 1954.
1438. Gough, J.: Diseases of the lung: The lungs in mitral stenosis. In: Harrison, C. V. (ed.): *Recent Advances in Pathology*. 7th ed. London, J. & A. Churchill, 1960, p. 57.
1439. Lendrum, A. C.: Pulmonary haemosiderosis: Pathological aspects. Proc. Roy. Soc. Med. (London), *53*:338, 1960.
1440. Heath, D., and Hicken, P.: The relation between atrial hypertension and lymphatic distension in lung biopsies. Thorax, *15*:54, 1960.
1441. Hicks, J. D.: Acute arterial necrosis in the lungs. J. Path. Bact., *65*:333, 1953.
1442. Whitaker, W., Black, A., and Warrack, A. J. N.: Pulmonary ossification in patients with mitral stenosis. J. Fac. Radiologists, *7*:29, 1955.
1443. Harrison, C. V.: Diseases of arteries: Pulmonary hypertension and arteriosclerosis. In: Harrison, C. V. (ed.): *Recent Advances in Pathology*. 7th ed. London, J. & A. Churchill, 1960, p. 160.
1444. Harrison, C. V.: IV. The pathology of the pulmonary vessels in pulmonary hypertension. In: *Pulmonary Hypertension: A Symposium*. Brit. J. Radiol., *31*:217, 1958.
1445. Heath, D., and Edwards, J. E.: The pathology of hypertensive pulmonary vascular disease. A description of six grades of structural changes in the pulmonary arteries with

special reference to congenital cardiac septal defects. Circulation, *18*:533, 1958.
1446. Bland, E. F., and Sweet, R. H.: A venous shunt for advanced mitral stenosis. J.A.M.A., *140*:1259, 1949.
1447. Ferguson, F. C., Kobilak, R. E., and Deitrick, J. E.: Varices of the bronchial veins as a source of hemoptysis in mitral stenosis. Am. Heart J., *28*:445, 1944.
1448. Broustet, P., Bricaut, H., and Mullon, P.: La circulation bronchique du poumon mitral. Arch. Mal. Coeur, *50*:522, 1957.
1449. Soulié, P., Baillet, J., Carlotti, J., Chiche, P., Picard, R., Servelle, M., and Voci, G.: Le poumon des mitraux. Essai de confrontation anatomo-physiologique. Arch. Mal. Coeur, *46*:393, 1953.
1450. Lewis, B. M., Gorlin, R., Houssay, H. E. J., Haynes, F. W., and Dexter, L.: Clinical and physiological correlations in patients with mitral stenosis. V. Am. Heart J., *43*:2, 1952.
1451. Ellis, L. B., Bloomfield, R. A., Graham, G. K., Greenberg, D. J., Hultgren, H. N., Kraus, H., Maresh, G., Mebane, J. G., Pfeiffer, P. H., Selverstone, L. A., and Taylor, J. A.: Studies in mitral stenosis. 1. A correlation of physiologic and clinical findings. A.M.A. Arch. Int. Med., *88*:515, 1951.
1452. Curti, P. C., Cohen, G., Castleman, B., Scannell, J. G., Friedlich, A. L., and Myers, G. S.: Respiratory and circulatory studies of patients with mitral stenosis. Circulation, *8*:893, 1953.
1453. Donald, K. W., Bishop, J. M., Wade, O. L., and Wormald, P. N.: Cardio-respiratory function two years after mitral valvotomy. Clin. Sci., *16*:325, 1957.
1454. Lammerant, J.: *Le Volume Sanguin des Poumons Chez l'Homme*. Brussels, Editions Arscia, 1957.
1455. Rapaport, E., Kuida, H., Haynes, F. W., and Dexter, L.: The pulmonary blood volume in mitral stenosis. J. Clin. Invest., *35*:1393, 1956.
1456. Ball, J. D., Kopelman, H., and Witham, A. C.: Circulatory changes in mitral stenosis at rest and on exercise. Brit. Heart J., *14*:363, 1952.
1457. Donald, K. W.: Exercise and heart disease. A study in regional circulation. Brit. Med. J., *1*:985, 1959.
1458. Charms, B. L., Brofman, B. L., and Kohn, P. M.: Pulmonary resistance in acquired heart disease. Circulation, *20*:850, 1959.
1459. Peabody, F. W.: Clinical studies on the respiration. III. A mechanical factor in the production of dyspnea in patients with cardiac disease. Arch. Int. Med., *20*:433, 1917.
1460. Krautwald, A., Garten, J., Hähnel, H., Kiessling, J., Kolmar, D., and Lichterfeld, A.: Ventilationsfunktion und Hämodynamik bei Mitralstenosen. Z. Kreislaufforsch., *50*:340, 1961.
1461. Palmer, W. H., Gee, J. B. L., Mills, F. C., and Bates, D. V.: Disturbances of pulmonary function in mitral valve disease. Canad. M. A. J., *89*:744, 1963.
1462. Englert, M., and Denolin, H.: Étude par la méthode a l'hélium de la ventilation pulmonaire interne dans la sténose mitrale. Acta Cardiol., *11*:365, 1965.
1463. Mürtz, R., and Eckern, E. T.: Zur Lungenfunktion bei Herz- und Lungenkranken unter besonderer Berücksichtigung der ventilatorischen Verteilungsstörung. Z. Kreislaufforsch., *50*:668, 1961.
1464. Friedman, B. L., Macias, J. J., and Yu, P. N.: Pulmonary function studies in patients with mitral stenosis. Am. Rev. Tuberc., *79*:265, 1959.
1465. Frank, N. R., Cugell, D. W., Gaensler, E. A., and Ellis, L. B.: Ventilatory studies in mitral stenosis. A comparison with findings in primary pulmonary disease. Am. J. Med., *15*:60, 1953.
1466. Garbagni, R., Angelino, P. F., Brusca, A., and Minetto, E.: Residual lung volume in mitral disease. Brit. Heart J., *20*:479, 1958.
1467. Dogliotti, G. C., Angelino, P. F., Brusca, A., Garbagni, R., Gavosto, F., Magri, G., and Minetto, E.: Pulmonary function in mitral valve disease. Hemodynamic and ventilatory studies. Am. J. Cardiol., *3*:28, 1959.
1468. Carroll, D., Cohn, J. E., and Riley, R. L.: Pulmonary function in mitral valvular disease: Distribution and diffusion characteristics in resting patients. J. Clin. Invest., *32*:510, 1953.
1469. Stock, J. P. P., and Kennedy, M. C. S.: The quantitative assessment of disability in mitral stenosis. Lancet, *2*:5, 1953.
1470. Lowther, C. P., and Turner, R. W. D.: Deterioration after mitral valvotomy. Brit. Med. J., *1*:1027, 1102, 1962.
1471. Bühlmann, A., Behn, H., and Schuppli, M.: Die Lungenfunktion bei chronischer Lungenstauung unter besonderer Berücksichtigung der Atemmechanik. Ein Beitrag zur Ätiologie der kardialen Dyspnoe. Schweiz. Med. Wchnschr., *89*:37, 1959.
1472. Turino, G. M., and Fishman, A. P.: The congested lung. J. Chron. Dis., *9*:510, 1959.
1473. Marshall, R., and Widdicombe, J. G.: The activity of pulmonary stretch receptors during congestion of the lungs. Quart. J. Exper. Physiol., *43*:320, 1958.
1474. Pauli, H. G., Noe, F. E., and Coates, E. O.: The ventilatory response to carbon dioxide in mitral disease. Brit. Heart J., *22*:255, 1960.
1475. Blount, S. G., Jr., McCord, M. C., and Anderson, L. L.: The alveolar-arterial oxygen pressure gradient in mitral stenosis. J. Clin. Invest., *31*:840, 1952.
1476. Miyamoto, S., Sezai, Y., Kanita, K., Hirota, Y., and Sakano, Y.: Disturbance of pulmonary diffusing capacity in mitral stenosis. Resp. Circ., *10*:233, 1962.
1477. Denolin, H., Englert, M., and De Coster, A.: La diffusion alvéolo-capillaire dans les cardiopathies. Poumon Coeur, *16*:1131, 1960.
1478. Kanagami, H., Katsuura, T., Shiroishi, K., Baba, K., Ogata, K., Tanaka, M., Watanabe, K., and Yanagihara, H.: CO pulmonary diffusing capacity in heart diseases. Resp. Circ., *10*:249, 1962.
1479. Fowler, N. O., Cubberly, R., and Dorney, E.: Pulmonary blood distribution and oxygen diffusion in mitral stenosis. Am. Heart J., *48*:1, 1954.
1480. Williams, M. H., Jr.: Pulmonary function studies in mitral stenosis before and after commissurotomy. J. Clin. Invest., *32*:1094, 1953.
1481. Cosby, R. S., Stowell, E. C., Jr., Hartwig, W. R., and Mayo, M.: Pulmonary function in left ventricular failure, including cardiac asthma. Circulation, *15*:492, 1957.
1482. Donald, K. W., Bishop, J. M., and Wade, O. L.: A study of minute to minute changes of arteriovenous oxygen content difference, oxygen uptake and cardiac output and rate of achievement of a steady state during exercise in rheumatic heart disease. J. Clin. Invest., *33*:1146, 1954.
1483. Lindgren, Å.: Studies on oxygen consumption, pulmonary ventilation and ventilation equivalent for oxygen at rest and after work in healthy persons and in cases of heart disease. Cardiologia, *23*:220, 1953.
1484. Ebnother, C. L., Selzer, A., Stone, A. O., and Feichtmier, T. V.: The ventilatory response to exercise in patients with mitral stenosis and its relationship to circulatory dynamics. Am. J. Med. Sci., *233*:46, 1957.
1485. Sinnott, J. C.: The control of pulmonary ventilation in physiological hyperpnea. Canad. M. A. J., *84*:471, 1961.
1486. Bishop, J. M., Harris, P., Bateman, M., and Raine, J. M.: Respiratory gas exchange in mitral stenosis at three levels of inspired oxygen before and after the infusion of acetylcholine. Clin. Sci., *22*:53, 1962.
1487. Bishop, J. M., Harris, P., Bateman, M., and Davidson, L. A. G.: The effect of acetylcholine upon respiratory gas exchange in mitral stenosis. J. Clin. Invest., *40*:105, 1961.
1488. Cook, C. D., Mead, J., Schreiner, G. L., Frank, N. R., and Craig, J. M.: Pulmonary mechanics during induced pulmonary edema in anesthetized dogs. J. Appl. Physiol., *14*:177, 1959.
1489. Braun, K.: Regulation of the pulmonary circulation in mitral stenosis. Acta Med. Orient., *16*:118, 1957.
1490. Söderholm, B., Werkö, L., and Widimský, J.: The effect of acetylcholine on pulmonary circulation and gas exchange in cases of mitral stenosis. Acta Med. Scand., *172*:95, 1962.
1491. Holling, H. E., and Venner, A.: Disability and circulatory changes in mitral stenosis. Brit. Heart J., *18*:103, 1956.
1492. Williams, M. H., Jr.: Effect of ANTU-induced pulmonary

edema on the alveolar arterial oxygen pressure gradient in dogs. Am. J. Physiol., *175*:84, 1953.
1493. Sharp, J. T., Bunnell, I. L., Griffith, G. T., and Greene, D. G.: The effects of therapy on pulmonary mechanics in human pulmonary edema. J. Clin. Invest., *40*:665, 1961.
1494. Sharp, J. T., Griffith, G. T., Bunnell, I. L., and Greene, D. G.: Ventilatory mechanics in pulmonary edema in man. J. Clin. Invest., *37*:111, 1958.
1495. von Basch, S.: Über cardiale Dyspnoe. In: *Verh. VIII Kongr. für innere Med., Wiesbaden, 1889*. Centralbl. Klin. Med., *10*: suppl. 28, p. 51, 1889.
1496. Cheyne, J.: A case of apoplexy in which the fleshy part of the heart was converted into fat. Dublin Hosp. Rep., *2*:216, 1818.
1497. Douglas, C. G., and Haldane, J. S.: The causes of periodic or Cheyne-Stokes breathing. J. Physiol. (London), *38*:401, 1909.
1498. Biot, J. B.: Mémoire sur la nature de l'air contenu dans la vessie natatoire des poissons. Mem. Phys. Chim. Soc. Arcueil, *1*:252, 1807.
1499. Pryor, W. W.: Cheyne-Stokes respiration in patients with cardiac enlargement and prolonged circulation time. Circulation, *4*:233, 1951.
1500. Mendel, D., and McIlroy, M. B.: The mechanical properties of the lungs in patients with periodic breathing. Brit. Heart J., *19*:399, 1957.
1501. Guyton, A. C., Crowell, J. W., and Moore, J. W.: Basic oscillating mechanism of Cheyne-Stokes breathing. Am. J. Physiol., *187*:395, 1956.
1502. Lange, R. L., and Hecht, H. H.: The mechanism of Cheyne-Stokes respiration. J. Clin. Invest., *41*:42, 1962.
1503. Stokes, W.: *The Diseases of the Heart and the Aorta*. Dublin, Hodges & Smith; Philadelphia, Lindsay & Blakiston, 1854, ch. 5, p. 302.
1504. Ebert, R. V.: The lung in congestive heart failure. Arch. Int. Med., *107*:450, 1961.
1505. Girgis, B.: Pulmonary heart disease due to bilharzia: the bilharzial cor pulmonale. A clinical study of twenty cases. Am. Heart J., *43*:606, 1952.
1506. Cortes, F. M., and Winters, W. L.: Schistosomiasis cor pulmonale. Am. J. Med., *31*:808, 1961.
1507. Rodríguez, H. F., and Rivera, E.: Pulmonary schistosomiasis. New Engl. J. Med., *258*:1196, 1958.
1508. Zaky, H. A., El-Heneidy, A. R., and Foda, M. T.: Haemodynamic shunts in schistosomal cor pulmonale. Brit. Med. J., *1*:367, 1962.
1509. Farid, Z., Greer, J. W., Ishak, K. G., El Nagah, A. M., LeGolvan, P. C., and Mousa, A. H.: Chronic pulmonary schistosomiasis. Am. Rev. Tuberc., *79*:119, 1959.
1510. Marchand, E. J., Marcial-Rojas, R. A., Rodríguez, R., Polanco, G., and Díaz-Rivera, R. S.: The pulmonary obstruction syndrome in Schistosoma mansoni pulmonary endarteritis: Report of five cases. A.M.A. Arch. Int. Med., *100*:965, 1957.
1511. Comroe, J. H., Jr.: Physiologic aspects of pulmonary embolism. In: Comroe, J. H., Jr., *et al.* (eds.): *Advances in Medicine and Surgery*. Philadelphia, W. B. Saunders Co., 1952, p. 238.
1512. Dunér, H., Pernow, B., and Rignér, K. G.: The prognosis of pulmonary embolism. A medical and physiological follow-up examination of patients treated at the Departments of Internal Medicine and Surgery, Karolinska Sjukhuset, in 1952–1958. Acta Med. Scand., *168*:381, 1960.
1513. Roh, C. E., Greene, D. G., Himmelstein, A., Humphreys, G. H., III, and Baldwin, E. de F.: Cardiopulmonary function studies in a patient with ligation of the left pulmonary artery. Am. J. Med., *6*:795, 1949.
1514. Landrigan, P. L., Purkis, I. E., Roy, D. E., and Cudkowicz, L.: Cardio-respiratory studies in a patient with an absent left pulmonary artery. Thorax, *18*:77, 1963.
1515. Robin, E. D., Forkner, C. E., Jr., Bromberg, P. A., Croteau, J. R., and Travis, D. M.: Alveolar gas exchange in clinical pulmonary embolism. New Engl. J. Med., *262*:283, 1960.
1516. Colp, C. R., and Williams, M. H., Jr.: Pulmonary function following pulmonary embolization. Am. Rev. Resp. Dis., *85*:799, 1962.
1517. Sadoul, P., Faivre, G., Gilgenkrantz, J. M., Cherrier, F., and Saunier, C.: Étude de la fonction respiratoire dans le cœur pulmonaire chronique post-embolique. L. Franc. Med. Chir. Thorac., *16*:433, 1962.
1518. McIlroy, M. B., and Apthorp, G. H.: Pulmonary function in pulmonary hypertension. Brit. Heart J., *20*:397, 1958.
1519. Robin, E. D.: Some aspects of the physiologic disturbances associated with pulmonary embolism. Med. Clin. N. Am., *44*:1269, 1960.
1520. Julian, D. G., Travis, D. M., Robin, E. D., and Crump, C. H.: Effect of pulmonary artery occlusion upon end-tidal CO_2 tension. J. Appl. Physiol., *15*:87, 1960.
1521. Yu, P. N.: Primary pulmonary hypertension: Report of six cases and review of literature. Ann. Int. Med., *49*:1138, 1958.
1522. Colebatch, H. J. H., and DeKock, M. A.: Histamine release in embolism of the lung with barium sulphate. Fed. Proc., *22*:282, 1963.
1523. Halmagyi, D. F. J., and Colebatch, H. J. H.: Cardiorespiratory effects of experimental lung embolism. J. Clin. Invest., *40*:1785, 1961.
1524. Jonsson, B., Linderholm, H., and Pinardi, G.: Atrial septal defect: A study of physical working capacity and hemodynamics during exercise. Acta Med. Scand., *159*:275, 1957.
1525. Bedell, G. N.: Comparison of pulmonary diffusing capacity in normal subjects and in patients with intracardiac septal defects. J. Lab. Clin. Med., *57*:269, 1961.
1526. Morse, M., and Cassels, D. E.: Arterial blood gases and acid-base balance in cyanotic congenital heart disease. J. Clin. Invest., *32*:837, 1953.
1527. Cruickshank, B.: Rheumatoid arthritis and rheumatoid disease. In: *Discussion on Rheumatoid Disease*. Proc. Roy. Soc. Med. (London), *50*:462, 1957.
1528. Baggenstoss, A. H., and Rosenberg, E. F.: Visceral lesions associated with chronic infectious (rheumatoid) arthritis. Arch. Path., *35*:503, 1943.
1529. Christie, G. S.: Pulmonary lesions in rheumatoid arthritis. Aust. Ann. Med., *3*:49, 1954.
1530. Bennett, G. A., Zeller, J. W., and Bauer, W.: Subcutaneous nodules of rheumatoid arthritis and rheumatic fever. A pathologic study. Arch. Path., *30*:70, 1940.
1531. Raven, R. W., Weber, F. P., and Price, L. W.: The necrobiotic nodules of rheumatoid arthritis. Case in which the scalp, abdominal wall (involving striped muscle), larynx, pericardium (involving myocardium), pleurae (involving lungs), and peritoneum were affected. Ann. Rheum. Dis., *7*:63, 1948.
1532. Caplan, A.: Certain unusual radiological appearances in the chest of coal-miners suffering from rheumatoid arthritis. Thorax, *8*:29, 1953.
1533. Caplan, A.: Rheumatoid disease and pneumoconiosis (Caplan's syndrome). Proc. Roy. Soc. Med. (London), *52*:1111, 1959.
1534. Gough, J., Rivers, D., and Seal, R. M. E.: Pathological studies of modified pneumoconiosis in coal-miners with rheumatoid arthritis (Caplan's syndrome). Thorax, *10*:9, 1955.
1535. Gray, A.: Maximum ventilatory capacity of Africans. Cent. Afr. J. Med., *2*:107, 1956.
1536. Papp, O. A.: Control of respiration: Role of the pressure in the atria and pulmonary artery. Thesis for Diploma in Internal Medicine, McGill University, Montreal, 1962.
1537. Sieker, H. O., Estes, E. H., Jr., Kelser, G. A., and McIntosh, H. D.: A cardiopulmonary syndrome associated with extreme obesity. J. Clin. Invest., *34*:916, 1955.
1538. Auchincloss, J. H., Jr., Cook, E., and Renzetti, A. D.: Clinical and physiological aspects of a case of obesity polycythemia and alveolar hypoventilation. J. Clin. Invest., *34*:1537, 1955.
1539. Carroll, D.: A peculiar type of cardiopulmonary failure associated with obesity. Am. J. Med., *21*:819, 1956.
1540. Ratto, O., Briscoe, W. A., Morton, J. W., and Comroe, J. H., Jr.: Anoxemia secondary to polycythemia and polycythemia secondary to anoxemia. Am. J. Med., *19*:958, 1955.
1541. Lambertsen, C. J.: Carbon dioxide and respiration in acid-base homeostasis. Anesthesiology, *21*:642, 1960.

1542. Fisher, J. M., Bedell, G. N., and Seebohm, P. M.: Differentiation of polycythemia vera and secondary polycythemia by arterial oxygen saturation and pulmonary function tests. J. Lab. Clin. Med., *50:*455, 1957.
1543. Rodman, T., Resnick, M. E., Berkowitz, R. D., Fennelly, J. F., and Olivia, J.: Alveolar hypoventilation due to involvement of the respiratory center by obscure disease of the central nervous system. Am. J. Med., *32:*208, 1962.
1544. Pare, P., and Lowenstein, L.: Polycythemia associated with disturbed function of the respiratory center. Blood, *11:*1077, 1956.
1545. Lawrence, L. T.: Idiopathic hypoventilation, polycythemia, and cor pulmonale. Am. Rev. Resp. Dis., *80:*575, 1959.
1546. Richter, T., West, J. R., and Fishman, A. P.: The syndrome of alveolar hypoventilation and diminished sensitivity of the respiratory center. New Engl. J. Med., *256:*1165, 1957.
1547. Garlind, T., and Linderholm, H.: Hypoventilation syndrome in a case of chronic epidemic encephalitis. Acta Med. Scand., *162:*333, 1958.
1548. Dalhamn, T.: Mucous flow and ciliary activity in the trachea of healthy rats and rats exposed to respiratory irritant gases (SO_2, H_3N, HCHO). A functional and morphologic (light microscopic and electron microscopic) study, with special reference to technique. Acta Physiol. Scand., *36:* suppl. 123, 1956.
1549. Frank, N. R., Amdur, M. O., Worcester, J., and Whittenberger, J. L.: Effects of acute controlled exposure to SO_2 on respiratory mechanics in healthy male adults. J. Appl. Physiol., *17:*252, 1962.
1550. Walker, J. E. C., and Wells, R. E., Jr.: Heat and water exchange in the respiratory tract. Am. J. Med., *30:*259, 1961.
1551. Wells, R. E., Jr., Walker, J. E. C., and Hickler, R. B.: Effects of cold air on respiratory airflow resistance in patients with respiratory-tract disease. New Engl. J. Med., *263:*268, 1960.
1552. Moyer, J. H., Glantz, G., and Brest, A. N.: Pulmonary arteriovenous fistulas. Physiologic and clinical considerations. Am. J. Med., *32:*417, 1962.
1553. Apthorp, G. H., and Bates, D. V.: Report of a case of pulmonary telangiectasia. Thorax, *12:*63, 1957.
1554. Rose, G. A., and Spencer, H.: Polyarteritis nodosa. Quart. J. Med., *(n.s.)26:*43, 1957.
1555. Zeek, P. M.: Periarteritis nodosa: A critical review. Am. J. Clin. Path., *22:*777, 1952.
1556. Churg, J., and Strauss, L.: Allergic granulomatosis, allergic angiitis, and periarteritis nodosa. Am. J. Path., *27:*277, 1951.
1557. von Meyenburg, H.: Das eosinophile Lungeninfiltrat: Pathologische Anatomie und Pathogenese. Schweiz. Med. Wchnschr., *72:*809, 1942.
1558. Soergel, K. H., and Sommers, S. C.: Idiopathic pulmonary hemosiderosis and related syndromes. Am. J. Med., *32:*499, 1962.
1559. McCaughey, W. T. E., and Thomas, B. J.: Pulmonary hemorrhage and glomerulonephritis. The relation of pulmonary hemorrhage to certain types of glomerular lesions. Am. J. Clin. Path., *38:*577, 1962.
1560. Rusby, N. L., and Wilson, C.: Lung purpura with nephritis. Quart. J. Med., *(n.s.)29:*501, 1960.
1561. Godman, G. C., and Churg, J.: Wegener's granulomatosis. Pathology and review of the literature. A.M.A. Arch. Path., *58:*533, 1954.
1562. Leggat, P. O., and Walton, E. W.: Wegener's granulomatosis. Thorax, *11:*94, 1956.
1563. Fahey, J. L., Leonard, E., Churg, J., and Godman, G.: Wegener's granulomatosis. Am. J. Med., *17:*168, 1954.
1564. Klinger, H.: Grenzformen der Periarteritis nodosa. Frankfurt, Z. Path., *42:*455, 1931.
1565. Wegener, F.: Über generalisierte, septische Gefässerkrankungen. Verh. Deutsch. Ges. Path., *29:*202, 1936.
1566. Thomas, A. M.: A case of Wegener's granulomatosis. J. Clin. Path., *11:*146, 1958.
1567. Richards, B. T., Razavi, M., and Leftwich, W. B.: Wegener's granulomatosis with severe hemoptysis. Am. Rev. Resp. Dis., *85:*890, 1962.
1568. Schuler, D.: Essential pulmonary hemosiderosis. Ann. Paediat., *192:*107, 1959.
1569. Smith, W. E., and Fienberg, R.: Early nonrecurrent idiopathic pulmonary hemosiderosis in an adult. Report of a case. New Engl. J. Med., *259:*808, 1958.
1570. Scheidegger, S., and Dreyfus, A.: Braune Lungeninduration des Kindes mit sekundärer Anämie. Ann. Paediat., *165:*2, 1945.
1571. Heptinstall, R. H., and Salmon, M. V.: Pulmonary haemorrhage with extensive glomerular disease of the kidney. J. Clin. Path., *12:*272, 1959.
1572. Soergel, K. H.: Idiopathic pulmonary hemosiderosis. Review and report of two cases. Pediatrics, *19:*1101, 1957.
1573. Glanzmann, E., and Walthard, B.: Idiopathische progressive braune Lungeninduration im Kindesalter mit hereditären Hämoptyse, intermittierender sekundärer Anämie und Eosinophilie und embolischer Herdnephritis. Monatsschr. Kinderheilk., *88:*1, 1941.
1574. Anspach, W. E.: Pulmonary hemosiderosis. Am. J. Roentgenol., *41:*592, 1939.
1575. Bruwer, A. J., Kennedy, R. L. J., and Edwards, J. E.: Recurrent pulmonary hemorrhage with hemosiderosis: so-called idiopathic pulmonary hemosiderosis. Am. J. Roentgenol., *76:*98, 1956.
1576. Steiner, B.: The value of splenectomy in the treatment of essential pulmonary haemosiderosis. Acta Med. Acad. Sci. Hung., *14:*211, 1959.
1577. Pilcher, J. D., and Eitzen, O. E.: Pulmonary hemosiderosis in a six year old boy. A clinical and pathologic report. Am. J. Dis. Child., *67:*387, 1944.
1578. Herzog, E.: Zum Wesen der sog. idiopathischen Haemosiderosis pulmonum. Ber. Oberheiss. Ges. Natur- Heilk. Giessen, Naturw. Abt. *27:*199, 1954.
1579. Doering, P., and Gothe, H. D.: Die idiopathische Lungenhämosiderose, klinische Beobachtungen und radiologische Untersuchungen mit Eisen[59] bei einem 17jährigen Patienten. Klin. Wchnschr., *35:*1105, 1957.
1580. Moersch, H. J., Purnell, D. C., and Good, C. A.: Pulmonary changes occurring in disseminated lupus erythematosus. Dis. Chest., *29:*166, 1956.
1581. Purnell, D. C., Baggenstoss, A. H., and Olsen, A. M.: Pulmonary lesions in disseminated lupus erythematosus. Ann. Int. Med., *42:*619, 1955.
1582. Teilum, G.: Pathogenetic studies on lupus erythematosus disseminatus and related diseases. Acta Med. Scand., *123:*126, 1946.
1583. Rakov, H. L., and Taylor, J. S.: Acute disseminated lupus erythematosus without cutaneous manifestations and with heretofore undescribed pulmonary lesions. Arch. Int. Med., *70:*88, 1942.
1584. Bader, M. E., Bader, R. A., and Selikoff, I. J.: Pulmonary function in asbestosis of the lungs. An alveolar-capillary block syndrome. Am. J. Med., *30:*235, 1961.
1585. Becklake, M. R., du Preez, L., and Lutz, W.: Lung function in silicosis of the Witwatersrand gold miner. Am. Rev. Tuberc., *77:*400, 1958.
1586. Bouhuys, A., Lindell, S. E., and Lundin, G.: Experimental studies on byssinosis. Brit. Med. J., *1:*324, 1960.
1587. Bruce, R. A., Lovejoy, F. W., Jr., Yu, P. N. G., Pearson, R., and McDowell, M.: Further observations on the pathological physiology of chronic pulmonary granulomatosis associated with beryllium workers. Am. Rev. Tuberc., *62:*29, 1950.
1588. Buechner, H. A., Prevatt, A. L., Thompson, J., and Blitz, O.: Bagassosis. A review, with further historical data, studies of pulmonary function, and results of adrenal steroid therapy. Am. J. Med., *25:*234, 1958.
1589. Gaensler, E. A., Verstraeten, J. M., Weil, W. B., Cugell, D. W., Marks, A., Cadigan, J. B., Jr., Jones, R. H., and Ellicott, M. F.: Respiratory pathophysiology in chronic beryllium disease. Review of thirty cases with some observations after long-term steroid therapy. A.M.A. Arch. Indust. Health, *19:*132, 1959.
1590. Gilson, J. C., Stott, H., Hopwood, B. E. C., Roach, S. A., McKerrow, C. B., and Schilling, R. S. F.: Byssinosis: The acute effect on ventilatory capacity of dusts in cotton ginneries, cotton, sisal, and jute mills. Brit. J. Indust. Med., *19:*9, 1962.

1591. Jordan, J. W.: Pulmonary fibrosis in a worker using an aluminum powder. Brit. J. Indust. Med., *18*:21, 1961.
1592. Kaltreider, N. L., and McCann, W. S.: Respiratory response during exercise in pulmonary fibrosis and emphysema. J. Clin. Invest., *16*:23, 1937.
1593. Oliner, H., Schwartz, R., Rubio, F., Jr., and Damashek, W.: Interstitial pulmonary fibrosis following busulfan therapy. Am. J. Med., *31*:134, 1961.
1594. Leathart, G. L.: The mechanical properties of the lung pneumoconiosis of coal-miners. Brit. J. Indust. Med., *16*:153, 1959.
1595. Leathart, G. L.: Clinical, bronchographic, radiological and physiological observations in ten cases of asbestosis. Brit. J. Indust. Med., *17*:213, 1960.
1596. McKerrow, C. B., McDermott, M., Gilson, J. C., and Schilling, R. S. F.: Respiratory function during the day in cotton workers: A study in byssinosis. Brit. J. Indust. Med., *15*:75, 1958.
1597. Robertson, A. J., Rivers, D., Nagelschmidt, G., and Duncumb, P.: Stannosis: Benign pneumoconiosis due to tin dioxide. Lancet, *1*:1089, 1961.
1598. Schilling, R. S. F.: Byssinosis in cotton and other textile workers. [Milroy Lectures.] Lancet, *2*:261, 319, 1956.
1599. Wright, G. W., and Filley, G. F.: Pulmonary fibrosis and respiratory function. Am. J. Med., *10*:642, 1951.
1600. Zohman, L. R., and Williams, M. H., Jr.: Cardiopulmonary function in pulmonary fibrosis. Am. Rev. Resp. Dis., *80*:700, 1959.
1601. Meiklejohn, A.: The origin of the term "pneumonokoniosis." Brit. J. Indust. Med., *17*:155, 1960.
1602. Enzer, N., and Sander, O. A.: Chronic lung changes in electric arc welders. J. Indust. Hyg. & Toxicol., *20*:333, 1938.
1603. Doig, A. T., and McLaughlin, A. I. G.: X ray appearances of the lungs of electric arc welders. Lancet, *1*:771, 1936.
1604. Young, W. A., Shaw, D. B., and Bates, D. V.: Pulmonary function in welders exposed to ozone. Arch. Environ. Health, *7*:337, 1963.
1605. Stewart, M. J., and Faulds, J. S.: The pulmonary fibrosis of haematite miners. J. Path. Bact., *39*:233, 1934.
1606. Gilson, J. C.: The disturbance of pulmonary function in industrial pulmonary disease. In: King, E. J., and Fletcher, C. M. (eds.): *A Symposium on Industrial Pulmonary Diseases.* London, J. & A. Churchill, 1960, p. 110.
1607. Pendergrass, E. P., and Leopold, S. S.: Benign pneumoconiosis. J.A.M.A., *127*:701, 1945.
1608. Heppleston, A. G.: The pathological anatomy of simple pneumokoniosis in coal workers. J. Path. Bact., *66*:235, 1953.
1609. Cochrane, A. L.: The attack rate of progressive massive fibrosis. Brit. J. Indust. Med., *19*:52, 1962.
1610. James, W. R. L.: The relationship of tuberculosis to the development of massive pneumokoniosis in coal workers. Brit. J. Tuberc., *48*:89, 1954.
1611. Carpenter, R. G., Cochrane, A. L., Gilson, J. C,, and Higgins, I. T. T.: The relationship between ventilatory capacity and simple pneumoconiosis in coalworkers. The effect of population selection. Brit. J. Indust. Med., *13*:166, 1956.
1612. Motley, H. L., Lang, L. P., and Gordon, B.: Pulmonary emphysema and ventilation measurements in one hundred anthracite coal miners with respiratory complaints. Am. Rev. Tuberc., *59*:270, 1949.
1613. Motley, H. L.: The pneumoconioses. In: Gordon, B. L. (ed.): *Clinical Cardiopulmonary Physiology.* 2nd rev. ed. New York, Grune & Stratton, 1960, p. 841.
1614. Motley, H. L., and Tomashefski, J. F.: Effect of high and low oxygen levels and intermittent positive pressure breathing on oxygen transport in the lungs in pulmonary fibrosis and emphysema. J. Appl. Physiol., *3*:189, 1950.
1615. Watson, A. J., Black, J., Doig, A. T., and Nagelschmidt, G.: Pneumoconiosis in carbon electrode makers. Brit. J. Indust. Med., *16*:274, 1959.
1616. Davies, C. N.: Pneumoconiosis, silicosis, and the physics and chemistry of dust. Ann. Rev. Med., *8*:323, 1957.
1617. King, E. J., and Nagelschmidt, G.: The physical and chemical properties of silica, silicates and modified forms of these in relation to pathogenic effects. In: Orenstein, A. J. (ed.): *Proceedings of the Pneumoconiosis Conference, Johannesburg, 1959.* London, J. & A. Churchill, 1960, p. 78.
1618. Gilson, J. C.: Industrial pulmonary disease. In: Schilling, R. S. F. (ed.): *Modern Trends in Occupational Health.* London, Butterworth & Co., 1960, p. 50.
1619. Vorwald, A. J.: Inhaled submicroscopic particles in the pathogenesis and pathology of silicosis. In: Orenstein, A. J. (ed.): *Proceedings of the Pneumoconiosis Conference, Johannesburg, 1959.* London, J. & A. Churchill, 1960, p. 137.
1620. Rossier, P. H., Bühlmann, A., and Luchsinger, P.: Die Pathophysiologie der Atmung bei der Silikose und die Begutachtung der Arbeitsfähigkeit. Deutsch. Med. Wchnschr., *80*:608, 1955.
1621. Lavenne, F.: Le retentissement cardio-vasculaire de la silicose et de l'anthraco-silicose. Contribution á l'étude du "cor pulmonale." Rev. Belge Path., *21*: suppl. 6, 1951.
1622. Lynch, K. M.: Pathology of asbestosis. A.M.A. Arch. Indust. Health, *11*:185, 1955.
1623. Beattie, J.: The asbestosis body. In: Davies, C. N. (ed.): *Inhaled Particles and Vapours.* New York, Pergamon Press, 1961, p. 434.
1624. Wagner, J. C., Sleggs, C. A., and Marchand, P.: Diffuse pleural mesothelioma and asbestos exposure in the northwestern Cape Province. Brit. J. Indust. Med., *17*:260, 1960.
1625. Williams, R., and Hugh-Jones, P.: The radiological diagnosis of asbestosis. Thorax, *15*:103, 1960.
1626. Wright, G. W.: Functional abnormalities of industrial pulmonary fibrosis. A.M.A. Arch. Indust. Health, *11*:196, 1955.
1627. Saltzman, H. A., Heyman, A., and Sieker, H. O.: Correlation of clinical and physiologic manifestations of sustained hyperventilation. New Engl. J. Med., *268*:1431, 1963.
1628. Fletcher, C. M., Hugh-Jones, P., McNicol, M. W., and Pride, N. B.: The diagnosis of pulmonary emphysema in the presence of chronic bronchitis. Quart. J. Med., *(n.s.)32*:33, 1963.
1629. Denny, J. J., Robson, W. D., and Irwin, D. A.: The prevention of silicosis by metallic aluminum. I. A preliminary report. Canad. M. A. J., *37*:1, 1937.
1630. Kennedy, M. C. S.: Aluminum powder inhalations in the treatment of silicosis of pottery workers and pneumoconiosis of coal miners. Brit. J. Indust. Med., *13*:85, 1956.
1631. Shaver, C. G., and Riddell, A. R.: Lung changes associated with the manufacture of alumina abrasives. J. Indust. Hyg. & Toxicol., *29*:145, 1947.
1632. Riddell, A. R. Shaver's Disease: Clinical aspects of Shaver's disease. In: Vorwald, A. J. (ed.): *Pneumoconiosis: Beryllium; Bauxite Fumes; Compensation: Sixth Saranac Symposium.* New York, Hoeber (Harper), 1950, part VI, ch. 30, p. 459.
1633. Hatch, T.: Respiratory dust retention and elimination. In: Orenstein, A. J. (ed.): *Proceedings of the Pneumoconiosis Conference, Johannesburg, 1959.* London, J. & A. Churchill, 1960, p. 113.
1634. Wyatt, J. P., and Riddell, A. C. R.: The morphology of bauxite-fume pneumoconiosis. Am. J. Path., *25*:447, 1949.
1635. Hardy, H. L.: Beryllium disease: A continuing diagnostic problem. Am. J. Med. Sci., *242*:150, 1961.
1636. Dudley, H. R.: The pathologic changes of chronic beryllium disease. A.M.A. Arch. Indust. Health, *19*:184, 1959.
1637. Williams, W. J.: A histological study of the lungs in 52 cases of chronic beryllium disease. Brit. J. Indust. Med., *15*:84, 1958.
1638. Vorwald, A. J.: The beryllium problem: The chronic or delayed disease: Pathologic aspects. In: Vorwald, A. J. (ed.): *Pneumoconiosis: Beryllium; Bauxite Fumes; Compensation: Sixth Saranac Symposium.* New York, Hoeber (Harper), 1950, part III, ch. 11, p. 190.
1639. Hardy, H. L.: Differential diagnosis between beryllium poisoning and sarcoidosis. Am. Rev. Tuberc., *74*:885, 1956.
1640. Kennedy, B. J., Pare, J. A. P., Pump, K. K., Beck, J. C., Johnson, L. G., Epstein, N. B., Venning, E. H., and Browne, J. S. L.: Effect of adrenocorticotropic hormone (ACTH) on beryllium granulomatosis and silicosis. Am. J. Med., *10*:134, 1951.

1641. Ferris, B. G., Jr., Affeldt, J. E., Kriete, H. A., and Whittenberger, J. L.: Pulmonary function in patients with pulmonary disease treated with ACTH. A.M.A. Arch. Indust. Hyg., *3*:603, 1951.
1642. Sodeman, W. A., and Pullen, R. L.: Bagasse disease of the lungs. Arch. Int. Med., *73*:365, 1944.
1643. Hunter, D., and Perry, K. M. A.: Bronchiolitis resulting from the handling of bagasse. Brit. J. Indust. Med., *3*:64, 1946.
1644. Stott, H.: Pulmonary disease amongst sisal workers. Brit. J. Indust. Med., *15*:23, 1958.
1645. Hunter, D.: *The Diseases of Occupations.* 2nd ed. London, English Universities Press, 1957, p. 960.
1646. Towey, J. W., Sweany, H. C., and Huron, W. H.: Severe bronchial asthma apparently due to fungus spores found in maple bark. J.A.M.A., *99*:453, 1932.
1647. Farmer's lung again [Annotation]. Brit. Med. J., *1*:727, 1961.
1648. Campbell, J. M.: Acute symptoms following work with hay. Brit. Med. J., *2*:1143, 1932.
1649. Cadham, F. T.: Asthma due to grain rusts. J.A.M.A., *83*:27, 1924.
1650. Dickie, H. A., and Rankin, J.: Farmer's lung. An acute granulomatous interstitial pneumonitis occurring in agricultural workers. J.A.M.A., *167*:1069, 1958.
1651. Totten, R. S., Reid, D. H. S., Davis, H. D., and Moran, T. J.: Farmer's lung. Report of two cases in which lung biopsies were performed. Am. J. Med., *25*:803, 1958.
1652. Farmer's lung [Annotation]. Brit. Med. J., *2*:98, 1958.
1653. Staines, F. H., and Forman, J. A. S.: Farmer's lung again [Letter to the Editor]. Brit. Med. J., *1*:1110, 1961.
1654. Frank, R. C.: Farmer's lung—a form of pneumoconiosis due to organic dusts. Am. J. Roentgenol., *79*:189, 1958.
1655. Quinlan, J. J., and Hiltz, J. E.: Farmer's lung or bronchomycosis fenisecarum. Canad. M. A. J., *80*:261, 1959.
1656. Baldus, W. P., and Peter, J. B.: Farmer's lung. Report of two cases. New Engl. J. Med., *262*:700, 1960.
1657. Williams, D. I., and Mulhall, P. P.: Farmer's lung in Radnor and North Breconshire. A report of ten cases. Brit. Med. J., *2*:1216, 1956.
1658. Lowry, T., and Schuman, L. M.: "Silo filler's disease"—a syndrome caused by nitrogen dioxide. J.A.M.A., *162*:153, 1956.
1659. Becklake, M. R., Goldman, H. I., Bosman, A. R., and Freed, C. C.: The long-term effects of exposure to nitrous fumes. Am. Rev. Tuberc., *76*:398, 1957.
1660. Darke, C. S., and Warrack, A. J. N.: Bronchiolitis from nitrous fumes. Thorax, *13*:327, 1958.
1661. Nichols, B. H.: The clinical effects of the inhalation of nitrogen dioxide. Am. J. Roentgenol., *23*:516, 1930.
1662. Lépine, C., and Soucy, R.: La bronchopneumopathie d'origine toxique. Évolution physio-pathologique. Union Med. Canada, *91*:7, 1962.
1663. Troisi, F. M.: Delayed death caused by gassing in a silo containing green forage. Brit. J. Indust. Med., *14*:56, 1957.
1664. LaFleche, L. R., Boivin, C., and Leonard, C.: Nitrogen dioxide—a respiratory irritant. Canad. M. A. J., *84*:1438, 1961.
1665. Grayson, R. R.: Silage gas poisoning: Nitrogen dioxide pneumonia, a new disease in agricultural workers. Ann. Int. Med., *45*:393, 1956.
1666. McAdams, A. J., Jr.: Bronchiolitis obliterans, Am. J. Med., *19*:314, 1955.
1667. Leib, G. M. P., Davis, W. N., Brown, T., and McQuiggan, M.: Chronic pulmonary insufficiency secondary to silo-filler's disease. Am. J. Med., *24*:471, 1958.
1668. Brille, D., Hatzfeld, C., and Laurent, R.: Emphysème pulmonaire après inhalation de vapeurs irritantes. (Ammoniaque en particulier.) Arch. Mal. Prof., *18*:320, 1957.
1669. Lane, R. E., and Campbell, A. C. P.: Fatal emphysema in two men making a copper cadmium alloy. Brit. J. Indust. Med., *11*:118, 1954.
1670. Thurlbeck, W. M., and Foley, F. D.: Experimental pulmonary emphysema. The effect of intratracheal injection of cadmium chloride solution in the guinea pig. Am. J. Path., *42*:431, 1963.
1671. Bonnell, J. A.: Emphysema and proteinuria in men casting copper-cadmium alloys. Brit. J. Indust. Med., *12*:181, 1955.
1672. *Proceedings of the National Conference on Air Pollution, Washington, 1958.* Washington, D.C. U.S. Department of Health, Education, and Welfare (Public Health Service Publication No. 654), 1959.
1673. Young, W. A., Shaw, D. B., and Bates, D. V.: Presence of ozone in aircraft flying at 35,000 feet. Aerospace Med., *33*:311, 1962.
1674. Jaffe, L. S., and Estes, H. D.: Ozone toxicity hazard in cabins of high altitude aircraft—A review and current program. Aerospace Med., *34*:633, 1963.
1675. Charr, R.: Pulmonary changes in welders: A report of three cases. Ann. Int. Med., *44*:806, 1946.
1676. Charr, R.: Respiratory disorders among welders. Am. Rev. Tuberc., *71*:877, 1955.
1677. Mann, B. T., and Lecutier, E. R.: Arc-welders' lung. Brit. Med. J., *2*:921, 1957.
1678. Challen, P. J. R., Hickish, D. E., and Bedford, J.: An investigation of some health hazards in an inert-gas tungsten-arc welding shop. Brit. J. Indust. Med., *15*:276, 1958.
1679. Young, W. A., and Shaw, D. B.: Effect of low concentrations of ozone on pulmonary function. Fed. Proc., *22*:396, 1963.
1680. Ainsworth, R. W.: Petrol-vapour poisoning. Brit. Med. J., *1*:1547, 1960.
1681. Gardner, A. M. N.: Aspiration of food and vomit. Quart. J. Med., *(n.s.)27*:227, 1958.
1682. Lister, W. B.: Carbon pneumoconiosis in a synthetic graphite worker. Brit. J. Indust. Med., *18*:114, 1961.
1683. Tschumy, W., Jr.: Pulmonary infiltration with eosinophilia (Löffler's syndrome) due to smoke inhalation: Report of a case and comment on pathogenesis. Ann. Int. Med., *49*:665, 1958.
1684. Bentivoglio, L. G., Beerel, F., Stewart, P. B., Bryan, A. C., Ball, W. C., Jr., and Bates, D. V.: Studies of regional ventilation and perfusion in pulmonary emphysema using xenon^{133}. Am. Rev. Resp. Dis., *88*:315, 1963.
1685. Harold, J. T.: Lymphangitis carcinomatosa of the lungs. Quart. J. Med., *(n.s.)21*:353, 1952.
1686. Hauser, T. E., and Steer, A.: Lymphangitic carcinomatosis of the lungs: Six case reports and a review of the literature. Ann. Int. Med., *34*:881, 1951.
1687. Resnick, M. E., Berkowitz, R. D., and Rodman, T.: Diffuse interstitial leukemic infiltration of the lungs producing the alveolar-capillary block syndrome. Report of a case, with studies of pulmonary function. Am. J. Med., *31*:149, 1961.
1688. Green, R. A., Nichols, N. J., and King, E. J.: Alveolar-capillary block due to leukemic infiltration of the lung: Case report. Am. Rev. Resp. Dis., *80*:895, 1959.
1689. Green, R. A., and Nichols, N. J.: Pulmonary involvement in leukemia. Am. Rev. Resp. Dis., *80*:833, 1959.
1690. Laios, N. C., and Lovelock, F. J.: Eosinophilic granuloma of the lung: Case report. Am. Rev. Resp. Dis., *83*:394, 1961.
1691. Arany, L. S., and Baumwell, M.: Primary pulmonary histiocytosis X: Case report. Am. Rev. Resp. Dis., *82*:873, 1960.
1692. Auld, D.: Pathology of eosinophilic granuloma of the lung. Arch. Path., *63*:113, 1957.
1693. Currens, J., and Popp, W. C.: Xanthomatosis—Hand-Schüller-Christian type: Report of a case with pulmonary fibrosis. Am. J. Med. Sci., *205*:780, 1943.
1694. Cunningham, G. J., and Parkinson, T.: Diffuse cystic lungs of granulomatous origin. A histological study of six cases. Thorax, *5*:43, 1950.
1695. Engelbreth-Holm, J., Teilum, G., and Christensen, E.: Eosinophilic granuloma of bone—Schüller-Christian's disease. Acta Med. Scand., *118*:292, 1944.
1696. McKeown, F.: Letterer-Siwe disease: A report of two cases. J. Path. Bact., *68*:147, 1954.
1697. Bickers, J. N., Buechner, H. A., and Ekman, P. J.: Pulmonary histiocytosis X. A case report. Am. Rev. Resp. Dis., *85*:211, 1962.
1698. Mengis, C. L.: Eosinophilic granuloma confined to the lung. Report of a case. A.M.A. Arch. Int. Med., *104*:580, 1959.

1699. Crisler, E. C., Durant, J. R., and Parker, T. M.: Pulmonary histiocytosis X. A case report. Am. J. Roentgenol., *85*:271, 1961.
1700. Hoffman, L., Cohn, J. E., and Gaensler, E. A.: Respiratory abnormalities in eosinophilic granuloma of the lung. Long-term study of five cases. New Engl. J. Med., *267*:577, 1962.
1701. Arnett, N. L., and Schulz, D. M.: Primary pulmonary eosinophilic granuloma. Radiology, *69*:224, 1957.
1702. Thompson, J., Buechner, H. A., and Fishman, R.: Eosinophilic granuloma of the lung. Am. Int. Med., *48*:1134, 1958.
1703. May, I. A., Garfinkle, J. M., and Dugan, D. J.: Eosinophilic granuloma of lung: Report of three cases. Ann. Int. Med., *40*:549, 1954.
1704. McClement, J. H., Renzetti, A. D., Jr., Carroll, D., Himmelstein, A., and Cournand, A.: Cardiopulmonary function in hematogenous pulmonary tuberculosis in patients receiving streptomycin therapy. Am. Rev. Tuberc., *64*:583, 1951.
1705. Becklake, M. R.: Pneumoconiosis. In: *Handbook of Physiology*, Respiration Sect., vol. I.: Washington, American Physiological Society, ch. 73: 1964.
1706. Gaensler, E. A., Hoffman, L., and Elliott, M. F.: Troubles de la diffusion en fibrose interstitielle dans la silicose. Poumon Coeur, *16*:1137, 1960.
1707. Söderholm, B.: The hemodynamics of the lesser circulation in pulmonary tuberculosis. Effect of exercise, temporarily unilateral pulmonary artery occlusion, and operation. Scand. J. Clin. Lab. Invest, *9*: suppl. 26, 1957.
1708. Schmidt, F.: Untersuchungen der Atemfunktion bei einseitiger Lungentuberkulose. Der Einfluss von Pleuraverschwartungen nach Pleuritis exsudativa und nach intrapleuralem Pneumothorax. Acta Tuberc. Scand., *33*:367, 1957.
1709. Simonin, P., Sadoul, P., Metz, J., and Durand, D.: Les perturbations fonctionnelles au cours de la tuberculose pulmonaire. Apports de l'exploration fonctionnelle pulmonaire. Rev. Tuberc., *22*:608, 1958.
1710. Birath, G.: Forms of chronic cardio-pulmonary insufficiency in pulmonary tuberculosis and their diagnosis. In: Fløystrup, T., *et al.* (eds.): *Papers Dedicated to Dr. K. Tørning on His Sixtieth Birthday.* Acta Tuberc. Scand., suppl. *47*:32, 1959.
1711. Orimoto, M.: Pulmonary disability of the far-advanced cases of tuberculosis. Jap. Circ. J., *25*:561, 1961.
1712. Loewen, D. F., Procknow, J. J., and Loosli, C. G.: Chronic active pulmonary histoplasmosis with cavitation. A clinical and laboratory study of thirteen cases. Am. J. Med., *28*:252, 1960.
1713. Simenstad, J. O., Galway, C. F., and MacLean, L. D.: The treatment of aspiration and atelectasis by tracheobronchial lavage. Surg. Gynec. Obstet., *115*:721, 1962.
1714. Binger, C. A. L., and Brown, G. R.: Studies on the respiratory mechanism in lobar pneumonia. A study of lung volume in relation to the clinical course of the disease. J. Exper. Med., *39*:677, 1924.
1715. Ryan, J. M., and Hickam, J. B.: The alveolar-arterial O_2 pressure gradient in anemia. J. Clin. Invest., *31*:188, 1952.
1716. Sproule, B. J., Mitchell, J. H., and Miller, W. F.: Cardiopulmonary physiological responses to heavy exercise in patients with anemia. J. Clin. Invest., *39*:378, 1960.
1717. Bishop, J. M., Donald, K. W., and Wade, O. L.: Circulatory dynamics at rest and on exercise in the hyperkinetic states. Clin. Sci., *14*:329, 1955.
1718. Burrows, B., and Niden, A. H.: Effect of anemia on CO diffusion in the perfused dog lung. Fed. Proc., *21*:443, 1962.
1719. McIlroy, M. B., Eldridge, F. L., and Stone, R. W.: The mechanical properties of the lungs in anoxia, anaemia and thyrotoxicosis. Clin. Sci., *15*:353, 1956.
1720. Balke, B., Grillo, G. P., Konecci, E. B., and Luft, U. C.: Work capacity after blood donation. J. Appl. Physiol., *7*:231, 1954.
1721. Schopp, R. T., Gilfoil, T. M., and Youmans, W. B.: Mechanisms of respiratory stimulation during hemorrhage. Am. J. Physiol., *189*:117, 1957.
1722. Calabresi, P., and Meyer, O. O.: Polycythemia vera. I. Clinical and laboratory manifestations. Ann. Int. Med., *50*:1182, 1959.
1723. Cassels, D. E., and Morse, M.: The arterial blood gases, the oxygen dissociation curve, and the acid base balance in polycythemia vera. J. Clin. Invest., *32*:52, 1953.
1724. Hornbein, T. F., and Roos, A.: Effect of polycythemia on respiration. J. Appl. Physiol., *12*:86, 1958.
1725. Hodgson, C. H., Burchell, H. B., Good, C. A., and Clagett, O. T.: Hereditary hemorrhagic telangiectasia and pulmonary arteriovenous fistula. Survey of a large family. New Engl. J. Med., *261*:625, 1959.
1726. Muri, J.: Arterio-venous aneurysma of the lung. Dis. Chest., *24*:49, 1953.
1727. Le Roux, B. T.: Pulmonary arteriovenous fistulae. Quart. J. Med., (*n.s.*)*28*:1, 1959.
1728. Salvesen, H. A., and Marstrander, F.: Arteriovenous fistula of the lung. Report of 4 cases, including an acyanotic case. Acta Med. Scand., *139*:167, 1951.
1729. Grung, P.: Teleangiectasia haemorrhagica hereditaria Osler with arteriovenous aneurysms of the lung and with hepatosplenomegaly. A case report. Acta Med. Scand., *150*:95, 1954.
1730. Pezza, N., and Pecchiai, L.: Un caso di angiomatosi ipossiemizzante (Malattia di Rendu-Osler a localizzazione prevalentemente polmonare). Folia Hered. Path., *7*:173, 1958; Exec. Med. XV, *12*: abstr. no. 1650: p. 420, 1959.
1731. André, R., Dreyfus, B., and Brille, D.: Anévrysme artério-veineux du poumon. Lobectomie. Guérison. Bull. Mem. Soc. Med. Hop. Paris, *68*:646, 1952.
1732. Denolin, H., Dumont, A., Duprez, A., Segers, M., De Coster, A., and Bollaert, A.: Un nouveau cas d'anévrysme artério-veineux pulmonaire. Acta Cardiol., *8*:420, 1953.
1733. Hauch, H. J., and Hertz, C. W.: Das arteriovenöse Lungenaneurysma. Thoraxchirurgie, *1*:411, 1954.
1734. Overholt, E. L.: Hereditary hemorrhagic telangiectasia in three families. Arch Int. Med., *99*:301, 1957.
1735. Weiss, E., and Gasul, B. M.: Pulmonary arteriovenous fistula and telangiectasia. Ann. Int. Med., *41*:989, 1954.
1736. Pierce, J. A., Reagan, W. P., and Kimball, R. W.: Unusual cases of pulmonary arteriovenous fistulas, with a note on thyroid carcinoma as a cause. New Engl. J. Med., *260*:901, 1959.
1737. Rydell, R., and Hoffbauer, F. W.: Multiple pulmonary arteriovenous fistulas in juvenile cirrhosis. Am. J. Med., *21*:450, 1956.
1738. Georg, J., Mellemgaard, K., Tygstrup, N., and Winkler, K.: Venoarterial shunts in cirrhosis of the liver. Lancet, *1*:852, 1960.
1739. Murray, J. F., Dawson, A. M., and Sherlock, S.: Circulatory changes in chronic liver disease. Am. J. Med., *24*:358, 1958.
1740. Bashour, F. A., Miller, W. F., and Chapman, C. B.: Pulmonary venoarterial shunting in hepatic cirrhosis, including a case with cirsoid aneurysm of the thoracic wall. Am. Heart J., *62*:350, 1961.
1741. Abelmann, W. H., Calabresi, P., Kramer, G., McNeely, W. F., and Gravallese, M. A., Jr.: Arterial unsaturation, venous admixture, and portopulmonary anastomoses in patients with cirrhosis of the liver [Abstract]. J. Clin. Invest., *34*:919, 1955.
1742. Schoenmackers, J., and Vieten, H.: Leber- und Ösophagusgefässe bei Leberveränderungen mit portalem Hochdruck. Arch. Kreislaufforsch., *25*:222, 1957.
1743. Williams, M. H., Jr.: Hypoxemia due to venous admixture in cirrhosis of the liver. J. Appl. Physiol., *15*:253, 1960.
1744. Rodman, T., Hurwitz, J. K., Pastor, B. H., and Close, H. P.: Cyanosis, clubbing and arterial oxygen unsaturation associated with Laennec's cirrhosis. Am. J. Med. Sci., *238*:534, 1959.
1745. Morrow, J. D., Schroeder, H. A., and Perry, H. M., Jr.: Studies on the control of hypertension by Hyphex. II. Toxic reactions and side effects. Circulation, *8*:829, 1953.
1746. Doniach, I., Morrison, B., and Steiner, R. E.: Lung changes during hexamethonium therapy for hypertension. Brit. Heart J., *16*:101, 1954.
1747. Park, W. W., and Cockersole, F. J.: Lung changes during methonium therapy. [Letter to the Editor.] Brit. Med. J., *2*:466, 1957.
1748. Hildeen, T., Krogsgaard, A. R., and Vimtrup, B.: Fatal pulmonary changes during the medical treatment of malignant hypertension. Lancet, *2*:830, 1958.

1749. Petersen, A. G., Dodge, M., and Helwig, F. C.: Pulmonary changes associated with hexamethonium therapy. A.M.A. Arch. Int. Med., *103*:285, 1959.

1750. Rosen, S. H., Castleman, B., and Liebow, A. A.: Pulmonary alveolar proteinosis. New Engl. J. Med., *258*:1123, 1958.

1751. Snider, T. H., Wilner, F. M., and Lewis, B. M.: Cardiopulmonary physiology in a case of pulmonary alveolar proteinosis. Ann. Int. Med., *52*:1318, 1960.

1752. Landis, F. B., Rose, H. D., and Sternlieb, R. O.: Pulmonary alveolar proteinosis. A case report with unusual clinical and laboratory manifestations. Am. Rev. Resp. Dis., *80*:249, 1959.

1753. Fraimow, W., Cathcart, R. T., Kirshner, J. J., and Taylor, R. C.: Pulmonary alveolar proteinosis. A correlation of pathological and physiological findings in a patient followed up with serial biopsies of the lung. Am. J. Med., *28*:458, 1960.

1754. Fraimow, W., Cathcart, R. T., and Taylor, R. C.: Physiologic and clinical aspects of pulmonary alveolar proteinosis. Ann. Int. Med., *52*:1177, 1960.

1755. Hall, G. F. M.: Pulmonary alveolar proteinosis. Lancet, *1*:1383, 1960.

1756. Williams, G. E. G., Medley, D. R. K., and Brown, R.: Pulmonary alveolar proteinosis. Lancet. *1*:1385, 1960.

1757. Lull, G. F., Jr., Beyer, J. C., Maier, J. G., and Morss, D. F., Jr.: Pulmonary alveolar proteinosis. Report of two cases. Am. J. Roentgenol., *82*:76, 1959.

1758. Christie, R. V.: Some types of respiration in the neuroses. Quart. J. Med., *(n.s.)4*:427, 1935.

1759. Bülow, K.: Lung function in cardiac neurosis. Acta Med. Scand., *169*:1, 1961.

1760. Lewis, B. I.: The hyperventilation syndrome. Ann. Int. Med., *38*:918, 1953.

1761. Holmgren, A., Jonsson, B., Levander, M., Linderholm, H., Sjöstrand, T., and Ström, G.: Low physical working capacity in suspected heart cases due to inadequate adjustment of peripheral blood flow (vasoregulatory asthenia). Acta Med. Scand., *158*:413, 1957.

1762. Holmgren, A., Jonsson, B., Levander-Lindgren, M., Linderholm, H., Mossfeldt, F., Sjöstrand, T., and Ström, G.: Vasoregulative Asthenie und deren Behandlung durch körperliches Training. Aerztl. Forsch., *12*, part I:425, 1958.

1763. Holmgren, A., Jonsson, B., Levander, M., Linderholm, H., Mossfeldt, F., Sjöstrand, T., and Ström, G.: Physical training of patients with vasoregulatory asthenia. Acta Med. Scand., *158*:437, 1957.

1764. Holmgren, A., Jonsson, B., Levander, M., Linderholm, H., Mossfeldt, F., Sjöstrand, T., and Ström, G.: Physical training of patients with vasoregulatory asthenia, in Da Costa's syndrome, and in neurosis without heart symptoms. Acta Med. Scand., *165*:89, 1959.

1765. Wilson, W. R., and Bedell, G. N.: The pulmonary abnormalities in myxedema. J. Clin. Invest., *39*:42, 1960.

1766. Wayne, E. J.: The diagnosis of thyrotoxicosis. [Bradshaw Lecture.] Brit. Med. J., *1*:411, 1954.

1767. Stein, M., Kimbel, P., and Johnson, R. L., Jr.: Pulmonary function in hyperthyroidism. J. Clin. Invest., *40*:348, 1961.

1768. Valtin, H., and Tenney, S. M.: Respiratory adaptation to hyperthyroidism. J. Appl. Physiol., *15*:1107, 1960.

1769. Sosman, M. C., Dodd, G. D., Jones, W. D., and Pillmore, G. U.: The familial occurrence of pulmonary alveolar microlithiasis. Am. J. Roentgenol., *77*:947, 1957.

1770. Badger, T. L., Gottlieb, L., and Gaensler, E. A.: Pulmonary alveolar microlithiasis, or calcinosis of the lungs. New Engl. J. Med., *253*:709, 1955.

1771. Thomson, W. B.: Pulmonary alveolar microlithiasis. Thorax, *14*:76, 1959.

1772. Svanberg, L.: Clinical value of analysis of lung function in some intrathoracic diseases. A spirometric, bronchospirometric and angiopneumonographic investigation. Acta Chir. Scand., *111*:169, 1956.

1773. Söderholm, B., and Widimský, J.: The effect of acetylcholine infusion on the pulmonary circulation in cases of impaired ventilation. Acta Med. Scand., *172*:219, 1962.

1774. Robin, E. D., Crump, C. H., and Wagman, R. J.: Low sedimentation rate, hypofibrinogenemia and restrictive pseudo-obstructive pulmonary disease associated with trichinosis. New Engl. J. Med., *262*:758, 1960.

1775. Connolly, J. J., Jr., Neu, H. C., Schwertley, F. W., Ladwig, H. A., and Brody, A. W.: Studies of pulmonary function in Parkinsonian patients [Abstract]. Physiologist, *2*/3:25, 1959.

1776. Boyd, M. W. J., and Grant, A. P.: Werner's syndrome (progeria of the adult). Further pathological and biochemical observations. Brit. Med. J., *2*:920, 1959.

1777. Miller, R. D., Mulder, D. W., Fowler, W. S., and Olsen, A. M.: Exertional dyspnea: A primary complaint in unusual cases of progressive muscular atrophy and amyotrophic lateral sclerosis. Ann. Int. Med., *46*:119, 1957.

1778. Vanamee, P., Poppell, J. W., Glicksman, A. S., Randall, H. T., and Roberts, K. E.: Respiratory alkalosis in hepatic coma. Arch. Int. Med., *97*:762, 1956.

1779. Comroe, J. H., Jr., and Botelho, S.: The unreliability of cyanosis in the recognition of arterial anoxemia. Am. J. Med. Sci., *214*:1, 1947.

1780. Nairn, J. R., and McNeill, R. S.: Adaptation of the Wright peak flow meter to measure inspiratory flow. Brit. Med. J., *1*:1321, 1963.

1781. Flint, F. J., and Khan, M. O.: Clinical use of peak flow meter. Brit. Med. J., *2*:1231, 1962.

1782. Priban, I. P.: An analysis of some short-term patterns of breathing in man at rest. J. Physiol. (London), *166*:425, 1963.

1783. Wright, B. M.: Discussion on measuring pulmonary ventilation. In: Harbord, R. P., and Woolmer, R. (eds.): *Symposium on Pulmonary Ventilation, Leeds, 1958*. Altrincham, England, John Sherratt & Son, 1959, p. 87.

1784. Lewinsohn, H. C., Capel, L. H., and Smart, J.: Changes in forced expiratory volumes throughout the day. Brit. Med. J., *1*:462, 1960.

1785. Barry, C. T.: The Snider match test. Lancet, *2*:964, 1962.

1786. Tierney, D. F., and Nadel, J. A.: Concurrent measurements of functional residual capacity by three methods. J. Appl. Physiol., *17*:871, 1962.

1787. DuBois, A. B., Botelho, S. Y., Bedell, G. N., Marshall, R., and Comroe, J. H., Jr.: A rapid plethysmographic method for measuring thoracic gas volume: A comparison with a nitrogen washout method for measuring functional residual capacity in normal subjects. J. Clin. Invest., *35*:322, 1956.

1788. Barnhard, H. J., Pierce, J. A., Joyce, J. W., and Bates, J. H.: Roentgenographic determination of total lung capacity. A new method evaluated in health, emphysema and congestive heart failure. Am. J. Med., *28*:51, 1960.

1789. Malmberg, R., Simonsson, B., and Berglund, E.: Airways obstruction and uneven gas distribution in the lung. Thorax, *18*:168, 1963.

1790. Young, A. C., Martin, C. J., and Pace, W. R., Jr.: Effect of expiratory flow patterns on lung emptying. J. Appl. Physiol., *18*:47, 1963.

1791. Kourilsky, R.: Une nouvelle méthode électronique d'investigation en pathologie respiratoire: la statidensigraphie (de Maurice Marchal). Bull. Acad. Nat. Med. (Paris), *138*:286, 1954.

1792. Kourilsky, R., Marchal, M., Brille, D., Marchal, M. T., and Hatzfeld, C.: Répartition de la capacité vitale entre les deux poumons. Comparaisons et mesures faites par la statidensigraphie et la spirométrie chez neuf malades. J. Franc. Med. Chir. Thorac., *11*:624, 1957.

1793. Defares, J. G., Wise, M. E., and Duyff, J. W.: New indirect Fick procedure for the determination of cardiac output. Nature, *192*:760, 1961.

1794. Defares, J. G.: Determination of Pv_{CO_2} from the exponential CO_2 rise during rebreathing. J. Appl. Physiol., *13*:159, 1958.

1795. Bouhuys, A., Lichtneckert, S., Lundgren, C., and Lundin, G.: Voluntary changes in breathing pattern and N_2 clearance from lungs. J. Appl. Physiol., *16*:1039, 1961.

1796. Kovach, J. C., Avedian, V., Morales, G., and Poulos, P.: Lung compartment determination. J. Thoracic Surg., *31*:452, 1956.

1797. Lenfant, C.: Nomogram for rapid determination of Pco_2 when in vivo temperature of blood is different from 37 C. J. Appl. Physiol., *16*:909, 1961.

1798. Siggaard-Andersen, O.: Blood acid-base alignment nomogram. Scales for pH, pCO_2, base excess of whole blood of different hemoglobin concentrations, plasma bicarbonate, and plasma total-CO_2. Scand. J. Clin. Lab. Invest., *15*:211, 1963.

1799. Raine, J. M., and Bishop, J. M.: A-a difference in O_2 tension and physiological dead space in normal man. J. Appl. Physiol., *18*:284, 1963.

1800. Farhi, L. E., Edwards, A. W. T., and Homma, T.: Determination of dissolved N_2 in blood by gas chromatography and (a–A) N_2 difference. J. Appl. Physiol., *18*:97, 1963.

1801. Hart, M. C., Orzalesi, M. M., and Cook, C. D.: Relation between anatomic respiratory dead space and body size and lung volume. J. Appl. Physiol., *18*:519, 1963.

1802. Lichtneckert, S. J. A., and Lundgren, C. E. G.: An index of alveolar ventilation. J. Appl. Physiol., *18*:639, 1963.

1803. Nelson, N. M., Prod'hom, L. S., Cherry, R. B., Lipsitz, P. J., and Smith, C. A.: Pulmonary function in the newborn infant: The alveolar-arterial oxygen gradient. J. Appl. Physiol., *18*:534, 1963.

1804. Bishop, J. M., and Cole, R. B.: The effects of inspired oxygen concentration, age and body position upon the alveolar-arterial oxygen tension difference (A–aD) and physiological dead space. J. Physiol. (London), *162*:60 *P*, 1962.

1805. Cain, S. M., and Otis, A. B.: Carbon dioxide transport in anesthetized dogs during inhibition of carbonic anhydrase. J. Appl. Physiol., *16*:1023, 1961.

1806. Cain, S. M., and Otis, A. B.: Effect of carbonic anhydrase inhibition on mixed venous CO_2 tension in anesthetized dogs. J. Appl. Physiol., *15*:390, 1960.

1807. Bartels, H., and Rodewald, G.: Der arterielle Sauerstoffdruck, die alveolär-arterielle Sauerstoffdruckdifferenz und weitere atmungsphysiologische Daten gesunder Männer. Arch. Ges. Physiol., *256*:113, 1952.

1808. Farhi, L. E., and Rahn, H.: A theoretical analysis of the alveolar-arterial O_2 difference with special reference to the distribution effect. J. Appl. Physiol., *7*:699, 1955.

1809. Young, A. C.: Dead space at rest and during exercise. J. Appl. Physiol., *8*:91, 1955.

1810. McGrath, M. W., and Hugh-Jones, P.: Some observations on the distribution of gas flow in the human bronchial tree. Clin. Sci., *24*:209, 1963.

1811. Gurtner, H. P., Briscoe, W. A., and Cournand, A.: Studies of the ventilation-perfusion relationships in the lungs of subjects with chronic pulmonary emphysema, following a single intravenous injection of radioactive krypton (Kr^{85}). I. Presentation and validation of a theoretical model. J. Clin. Invest., *39*:1080, 1960.

1812. Söderholm, B.: Investigation of the methodologic error in bronchospirometry. J. Lab. Clin. Med., *46*:298, 1955.

1813. Piiper, J., Haab, P., and Rahn, H.: Unequal distribution of pulmonary diffusing capacity in the anesthetized dog. J. Appl. Physiol., *16*:499, 1961.

1814. Leathart, G. L.: Steady-state diffusing capacity determined by a simplified method. Thorax, *17*:302, 1962.

1815. Marchal, M.: De l'enregistrement des pulsations invisibles du poumon à l'état normal et a l'état pathologique. Compt. Rend. Acad. Sci., *222*:1314, 1946.

1816. Mostyn, E. M., Helle, S., Gee, J. B. L., Bentivoglio, L. G., and Bates, D. V.: Pulmonary diffusing capacity of athletes. J. Appl. Physiol., *18*:687, 1963.

1817. Bohr, C.: Über die spezifische Tätigkeit der Lungen bei der respiratorischen Gasaufnahme und ihr Verhalten zu der durch die Alveolarwand stattfindenden Gasdiffusion. Skand. Arch. Physiol., *22*:221, 1909.

1818. Kreukniet, J., and Visser, B. F.: CO-diffusing capacity, fractional CO-uptake and unequal ventilation. Acta Physiol. Pharmacol. Neerl., *11*:386, 1962.

1819. Nye, R. E., Jr.: D_{Lco}. *Personal communication,* 1963.

1820. Feisal, K. A., Sackner, M. A., and DuBois, A. B.: Comparison between the time available and the time required for CO_2 equilibration in the lung. J. Clin. Invest., *42*:24, 1963.

1821. Soni, J., Feisal, K. A., and DuBois, A. B.: The rate of intrapulmonary blood gas exchange in living animals. J. Clin. Invest., *42*:16, 1963.

1822. Cain, S. M., and Otis, A. B.: CO_2 retention in anesthetized dogs after inhibition of carbonic anhydrase. Proc. Soc. Exper. Biol. Med., *103*:439, 1960.

1823. Edwards, A. W. T., Velasquez, T., and Farhi, L. E.: Determination of alveolar capillary temperature. J. Appl. Physiol., *18*:107, 1963.

1824. Chinard, F. P., Enns, T., and Nolan, M. F.: Diffusion and solubility factors in pulmonary inert gas exchanges. J. Appl. Physiol., *16*:831, 1961.

1825. Jameson, A. G.: Diffusion of gases from alveolus to precapillary arteries. Science, *139*:826, 1963.

1826. Ross, J. C., Ley, G. D., Coburn, R. F., Eller, J. L., and Forster, R. E.: Influence of suit inflation on pulmonary diffusing capacity in man. J. Appl. Physiol., *17*:259, 1962.

1827. Farhi, L. E., and Riley, R. L.: Graphic analysis of moment-to-moment changes in blood passing through the pulmonary capillary, including a demonstration of three graphic methods for estimating mean alveolar–capillary diffusion gradient (Bohr integration). J. Appl. Physiol., *10*:179, 1957.

1828. Durand, J., and Cournand, A.: Emploi d'un isotope du krypton (Kr^{85}) dans l'exploration fonctionnelle cardiovasculaire et pulmonaire. Rev. Franc. Etud. Clin. Biol., *7*:411, 1962.

1829. Fowler, K. T., and Read, J.: Cardiogenic oscillations as an index of pulmonary blood flow distribution. J. Appl. Physiol., *18*:233, 1963.

1830. Cotes, J. E.: Effect of variability in gas analysis on the reproducibility of the pulmonary diffusing capacity by the single breath method. Thorax, *18*:151, 1963.

1831. Gómez, D. M.: A mathematical treatment of the distribution of tidal volume throughout the lung. Proc. Nat. Acad. Sci. U.S.A., *49*:312, 1963.

1832. Burrows, B., and Harper, P. V., Jr.: Determination of pulmonary diffusing capacity from carbon monoxide equilibration curves. J. Appl. Physiol., *12*:283, 1958.

1833. Young, R. C., Jr., Nagano, H., Vaughan, T. R., Jr., and Staub, N. C.: Pulmonary capillary blood volume in dog: effects of 5-hydroxytryptamine. J. Appl. Physiol., *18*:264, 1963.

1834. Niden, A. H., Mittman, C., and Burrows, B.: Pulmonary diffusion in the dog lung. J. Appl. Physiol., *17*:885, 1962.

1835. Daly, J. J., and Roe, J. W.: Serial measurements of the pulmonary diffusing capacity for carbon monoxide in a group of men employed in industry. Thorax, *17*:298, 1962.

1836. Birath, G.: Airway and physiologic dead space in patients with obstructive emphysema. Med. Thorac., *19*:4, 1962.

1837. Birath, G., Kjellmer, I., and Sandqvist, L.: Spirometric studies in normal subjects. II. Ventilatory capacity tests in adults. Acta Med. Scand., *173*:193, 1963.

1838. Grimby, G., and Söderholm, B.: Spirometric studies in normal subjects. III. Static lung volumes and maximum voluntary ventilation in adults with a note on physical fitness. Acta Med. Scand., *173*:199, 1963.

1839. Hamer, N. A. J.: Variations in the components of the diffusing capacity as the lung expands. Clin. Sci., *24*:275, 1963.

1840. Fowler, K. T., and Read, J.: Cardiac oscillations in expired gas tensions, and regional pulmonary blood flow. J. Appl. Physiol., *16*:863, 1961.

1841. Burrows, B., and Niden, A. H.: Effects of anemia and hemorrhagic shock on pulmonary diffusion in the dog lung. J. Appl. Physiol., *18*:123, 1963.

1842. Ashton, C. H., and McHardy, G. J. R.: A rebreathing method for determining mixed venous P_{CO_2} during exercise. J. Appl. Physiol., *18*:668, 1963.

1843. Berglund, E., Birath, G., Bjure, J., Grimby, G., Kjellmer, I., Sandqvist, L., and Söderholm, B.: Spirometric studies in normal subjects. I. Forced expirograms in subjects between 7 and 70 years of age. Acta Med. Scand., *173*:185, 1963.

1844. Said, S. I., and Banerjee, C. M.: Venous admixture to the pulmonary circulation in human subjects breathing 100 per cent oxygen. J. Clin. Invest., *42*:507, 1963.

1845. Daly, W. J., and Bondurant, S.: Direct measurement of respiratory pleural pressure changes in normal man. J. Appl. Physiol., *18:*513, 1963.
1846. Ferris, B. G., Jr., and Pollard, D. S.: Effect of deep and quiet breathing on pulmonary compliance in man. J. Clin. Invest., *39:*143, 1960.
1847. Tenney, S. M., and Remmers, J. E.: Comparative quantitative morphology of the mammalian lung: diffusing area. Nature, *197:*54, 1963.
1848. Crofton, J., Douglas, A., Simpson, D., and Merchant, S.: The measurement of bronchial endomural or "squeeze" pressure. Thorax, *18:*68, 1963.
1849. Marshall, R., and Holden, W. S.: Changes in calibre of the smaller airways in man. Thorax, *18:*54, 1963.
1850. McIlroy, M. B., Tierney, D. F., and Nadel, J. A.: A new method for measurement of compliance and resistance of lungs and thorax. J. Appl. Physiol., *18:*424, 1963.
1851. Hyatt, R. E., and Wilcox, R. E.: Extrathoracic airway resistance in man. J. Appl. Physiol., *16:*326, 1961.
1852. Hyatt, R. E., and Wilcox, R. E.: The pressure-flow relationships of the intrathoracic airway in man. J. Clin. Invest., *42:*29, 1963.
1853. Dekker, E., Defares, J. G., and Heemstra, H.: Direct measurement of intrabronchial pressure. Its application to the location of the check-valve mechanism. J. Appl. Physiol., *13:*35, 1958.
1854. Wyss, F.: Influence du calibre de la trachée et des grosses bronches: Dyskinésie trachéo-bronchique (Changement physiologique et pathologique de la lumière bronchique pendant la respiration). In: *Proc. 10th Congr., Assoc. Intern. pour l'Etude des Bronches.* Bronches, *11:*11, 1961.
1855. Shephard, R. J.: Mechanical characteristics of the human airway in relation to use of the interrupter valve. Clin. Sci., *25:*263, 1963.
1856. Radford, E. P., Jr.: Mechanical stability of the lung. Arch. Environ. Health, *6:*128, 1963.
1857. Parker, J. C., Peters, R. M., and Barnett, T. B.: Carbon dioxide and the work of breathing. J. Clin. Invest., *42:*1362, 1963.
1858. Widdicombe, J. G., and Nadel, J. A.: Airway volume, airway resistance, and work and force of breathing: Theory. J. Appl. Physiol., *18:*863, 1963.
1859. Storey, W. F., and Staub, N. C.: Ventilation of terminal air units. J. Appl. Physiol., *18:*391, 1962.
1860. Colebatch, H. J. H., and Halmagyi, D. F. J.: Reflex airway reaction to fluid aspiration. J. Appl. Physiol., *17:*787, 1962.
1861. Kanagami, H., Baba, K., Katsura, T., and Shiroishi, K.: Studies on the pulmonary function during exercise in normal subjects—On the comparison of three different exercise tests. Resp. Circ., *9:*188, 1961.
1862. Erickson, L., Simonson, E., Taylor, H. L., Alexander, H., and Keys, A.: The energy cost of horizontal and grade walking on the motor-driven treadmill. Am. J. Physiol., *145:*391, 1946.
1863. Workman, J. M., and Armstrong, B. W.: Oxygen cost of treadmill walking. J. Appl. Physiol., *18:*798, 1963.
1864. Cavagna, G. A., Saibene, F. P., and Margaria, R.: External work in walking. J. Appl. Physiol., *18:*1, 1963.
1865. Rahn, H.: The role of N_2 gas in various biological processes with particular reference to the lung. Harvey Lect., *55:*173, 1961.
1866. Dulfano, M. J., and Di Rienzo, A.: Laminagraphic observations of the lung vasculature in chronic pulmonary emphysema. Am. J. Roentgenol., *88:*1043, 1962.
1867. De Clercq, F., De Coster, A., Bollaert, A., Denolin, H., and Englert, M.: Aspects angiopneumographiques de l'emphysème pulmonaire diffus. Acta Tuberc. Beige, *47*/3:194, 1956.
1868. Weibel, E. R.: Morphometrische Analyse von Zahl, Volumen und Oberfläche der Alveolen und Kapillaren der menschlichen Lunge. Z. Zellforsch., *57:*648, 1962.
1869. Gieseking, R.: Elektronenoptische Beobachtungen im Alveolarbereich der Lunge. Beitr. Path. Anat., *116:*177, 1956.
1870. Harris, P., Bateman, M., and Gloster, J.: Relations between the cardio-respiratory effects of exercise and the arterial concentration of lactate and pyruvate in patients with rheumatic heart disease. Clin. Sci., *23:*531, 1962.
1871. Hepper, G. G. N., Fowler, W. S., and Helmholz, H. F., Jr.: Relationship of height to lung volume in healthy men. Dis. Chest, *37:*314, 1960.
1872. Heller, S. S., Hicks, W. R., and Root, W. S.: Lung volumes of singers. J. Appl. Physiol., *15:*40, 1960.
1873. Robin, E. D., Whaley, R. D., Crump, C. H., and Travis, D. M.: Alveolar gas tensions, pulmonary ventilation and blood pH during physiologic sleep in normal subjects. J. Clin. Invest., *37:*981, 1958.
1874. Sieker, H. O., Heyman, A., and Birchfield, R. I.: The effects of natural sleep and hypersomnolent states on respiratory function. Ann. Int. Med., *52:*500, 1960.
1875. Heaf, P. J. D., and Prime, F. J.: The compliance of the thorax in normal human subjects. Clin. Sci., *15:*319, 1956.
1876. Rodman, T.: The effect of anesthesia and surgery on pulmonary and cardiac function. Am. J. Cardiol., *12:*444, 1963.
1877. Knuttgen, H. G.: Oxygen debt, lactate, pyruvate, and excess lactate after muscular work. J. Appl. Physiol., *17:*639, 1962.
1878. Bevegård, S., Holmgren, A., and Jonsson, B.: The effect of body position on the circulation at rest and during exercise, with special reference to the influence on the stroke volume. Acta Physiol. Scand., *49:*279, 1960.
1879. Hornbein, T. F., and Roos, A.: Effect of mild hypoxia on ventilation during exercise. J. Appl. Physiol., *17:*239, 1962.
1880. Åstrand, P. O., Hallbäck, I., Hedman, R., and Saltin, B.: Blood lactates after prolonged severe exercise. J. Appl. Physiol., *18:*619, 1963.
1881. Harris, P., Bailey, T., Bateman, M., Fitzgerald, M. G., Gloster, J., Harris, E. A., and Donald, K. W.: Lactate, pyruvate, glucose, and free fatty acid in mixed venous and arterial blood. J. Appl. Physiol., *18:*933, 1963.
1882. Wathen, R. L., Rostorfer, H. H., Robinson, S., Newton, J. L., and Bailie, M. D.: Changes in blood gases and acid-base balance in the exercising dog. J. Appl. Physiol., *17:*656, 1962.
1883. Lorentzen, F. V.: Lactic acid in blood after various combinations of exercise and hypoxia. J. Appl. Physiol., *17:*661, 1962.
1884. Downey, J. A., and Darling, R. C.: Effects of salicylates on exercise metabolism. J. Appl. Physiol., *17:*665, 1962.
1885. Huckabee, W. E.: Relationships of pyruvate and lactate during anaerobic metabolism. I. Effects of infusion of pyruvate or glucose and of hyperventilation. II. Exercise and formation of O_2-debt. III. Effect of breathing low-oxygen gases. J. Clin. Invest., *37:*244, 255, 264, 1958.
1886. Kirchhoff, H. W., Reindell, H., and Gebauer, A.: Untersuchungen über die Sauerstoffaufnahme, Kohlensäureabgabe, das Atemminutenvolumen, Atemäquivalent und den respiratorischen Quotienten während körperlicher Belastung bei Normalpersonen und Hochleistungssportlern. Deutsch. Arch. Klin. Med., *203:*423, 1956.
1887. Hinshelwood, C. N.: *The Chemical Kinetics of the Bacterial Cell.* Oxford, Clarendon Press, 1946.
1888. Shepard, R. H., Varnauskas, E., Martin, H. B., White, H. A., Permutt, S., Cotes, J. E., and Riley, R. L.: Relationship between cardiac output and apparent diffusing capacity of the lung in normal men during treadmill exercise. J. Appl. Physiol., *13:*205, 1958.
1889. Bannister, R. G., Cotes, J. E., Jones, R. S., and Meade, F.: Pulmonary diffusing capacity on exercise in athletes and non-athletic subjects. J. Physiol. (London), *152:*66 *P*, 1960.
1890. Turino, G. M., Bergofsky, E. H., Goldring, R. M., and Fishman, A. P.: Effect of exercise on pulmonary diffusing capacity. J. Appl. Physiol., *18:*447, 1963.
1891. Ross, J. C., Reinhart, R. W., Boxell, J. F., and King, L. H., Jr.: Relationship of increased breath-holding diffusing capacity to ventilation in exercise. J. Appl. Physiol., *18:*794, 1963.
1892. Widimský, J., Berglund, E., and Malmberg, R.: Effect of repeated exercise on the lesser circulation. J. Appl. Physiol., *18:*983, 1963.
1893. Damoiseau, J., Petit, J. M., Namur, M., and Lagneaux,

D.: Régime ventilatoire stable au cours de l'exercise musculaire prolongé chez l'individu sain. Arch. Int. Physiol., *69*:310, 1961.
1894. Åstrand, I., Åstrand, P. O., Christensen, E. H., and Hedman, R.: Circulatory and respiratory adaptation to severe muscular work. Acta Physiol. Scand., *50*:254, 1960.
1895. Åstrand, I.: Physiological methods for estimating the physical work capacity in workers especially of older age groups. Ergonomics, *1*:129, 1958.
1896. Åstrand, I.: Clinical and physiological studies of manual workers 50–64 years old at rest and during work. Acta Med. Scand., *162*:155, 1958.
1897. Åstrand, P. O., and Saltin, B.: Maximal oxygen uptake and heart rate in various types of muscular activity. J. Appl. Physiol., *16*:977, 1961.
1898. von Döbeln, W.: Maximal oxygen intake, body size, and total hemoglobin in normal man. Acta Physiol. Scand., *38*:193, 1956.
1899. Taylor, H. L., Buskirk, E., and Henschel, A.: Maximal oxygen uptake as an objective measure of cardio-respiratory performance. J. Appl. Physiol., *8*:73, 1955.
1900. Slonim, N. B., Gillespie, D. G., and Harold, W. H.: Peak oxygen uptake of healthy young men as determined by a treadmill method. J. Appl. Physiol., *10*:401, 1957.
1901. Perret, C.: Hyperoxie et régulation de la ventilation durant l'exercice musculaire. Helv. Physiol. Pharmacol. Acta, *18*:72, 1960.
1902. Bannister, R. G., and Cunningham, D. J. C.: The effects on the respiration and performance during exercise of adding oxygen to the inspired air. J. Physiol. (London), *125*:118, 1954.
1903. Cronin, R. F. P., and MacIntosh, D. J.: The effect of induced hypoxia on oxygen uptake during muscular exercise in normal subjects. Canad. J. Biochem. Physiol., *40*:717, 1962.
1904. Gudbjerg, C. E.: *Bronchiectasis: Radiological Diagnosis and Prognosis after Operative Treatment* (A. la Cour, translator). Acta Radiol., suppl. 143, 1957.
1905. Harris, E. A., and Thomson, J. G.: The pulmonary ventilation and heart rate during exercise in healthy old age. Clin. Sci., *17*:349, 1958.
1906. Åstrand, I., Åstrand, P. O., and Rodahl, K.: Maximal heart rate during work in older men. J. Appl. Physiol., *14*:562, 1959.
1907. Dill, D. B., and Consolazio, C. F.: Responses to exercise as related to age and environmental temperature. J. Appl. Physiol., *17*:645, 1962.
1908. Cohn, J. E., and Donoso, H. D.: Mechanical properties of lung in normal men over 60 years old. J. Clin. Invest., *42*:1406, 1963.
1909. Robin, E. D.: The aging lung—Functional aspects. Arch. Environ. Health, *6*:44, 1963.
1910. Bouhuys, A.: Pulmonary nitrogen clearance in relation to age in healthy males. J. Appl. Physiol., *18*:297, 1963.
1911. Auld, P. A. M., Nelson, N. M., Cherry, R. B., Rudolph, A. J., and Smith, C. A.: Measurement of thoracic gas volume in the newborn infant. J. Clin. Invest., *42*:476, 1963.
1912. Smythe, P. M.: Studies on neonatal tetanus, and on pulmonary compliance of the totally relaxed infant. Brit. Med. J., *1*:565, 1963.
1913. Cook, C. D., and Hamann, J. F.: Relation of lung volumes to height in healthy persons between the ages of 5 and 38 years. J. Pediat., *59*:710, 1961.
1914. Murray, A., and Cook, C. D.: Measurement of peak expiratory flow rates in 220 normal children from 4.5 to 18.5 years of age. J. Pediat., *62*:186, 1963.
1915. Bjure, J.: Spirometric studies in normal subjects. IV. Ventilatory capacities in healthy children 7–17 years of age. Acta Pediat., *52*:232, 1963.
1916. Gill, M. B., Milledge, J. S., Pugh, L. G. C. E., and West, J. B.: Alveolar gas composition at 21,000 to 25,700 ft. (6400–7830 m). J. Physiol. (London), *163*:373, 1962.
1917. Tenney, S. M.: Physiological adaptations to life at high altitude. Mod. Conc. Cardiov. Dis., *31*:713, 1962.
1918. Hultgren, H. N., Marticorena, E., and Miller, H.: Right ventricular hypertrophy in animals at high altitude. J. Appl. Physiol., *18*:913, 1963.
1919. Reeves, J. T., Grover, B., and Grover, R. F.: Circulatory responses to high altitude in the cat and rabbit. J. Appl. Physiol., *18*:575, 1963.
1920. Kuida, J., Hecht, H. H., Lange, R. L., Brown, A. M., Tsagaris, T. J., and Thorne, J. L.: Brisket disease. III. Spontaneous remission of pulmonary hypertension and recovery from heart failure. J. Clin. Invest., *42*:589, 1963.
1921. Grover, R. F., Reeves, J. T., Will, D. H., and Blount, S. G., Jr.: Pulmonary vasoconstriction in steers at high altitude. J. Appl. Physiol., *18*:567, 1963.
1922. Grover, R. F.: Basal oxygen uptake of man at high altitude. J. Appl. Physiol., *18*:909, 1963.
1923. Åstrand, P. O., and Åstrand, I.: Heart rate during muscular work in man exposed to prolonged hypoxia. J. Appl. Physiol., *13*:75, 1958.
1924. Dejours, P., Kellogg, R. H., and Pace, H.: Regulation of respiration and heart rate response in exercise during altitude acclimatization. J. Appl. Physiol., *18*:10, 1963.
1925. Margaria, R., Cerretelli, P., and Bordoni, U.: Regulation of pulmonary ventilation in acclimatization to altitude. Aerospace Med., *33*:799, 1962.
1926. Cerretelli, P.: Esistenza di una permanente stimolazione ipossica del centro respiratorio in individui acclimatati a quote di 5,000–7,500 m s.l.m. (Himalaya). In: *Proc. Internat. Congr. Aeronautical & Space Med., Rome, 1959*, vol. II. Rome, Tipografia del Senato, 1961, p. 866.
1927. Strang, L. B.: The ventilatory capacity of normal children. Thorax, *14*:305, 1959.
1928. Kennedy, M. C. S., Thursby-Pelham, D. C., and Oldham, P. D.: Pulmonary function studies in normal boys. Arch. Dis. Child., *32*:347, 1957.
1929. Oliver, T. K., Jr., Shaw, R. S., and Wheeler, W. E.: Pulmonary ventilation in infants under one year of age. A.M.A. J., Dis. Child., *97*:744, 1959.
1930. Morse, M., Schlutz, F. W., and Cassels, D. E.: The lung volume and its subdivisions in normal boys 10–17 years of age. J. Clin. Invest., *31*:380, 1952.
1931. Lyons, H. A., and Tanner, R. W.: Total lung volume and its subdivisions in children: Normal standards. J. Appl. Physiol., *17*:601, 1962.
1932. Ferris, B. G., Jr., and Smith, C. W.: Maximum breathing capacity and vital capacity in female children and adolescents. Pediatrics, *12*:341, 1953.
1933. Engström, I., Karlberg, P., and Kraepelien, S.: Respiratory studies in children; Lung volumes in healthy children, 6–14 years of age. Acta Paediat., *45*:277, 1956.
1934. Avery, M. E., Chernick, V., Dutton, R. E., and Permutt, S.: Ventilatory response to inspired carbon dioxide in infants and adults. J. Appl. Physiol., *18*:895, 1963.
1935. Bernstein, I. L., Fragge, R. G., Gueron, M., Kreindler, L., and Ghory, J. E.: Pulmonary function in children. I. Determination of norms. J. Allergy, *30*:514, 1959.
1936. Bakulin, S. A.: Gas exchange during muscular work in youths aged 14–17 years in different states of training. Sechenov Physiol. J., *45*/9:93, 1959 (Fiziol. Zh. SSSR Sechenov, *45*:1136, 1959).
1937. Holmgren, A., and Strandell, T.: The relationship between heart volume, total hemoglobin and physical working capacity in former athletes. Acta Med. Scand., *163*:149, 1959.
1938. *Symposium on Exercise Fitness Tests: Their Physiological Basis and Clinical Application to Pediatrics;* Los Angeles, Dec., 1962. Pediatrics, *32*:653, 1963.
1939. Harris, E. A.: Exercise-tolerance tests. Lancet, *2*:409, 1958.
1940. Durnin, J.V.G.A., and Mikulicic, V.: The influence of graded exercises on the oxygen consumption, pulmonary ventilation and heart rate of young and elderly men. Quart. J. Exper. Physiol., *41*:442, 1956.
1941. Voitkevich, V. I.: Dosvid visokogirnikh doslidzhen' za dopomogoiu oksigemometra. (High mountain investigations by means of the oxyhaemometer.] Fiziol. Zh. (Kiev), *1*:123, 1955; Referat. Zh. Biol. 1957, Abstr. No. 3275.
1942. Lacoste, J., and Schrijen, F.: Étude des variations du volume résiduel chez l'homme adulte en fonction de la morphologie. Compt. Rend. Soc. Biol. (Paris), *155*:374, 1961.
1943. Taylor, H. L., Henschel, A., Brožek, J., and Keys, A.:

Effects of bed rest on cardiovascular function and work performance. J. Appl. Physiol., *2*:223, 1949.
1944. Lagerlöf, H., Eliasch, H., Werkö, L., and Berglund, E.: Orthostatic changes of pulmonary and peripheral circulation in man. A preliminary report. Scand. J. Clin. Lab. Invest., *3*:85, 1951.
1945. Gilson, J. C.: Changes in lung function with age. In: Orenstein, A. J. (ed.): *Proceedings of the Pneumoconiosis Conference, Johannesburg, 1959*. London, J. & A. Churchill, 1960, p. 280.
1946. Bouhuys, A., and van Lennep, H. J.: Effect of body posture on gas distribution in the lungs. J. Appl. Physiol., *17*:38, 1962.
1947. Daly, I. de B.: Intrinsic mechanisms of the lung. Quart. J. Exper. Physiol., *43*:2, 1958.
1948. Liljestrand, G.: Regulation of pulmonary arterial blood pressure. Arch. Int. Med., *81*:162, 1948.
1949. Nisell, O.: The influence of blood gases on the pulmonary vessels of the cat. Acta Physiol. Scand., *23*:85, 1951.
1950. Nisell, O.: Reactions of the pulmonary venules of the cat with special reference to the effect of the pulmonary elastance. Acta Physiol. Scand., *23*:361, 1951.
1951. Duke, H. N.: Observations on the effects of hypoxia on the pulmonary vascular bed. J. Physiol. (London), *135*:45, 1957.
1952. Duke, H. N.: The action of carbon dioxide on isolated perfused dog lungs. Quart. J. Exper. Physiol., *35*:25, 1949–50.
1953. Dirken, M. N. J., and Heemstra, H.: Alveolar oxygen tension and lung circulation. Quart. J. Exper. Physiol., *34*:193, 1947–8.
1954. Dirken, M. N. J., and Heemstra, H.: The adaptation of the lung circulation to the ventilation. Quart. J. Exper. Physiol., *34*:213, 1947–8.
1955. Dirken, M. N. J., and Heemstra, H.: Agents acting on the lung circulation. Quart. J. Exper. Physiol., *34*:227, 1947–8.
1956. Peters, R. M., and Roos, A.: Effect of unilateral nitrogen breathing upon pulmonary blood flow. Am. J. Physiol., *171*:250, 1952.
1957. Rahn, H., and Bahnson, H. T.: Effect of unilateral hypoxia on gas exchange and calculated pulmonary blood flow in each lung. J. Appl. Physiol., *6*:105, 1953.
1958. Hall, P. W., III: Effects of anoxia on postarteriolar pulmonary vascular resistance. Circ. Res., *1*:238, 1953.
1959. Cournand, A.: Pulmonary circulation. Its control in man, with some remarks on methodology. Science, *125*:1231, 1957.
1960. Cournand, A., Fritts, H. W., Jr., Harris, P., and Himmelstein, A.: Preliminary observations on the effects in man of continuous perfusion with acetylcholine of one branch of the pulmonary artery upon the homolateral pulmonary blood flow. Tr. A. Am. Physicians, *69*:163, 1956.
1961. Cournand, A.: The mysterious influence of unilateral pulmonary hypoxia upon the circulation in man. Acta Cardiol., *10*:429, 1955.
1962. Fritts, H. W., Jr., Harris, P., Clauss, R. H., Odell, J. E., and Cournand, A.: The effect of acetylcholine on the human pulmonary circulation under normal and hypoxic conditions. J. Clin. Invest., *37*:99, 1958.
1963. Fishman, A. P., Fritts, H. W., Jr., and Cournand, A.: Effects of acute hypoxia and exercise on the pulmonary circulation. Circulation, *22*:204, 1960.
1964. Fishman, A. P., Fritts, H. W., Jr., and Cournand, A.: Effects of breathing carbon dioxide upon the pulmonary circulation. Circulation, *22*:220, 1960.
1965. Fritts, H. W., Jr., and Cournand, A.: Physiological factors regulating pressure, flow and distribution of blood in the pulmonary circulation. In: Adams, W. R., and Veith, I. (eds.): *Pulmonary Circulation: An International Symposuim, Chicago, 1958*. New York, Grune & Stratton, 1959, p. 62.
1966. Fritts, H. W., Jr., Odell, J. E., Harris, P., Braunwald, E. W., and Fishman, A. P.: Effects of acute hypoxia on the volume of blood in the thorax. Circulation, *22*:216, 1960.
1967. Himmelstein, A., Harris, P., Fritts, H. W., Jr., and Cournand, A.: Effect of severe unilateral hypoxia on the partition of pulmonary blood flow in man. J. Thoracic Surg., *36*:369, 1958.
1968. Goldring, R. M., Turino, G. M., Gohen, G., Jameson, A. G., Bass, B. G., and Fishman, A. P.: The catecholamines in the pulmonary arterial pressor response to acute hypoxia. J. Clin. Invest., *41*:1211, 1962.
1969. Bergofsky, E. H., Lehr, D. E., Tuller, M. A., Rigatto, M., and Fishman, A. P.: The effects of acute alkalosis and acidosis on the pulmonary circulation. Ann. N.Y. Acad. Sci., *92*:627, 1961.
1970. Bergofsky, E. H., Lehr, D. E., and Fishman, A. P.: The effect of changes in hydrogen ion concentration on the pulmonary circulation. J. Clin. Invest., *41*:1492, 1962.
1971. Löhr, B.: Der Einfluss gestörter Lungenbelüftung auf den kleinen Kreislauf. Pathophysiologie und Klinik. Muench. Med. Wchnschr., *98*:838, 1956.
1972. Arborelius, M., Jr., Defares, J., Lundin, G. Strömblad, B. C. R., and Svanberg, L.: Effect of hypoxia of one lung on the pulmonary circulation in man. J. Physiol. (London), *142*:38 *P*, 1958.
1973. Brofman, B. L., Charms, B. L., Kohn, P. M., Elder, J., Newman, R., and Rizika, M.: Unilateral pulmonary artery occlusion in man. Control studies. J. Thoracic Surg., *34*:206, 1957.
1974. Patel, D. J., Lange, R. L., and Hecht, H. H.: Some evidence for active constriction in the human pulmonary vascular bed. Circulation, *18*:19, 1958.
1975. Lanari-Zubiaur, F. J., and Hamilton, W. F.: Effect of unilateral anoxia on pulmonary circulation. Circ. Res., *6*:289, 1958.
1976. DuBois, A. B., and Marshall, R.: Measurements of pulmonary capillary blood flow and gas exchange throughout the respiratory cycle in man. J. Clin. Invest., *36*:1566, 1957.
1977. Feisal, K. A., Soni, J., and DuBois, A. B.: Pulmonary arterial circulation time, pulmonary arterial blood volume, and the ratio of gas to tissue volume in the lungs of dogs. J. Clin. Invest., *41*:390, 1962.
1978. Chinard, F. P., Enns, T., and Nolan, M. F.: Pulmonary extravascular water volumes from transit time and slope data. J. Appl. Physiol., *17*:179, 1962.
1979. Kuida, H., Hinshaw, L. B., Gilbert, R. P., and Vischer, M. B.: Effect of Gram-negative endotoxin on pulmonary circulation. Am. J. Physiol., *192*:335, 1958.
1980. Fowler, K. T., and Read, I.: Effect of alveolar hypoxia on zonal distribution of pulmonary blood flow. J. Appl. Physiol., *18*:244, 1963.
1981. Bergofsky, E. H., Bass, B. G., Ferretti, R., and Fishman, A. P.: Pulmonary vasoconstriction in response to precapillary hypoxemia. J. Clin. Invest., *42*:1201, 1963.
1982. Severinghaus, J. W., Swenson, E. W., Finley, T. N., Lategola, M. T., and Williams, J.: Unilateral hypoventilation produced in dogs by occluding one pulmonary artery, J. Appl. Physiol., *16*:53, 1961.
1983. Swenson, E. W., Finley, T. N., and Guzman, S. V.: Unilateral hypoventilation in man during temporary occlusion of one pulmonary artery. J. Clin. Invest., *40*:828, 1961.
1984. Shaw, D. B.: Compliance and inertance in the pulmonary arterial system. Clin. Sci., *25*:181, 1963.
1985. Ross, J. C., Maddock, G. E., and Ley, G. D.: Effect of pressure suit inflation on pulmonary capillary blood volume. J. Appl. Physiol., *16*:674, 1961.
1986. Greenfield, J. C., Jr., and Griggs, D. M., Jr.: Relation between pressure and diameter in main pulmonary artery of man. J. Appl. Physiol., *18*:557, 1963.
1987. Schreiner, B. F., Jr., Murphy, G. W., Glick, G., and Yu, P. N.: Effect of exercise on the pulmonary blood volume in patients with acquired heart disease. Circulation, *27*:559, 1963.
1988. Glick, G., Schreiner, B. F., Jr., Murphy, G. W., and Yu, P. N.: Effects of inhalation of 100 per cent oxygen on the pulmonary blood volume in patients with organic heart disease. Circulation, *27*:554, 1963.
1989. Yu, P. N., Glick, G., Schreiner, B. F., Jr., and Murphy, G. W.: Effects of acute hypoxia on the pulmonary vascular bed of patients with acquired heart disease. With special reference to the demonstration of active vasomotion. Circulation, *27*:541, 1963.

1990. Donato, L., Giuntini, C., Lewis, M. L., Durand, J., Rochester, D. F., Harvey, R. M., and Cournand, A.: Quantitative radiocardiograpy. I. Theoretical considerations. Circulation, *26:*174, 1962.

1991. Donato, L., Rochester, D. F., Lewis, M. L., Durand, J., Parker, J. O., and Harvey, R. M.: Quantitative radiocardiography. II. Technic and analysis of curves. Circulation, *26:*183, 1962.

1992. Lewis, M. L., Giuntini, C., Donato, L., Harvey, R. M., and Cournand, A.: Quantitative radiocardiography. III. Results and validation of theory and method. Circulation, *26:*189, 1962.

1993. Daly, W. J., Ross, J. C., and Behnke, R. H.: The effect of changes in the pulmonary vascular bed produced by atropine, pulmonary engorgement, and positive-pressure breathing on diffusing and mechanical properties of the lung. J. Clin. Invest., *42:*1083, 1963.

1994. Giuntini, C., Lewis, M. L., Luis, A. S., and Harvey, R. M.: A study of the pulmonary blood volume in man by quantitative radiocardiography. J. Clin. Invest., *42:*1589, 1963.

1995. Weissler, A. M., McCraw, B. H., and Warren, J. V.: Pulmonary blood volume determined by a radioactive tracer technique. J. Appl. Physiol., *14:*531, 1959.

1996. Messer, J. W., Peters, G. A., and Bennett, W. A.: Causes of death and pathologic findings in 304 cases of bronchial asthma. Dis. Chest, *38:*616, 1960.

1997. Thomson, W. B., and Hugh-Jones, P.: Forced expiratory volume as a test for successful treatment of asthma. Brit. Med. J., *1:*1093, 1958.

1998. Chapin, H. B., and Loeb, L.: Pulmonary ventilation function in patients with asthma. A study of mean maximal expiratory volume velocity (flow rate) as determined by a special apparatus. Canad. M. A. J., *84:*641, 1961.

1999. Fyles, T. W., Pare, J. A. P., and Rose, B.: The effect of corticotropin and cortisone on respiratory function in bronchial asthma. J. Allergy, *26:*340, 1955.

2000. Anthonisen, N. R.: Changes in compliance in rabbits subjected to acute bronchoconstriction. J. Appl. Physiol., *18:*539, 1963.

2001. The College of General Practitioners, Respiratory Diseases Study Group: Chronic bronchitis in Great Britain: A national survey. Brit. Med. J., *2:*973, 1961.

2002. Fletcher, C. M.: An account of chronic bronchitis in Great Britain with a comparison between British and American experience of the disease. Dis. Chest, *44:*1, 1963.

2003. Whitfield, A. G. W., Arnott, W. M., and Waterhouse, J. A. H.: The effect of tobacco on lung-volume. Quart. J. Med., *(n.s.)20:*141, 1951.

2004. Wilson, R. H., Meador, R. S., Jay, B. E., and Higgins, E.: The pulmonary pathologic physiology of persons who smoke cigarettes. New Engl. J. Med., *262:*956, 1960.

2005. Read, J., and Selby, T.: Tobacco smoking and ventilatory function of the lungs. Brit. Med. J., *2:*1104, 1961.

2006. Zamel, N., Youssef, H. H., and Prime, F. J.: Airway resistance and peak expiratory flow-rate in smokers and non-smokers. Lancet, *1:*1237, 1963.

2007. Martt, J. M.: Pulmonary diffusing capacity in cigarette smokers. Ann. Int. Med., *56:*39, 1962.

2008. Davies, G. M.: Fog bronchiolitis. Lancet, *1:*580, 1963.

2009. Campiche, M., Prod'hom, S., and Gautier, A.: Étude au microscope électronique du poumon de prématurés morts en détresse respiratoire. Ann. Paediat., *196:*81, 1961.

2010. Anderson, D. O.: Observations on the classification and distribution of pulmonary emphysema in Canada. Canad. M. A. J., *89:*709, 1963.

2011. Branscomb, B.: The application of the respiratory flow-volume loop in epidemiologic surveys. Am. Rev. Resp. Dis., *86:*697, 1962.

2012. Thurlbeck, W. M.: Pulmonary emphysema. Am. J. Med. Sci., *246:*332, 1963.

2013. American Thoracic Society, Committee on Diagnostic Standards for Non-tuberculous Respiratory Diseases: Definitions and classification of chronic bronchitis, asthma, and pulmonary emphysema. Am. Rev. Resp. Dis., *85:*762, 1962.

2014. Definition and diagnosis of pulmonary diseases with special reference to chronic bronchitis and emphysema. In: *Chronic Cor Pulmonale: Report of An Expert Committee.* Geneva, World Health Organization, Tech. Rep. Ser. No. 213, 1961, p. 15.

2015. Rainey, G.: On the minute anatomy of the emphysematous lung. Med. Chir. Trans., *31:*297, 1848.

2016. Whitfield, A. G. W., Smith, O. E., Richards, D. G. B., Waterhouse, J. A. H., and Arnott, W. H.: The correlation between the radiological appearances and the clinical and spirometric state in emphysema. Quart. J. Med. *(n.s.)20:*247, 1951.

2017. Pierce, J. A., Hocott, J. B., and Ebert, R. V.: The collagen and elastin content of the lung in emphysema. Ann. Int. Med., *55:*210, 1961.

2018. Hammond, J. D. S.: The work of breathing in patients with chronic cor pulmonale. Clin. Sci., *20:*107, 1961.

2019. Hickam, J. B., and Ross, J. C.: Respiratory acidosis in chronic pulmonary heart disease: Pathogenesis, clinical features and management. Progr. Cardiov. Dis., *1:*309, 1959.

2020. Robin, E. D.: Abnormalities of acid-base regulation in chronic pulmonary disease, with special reference to hypercapnia and extracellular alkalosis. New Engl. J. Med., *268:*917, 1963.

2021. Aber, G. M., Bayley, T. J., and Bishop, J. M.: Interrelationships between renal and cardiac function and respiratory gas exchange in obstructive airways disease. Clin. Sci., *25:*159, 1963.

2022. Cotes, J. E., and Rivers, D.: Relation entre la fonction alvéolo-capillaire, le pronostic et les découvertes d'autopsie dans les pneumopathies chroniques. Poumon Coeur, *16:*1121, 1960.

2023. Kellaway, G.: Acute anoxic cardiac failure in pulmonary heart-disease. Lancet, *2:*768, 1959.

2024. Charms, B. L., Brofman, B. L., Elder, J. C., and Kohn, P. M.: Unilateral pulmonary artery occlusion in man. II. Studies in patients with chronic pulmonary disease. J. Thoracic Surg., *35:*316, 1958.

2025. Kitchen, A. H., Lowther, C. P., and Matthews, M. B.: The effects of exercise and of breathing oxygen-enriched air on the pulmonary circulation in emphysema. Clin. Sci., *21:*93, 1961.

2026. Cotes, J. E., Pisa, Z., and Thomas, A. J.: Effect of breathing oxygen upon cardiac output, heart rate, ventilation, systemic and pulmonary blood pressure in patients with chronic lung disease. Clin. Sci., *25:*305, 1963.

2027. Hamm, J., and Gaensler, E. A.: Einseitig helle Lunge. Radiologe, *2:*333, 1962.

2028. Allison, S. T.: The vanishing lung: Report of a case of advanced bullous emphysema. Ann. Int. Med., *17:*139, 1942.

2029. Seebohm, P. M., and Bedell, G. N.: Primary pulmonary emphysema in young adults. Am. Rev. Resp. Dis., *87:*41, 1963.

2030. Borden, C. W., Wilson, R. H., Ebert, R. V., and Wells, H. S.: Pulmonary hypertension in chronic pulmonary emphysema. Am. J. Med., *8:*701, 1950.

2031. Whitcomb, W. H., Bird, R. M., Johnson, P. C., Hammarsten, J. F., and Moore, M.: The erythropoietic factor in hypoxic patients with emphysema without secondary polycythemia. A.M.A. Arch. Int. Med., *103:*871, 1959.

2032. Strawbridge, H. T. G.: Chronic pulmonary emphysema (An experimental study). I. Historical review. Am. J. Path., *37:*161, 1960.

2033. Strawbridge, H. T. G.: Chronic pulmonary emphysema (An experimental study). III. Experimental pulmonary emphysema. Am. J. Path., *37:*391, 1960.

2034. Baxter, S. G., and Meakins, J. F.: Developmental bronchial cysts. Ann. Int. Med., *38:*967, 1953.

2035. Perrott, E. A.: Cystic disease of the lungs. Brit. Med. J., *1:*436, 1956.

2036. Marchand, P., Gilroy, J. C., and Wilson, V. H.: An anatomical study of the bronchial vascular system and its variations in disease. Thorax, *5:*207, 1950.

2037. Holland, R. A. B., and Forster, R. E.: Effect of size of red cells on the kinetics of their oxygen uptake in different species [Abstract]. Fed. Proc., *21:*442, 1962.

2038. Turner-Warwick, M.: Systemic arterial patterns in the lung and clubbing of the fingers. Thorax, *18*:238, 1963.
2039. Clark, N. S.: Bronchiectasis in childhood. Brit. Med. J., *1*:80, 1963.
2040. Avery, M. E., Riley, M. C., and Weiss, A.: The course of bronchiectasis in childhood. Bull. Johns Hopkins Hosp., *109*:20, 1961.
2041. Kilburn, K. H.: Cardiorespiratory effects of large pneumothorax in conscious and anesthetized dogs. J. Appl. Physiol., *18*:279, 1963.
2042. Strang, C.: The fate of children with bronchiectasis. Ann. Int. Med., *44*:630, 1956.
2043. Sadoul, P., and Cherrier, F.: L'insuffisance respiratoire des gibbeux. J. Franc. Med. Chir. Thorac, *17*:167, 1963.
2044. Ogilvie, C., Harris, L. H., Meecham, J., and Ryder, G.: Ten years after pneumonectomy for carcinoma. Brit. Med. J., *1*:1111, 1963.
2045. Björk, V. O., and Hilty, H. J.: The arterial oxygen and carbon dioxide tension during the postoperative period in cases of pulmonary resections and thoracoplasties. J. Thoracic Surg., *27*:455, 1954.
2046. Björk, V. O., and Scrosoppi, F.: The arterial oxygen tension after resection with simultaneous osteoplastic thoracoplasty. J. Thoracic Surg., *29*:105, 1955.
2047. Swenson, E. W., Birath, G., Bergh, N. P., and Berglund, E.: Respiratory gas exchange in patients up to one year after pulmonary resection. Acta Tuberc. Scand., *41*:216, 1962.
2048. Herbert, F. A., Nahmias, B. B., Gaensler, E. A., and MacMahon, H. E.: Pathophysiology of interstitial pulmonary fibrosis. Report of 19 cases and follow-up with corticosteroids. Arch. Int. Med., *110*:628, 1962.
2049. Nahmias, B. B., Churchwell, A. G., and Bowles, F. N.: Diffuse interstitial pulmonary fibrosis (Hamman-Rich syndrome). A correlation of clinical, physiologic, roentgenologic and pathologic findings in a patient studied for three years, before and after adrenocorticosteroid treatment. Am. J. Med., *31*:154, 1961.
2050. Smith, K. V.: Chronic diffuse interstitial pneumonia and diffuse interstitial pulmonary fibrosis. Med. J. Aust., *2*:244, 1961.
2051. Read, J., Colebatch, H. J. H., and Smith, K. V.: Acute diffuse interstitial pulmonary fibrosis in scleroderma. Aust. Ann. Med., *9*:271, 1960.
2052. White, R. B., and Craighead, J. T.: Hamman-Rich syndrome (diffuse interstitial pulmonary fibrosis). Dis. Chest, *31*:335, 1957.
2053. Rubin, E. H.: Pulmonary lesions in "rheumatoid disease" with remarks on diffuse interstitial pulmonary fibrosis. Am. J. Med., *19*:569, 1955.
2054. Milliken, J. A., Waugh, D., and Kadish, M. E.: Acute interstitial pulmonary fibrosis caused by a smoke bomb. Canad. M. A. J., *88*:36, 1963.
2055. Dawson, J. J. Y.: Scleroderma with pulmonary involvement and chronic bronchitis. Proc. Roy. Soc. Med. (London), *48*:152, 1955.
2056. Bendixen, H. H., Hedley-Whyte, J., and Laver, M. B.: Impaired oxygenation in surgical patients during general anesthesia with controlled ventilation: A concept of atelectasis. New Engl. J. Med., *269*:991, 1963.
2057. Beaudry, P. H.: *Unpublished data.*
2058. Bernstein, I. L., Kreindler, L., Ghory, J. E., Fragge, R. G., and Gueron, M.: Pulmonary function in children. II. Preliminary studies in chronic intractable childhood asthma. J. Allergy, *30*:534, 1959.
2059. Andrewes, J. F., and Simmons, D. H.: Lung volumes of normal and asthmatic children. Pediatrics, *23*:507, 1959.
2060. Hamer, N. A. J.: Changes in the components of the diffusing capacity in pulmonary sarcoidosis. Thorax, *18*:275, 1963.
2061. Arnott, W. M.: The lungs in mitral stenosis. Brit. Med. J., *2*:765, 1963.
2062. Yu, P. N. G., Simpson, J. H., Lovejoy, F. W., Joos, H. A., and Nye, R. E., Jr.: Studies in pulmonary hypertension. IV. Pulmonary circulatory dynamics in patients with mitral stenosis at rest. Am. Heart J., *47*:330, 1954.
2063. Raine, J., and Bishop, J. M.: The distribution of alveolar ventilation in mitral stenosis at rest and after exercise. Clin. Sci., *24*:63, 1963.
2064. Bishop, J. M., and Wade, O. L.: Relationships between cardiac output and rhythm, pulmonary vascular pressures and disability in mitral stenosis. Clin. Sci., *24*:391, 1963.
2065. Donald, K. W., Gloster, J., Harris, E. A., Reeves, J., and Harris, P.: The production of lactic acid during exercise in normal subjects and in patients with rheumatic heart disease. Am. Heart J., *62*:494, 1961.
2066. Horres, A. D., and Bernthal, T.: Localized multiple minute pulmonary embolism and breathing. J. Appl. Physiol., *16*:842, 1961.
2067. Cahill, J. M., Attinger, E. O., and Byrne, J. J.: Ventilatory responses to embolization of lung. J. Appl. Physiol., *16*:469, 1961.
2068. Stein, M., Forkner, C. E., Jr., Robin, E. D., and Wessler, S.: Gas exchange after autologous pulmonary embolism in dogs. J. Appl. Physiol., *16*:488, 1961.
2069. Cain, S. M.: Effects of fat emulsion on O_2 transport and alveolar-arterial gas tensions. J. Appl. Physiol., *17*:263, 1962.
2070. Sabiston, D. C., Jr., Marshall, R., Dunnill, M. S., and Allison, P. R.: Experimental pulmonary embolism: Description of a method utilizing large venous thrombi. Surgery, *52*:9, 1962.
2071. Marshall, R.: Pulmonary embolism and thrombosis. Postgrad. Med. J., *38*:13, 1962.
2072. Cronin, R. F. P., and MacIntosh, D. J.: The relationship of oxygen uptake to muscular exercise in patients with mitral stenosis. Dis. Chest, *42*:508, 1962.
2073. Richards, P.: Pulmonary œdema and intracranial lesions. Brit. Med. J., *2*:83, 1963.
2074. Katz, A., Bernard, R., Denolin, H., Englert, M., and Lequime, J.: L'hypertension pulmonaire primitive. Étude clinque et physiopathologique. Acta Cardiol., *16*:507, 1961.
2075. Hughes, R., May, A. J., and Widdicombe, J. G.: Mechanical factors in the formation of oedema in perfused rabbits' lungs. J. Physiol. (London), *142*:292, 1958.
2076. Widdicombe, J. G.: The activity of pulmonary stretch receptors during bronchoconstriction, pulmonary oedema, atelectasis and breathing against a resistance. J. Physiol. (London), *159*:436, 1961.
2077. Bucci, G., and Cook, C. D.: Studies of respiratory physiology in children. VI. Lung diffusing capacity, diffusing capacity of the pulmonary membrane and pulmonary capillary blood volume in congenital heart disease. J. Clin. Invest., *40*:1431, 1961.
2078. Fraser, R. S., Sproule, B. J., and Dvorkin, J.: Hypoventilation, cyanosis and polycythemia in a thin man. Canad. M. A. J., *89*:1178, 1963.
2079. Gillam, P. M. S., and Mymin, D.: Hypoventilation and heart-disease. Lancet, *2*:853, 1961.
2080. Casey, T. R., Fast, B. B., and Cherniack, R. M.: Pseudo-pseudohypoparathyroidism. Report of a case with associated cardiopulmonary syndrome of obesity. J.A.M.A., *169*:1988, 1959.
2081. Zeidberg, L. D., Prindle, R. A., and Landau, E.: The Nashville air pollution study. I. Sulfur dioxide and bronchial asthma. A preliminary report. Am. Rev. Resp. Dis., *84*:489, 1961.
2082. Cochrane, A. L., and Higgins, I. T. T.: Pulmonary ventilatory functions of coalminers in various areas in relation to the X-ray category of pneumoconiosis. Brit. J. Prev. Soc. Med., *15*:1, 1961.
2083. Hunt, A. C.: Massive pulmonary fibrosis from the inhalation of talc. Thorax, *11*:287, 1956.
2084. Aluminum and the lung [Annotation]. Lancet, *1*:151, 1963.
2085. DeNardi, J. M., Van Ordstrand, H. S., and Carmody, M. G.: Chronic pulmonary granulomatosis. Report of ten cases. Am. J. Med., *7*:345, 1949.
2086. Bouhuys, A., and Lindell, S. E.: Release of histamine by cotton dust extracts from human lung tissue *in vitro*. Experientia, *17*:211, 1961.

2087. McKerrow, C. B., and Schilling, R. S. F.: A pilot enquiry into byssinosis in two cotton mills in the United States. J.A.M.A., *177*:850, 1961.
2088. Bouhuys, A.: Byssinosis in a cotton weaving mill. Arch. Environ. Health, *6*:465, 1963.
2089. Bouhuys, A., and Lindell, S. E.: World-wide byssinosis. Brit. Med. J., *2*:1396, 1962.
2090. Fuller, C. J.: Farmer's lung: A review of present knowledge. Thorax, *8*:59, 1953.
2091. Parish, W. E.: Farmer's lung. Part I. An immunological study of some antigenic components of mouldy foodstuffs. Thorax, *18*:83, 1963.
2092. Pepys, J., Riddell, R. W., Citron, K. M., and Clayton, Y. M.: Precipitins against extracts of hay and moulds in the serum of patients with farmer's lung, aspergillosis, asthma, and sarcoidosis. Thorax, *17*:366, 1962.
2093. Williams, J. V.: Pulmonary function studies in patients with farmer's lung. Thorax, *18*:255, 1963.
2094. Hughes, R., May, A. J., and Widdicombe, J. G.: The effect of pulmonary congestion and oedema on lung compliance. J. Physiol. (London), *142*:306, 1958.
2095. Brasseur, L.: *L'Exploration Fonctionnelle Pulmonaire dans la Pneumoconiose des Houilleurs.* Brussels, Editions Arscia; Paris, Librairie Maloine, 1963.
2096. Thomson, J. G., Kaschula, R. O. C., and MacDonald, R. R.: Asbestos as a modern urban hazard. S. African Med. J., *37*:77, 1963.
2097. U. S. Chemical Warfare Service: *Proceedings on a Board Appointed for the Purpose of Investigating Conditions Incident to the Disaster at the Cleveland Hospital Clinic, Cleveland, Ohio, on May 15, 1929.* (Lt. Col. W. C. Baker, C. W. S., Commanding, Edgewood Arsenal, Md.) Washington, D.C., U.S. Government Printing Office, 1929.
2098. Mendenhall, R. M., and Stokinger, H. E.: Films from lung washings as a mechanism model for lung injury by ozone. J. Appl. Physiol., *17*:28, 1962.
2099. Ellis, F. P.: Petrol-vapour poisoning [Letter to the Editor]. Brit. Med. J., *2*:1413, 1958.
2100. Waring, J. I.: Pneumonia in kerosene poisoning. Am. J. Med. Sci., *185*:325, 1933.
2101. Nunn, J. A., and Martin, F. M.: Gasoline and kerosene poisoning in children. J.A.M.A., *103*:472, 1934.
2102. Deichmann, W. B., Kitzmiller, K. V., Witherup, S., and Johansmann, R.: Kerosene intoxication. Ann. Int. Med., *21*:803, 1944.
2103. Steiner, M. M.: Syndromes of kerosene poisoning in children. Am. J. Dis. Child, *74*:32, 1947.
2104. Lesser, L. I., Weens, H. S., and McKey, J. D.: Pulmonary manifestations following ingestion of kerosene. J. Pediat., *23*:352, 1943.
2105. Richardson, J. A., and Pratt-Thomas, H. R.: Toxic effects of varying doses of kerosene administered by different routes. Am. J. Med. Sci., *221*:531, 1951.
2106. Kerosene (paraffin) poisoning [Annotation]. Brit. Med. J., *1*:208, 1963.
2107. Kazantzis, G.: Respiratory function in men casting cadmium alloys; assessment of respiratory function. Brit. J. Indust. Med., *13*:30, 1956.
2108. Bergmann, M., Flance, I. J., and Blumenthal, H. T.: Thesaurosis following inhalation of hair spray. A clinical and experimental study. New Engl. J. Med., *258*:471, 1958.
2109. Edelston, B. G.: Thesaurosis following inhalation of hair spray. Lancet, *2*:112, 1959.
2110. Bergmann, M., Flance, I. J., Cruz, P. T., Klam, N., Aronson, P. R., Joshi, R. A., and Blumenthal, H. T.: Thesaurosis due to inhalation of hair spray. Report of twelve new cases, including three autopsies. New Eng. J. Med., *266*:750, 1962.
2111. Trenchard, H. J., and Harris, W. C.: An outbreak of respiratory symptoms caused by toluene di-isocyanate. Lancet, *1*:404, 1963.
2112. Fleming, W. H., Szakacs, J. E., Hartney, T. C., and King, E. R.: Hyaline membrane following total body radiation. Relation to lung plasminogen activator. [Preliminary communication.] Lancet, *2*:1010, 1960.
2113. Emanuel, D. A., Lawton, B. R., and Wenzel, F. J.: Maple-bark disease. Pneumonitis due to *Coniosporium corticale.* New Engl. J. Med., *266*:333, 1962.
2114. West, J. R., Levin, S. M., and di Sant'Agnese, P. A.: Pulmonary function in cystic fibrosis of the pancreas. Pediatrics, *13*:155, 1954.
2115. May, C. D.: *Cystic Fibrosis of the Pancreas in Infants and Children.* (American Lecture Series, Publication No. 234; American Lectures in Pediatrics, edited by J. A. Anderson.) Springfield, Ill., Charles C Thomas, 1954.
2116. Shwachman, H., and Castleman, B.: Bronchiectasis in seven-year-old boy (Massachusetts General Hospital Case Record No. 81-1963). New Engl. J. Med., *269*:1427, 1963.
2117. Nadas, A. S., Cogan, G., Landing, B. H., and Shwachman, H.: Studies in pancreatic fibrosis. Cor pulmonale: clinical and pathologic observations. Pediatrics, *10*:319, 1952.
2118. Gandevia, B., and Anderson, C.: The effect of a bronchodilator aerosol on ventilatory capacity in fibrocystic disease of the pancreas. Arch. Dis. Child., *34*:511, 1959.
2119. Cook, C. D., Helliesen, P. J., Kulczycki, L., Barrie, H., Friendlander, L., Agathon, S., Harris, G. B. C., and Schwachman, H.: Studies of respiratory physiology in children. II. Lung volumes and mechanics of respiration in 64 patients with cystic fibrosis of the pancreas. Pediatrics, *24*:181, 1959.
2120. di Sant'Agnese, P. A.: Recent observations on pathogenesis of cystic fibrosis of the pancreas. Pediatrics, *24*:313, 1959.
2121. Roberts, G. B. S.: Fundamental defect in fibrocystic disease of the pancreas. Lancet, *2*:964, 1959.
2122. West, J. R., and di Sant'Agnese, A.: Studies of pulmonary function in cystic fibrosis of the pancreas. [Abstr.] A.M.A. J. Dis. Child., *86*:496, 1953.
2123. Freeman, J., and Nunn, J. F.: Ventilation-perfusion relationships after haemorrhage. Clin. Sci., *24*:135, 1963.
2124. Bartlett, D., Jr., and Tenney, S. M.: Tissue gas tensions in experimental anemia. J. Appl. Physiol., *18*:734, 1963.
2125. Burgess, J. H., and Bishop, J. M.: Pulmonary diffusing capacity and its subdivisions in polycythemia vera. J. Clin. Invest., *42*:997, 1963.
2126. Bedell, G. N., Sheets, R. F., Fischer, H. W., and Theilen, E. O.: Polycythemia: A manifestation of heart disease, lung disease or a primary blood dyscrasia. Circulation, *18*:107, 1958.
2127. Bland, E. F., and Castleman, B.: Polycythemia and pulmonary hypertension (Massachusetts General Hospital Case Record No. 59-1963). New Engl. J. Med., *269*:626, 1963.
2128. Jones, C. C.: Pulmonary alevolar proteinosis with unusual complicating infections. A report of two cases. Am. J. Med., *29*:713, 1960.
2129. Ray, R. L., and Salm, R.: A fatal case of pulmonary alveolar proteinosis. Thorax, *17*:257, 1962.
2130. McCredie, M., Lovejoy, F. W., Jr., and Kaltreider, N. L.: Pulmonary function in diaphragmatic paralysis. Thorax, *17*:213, 1962.
2131. Comroe, J. H., Jr., Wood, F. C., Kay, C. F., and Spoont, E. M.: Motor neuritis after tetanus anti-toxin with involvement of the muscles of respiration. Am. J. Med., *10*:786, 1951.
2132. Faerber, I., Liebert, P. B., and Suskind, M.: Loss of functional residual capacity in poliomyelitis. J. Appl. Physiol., *17*:289, 1962.
2133. Viswanathan, R.: Pulmonary alveolar microlithiasis. Thorax, *17*:251, 1962.
2134. Powell, V.: Pulmonary telangiectasis. Thorax, *13*:321, 1958.
2135. Armentrout, H. L., and Underwood, F. J.: Familial hemorrhagic telangiectasia with associated pulmonary arteriovenous aneurysm. Am. J. Med., *8*:246, 1950.
2136. Hultgren, H. N., and Gerbode, F.: Physiologic studies in a patient with a pulmonary arteriovenous fistula. Am. J. Med., *17*:126, 1954.
2137. Lange, K.: Capillary permeability in myxedema. Am. J. Med. Sci., *208*:5, 1944.

2138. Pauli, H. G., and Reubi, F.: Respiratory control in uremic acidosis. J. Appl. Physiol., *18*:717, 1963.
2139. Refsum, H. E.: Respiratory response to acute exercise in induced metabolic acidosis. Acta Physiol. Scand., *52*:32, 1961.
2140. Black, D. A. K., and Stanbury, S. W.: Renal insufficiency in terminal respiratory failure. Brit. Med. J., *1*:872, 1958.
2141. Eichenholz, A., Mulhausen, R. O., Anderson, W. E., and MacDonald, F. M.: Primary hypocapnia: a cause of metabolic acidosis. J. Appl. Physiol., *17*:283, 1962.
2142. Reeves, J. L., and Brown, E. B., Jr.: Respiratory compensation to metabolic alkalosis in dogs: Influence of high oxygen concentration. J. Appl. Physiol., *13*:179, 1958.
2143. Singer, R. B., Deering, R. C., and Clark, J. K.: The acute effects in man of a rapid intravenous infusion of hypertonic sodium bicarbonate solution. II. Changes in respiration and output of carbon dioxide. J. Clin. Invest., *35*:245, 1956.
2144. Roberts, K. E., Poppell, J. W., Vanamee, P., Beals, R., and Randall, H. T.: Evaluation of respiratory compensation in metabolic alkalosis. J. Clin. Invest., *35*:261, 1956.
2145. Stone, D. J.: Respiration in man during metabolic alkalosis. J. Appl. Physiol., *17*:33, 1962.
2146. Cander, L., and Hanowell, E.: The effects of fever on the pulmonary diffusing capacity and pulmonary mechanics in man [Abstract]. Fed. Proc., *19*:374, 1960.
2147. Moser, K. M., Perry, R. B., and Luchsinger, P. C.: Cardiopulmonary consequences of pyrogen-induced hyperpyrexia in man. J. Clin. Invest., *42*:626, 1963.
2148. Abelmann, W. H., Frank, N. R., Gaensler, E. A., and Cugell, D. W.: Effects of abdominal distension by ascites on lung volumes and ventilation. Arch. Int. Med., *93*:528, 1954.
2149. Renzetti, A. D., Jr., Harris, B. A., and Bowen, J. F.: Influence of ammonia on respiration. J. Appl. Physiol., *16*:703, 1961.
2150. Castillon du Perron, M., Liot, F., Vasselin, M., and Bechtel, P.: Étude de la fonction ventilatoire au cours des diminutions du calibre trachéal d'origine non tumorale. Bronches, *11*:33, 1961.
2151. Coulshed, N., and Jones, E. W.: Tracheal vascular ring causing dyspnœa. Brit. Heart J., *20*:147, 1958.
2152. Intensive care unit [Annotation]. Brit. Med. J., *1*:904, 1963.
2153. Forke, M. E., Schoemperlen, C. B., and Cherniack, R. M.: Alveolar ventilation during bronchoscopy. Dis. Chest, *42*:311, 1962.
2154. Hercus, V.: Planning a respiratory unit. Brit. Med. J., *2*:1604, 1962.
2155. Patterson, J. L., Jr., Mullinax, P. F., Jr., Bain, T., Kreuger, J. J., and Richardson, D. W.: Carbon dioxide-induced dyspnea in a patient with respiratory muscle paralysis. Am. J. Med., *32*:811, 1962.
2156. Smith, A. C., Schuster, E., and Spalding, J. M. K.: An end-tidal air sampler for use during artificial respiration. Lancet, *1*:277, 1959.
2157. Griggs, D. E., Hackney, J. D., Collier, C. R., and Affeldt, J. E.: The rapid diagnosis of ventilatory failure with the carbon dioxide analyzer. Am. J. Med., *25*:31, 1958.
2158. Geraci, J. E., and Wood, E. H.: The relationship of the arterial oxygen saturation to cyanosis. Med. Clin. N. Am., *35*:1185, 1951.
2159. Greene, N. M., and Phillips, A. D.: Metabolic response of dogs to hypoxia in the absence of circulating epinephrine and norepinehphrine. Am. J. Physiol., *189*:475, 1957.
2160. DuBois, A. B., Hyde, R. W., and Hendler, E.: Pulmonary mechanics and diffusing capacity following simulated space flight of 2 weeks' duration. J. Appl. Physiol., *18*:696, 1963.
2161. Donald, K. W.: Oxygen poisoning in man. Brit. Med. J., *1*:667, 1947.
2162. Yeomans, A., and Stueck, G. H., Jr.: Clinical-chemical studies of acid-base abnormalities. Changes in acid-base balance observed in renal and respiratory disease. Am. J. Med., *13*:183, 1952.
2163. Foster, C. A., and Churchill-Davidson, I.: Response to high pressure oxygen of conscious volunteers and patients. J. Appl. Physiol., *18*:492, 1963.
2164. Comroe, J. H., Jr., Dripps, R. D., Dumke, P. R., and Deming, M.: Oxygen toxicity. The effect of inhalation of high concentrations of oxygen for 24 hours on normal men at sea level and at a simulated altitude of 18,000 ft. J.A.M.A., *128*:710, 1945.
2165. Smith, C. W., Lehan, P. H., and Monks, J. J.: Cardiopulmonary manifestations with high O_2 tensions at atmospheric pressure. J. Appl. Physiol., *18*:849, 1963.
2166. Cedergren, B., Gyllensten, L., and Wersall, J.: Pulmonary damage caused by oxygen poisoning: An electron-microscopic study in mice. Acta Paediat., *48*:477, 1959.
2167. Griffo, Z. J., and Roos, A.: Effect of O_2 breathing on pulmonary compliance. J. Appl. Physiol., *17*:233, 1962.
2168. Doležal, V.: [The effect of long-lasting oxygen inhibition upon respiratory parameters in man.] Physiol. Bohemoslav., *11*:149, 1962 [Biol. Abstr., *39*:1812, 1962, abstr. no. 22918].
2169. Beecher, H. K., and Murphy, A. J.: Acidosis during thoracic surgery. J. Thoracic surg., *19*:50, 1950.
2170. Smith, T. C., Cook, F. D., DeKornfeld, T. J., and Siebecker, K. L.: Pulmonary function in the immediate postoperative period. Observations of vital capacity, timed vital capacity, and maximum expiratory flow rates in two groups of thoracotomy patients and a group of nonthoracotomy patients for seven postoperative days. J. Thorac. Cardiov. Surg., *39*:788, 1960.
2171. Thornton, J. A.: Physiological dead space. Changes during general anesthesia. Anaesthesia, *15*:381, 1960.
2172. Schultz, E. A., Buckley, J. J., Oswald, A. J., and Van Bergen, F. H.: Profound acidosis in an anesthetized human: Report of a case. Anesthesiology, *21*:285, 1960.
2173. Ellison, K. T., Yeh, T. J., Moretz, W. H., and Ellison, R. G.: Pulmonary diffusion studies in patients undergoing nonthoracic, thoracic, and cardiopulmonary bypass procedures. Ann. Surg., *157*:327, 1963.
2174. Gibbon, J. H., Jr., Allbritten, F. F., Jr., Stayman, J. W., Jr., and Judd, J. M.: A critical study of respiratory exchange during prolonged operations with an open thorax. Ann. Surg., *132*:611, 1950.
2175. Cooper, E. A., Smith, H., and Pask, E. A.: On the effieiency of intra-gastric oxygen. Anaesthesia, *15*:211, 1960.
2176. Effersöe, P., Kristensen, H. S., and Lassen, H. C. A.: Effect of oxygen therapy on oedema in patients with cor pulmonale. Brit. Med. J., *1*:1469, 1960.
2177. McNicol, M. W., Pride, N. B., Reynolds, E. O. R., and Semple, S. J. G.: Nikethamide for severe CO_2 retention in exacerbations of chronic bronchitis. Brit. Med. J., *1*:646, 1963.
2178. Milhaud, A., Poisvert, M., and Cara, M.: Une solution au difficile problème de l'humidification de l'air inspiré chez les patients trachéotomisés: Le nez artificiel. Vie Med., *43 (special)*:61, 1962.
2179. Cara, M.: Les respirateurs automatiques. Principes généraux et classification. Acta Anaesth. Belg., *11*/2(suppl.):311, 1960.
2180. Sadoul, P., Gay, R., and Peslin, R.: Ventilation instrumentale au cours de l'insuffisance respiratoire aiguë des pulmonaires chroniques. In: Sadoul, P., *et al.* (eds.): *Le Traitment de l'Insuffisance Respiratoire Aiguë des Pulmonaires Chroniques.* Prob. Reamination, *2*:–, 1962. (Doin; Nancy, Impr. Georges Thomas, 1963.)
2181. Shephard, R. J.: Ergonomics of the respirator. In: Davies, C. N. (ed.): *Design and Use of Respirators.* Oxford, Pergamon Press, 1962. p. 51.
2182. Tracheotomy in children [Annotation]. Lancet, *2*:1040, 1962.
2183. Hutchison, J. H., Kerr, M. M., McPhail, M. F. M., Douglas, T. A., Smith, G., Norman, J. N., and Bates, E. H.: Studies in the treatment of the pulmonary syndrome of the newborn. Lancet, *2*:465, 1962.
2184. Gribetz, I., Frank, N. R., and Avery, M. E.: Static volume-pressure relations of excised lungs of infants with

hyaline membrane disease, newborn and stillborn infants. J. Clin. Invest., *38:*2168, 1959.

2185. Glauser, E. M., McCance, R. A., and Widdowson, E. M.: Experimental respiratory embrarrassment in new-born piglets. J. Physiol. (London), *161:*313, 1962.
2186. The stove-in chest [Annotation]. Lancet, *1:*871, 1963.
2187. Sieker, H. O., Hickam, J. B., and Pryor, W. W.: The treatment of carbon dioxide narcosis by the use of an automatic positive-negative resuscitator. Am. Rev. Tuberc., *74:*309, 1956.
2188. Pare, J. A. P., Morton, J. W., and Rose, B.: Carbon dioxide narcosis and the management of advanced pulmonary insufficiency. Canad. M. A. J., *73:*278, 1955.
2189. Whittenberger, J. L. (ed.): *Artificial Respiration. Theory and Applications.* New York, Hoeber (Harper), 1962.
2190. Beer, R., Loeschcke, G., Schaudig, A., Pasini, M., Auberger, H. G., Ranz, H., and Borst, H. G.: Lungenfunktion nach Anwendung extrakorporaler Zirkulation. Thoraxchirurgie, *9:*427, 1961.
2191. Schramel, R. J., Cameron, R., Ziskind, M. M., Adam, M., and Creech, O., Jr.: Studies of pulmonary diffusion after open heart surgery. J. Thorac. Cardiov. Surg., *38:*281, 1959.
2192. Osborn, J. J., Popper, R. W., Kerth, W. J., and Gerbode, F.: Respiratory insufficiency following open heart surgery. Ann. Surg., *156:*638, 1962.
2193. Howatt, W. F., Talner, N. S., Sloan, H., and DeMuth, G. R.: Pulmonary function changes following repair of heart lesions with the aid of extra-corporal circulation. J. Thorac. Cardiov. Surg., *43:*649, 1962.
2194. Gardner, R. E., Finley, T. N., and Tooley, W. H.: The effect of cardiopulmonary bypass on surface activity of lung extracts. Bull. Soc. Int. Chir., *21:*542, 1962.
2195. Schramel, R., Schmidt, F., Davis, F., Palmisano, D., and Creech, O., Jr.: Pulmonary lesions produced by prolonged partial perfusion. Surgery, *54:*224, 1963.
2196. Hepps, S. A., Roe, B. B., Wright, R. F., and Gardner, R. E.: Amelioration of the pulmonary post-perfusion syndrome with hemodilution and low molecular weight dextran. Surgery, *54:*232, 1963.
2197. Galletti, P. M., and Salisbury, P. F.: Partial extra-corporeal circulation in closed-chest dogs. J. Appl. Physiol., *14:*684, 1959.
2198. Henderson, M., and Apthorp, G. H.: Rapid method for estimation of carbon monoxide in blood. Brit. Med. J., *2:*1853, 1960.
2199. Smith, G., Ledingham, I. M., Sharp, G. R., Norman, J. N., and Bates, E. H.: Treatment of coal-gas poisoning with oxygen at 2 atmospheres pressure. Lancet, *1:*816, 1962.
2200. Cournand, A.: Hémodynamique et échanges respiratoires dans le choc. In: Wollheim, E., and Schlegel, B. (eds.): *Proceedings of the VIIth International Congress on Internal Medicine, Munich, 1962.* Stuttgart, Thieme, 1963, p. 366.
2201. Acidosis in cardiac arrest [Annotation]. Lancet, *2:*976, 1962.
2202. Campiche, M., Jaccottet, M., and Juillard, E.: La pneumonose à membranes hyalines. Observations au microscope électronique. Ann. Paediat., *199:*74, 1962.
2203. Wright, G. W., and Kleinerman, J.: A consideration of the etiology of emphysema in terms of contemporary knowledge [Amberson Lecture, 1963]. Am. Rev. Resp. Dis., *88:*605, 1963.
2204. Crowell, J. W., and Kaufmann, B. N.: Changes in tissue pH after circulatory arrest. Am. J. Physiol., *200:*743, 1961.
2205. Ledingham, I. M., and Norman, J. N.: Acid-base studies in experimental circulatory arrest [Preliminary communication]. Lancet, *2:*967, 1962.
2206. Stewart, J. S. S., Stewart, W. K., and Gillies, H. G.: Cardiac arrest and acidosis. Lancet, *2:*967, 1962.
2207. Whitwam, J. G., and Norman, J.: A resuscitation service. Lancet, *1:*46, 1963.
2208. Brinkman, G. L., and Coates, E. O., Jr.: The effect of bronchitis, smoking and occupation on ventilation. Am. Rev. Resp. Dis., *87:*684, 1963.
2209. Prolongation of dying [Annotation]. Lancet, *2:*1205, 1962.
2210. Intensive care [Annotation]. Lancet, *2:*1314, 1962.
2211. Chapin, J. L., Otis, A. B., and Rahn, H.: Changes in the sensitivity of the respiratory center in man after prolonged exposure to 3% CO_2. In: Rahn, H., and Fenn, W. O. (eds.): *Studies in Respiratory Physiology,* 2nd ser. Wright Air Development Center, WADC T-R 55-357, 1955, p. 250.
2212. Cox, J. R., Davies-Jones, G. A. B., Leonard, P. J., and Singer, B.: The effect of positive pressure respiration on urinary aldosterone excretion. Clin. Sci., *24:*1, 1963.
2213. Lee, W. L., Jr., Caldwell, P. B., and Schildkraut, H. S.: Changes of lung volume, diffusing capacity and blood gases in oxygen toxicity in humans [Absract]. Fed. Proc., *22:*395, 1963.
2214. Campbell, E. J. M., and Howell, J. B. L.: The sensation of breathlessness. Brit. Med. Bull., *19:*36, 1963.
2215. Bromberg, P. A., and Robin, E. D.: Abnormalities of lung function in tuberculosis. Advances Tuberc. Res., *12:*1, 1963; Bibl. Tuberc., *17:*1, 1963.
2216. Gregoire, F., Soucy, R., Lépine, C., and Laberge, M. J.: Comparative physiological studies in chronic pulmonary diseases. Med. Serv. J. Can., *14:*617, 1958.
2217. Gaensler, E. A., Cugell, D. W., Lindgren, I.: Verstraeten, J. M., Smith, S. S., and Strieder, J. W.: The role of pulmonary insufficiency in mortality and invalidism following surgery for pulmonary tuberculosis. J. Thoracic Surg., *29:*163, 1955.
2218. Salyer, J. M., Harrison, H. N., Winn, D. F., Jr., and Taylor, R. R.: Chronic fibrous mediastinitis and superior vena caval obstruction due to histoplasmosis. Dis. Chest., *35:*364, 1959.
2219. Alexander, J. K., Takezawa, H., Abu-Nassar, H. J., and Yow, E. M.: Studies on pulmonary blood flow in pneumococcal pneumonia. Cardiov. Res. Cent. Bull., *1:*86, 1963.
2220. Colp, C. R., Park, S. S., and Williams, M. H., Jr.: Pulmonary function studies in pneumonia. Am. Rev. Resp. Dis., *85:*808, 1962.
2221. Reynolds, E. O. R.: Arterial blood gas tensions in acute disease of lower respiratory tract in infancy. Brit. Med. J., *1:*1192, 1963.
2222. Disney, M. E., Sandiford, B. R., Cragg, J., and Wolff, J.: Epidemic bronchiolitis in infants. Brit. Med. J., *1:*1407, 1960.
2223. Tuberculosis Society of Scotland, Research Committee: Prednisolone in the treatment of pulmonary tuberculosis: A controlled trial [Preliminary report]. Brit. Med. J., *2:*1131, 1957.
2224. Weibel, E. R.: *Morphometry of the Human Lung.* New York, Academic Press, 1963.
2225. Bjure, J., Söderholm, B., and Widimský, J.: Cardiolpulmonary function studies in workers dealing with asbestos and glasswool. Thorax, *19:*22, 1964.
2226. Hardy, J. D., Webb, W. R., Dalton, M. L., Jr., and Walker, G. R., Jr.: Lung homotransplantation in man. Report of the initial case. J.A.M.A., *186:*1065, 1963.
2227. Cassels, D. E., and Morse, M.: *Cardiopulmonary Data for Children and Young Adults.* Springfield, Ill., Charles C Thomas, 1962, p. 134.
2228. Coates, E. O., Jr., Brinkman, G. L., and Noe, F. E.: Hypoventilation syndrome: Physiologic studies in selected cases. Ann. Int. Med., *48:*50, 1958.
2229. Marshall, R., Sabiston, D. C., Allison, P. R., Bosman, A. R., and Dunnill, M. S.: Immediate and late effects of pulmonary embolism by large thrombi in dogs. Thorax, *18:*1, 1963.
2230. Permutt, S., and Riley, R. L.: Hemodynamics of collapsible vessels with tone: The vascular waterfall. J. Appl. Physiol., *18:*924, 1963.
2231. Kahana, L. M., Aronovitch, M., and Place, R.: A comparative study of the clinical and functional pattern in emphysematous patients with and without chronic respiratory failure. Am. Rev. Resp. Dis., *87:*699, 1963.
2232. Lloyd, T. C., Jr., and Wright, G. W.: Evaluation of methods used in detecting changes of airway resistance in man. Am. Rev. Resp. Dis., *87:*529, 1963.
2233. Massaro, D. J., Katz, S., and Luchsinger, P. C.: The use of a carbon dioxide buffer (trishydroxymethylaminometh-

ane) in the treatment of respiratory acidosis. Am. Rev. Resp. Dis,, *86*:353, 1962.
2234. Yeh, T. J., Ellison, L. T., and Ellison, R. G.: Functional evaluation of the autotransplanted lung in the dog. Am. Rev. Resp. Dis., *86*:791, 1962.
2235. Soergel, K. H., and Sommers, S. C.: The alveolar epithelial lesion in idiopathic pulmonary hemosiderosis. Am. Rev. Resp. Dis., *85*:540, 1962.
2236. Wynn-Williams, N., and Young, R. D.: Idiopathic pulmonary haemosiderosis in adults. Thorax, *11*:101, 1956.
2237. Gurewich, V., and Thomas, M. A.: Idiopathic pulmonary hemorrhage in pregnancy. Report of a case suggesting early pulmonary hemosiderosis with recovery after steroid therapy. New Engl. J. Med., *261*:1154, 1959.
2238. Sekelj, P., and Johnson, A.: Photoelectric method for estimation of the oxygen saturation of nonhemolyzed whole blood. J. Lab. Clin. Med., *49*:465, 1957.
2239. Fritts, H. W., Jr., Harris, P., Chidsey, C. A., III, Clauss, R. H., and Cournand, A.: Estimation of flow through bronchial-pulmonary vascular anastomoses with use of T-1824 dye. Circulation, *23*:390, 1961.
2240. Harmel, M. H., Elder, J. D., and Norlander, O.: Flow-pressure-volume characteristics of some different respirators. Acta Anaesth. Scand., suppl. 6, p. 62, 1960.
2241. Heaf, P. J. D., and Prime, F. J.: The mechanical aspects of artificial pneumothorax. Lancet, *2*:468, 1954.
2242. Herxheimer, H., and Stresemann, E.: Die Retention feuchter Aerosolteilchen in den Atemwegen bei Gesunden und Kranken mit Bronchialverengung. Arch. Exper. Path. Pharmakol., *241*:225, 1961.
2243. Chatgidakis, C. B.: Silicosis in South African white gold miners. A comparative study of the disease in different stages. Med. Proc., *9*:383, 1963.
2244. Caplan, A.: Correlation of radiological category with lung pathology in coal-workers' pneumoconiosis. Brit. J. Indust. Med., *19*:171, 1962.
2245. Arias-Stella, J., and Recavarren, S.: Right ventricular hypertrophy in native children living at high altitude. Am. J. Path., *41*:54, 1962.
2246. Thung, N., Herzog, P., Christlieb, I. I., Thompson, W. M., Jr., and Dammann, J. F., Jr.: The cost of respiratory effort in postoperative cardiac patients. Circulation, *28*:552, 1963.
2247. Perry, H. M., Jr., O'Neal, R. M., and Thomas, W. A.: Pulmonary disease following chronic chemical ganglionic blockade. A clinical and pathologic study. Am. J. Med., *22*:37, 1957.
2248. Robillard, R., Riopelle, J. L., Adamkiewicz, L., Tremblay, G., and Genest, J.: Pulmonary complications during treatment with hexamethonium. Canad. M. A. J., *72*:448, 1955.
2249. Mills, F. C., Parsons, W. D., Pare, J. A. P., and Bates, D. V.: The physical status of men in the lowest income group in the sixth decade of life. Canad. M. A. J., *89*:281, 1963.
2250. Shepard, R. H.: The influence of distribution of V_A/Q_C on the Filley D_{CO} in a two-alveolus model of the lung. [Abstr.] Fed. Proc., *23*:365, 1964.
2251. Holmgren, A., and McIlroy, M. B.: Effect of temperature on arterial blood gas tensions and pH during exercise. J. Appl. Physiol., *19*:243, 1964.
2252. Shaw, K. M., and Burton, N. A.: Experimental pulmonary reimplantation. Thorax, *19*:180, 1964.
2253. Goldring, R. M., and Heinemann, H. O.: Respiratory adjustments in induced metabolic alkalosis. [Abstr.] Fed. Proc., *23*:308, 1964.
2254. Gillam, P. M. S., Heaf, P. J. D., Kaufman, L., and Lucas, B. G. B.: Respiration in dystrophia myotonica. Thorax, *19*:112, 1964.
2255. Rossier, P. H.: Les épreuves fonctionnelles respiratoires pré-opératoires des cancers bronchiques primitifs. Bronches, *12*:473, 1962.
2256. Berg, W. C., and Tammeling, G. J.: Changes in pulmonary function resulting from bronchography. Koninkl. Ned. Verenig. Tuberk. Bestrij., *515*:72, 1963 [Excerpta Med. (XV), *16*:492, 1963].
2257. Ball, W. C., Jr.: Effect in a lung model of non-uniformity on estimates of CO diffusing capacity by Filley and Bates techniques. [Abstr.] Fed. Proc., *23*:365, 1964.
2258. Marcelle, R.: Aérosol d'histamine et résistance dynamique pulmonaire de l'homme. Int. Arch. Allergy, *22*:45, 1963.
2259. Gotsman, M. S., and Whitby, J. L.: Respiratory infection following tracheostomy. Thorax, *19*:89, 1964.
2260. Terman, J. W., and Newton, J. L.: Changes in alveolar and arterial gas tensions as related to altitude and age. J. Appl. Physiol., *19*:21, 1964.
2261. Flenley, D. C., Hutchison, D. C. S., and Donald, K. W.: Behaviour of apparatus for oxygen administration. Brit. Med. J., *2*:1081, 1963.
2262. Milic-Emili, J., Orzalesi, M. M., Cook, C. D., and Turner, J. M.: Respiratory thoraco-abdominal mechanics in man. J. Appl. Physiol., *19*:217, 1964.
2263. Bernstein, I. L., and Kreindler, A.: Lung compliance and pulmonary flow resistance. I. Clinical studies in symptomatic and asymptomatic asthmatic children. J. Allergy, *34*:127, 1963.
2264. Shapiro, W., Johnston, C. E., Dameron, R. A., Jr., and Patterson, J. L., Jr.: Maximum ventilatory performance and its limiting factors. J. Appl. Physiol., *19*:199, 1964.
2265. Jaeger, M. J., and Otis, A. B.: Effects of compressibility of alveolar gas on dynamics and work of breathing. J. Appl. Physiol., *19*:83, 1964.
2266. Severinghaus, J. W., Mitchell, R. A., Richardson, B. W., and Singer, M. M.: Respiratory control at high altitude suggesting active transport regulation of CSF pH. J. Appl. Physiol., *18*:1155, 1963.
2267. Vogel, J. H. K., Weaver, W. F., Rose, R. L., Blount, S. G., Jr., and Grover, R. F.: Pulmonary hypertension on exertion in normal man living at 10,150 feet (Leadville, Colorado). Med. Thorac., *19*:461, 1962.
2268. Lenfant, C.: Measurement of ventilation/perfusion distribution with alveolar-arterial differences. J. Appl. Physiol., *18*:1090, 1963.
2269. Bergman, N. A.: Distribution of inspired gas during anesthesia and artificial ventilation. J. Appl. Physiol., *18*:1085, 1963.
2270. Schramel, R. J., Tyler, J., Kirkpatrick, J. L., Ziskind, M. M., and Creech, O., Jr.: Studies of respiratory function after thoracic injuries. J. Trauma, *3*:206, 1963.
2271. Ayres, S. M., Criscitiello, A., and Grabovsky, E.: Components of alveolar-arterial O_2 difference in normal man. J. Appl. Physiol., *19*:43, 1964.
2272. Gandevia, B.: The spirogram of gross expiratory tracheobronchial collapse in emphysema. Quart. J. Med., (*n.s.*) *32*:23, 1963.
2273. Dysinger, P. W., Lemon, F. R., Crenshaw, G. L., and Walden, R. T.: Pulmonary emphysema in a non-smoking population. Dis. Chest, *43*:17, 1963.
2274. Montgomery, R. D., Stirling, G. A., and Hamer, N. A. J.: Bronchiolar carcinoma in progressive systemic sclerosis. Lancet, *1*:586, 1964.
2275. Kennedy, A. C., Luke, R. G., Campbell, D., and Cannon, R. N.: Combined renal and respiratory failure after trauma. Lancet, *2*:1304, 1963.
2276. Cohen, B. M.: The helium-mixing curve low point as an index of pulmonary disability: A study of 496 patients. Dis. Chest. *43*:496, 1963.
2277. Liver and lung transplantation. [Annotation.] Brit. Med. J., *1*:514, 1964.
2278. MacPhee, I. W., and Wright, E. S.: Experimental lung transplantation. Lancet, *1*:192, 1964.
2279. Workman, J. M., and Armstrong, B. W.: A nomogram for predicting treadmill-walking oxygen consumption. J. Appl. Physiol., *19*:150, 1964.
2280. Hale, F. C., Cohen, A. A., and Hemingway, A.: Reliability of the estimation of functional residual capacity in the emphysematous patient. Am. Rev. Resp. Dis., *87*:820, 1963.
2281. Cavagna, G. A., Saibene, F. P., and Margaria, R.: Mechanical work in running. J. Appl. Physiol., *19*:249, 1964.
2282. Aber, G. M., Harris, A. M., and Bishop, J. M.: The effect of acute changes in inspired oxygen concentration on cardiac, respiratory and renal function in patients with chronic obstructive airways disease. Clin. Sci., *26*:133, 1964.
2283. Schaefer, K. E., Hastings, B. J., Carey, C. R., and Nichols, G., Jr.: Respiratory acclimatization to carbon dioxide. J. Appl. Physiol., *18*:1071, 1963.

2284. Daly, W. J., Giammona, S. T., Ross, J. C., and Feigenbaum, H.: Effects of pulmonary vascular congestion on the postural changes in the perfusion and filling of the pulmonary vascular bed. J. Clin. Invest., *43:*68, 1964.
2285. Nelson, N. M., Prod'hom, L. S., Cherry, R. B., Lipsitz, P. J., and Smith, C. A.: Pulmonary function in the newborn infant. II. Perfusion–Estimation by analysis of the arterial-alveolar carbon dioxide difference. Pediatrics, *30:*975, 1962.
2286. Åstrand, P. O., Cuddy, T. E., Saltin, B., and Stenberg, J.: Cardiac output during submaximal and maximal work. J. Appl. Physiol., *19:*268, 1964.
2287. Charlton, G., Read, D., and Read, J.: Continuous intra-arterial P_{O_2} in normal man using a flexible microelectrode. J. Appl. Physiol., *18:*1247, 1963.
2288. Flatley, F. J., Constantine, H., McCredie, R. M., and Yu, P. N.: Pulmonary diffusing capacity and pulmonary capillary blood volume in normal subjects and in cardiac patients. Am. Heart J., *64:*159, 1962.
2289. Whitwam, J. G., and Norman, J.: Hypoxaemia after crush injury of the chest. Brit. Med. J., *1:*349, 1964.
2290. Sølvsteen, P.: Measurement of lung diffusing capacity by means of $C^{14}O$ in a closed system. J. Appl. Physiol., *19:*59, 1964.
2291. Elder, J. D., Jr., Duncalf, D., Binder, L. S., and Harmel, M. H.: An evaluation of mechanical ventilating devices. Anesthesiology, *24:*95, 1963.
2292. Fatt, I.: An ultramicro oxygen electrode. J. Appl. Physiol., *19:*326, 1964.
2293. Milic-Emili, J., Mead, J., Turner, J. M., and Glauser, E. M.: Improved technique for estimating pleural pressure from esophageal balloons. J. Appl. Physiol., *19:*207, 1964.
2294. Cole, R. B., and Bishop, J. M.: Effect of varying inspired O_2 tension on alveolar-arterial O_2 tension difference in man. J. Appl. Physiol., *18:*1043, 1963.
2295. Simpson, T., Heard, B., and Laws, J. W.: Severe irreversible airways obstruction without emphysema. Thorax, *18:*361, 1963.
2296. Livingstone, J. L., Lewis, J. G., Reid, L., and Jefferson, K. E.: Diffuse interstitial pulmonary fibrosis. A clinical, radiological, and pathological study based on 45 patients. Quart. J. Med., (*n.s.*) *33:*71, 1964.
2297. Nelson, N. M., Prod'hom, L. S., Cherry, R. B., Lipsitz, P. J., and Smith, C. A.: Pulmonary function in the newborn infant. V. Trapped gas in the normal infant's lung. J. Clin. Invest., *42:*1850, 1963.
2298. Sanders, J. S., and Martt, J. M.: Pulmonary function in "farmer's lung" and related conditions. Missouri Med., *60:*429, 1963.
2299. Kanagami, H., Baba, K., Katsura, T., Shiroishi, K., Ogata, K., and Tanaka, M.: [Measurement of CO pulmonary diffusing capacity in normal subjects during exercise by single-breath method. (Jap.)] Resp. Circ., *11:*381, 1963. [Excerpta Med. (XV), *16:*620, 1963.]
2300. Craig, F. N., Cummings, E. G., and Blevins, W. V.: Regulation of breathing at beginning of exercise. J. Physiol., London, *18:*1183, 1963.
2301. Rowell, L. B., Taylor, H. L., Wang, Y., and Carlson, W. S.: Saturation of arterial blood with oxygen during maximal exercise. J. Appl. Physiol., *19:*284, 1964.
2302. Bryan, A. C., Bentivoglio, L. G., Beerel, F., MacLeish, H., Zidulka, A., and Bates, D. V.: Factors affecting regional distribution of ventilation and perfusion in the lung. J. Appl. Physiol., *19:*395, 1964.
2303. Morgan, W. K. C., and Kerr, H. D.: Pathologic and physiologic studies of welders' siderosis. Ann. Int. Med., *58:*293, 1963.
2304. Dollery, C. T., and Gillam, P. M. S.: The distribution of blood and gas within the lungs measured by scanning after administration of ^{133}Xe. Thorax, *18:*316, 1963.
2305. Bradfield, W.: Disposable tracheostomy tube. [New invention.] Lancet, *1:*416, 1964.
2306. Milic-Emili, J., Mead, J., and Turner, J. M.: Topography of esophageal pressure as a function of posture in man. J. Appl. Physiol., *19:*212, 1964.
2307. The postoperative chest. [Annotation.] Lancet, *1:*153, 1964.
2308. Cumming, G. R., and Cumming, P. M.: Working capacity of normal children tested on a bicycle ergometer. Canad. M. A. J., *88:*351, 1963.
2309. Rosenblatt, G., Alkalay, I., McCann, P. D., and Stein, M.: The correlation of peak flow rate with maximal expiratory flow rate, one-second forced expiratory volume, and maximal breathing capacity. Am. Rev. Resp. Dis., *87:*589, 1963.
2310. Williams, M. H., Jr., and Kane, C.: Effect of simulated breath sounds on ventilation. J. Appl. Physiol., *19:*233, 1964.
2311. Ritchie, B.: Pulmonary function in scleroderma. Thorax, *19:*28, 1964.
2312. Kreuzer, F., Tenney, S. M., Mithoefer, J. C., and Remmers, J.: Alveolar-arterial oxygen gradient in Andean natives at high altitude. J. Appl. Physiol., *19:*13, 1964.
2313. Refsum, H. E.: Relationship between state of consciousness and arterial hypoxaemia and hypercapnia in patients with pulmonary insufficiency, breathing air. Clin. Sci., *25:*361, 1963.
2314. Nye, R. E., Jr.: Influence of inequalities of $\dot{V}_A/\dot{Q}$ ratio on the measurement of $D_{L_{CO}}$ by the steady state technique. [Abstr.] Fed. Proc., *23:*365, 1964.
2315. Pepys, J., Jenkins, P. A., Festenstein, G. N., Gregory, P. H., Lacey, M., and Skinner, F. A.: Farmer's lung. Thermophilic actinomycetes as a source of "farmer's lung hay" antigen. Lancet, *2:*607, 1963.
2316. Yarington, C. T., Jr.: Unilateral primary interstitial pulmonary fibrosis. Unknown etiology. Arch. Int. Med., *111:*612, 1963.
2317. Bolt, W.: Examen de la fonction respiratoire dans le diagnostic pré-opératoire des carcinomes bronchiques primitifs. Bronches, *12:*494, 1962.
2318. Milic-Emili, J., and Henderson, J. A. M.: Studies of regional pulmonary ventilation using Xe^{133}. [Abstr.] Fed. Proc., *23:*117, 1964.
2319. International Council of Sport and Physical Education and the Swedish Sport Federation: *Physical Fitness in Relation to Age and Sex; Scientific Seminar, Stockholm, 1962.* Stockholm: Riksidrottsförbundets Poliklinikkommitté, 1962.
2320. Severinghaus, J. W.: Electrodes for blood and gas Pco_2, Po_2 and blood pH. Acta Anaesthesiol. Scand., suppl. *11:*207, 1962.
2321. Tornvall, G.: Assessment of physical capabilities. With special reference to the evaluation of maximal voluntary isometric muscle strength and maximal working capacity. An experimental study on civilian and military subject groups. Acta Physiol. Scand., *58:*suppl. 201, 1963.
2322. Ross, J. C., Eller, J. L., Ley, G. D., and King, R. D.: Alterations in lung volume and intrapulmonary gas mixing after inguinal herniorrhaphy in patients with normal lung function and in patients with emphysema. Am. Rev. Resp. Dis., *88:*213, 1963.
2323. Moret, P. R.: Circulation pulmonaire. Étude de la relation entre pression, débit et résistance et de l'influence de l'hypoxie, de l'hypercapnie et de l'acidose sur la circulation pulmonaire. Études expérimentales et données récentres. Helv. Med. Acta, *30:*suppl. 43, 1963.
2324. Sanchez-Salazar, A. A., Pembleton, W. E., and Banerjee, C. M.: Doxapram hydrochloride as a respiratory stimulant in anesthetized man. Anesthesiology, *24:*808, 1963.
2325. Matell, G.: Time-courses of changes in ventilation and arterial gas tensions in man induced by moderate exercise. Acta Physiol. Scand., *58:*suppl. 206, 1963.
2326. Valdivia, E., Watson, M., and Dass, C. M.: Histologic alterations in muscles of guinea pigs during chronic hypoxia. A.M.A. Arch. Pathol., *69:*199, 1960.
2327. Volkov, N. I.: Potreblenie kisloroda i soderžanię moločnoi kisloty v krovi pri napriažennoĭ myšečnoĭ rabote. [Oxygen uptake and blood lactic acid during strenuous muscle exercise.] Fiziol. Z. SSSR Sechenova, *48*/3:314, 1962. [Fed. Proc. *22:*T118, 1963.]
2328. Ivanov, Y. N.: Izmenenie biozlektričeskoĭ aktivnostį različnyh otdelov golovnogo mozga košek i sobak pri deistvii uglekislogo gaza. [Changes in electrical activity of differ-

ent brain regions in cats and dogs on exposure to carbon dioxide.] Fiziol. Z. SSSR Sechenova, *48/3:*279, 1962. [Fed. Proc., *22:*T13, 1963.]
2329. Stuart-Harris, C. H.: Shortness of breath. Brit. Med. J., *1:*1203, 1964.
2330. Wright, G., Lloyd, T. C., Hamill, P., and Prindle, R.: Epidemiologic study of obstructive pulmonary disease in two small towns. A consideration of pulmonary function measurements. Am. Rev. Resp. Dis., *86:*713, 1962.
2331. Staub, N. C.: The interdependence of pulmonary structure and function. Anesthesiology, *24:*831, 1963.
2332. Robin, E. D., and O'Neill, R. P.: The fighter versus the nonfighter. Control of ventilation in chronic obstructive pulmonary disease. Arch. Environ. Health, *7:*125, 1963.
2333. Wilhelmsen, L., Selander, S., Söderholm, B., Paulin, S., Varnauskas, E., and Werkö, L.: Recurrent pulmonary embolism. Medicine, *42:*335, 1963.
2334. Polgar, G.: The first breath: A turbulent period of physiologic adjustment. Clin. Pediat., *2:*562, 1963.
2335. Margaria, R., Cerretelli, P., diPrampero, P. E., Massari, C., and Torelli, G.: Kinetics and mechanism of oxygen debt contraction in man. J. Appl. Physiol., *18:*371, 1963.
2336. Margaria, R.: A historical review of the physiology of oxygen debt and steady state in relation to lactic acid formation and removal. Med. Sport [Roma], *3:*637, 1963.
2337. Johnstone, M. C. (ed.): Problems in cystic fibrosis. Ann. N. Y. Acad. Sci., *93:*485, 1962.
2338. Finley, T. N., Tooley, W. H., Swenson, E. W., Gardner, R. E., and Clements, J. A.: Pulmonary surface tension in experimental atelectasis. Am. Rev. Resp. Dis., *89:*372, 1964.
2339. Margaria, R., and Cerretelli, P.: Physiological aspects of life at extreme altitudes. *In:* Tromp, S. W. (ed.): *Biometeorology; Proc. II Internat. Bioclimatological Congress, London, 1960.* Oxford & New York, Pergamon Press, 1962.
2340. Whitfield, A. G. W., Bond, W. H., and Kunkler, P. B.: Radiation damage to thoracic tissues. Thorax, *18:*371, 1963.
2341. Petersen, E. S.: Gas-mixing in the lungs. A study of the clinical applicability of the so-called Becklake-index. Acta Med. Scand., *174:*507, 1963.
2342. Avery, M. E.: *The Lung and Its Disorders in the Newborn Infant.* (Vol. I in series *Major Problems in Clinical Pediatrics;* A. J. Schaffer, consult. ed.) Philadelphia, W. B. Saunders Co., 1964.
2343. Leopold, J. G., and Gough, J.: Post-mortem bronchography in the study of bronchitis and emphysema. Thorax, *18:*172, 1963.
2344. Rosenzweig, D. Y., and Filley, G. F.: Postmortem lung studies. Mechanical and bronchographic properties. Am. Rev. Resp. Dis., *88:*6, 1963.
2345. Heard, B. E.: Photographs of serial sections of the lung projected rapidly in sequence using 16-mm film. Nature, *174:*319, 1954.
2346. Kleinerman, J., and Cowdrey, C. R.: The use of cinephotomicrography of serial sections in the study of lung pathology. Am. Rev. Resp. Dis., *89:*200, 1964.
2347. Turner-Warwick, M.: Precapillary systemic-pulmonary anastomoses. Thorax, *18:*225, 1963.
2348. Richards, R. L., and Milne, J. A.: Cancer of the lung in progressive systemic sclerosis. Thorax, *13:*238, 1958.
2349. Bishop, J. M., Melnick, S. C., and Raine, J.: Farmer's lung: Studies of pulmonary function and aetiology. Quart. J. Med., (*n.s.*) *32:*257, 1963.
2350. Hatch, T. F., and Gross, P.: *Pulmonary Deposition and Retention of Inhaled Aerosols.* New York, Academic Press, 1964.
2351. McLaughlin, A. I. G., Kazantzis, G., King, E., Teare, D., Porter, R. J., and Owen, R.: Pulmonary fibrosis and encephalopathy associated with the inhalation of aluminum dust. Brit. J. Industr. Med., *19:*253, 1962.
2352. McLaughlin, A. I. G., Bidstrup, P. L., and Konstam, M.: *Quoted in reference No. 2353.* Food Cosmet. Toxicol., *1:*171, 1963.
2353. Hair-sprays. [Annotation.] Lancet, *1:*709, 1964.
2354. Rankin, J., Jaeschke, W. H., Callies, Q. C., and Dickie, A.: Farmer's lung. Physiopathologic features of the acute interstitial granulomatous pneumonitis of agricultural workers. Ann. Int. Med., *57:*606, 1962.
2355. National Academy of Sciences—National Research Council, Committee on Anesthesia: Workshop on intensive care units, Washington, 1963. Anesthesiology, *25/2:*192, 1964.
2356. Bradley, R. D., Spencer, G. T., and Semple, S. J. G.: Tracheostomy and artificial ventilation in the treatment of acute exacerbations of chronic lung disease. A study in twenty-nine patients. Lancet, *1:*854, 1964.
2357. Heese, H. de V., and Freeseman, C.: Determination of mixed venous Pco_2 in infants and children. Brit. Med. J., *1:*1290, 1964.
2358. Taylor, S. H., Scott, D. B., and Donald, K. W.: Respiratory effects of general anaesthesia. Lancet, *1:*841, 1964.
2359. Brumley, G. W., Chernick, V., Hodson, W. A., Normand, C., Fenner, A., and Avery, M. E.: Correlations of mechanical stability, morphology, pulmonary surfactant, and phospholipid content in the developing lamb lung. J. Clin. Invest., *46:*863–873, 1967.
2360. Conference on Ciliary Function. Amer. Rev. Resp. Dis., *93:*No. 3, Part 2, 1966.
2361. Horsfield, K., and Cumming, G.: Angles of branching and diameters of branches in the human bronchial tree. Bull. Math. Biophys., *29:*245–259, 1967.
2362. Horsfield, K., and Cumming, G.: Morphology of the bronchial tree in man. J. Appl. Physiol., *24:*373–383, 1968.
2363. Azzopardi, A., and Thurlbeck, W. M.: The histochemistry of the nonciliated bronchiolar epithelial cell. Amer. Rev. Resp. Dis., *99:*516–525, 1969.
2364. Niden, A. H.: Bronchiolar and large alveolar cell in pulmonary phospholipid metabolism. Science, *158:*1323, 1967.
2365. Fung, Y. C., and Sobin, S. S.: Theory of sheet flow in lung alveoli, J. Appl. Physiol., *26:*472–488, 1969.
2366. Berlyne, G. M., Lee, H. A., Ralston, A. J., and Woolcock, J. A.: Pulmonary complications of peritoneal dialysis. Lancet, *2:*75–78, 1966.
2367. Cotes, J. E., Rossiter, C. E., Higgins, I. T. T., and Gilson, J. C.: Average normal values for the forced expiratory volume in white Caucasian males. Brit. Med. J., *1:*1016–1019, 1966.
2368. Alpers, J. H., and Guyatt, A. R.: Significance of a looped appearance of the flow:alveolar pressure relationship of the lung as examined by the whole body plethysmograph. Clin. Sci., *33:*1–10, 1967.
2369. Gildenhorn, H. L., and Hallett, W. Y.: An evaluation of radiological methods for the determination of lung volume. Radiology, *84:*754–756, 1965.
2370. Loyd, H. M., String, S. T., and DuBois, A. B.: Radiographic and plethysmographic determination of total lung capacity. Radiology, *86:*7–14, 1966.
2371. Bendixen, H. H., Smith, G. M., and Mead, J.: Patterns of ventilation in young adults. J. Appl. Physiol., *19:*195–198, 1964.
2372. Mead, J.: A model of lung elasticity and some of its implications. In: *Form and Function of the Human Lung.* Proc. of Symposium on Breathlessness (G. Cumming and L. B. Hunt, editors). Edinburgh, E. S. Livingstone, 1968, pp. 47–65.
2373. Mead, J., Peterson, N., Grimby, G., and Mead, J.: Pulmonary ventilation measured from body surface movements. Science, *156:*1383–1384, 1967.
2374. Cumming, G., Crank, J., Horsfield, K., and Parker, I.: Gaseous diffusion in the airways of the human lung. Resp. Physiol., *1:*58–74, 1966.
2375. Cumming, G., Horsefield, K., Jones, J. G., and Muir, D. C. F.: The influence of gaseous diffusion on the alveolar plateau at different lung volumes. Resp. Physiol., *2:*386–398, 1967.
2376. Staub, N. C.: *Annual Review of Physiology: Respiration, 31:*173–202, 1969.
2377. Sikand, R., Cerretelli, P., and Farhi, L. E.: Effects of V_A and V_A/Q distribution and of time on the alveolar plateau. J. Appl. Physiol., *21:*1331–1337, 1966.
2378. Georg, J., Lassen, N. A., Mellemgaard, K., and Vinther, A.: Diffusion in the gas phase of the lungs in normal and emphysematous subjects. Clin. Sci., *29:*525–532, 1965.

2379. Guyatt, A. R., and Alpers, J. H.: Factors affecting airways conductance: a study of 752 working men. J. Appl. Physiol., *24*:310–316, 1968.
2380. Turner, J. M., Mead, J., and Wohl, M. E.: Elasticity of human lungs in relation to age. J. Appl. Physiol., *25*:664–671, 1968.
2381. Finucane, K. E., and Colebatch, H. J. H.: Elastic behaviour of lungs in patients with airway obstruction. J. Appl. Physiol., *26*:330–338, 1969.
2382. Wilhelmsen, L.: Lung mechanics in rheumatic valvular disease. Acta Med. Scand., Supplement *489*:1–114, 1968.
2383. Wood, T. E., Anthonisen, N. R., and Macklem, P. T.: *Unpublished data.*
2384. Woolcock, A. J., and Mead, J.: The static elastic properties of the lungs in asthma. Amer. Rev. Resp. Dis., *98*:788–794, 1968.
2385. Brunes, L., and Holmgren, A.: Total airway resistance and its relationship to body size and lung volumes in healthy young women. Scand. J. Clin. Lab. Invest., *18*:316–324, 1966.
2386. Zapletal, A., Motoyama, E. K., Van de Woestijne, K. P., Hunt, V. R., and Bouhuys, A.: Maximum expiratory flow-volume curves and airway conductance in children and adolescents. J. Appl. Physiol., *26*:308–316, 1969.
2387. Macklem, P. T., Woolcock, A. J., Hogg, J. C., Nadel, J. A., and Wilson, N. J.: Partitioning of pulmonary resistance in the dog. J. Appl. Physiol., *26*:798–805, 1969.
2388. Horsfield, K., and Cumming, G.: Functional consequences of airway morphology. J. Appl. Physiol., *24*:384–390, 1968.
2389. Bachofen, H.: Lung tissue resistance and pulmonary hysteresis. J. Appl. Physiol., *24*:296–314, 1968.
2390. Woolcock, A. J., Macklem, P. T., Hogg, J. C., Wilson, N. J., Nadel, J. A., Frank, N. R., and Brain, J.: Effect of vagal stimulation on central and peripheral airways in dogs. J. Appl. Physiol., *26*:806–813, 1969.
2391. Woolcock, A. J., Macklem, P. T., Hogg, J. C., and Wilson, N. J.: Influence of autonomic nervous system on airway resistance and elastic recoil. J. Appl. Physiol., *26*:814–818, 1969.
2392. Cavagna, G. A., Stemmler, E. J., and DuBois, A. B.: Alveolar resistance to atelectasis. J. Appl. Physiol., *22*:441–453, 1967.
2393. Grimby, G., Takashima, T., Graham, W., Macklem, P., and Mead, J.: Frequency dependence of flow resistance in patients with obstructive lung disease. J. Clin. Invest., *47*:1455–1465, 1968.
2394. Fisher, A. B., DuBois, A. B., and Hyde, R. W.: Evaluation of the forced oscillation technique for the determination of resistance to breathing. J. Clin. Invest., *47*:2045–2051, 1968.
2395. Hyatt, R. E., and Flath, R. E.: Influence of lung parenchyma on pressure–diameter behaviour of dog bronchi. J. Appl. Physiol., *21*:1448–1452, 1966.
2396. Vincent, N. J., Knudson, R., Leith, D., Macklem, P. T., and Mead, J.: Factors influencing pulmonary resistance. J. Appl. Physiol., *29*:236–243, 1970.
2397. Ferris, B. G., Mead, J., and Opie, L. H.: Partitioning of respiratory flow resistance in man. J. Appl. Physiol., *19*:653–658, 1964.
2398. Woolcock, A. J., Vincent, N. J., and Macklem, P. T.: Frequency dependence of compliance as a test for obstruction in small airways. J. Clin. Invest., *48*:1097–1107, 1969.
2399. Brown, R., Woolcock, A. J., Vincent, N. J., and Macklem, P. T.: Physiological effects of experimental airway obstruction with beads. J. Appl. Physiol., *27*:328–335, 1969.
2400. Green, M.: How big are the bronchioles? St. Thomas' Hosp. Gaz., *63*:136–139, 1964.
2401. Mead, J., Takashima, T., and Leith, D.: Mechanical interdependence of distensible units in the lungs. Fed. Proc., *26*:551, 1967.
2402. Hogg, J. C., Macklem, P. T., and Thurlbeck, W. M.: Resistance to collateral flow in excised human lungs. J. Clin. Invest., *48*:421–431, 1969.
2403. Woolcock, A. J., and Macklem, P. T.: Mechanical factors influencing collateral ventilation in human, dog, and pig lungs. J. Appl. Physiol., *30*:99–115, 1971.
2404. Hyatt, R. E., and Flath, R. E.: Relationship of airflow to pressure during maximal respiratory effort in man. J. Appl. Physiol., *21*:477–482, 1966.
2405. Olafsson, S., and Hyatt, R. E.: Ventilatory mechanics in normal subjects during exercise. Fed. Proc., *26*:722, 1967.
2406. Mead, J., Turner, J. M., Macklem, P. T., and Little, J. B.: Significance of the relationship between lung recoil and maximum expiratory flow. J. Appl. Physiol., *22*:95–109, 1967.
2407. Pride, N. B., Permutt, S., Riley, R. L., and Bomberger-Barnea, B.: Determinants of maximal expiratory flow from the lungs. J. Appl. Physiol., *23*:646–662, 1967.
2408. Macklem, P. T., and Wilson, N. J.: Measurement of intrabronchial pressure in man. J. Appl. Physiol., *20*:653–663, 1965.
2409. Macklem, P. T., Proctor, D. F., and Hogg, J. C.: The stability of the peripheral airways. Resp. Physiol., *8*:191–203, 1970.
2410. Hogg, J. C., Nepszy, S. J., Macklem, P. T., and Thurlbeck, W. M.: Elastic properties of the centrilobular emphysematous spaces. J. Clin. Invest., *48*:1306–1313, 1969.
2411. Krieger, I.: Studies on mechanics of respiration in infancy. Amer. J. Dis. Child., *105*:439–448, 1963.
2412. Swyer, P. R., Reiman, R. C., and Wright, J. J.: Ventilation and ventilatory mechanics in the newborn. J. Pediat., *56*:612–622, 1960.
2413. Mead, J.: Measurement of the inertia of the lungs at increased ambient pressure. J. Appl. Physiol., *9*:208, 1956.
2414. Einthoven, W.: Ueber die Wirkung der Bronchialmuskeln, nach einer neuen Methode untersucht, und ueber Asthma Nervosum. Arch. Ges. Physiol., *51*:367, 1892.
2415. Shephard, R. J., and Seliger, V.: On the estimation of total lung capacity from chest X rays. Radiographic and helium dilution estimates on children aged 10–12 years. Respiration, *26*:327–336, 1969.
2416. Hamilton, L. H., Beard, J. D., and Kory, R. C.: Impedance measurement of tidal volume and ventilation. J. Appl. Physiol., *20*:565–568, 1965.
2417. Davidson, L.: Repeatability of respiratory data in the individual subject. Thorax, *21*:47, 1966.
2418. Stein, M., Tanabe, G., Rege, V., and Khan, M.: Evaluation of spirometric methods used to assess abnormalities in airway resistance. Amer. Rev. Resp. Dis., *93*:257–263, 1966.
2419. Dawson, A.: Reproducibility of spirometric measurements in normal subjects. Amer. Rev. Resp. Dis., *93*:264–268, 1966.
2420. Blide, R. W., Kerr, H. D., and Spicer, W. S., Jr.: Measurement of upper and lower airway resistance and conductance in man. J. Appl. Physiol., *19*:1059–1069, 1964.
2421. Salazar, E., and Knowles, J. H.: Analysis of pressure–volume characteristics of lungs. J. Appl. Physiol., *19*:97–104, 1964.
2422. Holmes, E. L., and Nyboer, J.: Volumetric dynamics of respiration as measured by electrical impedance plethysmography. J. Appl. Physiol., *9*:166–173, 1964.
2423. Mills, R. J., and Harris, P.: Factors influencing concentration of expired N_2 after a breath of oxygen. J. Appl. Physiol., *20*:103–109, 1965.
2424. Cherniack, R. M., and Brown, E. Simple method for measuring total respiratory compliance: normal values for males. J. Appl. Physiol., *20*:87–91, 1965.
2425. Okubo, T., and Lenfant, C.: Distribution factor of lung volume and ventilation determined by lung N_2 washout. J. Appl. Physiol., *24*:658–667, 1968.
2426. Norris, R. M.: Effect of breath-holding on anatomical dead space. Clin. Sci., *33*:549–557, 1967.
2427. Leith, D. E., and Mead, J.: Mechanisms determining residual volume of lungs in normal subjects. J. Appl. Physiol., *2*:221–227, 1967.
2428. Guyatt, A. R., Alpers, J. H., Hill, I. D., and Bramley, A. C.: Variability of plethysmographic measurements of airway resistance in man. J. Appl. Physiol., *22*:383–389, 1967.
2429. Scarpelli, E. M.: *The Surfactant System of the Lung.* Philadelphia, Lea and Febiger, 1968, p. 269.
2430. Edelman, N. H., Mittman, C., Norris, A. H., and Shock,

N. W.: Effects of respiratory pattern on age differences in ventilation uniformity. J. Appl. Physiol., *24*:49–53, 1968.
2431. Dollfuss, R. E., Milic-Emili, J., and Bates, D. V.: Regional ventilation of the lung studied with boluses of xenon^{133}. Resp. Physiol., *2*:234–246, 1967.
2432. Regional distribution of pulmonary ventilation and perfusion in elderly subjects. J. Clin. Invest., *47*:81–92, 1968.
2433. Gréhant, N.: Recherches physiques sur la respiration de l'homme. Journal de l'Anatomie et de la Physiologie normale et Pathologique de l'Homme et des Animaux, *1*:523–555, 1864.
2434. *Handbook of Physiology*. Section 3, Vol. I and II. Respiration Section. Washington, D. C., American Physiological Society, 1964.
2435. Ouellet, Y., Poh, S. C., and Becklake, M. R.: Circulatory factors limiting maximal aerobic capacity. J. Appl. Physiol., *27*:874–880, 1969.
2436. Levison, H., Aspin, N., Bryan, A. C., and Weng, T. R.: The measurement of regional ventilation to perfusion ratios in man uxing xenon^{133} and a scintillation camera. Proc. Can. Fed. Biol. Soc., *10*:67–68, 1967.
2437. Regional lung function. *Scandinavian Journal of Respiratory Diseases*. Supplement 62, Munksgaard, Copenhagen, 1966.
2438. Newhouse, M. T., Wright, F. J., Ingham, G. K., Archer, N. P., Hughes, L. B., and Hopkins, O. L.: Use of scintillation camera and xenon^{135} for study of topographic lung function. Resp. Physiol., *4*:141–153, 1968.
2439. Abernethy, J. D., Maurizi, J. J., and Farhi, L. E.: Diurnal variations in urinary-alveolar N_2 difference and effects of recumbency. J. Appl. Physiol., *23*:875–879, 1967.
2440. Glaister, D. H.: The effect of posture on the distribution of ventilation and blood flow in the normal lung. Clin. Sci., *33*:391–398, 1967.
2441. Glazier, J. B., Hughes, J. M. B., Maloney, J. E., and West, J. B.: Vertical gradient of alveolar size in lungs of dogs frozen intact. J. Appl. Physiol., *23*:694–705, 1967.
2442. Kaneko, K., Milic-Emili, J., Dolovich, M. B., Dawson, A., and Bates, D. V.: Regional distribution of ventilation and perfusion as a function of body position. J. Appl. Physiol., *21*:767–777, 1966.
2443. Kreuger, J. J., Bain, T., and Patterson, J. L., Jr.: Elevation gradient of intrathoracic pressure. J. Appl. Physiol., *16*:465–468, 1961.
2444. Milic-Emili, J., Henderson, J. A. M., Dolovich, M. B., Trop, D., and Kaneko, K.: Regional distribution of inspired gas in the lung. J. Appl. Physiol., *21*:749–759, 1966.
2445. Milic-Emili, J., Henderson, J. A. M., and Kaneko, K.: Distribution of ventilation as investigated with radioactive gases. J. Nucl. Biol. Med., *11*:63–68, 1967.
2446. Robertson, P. C., Anthonisen, N. R., and Ross, D.: Effect of inspiratory flow rate on regional distribution of inspired gas. J. Appl. Physiol., *26*:438–443, 1969.
2447. Millette, B., Robertson, P. C., Ross, W. R. D., and Anthonisen, N. R.: Effect of expiratory flow rate on emptying of lung regions. J. Appl. Physiol., *27*:587–591, 1969.
2448. Rutishauser, W. J., Banchero, N., Tsakiris, A. S., Edmundowicz, A. C., and Wood, E. H.: Pleural pressures at dorsal and ventral sites in supine and prone body positions. J. Appl. Physiol., *21*:1500–1510, 1966.
2449. Suprenant, E. L., and Rodbard, S.: A hydrostatic pressure gradient in the pleural sac. Amer. Heart J., *66*:215–220, 1963.
2450. Sutherland, P. W., Katsura, T., and Milic-Emili, J.: Previous volume history of the lung and regional distribution of gas. J. Appl. Physiol., *25*:566–574, 1968.
2451. Wood, E. H., Nolan, A. C., Donald, D. E., and Cronin, L.: Influence of acceleration on pulmonary physiology. Fed. Proc., *22*:1024–1034, 1963.
2452. Zardini, P., and West, J. B.: Topographical distribution of ventilation in isolated lung. J. Appl. Physiol., *21*:794–802, 1966.
2453. Hoppin, F. G. Jr., Green, I. D., and Mead, J.: Distribution of pleural pressure in dogs. J. Appl. Physiol., *27*:863–873, 1969.
2454. McMahon, S. M., Proctor, D. F., and Permutt, S.: Pleural surface pressure in dogs. J. Appl. Physiol., *27*:881–885, 1969.
2455. Anthonisen, N. R., Danson, J., Robertson, P. C., and Ross, W. R. D.: Airway closure as a function of age. Resp. Physiol., *8*:58–65, 1969.
2456. Bates, D. V., Ball, W. C., Jr., and Bryan, A. C.: Use of xenon^{133} in studying the ventilation and perfusion of the lung. In: *Dynamic Clinical Studies with Radioiosotopes*. U.S. Atomic Energy Commission, June, 1964.
2457. Nairn, J. R., Prime, F. J., and Simon, G.: Association between radiological findings and total and regional function in emphysema. Thorax, *24*:218–227, 1969.
2458. Kingaby, G. P., Glazier, J. B., Hughes, J. M. B., Maloney, J. E., and West, J. B.: Automation of data collection and analysis in lung scanning with radioisotopes. Med. Electron. Biol. Engin., *6*:403–408, 1968.
2459. West, J. B.: Pulmonary function studies with radioactive gases. Ann. Rev. Med., *18*:459–470, 1967.
2460. Widimský, J., Oppelt, A., and Stanek, V.: Examination of regional pulmonary ventilation by means of radioactive xenon^{133}. Cas. Lek. Cesk., *105*:695–698, 1966.
2461. Dale, K.: Xenon^{133} radiospirometry in rabbits with some observations on unilateral hypoxia. Acta. Physiol. Scand., *71*:163–167, 1967.
2462. D'Angelo, E., Bonanni, M. V., Michelini, S., and Agostoni, E.: Topography of the pleural surface pressure in rabbits and dogs. Resp. Physiol., *8*:204–229, 1970.
2463. Levine, G., Housley, E., MaLeod, P., and Macklem, P. T.: Gas exchange abnormalities in mild bronchitis and asymptomatic asthma. New Eng. J. Med., *282*:1277–1282, 1970.
2464. Holley, H. S., Milic-Emili, J., Becklake, M. R., and Bates, D. V.: Regional distribution of pulmonary ventilation and perfusion in obesity. J. Clin. Invest., *46*:475–481, 1967.
2465. Picken, J. J., Couture, J., Bates, D. V., and Milic-Emili, J.: Effect of recumbency on ventilation distribution in the normal human lung. *Submitted for publication.*
2466. Anthonisen, N. R., and Milic-Emili, J.: Distribution of pulmonary perfusion in erect man. J. Appl. Physiol., *21*: 760–766, 1966.
2467. West, J. B., Dollery, C. T., and Naimark, A.: Distribution of blood flow in isolated lung; relation to vascular and alveolar pressures. J. Appl. Physiol., *19*:713–724, 1964.
2468. Gorsky, B. H., and Lloyd, T. C., Jr.: Effects of perfusate composition on hypoxic vasoconstriction in isolated lung lobes. J. Appl. Physiol., *23*:683–686, 1967.
2469. Dugard, A., and Naimark, A.: Effect of hypoxia on distribution of pulmonary blood flow. J. Appl. Physiol., *23*:663–671, 1967.
2470. Aviado, D. M.: *The Lung Circulation*. (2 vols.). New York, Pergamon Press, 1965.
2471. Lloyd, T. C., Jr.: Effect of alveolar hypoxia on pulmonary vascular resistance. J. Appl. Physiol., *19*:1086–1094, 1964.
2472. Johnson, R. L., Jr., and Miller, J. M.: Distribution of ventilation, blood flow and gas transfer coefficients in the lung. J. Appl. Physiol., *25*:1–15, 1968.
2473. Ranson-Bitker, B., LeRoy Ladurie, M., and Durand, J.: Measurement of blood flow distribution of the right and left lungs by bronchospirometry and excretion of a radioactive isotope of Krypton (Kr^{85}). Respiration, *25*:395–404, 1968.
2474. Askrog, V.: Changes in (a - A) CO_2 difference and pulmonary artery pressure in anesthetized man. J. Appl. Physiol., *21*:1299–1305, 1966.
2475. Fishman, A. P.: Editorial: The volume of blood in the lungs. Circulation, *33*:835–838, 1966.
2476. Haas, F., and Bergofsky, E. H.: Effect of pulmonary vasoconstriction on balance between alveolar ventilation and perfusion. J. Appl. Physiol., *24*:491–497, 1968.
2477. Hughes, J. M. B., Glazier, J. B., Maloney, J. E., and West, J. B.: Effect of interstitial pressure on pulmonary blood flow. Lancet, *1*:192–193, 1967.
2478. Temple, J. R., Pircher, F. J., and Sieker, H. O.: Pulmonary blood flow characteristics studied by lung scanning. Amer. Rev. Resp. Dis., *93*:234–237, 1966.
2479. Holley, H. S., Dawson, A., Bryan, A. C., Milic-Emili, J., and Bates, D. V.: Effect of oxygen on the regional distri-

bution of ventilation and perfusion in the lung. Canad. J. Physiol. Pharm. *44*:89–93, 1966.

2480. Lopez-Muniz, R., Stephens, N. L., Bromberger-Barnea, B., Permutt, S., and Riley, R. L.: Critical closure of pulmonary vessels analysed in terms of a Starling resistor model. J. Appl. Physiol., *24*:625–635, 1968.
2481. West, J. B., Dollery, C. T., and Heard, B. E.: Increased pulmonary vascular resistance in the dependent zone of the isolated dog lung caused by perivascular edema. Cir. Res., *17*:191–206, 1965.
2482. Permutt, S., Bromberger-Barnea, B., and Bane, H. N.: Alveolar pressure, pulmonary venous pressure, and the vascular waterfall. Med. Thorac., *19*:239–260, 1962.
2483. Banister, J., and Torrance, R. W.: The effects of the tracheal pressure upon flow: pressure relations in the vascular bed of isolated lungs. Quart. J. Exp. Physiol., *45*:352–367, 1960.
2484. Glaister, D. H.: Effect of positive centrifugal acceleration upon the distribution of ventilation and perfusion within the human lung, and its relation to pulmonary arterial and intra-oesophageal pressures. Proc. Roy. Soc. (B), *168*:311–334, 1967.
2485. Vane, J. R.: The release and fate of vaso-active hormones in the circulation. Brit. J. Pharmacol. *35*:209–242, 1969.
2486. Heinemann, H. O., and Fishman, A. P.: Nonrespiratory functions of mammalian lung. Physiol. Rev., *49*:1–47, 1969.
2487. Cotes, J. E.: *Lung Function: Assessment and Application in Medicine*. 2nd ed. Oxford, Blackwell Scientific Publications, 1968.
2488. West, J. B.: *Ventilation/Blood Flow and Gas Exchange*. Oxford, Blackwell Scientific Publications, 1965.
2489. Farhi, L. E.: Ventilation–perfusion relationship and its role in alveolar gas exchange. In: *Recent Advances in Respiratory Physiology*, edited by C. Caro. London, W. H. Arnold, 1965.
2490. Rahn, H., and Farhi, L. E.: Ventilation, perfusion, and gas exchange–the V_A/Q concept. In: *Handbook of Physiology*, vol. 1, sec. 3, edited by W. O. Fenn and H. Rahn. Washington, D.C., American Physiological Society, 1964, pp. 735–765.
2491. Otis, A. B.: Quantitative relationships in steady-stage gas exchange. In: *Handbook of Physiology*, vol. 1, sec. 3, edited by W. O. Fenn and H. Rahn. Washington, D.C., American Physiological Society, 1964, pp. 681–698.
2492. Roughton, F. J. W.: Transport of oxygen and carbon dioxide. In: *Handbook of Physiology*, vol. 1, sec. 3, edited by W. O. Fenn and H. Rahn. Washington, D.C., American Physiological Society, 1964, pp. 767–825.
2493. Forster, R. E.: Rate of gas uptake by red cells. In: *Handbook of Physiology*, vol. 1, sec. 3, edited by W. O. Fenn and H. Rahn. Washington, D.C., American Physiological Society, 1964, pp. 827–837.
2494. Peters, J. P., and Van Slyke, D. D.: *Quantitative Clinical Chemistry*. Vol. 2: *Methods*. Baltimore, Williams & Wilkins Company, 1932.
2495. Campbell, E. J. M.: Annual Review of Physiology: Respiration. *30*:105–132, 1968.
2496. Pierce, J. A. *Biochemistry of Aging in the Lung*. Hahnemann Conference on Aging in the Lung. edited by Cander. New York and London, Grune & Stratton, 1964, pp. 61–69.
2497. Pierce, J. A., and Ebert, R. V.: Fibrous network of the lung and its change with age. Thorax, *20*:469–476, 1965.
2498. Hodson, W. A., Chernick, V., and Avery, M. E.: A rebreathing method for measurement of arterial carbon dioxide tension in newborn infants and children. Lancet, *1*:515–517, 1966.
2499. *Acid Base Terminology*. Report by an ad-hoc Committee of the New York Academy of Sciences Conference. Lancet, *2*:1010–1012, 1965.
2500. *Medical Research Council: Definition and classification of chronic bronchitis for clinical and epidemiological purposes:* Report by Committee on Aetiology of Chronic Bronchitis. Lancet, *1*:775–779, 1965.
2501. McNicol, M. W., and Pride, N. B.: Unexplained underventilation of the lungs. Thorax, *20*:53–65, 1965.
2502. Burrows, B.: Chronic obstructive lung disease (Bronchitis–emphysema syndrome). Diagnosis and physiologic effects. Postgrad. Med., *39*:105–112, 1966.
2503. Mitchell, R. S., Ryan, S. F., Petty, T. L., and Filley, G. F.: Significance of morphologic chronic hyperplastic bronchitis. Amer. Rev. Resp. Dis., *93*:720–729, 1966.
2504. Burrows, B., Fletcher, C. M., Heard, B. E., Jones, N. L., and Wootliff, J. S.: Emphysematous and bronchial types of chronic airways obstruction: clinicopathological study of patients in London and Chicago. Lancet, *1*:830–835, 1966.
2505. Jones, N. L.: Pulmonary gas exchange during exercise in patients with chronic airway obstruction. Clin. Sci., *31*:39–50, 1966.
2506. Thurlbeck, W. M. Internal surface area and other measurements in emphysema. Thorax, *22*:483–496, 1967.
2507. Thurlbeck, W. M., and Angus, G. E.: Variation of Reid index measurements within the major bronchial tree. Amer. Rev. Resp. Dis., *95*:551–555, 1967.
2508. Reid, L.: *The Pathology of Emphysema*. Chicago, Year Book Medical Publishers, 1967.
2509. Mitchell, R. S., Filley, G. F., and Read, J. A.: Postscript. Proceedings of Tenth Aspen Conference (U.S. Public Health Service Publication No. 1717), pp. 517–520. 1967.
2510. Filley, G. F., Beckwitt, H. J., Reeves, J. T., and Mitchell, R. S.: Chronic obstructive bronchopulmonary disease. II. Oxygen transport in two clinical types. Amer. J. Med., *44*:26–38, 1968.
2511. Greenberg, S. D., Boushy, S. F., and Jenkins, D. E.: Differences in the lobar distribution of emphysema and chronic bronchitis in the lung. In: *Current Research in Chronic Airways Obstruction* (U.S. Public Health Service Publication No. 1717), May, 1968, pp. 101–108.
2512. Bates, D. V., Gordon, C. A., Paul, G. I., Place, R. E. G., Snidal, D. P., and Woolf, C. R.: *Chronic Bronchitis*. Report on the Third and Fourth Stages of the Co-ordinated Study of Chronic Bronchitis in the Department of Veteran's Affairs, Canada. Med. Serv. J. Canada, *22*:5–59, 1966.
2513. Heard, B. E., and Izukawa, T.: Pulmonary emphysema in fifty consecutive male necropsies in London. J. Path. Bact., *88*:423–431, 1964.
2514. Jones, N. L., Burrows, B., and Fletcher, C. M.: Serial studies of 100 patients with chronic airway obstruction in London and Chicago. Thorax, *22*:327–335, 1967.
2515. Thurlbeck, W. M., and Angus, G. E.: Distribution curve for chronic bronchitis. Thorax, *19*:436–442, 1964.
2516. Bedell, G. N., and Ostiguy, G. L.: Transfer factor for carbon monoxide in patients with airways obstruction. Clin. Sci., *32*:239–248, 1967.
2517. Thurlbeck, W. M.: Chronic obstructive lung disease. In: *Pathology Annual 1968*, edited by S. Somers, pp. 367–398.
2518. Greenberg, S. D., Boushy, S. F., and Jenkins, D. E.: Chronic bronchitis and emphysema: Correlation of pathologic findings. Amer. Rev. Resp. Dis., *96*:918–928, 1967.
2519. Filley, G. F., Dart, G. A., and Mitchell, R. S.: Emphysema and chronic bronchitis: clinical manifestations and their physiological significance. In: *Current Research in Chronic Airways Obstruction* (U.S. Public Health Service Publication No. 1717), May, 1968, pp. 339–349.
2520. Dunnill, M. S.: In: *Form and Function in the Human Lung*, edited by G. Cumming and L. B. Hunt. Baltimore, Williams & Wilkins Company, 1968, p. 241.
2521. Horsfield, K., Cumming, G., and Hicken, P.: A morphologic study of airway disease using bronchial casts. Amer. Rev. Resp. Dis., *93*:900–906, 1966.
2522. Fletcher, C. M., Jones, N. L., and Campbell, E. J. M.: Research into bronchitis and emphysema. Postgrad. Med. J., *44*:48–52, 1968. (Festschrift for Sir J. McMichael.)
2523. Scadding, J. G.: *Early stages of chronic bronchitis*. Symposium of College of General Practitioners. Brit. Med. J., *2*:1118–1119, 1965.
2524. Thurlbeck, W. M., Henderson, J. A. M., Fraser, R. G., and Bates, D. V.: Chronic obstructive lung disease: a comparison between clinical, roentgenologic, functional, and morphologic criteria in chronic bronchitis, emphy-

sema, asthma, and bronchiectasis. Medicine, *49*:81-145, 1970.

2525. Briscoe, W. A., and King, T. K. C.: Bohr integral isopleths and their use to study the diffusing capacity of the lung in obstructive disease. In: *Current Research in Chronic Airways Obstruction.* (U.S. Public Health Service Publication No. 1717), May, 1968, pp. 351-363.
2526. Burrows, B.: The bronchial and emphysematous types of chronic obstructive lung disease in London and Chicago. In: *Current Research in Chronic Airways Obstruction.* (U.S. Public Health Service Publication No. 1717), May, 1968, pp. 327-338.
2527. *Editorial: British Medical Journal.* Obstructive airways disease. Brit. Med., J., *2*:436, 1967.
2528. Thurlbeck, W. M.: The geographic pathology of pulmonary emphysema and chronic bronchitis. Arch. Environ. Health, *14*:21-30, 1967.
2529. Simpson, T.: The emphysema problem. Brit. J. Dis. Chest, *62*:188-194, 1968.
2530. King, T. K. C., and Briscoe, W. A.: The distribution of ventilation, perfusion, lung volume, and transfer factor (diffusing capacity) in patients with obstructive lung disease. Clin. Sci., *35*:153-170, 1968.
2531. Gough, J.: Letter to Editor: Chronic bronchitis and occupation. Brit. Med. J., *1*:480, 1966.
2532. Anthonisen, N. R., Bass, H., Oriol, A., Place, R. E. G., and Bates, D. V.: Regional lung function in patients with chronic bronchitis. Clin. Sci., *35*:495-512, 1968.
2533. Davis, A. L., and McClement, J. H.: The course and prognosis of chronic obstructive pulmonary disease. In: *Current Research in Chronic Airways Obstruction.* (U.S. Public Health Service Publication No. 1717), May, 1968, pp. 219-232.
2534. Clark, T. J. H., Freedman, S., Campbell, E. J. M., and Winn, R. R.: The ventilatory capacity of patients with chronic airways obstruction. Clin. Sci., *36*:307-316, 1969.
2535. Vandenbergh, E., Van de Woestijne, K. P., and Gyselen, A.: Chronic bronchitis and obstructive emphysema. Clinical aspects and course. T. Soc. Geneesk., *22*:24-40, 1966.
2536. Burrows, B., Saksena, F. B., and Diener, C. F.: Carbon dioxide tension and ventilatory mechanics in chronic obstructive lung disease. Ann. Intern. Med., *65*:685-700, 1966.
2537. Mitchell, R. S., Petty, T. L., Ryan, S. F., and Filley, G. F.: Morphologic vs clinical chronic bronchitis. Med. Thorac., *24*:75-76, 1967.
2538. Thurlbeck, W. M.: Measurement of pulmonary emphysema. Amer. Rev. Resp. Dis., *95*:752-764, 1967.
2539. Nicklaus, T. M., Watanabe, S., Mitchell, M. M., and Renzetti, A. D., Jr.: Roentgenologic, physiologic and structural estimations of the total lung capacity in normal and emphysematous subjects. Amer. J. Med., *42*:547-553, 1967.
2540. King, T. K. C., and Briscoe, W. A.: Blood gas exchange in emphysema: an example illustrating method of calculation. J. Appl. Physiol., *23*:672-682, 1967.
2541. Galy, P.: Chronic bronchitis and emphysema. The differentiation of diseases which present with chronic ventilatory obstruction. Poumon Coeur, *24*:147-168, 1968.
2542. Khoury, F., Bignon, J., Even, P., and Brouet, G.: A comparative study of the anatomical and radiological findings in emphysema and in chronic obstructive bronchopneumopathies. Rev. Tuberc., *32*:245-260, 1968.
2543. Levame, M., Brille, D., and Hatzfeld, C.: An analysis of the bronchial and pulmonary lesions and a quantitative estimate of emphysematous destruction in chronic obstructive bronchopneumopathy. Rev. Tuberc., *32*:281-298, 1968.
2544. Hogg, J. C., Macklem, P. T., and Thurlbeck, W. M.: Site and nature of airway obstruction in chronic obstructive lung disease. New Engl. J. Med., *278*:1355-1360, 1968.
2545. Kelling, H. W.: Secretolytic and antibiotic treatment with longterm prophylaxis in chronic asthmatoid emphysematous bronchitis. Med. Mschr., *21*:420-424, 1967.
2546. Mitchell, R. S., Silvers, G. W., Dart, G. A., Petty, T. L., Vincent, T. N., Ryan, S. F., and Filley, G. W.: Clinical and morphologic correlations in chronic airway obstruction. Amer. Rev. Resp. Dis., *97*:54-62, 1968.
2547. Burrows, B., Niden, A. H., Barclay, W. R., and Kasik, J. E.: Chronic obstructive lung disease. II. Relationship of clinical and physiologic findings to the severity of airways obstruction. Amer. Rev. Resp. Dis., *91*:665-678, 1965.
2548. Gough, J.: The pathology of emphysema. Postgrad. Med. J., *41*:392-400, 1965.
2549. Watanabe, S., Mitchell, M., and Renzetti, A. D., Jr.: Correlation of structure and function in chronic pulmonary emphysema. Amer. Rev. Resp. Dis., *92*:221-227, 1965.
2550. Kreukniet, J.: Pulmonary emphysema and lung function studies in patients with chronic non-specific lung diseases (C.N.S.L.D.). Med. Thorac, *22*:433-449, 1965.
2551. Briscoe, W. A., and Nash, E. S.: Slow space in chronic obstructive pulmonary disease. Ann. N.Y. Acad. Sci., *121*:706-722, 1965.
2552. Nash, E. S., Briscoe, W. A., and Cournand, A.: Relationship between clinical and physiological findings in chronic obstructive disease of the lungs. Med. Thorac., *22*:305-327, 1965.
2553. Filley, G. F.: Emphysema and chronic bronchitis: clinical manifestations and their physiologic significance. Med. Clin. N. Amer., *51*:283-292, 1967.
2554. Lenfant, C., and Pace, W. R., Jr.: Alterations of ventilation to perfusion ratios distribution associated with successive clinical stages of pulmonary emphysema. J. Clin. Invest., *44*:1566-1581, 1965.
2555. Ashcroft, T.: Daily variations in sputum volume in chronic bronchitis. Brit. Med. J., *1*:288-290, 1965.
2556. Jenkins, D. E., Greenberg, D., Boushy, S. F., Schweppe, H. I., and O'Neal, R. M.: Correlation of morphologic emphysema with pulmonary function parameters. Trans. Assoc. Amer. Physicians, *78*:218-230, 1965.
2557. Bates, D. V.: Chronic bronchitis and emphysema. New Eng. J. Med., *278*:546-551, 600-604, 1968.
2558. Dunnill, M. S.: *The Pathology of Asthma.* Transactions of World Asthma Conference, March, 1965.
2559. Bjure, J., Söderholm, B., and Widimský, J.: The effect of histamine infusion on pulmonary hemodynamics and diffusing capacity. Scand. J. Resp. Dis., *47*:53-63, 1966.
2560. Rees, H. A., Borthwick, R. C., Millar, J. S., and Donald, K. W.: Aminophylline in bronchial asthma. Lancet, *2*:1167-1169, 1967.
2561. Rees, H. A., Millar, J. S., and Donald, K. W.: Adrenaline in bronchial asthma. Lancet, *2*:1164-1167, 1967.
2562. Palmer, K. N. V., and Diament, M. L.: Effect of aerosol isoprenaline on blood-gas tensions in severe bronchial asthma. Lancet, *2*:1532-1533, 1967.
2563. Nadel, J. A.: Mechanisms of airway response to inhaled substances. Arch. Environ. Health, *16*:171-174, 1968.
2564. Simonsson, B. G., Jacobs, F. M., and Nadel, J. A.: Role of autonomic nervous system and the cough reflex in the increased responsiveness of airways in patients with obstructive airway disease. J. Clin. Invest., *46*:1812-1818, 1967.
2565. Field, G. B.: The effects of posture, oxygen, isoproterenol and atropine on ventilation-perfusion relationships in the lung in asthma. Clin. Sci., *32*:279-288, 1967.
2566. Amdur, M. O.: The respiratory responses of guinea pigs to histamine aerosol. Arch. Environ. Health, *13*:29-37, 1966.
2567. Millar, J. S., Nairn, J. R., Unkles, R. D., and McNeill, R. S.: Cold air and ventilatory function. Brit. J. Dis. Chest, *59*:23-27, 1965.
2568. Tai, E., and Read, J.: Response of blood gas tensions to aminophylline and isoprenalin in patients with asthma. Thorax, *22*:543-550, 1967.
2569. Nadel, J. A., Salem, H., Tamplin, B., and Tokiwa, Y.: Mechanism of bronchoconstriction. Arch. Environ. Health, *10*:175-178, 1965.
2570. Sterling, G. M.: Mechanism of bronchoconstriction caused by cigarette smoking. Brit. Med. J., *3*:275-277, 1967.
2571. Sterling, G. M.: Asthma due to aluminum soldering flux. Thorax, *22*:533-537, 1967.
2572. Heckscher, T., Bass, H., Oriol, A., Rose, B., Anthonisen, N. R., and Bates, D. V.: Regional lung function in patients with bronchial asthma. J. Clin. Invest., *47*:1063-1070, 1968.

2573. Woolcock, A. J., and Read, J.: Improvement in bronchial asthma not reflected in forced expiratory volume. Lancet, *2*:1323–1325, 1965.
2574. Valabhji, P.: Gas exchange in the acute and asymptomatic phases of asthma breathing air and oxygen. Clin. Sci., *34*:431–440, 1968.
2575. LeRoy, N. B., and Guerrant, J. L.: Breathing mechanics in asthma. Ann. Intern. Med., *63*:572–582, 1965.
2576. Lecks, H. I., Wood, D. W., and Downes, J.: Segmental atelectasis and pulmonary shunting in acute bronchial asthma and status asthmaticus. Ann. Allerg., *23*:636–640, 1965.
2577. Woolcock, A. J., and Read, J.: Lung volumes in exacerbations of asthma. Amer. J. Med., *41*:259–272, 1966.
2578. Gervais, P.: Occupational asthma in the plastic-material industry. Poumon Coeur, *22*:497–511, 1966.
2579. Helander, E., Lindell, S-E., Soderholm, B., and Westling, H.: The pulmonary circulation and ventilation in bronchial asthma. Acta Allerg. (Kobenhavn), *21*:441–465, 1966.
2580. Woolcock, A. J., McRae, J., Morris, J. G., and Read, J.: Abnormal pulmonary blood flow distribution in bronchial asthma. Aust. Ann. Med., *15*:196–203, 1966.
2581. Mishkin, F. S., Wagner, H. N., Jr., and Tow, D. E.: Regional distribution of pulmonary arterial blood flow in acute asthma. J.A.M.A., *203*:1019–1021, 1968.
2582. Pecora, L. J., Bernstein, I. L., and Feldman, D. P.: Pulmonary diffusing capacity, membrane diffusing capacity, and capillary blood volume in children with intractable asthma with and without chronic overinflation of the lungs. J. Allerg., *37*:204–215, 1966.
2583. Mishkin, F., and Wagner, H. N., Jr.: Regional abnormalities in pulmonary arterial blood flow during acute asthmatic attacks. Radiology *88*:142–144, 1967.
2584. Graham, W. G. B., Heim, E., and Constantine, H. P.: Measurement of airway variation and bronchial reactivity in normal and asthmatic subjects. Amer. Rev. Resp. Dis., *96*:266–274, 1967.
2585. Gold, W. M., Kaufman, H. S., and Nadel, J. A.: Elastic recoil of the lungs in chronic asthmatic patients before and after therapy. J. Appl. Physiol., *23*:433–438, 1967.
2586. Meisner, P., and Hugh-Jones, P.: Pulmonary function in bronchial asthma. Brit. Med. J., *1*:470–475, 1968.
2587. Lynne-Davies, P., and Sproule, B. J.: Comparative studies of lung function in airway obstruction. Amer. Rev. Resp. Dis., *97*:610–616, 1968.
2588. Gayrard, P.: The role of the main bronchi in the asthmatic attack. Rev. Franc. Allerg., *8*:34–49, 1968.
2589. Backlund, L., and Irnell, L.: Compliance in bronchial asthma. Acta Med. Scand., *183*:281–287, 1968.
2590. Mellins, R. B., Lord, G. P., and Fishman, A. P.: Dynamic behaviour of the lung in acute asthma. Med. Thorac., *24*:81–144, 1967.
2591. Helander, E., Lindell, S-E., Soderholm, B., and Westling, H.: Observations on the pulmonary circulation during induced bronchial asthma. Acta Allerg. (Kobhenhavn)., *17*:112–119, 1962.
2592. Palmer, K. N. V., and Diament, M. L.: Dynamic and static lung volumes and blood-gas tensions in bronchial asthma. Lancet, *1*:591–593, 1969.
2593. Waddell, J. A., Emerson, P. A., and Gunstone, R. F.: Hypoxia in bronchial asthma. Brit. Med. J., *2*:402–404, 1967.
2594. Palmer, K. N. V., and Diament, M. L.: Spirometry and blood-gas tensions in bronchial asthma and chronic bronchitis. Lancet, *2*:383–384, 1967.
2595. Palmer, K. N. V., and Diament, M. L.: Hypoxaemia in bronchial asthma. Lancet, *1*:318–319, 1968.
2596. McFadden, E. R., Jr., and Lyons, H. A.: Arterial blood gas tension in asthma. New Engl. J. Med., *278*:1027–1032, 1968.
2597. Simpson, H., Forfar, J. O., and Grubb, D. J.: Arterial blood gas tensions and pH in acute asthma in childhood. Brit. Med. J., *2*:460–464, 1968.
2598. Rees, H. A., Millar, J. S., and Donald, K. W.: A study of the clinical course and arterial blood gas tensions of patients in status asthmaticus. Quart. J. Med., *38*:541–561, 1968.
2599. McNeill, R. S., Nairn, J. R., Millar, J. S., and Ingram, C. G.: Exercise-induced asthma. Quart. J. Med., *35*:55–67, 1966.
2600. Itkin, I. H., and Nacman, M.: The effect of exercise on the hospitalized asthmatic patient. J. Allerg., *37*:253–263, 1966.
2601. Irnell, L., and Swartling, S.: Maximal expiratory flow at rest and during muscular work in patients with bronchial asthma. Scand. J. Resp. Dis., *47*:103–113, 1966.
2602. Beaudry, P. H., Wise, M. B., and Seely, J. E.: Respiratory gas exchange at rest and during exercise in normal and asthmatic children. Amer. Rev. Resp. Dis., *95*:248–254, 1967.
2603. Jones, R. H. T., and Jones, R. S.: Ventilatory capacity in young adults with a history of asthma in childhood. Brit. Med. J., *2*:976–978, 1966.
2604. Crompton, G. K.: An unusual example of exercise-induced asthma. Thorax, *23*:165–167, 1968.
2605. Rebuck, A. S., and Read, J.: Exercise-induced asthma. Lancet, *2*:429–431, 1968.
2606. Atakova, E. E., and Nemirovskaya, N. A.: Death during an attack of bronchial asthma. Ter. Arkh., *37*:113–116, 1965.
2607. Roe, P. F.: Sudden death in asthma. Brit. J. Dis. Chest, *59*:158–163, 1965.
2608. Shapiro, J. B., and Tate, C. F.: Death in status asthmaticus: a clinical analysis of eighteeen cases. Dis. Chest, *48*:484–489, 1965.
2609. Marchand, P., and Van Hasselt, H.: Last-resort treatment of status asthmaticus. Lancet, *1*:227–230, 1966.
2610. Beam, L. R., Marcy, J. H., and Mansmann, H., Jr.: Medically irreversible status asthmaticus in children. Report of three cases treated with paralysis and controlled respiration. J.A.M.A., *194*:968–972, 1965.
2611. Williams, M. H., Jr., and Levin, M.: Sudden death from bronchial asthma. Amer. Rev. Resp. Dis., *94*:608–611, 1966.
2612. Reisman, R. E., Friedman, I., and Arbesman, C. E.: Severe status asthmaticus: prolonged treatment with assisted ventilation. J. Allerg., *41*:37–48, 1968.
2613. Ghannam, R. D., Schreier, L., and Vanselow, N. A.: Fatal bronchial asthma: an analysis of terminal treatment in twenty cases. Ann. Allerg., *26*:194–205, 1968.
2614. Gregory, J. J., Ayres, S. M., Gianelli, S., Jr., and Conklin, E. F.: Treatment of acute respiratory acidosis complicating status asthmaticus. J. Thorac. Cardiov. Surg., *55*:426–430, 1968.
2615. Speizer, F. E., Doll, R., and Heaf, P.: Observations on recent increase in mortality from asthma. Brit. Med. J., *1*:335–339, 1968.
2616. Busey, J. F., Fenger, E. P. K., Hepper, N. G., Kent, D. C., Kilburn, K. H., Matthews, L. W., Simpson, D. G., and Gryzbowski, S.: Management of status asthmaticus. Amer. Rev. Resp. Dis., *97*:735–736, 1968.
2617. Gandevia, B.: The changing pattern of mortality from asthma in Australia. Med. J. Aust., *55*:747–752, 1968.
2618. Read, J.: The reported increase in mortality from asthma: A clinico-functional analysis. Med. J. Aust., *1*:879–884, 1968.
2619. Gandevia, B.: The changing pattern of mortality from asthma in Australia. II. Mortality and modern therapy. Med. J. Aust., *1*:884–891, 1968.
2620. Leading Article: Death from Asthma. Lancet, *1*:1412–1413, 1968.
2621. Mithoefer, J. C., Porter, W. F., and Karetzky, M. S.: Indications for the use of sodium bicarbonate in the treatment of intractable asthma. Respiration, *25*:201–215, 1968.
2622. Annotation: Controlled respiration in status asthmaticus. Lancet, *1*:247–248, 1966.
2623. James, G.: Health challenges today: public health vision. Amer. Rev. Resp. Dis., *90*:349–358, 1964.
2624. McGowan, A. T.: Chronic bronchitis. J. Roy. Inst. Public Health, *29*:2, 1966.
2625. Esipova, I. K.: Chronic bronchitis and pulmonary emphysema. Arkh. Pat., *26*:3–18, 1964.
2626. Stuart-Harris, C. H.: The pathogenesis of chronic bronchitis and emphysema. Scot. Med. J., *10*:93–107, 1965.
2627. Simonsson, B. G.: Clinical and physiological studies on

chronic bronchitis. I. Clinical description of the patient material. Acta Allerg. (Kobenhavn) *20:*257–300, 1965.
2628. Simonsson, B. G.: *Studies on Chronic Bronchitis.* Goteborg, Orstadius Boktryckeri Aktiebolag, 1965.
2629. Kreukniet, J., and Young, E.: Criteria of allergy in patients with chronic non-specific lung diseases (C.N.S.L.D.). Med. Thorac., *21:*284–294, 1964.
2630. Charpin, J., Zafiropoulo, A., Aubert, J., and Laurendeau, O.: Quelle est la place de l'allergie dans l'étiologie des bronchites chroniques de l'adulte? Poumon Coeur, *20:*691–698, 1964.
2631. Rose, B., and Phills, J. A.: Immune reaction in pulmonary disease. Arch. Environ. Health, *14:*97–106, 1967.
2632. Simonsson, B. G.: Clinical and physiological studies on chronic bronchitis. III. Bronchial reactivity to inhaled acetylcholine. Acta Allerg. (Kobenhavn), *20:*325–348, 1965.
2633. Bariéty, M., and Milochevitch, R.: Bronchopulmonary excitability in chronic bronchitis with spasm. Poumon Coeur, *21:*245–254, 1965.
2634. Salvati, F., Spina, G., and Cramiccioni, E.: Role of allergic factors in chronic bronchitis. Riv. Sicilia Tuberc., *12:*311–348, 1964.
2635. Fletcher, C. M.: Bronchial infection and reactivity in chronic bronchitis. J. Roy. Coll. Phys. London, *2:*183–190, 1968.
2636. Brouet, G., Chrétien, J., and Lemoine J-M: The anatomical alterations of the trachea and the large bronchi during "chronic bronchitis." Bull. Soc. Med. Hôp. Paris. *115:*51–56, 1964.
2637. Restrepo, G. L., and Heard, B. E.: Air trapping in chronic bronchitis and emphysema. Measurements of the bronchial cartilage. Amer. Rev. Resp. Dis., *90:*395–400, 1964.
2638. Schmidt, O. P., Gunther, W., and Bottke, H.: *Das bronchitische Syndrom.* Munchen, J. F. Lehmans Verlag, 1965, p. 334.
2639. Hosogaya, M.: Studies on chronic bronchitis. I. Pathomorphological classification of chronic bronchitis by bronchial biopsy. Shinshu Med. J., *13:*633–644, 1964.
2640. Hosogaya, M.: Studies on chronic bronchitis. II. Correlation between the clinical features and bronchial biopsy. Shinshu Med. J., *13:*645–651, 1964.
2641. Hernandez, J. A., Anderson, A. E., Jr., Holmes, W. L., Morrone, N., and Foraker, A. G.: The bronchial glands in aging. J. Amer. Geriat. Soc., *13:*799–804, 1965.
2642. De Haller, R., and Reid, L.: Adult chronic bronchitis. Morphology, histochemistry and vascularisation of the bronchial mucous glands. Med. Thorac., *22:*549–567, 1965.
2643. Field, W. E. H., Davey, E. N., Reid, L., and Roe, F. J. C.: Bronchial mucus gland hypertrophy: its relation to symptoms and environment. Brit. J. Dis. Chest, *60:*66–80, 1966.
2644. Cumming, G., and Hunt, L. B. (eds.): *Form and Function in the Human Lung.* Baltimore, Williams & Wilkins Company, 1968, p. 259.
2645. Levame, M., Brille, D., and Hatzfeld, C.: An analysis of the bronchial and pulmonary lesions and a quantitative estimate of emphysematous destruction in chronic obstructive bronchopneumopathy. Rev. Tuberc., *32:*281–298, 1968.
2646. Simon, G.: Radiology and emphysema. Clin. Radiol., *15:*293–306, 1964.
2647. Reid, L., and Millard, F. J.: Correlation between radiological diagnosis and structural lung changes in emphysema. Clin. Radiol., *15:*307–311, 1964.
2648. Sutinen, S., Christoforidis, A. J., Klugh, G. A., and Pratt, P. C.: Roentgenologic criteria for the recognition of nonsymptomatic pulmonary emphysema. Correlation between roentgenologic findings and pulmonary pathology. Amer. Rev. Resp. Dis., *91:*69–76, 1965.
2649. Nicklaus, T. M., Stowell, D. W., Christiansen, W. R., and Renzetti, A. D.: Accuracy of roentgenologic diagnosis of chronic pulmonary emphysema. Amer. Rev. Resp. Dis., *93:*889–899, 1966.
2650. Redi, L.: Mucus secretion and chronic bronchitis. Med. Thorac., *24:*40–43, 1967.
2651. Gernez-Rieux, Ch., Biserte, G., Havez, R., Voisin, C., and Cuvelier, R.: Etude biochimique de l'expectoration bronchique. Path. Biol. (Paris), *11:*729–741, 1963.
2652. Masson, P. L., Heremans, J. F., and Prignot, J.: Studies on proteins of human bronchial secretions. Biochim. Biophys. Acta, *111:*466–478, 1965.
2653. Bonomo, L., and D'Addabbo, A.: (I^{131}) Albumin turnover and loss of protein into sputum in chronic bronchitis. Clin. Chim. Acta, *10:*214–222, 1964.
2654. Zeilhofer, R., and Friebel, H.: Untersuchungen über die Elektrolytkonzentration im Bronchialsekret bei chronischer Bronchitis. Klin. Wchnschr., *43:*32–37, 1965.
2655. Storey. P. B., Morgan, W. K. C., Diaz, A. J., Klaff, J. L., and Spicer, W. S., Jr.: Chronic obstructive airway disease: bacterial and cellular content of sputum. Amer. Rev. Resp. Dis., *90:*730–735, 1964.
2656. Ross, C. A. C., McMichael, S., Eadie, M. B., Lees, A. W., Murray, E. A., and Pinkerton, I.: Infective agents and chronic bronchitis. Thorax, *21:*461–464, 1966.
2657. Burns, M. W., and May, J. R.: Haemophilus influenzae precipitins in the serum of patients with chronic bronchial disorders. Lancet, *1:*354–358, 1967.
2658. Mimica, M., Palecek, I., and Zagar, Z.: The significance of haemophilus influenzae in chronic bronchitis and bronchial asthma. Allerg. Asthmaforsch., *11:*176–180, 1965.
2659. Galzigna, L., Terribile, P., and Berra, A.: Certain characteristic features of the bronchial secretion in chronic bronchitis. Minerva Med., *57:*2229–2232, 1966.
2660. Sharp, J. T., Paul, O., Lepper, M. H., McKean, H., and Saxton, G. A.: Prevalence of chronic bronchitis in American male urban industrial population. Amer. Rev. Resp. Dis., *91:*510–520, 1965.
2661. Sami, A. A., Abdel-Hakeem, M., Soliman, O., and Yousri, S.: Chronic bronchitis and emphysema in Egypt. Geriatrics, *20:*510–516, 1965.
2662. Huhti, E.: Chronic respiratory disease among old people in a Finnish rural area. Ann. Med. Intern. Fenn., *55:*99–105, 1966.
2663. Jensen, V.: Lung diseases in rural general practice. T. Norske Laegeforen. *87:*558, 1967.
2664. Akgün, N., and Özgönül, H.: Lung volumes in wind instrument (Zurna) players. Amer. Rev. Resp. Dis., *96:*946–951, 1967.
2665. Anderson, D. O., Ferris, B. G., Jr., and Zickmantel, R.: *The Chilliwack Respiratory Survey, 1963:* III. The prevalence of respiratory disease in a rural Canadian town. Canad. Med. Assoc. J., *92:*1007–1016, 1965.
2666. Poppius, H., Lehtinen, M., and Patiala, J.: Chronic bronchitis in forest workers in Finland. Duodecim (Helsinki), *81:*881–894, 1965.
2667. Neilson, M. G. C., and Crofton, E.: *The Social Effects of Chronic Bronchitis. A Scottish Study.* Edinburgh, Chest and Heart Association 1965, p. 72.
2668. Holland, W. W., and Stone, R. W.: Respiratory disorders in United States east coast telephone men. Amer. J. Epidemiol., *82:*92–101, 1965.
2669. Huhti, E.: Prevalence of respiratory symptoms, chronic bronchitis and pulmonary emphysema in a Finnish rural population. Acta Tuberc. Scand., (Supplement 61), 1965.
2670. Crofton, E. C.: A comparison of the mortality from bronchitis in Scotland and in England and Wales. Brit. Med. J., *1:*1635–1639, 1965.
2671. Meadows, S. H., Wood, C. H., and Schilling, R. S. F.: Respiratory symptoms and smoking habits of senior industrial staff. Brit. J. Industr. Med., *22:*149–153, 1965.
2672. Caplin, M., Capel, L. H., and Wheeler, W. F.: A bronchitis registry in East London. A report on the first year's work. Brit. J. Dis. Chest, *58:*97–111, 1964.
2673. Caplin, M. M., Capel, L. H., and Wheeler, W. F.: A bronchitis registry in East London. Brit. J. Dis. Chest, *58:*112–118, 1964.
2674. Leading Article: Cardiorespiratory comparisons. Lancet, *2:*1401–1402, 1967.
2675. Burrows, B., Niden, A. H., Fletcher, C. M., and Jones, N. L.: Clinical types of chronic obstructive lung disease in London and Chicago. A study of one hundred patients. Amer. Rev. Resp. Dis., *90:*14–27, 1964.
2676. Reid, D. D., Anderson, D. O., Ferris, B. G., and Fletcher,

C. M.: An Anglo-American comparison of the prevalence of bronchitis. Brit. Med. J., *2:*1487–1491, 1964.

2677. Doll, R., Fisher, R. E. W., Gammon, E. J., Gunn, W., Hughes, G. O., Tyrer, F. H., and Wilson, W.: Mortality of gasworkers with special reference to cancers of the lung and bladder, chronic bronchitis, and pneumoconiosis. Brit. J. Industr. Med., *22:*1–12, 1965.
2678. Holland, W. W., and Reid, D. D.: Urban factor in chronic bronchitis. Lancet, *1:*445–448, 1965.
2679. Kourilsky, R., Brille, D., and Hatte, J.: The physiognomy of chronic bronchitis, as revealed by an epidemiological investigation of 5,467 workers from the Paris region. Bull. Acad. Nat. Med. (Paris), *150:*168–178, 1966.
2680. Staněk, V., Fodor, J., Hejl, Z., Widimský, J., Charvát, P., Santrůček, M., Zajíc, F., and Vavřík, M.: A contribution to the epidemiology of chronic bronchitis. Acta Med. Scand., *179:*737–746, 1966.
2681. Holland, W. W., Ashford, J. R., Colley, J. R. T., Morgan, D. C., and Pearson, N. J.: A comparison of two respiratory symptoms questionnaires. Brit. J. Prev. Soc. Med., *20:*76–96, 1966.
2682. Sikand, B. K., Pamra, S. P., and Mathur, G. P.: Chronic bronchitis in Delhi as revealed by mass survey. Indian J. Tuberc., *13:*94–101, 1966.
2683. Langlands, J.: The dynamics of cough in health and in chronic bronchitis. Thorax, *22:*88–96, 1967.
2684. Huhti, E.: Chronic respiratory disease among old people in a Finnish rural area. Ann. Med. Intern. Fenn., *55:*99–105, 1966.
2685. Walshe, M. M., and Hayes, J. A.: Respiratory symptoms and smoking habits in Jamaica. Amer. Rev. Resp. Dis., *96:*640–644, 1967.
2686. Fréour, P., and Coudray, P.: An epidemiological study of the bronchorespiratory disorders in a large urban agglomeration. Bull. Inst. Nat. Sante Rech. Med., *22:*901–926, 1967.
2687. Best, E. W. R., Walker, C. B., Baker, P. M., Delaquis, F. M., McGregor, J. T., and McKenzie, A. C.: Summary of a Canadian study of smoking and health. Canad. Med. Assoc. J., *96:*1104–1108, 1967.
2688. Meluzin, J.: The smoking habit and chronic bronchitis. Rozhl. Tuberk., *28:*119–125, 1968.
2689. Oshima, Y., Ishizaki, T., Miyamoto, T., Shimuzu, T., Shida, T., and Kabe, J.: Air pollution and respiratory diseases in the Tokyo-Yokohama Area. Amer. Rev. Resp. Dis., *90:*572–581, 632–634, 1964.
2690. Ishizaki, T., et al.: The influence of air pollution on the respiratory function of man. I. Results of the mass examination conducted in the Tokyo and Yokohama districts. Jap. J. Public Health, *11:*945–953, 1964.
2691. Wynder, E. L., Lemon, F. R., and Mantel, N.: Epidemiology of persistent cough. Amer. Rev. Resp. Dis., *91:*679–700, 1965.
2692. Winkelstein, W., Jr., Kanter, S., Davis, E. W., Maneri, C. S., and Mosher, W. E.: Relationship of air pollution and economic status to total mortality and selected respiratory system mortality in men. Arch. Environ. Health, *14:*162–171, 1967.
2693. Seventh Annual Air Pollution Medical Research Conference Los Angeles, February 10–11, 1964. Arch. Environ. Health, *10:*143–388, 1965.
2694. Angel, J. H., Fletcher, C. M., Hill, I. D., and Tinker, C. M.: Respiratory illness in factory and office workers. A study of minor respiratory illnesses in relation to changes in ventilatory capacity, sputum characteristics, and atmospheric pollution. Brit. J. Dis. Chest, *59:*66–80, 1965.
2695. Spotnitz, M.: The significance of Yokohama asthma. Amer. Rev. Resp. Dis., *92:*371–375, 1965.
2696. Miyamoto, T., Makino, S., Kabe, J., Kodama, T., and Shiraishi, T.: Pulmonary diffusing capacity among Japanese patients with clinical features similar to Tokyo-Yokohama asthma. Amer. Rev. Resp. Dis., *94:*734–740, 1966.
2697. Sekimoto, T.: Effect of air pollution on chronic respiratory disease. J. Keio Med. Soc., *43:*215–226, 1966.
2698. Lawther, P. J.: Air pollution and chronic bronchitis. Med. Thorac., *24:*44–52, 1967.
2699. Ogilvie, A. G.: Observations on exacerbations of bronchitis. Med. Thorac., *24:*53–62, 1967.
2700. Zeidberg, L. D., Horton, R. J. M., and Landau, E.: The Nashville air pollution study. V. Mortality from diseases of the respiratory system in relation to air pollution. Arch. Environ. Health, *15:*214–224, 1967.
2701. *Medical and Epidemiological aspects of Air Pollution: Symposium Number 6.* Proc. Roy. Soc. Med., *57:*965–1040, 1964.
2702. McKerrow, C. B.: Chronic respiratory disease in Great Britain. Arch. Environ. Health, *8:*174–179, 1964.
2703. Jaffe, L. S.: Photochemical air pollutants and their effects on men and animals. Arch. Environ. Health, *15:*782–791, 1967, *16:*241–255, 1968.
2704. Hamming, W. J., MacBeth, W. G., and Chass, R. L.: The photochemical air pollution syndrome. Arch. Environ. Health, *14:*137–149, 1967.
2705. Toyama, T.: Air pollution and its health effects in Japan. Arch. Environ. Health, *8:*153–173, 1964.
2706. Stokinger, H. F.: Ozone toxicology. Arch. Environ. Health, *10:*719–731, 1965.
2707. Kelsey, J. L., Mood, E. W., and Acheson, R. M.: Population mobility and epidemiology of chronic bronchitis in Connecticut. Arch. Environ. Health, *16:*853–861, 1968.
2708. Hong, C. S., Gandevia, B., and Lovell, H.: Ventilatory capacity in a series of male adults and the effect of respiratory symptoms, productive cough, smoking habit and occupation. Med. J. Aust., *1:*169–172, 1967.
2709. Ingram, W., McCarroll, J. R., Cassell, E. J., and Wolter, D.: Health and the urban environment. Arch. Environ. Health, *10:*364–366, 1965.
2710. Cassell, E. J., McCarroll, J. R., Ingram, W., and Wolter, D.: Health and the urban environment. Arch. Environ. Health, *10:*367–369, 1965.
2711. Cederlof, R.: Urban factor and prevalence of respiratory symptoms and angina pectoris. Arch. Environ. Health, *13:*743–748, 1966.
2712. Becker, W. H., Schilling, F. J., and Verma, M. P.: The effect on health of the 1966 eastern seabord air pollution episode. Arch. Environ. Health, *16:*414–419, 1968.
2713. Cullen, K. J., Stenhouse, N. S., Welborn, T. A., McCall, M. G., and Curnow, D. H.: Chronic respiratory disease in a rural community. Lancet, *2:*657–660, 1968.
2714. Spodnik, M. J., Cushman, G. D., Kerr, D. H., Blide, R. W., and Spicer, W. S.: Effects of environment on respiratory function. Arch. Environ. Health, *13:*243–254, 1966.
2715. Petrilli, F. L., Agnese, G., and Kanitz, S.: Epidemiologic studies of air pollution effects in Genoa, Italy. Arch. Environ. Health, *12:*733–740, 1966.
2716. Tipton, I. H., and Shafer, J. J.: Statistical analysis of lung trace element levels. Arch. Environ. Health, *8:*58–67, 1964.
2717. Frank, N. R., and Speizer, F. E.: SO_2 effects on the respiratory system of dogs. Arch. Environ. Health, *11:*624–634, 1965.
2718. Speizer, F. E., and Frank, N. R.: The uptake and release of SO_2 by the human nose. Arch. Environ. Health, *12:*725–728, 1966.
2719. Larsen, R. I.: United States air quality. Arch. Environ. Health, *8:*325–333, 1964.
2720. Lawther, P. J., Ellison, J. McK., and Waller, R. E.: Some medical aspects of aerosol research. Proc. Roy. Soc. (A) *307:*223–234, 1968.
2721. Holland, W. W., Reid, D. D., Seltser, R., and Stone, R. W.: Respiratory disease in England and the United States. Arch. Environ. Health, *10:*338–343, 1965.
2722. Ferris, B. G.: Epidemiological studies on air pollution and health. Arch. Environ. Health, *16:*541–555, 1968.
2723. Lowe, C. R.: Industrial bronchitis. Brit. Med. J., *1:*463–468, 1969.
2724. Douglas, J. W. B., and Waller, R. E.: Air pollution and respiratory infection in children. Brit. J. Prev. Soc. Med., *20:*1–8, 1966.
2725. Lunn, J. E., Knowelden, J., and Handyside, A. J.: Patterns of respiratory illness in Sheffield schoolchildren. Brit. J. Prev. Soc. Med., *21:*7–16, 1967.
2726. Glasser, M., Greenburg, L., and Field, F.: Mortality and

morbidity during a period of high levels of air pollution. Arch. Environ. Health, *15*:684–694, 1967.

2727. Schleusner, A.: Quantitative assessment of small airways. *Personal Communication.*
2728. Fletcher, C. M., Jones, N. L., Burrows, B., and Niden, A. H.: American emphysema and British bronchitis: standardised comparative study. Amer. Rev. Resp. Dis., *99*:1–13, 1964.
2729. Monograph: *Air Conservation:* American Association for the Advancement of Science (Publication No. 80), 1965.
2730. Stern, A. C.: *Air Pollution.* Vol. I, II, and III. New York and London, Academic Press, 1968.
2731. Proceedings of Committee of Senate (Public Works). *Air and Water Pollution* (Senator E. S. Muskie). 90th Congress, 2d Session, May, 1968. (CJ NITE MONO-1.)
2732. Bates, D. V.: Air Pollution in perspective. McGill News, *49*:6–9, 1968.
2733. Haydon, G. B., Freeman, G., and Furiosi, N. J.: Covert pathogenesis of NO_2 induced emphysema in the rat. Arch. Environ. Health, *11*:776–783, 1965.
2734. Molokhia, M. M., and Smith, H.: Trace elements in the lung. Arch. Environ. Health, *15*:745–750, 1967.
2735. Cachovan, M.: The effect of a single stay in the High Tatra mountain climate on the vegetative equilibirum of chronic bronchitis. Bratisl. Lek. Listy, *44*:273–280, 1964.
2736. The Health Consequences of Smoking: 1968 supplement to the 1967 Public Health Service Review (U.S. Public Health Service Publication No. 1696), p. 66.
2737. Pastor, J., Charpin, J., and Dumon, G.: Study of the "Sweat Test" in a group of chronic bronchitics. Poumon Coeur, *21*:301–307, 1965.
2738. Larson, R. K., and Barman, M. L.: The familial occurrence of chronic obstructive pulmonary disease. Ann. Intern. Med., *63*:1001–1008, 1965.
2739. Hole, B. V., and Wasserman, K.: Familial emphysema. Ann. Intern. Med., *63*:1009–1017.
2740. Jacobson, G., Turner, A. F., Balchum, O., and Judge, C.: Pulmonary arteriovenous shunts in emphysema demonstrated by wedge arteriography. Amer. J. Roentgen., *93*:868–878, 1965.
2741. Gilbert, R., Keighley, J., and Auchincloss, J. H., Jr.: Mechanisms of chronic carbon dioxide retention in patients with obstructive pulmonary disease. Amer. J. Med., *38*:217–225, 1965.
2742. Simonsson, B. G.: Clinical and physiological studies in chronic bronchitis. I. Clinical description of the patient material. Acta Allerg. (Kobenhavn), *20*:257–300, 1965.
2743. Abernethy, J. D.: Effects of inhalation of an artificial fog. Thorax, *23*:421–426, 1968.
2744. Macklem, P. T., and Mead, J.: Resistance of central and peripheral airways measured by retrograde catheter. J. Appl. Physiol., *22*:395–401, 1967.
2745. Ingram, R. H., Jr., and Schilder, D. P.: Association of a decrease in dynamic compliance with a change in gas distribution. J. Appl. Physiol., *23*:911–916, 1967.
2746. Fletcher, C. M., Jones, N. L., and Campbell, E. J. M.: Research into bronchitis and emphysema. Postgrad. Med. J., *44*:48–52, 1968. (Festschrift for Sir J. McMichael.)
2747. Lane, D. J., Howell, J. B. L., and Giblin, B.: Relation between airways obstruction and CO_2 tension in chronic obstructive airways disease. Brit. Med. J., *2*:707–709, 1968.
2748. Oswald, N. C.: Follow-up in chronic bronchitis. Med. Thorac., *24*:74, 1967.
2749. Brinkman, G. L., and Block, D. L.: The prognosis in chronic bronchitis. In: *Current Research in Chronic Airways Obstruction* (U.S. Dept. of Health, Education and Welfare Publication No. 1717), 1968, pp. 317–326.
2750. Brinkman, G. L., and Block, D. L.: The prognosis in chronic bronchitis. J.A.M.A., *197*:1–7, 1966.
2751. Renzetti, A. D., McClement, J. H., and Litt, B. D.: Mortality in relation to respiratory function in chronic obstructive pulmonary disease. In: *Current Research in Chronic Airways Obstruction.* (U.S. Dept. of Health, Education and Welfare Publication No. 1717), 1968, pp. 367–378.
2752. Fletcher, C. M.: Prognosis in chronic bronchitis. In: *Current Research in Chronic Airways Obstruction.* (U.S. Dept. of Health, Education and Welfare Publication No. 1717), 1968, pp. 309–315.
2753. Jones, N. L., Burrows, B., and Fletcher, C. M.: Serial studies of 100 patients with chronic airway obstruction in London and Chicago. Thorax, *22*:327–335, 1967.
2754. Gregg, I.: A study of the causes of progressive airways obstruction in chronic bronchitis. In: *Current Research in Chronic Airways Obstruction.* (U.S. Dept. of Health, Education and Welfare Publication No. 1717), 1968, pp. 235–246.
2755. Simonsson, B. G.: Clinical and physiological studies on chronic bronchitis. II. Classification according to spirometric findings and effect of bronchodilators. Acta Allerg. (Kobenhavn), *20*:301–324, 1965.
2756. Rosenzweig, D. Y., Arkins, J. A., and Schrock, L. G.: Ventilation studies on a normal population after a seven year interval. Amer. Rev. Resp. Dis., *94*:74–78, 1966.
2757. Kreukniet, J., and Bangma, P. J.: The course of pulmonary function in patients with chronic non-specific lung diseases (CNSLD). Scand. J. Resp. Dis., *47*:173–181, 1966.
2758. Oswald, N. C., Medvei, V. C., and Waller, R. E.: Chronic bronchitis: A 10-year follow-up. Thorax, *22*:279–285, 1967.
2759. Simpson, T.: Chronic bronchitis and emphysema with special reference to prognosis. Brit. J. Dis. Chest, *62*:57–69, 1968.
2760. Simpson, T.: Chronic bronchitis and emphysema with special reference to treatment. Brit. J. Dis. Chest, *62*:70–80, 1968.
2761. Ross, J. C., Ley, G. D., Krumholz, R. A., and Rahbari, H.: Technique for evaluation of gas mixing in the lung: studies in cigarette smokers and non-smokers. Amer. Rev. Resp. Dis., *95*:447–453, 1967.
2762. Haynes, W. F., Jr., Krstulovic, V. J., and Loomis Bell, A. L., Jr.: Smoking habit and incidence of respiratory tract infections in a group of adolescent males. Amer. Rev. Resp. Dis., *93*:730–735, 1966.
2763. Parnell, J. L., Anderson, D. O., and Kinnis, C.: Cigarette smoking and respiratory infections in a class of student nurses. New Engl. J. Med., *274*:979–984, 1966.
2764. McDermott, M., and Collins, M. M.: Acute effects of smoking on lung airways resistance in normal and bronchitic subjects. Thorax, *20*:562–569, 1965.
2765. Krumholz, R. A., Chevalier, R. B., and Ross, J. C.: A comparison of pulmonary compliance in young smokers and nonsmokers. Amer. Rev. Resp. Dis., *92*:102–107, 1965.
2766. Dawson, A.: Reproducibility of spirometric measurements in normal subjects. Amer. Rev. Resp. Dis., *93*:264–268, 1966.
2767. Pelzer, A. M., and Thomson, M. L.: Effect of age, sex, stature, and smoking habits on human airway conductance. J. Appl. Physiol., *21*:469–476, 1966.
2768. Krumholz, R. A., Chevalier, R. B., and Ross, J. C.: Changes in cardiopulmonary functions related to abstinence from smoking. Studies in young cigarette smokers at rest and exercise at 3 and 6 weeks of abstinence. Ann. Intern. Med., *62*:197–207, 1965.
2769. Krumholz, R. A., Chevalier, R. B., and Ross, J. C.: Cardiopulmonary function in young smokers. Ann. Intern. Med., *60*:603–610, 1964.
2770. Aviado, D. M., and Samanek, M.: Bronchopulmonary effects of tobacco and related substances. Arch. Environ. Health, *11*:141–151, 1965.
2771. Holland, W. W., and Elliott, A.: Cigarette smoking, respiratory symptoms, and anti-smoking propaganda. Lancet, *1*:41–43, 1968.
2772. Stanescu, D. C., Teculescu, D. B., Pacuraru, R., and Gavrilescu, N.: Chronic effect of smoking upon pulmonary distribution of ventilation in healthy males. Respiration, *25*:497–504, 1968.
2773. Petty, T. L., Ryan, S. F., and Mitchell, R. S.: Cigarette smoking and the lungs. Arch. Environ. Health, *14*:172–177, 1967.

2774. Rankin, J., Gee, J. B. L., and Chosy, L. W.: Influence of age and smoking on pulmonary diffusing capacity of healthy subjects. Med. Thorac., *22*:366–374, 1965.
2775. Peterson, D. I., Lonergan, L. H., and Hardinge, M. G.: Smoking and pulmonary function. Arch. Environ. Health, *16*:215–218, 1968.
2776. Dunnill, M. S.: Evaluation of a simple method of sampling the lung for quantitative histological analysis. Thorax, *19*:443–448, 1964.
2777. Thurlbeck, W. M.: The diagnosis of emphysema. Thorax, *19*:571–574, 1964.
2778. Duguid, J. B., Young, A., Cauna, D., and Lambert, M. W.: The internal surface area of the lung in emphysema. J. Path. Bact., *88*:405–421, 1964.
2779. Giese, W., and Hartung, W.: Pulmonary emphysema; pathogenetic classification and clinico-pathologic correlation. Med. Thorac., *21*:193–203, 1964.
2780. Smith, K. V.: A survey of the types and severity of emphysema in routine autopsies. Aust. Ann. Med., *14*:28–34, 1965.
2781. Silverton, R. E.: Gross fixation methods used in the study of pulmonary emphysema. Thorax, *20*:289–297, 1965.
2782. Anderson, J. A., and Dunnill, M. S.: Observations on the estimation of the quantity of emphysema in the lungs by the point-sampling method. Thorax, *20*:462–466, 1965.
2783. Gross, P., Pfitzer, E. A., Tolker, E., Babyak, M. A., and Kaschak, M.: Experimental emphysema. Its production with papain in normal and silicotic rats. Arch. Environ. Health, *11*:50–58, 1965.
2784. McLaughlin, R. F., Jr., Tyler, W. S., Edwards, D. W., Crenshaw, G. L., Canada, R. O., Fowler, M. A., Parker, E. A., and Reifenstein, G. H.: Chlorpromazine-induced emphysema. Results of an initial study in the horse. Amer. Rev. Resp. Dis., *92*:597–608, 1965.
2785. Edge, J., Simon, G., and Reid, L.: Peri-acinar (paraseptal) emphysema: its clinical, radiological, and physiological features. Brit. J. Dis. Chest, *60*:10–18, 1966.
2786. Kory, R. C., Rauterkus, L. T., Korthy, A. L., and Côté, R. A.: Quantitative estimation of pulmonary emphysema in lung macrosections by photoelectric measurement of transmitted light. Amer. Rev. Resp. Dis., *93*:758–768, 1966.
2787. Vosskuhler, P.: The role of obstruction in the development of "obstructive" emphysema. Prax. Pneumol., *20*:13–20, 1966.
2788. Hernandez, J. A., Anderson, A. E., Jr., Holmes, W. L., and Foraker, A. G.: Macroscopic relations in emphysematous and aging lungs. Geriatrics, *21*:155–166, 1966.
2789. Anderson, A. E., Jr., Hernandez, J. A., Holmes, W. L., and Foraker, A. G.: Pulmonary emphysema. Prevalence, severity, and anatomical patterns in macrosections, with respect to smoking habits. Arch. Environ. Health, *12*:569–577, 1966.
2790. Longfield, A. N., and Hentel, W.: Lung destruction measured by energy transmission through fume fixed lungs. Dis. Chest, *50*:225–231, 1966.
2791. Bignon, J., Got, C., Khoury, F., and Brouet, G.: Method for the fixation of entire lungs for the quantitative macroscopic and microscopic study of progressive respiratory failure. Presse Méd., *74*:2461–2463, 1966.
2792. Thurlbeck, W. M.: The internal surface area of non-emphysematous lungs. Amer. Rev. Resp. Dis., *95*:765–773, 1967.
2793. Hicken, P., Heath, D., and Brewer, D.: The relation between the weight of the right ventricle and the percentage of abnormal air space in the lung in emphysema. J. Path. Bact., *92*:519–528, 1966.
2794. Hicken, P., Brewer, D., and Heath, D.: The relation between the weight of the right ventricle of the heart and the internal surface area and number of alveoli in the human lung in emphysema. J. Path. Bact., *92*:529–546, 1966.
2795. Sherwin, R. P., Levenson, M., and Balchum, O.: The quantitative measurement of emphysema using diazo replication and the particle analyzer. Amer. Rev. Resp. Dis., *95*:986–997, 1967.
2796. Fitzpatrick, M.: Studies of human pulmonary connective tissue. III. Chemical changes in structural proteins with emphysema. Amer. Rev. Resp. Dis., *96*:254–265, 1967.
2797. Pratt, P. C., and Klugh, G. A.: Chronic expiratory airflow obstruction: cause or effect of centrilobular emphysema? Dis. Chest, *52*:342–349, 1967.
2798. Colp, C., Coppola, A., and Buchberg, A. S.: Diffuse emphysema as a result of nonobstructive interstitial pulmonary disease. Amer. Rev. Resp. Dis., *96*:788–794, 1967.
2799. Strieder, D. J., and Kazemi, H.: Hypoxemia in young asymptomatic cigarette smokers. Ann. Thorac. Surg., *4*:523–531, 1967.
2800. Boushy, S. F., Greenberg, S. D., and Jenkins, D. E.: The prevalence of emphysema in 67 unselected male necropsies. Dis. Chest, *53*:497–501, 1968.
2801. Gough, J., Ryder, R. C., Otto, H., and Heller, G.: Comparative morphological studies on the frequency of pulmonary emphysema. Frankfurt. Z. Path., *77*:317–327, 1967.
2802. Hasleton, P. S., Heath, D., and Brewer, D. B.: Hypertensive pulmonary vascular disease in states of chronic hypoxia. J. Path. Bact., *95*:431–440, 1968.
2803. Rochemaure, J., Bignon, J., Khoury, F., and Brouet, G.: A comparative study of the anatomical and ECG findings in 50 patients with chronic bronchopneumopathy. Rev. Tuberc. (Paris), *32*:261–268, 1968.
2804. Wright, R. R., and Stuart, C. M.: Chronic bronchitis with emphysema: a pathological study of the bronchi. Med. Thorac., *22*:210–218, 1965.
2805. Bignon, J., Khoury, F., Even, P., André, J., and Brouet, G.: Quantitative anatomic study of chronic obstructive bronchopneumopathy. Rev. Tuberc. (Paris), *32*:207–244, 1968.
2806. Laennec, R. T. H.: *De l'Auscultation Médiate ou Traité du Diagnostic des Maladies des Poumons et du Coeur, fondé Principalement sur ce Nouveau Moyen d'Exploration* (2 tomes). 8°, Paris, 1819.
2807. Fluck, D. C., Chandrasekar, R. G., and Gardner, F. V.: Left ventricular hypertrophy in chronic bronchitis. Brit. Heart J., *28*:92–97, 1966.
2808. Mori, P. A., Anderson, A. E., Jr., and Eckert, P.: The radiological spectrum of aging and emphysematous lungs. Radiology, *83*:48–57, 1964.
2809. Millard, F. J. C., Edge, J. R., Reid, L., and Simon, G.: The radiographic appearances of the chest in persons of advanced age. Brit. J. Radiol., *37*:769–774, 1964.
2810. Simon, G.: Radiology and emphysema. Clin. Radiol., *15*:307–311, 1964.
2811. Lopez-Majano, V., Tow, D. E., and Wagner, H. N., Jr.: Regional distribution of pulmonary blood flow in emphysema. J.A.M.A., *197*:81–84, 1966.
2812. Ritchie, B., and Hugh-Jones, P.: Studies of lobar function in the lungs of patients with emphysema. Scand. J. Resp. Dis. Supplement *62*:83–90, 1966.
2813. Jacobson, G., Turner, A. F., Balchum, O. J., and Jung, R.: Vascular changes in pulmonary emphysema. The radiologic evaluation by selective and peripheral pulmonary wedge angiography. Amer. J. Roentgen., *100*:374–396, 1967.
2814. Galy, P., and Loire, R.: L'emphysème pulmonaire diffus et la bronchite chronique. Bull. Physio-Path. Resp., *3*:179–235, 1967.
2815. Pain, M. C. F., Glazier, J. B., Simon, H., and West, J. B.: Regional and overall inequality of ventilation and blood flow in patients with chronic airflow obstruction. Thorax, *22*:453–461, 1967.
2816. Katsura, S. and Martin, C. J.: The roentgenologic diagnosis of anatomic emphysema. Amer. Rev. Resp. Dis., *96*:700–706, 1967.
2817. Even, P., Duroux, P., Ferrane, J., Bignon, J., and Leconte, A.: Evaluation radiologique, fonctionelle, et anatomique de la capacité pulmonaire totale, chez les sujets normaux et au cours des broncho-pneumopathies chroniques. Rev. Tuberc. (Paris), *32*:269–280, 1968.
2818. Cordasco, E. M., Beerel, F. R., Vance, J. W., Wende, R. W., and Tottolo, R. R.: Newer aspects of the pulmonary vasculature in chronic lung disease. A comparative study. Angiology, *19*:399–407, 1968.

2819. Godfrey, S., Edwards, R. H. T., Campbell, E. J. M., Armitage, P., and Oppenheimer, E. A.: Repeatability of physical signs in airways obstruction. Thorax, *24:*4–9, 1969.
2820. Campbell, E. J. M.: Physical signs of diffuse airways obstruction and lung distension. Thorax, *24:*1–3, 1969.
2821. Schneider, I. C., and Anderson, A. E., Jr.: Correlation of clinical signs with ventilatory function in obstructive lung disease. Ann. Intern. Med., *62:*477–485, 1965.
2822. Smyllie, H. C., Blendis, L. M., and Armitage, P.: Observer disagreement in physical signs of the respiratory system. Lancet, *2:*412–413, 1965.
2823. Forgacs, P.: Crackles and wheezes. Lancet, *2:*203–205, 1967.
2824. Leiner, G. C., Abramowitz, S., and Small, M. J.: The vital capacity in pulmonary emphysema. Ann. Intern. Med., *60:*61–65, 1964.
2825. Lim, T. P. K., and Brownlee, W. E.: Diffusion impairment in obstructive pulmonary emphysema. Amer. Rev. Resp. Dis., *90:*213–222, 1964.
2826. Gilbert, R., Keighley, J., and Auchincloss, J. H., Jr.: Disability in patients with obstructive pulmonary disease. Amer. Rev. Resp. Dis., *90:*383–394, 1964.
2827. Refsum, H. E.: Acid-base status in patients with chronic hypercapnia and hypoxemia. Clin. Sci., *27:*407–415, 1964.
2828. Sølvsteen, P.: Lung diffusing capacity: Rebreathing method, applicability in nonuniform ventilation. J. Appl. Physiol., *20:*99–102, 1965.
2829. Burrows, B., Niden, A. H., Barclay, W. R., and Kasik, J. E.: Chronic obstructive lung disease. I. Clinical and physiologic findings in 175 patients and their relationship to age and sex. Amer. Rev. Resp. Dis., *91:*521–540, 1965.
2830. Schilder, D. P., Roberts, A., Greenfield, J. C., Jr., and Fry, D. L.: Regional distribution of intraesophageal pressure in normal and emphysematous subjects. J. Appl. Physiol., *20:*209–214, 1965.
2831. Matthews, C. M. E., and Dollery, C. T.: Interpretation of ^{133}Xe lung wash-in and wash-out curves using an analogue computer. Clin. Sci., *28:*573–590, 1965.
2832. Park, S. S.: Factors responsible for carbon dioxide retention in chronic obstructive lung disease. Amer. Rev. Resp. Dis., *92:*245–254, 1965.
2833. Burrows, B., Strauss, R. H., and Niden, A. H.: Chronic Obstructive Lung Disease. III. Interrelationships of pulmonary function test data. Amer. Rev. Resp. Dis., *91:*861–868, 1965.
2834. Anderson, G., and Capel, L. H.: The diurnal variations in arterial pCO_2 in chronic airways obstruction. Brit. J. Dis. Chest, *59:*113–115, 1965.
2835. Fuleihan, F. J. D., and Abboud, R. T.: Diurnal variation in pulmonary function in patients with airway obstructive disease. Amer. Rev. Resp. Dis., *98:*101–103, 1968.
2836. Williams, M. H., Jr., and Park, S. S.: Diffusion of gases within the lungs of patients with chronic obstructive pulmonary disease. Amer. Rev. Resp. Dis., *98:*210–216, 1968.
2837. Macklem, P. T., Fraser, R. G., and Brown, W. G.: Bronchial pressure measurements in emphysema and bronchitis. J. Clin. Invest., *44:*897–905, 1965.
2838. Nakhjavan, F. K., Palmer, W. H., and McGregor, M.: Influence of respiration on venous return in pulmonary emphysema. Circulation, *33:*8–16, 1966.
2839. Brody, J. S., and Glazier, J. B.: The effect of position on pulmonary function in chronic obstructive lung disease. Amer. Rev. Resp. Dis., *92:*579–588, 1965.
2840. Ayres, S. M., and Gianelli, S., Jr.: Causes of arterial hypoxemia in patients with obstructive pulmonary emphysema. Amer. J. Med., *39:*422–428, 1965.
2841. Read, J., Read, D. J. C., and Pain, M. C. F.: Influence of non-uniformity of the lungs on measurement of pulmonary diffusing capacity. Clin. Sci., *29:*107–118, 1965.
2842. Beerel, F. R., and Vance, J. W.: Daily pCO_2 and pH fluctuations in pulmonary emphysema with carbon dioxide retention. Amer. Rev. Resp. Dis., *92:*894–899, 1965.
2843. Bates, D. V., Gee, J. B. L., Bentivoglio, L. G., and Mostyn, E. Diffusion as a limiting factor in exercise. In: *International Symposium on the Cardiovascular and Respiratory Effects of Hypoxia.* Basel (Switzerland), S. Karger and Sons, 1966.
2844. Pain, M. C. F., Read, D. J. C., and Read, J.: Changes of arterial carbon-dioxide tension in patients with chronic lung disease breathing oxygen. Aust. Ann. Med., *14:*195–204, 1965.
2845. Penman, R. W. B., and Howard, P.: Distribution of pulmonary ventilation and blood flow in normal subjects and patients with chronic bronchitis. Clin. Sci., *30:*63–78, 1966.
2846. Hanson, J. S., and Tabakin, B. S.: Correlation of vital capacity with other indices of disease in obstructive emphysema. Dis. Chest, *49:*52–56, 1966.
2847. Adyshirin-Zade, E. A.: The state of the capillary sector of the vascular circuit of the emphysematous lung. Trudy Kuibyshevsk. Med. Inst., *35:*110–115, 1965.
2848. Tulou, P. P.: Distribution of ventilation; clinical evaluation by rapid CO_2 analysis. Dis. Chest, *49:*139–146, 1966.
2849. Stein, M., Tanabe, G., Rege, V., and Khan, M.: Evaluation of spirometric methods used to assess abnormalities in airway resistance. Amer. Rev. Resp. Dis., *93:*257–263, 1966.
2850. Nakamura, T., Taskashima, T., Okubo, T., Sasaki, T., and Takahashi, H.: Distribution function of the clearance time constant in lungs. J. Appl. Physiol., *21:*227–232, 1966.
2851. Sølvsteen, P.: Lung diffusing capacities. *Thesis,* Munksgaard, Copenhagen, 1966.
2852. Piiper, J., and Sikand, R. S.: Determination of D_{CO} by the single breath method in inhomogeneous lungs: Theory. Resp. Physiol., *1:*75–87, 1966.
2853. Paul, G., Eldridge, F., Mitchell, J., and Fiene, T.: Some effects of slowing respiration rate in chronic emphysema and bronchitis. J. Appl. Physiol., *21:*877–882, 1966.
2854. Erwin, W. S., Zolov, D., and Bickerman, H. A.: The effect of posture on respiratory function in patients with obstructive pulmonary emphysema. Amer. Rev. Resp. Dis., *94:*865–872, 1966.
2855. Emmanuel, G. E., and Moreno, F.: Distribution of ventilation and blood flow during exercise in emphysema. J. Appl. Physiol., *21:*1532–1544, 1966.
2856. Howard, P., and Penman, R. W. B.: The effect of breathing 30 per cent oxygen on pulmonary ventilation–perfusion inequality in normal subjects and patients with chronic lung disease. Clin. Sci., *32:*127–137, 1967.
2857. Astin, T. W., and Penman, R. W. B.: Airway obstruction due to hypoxemia in patients with chronic lung disease. Amer. Rev. Resp. Dis., *95:*567–575, 1967.
2858. Pain, M. C. F., Charlton, G. C., and Read, J.: Effect of intravenous aminophylline on distribution of pulmonary blood flow in obstructive lung disease. Amer. Rev. Resp. Dis., *95:*1005–1014, 1967.
2859. Cumming, G.: Gas mixing efficiency in the human lung. Resp. Physiol., *2:*213–224, 1967.
2860. Cohn, J. E., and Donoso, H. D.: Exercise and intrapulmonary ventilation–perfusion relationships in chronic obstructive airway disease. Amer. Rev. Resp. Dis., *95:*1015–1025, 1967.
2861. Sølvsteen, P.: Lung diffusing capacity with particular reference to its determination in patients with uneven ventilation. Danish Med. Bull., *14:*142–150, 1967.
2862. Mellemgaard, K.: The alveolar–arterial oxygen difference in chronic obstructive lung disease. Scand. J. Resp. Dis., *48:*23–39, 1967.
2863. Balchum, O. J., Jung, R. C., Turner, A. F., and Jacobson, G.: Pulmonary artery to vein shunts in obstructive pulmonary disease. Amer. J. Med., *43:*178–185, 1967.
2864. Flenley, D. C., and Millar, J. S.: Ventilatory response to oxygen and carbon dioxide in chronic respiratory failure. Clin. Sci., *33:*319–334, 1967.
2865. Schleuter, D. P., Immekus, J., and Stead, W. W.: Relationship between maximal inspiratory pressure and total lung capacity (coefficient of retraction) in normal subjects and in patients with emphysema, asthma, and diffuse pulmonary infiltration. Amer. Rev. Resp. Dis., *96:*656–665, 1967.
2866. Mitchell, M., Watanabe, S., and Renzetti, A. D., Jr.: Evaluation of airway conductance measurements in normal

subjects and patients with chronic obstructive pulmonary disease. Amer. Rev. Resp. Dis., *96:*685–691, 1967.

2867. Galy, P., Brune, J., Wiesendanger, T., and Brune, A.: A study of the diffusion capacity in obstructive chronic bronchopneumopathy of the adult. Its value as a "functional" test of emphysema. J. Franc. Med. Chir. Thorac., *21:*537–554, 1967.

2868. Hatzfeld, C., Wiener, F., and Briscoe, W. A.: Effects of uneven ventilation-diffusion ratios on pulmonary diffusing capacity in disease. J. Appl. Physiol., *23:*1–10, 1967.

2869. Mittman, C.: Nonuniform pulmonary diffusing capacity measured by sequential CO uptake and washout. J. Appl. Physiol., *23:*131–138, 1967.

2870. Giuntini, C., Guerini, C., Mariani, M., Maseri, A., and Menichini, G.: Changes of air and blood distribution to the lung assessed by tritium. J. Nucl. Biol. Med., *11:*40–46, 1967.

2871. Sølysteen, P.: A simple index for uneven ventilation: with use of a closed circuit system. Acta Med. Scand., *182:*219–224, 1967.

2872. Wiener, F., Hatzfeld, C., and Briscoe, W. A.: Limits to arterial nitrogen tension in unevenly ventilated and perfused human lungs. J. Appl. Physiol., *23:*439–456, 1967.

2873. Anthonisen, N. R., Bass, H., Heckscher, T., Oriol, A., and Bates, D. V.: Recent observations on the measurement of regional $\dot{V}/\dot{Q}$ ratios in chronic lung disease. J. Nucl. Biol. Med., *11:*73–79, 1967.

2874. Takashima, T., Grimby, G., Graham, W., Knudson, R., Macklem, P. T., and Mead, J.: Flow-volume curves during quiet breathing, maximum voluntary ventilation, and forced vital capacities in patients with obstructive lung disease. Scand. J. Resp. Dis., *48:*384–393, 1967.

2875. Cellerino, A. F., Gaetini, A., Rosso, F., and Banaudi, C.: Unevenness of blood and air distribution to the lungs studied by a combined radiokrypton and helium method. J. Nucl. Biol. Med., *11:*32–39, 1967.

2876. Gonzalez, E., Weill, H., Ziskind, M. M., and George, R. B.: The value of the single breath diffusing capacity in separating chronic bronchitis from pulmonary emphysema. Dis. Chest, *53:*229–236, 1968.

2877. Schlie, G.: States of extreme hypoxemia in obstructive pulmonary emphysema. Respiration, *25:*173–183, 1968.

2878. Gurtner, H. P.: The distribution of the pulmonary circulation in chronic emphysema. A contribution to the technique of studying abnormal distributions. Bern, Verlag Hans Huber, 1968.

2879. Samad, I. A., Sanders, D. E., Suero, J. T., and Woolf, C. R.: The relationship between tracheo-bronchial collapse and pulmonary function in chronic obstructive pulmonary disease. Dis. Chest, *53:*407–412, 1968.

2880. Bryant, L. R., Cohn, J. E., O'Neill, R. P., Danielson, G. K., and Greenlaw, R. H.: Pulmonary blood flow distribution in chronic obstructive airway disease. Lung scintiscanning and pulmonary arteriography. Amer. Rev. Resp. Dis., *97:*832–842, 1968.

2881. Sobol, B. J., Emirgil, C., Garcia, F., and Goyal, P.: Tests of ventilatory function not requiring maximal subject effort. I. The single breath nitrogen washout. Amer. Rev. Resp. Dis., *97:*859–867, 1968.

2882. Pevny, E., and Scheida, N.: Tolerance curves of carbon dioxide during rebreathing in normal subjects, pulmonary emphysema and obesity. Dis. Chest, *53:*470–475, 1968.

2883. Fruhmann, G.: The diffusion capacity for oxygen in disorders of the lungs. Respiration, *25:*323–333, 1968.

2884. Krumholz, R. A., and Albright, C. D.: The compliance of the chest wall and thorax in emphysema. Amer. Rev. Resp. Dis., *97:*827–831, 1968.

2885. Van Heijst, A. N. P.: The acid-base balance in blood and cerebrospinal fluid in normal subjects and patients suffering from emphysema, with special reference to control of ventilation and cerebral circulation. Thesis, Utrecht, 1968.

2886. Alroy, G. G., and Flenley, D. C.: The acidity of the cerebrospinal fluid in man with particular reference to chronic ventilatory failure. Clin. Sci., *33:*335–343, 1967.

2887. Ayres, S. M., Buehler, M. E., and Armstrong, R. G.: Diffusing capacity of the lung in pulmonary emphysema. J. Appl. Physiol., *19:*981–989, 1964.

2888. Flenley, D. C., and Millar, J. S.: The effects of carbon dioxide inhalation on the inspiratory work of breathing in chronic ventilatory failure. Clin. Sci., *34:*385–395, 1968.

2889. Huang, C. T., and Lyons, H. A.: The maintenance of acid-base balance between cerebrospinal fluid and arterial blood in patients with chronic respiratory disorders. Clin. Sci., *31:*273–284, 1966.

2890. Campbell, A. H., and Faulks, L. W.: Bronchial pressure measurements in patients with tracheobronchial collapse. Respiration, *26:*23–27, 1969.

2891. Clark, T. J. H.: Ventilatory response to CO_2 in chronic airways obstruction measured by a rebreathing method. Clin. Sci., *34:*559–568, 1968.

2892. Aber, G. M., and Bishop, J. M.: Serial changes in renal function, arterial gas tensions, and the acid-base state in patients with chronic bronchitis and oedema. Clin. Sci., *28:*511–525, 1965.

2893. Sølvsteen, P.: Lung diffusing capacity: cyclically and continuously ventilated closed systems. J. Appl. Physiol., *20:*92–98, 1965.

2894. Anthonisen, N. R., Dolovich, M. B., and Bates, D. V.: Steady state measurement of regional ventilation to perfusion ratios in normal man. J. Clin. Invest., *45:*1349–1356, 1966.

2895. Williams, J. F., and Behnke, R. H.: The effect of pulmonary emphysema upon cardiopulmonary hemodynamics at rest and during exercise. Ann. Intern. Med., *60:*824–842, 1964.

2896. Nairn, J. R., and Prime, F. J.: A physiological study of MacLeod's syndrome. Thorax, *22:*148–155, 1967.

2897. Weg, J. G., Krumholz, R. A., and Hackleroad, L. E.: Unilateral hyperlucent lung. Ann. Intern. Med., *62:*675–684, 1965.

2898. Eriksson, S.: Studies in α-antitrypsin deficiency. Acta Med. Scand., *177* (Supplement 432): 1–85, 1965.

2899. Briscoe, W. A., Kueppers, F., Davis, A. L., and Bearn, A. G.: Case of inherited deficiency of serum $alpha_1$-antitrypsin associated with pulmonary emphysema. Amer. Rev. Resp. Dis., *94:*529–539, 1966.

2900. Talamo, R. C., Blennerhassett, J. B., and Austen, K. F.: Current concepts: familial emphysema and $alpha_1$-antitrypsin deficiency. New Engl. J. Med., *275:*1301–1304, 1966.

2901. Talamo, R. C., Austen, K. F., and Allen, J. D.: Familial emphysema and $alpha_1$-antitrypsin deficiency. (U.S. Public Health Service Publication No. 1717) May, 1968, pp. 491–495.

2902. Kueppers, F., and Bearn, A. G.: Possible experimental approach to association of hereditary $alpha_1$ antitrypsin deficiency and pulmonary emphysema. Proc. Soc. Exp. Biol. Med., *121:*1207–1209, 1966.

2903. Kueppers, F., Briscoe, W. A., and Bearn, A. G.: Hereditary deficiency of serum α_1-antitrypsin. Science, *146:*1678, 1964.

2904. Cullen, J. H., Katz, H. L., and Kaemmerlen, J. T.: Chronic diffuse pulmonary infiltration and airway obstruction. Amer. Rev. Resp. Dis., *92:*775–780, 1965.

2905. Christie, D.: Physical training in chronic obstructive lung disease. Brit. Med. J., *2:*150–151, 1968.

2906. Saunders, K. B., and White, J. E.: Controlled trial of breathing exercises. Brit. Med. J., *2:*680–682, 1965.

2907. Ham, J. C.: Acute infectious obstructing bronchiolitis. Ann. Intern. Med., *60:*47–60, 1964.

2908. Goldberg, I., and Cherniack, R. M.: The effect of nebulized bronchodilator delivered with and without IPPB on ventilatory function in chronic obstructive emphysema. Amer. Rev. Resp. Dis., *91:*13–20, 1965.

2909. Hugh-Jones, P., Ritchie, B. C., and Dollery, C. T.: Surgical treatment of emphysema. Brit. Med. J., *2:*1133–1138, 1966.

2910. Massaro, D., Cusick, A. M., and Katz, S.: Erythropoiesis in subjects with chronic bronchitis. Amer. Rev. Resp. Dis., *91:*541–551, 1965.

2911. Massaro, D., and Katz, S.: Effect of venesection on arterial gas values and ventilatory function in patients with chronic bronchitis. Thorax, *20:*441–446, 1965.

2912. Hume, R., and Goldberg, A.: Actual and predicted normal red-cell and plasma volumes in primary and secondary polycythemia. Clin. Sci., *26:*499-508, 1964.

2913. Finley, T. N., Simson, G., McKay, M. B., and Lovekin, W. S.: Effect of high hematocrit states on ventilation at 5,317 feet. In: *Current Research on Chronic Airways Disease* (U.S. Public Health Service Publication No. 1717), May, 1968, pp. 149-161.
2914. Saunier, C., Aug-Laxenaire, M-C., Schibi, M., and Sadoul, P.: Acid base and electrolyte equilibrium of arterial blood and cerebro-spinal fluid in respiratory insufficiency. Respiration, *26:*81-101, 1969.
2915. Jaikin, A., and Agrest, A.: Cerebrospinal fluid glutamine concentration in patients with chronic hypercapnia. Clin. Sci., *36:*11-14, 1969.
2916. Brun, J., Biot, N., Kofman, J., and Perrin-Fayolle, M.: Deficiency of α_1-antitrypsin associated with chronic respiratory disease and emphysema. Poumon Coeur, *23:*1119-1130, 1967.
2917. Hume, R.: Blood volume changes in chronic bronchitis and emphysema. Brit. J. Haemat., *15:*131-139, 1968.
2918. Tarkoff, M. P., Kueppers, F., and Miller, W. F.: Pulmonary emphysema and alpha$_1$-antitrypsin deficiency. Amer. J. Med., *45:*220-228, 1968.
2919. Mazodier, P.: Constitutional deficiency of α_1-antitrypsin. Its relationship to chronic bronchopulmonary disorders of the obstructive type. J. Franc. Med. Chir. Thorac., *20:*247-258, 1966.
2920. Prowse, C. M., Fuchs, J. E., Kaufman, S. A., and Gaensler, E. A.: Chronic obstructive pseudoemphysema. A rare cause of unilateral hyperlucent lung. New Engl. J. Med., *271:*127-132, 1964.
2921. Gallouédec, C., Binet, J-P., and Brocard, H.: Giant lobar emphysema in adults. J. Franc. Med. Chir. Thorac, *18:*553-568, 1964.
2922. Ueda, H., Kaihara, S., Iio, M., and Togashi, M.: Abnormal transradiancy of one lung studied by pulmonary scintiscanning. Jap. Heart J., *6:*262-272, 1965.
2923. Hendren, W. H., and McKee, D. M.: Lobar emphysema of infancy. J. Pediat. Surg., *1:*24-39, 1966.
2924. Reid, J. M., Barclay, R. S., Stevenson, J. G., and Welsh, T. M.: Congenital obstructive lobar emphysema. Dis. Chest, *49:*359-361, 1966.
2925. Staple, T. W., Hudson, H. H., Hartmann, A. F., Jr., and McAlister, W. H.: The angiographic findings in four cases of infantile lobar emphysema. Amer. J. Roentgen., *97:*195-202, 1966.
2926. Paplow, B.: Lobar emphysema in infancy. Zbl. Chir., *91:*1377-1387, 1966.
2927. Franken, E. A., Jr., and Buchl, I.: Infantile lobar emphysema. Report of two cases with unusual roentgenographic manifestation. Amer. J. Roentgen., *98:*354-357, 1966.
2928. Houk, V. N., Kent, D. C., and Fosburg, R. G.: Unilateral hyperlucent lung: a study in pathophysiology and etiology. Amer. J. Med. Sci., *253:*406-416, 1967.
2929. Reid, L., Simon, G., Zorab, P. A., and Seidelin, R.: The development of unilateral hypertransradiancy of the lung. Brit. J. Dis. Chest, *61:*190-192, 1967.
2930. Brunner, S.: Lung cysts. A clinical radiological study. Thesis, Munksgaard, Copenhagen, 1964.
2931. Rosso, C., Vento, R., and De Cecco, C.: A rare case of intrathoracic bronchogenic cyst in a 45 day old infant. Minerva Pediat., *16:*892-897, 1964.
2932. Herzog, K. H.: Congenital pulmonary cysts. Chirurg., *35:*241-247, 1964.
2933. Massaro, D., Katz, S., Matthews, M. J., and Higgins, C.: Von Recklinghausen's neurofibromatosis associated with cystic lung disease. Amer. J. Med., *38:*233-240, 1965.
2934. Jones, J. C., Almond, C. H., Snyder, H. M., and Meyer, B. W.: Congenital pulmonary cysts in infants and children. Ann. Thorac. Surg., *3:*297-306, 1967.
2935. DeRosario, J. L., Braaten, V., and Dawkins, W.: Int. Surg. (Chicago), *46:*147-151, 1966.
2936. Fain, W. R., Conn, J. H., Campbell, G. D., Chavez, C. M., Gee, H. L., and Hardy, J. D.: Excision of giant pulmonary emphysematous cysts; report of 20 cases without deaths. Surgery, *62:*552-559, 1967.
2937. Chavez, C. M., Fain, W. R., and Conn, J. H.: Angiography in giant cystic disease of the lung. J. Thorac. Cardiov. Surg., *55:*638-641, 1968.
2938. Ossowska, K., and Pawlicka, L.: Radiological evaluation of the results of surgical treatment in cases of primary bronchiectasis. Pol. Przegl. Radiol., *28:*31-44, 1964.
2939. Glauser, E. M., Cook, C. D., and Harris, G. B. C.: Bronchiectasis: A review of 187 cases in children with follow-up pulmonary function studies in 58. Acta Paediat. Scand. (Uppsala) Supplement *165:*1-16, 1966.
2940. Marland, P., Descomps, H., Wache, M., and Rigaut, J. P.: The Kartagener syndrome and the etiopathogenetic problem of idiopathic bronchiectasis. Poumon Coeur, *23:*41-68, 1967.
2941. Glantsberg, N. A., and Sokolov, R. V.: The remote results of pneumonectomy in adolescents suffering from bronchiectasis. Pediatriya, *2:*37-41, 1967.
2942. Cherniack, N. S., and Carton, R. W.: Factors associated with respiratory insufficiency in bronchiectasis. Amer. J. Med., *41:*562-571, 1966.
2943. Cherniack, N. S.. Dowling, H. F., Carton, R. W., and McBryde, V. E.: The role of acute lower respiratory infection in causing pulmonary insufficiency in bronchiectasis. Ann. Intern. Med., *66:*489-497, 1967.
2944. Hasimoto, K.: Studies on bronchiectasis. I. Pulmonary function and circulation tests in bronchiectasis. Bull. Kobe Med. Coll, *27:*132-160, 1965.
2945. Bass, H., Henderson, J. A. M., Heckscher, T., Oriol, A., and Anthonisen, N. R.: Regional structure and function in bronchiectasis. A correlative study using bronchography and Xe^{133}. Amer. Rev. Resp. Dis., *97:*598-609, 1968.
2946. Hutchin, P., Terzi, R. G. G., and Peters, R. M.: Bronchial-pulmonary artery reverse flow. Angiographic demonstration in bronchiectasis. Ann. Thorac. Surg., *4:*391-398, 1967.
2947. Nagy, M., and Mészaros, G.: Long-term results of the conservative treatment of bronchiectasis in adults. Z. Tuberk., *127:*283-290, 1967.
2948. Dollery, C. T., Gillam, P. M. S., Hugh-Jones, P., and Zorab, P. A.: Regional lung function in kyphoscoliosis. Thorax, *20:*175-181, 1965.
2949. Galimberti, A.: Importance of evaluating respiratory function in kyphoscoliosis. Minerva Ortop., *18:*540-543, 1967.
2950. Sharp, J. T., Sweany, S. K., Henry, J. P., Pietras, R. J., Meadows, W. R., Amaral, E., and Rubinstein, H. M.: Lung and thoracic compliances in ankylosing spondylitis. J. Lab. Clin. Med., *63:*254-263, 1964.
2951. Sharp, J. T., Sweany, S. K., Henry, J. P., Pietras, R. J., Meadows, W. R., and Amaral, E.: Lung and thoracic compliances in ankylosing spondylitis. J. Lab. Clin. Med., *62:*1015-1016, 1963.
2952. Miller, J. M., and Sproule, B. J.: Pulmonary function in ankylosing spondylitis. Amer. Rev. Resp. Dis., *90:*376-382, 1964.
2953. Randowa, D., and Roslawski, A.: Studies on lung ventilation in patients with ankylosing spondylitis. Pol. Tyg. Lek., *21:*383-384, 1966.
2954. Verhaeghe, A., Lemaitre, G., Lebeurre, R., Delcambre, B., and Hennion, M.: Le "poumon de la spondylarthrite ankylosante" existe-t-il? Rev. Rhum., *34:*123-126, 1967.
2955. Weg, J. G., Krumholz, R. A., and Harkleroad, L. E.: Pulmonary dysfunction in pectus excavatum. Amer. Rev. Resp. Dis., *96:*936-945, 1967.
2956. Unnerus, C-E.: Basal lamellary atelectases as an indication of a pathological condition in the abdomen. Ann. Med. Intern. Fenn., *53:*129-136, 1964.
2957. Niden, A. H.: The acute effects of atelectasis on the pulmonary circulation. J. Clin. Invest., *43:*810-824, 1964.
2958. Sutnick, A., and Soloff, L. A.: Pulmonary surfactant and atelectasis. Anesthesiology, *25:*676-681, 1964.
2959. Levine, B. E., and Johnson, R. P.: Effects of atelectasis on pulmonary surfactant and quasi-static lung mechanics. J. Appl. Physiol., *20:*859-864, 1965.
2960. Cranz, H. J., and Pribram, H. F. W.: The pulmonary vessels in the diagnosis of lobar collapse. Amer. J. Roentgen., *94:*665-673, 1965.
2961. Gibson, R. M., Jr., Greenberg, S. D., and Hallman, G. L.:

Alterations in lung distal to total exclusion of a lobar bronchus. An experimental study in dogs. Amer. Rev. Resp. Dis., *94:*217-224, 1966.

2962. Williams, J. V., Tierney, D. F., and Parker, H. R.: Surface forces in the lung, atelectasis, and transpulmonary pressure. J. Appl. Physiol., *21:*819-827, 1966.
2963. DuBois, A. B., Turaids, T., Mammen, R. E., and Nobrega, F. T.: Pulmonary atelectasis in subjects breathing oxygen at sea level or at simulated altitude. J. Appl. Physiol., *21:*828-836, 1966.
2964. Yeh, T. J., Manning, H., Ellison, L. T., and Ellison, R. G.: Alevolar surfactant in chronic experimental atelectasis. Amer. Rev. Resp. Dis., *93:*953-956, 1966.
2965. Giese, W.: Pathologic-anatomic aspects of surgical diseases of the lung, surface forces and pulmonary atelectasis. Thoraxchirurgie, *15:*466-473, 1967.
2966. Sutnick, A. I., Soloff, L. A., and Sethi, R. S.: Influence of alveolar collapse upon surface activity of lung extracts. Dis. Chest, *53:*257-262, 1968.
2967. Sekulic, S. M., Hamlin, J. T., Ellison, R. G., and Ellison, L. T.: Pulmonary surfactant and lung circulation in experimental atelectasis. Amer. Rev. Resp. Dis., *97:*69-75, 1968.
2968. Edmunds, L H., Jr., and Holm, J. C.: Effect of atelectasis on lung changes after pulmonary arterial ligation. J. Appl. Physiol., *25:*115-123, 1968.
2969. Burger, E. J., Jr., and Macklem, P. T.: Airway closure: demonstration by breathing 100% O_2 at low lung volumes and by N_2 washout. J. Appl. Physiol., *25:*139-148, 1968.
2970. Norris, R. M., Jones, J. G., and Bishop, J. M.: Respiratory gas exchange in patients with spontaneous pneumothorax. Thorax, *23:*427-433, 1968.
2971. Williams, M. H., Jr., and Kane, C.: Pulmonary function in patients who have recovered from spontaneous pneumothorax. Dis. Chest, *47:*153-156, 1965.
2972. Rullière, R., and Capronnier, C.: Acute cor pulmonale in spontaneous pneumothorax. Coeur Med. Intern., *5:*149-155, 1966.
2973. Lenggenhager, K.: The blood circulation in the presence of pneumothorax. The causation of spontaneous pneumothorax. Thoraxchirurgie, *14:*338-344, 1966.
2974. Condon, R. E.: Spontaneous resolution of experimental clotted hemothorax. Surg. Gynec. Obstet., *126:*505-515, 1968.
2975. Dwyer, E. M., and Troncale, F.: Spontaneous pneumothorax and pulmonary disease in the Marfan syndrome. Ann. Intern. Med., *62:*1285-1292, 1965.
2976. Cran, I. R., and Rumball, C. A.: Survey of spontaneous pneumothoraces in the Royal Air Force. Thorax, *22:*462-465, 1967.
2977. Kamo, N., and Kawamoto, S.: Pulmonary function shortly after pulmonary resection. Jap. J. Thorac. Surg., *16:*763-767, 1963.
2978. Shimuzu, T., and Lewis, F. J.: An experimental study of respiratory mechanics following chest surgery. J. Thorac. Cardiov. Surg., *52:*68-75, 1966.
2979. Virtue, R. W., Permutt, S., Tanaka, R., Pearcy, C., Bane, H. N., and Bromberger-Barnea, B.: Ventilation-perfusion changes during thoracotomy. Anesthesiology, *27:*132-146, 1966.
2980. Hagiwara, N., Suzuki, K., Oshibe, K., and Hirama, J.: Cardio-pulmonary function in the late postoperative period of patients treated by unilateral pneumonectomy. Tuberc. Leprosy, *16:*469-474, 1963.
2981. Wiederanders, R. E., White, S. M., and Saichek, H. B.: The effect of pulmonary resection on pulmonary artery pressures. Ann. Surg., *160:*889-896, 1964.
2982. Ellison, L. T., and Ellison, R. G.: Surgery of bullae, blebs, and cysts of the lung: a six-year review of cases. Amer. Surg., *30:*774-779, 1964.
2983. Filler, J., Gomez, D. M., and Stone, S.: Effects upon pulmonary function of pneumonectomy performed during childhood. Amer. Rev. Resp. Dis., *93:*184-193, 1966.
2984. Aleksandrovskii, V. P., Vorobev, M. F., and Deduchenko, V. I.: Clinico-roentgenological and functional findings in patients with one lung at 9-10 years after pneumonectomy. Probl. Tuberk., *2:*23-28, 1965.
2985. De Coster, A., Denolin, H., Englert, M., Degré, S., Kornitzer, M., and Dumont, A.: Répercussions ventilatoires et circulatoires de la pneumonectomie. Poumon Coeur, *21:*781-817, 1965.
2986. Birath, G., Malmberg, R., and Simonsson, B. G.: Lung function after pneumonectomy in man. Clin. Sci., *29:*59-72, 1965.
2987. DeGraff, A. C., Jr., Taylor, H. F., Ord, J. W., Chuang, T. H., and Johnson, R. L., Jr.: Exercise limitation following extensive pulmonary resection. J. Clin. Invest., *44:*1514-1522, 1965.
2988. Lejawka, W., and Rzepecki, W.: Partial resection of the sole remaining lung. Gruzlica, *34:*483-489, 1966.
2989. Semisch, R.: Morphological and functional changes in the lung remnant following pulmonary resection. Bruns Beitr. Klin. Chir., *214:*126-136, 1967.
2990. Fry, W. A., Archer, F. A., and Adams, W. E.: Long-term clinical-pathologic study of the pneumonectomy patient. Dis. Chest, *52:*720-726, 1967.
2991. Bennike, K-A.: PO_2 and PCO_2 in the arterial blood after pneumonectomy. Anaesthetist, *17:*34-38, 1968.
2992. Massion, W. H., and Schilling, J. A.: Physiological effects of lung resection in adult and puppy dogs. J. Thorac. Cardiov. Surg., *48:*239-250, 1964.
2993. Ranson-Bitker, B.: Predictability of operative hazard in thoracic surgery. Bull. Physio-path. Resp., *2:*15-24, 1966.
2994. Larsen, M. C., and Cliffton, E. E.: The prognostic value of preoperative evaluation of patients undergoing thoracic surgery. Dis. Chest, *47:*589-594, 1965.
2995. Dolina, O. A.: Prevention and treatment of acute respiratory failure after operations on the lungs. Khirurgiya, *8:*30-35, 1965.
2996. Laros, C. D., and Swierenga, J.: Temporary unilateral pulmonary artery occlusion in the preoperative evaluation of patients with bronchial carcinoma. Med. Thorac., *24:*269-283, 1967.
2997. Wildevuur, C. R. H.: Lung reimplantation in dogs. Thesis, Groningen, 1967.
2998. Matthew, H., Logan, A., Woodruff, M. F. A., and Heard, B.: Paraquat poisoning—lung transplantation. Brit. Med. J., *2:*759-763, 1968.
2999. Hardy, J. D., Eraslan, S., and Webb, W. R.: Transplantation of the lung. Ann. Surg., *160:*440-448, 1964.
3000. Borrie, J., and Lichter, I.: Lung transplantation: technical problems. Thorax, *19:*383-396, 1964.
3001. Slim, M. S., Yacoubian, H. D., Wilson, J. L., Rubeiz, G. A., and Ghandur-Manymneh, L.: Successful bilateral reimplantation of canine lungs. Surgery, *55:*676-683, 1964.
3002. Gago, O., Benfield, J. R., Nigro, S. L., and Adams, W. E.: Left lower pulmonary lobe transplantation. J.A.M.A., *191:*306-310, 1965.
3003. Trummer, M. J., and Christiansen, K. H.: Radiographic and functional changes following autotransplantation of the lung. J. Thorac. Cardiov. Surg., *49:*1006-1014, 1965.
3004. Suzuki, C., Nakada, T., Furusawa, A., Watanabe, A., and Hirose, M.: Experimental reimplantation of the lung. Z. Tuberk., *123:*195-202, 1965.
3005. Largiader, F., Manax, W., Lyons, G. W., and Lillehei, R. C.: Experimental homotransplantation of preserved lungs. Schweiz. Med. Wschr., *95:*1151-1154, 1965.
3006. Davies, L. G., Rosser, T. H. L., and West, L. R.: Autotransplantation of the lung in sheep. Thorax, *20:*481-494, 1965.
3007. Portnoi, V. F., and Adamyan, A. A.: Transplantation of the lung. Eksp. Khir. Anest., *4:*3-9, 1965.
3008. Guilmet, D., Brunet, A., Krakora, P., Leiva, A., and Weiss, M.: Reimplantation of the lung in dogs. Rozhl. Chir., *45:*275-279, 1966.
3009. Tsuji, Y., Tomito, M., Kawashime, N., Shegematsu, S., Miure, T., Hamesaki, A., Makashime, M., and Fukuda, M.: Experimental studies of lung transplantation; preservation of the canine lung by means of cold perfusion. Acta Med. Nagasaki, *9:*22-28, 1964.
3010. Shinoi, K., Hayata, Y., Aoki, H., Kozaki, M., Yoshioka, K., Shinoda, A., Iwahashi, H., Ito, M., and Endo, M.: Pulmonary lobe transplantation in human subjects. Amer. J. Surg., *111:*617-628, 1966.

3011. Sharma, A. N., Soroff, H. S., Bellas, A. E., Harrison, H. N., Sherman, J., and Deterling, R. A., Jr.: Experimental studies of the autotransplantation of pulmonary tissue. Surg. Gynec. Obstet., *123*:295–302, 1966.
3012. Pain, M. C. F., De Bono, A. H., Glazier, J. B., Maloney, J. E., and West, J. B.: Measurement of function of the transplanted lung in the dog with the use of Xenon 133. J. Thorac. Cardiov. Surg., *53*:707–715, 1967.
3013. Trimble, A. S., Kim, J-P., Bharadwaj, B., Bedard, P., and Wells, C.: Changes in alveolar surfactant after lung reimplantation. J. Thorac. Cardiov. Surg., *52*:271–276, 1966.
3014. Sharma, A. N., Soroff, H. S., Bellas, A. E., Sachs, B. F., Nettleblad, S. C., and Deterling, R. A., Jr.: Experimental studies of the homotransplantation of pulmonary tissue. Surg. Gynec. Obstet., *123*:1001–1009, 1966.
3015. Didenko, V. I.: Morphology and histochemistry of the pulmonary nervous system after complete division of its external nervous connections following autotransplantation. Arkh. Anat., *51*:60–68, 1966.
3016. Eraslan, S., and Hardy, J. D.: Differential division of hilar tissue: effects upon lung function in the dog. Dis. Chest, *50*:449–455, 1966.
3017. Hedley-Jones, W.: The application of bronchostomy to the experimental study of transplanted pulmonary tissue. Thorax, *21*:405–412, 1966.
3018. White, J. J., Tanser, P. H., Anthonisen, N. R., Wynands, J. E., Pare, J. A. P., Becklake, M. R., Munro, D. D., and MacLean, L. D.: Human lung homotransplantation. Canad. Med. Assoc. J., *94*:1199–1209, 1966.
3019. Marshall, R., and Gunning, A. J.: The long-term physiological effects of lung reimplantation in the dog. J. Surg. Res., *6*:185–195, 1966.
3020. Eraslan, S., Hardy, J. D., and Elliott, R. L.: Lung replantation. Respiratory reflexes, vagal integrity, and lung function in chronic dogs. J. Surg. Res., *6*:383–388, 1966.
3021. Trimble, A. S., Bharadwaj, B., and Bedard, P.: Successful bilateral lung reimplantation in the dog. Canad. J. Surg., *10*:89–93, 1967.
3022. Lyager, S., Mouritzen, C., Ottosen, P., and Boye, E.: Lung transplantation. Pathophysiologic aspects in dogs with a reimplanted left lung. Scand. J. Cardiov. Surg., *1*:93–100, 1967.
3023. Waldhausen, J. A., Daly, W. J., Baez, M., and Giammona, S. T.: Physiologic changes associated with autotransplantation of the lung. Ann. Surg., *165*:580–589, 1967.
3024. Strieder, D. J., Barnes, B. A., Aronow, S., Russell, P. S., and Kazemi, H.: Xenon^{133} study of ventilation and perfusion in normal and transplanted dog lungs. J. Appl. Physiol., *23*:359–366, 1967.
3025. Webb, W. R., Cook, W. A., Unal, M. O., Theodorides, T., and Nakae, S.: Growth and function of the reimplanted dog lung. Surgery, *62*:227–231, 1967.
3026. Greenfield, L. J., Chernick, V., Hodson, W. A., and Brumley, G. W.: Alterations in pulmonary surfactant following compression atelectasis, pulmonary artery ligation, and reimplantation of the lung. Ann. Surg., *166*:109–116, 1967.
3027. Brownlee, R. T., and Couves, C. M.: Factors concerned in the maintenance of viability in pulmonary transplants. Ann. Thorac. Surg., *5*:112–121, 1968.
3028. Brownlee, R. T., Couves, C. M., Dritsas, K. G., and Kowalewski, K.: Metabolic alterations in pulmonary tissue preserved for transplantation. Canad. J. Surg., *11*:237–245, 1968.
3029. Garzon, A. A., Cheng, C., Pangan, J., and Karlson, K. E.: Hypothermic hyperbaric lung preservation for twenty-four hours with replantation. J. Thorac. Cardiov. Surg., *55*:546–554, 1968.
3030. Hill, P. M., and Shaw, K. M.: Long-term survival of dogs after experimental pulmonary reimplantation and stage contralateral pneumonectomy. Thorax, *23*:408–413, 1968.
3031. Vermeire, P.: Prolonged survival after human lung transplantation. Thorax, *24*:508, 1969.
3032. Keene, C. H.: *The social organisation of medicine*. Harvard Public Health Bulletin (Supplement). *22*:1–12, 1965.
3033. Hooft, C., Van den Brande, J-L., Van der Straeten, M., and Delbeke, M. J.: Diffuse idiopathic pulmonary interstitial fibrosis of chronic evolution in children. Sem. Hop. Paris (Ann. Pediat.), *38*:3400–3407, 1962.
3034. Arminte de Oliviera Penna, H., Araujo Ramos, J. L., Fabio Lion, M., Manissadjian, A., Aleixo de Paula, E., and Rubens Montenegro, M.: Progressive diffuse interstitial fibrosis of the lungs. Rev. Paul. Med., *66*:74–86, 1965.
3035. Chyrek-Borowska, S., Poniecki, A., and Stasiewicz, A. I.: The occurrence of pleuro-pulmonic changes in rheumatoid arthritis. Reumatologia, *6*:209–216, 1968.
3036. Gregoire, F., Comeau, M., Rou, L., Ventura, J., and Soucy, R.: A study of the Hamman-Rich Syndrome, or idiopathic diffuse, and progressive pulmonary interstitial fibrosis. Un. Med. Canada, *95*:9–14, 1966.
3037. Daum, S., and Levinsky, L.: Diffusing capacity of the lungs and its components in interstitial idiopathic Hamman-Rich fibrosis in adults. Rev. Czech. Med., *12*:188–200, 1966.
3038. Kuisk, H., and Sanchez, J. S.: Diffuse bronchiolectasis with muscular hyperplasia ("muscular cirrhosis of the lung"). Amer. J. Roentgen., *96*:979–990, 1966.
3039. Scadding, J. G., and Hinson, K. F. W.: Diffuse fibrosing alveolitis (diffuse interstitial fibrosis of the lungs). Thorax, *22*:291–304, 1967.
3040. Hughes, E. W.: Familial interstitial fibrosis. Thorax, *19*:515–525, 1964.
3041. Hamer, J.: Cause of low arterial oxygen saturation in pulmonary fibrosis. Thorax, *19*:507–513, 1964.
3042. Israel-Asselain, R., Chebat, J., Sors, Ch., Basset, F., and Le Rolland, A.: Diffuse interstitial fibrosis in a mother and son with Von Recklinghausen's disease. Thorax, *20*:153–157, 1965.
3043. Pimentel, J. C.: Tridimensional photographic reconstruction in a study of the pathogenesis of honeycomb lung. Thorax, *22*:444–452, 1967.
3044. Reid, J. M., Cuthbert, J., and Craik, J. E.: Chronic diffuse idiopathic fibrosing alveolitis. Brit. J. Dis. Chest, *59*:194–201, 1965.
3045. Young, R. C., Jr., Jackson, M. A., and Bell, H. D.: Desquamative interstitial pneumonia. Report of a case of a recently described entity. Med. Ann. D. C., *35*:535–540, 1966.
3046. Persaud, V., Bateson, E. M., Ling, J. A., and Hayes, J. A.: Desquamative interstitial pneumonia. Brit. J. Dis. Chest, *61*:159–162, 1967.
3047. Kapanci, Y., and Chauvet, M.: Desquamative interstitial pneumonia. Schweiz. Med. Wschr., *97*:1199–1208, 1967.
3048. Schneider, R. M., Nevius, D. B., and Brown, H. Z.: Desquamative interstitial pneumonia in a four-year-old child. New Engl. J. Med., *277*:1056–1058, 1967.
3049. Wilson, R. J., Rodnan, G. P., and Robin, E. D.: An early pulmonary physiologic abnormality in progressive systemic sclerosis (diffuse scleroderma). Amer. J. Med., *36*:361–369, 1964.
3050. Morgan, W. K. C., and Wolfel, D. A.: The lungs and pleura in rheumatoid arthritis. Amer. J. Roentgen., *98*:334–342, 1966.
3051. Scarff, M. A.: Progressive systemic sclerosis with severe pulmonary involvement (honeycomb lung). Harper Hosp. Bull., *21*:172–179, 1963.
3052. Israel-Asselin, R., Chebat, J., Menkes, J., Lechien, J., and Basset, F.: Diffuse pulmonary interstitial fibrosis and scleroderma. Bull. Soc. Med. Hop. Paris, *115*:503–524, 1964.
3053. Sackner, M. A., Akgun, N., Kimbel, P., and Lewis, D. H.: The pathophysiology of scleroderma involving the heart and respiratory system. Ann. Intern. Med., *60*:611–630, 1964.
3054. Polleri, A., Canepe, F., and De Gaetani, G.: Carbon monoxide diffusion in rheumatoid arthritis, scleroderma, systemic erythematosus and dermatomyositis. Arch. Maragliano Pat. Clin., *21*:41–46, 1965.
3055. Catterall, M., and Rowell, N. R.: Respiratory function studies in patients with certain connective tissue diseases. Brit. J. Derm., *77*:221–225, 1965.
3056. Guglielmetti, P., and Catenacci, G.: Pneumopathy in scleroderma. G. Clin. Med., *46*:270–277, 1965.
3057. Huang, C. T., and Lyons, H. A.: Comparison of pulmo-

nary function in patients with systemic lupus erythematosus, scleroderma, and rheumatoid arthritis. Amer. Rev. Resp. Dis., *93*:865-874, 1966.
3058. Weaver, A. L., Divertie, M. B., and Titus, J. L.: The lung in slceroderma. Mayo Clin. Proc., *42*:754-766, 1967.
3059. Stack, B. H. R., and Grant, I. W. B.: Rheumatoid interstitial lung disease. Brit. J. Dis. Chest, *59*:202-211, 1965.
3060. Scadding, J. G.: The lungs in rheumatoid arthritis. Proc. Roy. Soc. Med., *62*:227-238, 1969.
3061. Patterson, C. D., Harville, W. E., and Pierce, J. A.: Rheumatoid lung disease. Ann. Intern. Med., *62*:685-697, 1965.
3062. Jordan, J. D., and Snyder, C. H.: Rheumatoid disease of the lung and cor pulmonale. Observations in a child. Amer. J. Dis. Child, *108*:174-180, 1964.
3063. Sievers, K., Aho, K., Hurri, L., and Perttala, Y.: Studies of rheumatoid pulmonary disease. Acta Tuberc. Scand., *45*:21-34, 1964.
3064. Verhaeghe, A., Lemaître, G., Lebeurre, R., Defouilly, A., and Delcambre, B.: Radiologic aspects of the pleura and the lungs in rheumatoid arthritis of the adult. J. Belg. Med. Phys. Rhum., *21*:262-279, 1966.
3065. Georgesco, A., Catoiu-Vulpesco, S., Ciobanu, V., Stroesco, O., and Nuta, M.: Clinical and radiologic study of the lung in rheumatoid arthritis. Rev. Roum. Med. Interne, *2*:307-313, 1965.
3066. Krauze, J.: A contribution on the frequency of lung involvement in rheumatoid arthritis. Reumatologia, *4*:347-349, 1966.
3067. Petty, T. L., and Wilkins, M.: The five manifestations of rheumatoid lung. Dis. Chest, *49*:75-82, 1966.
3068. Brannan, H. M., Good, C. A., Divertie, M., and Baggenstoss, A. H.: Pulmonary disease associated with rheumatoid arthritis. J.A.M.A., *189*:914-918, 1964.
3069. Fouquet, J., Jais, M., Renault, P., and Castelain, G.: Uncommon evolution of an acute pneumopathy during chronic evolutive polyarthritis. Bull. Soc. Med. Hop. Paris, *115*:175-181, 1964.
3070. Portner, M. M., and Gracie, W. A., Jr.: Rheumatoid lung disease with cavitary nodules, pneumothorax and eosinophilia. New Engl. J. Med., *275*:697-700, 1966.
3071. Coltorti, M., Di Simone, A., Vitale, P., and Scognamillo, A.: Rheumatoid arthritis with diffuse lung fibrosis in homozygotic twins. Policlinico. [Med.], *74*:8-33, 1967.
3072. Onodera, S., and Hill, J. R.: Pulmonary hypertension. Report of a case in association with rheumatoid arthritis. Ohio Med. J., *61*:141-144, 1965.
3073. Caplan, A.: Rheumatoid pneumoconiosis syndrome. Med. Lavoro, *56*:494-499, 1965.
3074. Liebow, A. A., Steer, A., and Billingsley, J. G.: Desquamative interstitial pneumonia. Amer. J. Med., *39*:369-404, 1965.
3075. Sandbank, M., Grunebaum, M., and Katzenellenbogen, I.: Dermatomyositis associated with subacute pulmonary fibrosis. Arch. Derm., *94*:432-435, 1966.
3076. Boushy, S. F., Kurtzmann, R. S., Martin, N. D., and Lewis, B. M.: The course of pulmonary function in sarcoidosis. Ann. Intern. Med., *62*:939-955, 1965.
3077. Foss Abrahamsen, A., Erikson, H., and Refsum, H. E.: Cardio-pulmonary function in sarcoidosis of the lungs. Acta Tuberc. Scand., *44*:138-144, 1964.
3078. Reindell, H., Doll, E., and Wurm, K.: Functional radiological study of lung diseases. Fortschr. Roentgenstr., *100*:342-358, 1964.
3079. Gamain, B., Coby, J., Lambard, D., Chambatte, C., Ledédenté, A., and Kermarec, J.: La fonction respiratoire au cours de la sarcoidose. Poumon *20*:857-873, 1964.
3080. Kent, D. C., and Spence, W.: Physiologic abnormalities in pulmonary sarcoidosis. Dis. Chest, *46*:680-691, 1964.
3081. Doll, E., Reindell, H., Wurm, K., and Rinke, C.: Oxygen transport in the lung in pulmonary sarcoidosis. Deutsch Arch. Klin. Med., *209*:501-516, 1964.
3082. Turiaf, J.: Unexpected radiographic aspects of pulmonary sarcoidosis. Rev. Tuberc., *28*:971-996, 1964.
3083. Sellers, R. D., and Siebens, A. A.: The effects of sarcoidosis on pulmonary function with particular reference to changes in pulmonary compliance. Amer. Rev. Resp. Dis., *91*:660-664, 1965.
3084. Richert, J. H., and Klocke, R. A.: Sarcoidosis. Long-term follow-up of pulmonary function. Med. Ann. D.C., *35*:188-191, 1966.
3085. Ting, E. Y., and Williams, M. H., Jr.: Mechanics of breathing in sarçoidosis of lung. J.A.M.A., *192*:619-624, 1965.
3086. Sharma, O. P., Colp, C., and Williams, M. H., Jr.: Course of pulmonary sarcoidosis with and without corticosteroid therapy as determined by pulmonary function studies. Amer. J. Med., *41*:541-551, 1966.
3087. Young, R. C., Jr., Carr, C., Shelton, T. G., Mann, M., Ferrin, A., Laurey, J. R., and Harden, K. A.: Sarcoidosis: Relationship between changes in lung structure and function. Amer. Rev. Resp. Dis., *95*:224-238, 1967.
3088. Schermuly, W., Behrend, H., Hamm, J., Fabel, H., and Wilke, K. H.: Radiologically recognizable morphologic features of altered pulmonary function in patients with sarcoidosis. Fortschr. Roentgenstr., *104*:206-226, 1966.
3089. Sharma, O. P., Colp, C., and Williams, M. H., Jr.: Pulmonary function studies in patients with bilateral sarcoidosis of hilar lymph glands. Arch. Intern. Med., *117*:436-439, 1966.
3090. Harden, K. A., Young, R. C., Jr., Carr., C., and Laurey, J. R.: Oxygen cost of breathing. II. Studies in patients with sarcoidosis. Amer. Rev. Resp. Dis., *97*:1127-1130, 1968.
3091. Kotler, M. N., Zwi, S., and Goldman, H. I.: Pulmonary function in sarcoidosis and the effect of steroid treatment. S. Afr. Med. J., *41*:625-629, 1967.
3092. Cullen, J. H., Katz, H. L., and Kaemmerlen, J. T.: Chronic diffuse pulmonary infiltration and airway obstruction. Amer. Rev. Resp. Dis., *92*:775-780, 1965.
3093. Gurevich, M. A., and Kruk, S. I.: Pulmonary changes in periarteritis nodosa. Ter. Arkh., *36*:79-82, 1964.
3094. Wanke, M.: Isolated periarteritis nodosa of the lung, with a comment on so-called inflammatory arteriosclerosis. Z. Kreislauforsch., *54*:235-245, 1965.
3095. Krauter, S., and Braun, O.: Infiltration of the lungs in polyarteritis nodosa. Wien. Klin. Wschr., *78*:99-105, 1966.
3096. Glay, A., and Rona, G.: The pulmonary-renal syndrome of Goodpasture: case report. Radiology, *83*:314-318, 1964.
3097. O'Connell, E. J., Dower, J. C., Burke, E. C., Brown, A. L., Jr., and McCaughey, W. T. E.: Pulmonary hemorrhage-glomerulonephritis syndrome. Amer. J. Dis. Child., *108*:302-308, 1964.
3098. Azen, E. A., and Clatanoff, D. V.: Prolonged survival in Goodpasture's syndrome. Arch. Intern. Med., *114*:453-460, 1964.
3099. Benoit, F. L., Rulon, D. B., Theil, G. B., Doolan, P. D., and Watten, R. H.: Goodpasture's syndrome. A clinicopathological entity. Amer. J. Med., *37*:424-444, 1964.
3100. Botting, A. J., Brown, A. L., Jr., and Divertie, M. B.: The pulmonary lesion in a patient with Goodpasture's syndrome as studied with the electron microscope. Amer. J. Clin. Path., *42*:387-394, 1964.
3101. Sybers, R. G., Sybers, J. L., Dickie, H. A., and Paul, L. W.: Roentgenographic aspects of hemorrhagic pulmonary-renal disease (Goodpasture's syndrome). Amer. J. Roentgen., *94*:674-680, 1965.
3102. Pfeiffer, S. H., Desforges, G., and Gaensler, E. A.: Pulmonary hemosiderosis and glomerular kidney disease: Goodpasture's syndrome. Med. Thorac., *22*:470-479, 1965.
3103. Elder, J. L., Kirk, G. M., and Smith, W. G.: Idiopathic pulmonary hemosiderosis and the Goodpasture syndrome. Brit. Med. J., *2*:1152-1155, 1965.
3104. Otto, H., and Breining, H.: Involvement of the lungs in rheumatoid diseases with special emphasis on the Goodpasture syndrome. Prax. Pneumol., *20*:593-600, 1966.
3105. Davidson, M. B., Cutler, R. E., and Schuldberg, I. I.: Goodpasture's syndrome in a 78-year-old woman. Arch. Intern. Med., *117*:652-657, 1966.
3106. Wilde, W. T.: Goodpasture syndrome. Amer. Rev. Resp. Dis., *94*:773-776, 1966.

3107. Sirak, H. D., Sartawi, I. A., and Kim, Y. T.: The hemorrhagic pulmonary-renal syndrome of Goodpasture. J. Thorac. Cardiov. Surg., *52*:54–60, 1966.

3108. Leak, D., and Clein, G. P.: Acute Wegener's granulomatosis. Thorax, *22*:437–443, 1967.

3109. McIlvanie, S. K.: Wegener's granulomatosis. Successful treatment with chlorambucil. J.A.M.A., *197*:90–132, 1966.

3110. Constantine, H., Desforges, G., and Gaensler, E. A.: Noninfectious necrotizing granulomatosis of the lung. Wegener's syndrome. Med. Thorac., *23*:115–126, 1966.

3111. Kuntz, E., Beneke, G., and Knoth, W.: Wegener's granulomatosis. Med. Welt, *6*:296–304, 1967.

3112. Buerger, L., and Hathaway, J.: Idiopathic pulmonary haemosiderosis with allergic pulmonary vasculitis. Thorax, *19*:311–315, 1964.

3113. Golitsyna, L. V., and Timasheva, E. D.: Idiopathic hemosiderosis of the lungs. Probl. Tuberk., *42*:77, 1964.

3114. Sakharova, V. M., and Kheifets, S. I.: Chronic idiopathic hemosiderosis of the lungs. Probl. Tuberk., *42*:79–80, 1964.

3115. Vezendi, S., Mandi, L., Kormos, M., Papp, A., and Sashegyi, B.: Essential pulmonary hemosiderosis in adults. Prax. Pneumol., *21*:472–478, 1967.

3116. Fuleihan, F. J. D., Abboud, R. T., and Hubaytar, R.: Idiopathic pulmonary hemosiderosis. Case report with pulmonary function tests and review of the literature. Amer. Rev. Resp. Dis., *98*:93–97, 1968.

3117. Kovacs, B., Bencze, G., and Lakatos, L.: Respiratory functional examinations in systemic lupus erythematosus and rheumatoid arthritis. Magy. Belorv. Arch., *17*:70–71, 1964.

3118. Newcomer, A. D., Miller, R. D., Hepper, N. G. G., and Carter, E. T.: Pulmonary dysfunction in rheumatoid arthritis and systemic lupus erythematosus. Dis. Chest, *46*:562–570, 1964.

3119. Huang, C. T., Hennigar, G. R., and Lyons, H. A.: Pulmonary dysfunction in systemic lupus erythematosus. New Engl. J. Med., *272*:288–293, 1965.

3120. Gold, W. M., and Jennings, D. B.: Pulmonary function in patients with systemic lupus erythematosus. Amer. Rev. Resp. Dis., *93*:556–567, 1966.

3121. Hoffbrand, B. I.: 'Unexplained' dyspnoea and shrinking lungs in systemic lupus erythematosus. Brit. Med. J., *1*:1273–1277, 1965.

3122. Vuorinen, P., and Kalliomaki, J. L.: Radiological chest changes in disseminated lupus erythematosus. Rontgenblatter., *18*:520–523, 1965.

3123. Bohme, H., and Luther, T.: The pulmonary form of disseminated lupus erythematosus. Z. Ges. Inn. Med., *22*:732–735, 1967.

3124. Roy, S. B., Bhardwaj, P., and Bhatia, M. L.: Pulmonary blood volume in mitral stenosis. Brit. Med. J., *2*:1466–1469, 1965.

3125. Aber, C. P., and Campbell, J. A.: Significance of changes in the pulmonary diffusing capacity in mitral stenosis. Thorax, *20*:135–145, 1965.

3126. Bjure, J., Korsgren, M., and Varnauskas, E.: Pulmonary blood volume and diffusing capacity in cardiopulmonary disease. Clin. Sci., *33*:225–232, 1967.

3127. Hamm, J., and Scholmerich, P.: Über Lungenschwellung und Lungenstarrheit: Atemmechanische Untersuchungen an 100 Mitralstenosen. Klin. Wschr., *42*:1108–1117, 1964.

3128. McCredie, R. M.: The diffusing capacity characteristics of the pulmonary capillary bed in mitral valve disease. J. Clin. Invest., *43*:2279–2289, 1964.

3129. Woolf, C. R.: The relationships between dyspnea, pulmonary function and intracardiac pressures in adults with left heart valve lesions. Dis. Chest, *49*:225–240, 1966.

3130. Mudd, J. G., and Wyatt, J. P.: Pulmonary vascular alterations in mitral stenosis. Missouri Med., *62*:996–1003, 1965.

3131. Dawson, A., Kaneko, K., and McGregor, M.: Regional lung function in patients with mitral stenosis studied with Xenon^{133} during air and oxygen breathing. J. Clin. Invest., *44*:999–1008, 1965.

3132. Jordan, S. C., Hicken, P., Watson, D. A., Heath, D., and Whitaker, W.: Pathology of the lungs in mitral stenosis in relation to respiratory function and pulmonary haemodynamics. Brit. Heart J., *28*:101–107, 1966.

3133. Olsen, E. J. G.: Perivascular fibrosis in lungs in mitral valve disease. A possible mechanism of production. Brit. J. Dis. Chest, *60*:129–136, 1966.

3134. Camerini, F., Manfredi, F., and Guerra, S.: Radiologic diagnosis of pulmonary hypertension in mitral stenosis (a correlative radiologic and hemodynamic study). Radiol. Med., *53*:972–986, 1967.

3135. Hughes, J. M. B., Glazier, J. B., Maloney, J. E., and West, J. B.: Effect of lung volume on the distribution of pulmonary blood flow in man. Resp. Physiol., *4*:58–72, 1968.

3136. Hepper, N. G. G., Black, L. F., and Fowler, W. S.: Relationship of lung volume to height and arm span in normal subjects and in patients with spinal deformity. Amer. Rev. Resp. Dis., *91*:356–362, 1965.

3137. Rosenthal, R., and Doyle, J. T.: Pulmonary compliance in preclinical heart disease. Dis. Chest, *48*:193–198, 1965.

3138. Saunders, K. B.: Physiological dead space in left ventricular failure. Clin. Sci., *31*:145–151, 1966.

3139. Wilhelmsen, L., and Varnauskas, E.: Effects of acute plasma expansion on the mechanics of breathing. Clin. Sci., *33*:29–38, 1967.

3140. Tanser, A. R.: Impedance pneumograph studies in left ventricular failure. Thorax, *22*:550–554, 1967.

3141. Mauck, H. P., Jr., Shapiro, W., and Patterson, J. L., Jr.: Pulmonary venous (wedge) pressure. Correlation with onset and disappearance of dyspnea in acute left ventricular heart failure. Amer. J. Cardiol., *13*:301–309, 1964.

3142. Said, S. I., Longacher, J. W., Jr., Davis, R. K., Banerjee, C. M., Davis, W. M., and Wooddell, W. J.: Pulmonary gas exchange during induction of pulmonary edema in anaesthetized dogs. J. Appl. Physiol., *19*:403–407, 1964.

3143. Staub, N. C., Nagano, H., and Pearce, M. E.: Pulmonary edema in dogs, especially sequence of fluid accumulation in lungs. J. Appl. Physiol., *22*:227–240, 1967.

3144. McCredie, R. M., Lovejoy, F. W., Jr., and Yu, P. N.: Pulmonary diffusing capacity and pulmonary capillary blood volume in patients with intracardiac shunts. J. Lab. Clin. Med., *63*:914–923, 1964.

3145. Sloman, G., and Gandevia, B.: Ventilatory capacity and exercise ventilation in congenital and acquired cardiac disease. Brit. Heart. J., *26*:121–128, 1964.

3146. Rao, B. S., Cohn, K. E., Eldridge, F. L., and Hancock, E. W.: Left ventricular failure secondary to chronic pulmonary disease. Amer. J. Med., *45*:229–241, 1968.

3147. Anthonisen, N. R., and Smith, H. J. Respiratory acidosis as a consequence of pulmonary edema. Ann. Intern. Med., *62*:991–999, 1965.

3148. Petersen, E. S.: Lung function and respiratory changes in patients with arteriosclerotic heart disease. Thesis, Aarhus, 1968.

3149. Heard, B. E., Steiner, R. E., Herdan, A., and Gleason, D.: Oedema and fibrosis of the lungs in left ventricular failure. Brit. J. Radiol., *41*:161–171, 1968.

3150. Luisada, A. A.: Mechanism of neurogenic pulmonary edema. Amer. J. Cardiol., *20*:66–68, 1967.

3151. Ducker, T. B.: Increased intracranial pressure and pulmonary oedema. I. Clinical study of 11 patients. J. Neurosurg., *28*:112–117, 1968.

3152. Massumi, R. A., and Nutter, D. O.: Cardiac arrhythmias associated with Cheyne-Stokes respiration: A note on the possible mechanism. Dis. Chest, *54*:21–32, 1968.

3153. Dowell, A. R., Heyman, A., Sieker, H. O., and Tripathy, K.: Effect of aminophylline on respiratory-center sensitivity in Cheyne-Stokes respiration and in pulmonary emphysema. New Engl. J. Med., *273*:1447–1453, 1965.

3154. Higgs, B. E.: Factors affecting pulmonary gas exchange during the acute stages of myocardial infarction. Clin. Sci., *35*:115–122, 1968.

3155. Higgs, B. E., Clode, M., and Campbell, E. J. M.: Changes in ventilation, gas exchange, and circulation during exercise after recovery from myocardial infarction. Lancet, *2*:793–795, 1968.

3156. Lal, S., Savidge, R. S., and Chhabra, G. P.: Cardiovascular and respiratory effects of morphine and pentazocine in patients with myocardial infarction. Lancet, *1*:379-381, 1969.

3157. McNicol, M. W., Kirby, B. J., Bhoola, K. D., Everest, M. E., Price, H. V., and Freedman, S. F.: Pulmonary function in acute myocardial infarction. Brit. Med. J., *2*:1270-1273, 1965.
3158. McNicol, M. W., Kirby, B. J., Bhoola, K. D., Fulton, P. M., and Tattersfield, A. E.: Changes in pulmonary function 6-12 months after recovery from myocardial infarction. Lancet, *2*:1441-1443, 1966.
3159. Zaky, H. A., El Heneidy, R. E., Foda, M., Khalil, M., and Tarabeih, A. A.: Cardiopulmonary Bilharziasis. *Bilharziasis* (edited by F. K. Mostofi). Berlin, Springer-Verlag, 1967, pp. 30-38.
3160. Zaky, H. A., El Heneidy, A. R., and El Maksoud Tarabeih, A. A.: Hyperventilation and effort dyspnoea in porto-pulmonary bilharziasis. Dis. Chest, *53*:162-171, 1968.
3161. Wessel, H. U., Sommers, H. M., Cugell, D. W., and Paul, M. H.: Variants of cardiopulmonary manifestations of Manson's schistosomiasis. Ann. Intern. Med., *62*:757-766, 1965.
3162. Chaves, E.: Schistosomal arteritis of the lung. Hospital (Rio), *66*:1335-1346, 1964.
3163. Frayser, R., and De Alonso, A. E.: Studies of pulmonary function in patients with schistosomiasis mansoni. Amer. Rev. Resp. Dis., *95*:1036-1040, 1967.
3164. Weisberg, H., Lopez, J. F., Luria, M. H., and Katz, L. N.: Persistence of lung edema and arterial pressure rise in dogs after lung emboli. Amer. J. Physiol., *207*:641-646, 1964.
3165. Sabiston, D. C., and Wagner, H. N., Jr.: The diagnosis of pulmonary embolism by radioisotope scanning. Ann. Surg., *160*:575-588, 1964.
3166. Wagner, H. N., Jr., Sabiston, D. C., Jr., McAfee, J. G., Tow, D., and Stern, H. S.: Diagnosis of massive pulmonary embolism in man by radioisotope scanning. New Engl. J. Med., *271*:377-384, 1964.
3167. Petersen, E. S.: The pathophysiological disturbances in arterial pulmonary embolism. Ugeskr. Laeg., *126*:1014-1016, 1964.
3168. Dunnill, M. S.: The pathology of pulmonary embolism. Brit. J. Surg., *55*:790-794, 1968.
3169. Jones, N. L., and Goodwin, J. F.: Respiratory function in pulmonary thromboembolic disorders. Brit. Med. J., *1*:1089-1093, 1965.
3170. Greenberg, H. B.: Refractory dyspnea—a symptom of recurrent pulmonary embolism. J. Amer. Geriat. Soc., *13*:748-755, 1965.
3171. Llamas, R., and Swenson, E. W.: Diagnostic clues in pulmonary thrombo-embolism evaluated by angiographic and ventilation-blood flow studies. Thorax, *20*:327-336, 1965.
3172. Levy, S. E., Stein, M., Totten, R. S., Bruderman, I., Wessler, S., and Robin, E. D.: Ventilation-perfusion abnormalities in experimental pulmonary embolism. J. Clin. Invest., *44*:1699-1706, 1965.
3173. West, J. B., Dollery, C. T., and Heard, B. E.: Increased pulmonary vascular resistance in the dependent zone of the isolated dog lung caused by perivascular edema. Circ. Res., *17*:191-206, 1965.
3174. Nadel, J. A., Gold, W. M., Jennings, D. B., Wright, R. R., and Fudenberg, H. H.: Unusual disease of pulmonary arteries with dyspnea. Structure-function relationships. Amer. J. Med., *41*:440-447, 1966.
3175. Fowler, N. O., Black-Schaffer, B., Scott, R. C., and Gueron, M.: Idiopathic and thromboembolic pulmonary hypertension. Amer. J. Med., *40*:331-345, 1966.
3176. McCredie, R. M.: The pulmonary capillary bed in various forms of pulmonary hypertension. Circulation, *33*:854-861, 1966.
3177. Nutter, D. O., and Massumi, R. A.: The arterial-alveolar carbon dioxide tension gradient in diagnosis of pulmonary embolus. Dis. Chest, *50*:380-387, 1966.
3178. Moser, K. M., Tisi, G. M., Rhodes, P. G., Landis, G. A., and Miale, A., Jr. Correlation of lung photoscans with pulmonary angiography in pulmonary embolism. Amer. J. Cardiol., *18*:810-820, 1966.
3179. Fred, H. L., Burdine, J. A., Jr., Gonzalez, D. A., Lockhart, R. W., Peabody, C. A., and Alexander, J. K.: Arteriographic assessment of lung scanning in the diagnosis of pulmonary thromboembolism. New Engl. J. Med., *275*:1025-1032, 1966.
3180. Bjure, J., Paulin, S., Soderholm, B., and Wilhelmsen, L.: Pulmonary gas exchange and hemodynamics in patients with recurrent pulmonary embolism and polycythemia vera. Cor Vasa (Praha), *9*:34-47, 1967.
3181. Ferris, E. J., Stanzler, R. M., Rourke, J. A., Blumenthal, J., and Messer, J. V.: Pulmonary angiography in pulmonary embolic disease. J. Roentgen., *100*:355-363, 1967.
3182. Chait, A., Summers, D., Krasnow, N., and Wechsler, B. M.: Observations on the fate of large pulmonary emboli. Amer. J. Roentgen., *100*:364-373, 1967.
3183. Leibendgut, B.: Pulmonary embolism (a follow-up study of 118 cases). Arch. Kreisl. Forsch., *52*:190-206, 1967.
3184. Bass, H., Heckscher, T., and Anthonisen, N. R.: Regional pulmonary gas exchange in patients with pulmonary embolism. Clin. Sci., *33*:355-364, 1967.
3185. Takahashi, M., and Abrams, H. L.: Arborizing pulmonary embolization following lymphangiography. Report of three cases and an experimental study. Radiology, *89*:633-638, 1967.
3186. Nikodymova, L., Daum, S., Stiksa, J., and Widimsky, J.: Respiratory changes in thromboembolic disease. Respiration, *25*:51-66, 1968.
3187. Janota, M., Widimsky, J., Hurych, J., and Stanek, V.: The alveolar dead space during pulmonary artery occlusion. Respiration, *25*:292-305, 1968.
3188. Daum, S.: The diffusing capacity of the lungs in pulmonary embolism. Respiration, *26*:8-15, 1969.
3189. Rosenberg, S. A.: A study of the etiological basis of primary pulmonary hypertension. Amer. Heart J., *68*:484-489, 1964.
3190. Wessel, H. U., Kezdi, P., and Cugell, D. W.: Respiratory and cardiovascular function in patients with severe pulmonary hypertension. Circulation, *29*:825-832, 1964.
3191. Secker-Walker, R. H.: Scintillation scanning of lungs in diagnosis of pulmonary embolism. Brit. Med. J., *1*:206-208, 1968.
3192. Braun, K., and Stern, S.: Functional significance of the pulmonary venous system. Amer. J. Cardiol., *20*:56-65, 1967.
3193. Heath, D., Segal, N., and Bishop, J.: Pulmonary veno-occlusive disease. Circulation, *34*:242-248, 1966.
3194. Brown, C. H., and Harrison, C. V.: Pulmonary veno-occlusive disease. Lancet, *2*:61-66, 1966.
3195. Stovin, P. G. I., and Mitchison, M. J.: Pulmonary hypertension due to obstruction of the intra-pulmonary veins. Thorax, *20*:106-113, 1965.
3196. Lees, M. H., Way, R. C., and Ross, B. B.: Ventilation and respiratory gas transfer of infants with increased pulmonary blood flow. Pediatrics, *40*:259-271, 1967.
3197. Crawford, D. W., Simpson, E., and McIlroy, M. B.: Cardiopulmonary function in Fallot's tetralogy after palliative shunting operations. Amer. Heart J., *74*:463-472, 1967.
3198. Estevez, J. A., Isoardi, O., Patrito, L., Dorado, A., and Podio, R. B.: Pulmonary function in congenital heart diseases. Prensa. Med. Argent., *54*:106-108, 1967.
3199. Linde, L. M., Siegel, S. I., Martelle, R. R., and Simmons, D. H.: Lung function in congenital heart disease. Dis. Chest, *46*:46-50, 1964.
3200. Hamilton, R. W., Jr., Hustead, R. F., and Peltier, L. F.: Fat embolism: the effect of particulate embolism on lung surfactant. Surgery, *56*:53-56, 1964.
3201. Smith, D. E., Downes, H., Caskie, J. D., and Van Norman, R. W.: Intermittent positive pressure breathing in the treatment of fat embolism. J. Trauma, *5*:761-774, 1965.
3202. Wiener, L., and Forsyth, D.: Pulmonary pathophysiology of fat embolism. Amer. Rev. Resp. Dis., *92*:113-118, 1965.
3203. Kapanci, Y., and Koralnik, O.: Recurrent fat embolism of

the lung. A study of the alveolar lesions resulting from a decrease of the perfusion. Helv. Med. Acta, *32*:47–66, 1965.
3204. Gigon, J. P., Enderlin, F., and Scheidegger, S.: The fate of infused fat emulsions in the human lung. Schweiz. Med. Wschr., *96*:71–75, 1966.
3205. Henzel, J. H., Smith, J. L., Pories, W. J., and Burget, D. E.: Fat embolism. Diagnostic challenge of a potentially lethal clinical entity. Amer. J. Surg., *113*:525–532, 1967.
3206. Hupe, K.: Fat embolism. Clinical studies and experiments in animals. Fortschr. Med., *85*:663–666, 1967.
3207. Acker, S. E., and Greenberg, H. B.: Pulmonary injury from post-traumatic fat embolism. Amer. Rev. Resp. Dis., *97*:423–428, 1968.
3208. Gold, W. M., Youker, J., Anderson, S., and Nadel, J. A.: Pulmonary function abnormalities after lymphangiography. New Engl. J. Med., *273*:519–524, 1965.
3209. Clouse, M. E., Hallgrimsson, J., and Wenlund, D. E.: Complications following lymphography with particular reference to pulmonary oil embolization. Amer. J. Radiol., *96*:972–978, 1966.
3210. Richardson, P., Crosby, E. H., Bean, H. A., and Dexter, D.: Pulmonary oil deposition in patients subjected to lymphography. Canad. Med. Assoc. J., *94*:1086–1091, 1966.
3211. Koehler, P. R.: Typical fatal reactions after lymphography. Cancer Chemother. Rep., *52*:113–118, 1968.
3212. Threefoot, S. A.: Pulmonary hazards of lymphography. Cancer Chemother. Rep., *52*:107–111, 1968.
3213. Fabel, H., Kunitsch, G., and Stender, H. S.: Disorders of lung function after lymphography. Fortschr. Rontgenstr., *107*:609–618, 1967.
3214. Fabel, H., Kunitsch, G., and Stender, H. S.: Changes in the pulmonary circulation and gas exchange due to oil embolism following lymphography. Z. Ges. Exp. Med., *147*:143–153, 1968.
3215. Weg, J. G., and Harkleroad, L. E.: Aberrations in pulmonary function due to lymphangiography. Dis. Chest, *53*:534–540, 1968.
3216. Pain, M. C. F., Stannard, M., and Sloman, G.: Disturbances of pulmonary function after acute myocardial infarction. Brit. Med. J., *2*:591–594, 1967.
3217. Falsetti, H. L., Hanson, J. S., and Tabakin, B. S.: Obesity-hypoventilation syndrome in siblings. Amer. Rev. Resp. Dis., *90*:105–110, 1964.
3218. Galy, P., Brune, J., Lheureux, P., and Brune, A.: A propos des troubles respiratoires des obèses. Rev. Tuberc., 28:281–288, 1964.
3219. Schonthal, H.: Ein Beitrag zum Pickwickian-syndrom. Deutsch. Arch. Klin. Med., *209*:277–288, 1964.
3220. Lopez, M. V., Chulia, O. F., and Romar, M. A.: Sindrome de Pickwick. Rev. Clin. Esp., *95*:164–173, 1964.
3221. Scherrer, M., and Haldimann, C.: Zur Genese des Pickwick-syndroms. Helv. Med. Acta, *31*:512–517, 1964.
3222. Fishman, L. S., Samson, J. H., and Sperling, D. R.: Primary alveolar hypoventilation syndrome (Ondine's curse). Association with manifestations of hypothalamic disease. Amer. J. Dis. Child., *110*:155–161, 1965.
3223. Atlan, G., and Brille, D.: The role of a clinical or latent bronchial factor in the mechanism of alveolar hypoventilation in obese persons. J. Franc. Med. Chir. Thorac., *20*:229–235, 1966.
3224. Kretschy, A., and Muhar, F.: The cause of the alveolar hypoventilation in the Pickwick syndrome. Wien. Klin. Wschr., *77*:286–289, 1965.
3225. Tsitouris, G., and Fertakis, A.: Alveolar hypoventilation due to respiratory center dysfunction of unknown cause. Amer. J. Med., *39*:173–178, 1965.
3226. Fontana, G., Morino, A., Puviani, G., Tincani, G. P., and Soro, A.: La sindrome di Pickwick. Osservazioni su 6 casi clinici. G. Clin. Med., *47*:1191–1216, 1966.
3227. Abrahamsen, A. M., and Nitter-Hauge, S.: Extreme obesity with respiratory failure, necessitating artificial ventilation. Acta Med. Scand., *180*:113–116, 1966.
3228. Mannhart, M., Kostyal, A., Baumann, H. R., and Herzog, H.: Central alveolar hypoventilation during exertion with normal arterial blood gas tensions at rest. Helv. Med. Acta., *33*:479–486, 1967.
3229. Watts, R. S., and Curran, W. S.: Hypoventilation and myxedema. Rocky Mountain Med. J., *64*:54–57, 1967.
3230. Dowell, A. R., Sieker, H. O., and Schwartzmann, R.: Atypical periodic respiration in an obese patient. Arch. Intern. Med., *120*:591–598, 1967.
3231. Lyons, H. A., and Huang, C. T.: Therapeutic use of progesterone in alveolar hypoventilation associated with obesity. Amer. J. Med., *44*:881–888, 1968.
3232. Nitzan, M., Spitzer, S., and Elian, E.: Obesity-hypoventilation (Pickwickian) syndrome in a child. Israel J. Med. Sci., *4*:264–269, 1968.
3233. Escande, J. P., Schwartz, B. A., Gentilini, M., Hazard, J., Choubrac, P., and Domart, A.: The Pickwick syndrome. Bull. Soc. Med. Hop., *118*:273–294, 1967.
3234. Hughes, J. M. B.: Central respiratory failure reversed by treatment. Brain, *90 (Part III)*:675–680, 1967.
3235. Kleinfeld, M., Messite, J., Shapiro, J., Kooyman, O., and Levin, E.: A clinical, roentgenological, and physiological study of magnetite workers. Arch. Environ. Health., *16*:392–397, 1968.
3236. Zorn, O.: Barytosis and tin-oxide lung. Zbl. Arbeitsmed., *16*:133–135, 1966.
3237. Cooper, D. A., Pendergrass, E. P., Vorwald, A. J., Mayock, L., and Brieger, H.: Pneumoconiosis among workers in an antimony industry. Amer. J. Roentgen., *103*:495–508, 1968.
3238. Wright, G. W.: Airborne fibrous glass particles. Arch. Environ. Health, *16*:175–181, 1968.
3239. Zakova, N., and Svoboda, M.: Morphological changes in the lungs following bronchography with barium sulphate. Acta Univ. Carol., *11*:125–135, 1965.
3240. Levi-Valensi, P., Drif, M., Dat, A., and Hadjadj, G.: Fifty-seven cases of barytosis of the lungs (the results of systematic examination of workers in a barium factory). J. Franc. Med. Chir. Thorac., *20*:443–455, 1966.
3241. Duguid, J. B., and Lambert, M. W.: The pathogenesis of coal miner's pneumoconiosis. J. Path. Bact., *88*:389–403, 1964.
3242. Nissardi, G. P., Sanna-Randaccio, F., Torrazza, P. L., and Casciu, L.: Studies of lung diffusing capacity at rest in silicotic patients. Lav. Umano, *17*:367–378, 1964.
3243. Muysers, K., Siehoff, F., Worth, G., Gasthaus, L., and Smidt, U.: Recent studies of respiratory physiology in coal miners with reference to silicosis, bronchitis, and emphysema. Int. Arch. Gewerbepath., *22*:215–224, 1966.
3244. Grailles, M., and Collet, A.: The site and development of initial pneumoconiotic deposits in the lungs of coal miners. Rev. Tuberc. (Paris), *30*:489–504, 1966.
3245. Nicaise, R., Vereerstraeten, J., and De Clercq, F.: The diffusion capacity at rest and during exercise in pneumoconiosis. Select. Papers, *10*:70–79, 1967.
3246. Ogilvie, C., Brown, K., and Kearns, W. E.: Overinflation of the lungs of coal miners. Brit. Med. J., *2*:10–14, 1967.
3247. Boren, H. G.: Pulmonary response to inhaled carbon: a model of lung injury. Yale J. Biol. Med., *40*:364–388, 1968.
3248. Rasmussen, D. L., Laqeur, W. A., Futterman, P., Warren, H. D., and Nelson, C. W.: Pulmonary impairment in Southern West Virginia coal miners. Amer. Rev. Resp. Dis., *98*:658–667, 1968.
3249. Muysers, K., Siehoff, F., Worth, G., and Gasthaus, L.: Pulmonary function in bronchitis with special reference to occupational exposure to air pollution. Med. Thorac., *23*:265–282, 1966.
3250. Fourteenth International Congress on Occupational Medicine, Madrid, 1963. Practical value of functional respiratory exploration in assessment of silicosis. Arch. Mal. Prof., *25*:541–552, 1964.
3251. Nissardi, G. P., Sanna-Randaccio, F., Torrazza, P. L., and Gariel, G.: Lung diffusing capacity on effort in normal and silicotic subjects. Lav. Umano, *17*:397–414, 1965.
3252. Podlesch, I., Stevanovic, M., and Ulmer, W. T.: The diffusing capacity of the lungs in silicosis. Med. Thorac., *23*:283–293, 1966.
3253. Vecchione, C., and Mole, R.: The compliance in the silicotic subject. Poumon Coeur, *23*:713–719, 1967.

3254. Teculescu, D. B., Stanescu, D. C., and Pilat, L.: Pulmonary mechanics in silicosis. Arch. Environ. Health, *14:* 461–468, 1967.
3255. Sartorelli, E.: A study of the ventilation/perfusion ratio in silicosis by measurement of the arterioalveolar P_{CO_2} gradient during rest and exercise. Acta Geront., *17*:38–42, 1967.
3256. Kleinfeld, M., Messite, J. Shapiro, J., Kooyman, O., and Swencicki, R.: Lung function in talc workers. Arch. Environ. Health, *9*:559–566, 1964.
3257. Kleinfeld, M., Messite, J., Shapiro, J., and Swencicki, R.: Effect of talc dust inhalation on lung function. Arch. Environ. Health, *10*:431–437, 1965.
3258. Capodaglio, E., Salvadeo, A., Catenacci, G., and Pezzagno, G.: Changes in pulmonary function and chest radiographs of brick-furnace workers. Med. Lavoro, *55*:414–423, 1964.
3259. *Asbestosis: A bibliography of the world's literature abstracted and indexed 1960–1968.* Pneumoconiosis Research Unit, Council for Scientific and Industrial Research, South African Institute for Medical Research. Johannesburg, 1969.
3260. Brodeur, P.: A reporter at large: the magic mineral. New Yorker, *44*:117–165, 1968.
3261. Kleinfeld, M., Messite, J., Kooyman, O., and Sarfaty, J.: Effect of asbestos dust inhalation on lung function. Arch. Environ. Health, *12*:741–746, 1966.
3262. Vaerenberg, C.: Respiratory asbestosis. Lung function in pulmonary asbestosis. Acta Tuberc. Belg., *55*:92–101, 1964.
3263. Cauna, D., Totten, R. S., and Gross, P.: Asbestos bodies in human lungs at autopsy. J.A.M.A., *192*:371–373, 1965.
3264. Hardy, H. L.: Asbestos related disease. Amer. J. Med. Sci., *250*:381–389, 1965.
3265. Hunt, R.: Routine lung function studies on 830 employees in an asbestos processing factory. Ann. N. Y. Acad. Sci., *132*:406–420, 1965.
3266. Hany, A., Burckhardt, P., and Buhlmann, A.: The clinical features and pathophysiology of pulmonary asbestosis. Schweiz. Med. Wschr., *97*:597–603, 1967.
3267. Davis, J. M. G.: Electron-microscope studies of asbestosis in man and animals. Ann. N. Y. Acad. Sci., *132*:98–111, 1965.
3268. Enterline, P. E., and Kendrick, M. A.: Asbestos-dust exposures at various levels and mortality. Arch. Environ. Health, *15*:181–186, 1967.
3269. Ghezzi, I., Molteni, G., and Puccetti, U.: Asbestos bodies in the lungs of inhabitants of Milan. Med. Lavoro, *58*:223–227, 1967.
3270. Polliack, A., and Sacks, M. I.: Prevalence of asbestos bodies in basal lung smears. Israel J. Med. Sci., *4*:223–226, 1968.
3271. Freour, P., Germouty, J., Jault, D., Plancel, F., and Warin, J.: A case of pneumoconiosis due to aluminum dust. Presse Méd., *74*:2547–2549, 1966.
3272. Redding, R. A., Hardy, H. L., and Gaensler, E. A.: Beryllium disease: a 16 year follow up case study. Respiration, *25*:263–278, 1968.
3273. Van Ordstrand, H. S., DeNardi, J. M., and Zielinski, J. F.: Beryllium lung disease and its registry. Postgrad. Med., *36*:499–504, 1964.
3274. Loulergue, J.: A case of acute beryllium pneumonia. Recovery without sequelae. Arch. Mal. Prof., *27*:237–238, 1966.
3275. Pretl, K.: An unusual fatal case of chronic pulmonary beryllium damage. Wien. Klin. Wschr., *77*:771–775, 1965.
3276. Bouhuys, A., Barbero, A., Lindell, S-E., Roach, S. A., and Schilling, R. S. F.: Byssinosis in hemp workers. Arch. Environ. Health, *14*:533–544, 1967.
3277. Schilling, R. S. F.: Epidemiological studies of chronic respiratory disease among cotton operatives. Yale J. Biol. Med., *37*:55–74, 1964.
3278. Massoud, A., and Taylor, G.: Byssinosis: antibody to cotton antigens in normal subjects and in cotton cardroom workers. Lancet, *2*:607–610, 1964.
3279. Belin, L., Bouhuys, A., Hoekstra, W., Johansson, M-B., Lindell, S-E., and Pool, J.: Byssinosis in cardroom workers in Swedish cotton mills. Brit. J. Industr. Med., *22*:101–108, 1965.
3280. Gandevia, B., and Milne, J.: Ventilatory capacity changes on exposure to cotton dust and their relevance to byssinosis in Australia. Brit. J. Industr. Med., *22*:295–304, 1965.
3281. Bouhuys, A.: Response to inhaled histamine in bronchial asthma and in byssinosis. Amer. Rev. Resp. Dis., *95*:89–93, 1967.
3282. Massoud, A. A. E., Altounyan, R. E. C., Howell, J. B. L., and Lane, R. E.: Effects of histamine aerosol in byssinotic subjects. Brit. J. Industr. Med., *24*:38–40, 1967.
3283. Vuylsteek, K., Van Ganse, W., De Sweemer, C., Eylenbosch, W., Stevens, J., Debusscher, P., and Van Cauteren, G.: Byssinosis: an epidemiological study in the flax industry. T. Soc. Geneesk., *46*:134–140, 1968.
3284. Pierce, A. K., Nicholson, D. P., Miller, J. M., and Johnson, R. L., Jr.: Pulmonary function in Bagasse worker's lung disease. Amer. Rev. Resp. Dis., *97*:561–570, 1968.
3285. Weill, H., Buechner, H. A., Gonzalez, E., Herbert, S. J., Aucoin, E., and Ziskind, M. M.: Bagassosis: a study of pulmonary function in 20 cases. Ann. Intern. Med., *64*:737–747, 1966.
3286. Nicholson, D. P.: Bagasse worker's lung. Amer. Rev. Resp. Dis., *97*:546–560, 1968.
3287. Wenzel, F. J., and Emanuel, D. A.: The epidemiology of maple bark disease. Arch. Environ. Health, *14*:385–389, 1967.
3288. Emanuel, D. A., Wenzel, F. J., and Lawton, B. R.: Pneumonitis due to cryptostroma corticale (maple-bark disease). New Engl. J. Med., *274*:1413–1418, 1966.
3289. Pepys, J., and Jenkins, P. A.: Precipitin (FLH) test in farmer's lung. Thorax, *20*:21–35, 1965.
3290. Van Wormer, D. E.: Farmer's lung. Arch. Environ. Health, *10*:71–78, 1965.
3291. Wenzel, F. J., and Emanuel, D. A.: Experimental studies of farmer's lung. N. Y. J. Med., *65*:3032–3036, 1965.
3292. Johnson, J. E.: Farmer's lung in Maryland Clinical, microbiological, and immunological studies. Ann. Intern. Med., *64*:860–872, 1966.
3293. Hilvering, C., De Vries, K., and Orie, N. G. M.: Farmer's lung. Nederl. T. Geneesk., *110*:1297–1306, 1966.
3294. Blackburn, C. R. B., and Green, W.: Precipitins against extracts of thatched roofs in the sera of New Guinea natives with chronic lung disease. Lancet, *2*:1396–1397, 1966.
3295. Morawetz, F., and Meczoch, F.: Die "Farmerlunge," Wien. Klin. Wschr., *80*:313–320, 1968.
3296. Maier, A., Batzenschlager, A., Roos, C., and Orion, B.: Le poumon de fermier. Arch. Mal. Prof., *28*:833–849, 1967.
3297. Barbee, R. A., Callies, Q., Dickie, H. A., and Rankin, J.: Amer. Rev. Resp. Dis., *97*:223–231, 1968.
3298. Hapke, E. J., Seal, R. M. E., and Thomas, G. O.: Farmer's lung. A clinical, radiographic, functional, and serological correlation of acute and chronic stages. Thorax, *23*:451–468, 1968.
3299. Seal, R. M. E., Hapke, E. J., and Thomas, G. O.: The pathology of the acute and chronic stages of farmer's lung. Thorax, *23*:469–489, 1968.
3300. Barrowcliff, D. F., and Arblaster, P. G.: Farmer's lung: a study of an early acute fatal case. Thorax, *23*:490–500, 1968.
3301. Ashcroft, T.: Asbestos bodies in routine necropsies on Tyneside: a pathological and social study. Brit. Med. J., *1*:614–618, 1968.
3302. Gandevia, B.: Pulmonary function in asbestos workers. Amer. Rev. Resp. Dis., *96*:420–427, 1967.
3303. MacPherson, P., and Davidson, J. K.: Correlation between lung asbestos count at necropsy and radiological appearances. Brit. Med. J., *1*:355–357, 1969.
3304. Lyons, J. P., Clarke, W. G., Hall, A. M., and Cotes, J. E.: Transfer factor (diffusing capacity) for the lung in simple pneumoconiosis of coal workers. Brit. Med. J., *2*:772–774, 1967.
3305. Anjilvel, L., and Thurlbeck, W. M.: The incidence of asbestos bodies in the lungs at random necropsies in Montreal. Canad. Med. Assoc. J., *95*:1179–1182, 1966.

3306. Hargreave, F. E., Pepys, J., Longbottom, J. L., and Wraith, D. G.: Bird breeder's (fancier's) lung. Lancet, *1*:445–449, 1966.
3307. Reed, C. E., Sosman, A., and Barbee, R. A.: Pigeon-breeder's lung. A newly observed interstitial pulmonary disease. J.A.M.A., *193*:261–265, 1965.
3308. Villar, T. G., De Padua, F., De Avila, R., and Araujo, J.: A "Pigeon breeder's Lung." Soc. Cienc. Med. Lisboa, *130*:181–195, 1966.
3309. Nash, E. S., Vogelpoel, L., and Becker, W. B.: Pigeon breeder's lung. A case report. S. Afr. Med. J., *41*:191–193, 1967.
3310. Boyd, G., Dick, H. W., Lorimer, A. R., and Moran, F.: Bird breeder's lung. Scot. Med. J., *12*:69–71, 1967.
3311. Eyckmans, L., Gyselen, A., Lauwerijns, J., Cosemans, J., Wildiers, J., and Willems, J.: Pigeon breeder's lung. Report of three cases. Dis. Chest, *53*:358–364, 1968.
3312. Verbeke, R., Tasson, J., Lameire, N., and De Vis, R.: Two cases of "Pigeon breeder's lung." T. Soc. Geneesk., *24*:417–423, 1968.
3313. Fink, J. N., Sosman, A. J., Barboriak, J. J., Schlueter, D. P., and Holmes, R. A.: Pigeon breeder's disease. A clinical study of a hypersensitivity pneumonitis. Ann. Intern. Med., *68*:1205–1219, 1968.
3314. Mahon, W. E., Scott, D. J., Ansell, G., Manson, G. L., and Fraser, R.: Hypersensitivity to pituitary snuff with miliary shadowing in the lungs. Thorax, *22*:13–20, 1967.
3315. Kleinfeld, M., Messite, J., Swencicki, R. E., and Shapiro, J.: A clinical and physiologic study of grain handlers. Arch. Environ. Health, *16*:380–391, 1968.
3316. Riddle, H. F. V., Channell, S., Blyth, W., Weir, D. M., Lloyd, M., Amos, W. M. G., and Grant I. W. B.: Allergic alveolitis in a malt worker. Thorax, *23*:271–280, 1968.
3317. Freeman, G., and Haydon, G. B.: Emphysema after low level exposure to NO_2. Arch. Environ. Health, *8*:125–128, 1964.
3318. Van Mechelen, J., and Prignot, J.: Group poisoning with nitrous gases. Acta Tuberc. Belg., *56*:68–79, 1965.
3319. Davidson, J. T., Lillington, G. A., Haydon, G. B., and Wasserman, K.: Physiologic changes in the lungs of rabbits continuously exposed to nitrogen dioxide. Amer. Rev. Resp. Dis., *95*:790–796, 1967.
3320. Haydon, G. B., Davidson, J. T., Lillington, G. A., and Wasserman, K.: Nitrogen dioxide induced emphysema in rabbits. Amer. Rev. Resp. Dis., *95*:797–805, 1967.
3321. Dillmann, G., Henschler, D., and Thoenes, W.: Effects of nitrogen peroxide on pulmonary alveoli in mouse. Arch. Toxik., *23*:55–65, 1967.
3322. Sherwin, R. P., Richters, V., Brooks, M., and Buckley, R. D.: The phenomenon of macrophage congregation in vitro and its relationship to in vivo NO_2 exposure of guinea pigs. Lab. Invest., *18*:269–277, 1968.
3323. Gaultier, M., Fournier, E., Gervais, P., and Bodin, F.: Three cases of acute ammonia poisoning. Ann. Med. Leg., *44*:357–361, 1964.
3324. Larsen, R. I.: United States air quality. Arch. Environ. Health, *8*:325–333, 1964.
3325. Greenburg, L., Field, F., Erhardt, C. L., Glasser, M., and Reed, J. I.: Air pollution, influenza and mortality in New York City. Arch. Environ. Health, *15*:430–438, 1967.
3326. Nadel, J. A., Salem, H., Tamplin, B., and Tokiwa, Y.: Mechanism of bronchoconstriction during inhalation of sulfur dioxide. J. Appl. Physiol., *20*:164–167, 1965.
3327. Frada, G., Mentesana, G., and Rizzo, A.: A clinical and physiological description of chronic bronchopneumonia in sulfur workers. Folia Med., *47*:937–951, 1964.
3328. Speizer, F. E., and Frank, N. R.: A comparison of changes in pulmonary flow resistance in healthy volunteers acutely exposed to SO_2 by mouth and by nose. Brit. J. Industr. Med., *23*:75–78, 1966.
3329. Kahana, L. M., and Aronovitch, M.: Effects of sulfur dioxide on surface properties of the lung. Amer. Rev. Resp. Dis., *94*:201–207, 1966.
3330. Kowitz, T. A., Reba, R. C., Parker, R. T., and Spicer, W. S.: Effects of chlorine gas upon respiratory function. Arch. Environ. Health, *14*:545–563, 1967.
3331. Ferris, B. G., Jr., Burgess, W. A., and Worcester, J.: Prevalence of chronic respiratory disease in a pulp mill and a paper mill in the United States. Brit. J. Industr. Med., *24*:26–37, 1967.
3332. Gross, P., Rinehart, W. E., and Hatch, T.: Chronic pneumonitis caused by phosgene. An experimental study. Arch. Environ. Health, *10*:768–775, 1965.
3333. Heully, F., Gautheir, G., and De Ren: Intoxication sévère d'origine professionnelle par vapeurs de cadmium avec manifestations broncho-pulmonaires consécutives. (Severe occupational poisoning with cadmium vapor.) Arch. Mal. Prof., *27*:215–220, 1966.
3334. Townshend, R. H.: A case of acute cadmium pneumonitis: lung function tests during a four-year follow-up. Brit. J. Industr. Med., *25*:68–71, 1968.
3335. Easton, R. E., and Murphy, S. D.: Experimental ozone pre-exposure and histamine. Arch. Environ. Health, *15*:160–166, 1967.
3336. Hallett, W. Y.: Effect of ozone and cigarette smoke on lung function. Arch. Environ. Health, *10*:295–302, 1965.
3337. Jaffe, L. S.: Photochemical air pollutants and their effects on men and animals. Arch. Environ. Health, *16*:241–255, 1968.
3338. Kelly, F. J., Whiting, I., and Gill, W. E.: Ozone poisoning. Arch. Environ. Health, *10*:517–519, 1965.
3339. Goldsmith, J. R., and Nadel, J. A.: Experimental exposure of human subjects to ozone. J. Air Pollut. Contr. Assoc., *19*:329–330, 1969.
3340. Dixon, J. R., Wagner, W. D., Martin, T. D., Keenan, R. G., and Stokinger, H. E.: Metal shifts as early indicators of response from low grade pulmonary irritation. Toxic. Appl. Pharmacol., *9*:225–233, 1966.
3341. Coffin, D. L., Gardner, D. E., Holzman, R. S., and Wolock, F. J.: Influence of ozone on pulmonary cells. Arch. Environ. Health, *16*:633–636, 1968.
3342. Baldachin, B. J., and Melmed, R. N.: Clinical and therapeutic aspects of kerosene poisoning: a series of 200 cases. Brit. Med. J., *11*:28–30, 1964.
3343. Schwartz, S. I., Breslau, R. C., Kutner, F., and Smith, D.: Effects of drugs and hyperbaric oxygen environment on experimental kerosene pneumonitis. Dis. Chest, *47*:353–359, 1965.
3344. Sharma, O. P., and Williams, M. H.: Thesaurosis. Arch. Environ. Health, *13*:616–618, 1966.
3345. Garibaldi, R., and Caprotti, M.: Clinical investigation of a group of subjects exposed to the inhalation of hair-sprays. Med. Lavoro, *55*:424–433, 1964.
3346. Giovacchini, R. P., Becker, G. H., Brunner, M. J., and Dunlap, F. E.: Pulmonary disease and hair-spray polymers. Effects of long term exposure in dogs. J.A.M.A., *193*:298–299, 1965.
3347. Cares, R. M.: Thesaurosis from inhaled hair spray. Arch. Environ. Health, *11*:82–85, 1965.
3348. Maxon, F. C.: Respiratory irritation from toluene diisocyanate. Arch. Environ. Health, *8*:755–758, 1964.
3349. Swensson, A., Holmqvist, C., and Lundgren, K.: Injury to the respiratory tract by isocyanates used in making lacquers. Brit. J. Industr. Med., *12*:50–53, 1955.
3350. Exarhos, N. D., Logan, W. D., Jr., Abbott, O. A., and Hatcher, C. R., Jr.: The importance of pH and volume in tracheobronchial aspiration. Dis. Chest, *47*:167–169, 1965.
3351. Batzenschlager, A., and John, S.: Mendelson's syndrome. Morphology and course in humans. Presse Méd., *76*:423–426, 1968.
3352. Taylor, G., and Pryse-Davies, J.: Evaluation of endotracheal steroid therapy in acid pulmonary aspiration syndrome (Mendelson's syndrome). Anesthesiology, *29*:17–21, 1968.
3353. Wellington, J. L., and Lynn, R. B.: Effects of irradiation on lung function. Canad. Med. Assoc. J., *90*:1341–1344, 1964.
3354. Hoffbrand, B. I., Gillam, P. M. S., and Heaf, P. J. D.: Effect of chronic bronchitis on changes in pulmonary function caused by irradiation of the lungs. Thorax, *20*:303–308, 1965.
3355. Teates, C. D.: Effects of unilateral thoracic irradiation on lung function. J. Appl. Physiol., *20*:628–636, 1965.

3356. Hunnicutt, T. N., Jr., Cracovaner, D. J., and Myles, J. T.: Spirometric measurements in welders. Arch. Environ. Health, *8*:661–669, 1964.

3357. Meyer, E. C., Kratzinger, S. F., and Miller, W. H.: Pulmonary fibrosis in an arc welder. Arch. Environ. Health, *15*:462–469, 1967.

3358. Marchand, M., Jacob, M., and Lefebvre, J.: The pneumopathy of arc-welders. Lille Med., *9*:139–145, 1964.

3359. Stanescu, D. C., Pilat, L., Gavrilescu, N., Teculescu, D. B., and Cristescu, I.: Aspects of pulmonary mechanics in arc welders' siderosis. Brit. J. Industr. Med., *24*:143–147, 1967.

3360. Molokhia, M. M., and Smith, H.: Trace elements in the lung. Arch. Environ. Health, *15*:745–750, 1967.

3361. Dubos, R.: Environmental biology. Bioscience, *14*:11–14, 1964.

3362. Bates, D. V., Fish, B. R., Hatch, T. F., Mercer, T. T., and Morrow, P. E.: Deposition and retention models for internal dosimetry of the human respiratory tract. Task group on lung dynamics. Health Phys., *12*:173–208, 1966.

3363. *Circulatory and Respiratory Mass Transport.* A Ciba Foundation Symposium (edited by G. E. W. Wolstenholme and J. Knight). London, J. and A. Churchill Ltd., 1969, p. 310.

3364. Pepys, J.: Hypersensitivity diseases of the lungs due to fungi and organic dusts. Basel, Switzerland, S. Karger, 1969, p. 147.

3365. *Air Quality Criteria for Sulfur Oxides.* National Air Pollution Control Administration (Publication No. AP-50.) U.S. Dept. of Health, Education and Welfare. January, 1969.

3366. Bates, D. V.: Health effects of oxidants. J. Occup. Med., *10*:480–482, 1968.

3367. McCormick, P. W., Hay, R. G., and Griffin, R. W.: Pulmonary aspiration of gastric contents in obstetric patients. Lancet, *1*:1127–1130, 1966.

3368. Knudson, R. J., Badger, T. L., and Gaensler, E. A.: Eosinophilic granuloma of the lung. Med. Thorac., *23*:248–262, 1966.

3369. Stewart, T. W.: Dermatomyositis with alveolar cell carcinoma. Acta Dermatovener., *44*:118–121, 1964.

3370. Ellis, R. H.: Leukaemic infiltrations of the lungs. Brit. J. Dis. Chest, *59*:37–38, 1965.

3371. Lewis, J. G.: Eosinophilic granuloma and its variants with special reference to lung involvement. A report of 12 patients. Quart. J. Med., *33*:337–359, 1964.

3372. Beumer, H. M., and Porton, W. M.: Diffuse eosinophilic granuloma of the lungs. Acta Tuberc. Scand., *46*:153–158, 1965.

3373. Chusid, E. L.: Pulmonary eosinophilic granuloma. Aspects of pulmonary function. J. Mount Sinai Hosp., *33*:116–124, 1966.

3374. Ussher, C. W. J.: Primary pulmonary eosinophilic granuloma. A report of two patients. J. Roy. Nav. Med. Serv., *51*:241–248, 1965.

3375. Hutas, I.: Respiratory function in lung tumors. Prax. Pneumol., *18*:396–403, 1964.

3376. Mechir, J., and Cunderlik, J.: Visco-elastic properties of the lungs in lung carcinoma. Rozhl. Tuberk., *26*:42–50, 1966.

3377. Brady, L. W., Germon, P. A., and Cander, L.: The effects of radiation therapy on pulmonary function in carcinoma of the lung. Radiology, *85*:130–134, 1965.

3378. Pudelski, J., Oklek, K., and Moszner, S.: Study of ventilation in patients with carcinoma of the lung. Gruzlica, *36*:623–630, 1968.

3379. Spiegel, J. A.: Endoarterial choriocarcinoma of the lung. Report of a case and review of the literature. Obstet. Gynec., *24*:740–748, 1964.

3380. Winterbauer, R. H., Elfenbein, I. B., and Ball, W. C., Jr.: Incidence and clinical significance of tumor embolization to the lungs. Amer. J. Med., *45*:271–290, 1968.

3381. Nicodemowicz, E., Saunier, C., and Sadoul, P.: Respiratory exchange in patients with chronic pulmonary tuberculosis. Rev. Tuberc., *30*:55–70, 1966.

3382. Abe, M.: Studies of pulmonary function in pulmonary tuberculosis. Sapporo Med. J., *28*:127–143, 1965.

3383. Koike, S., Shiozawa, M., Kobayashi, E., Yajima, R., Imura, I., and Niwaji, F.: Pulmonary function in senile tuberculosis. Jap. J. Chest Dis., *26*:22–30, 1967.

3384. Martin, C. J., Cochran, T. H., and Katsura, S.: Tuberculosis, emphysema, and bronchitis. Amer. Rev. Resp. Dis., *97*:1089–1094, 1968.

3385. Kjellman, B.: Regional lung function studied with Xe^{133} in children with pneumonia. Acta Paediat. Scand., *56*:467–476, 1967.

3386. Tyrrell, D. A. J.: Acute respiratory diseases. Symposium organised by the College of Pathologists, London 1968. London, B.M.A. House, 1968, p. 134.

3387. Jones, R. S., Owen-Thomas, J. B., and Bouton, M. J.: Severe bronchopneumonia in the young child. Arch. Dis. Child., *43*:415–422, 1968.

3388. Knyvett, A. F.: Pulmonary calcifications following varicella. Amer. Rev. Resp. Dis., *92*:210–214, 1965.

3389. Sargent, E. N., Carson, M. J., and Reilly, E. D.: Varicella pneumonia. A report of 20 cases, with postmortem examination in six. Calif. Med., *107*:141–148, 1967.

3390. Triebwasser, J. H., Harris, R. E., Bryant, R. E., and Phoades, E. R.: Varicella pneumonia in adults. Report of seven cases and a review of the literature. Medicine, *46*:409–423, 1967.

3391. Van Gastel, C., Bangma, P. J., and Kreukniet, J.: Oxygen diffusion impairment as a sequel in a case of varicella pneumonia treated with adrenocortical steroids. Folia Med. Neerl., *11*:35–39, 1968.

3392. Krieger, I., and Whitten, C. F.: Work of respiration in bronchiolitis. Amer. J. Dis. Child., *107*:386–392, 1964.

3393. Simpson, H., and Flenley, D. C.: Arterial blood-gas tensions and pH in acute lower respiratory tract infections in infancy and childhood. Lancet, *1*:7–12, 1967.

3394. Phelan, P. D., Williams, H. E., and Freeman, M.: The disturbances of ventilation in acute viral bronchiolitis. Aust. Paediat. J., *4*:96–104, 1968.

3395. Klocke, R. A., Artenstein, M. S., Green, R. W., Dennery, J. J., and Richert, J. H.: The effect of acute respiratory infection on pulmonary function in military recruits. Amer. Rev. Resp. Dis., *93*:549–555, 1966.

3396. Acute infections of the lower respiratory tract in infancy. (Lancet leading article.) Lancet, *1*:354–355, 1969.

3397. Bocles, J. S., Ehrenkranz, N. J., and Marks, A.: Abnormalities of respiratory function in varicella pneumonia. Ann. Intern. Med., *60*:183–195, 1964.

3398. Manfredi, F.: Extracellular and intracellular acid-base relations in patients with chronic anemia. Amer. Rev. Resp. Dis., *92*:617–623, 1965.

3399. Housley, E.: Respiratory gas exchange in chronic anaemia. Clin. Sci., *32*:19–26, 1967.

3400. Lertzmann, M., Frome, B. M., Israels, L. G., and Cherniack, R. M.: Hypoxia in polycythemia vera. Ann. Intern. Med., *60*:409–417, 1964.

3401. Murray, J. F.: Arterial studies in primary and secondary polycythemic disorders. Amer. Rev. Resp. Dis., *92*:435–449, 1965.

3402. Bjure, J., Paulin, S., Soderholm, B., and Wilhelmsen, L.: Pulmonary gas exchange and hemodynamics in patients with recurrent pulmonary embolism and polycythemia vera. Cor Vasa, *9*:34–47, 1967.

3403. Larson, R. K., and Gordinier, R.: Pulmonary alveolar proteinosis. Ann. Intern. Med., *62*:292–312, 1965.

3404. Ramirez, R. J., and Campbell, G. D.: Pulmonary alveolar proteinosis. Endobronchial treatment. Ann. Intern. Med., *63*:429–441, 1965.

3405. Fujimoto, K.: An autopsy case of chronic pneumonitis with alveolar lipoid-proteinosis. J. Kumamoto Med. Soc., *39*:40–55, 1964.

3406. Divertie, M. B., Brown, A. L., Jr., and Harrison, E. G., Jr.: Pulmonary alveolar proteinosis. Two cases studied by electron microscopy. Amer. J. Med., *40*:351–359, 1966.

3407. Ramirez, R. J.: Bronchopulmonary lavage. New techniques and observations. Dis. Chest, *50*:581–588, 1966.

3408. Ramirez, R. J.: Pulmonary alveolar proteinosis. Treatment by massive bronchopulmonary lavage. Arch. Intern. Med., *119*:147–156, 1967.

3409. Wasserman, K., Blank, N., and Fletcher, G.: Lung lavage (alveolar washing) in alveolar proteinosis. Amer. J. Med., *44*:611–617, 1968.

3410. Heard, B. E., and Cooke, R. A.: Busulphan lung. Thorax, *23*:187–193, 1968.
3411. Littler, W. A., Kay, J. M., Hasleton, P. S., and Heath, D.: Busulphan lung. Thorax, *24*:639–655, 1969.
3412. Keltz, H.: The effect of respiratory muscle dysfunction on pulmonary function. Amer. Rev. Resp. Dis., *91*:934–938, 1965.
3413. Davis, J. N.: Contribution of somatic receptors in the chest wall to detection of added inspiratory airway resistance. Clin. Sci., *33*:249–260, 1967.
3414. Fluck, D. C.: Chest movements in hemiplegia. Clin. Sci., *31*:383–388, 1966.
3415. Gould, L., Kaplan, S., McElhinney, A. J., and Stone, D. J.: A method for the production of hemidiaphragmatic paralysis. Its application to the study of lung function in normal man. Amer. Rev. Resp. Dis., *96*:812–814, 1967.
3416. Siegfried, J., and Pitteloud, J.: Study of pulmonary function in Parkinsonian patients prior to and following stereotaxic operations on the thalamus. Confin. Neurol., *25*:227–233, 1965.
3417. Neu, H. C., Connolly, J. J., Jr., Schwertley, F. W., Ladwig, H. A., and Brody, A. W.: Obstructive respiratory dysfunction in Parkinsonian patients. Amer. Rev. Resp. Dis., *95*:33–47, 1967.
3418. Buchsbaum, H. W., Martin, W. A., Turino, G. M., and Rowland, L. P.: Chronic alveolar hypoventilation due to muscular dystrophy. Neurology, *18*:319–327, 1968.
3419. Haas, A., Rusk, H. A., Pelesof, H., and Adam, J. R.: Respiratory function in hemiplegic patients. Arch. Phys. Med., *48*:174–179, 1967.
3420. Januszkiewicz, J.: Involvement of the respiratory tract in trichinosis. Przegl. Epidem., *21*:307–316, 1967.
3421. Fuleihan, F. J. D., Abboud, R. T., Balikian, J. P., and Nucho, C. K. N.: Pulmonary alveolar microlithiasis: lung function in five cases. Thorax, *24*:84–90, 1969.
3422. Portnoy, L. M., Amadeo, B., and Hennigar, G. R.: Pulmonary alveolar microlithiasis. An unusual case (associated with milk-alkali syndrome). Amer. J. Clin. Path., *41*:194–201, 1964.
3423. Rotem, Y., Solomon, M., and Hertz-Frankenhuis, M.: Pulmonary alveolar microlithiasis. Ann. Paediat., *201*:4–12, 1963.
3424. Roher, H.: Mikrolithiasis alveolaris pulmonum. Med. Welt, *42*:2395–2400, 1965.
3425. Oka, S., Shiraishi, K., Ogata, K., Goto, Y., Yasuda, T., and Yanagihara, H.: Pulmonary alveolar microlithiasis. Report of three cases. Amer. Rev. Resp. Dis., *93*:612–616, 1966.
3426. Kamada, T.: Pulmonary alveolar microlithiasis. Hiroshima J. Med. Sci., *15*:95–102, 1966.
3427. Burguet, W., and Reginster, A.: The heredity of alveolar microlithiasis of the lungs, with a report of a new familial case. Ann. Genet., *10*:75–81, 1967.
3428. Mariani, B., and Bassi, A.: Current knowledge of pulmonary alveolar microlithiasis (Malpighi's Disease). Minerva Med., *58*:3761–3766, 1967.
3429. Morandi, D.: Pneumolithiasis (Microlithiasis alveolaris pulmonum). Respiration, *25*:184–199, 1968.
3430. Jach, S.: Venous acinar angioma of the lung. Pol. Przegl. Radiol., *28*:45–52, 1964.
3431. Duprez, A.: Pulmonary arteriovenous communications. Acta Chir. Belg., *62*:1013–1026, 1963.
3432. Meissner, F., and Schippan, R.: Arteriovenous pulmonary fistulas in childhood. Paediat. Grenzgeb., *4*:149–166, 1965.
3433. Jeresaty, R. M., Knight, H. F., and Hart, W. E.: Pulmonary arteriovenous fistulas in childhood. Amer. J. Dis. Child., *111*:256–261, 1966.
3434. Gautam, H. P.: Pulmonary arteriovenous fistula. Intern. Surg., *46*:168–175, 1966.
3435. Beresford, O. D.: Hereditary haemorrhagic telangiectasia with pulmonary arteriovenous fistula. Brit. J. Dis. Chest., *61*:219–220, 1967.
3436. Shields, L. H.: A case report of mediastinal neurogenic neoplasm containing arteriovenous fistulas. Dis. Chest, *4*:441–449, 1967.
3437. Krebs, T., and Buhlmeyer, K.: Pulmonary arteriovenous fistula in childhood and its complications. Mschr. Kinderheilk., *116*:459–465, 1968.
3438. Massumi, R. A., and Winnaker, J. L.: Severe depression of the respiratory center in myxedema. Amer. J. Med., *36*:876–882, 1964.
3439. Watts, R. S., and Curran, W. S.: Hypoventilation and myxedema. Rocky Mountain Med. J., *64*:54–57, 1967.
3440. Massey, D. G., Becklake, M. R., McKenzie, J. M., and Bates, D. V.: Circulatory and ventilatory response to exercise in thyrotoxicosis. New Engl. J. Med., *276*:1104–1112, 1967.
3441. Bukhman, A. I., and Balabolkin, M. I.: Clinical and X-ray examination of the external respiratory apparatus in patients with Itsenko-Cushing's Disease. Probl. Endokr. Gormonoter., *12*:20–26, 1966.
3442. Karlish, A. J., Marshall, R., Reid, L., and Sherlock, S.: Cyanosis with hepatic cirrhosis. Thorax, *22*:555–561, 1967.
3443. Ruff, F., Picken, J. J., Aronoff, A., Milic-Emili, J., and Bates, D. V.: Regional distribution of pulmonary ventilation and perfusion in patients with liver cirrhosis. (Abstract). J. Clin. Invest., *48*:71a, 1969.
3444. Cotes, J. E., Field, G. B., Brown, G. J. A., and Read, A. E.: Impairment of lung function after portacaval anastomosis. Lancet, *1*:952–955, 1968.
3445. Berthelot, P., Walker, J. G., Sherlock, S., and Reid, L.: Arterial changes in the lungs in cirrhosis of the liver–lung spider naevi. New Engl. J. Med., *274*:291–298, 1966.
3446. Karetzky, M. S., and Mithoefer, J. C.: The cause of hyperventilation and arterial hypoxia in patients with cirrhosis of the liver. Amer. J. Med. Sci., *254*:797–804, 1967.
3447. Wilder, C. E., Morrison, R. S., and Tyler, J. M.: Relationship between serum sodium and hyperventilation in cirrhosis. Amer. Rev. Resp. Dis., *96*:971–976, 1967.
3448. Jordanoglou, J., and Pride, N. B.: A comparison of maximum inspiratory and expiratory flow in health and in lung disease. Thorax, *23*:38–45, 1968.
3449. Simonsson, B. G., and Malmberg, R.: Differentiation between localized and generalized airway obstruction. Thorax, *19*:416–419, 1964.
3450. Cantrell, J. R., and Guild, H. G.: Congenital stenosis of the trachea. Amer. J. Surg., *108*:297–305, 1964.
3451. Illig, H.: The hyperventilation syndrome. Munchen Med. Wschr., *106*:1276–1281, 1964.
3452. Suzuki, K., et al.: A case of hyperventilation syndrome. Resp. Circulat., *12*:597–603, 1964.
3453. Weimann, G., and Georg, D.: The prognosis of the hyperventilation syndrome. Med. Welt, *11*:710–715, 1968.
3454. *Current Concepts of acid-base measurement.* Ann. N.Y. Acad. Sci., *133*, 1966.
3455. Bartels, H., Bucherl, E., Hertz, C. W., Rodewald, G., and Schwab, M.: Methods in Pulmonary Physiology (translated by J. M. Workman). New York, Hofner Publishing Co. Inc., 1963.
3456. Brockett, N. C., Jr., Cohen, J. J., and Schwartz, W. B.: Carbon dioxide titration curve of normal man. New Engl. J. Med., *272*:6–12, 1965.
3457. Michel, C. C., Lloyd, B. B., and Cunningham, D. J. C.: The in vivo carbon dioxide dissociation curve of the plasma. Resp. Physiol., *1*:121–137, 1966.
3458. Prys-Roberts, C., Kelman, G. R., and Nunn, J. F.: Determination of the in vivo carbon dioxide titration curve of anaesthetized man. Brit. J. Anaesth., *38*:500–509, 1966.
3459. Lenfant, C., Ways, P., Aucutt, C., and Cruz, J.: Effect of chronic hypoxic hypoxia on the O_2Hb Dissociation curve and respiratory gas transport in man. Resp. Physiol., *7*:7–29, 1969.
3460. Berglund, E., Malmberg, R., Simonsson, B., and Stenhagen, S.: Different methods for estimating arterial oxygen tension in man. Scand. J. Resp. Dis., *47*:209–214, 1966.
3461. Kelman, G. R.: Computer programme for the production of O_2–CO_2 diagrams. Resp. Physiol., *4*:260–269, 1968.
3462. Holling, H. E., McDonald, I., O'Halloren, J. A., and Venner, A.: Reliability of a spectrophotometric method of estimating blood oxygen. J. Appl. Physiol., *8*:249–254, 1955.
3463. Bjure, J., and Nilsson, N. J.: Spectrophotometric determi-

nation of oxygen saturation of hemoglobin in the presence of carboxyhemoglobin. Scand. J. Lab. Invest., *17*:491-500, 1965.

3464. Stainsby, W. N., Fales, J. T., and Lilienthal, J. L., Jr.: A rapid spectrophotometric method for determining oxygen content of dog's blood. J. Appl. Physiol., *7*:577-579, 1955.

3465. McIlroy, M. B., Crawford, D. W., Jennings, D. B., and Naimark, A.: Assessment of cardiac function using resaturation curves. J. Appl. Physiol., *21*:1561-1567, 1966.

3466. Wood, E. H.: Diagnostic applications of indicator-dilution techniques in congenital heart disease. Circ. Res., *10*:531-568, 1962.

3467. Nakamura, T., Katori, R., Watanabe, T., Miyazawa, K., Murai, M., Oda, J., and Ishikawa, K.: Quantitation of left-to-right shunt from a single earpiece dye-dilution curve. J. Appl. Physiol., *22*:1156-1160, 1967.

3468. McCredie, R. M., and Jose, A. D.: Analysis of carbon monoxide and oxygen by gas chromatography. J. Appl. Physiol., *22*:863-866, 1967.

3469. Ayers, S. M., Criscitiello, A., and Giannelli, S., Jr.: Determination of blood carbon monoxide content by gas chromatography. J. Appl. Physiol., *21*:1368-1370, 1966.

3470. Albers, C., and Farhi, L. E.: In: *Lectures on Gas Chromatography: Agricultural and Biological Applications* (1964) (edited by L. R. Mottick and H. A. Szymonski). New York, 1965.

3471. Albers, C., and Farhi, L. E.: Resche und zuverlässige Bestimmung des Sauerstoffgehaltes in Blut mittels Gaschromatographie. Z. Ges. Exp. Med., *139*:485-505, 1965.

3472. Lenfant, C., and Aucutt, C.: Measurement of blood gases by chromatography. Resp. Physiol., *1*:398-407, 1966.

3473. Ortega, F. G., Orie, S. A. M., and Tammeling, G. J.: Determination of carbon dioxide content of blood by infrared analysis. J. Appl. Physiol., *21*:1377-1380, 1966.

3474. Mayers, L. B., and Forster, R. E.: A rapid method for measuring blood oxygen content utilizing the oxygen electrode. J. Appl. Physiol., *21*:1393-1396, 1966.

3475. Laver, M. B., Murphy, A. J., Seifen, A., and Radford, E. P., Jr.: Blood O_2 content measurements using the oxygen electrode. J. Appl. Physiol., *22*:1063-1069, 1967.

3476. Laver, M. B.: Blood O_2 content measured with the Po_2 electrode: a modification. J. Appl. Physiol., *22*:1017-1019, 1967.

3477. Tucker, V. A.: Method for oxygen content and dissociation curves on microliter blood samples. J. Appl. Physiol., *23*:410-414, 1967.

3478. Theye, R. A.: Blood O_2 content measuring using the O_2 electrode. Anesthesiology, *28*:773-775, 1967.

3479. Klingenmaier, C. H., Behar, M. G., and Smith, T. C.: Blood oxygen content measured by oxygen tension after release by carbon monoxide. J. Appl. Physiol., *26*:653-655, 1969.

3480. Maio, D. A., and Neville, J. R.: Polarographic determination of oxygen content and capacity in a single blood sample. J. Appl. Physiol., *20*:774-778, 1965.

3481. Silver, I. A.: A simple micro-cathode for measuring Po_2 in gas or fluid. Med. Electron. Biol. Engin., *1*:547-551, 1963.

3482. Fatt, I.: An ultramicro oxygen electrode. J. Appl. Physiol., *19*:326-329, 1964.

3483. Saito, Y.: A sputtered Pt film electrode for polarographic O_2 measurement. J. Appl. Physiol., *23*:979-983, 1967.

3484. Hedley-Whyte, J., Radford, E. P., Jr., and Laver, M. B.: Nomogram for temperature correction of electrode calibration during Po_2 measurements. J. Appl. Physiol., *20*:785-786, 1965.

3485. LeFevre, M. E.: Calibration of Clark oxygen electrode for use in aqueous solutions. J. Appl. Physiol., *26*:844-846, 1969.

3486. Bishop, J. M., Pincock, A. C., Hollyhock, A., Raine, J., and Cole, R. B.: Factors affecting the measurement of the partial pressure of oxygen in blood using a covered electrode system. Res. Physiol. *1*:225-237, 1966.

3487. Heitmann, H., Buckles, R. G., and Laver, M. B.: Blood Po_2 measurements: performance of microelectrodes. Resp. Physiol., *3*:380-395, 1967.

3488. Flenley, D. C., Millar, J. S., and Rees, H. A.: Accuracy of oxygen and carbon dioxide electrodes. Brit. Med. J., *2*:349-352, 1967.

3489. Moran, F., Kettel, L. J., and Cugell, D. W.: Measurement of blood Po_2 with the microcathode electrode. J. Appl. Physiol., *21*:725-728, 1966.

3490. Rhodes, P. G., and Moser, K. M.: Sources of error in oxygen tension measurement. J. Appl. Physiol., *21*:729-734, 1966.

3491. Schuler, R., and Kreuzer, F.: Rapid polarographic in vivo oxygen catheter electrodes. Resp. Physiol., *3*:90-110, 1967.

3492. Kelman, G. R., and Nunn, J. F.: Nomograms for correction of blood Po_2, Pco_2, pH, and base excess for time and temperature. J. Appl. Physiol., *21*:1484-1490, 1966.

3493. Hedley-Whyte, J., and Laver, M. B.: O_2 solubility in blood and temperature correction factors for Po_2. J. Appl. Physiol., *19*:901-906, 1964.

3494. Kelman, G. R.: A theoretical study of factors affecting the in vivo Po_2 temperature coefficient. Resp. Physiol., *4*:301-308, 1968.

3495. Woldring, B., Owens, G., and Woolford, D. C.: Blood gases: continuous in vivo recording of partial pressures by mass spectrography. Science, *153*:885-887, 1966.

3496. Bioelectrodes (edited by W. Feder). Ann. N.Y. Acad. Sci., *148*:287, 1968.

3497. Burwell, S. C., and Robinson, G. C.: A method for the determination of the amount of oxygen and carbon dioxide in mixed venous blood of man. J. Clin. Invest., *1*:47-63, 1924.

3498. Cerretelli, P., Sikand, R., and Farhi, L. E.: Readjustments in cardiac output and gas exchange during onset of exercise and recovery. J. Appl. Physiol., *21*:1345-1350, 1966.

3499. Cerretelli, P., Cruz, J. C., Farhi, L. E., and Rahn, H.: Determination of mixed venous O_2 and CO_2 tensions and cardiac output by a rebreathing method. Resp. Physiol., *1*:258-264, 1966.

3500. Farhi, L. E., and Haab, P.: Mixed venous blood gas tensions and cardiac output by "bloodless" methods; recent developments and appraisal. Resp. Physiol., *2*:225-233, 1967.

3501. Jones, N. L., Campbell, E. J. M., McHardy, G. J. R., Higgs, B. E., and Clode, M.: The estimation of carbon dioxide pressure of mixed venous blood during exercise. Clin. Sci., *32*:311-327, 1967.

3502. Kim, T. S., Rahn, H., and Farhi, L. E.: Estimation of the venous and arterial Pco_2 by gas analysis of a single breath. J. Appl. Physiol., *21*:1338-1344, 1966.

3503. Gurtner, G. H., Song, S. H., and Farhi, L. E.: Alveolar to mixed venous Pco_2 difference under conditions of no gas exchange. Resp. Physiol., *7*:173-187, 1969.

3504. Jones, N. J., Campbell, E. J. M., Edwards, R. H. T., and Wilkoff, W. G.: Alveolar to blood Pco_2 difference during rebreathing in exercise. J. Appl. Physiol., *27*:356-360, 1969.

3505. Denison, D., Edwards, R. H. T., Jones, G., and Pope, H.: Direct and rebreathing estimates of the O_2 and CO_2 pressure in mixed venous blood. Resp. Physiol., *7*:326-334, 1969.

3506. Owen, J. A. Dudley, H. A. F., and Masterton, J. P.: Acid-base status assessed from measurements of hydrogen ion concentration and Pco_2. Lancet, *2*:660-661, 1965.

3507. Lal, S., Gebbie, T., and Campbell, E. J. M.: Simple methods for improving the value of oximetry in the study of pulmonary oxygen uptake. Thorax, *21*:50-56, 1966.

3508. Miller, J. N., and Tutt, P.: A comparison of four blood gas analysis systems in working conditions. Biomed. Engin., *2*:456-460, 1967.

3509. Eldridge, F., and Fretwell, L. K.: Change in O_2 tension of shed blood at various temperatures. J. Appl. Physiol., *20*:790-792, 1965.

3510. MacIntyre, J., Norman, J. N., and Smith, G.: Use of capillary blood in measurement of arterial Po_2. Brit. Med. J., *2*:640-643, 1968.

3511. Sinclair, M. J., Hart, R. A., Pope, H. M., and Campbell, E. J. M.: The use of the Henderson-Hasselbalch equation in routine medical practice. Clin. Chim. Acta, *19*:63-69, 1968.

3512. Ortega, F. G., and Tammeling, G. J.: A recirculation system for the determination of blood gases by gas chromatography. J. Appl. Physiol., *24*:119–123, 1968.
3513. Sorbini, C. A., Grassi, V., Solinas, E., and Muiesan, G.: Arterial oxygen tension in relation to age in healthy subjects. Respiration, *25*:3–10, 1968.
3514. Coburn, R. F., Blakemore, W. S., and Forster, R. E.: Endogenous carbon monoxide production in man. J. Clin. Invest., *42*:1172–1178, 1963.
3515. Coburn, R. F., Danielson, G. K., Blakemore, W. S., and Forster, R. E.: Carbon monoxide in blood: analytical method and sources of error. J. Appl. Physiol., *19*:510–515, 1964.
3516. *Aging of the Lung*. The Tenth Hahnemann Symposium (edited by L. Cander). New York and London, Grune and Stratton, p. 371.
3517. Anderson, T. W., Brown, J. R., Hall, J. W., and Shephard, J. T.: The limitations of linear regressions for the prediction of vital capacity and forced expiratory volume. Respiration, *25*:140–158, 1968.
3518. Anderson, T. W., and Shephard, R. J.: Normal values for single breath diffusing capacity—the influence of age, body size, and smoking habits. Respiration, *26*:1–7, 1969.
3519. Armstrong, B. W., Hurt, H. H., Jr., Palumbo, L., Workman, J. M., and Hanes, B.: Normal pulmonary D_{O_2}; a 10-year follow-up and an analysis of its errors. J. Appl. Physiol., *23*:902–910, 1967.
3520. Cotes, J. E., Rossiter, C. E., Higgins, I.T.T., and Gilson, J. C.: Average normal values for the forced expiratory volume in white Caucasian males. Brit. Med. J., *1*:1016–1019, 1966.
3521. Diament, M. L., and Palmer, K. N. V.: An analysis of preoperative Pa_{O_2} in a general surgical population. Thorax, *24*:126–128, 1969.
3522. Edelman, N. H., Mittman, C., Norris, A. H., and Shock, N. W.: Effects of respiratory pattern on age differences in ventilation uniformity. J. Appl. Physiol., *24*:49–53, 1968.
3523. Hoffbrand, B. I.: The expiratory capnogram: a measure of ventilation-perfusion inequalities. Thorax, *21*:518–523, 1966.
3524. Loew, P. G., and Thews, G.: Die Altersabhängigkeit des arteriellen Sauerstoffdruckes bei der berufstätigen Bevölkerung. Klin. Wschr., *40*:1093–1098, 1962.
3525. McClements, B., and Bodman, R.: Blood gas measurement. Lancet, *2*:112, 1968.
3526. Mellemgaard, K.: Alveolar-arterial oxygen difference: size and components in normal man. Acta Physiol. Scand., *67*:10–20, 1966.
3527. Pierce, J. A.: Tensile strength of human lung. J. Lab. Clin. Med., *66*:652–658, 1965.
3528. Podlesch, I., and Stevanovic, M.: Die Altersabhängigkeit der Diffusionskapazität der Lunge in Ruhe und während Belastung. Med. Thor., *23*:144–159, 1966.
3529. Pyorala, K., Heinonen, A. O., and Karvonen, M. J.: Pulmonary function in former endurance athletes. Acta Med. Scand., *183*:263–273, 1968.
3530. Shephard, R. J.: World standards of cardiorespiratory performance. Arch. Environ. Health, *13*:664–672, 1966.
3531. Sherrer, M., and Birchler, A.: Altersabhängigkeit des alveolo-arteriellen O_2—Partialdruckgradienten bei Schewarbeit in Normoxie, Hypoxie und Hyperoxie. Med. Thorac., *24*:99–117, 1967.
3532. Stanescu, S., Dutu, S. T., Jienescu, Z., Hartia, L., Nicolescu, N., and Sacerdoteanu, F.: Investigations into changes of pulmonary function in the aged. Respiration, *25*:232–242, 1968.
3533. Tlustý, L.: Physical fitness in old age. Respiration, *26*:161–182, 1969.
3534. von Dobeln, W., Astrand, I., and Bergstrom, A.: Analysis of age and other factors related to maximal oxygen uptake. J. Appl. Physiol., *22*:934–938, 1967.
3535. Kohn, R. H.: Changes in connective tissue. *In: Aging of the Lung (see* reference 3516).
3536. Anderson, T. W., and Shephard, R. J.: Physical training and exercise diffusing capacity. Int. Z. Angew. Physiol., *25*:198–209, 1968.
3537. Anderson, T. W., and Shephard, R. J.: The effects of hyperventilation and exercise upon the pulmonary diffusing capacity. Respiration, *25*:465–484, 1968.
3538. Anderson, T. W., and Shephard, R. J.: A theoretical study of some errors in the measurement of pulmonary diffusing capacity. Respiration, *26*:102–115, 1969.
3539. Arndt, H., King, T. K. C., and Briscoe, W. A.: Diffusing capacities and ventilation:perfusion ratios in patients with the clinical syndrome of alveolar capillary block. J. Clin. Invest., *49*:408–422, 1970.
3540. Arndt, H., Buchta, I., and Baltzer, G.: Die anderung der Blutgas—Partialdrucke und des pH im menschliche Blut während der Aufbewahrung bei verscheidenen Temperaturen. Respiration, *25*:306–322, 1968.
3541. Auchincloss, J. H., Jr., Gilbert, R., and Baule, G. H.: Unsteady-state measurement of oxygen transfer during treadmill exercise. J. Appl. Physiol., *25*:283–293, 1968.
3542. Bosman, A. R., Lee, G. de J., and Marshall, R.: The effect of pulsatile capillary blood flow upon gas exchange within the lungs of man. Clin. Sci., *28*:295–309, 1965.
3543. Brashear, R. E., Ross, J. C., and Daly, W. J.: Pulmonary diffusion and capillary blood volume in dogs at rest and with exercise. J. Appl. Physiol., *21*:516–520, 1966.
3544. Burgess, J. H., Gillespie, J., Graf, P. D., and Nadel, J. A.: Effect of pulmonary vascular pressures on single breath CO diffusing capacity. J. Appl. Physiol., *24*:692–696, 1968.
3545. Cerretelli, P., Sikand, R. S., and Farhi, L. E.: Effect of increased airway resistance on ventilation and gas exchange during exercise. J. Appl. Physiol., *27*:597–600, 1969.
3546. Cinkotai, F. F., and Thomson, M. L.: Diurnal variation in pulmonary diffusing capacity for carbon monoxide. J. Appl. Physiol., *21*:539–542, 1966.
3547. Cole, R. B., and Bishop, J. M.: Variation in alveolar-arterial O_2 tension difference at high levels of alveolar O_2 tension. J. Appl. Physiol., *22*:685–693, 1967.
3548. Cree, E. M., Benfield, J. R., and Rasmussen, H. K.: Differential lung diffusion, capillary volume and compliance in dogs. J. Appl. Physiol., *25*:186–190, 1968.
3549. Danzer, L. A., Cohn, J. E., and Zechman, W. F.: Relationship of D_M and Y_c to pulmonary diffusing capacity during exercise. Resp. Physiol., *5*:250–258, 1968.
3550. De Graff, A. C., Jr., and Romans, W.: Programmed valve sequencer and alveolar gas sampler for lung CO diffusing capacity measurements. J. Appl. Physiol., *23*:415–418, 1967.
3551. Di Prampero, P. E., and Margaria, R.: Relationship between O_2 consumption, high energy phosphates, and the kinetics of O_2 debt in exercise. Pflüger. Arch. Ges. Physiol., *304*:11–19, 1968.
3552. Downes, J. J., and Lambertsen, C. J.: Dynamic characteristics of ventilatory depression in man on abrupt administration of O_2. J. Appl. Physiol., *21*:447–453, 1966.
3553. Dunnill, M. S.: Effect of lung inflation on alveolar surface area in dog. Nature, *214*:1013–1014, 1967.
3554. Farhi, L. E., and Yokoyama, T.: The effects of ventilation/perfusion inequality on the elimination of inert gases. Resp. Physiol., *3*:12–20, 1967.
3555. Ferris, B. G., Jr., Anderson, D. O., and Zickmantel, R.: Prediction values for screening tests of pulmonary function. Amer. Rev. Resp. Dis., *91*:252–261, 1965.
3556. Filley, G. F., Bigelow, D. B., Olson, D. E., and Lacquet, L. M.: Pulmonary gas transport. A mathematical model of the lung. Amer. Rev. Resp. Dis., *98*:480–489, 1968.
3557. Frech, W. E., Schulte-Hinrichs, D., Vogel, H. R., and Thews, G.: Experiments on models to determine exchange of respiratory gases. Pflüger. Archiv. Ges Physiol., *301*:293–301, 1968.
3558. Freyschuss, U., and Holmgren, A.: Variation of $D_{L_{CO}}$ with increasing oxygen uptake during exercise in healthy ordinarily untrained young men and women. Acta Physiol. Scand., *65*:193–206, 1965.
3559. Gaensler, E. A., and Wright, G. W.: Evaluation of respiratory impairment. Arch. Environ. Health, *12*:146–189, 1966.
3560. Giammona, S. T., and Daly, W. J.: Pulmonary diffusing capacity in normal children ages 4 to 13. Amer. J. Dis. Child., *110*:144–151, 1965.
3561. Golbert, R., Auchincloss, J. H., and Baule, G. H.: Metabolic and circulatory adjustments to unsteady-state exercise. J. Appl. Physiol., *22*:905–912, 1967.

3562. Grover, R. F., and Reeves, J. T.: Exercise performance of athletes at sea level and 3100 meters altitude. Med. Thorac., *23:*129–143, 1966.
3563. Grover, R. F., Reeves, J. T., Grover, E. B., and Leathers, J. E.: Muscular exercise in young men native to 3100 meter altitude. J. Appl. Physiol., *22:*555–564, 1967.
3564. Guyatt, A. R., Newman, F., Cinkotai, F. F., Palmer, J. I., and Thomson, M. L.: Pulmonary diffusing capacity in man during immersion in water. J. Appl. Physiol., *20:*878–881, 1965.
3565. Hesser, C. M., and Matell, G.: Effect of light and moderate exercise on alveolar–arterial O_2 tension difference in man. Acta Physiol. Scand., *63:*247–256, 1965.
3566. Holmgren, A.: Measurements of the diffusing capacity of the lung for carbon monoxide. Scand. J. Clin. Lab. Invest., *17:*110–116, 117–122, 123–129, 1965.
3567. Holmgren, A.: Variation of D_{Lco} with increasing oxygen uptake during exercise in healthy trained young men and women. Acta Physiol. Scand., *65:*207–220, 1965.
3568. Holmgren, A., and Astrand, P.: D_L and dimensions and functional capacities of the O_2 transport system in humans. J. Appl. Physiol., *21:*1463–1470, 1966.
3569. Johnson, R. L.: Pulmonary diffusion as a limiting factor in exercise stress. Supplement 1 to Circulation Research, Vols. 20 and 21, 1967.
3570. Jones, N. L.: Exercise testing. Brit. J. Dis. Chest, *61:*169–189, 1967.
3571. Jouasset-Strieder, D., Cahill, J. M., Byrne, J. J., and Gaensler, E. A.: Pulmonary diffusing capacity and capillary blood volume in normal and anemic dogs. J. Appl. Physiol., *20:*113–116, 1965.
3572. Meade, F., Saunders, M. J., Hyett, F., Reynolds, J. A., Pearl, N., and Cotes, J. E.: Automatic measurement of lung function. Lancet, *2:*573–575, 1965.
3573. Menkes, H. A., Sera, K., Rogers, R. M., Hyde, R. W., Forster, R. E., and DuBois, A. B.: Pulsatile uptake of CO in the human lung. J. Clin. Invest., *49:*335–345, 1970.
3574. Miller, J. M., and Johnson, R. L.: Effect of lung inflation on pulmonary diffusing capacity at rest and exercise. J. Clin. Invest., *45:*493–500, 1966.
3575. Mittman, C.: Non-uniform pulmonary diffusing capacity measured by sequential CO uptake and washout. J. Appl. Physiol., *23:*131, 1967.
3576. Nairn, J., Power, C., Hyde, R., Forster, R. E., Lambertsen, C. J., and Dickson, J.: Diffusing capacity (D_{Lco}) and pulmonary capillary blood flow (F_c) at hyperbaric pressures. J. Clin. Invest., *44:*1591–1600, 1965.
3577. Piiper, J., and Sikand, R.: Diffusing capacity for CO by single breath method in inhomogeneous lungs. Resp. Physiol., *1:*75–87, 1966.
3578. Puy, R. J. M., Hyde, R. W., Fisher, A. B., Clark, J. M., Dickson, J., and Lambertsen, C. J.: Alterations in the pulmonary capillary bed during early O_2 toxicity in man. J. Appl. Physiol., *24:*537–543, 1968.
3579. Remmers, J. E., and Mithoefer, J. C.: The carbon monoxide diffusing capacity in permanent residents at high altitudes. Resp. Physiol., *6:*233–244, 1969.
3580. Reuschlein, P. S., Reddan, W. G., Burpee, J., Gee, J. B. L., and Rankin, J.: Effect of physical training on the pulmonary diffusing capacity during submaximal work. J. Appl. Physiol., *24:*152–158, 1968.
3581. Rochester, D. F., Brown, R. A., Wichern, W. A., and Fritts, H. W.: Comparison of alveolar and arterial concentrations of ^{85}Kr and ^{133}Xe infused intravenously in man. J. Appl. Physiol., *22:*423–430, 1967.
3582. Rosenberg, E., and MacLean, L. D.: Effect of high oxygen tensions on diffusing capacity for CO and Krogh's K. J. Appl. Physiol., *23:*11–17, 1967.
3583. Rowell, L. B., Taylor, H. L., Wang, Y., and Carlson, W. S.: Saturation of arterial blood with oxygen during maximal exercise. J. Appl. Physiol., *19:*284–286, 1964.
3584. Saltin, B., and Astrand, P.: Maximal oxygen uptake in athletes. J. Appl. Physiol., *23:*353–358, 1967.
3585. Schulte-Hinrichs, D., Vogel, H. R., and Thews, G.: Time course of the Bohr effect. Pflüger. Arch. Ges. Physiol., *301:*302–310, 1968.
3586. Shephard, R. J.: The oxygen cost of breathing during vigorous exercise. Quart. J. Exp. Physiol., *51:*336–350, 1966.
3587. Shephard, R. J.: Physiological determinants of cardiorespiratory fitness. J. Sport. Med., *7:*111–134, 1967.
3588. Smith, T. C., and Rankin, J.: Pulmonary diffusing capacity and the capillary bed during Valsalva and Muller maneuvres. J. Appl. Physiol., *27:*826–833, 1969.
3589. Zechman, F. W., Musgrave, F. S., Mains, R. C., and Cohn, J. E.: Respiratory mechanics and pulmonary diffusing capacity with lower body negative pressure. J. Appl. Physiol., *22:*247–250, 1967.
3590. Steiner, S., Frayser, R., and Ross, J.: Alterations in pulmonary diffsing capacity (D_L) and pulmonary capillary blood volume (V_C) with negative pressure breathing. J. Clin. Invest., *44:*1623–1631, 1965.
3591. Tenney, S. M., and Reese, R. E.: The abiilty to sustain great breathing efforts. Resp. Physiol., *5:*187–201, 1968.
3592. Thews, G., and Vogel, H. R.: Distribution analysis of ventilation/perfusion and O_2 diffusing capacity in lung, through concentration changes for three inspiratory gases. I. Theory. Pflüger. Archiv. Europ. J. Physiol., *303:*195–205, 1968.
3593. Vogel, H. R., and Thews, G.: II. Method. (*See* reference 3592.) Pflüger. Archiv. Europ. J. Physiol., *303:*206–217, 1968.
3594. Vandenbergh, E., Billiet, L., Van de Woestijne, K. P., and Gyselen, A.: Relation between single breath diffusing capacity and arterial blood gases in chronic obstructive lung disease. Scand. J. Resp. Dis., *49:*92–101, 1968.
3595. West, J. B.: Exercise limitations at increased altitudes. Med. Thorac., *24:*333–337, 1967.
3596. Wyndham, C. H., Williams, C. G., von Rahden, M. J. E., Kok, R., Strydom, N. B., and Zwi, S.: Effect on partial pressure of oxygen in arterial blood of exercise up to individual's maximum at medium altitude. Life Sci., *6:*919–924, 1967.
3597. Lefrancois, R., Gautier, H., and Pasquis, P.: Ventilatory oxygen drive in acute and chronic hypoxia. Resp. Physiol., *4:*217–228, 1968.
3598. Brooks, J. G., and Tenney, S. M.: Ventilatory response of llama to hypoxia at sea level and at altitude. Resp. Physiol., *5:*269–278, 1968.
3599. Acosta, I.: The naturall and morall historie of the East and West Indies. London, 1604, p. 550. (Cited by R. H. Kellogg; *see* ref. 3602.)
3600. Hurtado, A.: Animals at high altitudes. *Handbook of Physiology.* Section 4. Adaptation to the Environment. Washington, D.C., American Physiological Society, 1964.
3601. Pugh, L. G. C. E.: Animals at high altitudes. *Handbook of Physiology.* Section 4. Adaptation to the Environment. Washington, D. C., American Physiological Society, 1964.
3602. Kellogg, R. H.: Altitude acclimatization, a historical introduction emphasizing the regulation of breathing. Physiologist, *11:*37–57, 1968.
3603. Hultgren, H. N., and Grover, R. F.: Circulatory adaptation to high altitude. Ann. Rev. Med., *19:*119–152, 1968.
3604. *Effects of Altitude on Physical Performance.* International Symposium, the Athletic Institute, Albuquerque, New Mexico, 1967.
3605. *Exercise at Altitude* (edited by R. Margaria). Excerpta Medica Foundation, Amsterdam, 1967.
3606. Severinghaus, J. W., and Carcelen, B.: Cerebrospinal fluid in man native to high altitude. J. Appl. Physiol., *19:*319–321, 1964.
3607. Lahiri, S.: Alveolar gas pressures in man with life-time hypoxia. Resp. Physiol., *4:*373–386, 1968.
3608. Severinghaus, J. W., Bainton, C. R., and Carcelen, A.: Respiratory sensitivity to hypoxia in chronically hypoxic man. Resp. Physiol., *1:*308–334, 1966.
3609. Milledge, J. S., and Lahiri, S.: Respiratory control in lowlanders and Sherpa highlanders at altitude. Resp. Physiol., *2:*310–322, 1967.
3610. Sorenson, S. C., and Severinghaus, J. W.: Respiratory sensitivity to acute hypoxia in man born at sea level living at altitude. J. Appl. Physiol., *25:*211–216, 1968.
3611. Lahiri, S., Kao, F. F., Velasquez, T., Martinez, C., and

Pezzia, W.: Irreversible blunted sensitivity to hypoxia in high altitude natives. Resp. Physiol., *6:*360–364, 1969.

3612. Sorenson, S. C., and Severinghaus, J. W.: Irreversible insensitivity to acute hypoxia in man born at high altitude. J. Appl. Physiol., *25:*217–220, 1968.
3613. Edelman, N. H., Cherniack, N., Lahiri, S., and Fishman, A. P.: The ventilatory response to hypoxia in cyanotic congenital heart disease. Clin. Res., *16:*369, 1968.
3614. Sorenson, S. C., and Severinghaus, J. W.: Respiratory insensitivity to hypoxia persisting after correction of tetralogy of Fallot. J. Appl. Physiol., *25:*221–223, 1968.
3615. Reynafarje, C.: Humoral control of erythropoiesis at altitude. (*See* reference 3605.)
3616. Lenfant, C., Torrance, J., English, E., Finch, C. A., Reynafarje, C., Ramas, J., and Faura, J.: Effect of altitude on oxygen binding by hemoglobin. J. Clin. Invest., *47:*2652–2656, 1968.
3617. Lenfant, C., Ways, P., Aucutt, C., and Crug, J.: Effect of chronic hypoxia on the O_2 Hb dissociation curve and respiratory gas transport in man. Resp. Physiol., *7:*7–29, 1969.
3618. Staub, N. C.: Site of action of unilateral hypoxia on the pulmonary vascular bed. Amer. Rev. Resp. Dis., *88:*127, 1963.
3619. Arias-Stella, J., and Goldona, M.: The terminal portion of the pulmonary arterial tree in people native to high altitudes. Circulation, *28:*915–925, 1963.
3620. Pugh, L. G. C. E.: Athletes at altitude. J. Physiol., *192:*619–646, 1967.
3621. Haab, P., Held, D. R., Rust, H. E., and Farhi, L. E.: Ventilation-perfusion relationships during high altitude adaptation. J. Appl. Physiol., *26:*77–81, 1969.
3622. Dill, D. B.: Physiological adjustments to altitude changes. J.A.M.A., *205:*123, 1968.
3623. Kollias, J., Buskirk, E. R., Akers, R. F., Prokop, E. R., Baker, P. T., and Picon-Reatagui, E.: Work capacity of long term residents and newcomers to altitude. J. Appl. Physiol., *24:*792–799, 1968.
3624. Lahiri, S., Milledge, J. S., Chattopadhyay, H. P., Bhattacharyya, A. K., and Sinha, A. K.: Respiratory and heart rate of Sherpa highlanders during exercise. J. Appl. Physiol., *23:*545–554, 1967.
3625. Singh, I., Khanna, P. K., Srivastava, M. C., Lal, M., Roy, S. B., and Subramanyam, C. S. V.: Acute mountain sickness. New Engl. J. Med., *280:*175–184, 1969.
3626. Kronenberg, R. S., and Cain, S. M.: Effects of acetazolamide and hypoxia on cerebrospinal fluid bicarbonate. J. Appl. Physiol., *24:*17–20, 1968.
3627. Cain, S. M., and Dunn, J. E., II: Low doses of acetazolamide to aid accommodation of men to altitude. J. Appl. Physiol., *21:*1195–1200, 1966.
3628. Forward, S. A., Landowne, M., Follansbee, J. N., and Hansen, J. E.: Effect of acetazolamide on acute mountain sickness. New Engl. J. Med., *279:*839–845, 1968.
3629. Menon, N. D.: High altitude pulmonary edema. New Engl. J. Med., *273:*66–73, 1965.
3630. Singh, I., Kapila, C. C., Khanna, P. K., Nanda, N. B., and Rao, B. D. P.: High altitude pulmonary edema. Lancet, *1:*229–234, 1965.
3631. Wayne, T. F., Jr., and Severinghaus, J. W.: Experimental hypoxic pulmonary edema in the rat. J. Appl. Physiol., *25:*729–732, 1968.
3632. Hultgren, H. N.: (*See* International symposium reference 3604.)
3633. West, J. B.: Ventilation–perfusion inequality and overall gas exchange in computer models of the lung. Resp. Physiol., *7:*88–110, 1969.
3634. Ward, R. J., Tolas, A. G., Benveniste, R. J., Hansen, J. M., and Bonica, J. J.: Effect of posture on normal arterial blood gas tensions in the aged. Geriatrics, *21:*139–143, 1966.
3635. Leblanc, P., Ruff, F., and Milic-Emili, J.: Effects of age and body position on "airway closure" in man. J. Appl. Physiol., *28:*448–451, 1970.
3636. *Mass Spectrometer Applied to Lung Physiology* (edited by P. Sadoul and J. E. Cotes). Bull. Physiol-Path. Resp., *3:*279–538, 1967.
3637. Severinghaus, J. W.: High temperature operation of oxygen electrode giving fast response for respiratory gas sampling. Clin. Chem., *9:*727–733, 1963.
3638. Elliott, S. E., Segger, F. J., and Osborn, J. J.: A modified oxygen gauge for the rapid measurement of P_{O_2} in respiratory gases. J. Appl. Physiol., *21:*1672–1674, 1966.
3639. Canfield, R. E., and Rahn, H.: Arterial–alveolar N_2 gas pressure differences due to ventilation–perfusion variations. J. Appl. Physiol., *10:*165–172, 1957.
3640. Lenfant, C.: Measurement of ventilation/perfusion distribution with alveolar–arterial differences. J. Appl. Physiol., *18:*1090–1094, 1963.
3641. Lenfant, C.: Measurements of factors impairing gas exchange in man with hyperbaric pressure. J. Appl. Physiol., *19:*189–194, 1964.
3642. Arborelius, M., Jr.: Influence of moderate hypoxia in one lung on the distribution of the pulmonary circulation and ventilation. Scand. J. Clin. Lab. Invest., *17:*257–259, 1965.
3643. King, T. K. C., and Briscoe, W. A.: Bohr integral isopleths in the study of blood gas exchange in the lung. J. Appl. Physiol., *22:*659–674, 1967.
3644. Klocke, F. J., and Rahn, H.: The arterial–alveolar inert gas ("N_2") difference in normal and emphysematous subjects, as indicated by the analysis of urine. J. Clin. Invest., *40:*286–294, 1961.
3645. Briscoe, W. A., and Gurtner, H. P.: The alveolar–urinary N_2 partial pressure difference compared to other measures of the distribution of ventilation and perfusion within the lung. Fed. Proc., *19:*381, 1960.
3646. Cardus, D.: O_2 alveolar–arterial tension difference after 10 days recumbency in man. J. Appl. Physiol., *23:*934–937, 1967.
3647. Lenfant, C.: Time-dependent variations of pulmonary gas exchange in normal man at rest. J. Appl. Physiol., *22:*675–684, 1967.
3648. Benken-Kolmer, H. H., and Kreuzer, F.: Continuous polarographic recording of oxygen pressure in respiratory air. Resp. Physiol., *4:*109–117, 1968.
3649. Koch, G. Alveolar ventilation, diffusing capacity and the A–a P_{O_2} difference in the newborn infant. Resp. Physiol., *4:*168–192, 1968.
3650. Aksnes, E. C.: Determinations of physiological dead space and alveolar–arterial oxygen gradients by the indirect method of Riley and Enghoff. I. Studies on the experimental error of the method and on the variations observed in normal individuals. Scand. J. Clin. Lab. Invest., *14:*443–452, 1962.
3651. Overfield, E. M., and Kylstra, J. A.: Distribution component of alveolar–arterial oxygen pressure difference in man. J. Appl. Physiol., *27:*634–636, 1969.
3652. Bates, D. V.: Measurement of regional ventilation and blood flow distribution. In: *Handbook of Physiology,* Vol. 2, Section 3, pp. 1425–1436, 1965.
3653. Cumming, G., Jones, J. G., and Horsfield, K.: Inhaled argon boluses in man. J. Appl. Physiol., *27:*447–451, 1969.
3654. Klocke, R. A., and Farhi, L. E.: Simple method for determination of perfusion and ventilation perfusion ratio of the underventilated elements (the slow compartment) of the lung. J. Clin. Invest., *43:*2227–2232, 1964.
3655. Farhi, L. E.: Elimination of inert gas by the lung. Resp. Physiol., *3:*1–11, 1967.
3656. Lenfant, C., and Okubo, T.: Distribution function of pulmonary blood flow and ventilation–perfusion ratio in man. J. Appl. Physiol., *24:*668–677, 1968.
3657. Farhi, L. E., and Olszowka, A. J.: Analysis of alveolar gas exchange in the presence of soluble inert gases. Resp. Physiol., *5:*53–67, 1968.
3658. Hartley, L. H., Alexander, J. K., Modelski, M., and Grover, R. F.: Subnormal cardiac output at rest and during exercise in residents at 3,100 m. altitude. J. Appl. Physiol., *23:*839–848, 1967.
3659. Alexander, J. K., Hartley, L. H., Modelski, M., and Grover, R. F.: Reduction of stroke volume during exercise in man following ascent to 3,100 m. altitude. J. Appl. Physiol., *23:*849–858, 1967.

3660. *International Symposium on the Cardiovascular and Respiratory Effects of Hypoxia.* Basel, Switzerland, S. Karger, 1966, p. 406.
3661. Berggren, S. M.: The oxygen deficit of arterial blood caused by nonventilating parts of the lung. Acta Physiol. Scand., *4:* Suppl. 11, 1942.
3662. Bartels, H. E., Bucherl, M., Mochizuki, M., and Niemann, G.: Bestimmung der via venae thebesii in der linken Ventrikel fliessenden Blutmenge durch Messung des O_2 Druckes im Blut des linken Vorhofs und einer Arterie beim Menschen. Pflüger. Arch. Ges. Physiol., *262:*478–483, 1956.
3663. Bjork, V. O., Malmstrom, G., and Uggla, L. G.: Comparison of the oxygen tension in blood from the left atrium and a systemic artery. Amer. Heart J., *48:*8–12, 1954.
3664. Jose, A. D., and Milnor, W. R.: The demonstration of pulmonary arteriovenous shunts in normal human subjects, and their increase in certain disease states. J. Clin. Invest., *38:*1915–1923.
3665. Calabresi, P., and Abelmann, W. H.: Porto-caval and porto-pulmonary anastomosis in Laennec's cirrhosis and in heart failure. J. Clin. Invest., *36:*1257–1265, 1957.
3666. Shaldon, S., Caesar, J., Chiandussi, L., Williams, H. S., Sheville, E., and Sherlock, S.: Demonstration of porto-pulmonary anastomosis in portal cirrhosis with the use of radioactive krypton (Kr^{85}). New Engl. J. Med., *265:*410–414, 1961.
3667. Lassen, N. A., Mellemgaard, K., and Georg, J.: Tritium used for estimation of right-to-left shunts. J. Appl. Physiol., *16:*321–325, 1961.
3668. Mellemgaard, K., Lassen, N. A., and Georg, J.: Right-to-left shunt in normal man determined by the use of tritium and krypton.[85] J. Appl. Physiol., *17:*778–782, 1962.
3669. Georg, J., Hornum, I., and Mellemgaard, K.: The mechanism of hypoxaemia after laparotomy. Thorax, *22:*382–386, 1967.
3670. Oxygen pressure recording in gases, fluids, and tissues. (edited by F. Kreuzer). *Progress in Respiration Research.* Basel and New York, S. Karger, 1969.
3671. Kabe, J., and Beaudry, P. H.: A manometric determination of nitrogen in small samples of blood. Application to measurement of arterial–alveolar nitrogen difference in man. Canad. J. Physiol. Pharmacol., *46:*795–801, 1968.
3672. Sodal, I. E., Bowman, R. R., and Filley, G. F.: A fast-response oxygen analyser with high accuracy for respiratory gas measurement. J. Appl. Physiol., *25:*181–183, 1968.
3673. Bragg, Sir Lawrence: The white-coated worker. Punch, *225:*352–354, 1968.
3674. Downes, J. J., Wood, D. W., Striker, T. W., and Pittman, J. C.: Arterial blood gas and acid-base disorders in infants and children with status asthmaticus. Pediatrics, *42:*238–249, 1968.
3675. McFadden, E. R., Jr., and Lyons, H. A.: Airway resistance and uneven ventilation in bronchial asthma. J. Appl. Physiol., *25:*365–370, 1968.
3676. Davies, S. E.: Effect of disodium cromoglycate on exercise-induced asthma. Brit. Med. J., *3:*593–594, 1968.
3677. Cheney, F. W., Jr., and Butler, J.: The effects of ultrasonically produced aerosols on airway resistance in man. Anesthesiology, *29:*1099–1106, 1968.
3678. Stanescu, D. C., and Teculescu, D. B.: Effect of acetylcholine aerosols on diffusing capacity in asthmatic and normal subjects. J. Appl. Physiol., *26:*197–202, 1969.
3679. Gregg, I., and Batten, J.: Sudden death in a young asthmatic. Brit. Med. J., *1:*29–30, 1969.
3680. Hsieh, Y-C., Frayser, R., and Ross, J. C.: The effect of cold air inhalation on ventilation in normal subjects and in patients with chronic obstructive pulmonary disease. Amer. Rev. Resp. Dis., *98:*613–622, 1968.
3681. Dunnill, M. S., Massarella, G. R., and Anderson, J. A.: A comparison of the quantitative anatomy of the bronchi in normal subjects, in status asthmaticus, in chronic bronchitis, and in emphysema. Thorax, *24:*176–179, 1969.
3682. Ishikawa, S., Bowden, D. H., Fisher, V., and Wyatt, J. P.: The emphysema profile in two midwestern cities in North America. Arch. Environ. Health, *18:*660–666, 1969.
3683. Ekstam, G., Kiviloog, J., and Ostling, E.: α_1-antitrypsin deficiency and chronic pulmonary disease. Scand. J. Resp. Dis., *49:*311–321, 1968.
3684. Guenter, C. A., Welch, M. H., Russell, T. R., Hyde, R. M., and Hammarsten, J. F.: The pattern of lung disease associated with $alpha_1$ antitrypsin deficiency. Arch. Intern. Med., *122:*254–257, 1968.
3685. Schleusener, A., Talamo, R. C., Paré, J. A. P., and Thurlbeck, W. M.: Familial emphysema. Amer. Rev. Resp. Dis., *98:*692–696, 1968.
3686. Otto, H., Orell, S. R., and Guettich, R.: Comparative studies on the epidemiology of pulmonary emphysema. Prax. Pneumol., *22:*481–487, 1968.
3687. Pecora, L. J., Bernstein, I. L., and Feldman, D. P.: Comparison of the components of diffusing capacity utilizing the effective alveolar volume in patients with emphysema and chronic asthma. Amer. J. Med. Sci., *256:*69–80, 1968.
3688. Fraser, R. G., and Paré, J. A. P.: *Diagnosis of Diseases of the Chest.* 2 vols. Philadelphia, W. B. Saunders Co., 1970, p. 1388.
3689. Pride, N. B., Hugh-Jones, P., O'Brien, E. N., and Smith, L. A.: Changes in lung function following the surgical treatment of bullous emphysema. Quart. J. Med., *39:*49–69, 1970.
3690. Wentworth, P., Gough, J., and Wentworth, J. E.: Pulmonary changes and cor pulmonale in mucoviscidosis. Thorax, *23:*582–589, 1968.
3691. Esterly, J. R., and Oppenheimer, E. H.: Cystic fibrosis of the pancreas: structural changes in the peripheral airways. Thorax, *23:*670–675, 1968.
3692. di Sant'Agnese, P. A., and Talamo, R. C.: Pathogenesis and physiopathology of cystic fibrosis of the pancreas. New Engl. J. Med., *277:*1287–1294, 1344–1352, 1399–1408, 1967.
3693. Andersen, D. H.: Pathology of cystic fibrosis. Ann. N.Y. Acad. Sci., *93:*500–517, 1962.
3694. Bodian, M.: Fibrocystic disease of the pancreas: a congenital disorder of mucous production. London, Heinemann & Co., 1952, p. 244.
3695. Goldring, R. M., Fishman, A. P., Turino, G. M., Cohen, H. I., Denning, C. R., and Anderson, D. H.: Pulmonary hypertension and cor pulmonale in cystic fibrosis of the pancreas. J. Pediat., *65:*501–524, 1964.
3696. Bowden, D. H., Fisher, V. W., and Wyatt, J. P.: Cor pulmonale in cystic fibrosis: morphometric analysis. Amer. J. Med., *38:*226–232, 1965.
3697. Huang, N. H., Van Loon, E. L., and Sheng, K. T.: The flora of the respiratory tract of patients with cystic fibrosis of the pancreas. J. Pediat., *59:*512–521, 1959.
3698. Matthews, L. W., and Doershuk, C. F.: Measurements of pulmonary function in cystic fibrosis. Bibl. Paediat., *86:*237–246, 1967.
3699. Beier, F. R., Renzetti, A. D., Jr., Mitchell, M., and Watanabe, S.: Pulmonary pathophysiology in cystic fibrosis. Amer. Rev. Resp. Dis., *94:*430–440, 1966.
3700. De Muth, C. R., Howatt, W. F., and Talner, W. S.: Intrapulmonary gas distribution in cystic fibrosis. Amer. J. Dis. Child., *103:*129–135, 1962.
3701. West, J. R., and di Sant'Agnese, P. A.: Studies of pulmonary function in cystic fibrosis of the pancreas. Amer. J. Dis. Child, *86:*496, 1953.
3702. Wise, M. B., and Beaudry, P. H.: Blood gas studies in the evaluation of children with cystic fibrosis. Proc. XII International Congress of Pediatrics. Mexico City, Mexico, December, *Vol. III:* 464, 1968.
3703. Waring, W. W.: Ventilation-blood flow relationship in the lungs of children. Amer. Rev. Resp. Dis., *91:*77–85, 1965.
3704. Beaudry, P. H., Wise, M. B., and Kabe, J.: Obstructive airway impairment and ventilation–perfusion disturbances in children with cystic fibrosis. Cystic Fibrosis Conference, Atlantic City, 1960, p. 26.
3705. Moss, A. J., Harper, W. H., Dooley, R. R., Murray, J. F., and Mack, J. F.: Cor pulmonale in cystic fibrosis of the pancreas. J. Pediat., *67:*797–807, 1965.
3706. Kelminson, L. L., Cotton, E. K., and Vogel, J. H. K.: Reversibility of pulmonary hypertension in patients with cystic fibrosis; observations on effects of tolazoline hydrochloride. Pediatrics, *39:*24–35, 1967.
3707. Symchych, P. A., and Blanc, W. A.: Morphometry of the

pulmonary arterial tree in cor pulmonale in cystic fibrosis. Cystic Fibrosis Conference, Atlantic City, 1967, p. 33.

3708. Doerschuk, C. P., Tucker, A. S., Spector, S., and Matthews, L. W.: Pulmonary function and clinical evaluation of a prophylactic approach to therapy of cystic fibrosis. J. Pediat., *65:*1112–1114, 1964.

3709. Wolfsdorf, J., Swift, D. L., and Avery, M. E.: Mist therapy reconsidered; an evaluation of the respiratory deposition of labelled water aerosols produced by jet and ultrasonic nebulizers. Pediat., *43:*799–808, 1969.

3710. Chisholm, J. C., Cherniack, N. S., and Carton, R. W.: Results of pulmonary function testing in five persons with Marfan syndrome. J. Lab. Clin. Med., *71:*25–28, 1968.

3711. Bachofen, H., and Scherrer, M.: Lung tissue resistance in diffuse interstitial pulmonary fibrosis. J. Clin. Invest., *46:*133–140, 1967.

3712. Graham, J. R.: Cardiac and pulmonary fibrosis during methysergide therapy for headache. Amer. J. Med. Sci., *254:*1–12, 1967.

3713. Cruz, E., Rodriguez, J., Lisboa, C., and Ferretti, R.: Desquamative alveolar disease (desquamative interstitial pneumonia); case report. Thorax, *24:*186–191, 1969.

3714. Shortland, J. R., Darke, C. S., and Crane, W. A. J.: Electron microscopy of desquamative interstitial pneumonia. Thorax, *24:*192–208, 1969.

3715. Pimentel, J. C., and Marques, F.: "Vineyard Sprayer's Lung": a new occupational disease. Thorax, *24:*678–688, 1969.

3716. Godfrey, S., Bluestone, R., and Higgs, B. E.: Lung function and the response to exercise in systemic sclerosis. Thorax, *24:*427–434, 1969.

3717. Glaister, D. H.: The effect of posture on the distribution of ventilation and blood flow in the normal lung. Clin. Sci., *33:*391–398, 1967.

3718. Power, G. G.: Gaseous diffusion between airways and alveoli in the human lung. J. Appl. Physiol., *27:*701–709, 1969.

3719. Bates, D. V.: *The Other Lung.* (Editorial.) New Engl. J. Med., *282:*277, 1970.

3720. Vadas, G., Paré, J. A. P., and Thurlbeck, W. M.: Pulmonary and lymph node myomatosis. Canad. Med. Assoc. J., *96:*420–424, 1967.

3721. Maier, A., and Orion, B.: Pneumonie interstitielle desquamative. Poumon Coeur, *24:*1171–1183, 1968.

3722. Turiaf, J., Basset, G., and Georges, R.: Prognosis of patients who have been cured of pulmonary sarcoidosis, from functional respiratory exploration data. Poumon Coeur, *25:*1–15, 1969.

3723. Swaye, P., Van Ordstrand, H. S., McCormoack, L. J., and Wolpaw, S. E.: Familial Hamman-Rich syndrome. Report of eight cases. Dis. Chest, *55:*7–12, 1969.

3724. Mithoefer, J. C., Bossman, O. G., Thibeault, D. W., and Mead, G. D.: The clinical estimation of alveolar ventilation. Amer. Rev. Resp. Dis., *98:*868–871, 1968.

3725. Tanpaichitr, V., and Sukulmalchantra, Y., Tongmitr, V., and Jumbala, B.: Primary alveolar hypoventilation. A case report with hemodynamic study. Amer. Rev. Resp. Dis., *98:*1037–1043, 1968.

3726. Hiroka, M., Inaba, Y., and Ohno, T.: The Pickwickian syndrome in a child. Tohoku J. Exp. Med., *98:*363–372, 1969.

3727. Doll, E., Kuhlo, W., Steim, H., and Keul, J.: The genesis of cor pulmonale in the Pickwick syndrome. Deutsch Med. Wschr., *93:*2361–2365, 1968.

3728. Obrecht, H. G., Scherrer, M., and Gurtner, H. P.: Pulmonary gas exchange in the primary vascular form of cor pulmonale. Schweiz. Med. Wschr., *98:*1999–2007, 1968.

3729. Gazetopoulos, N., and Davies, H.: Ventilatory response to exercise in patients with left to right shunts. Brit. Heart J., *28:*590–598, 1966.

3730. Valentine, P. A., Fluck, D. C., Mounsey, J. P. D., Reid, D., Shillingford, J. P., and Steiner, R. E.: Blood-gas changes after acute myocardial infarction. Lancet, *2:*837–841, 1966.

3731. Davies, H., and Gazetopoulos, N.: Lung function in patients with left to right shunts. Brit. Heart J., *29:*317–326, 1967.

3732. Mürtz, R.: Effect of low O_2 pressure on respiration in chronic hypoxaemia. Z. Ges. Exp. Med., *139:*58–69, 1965.

3733. Gianelli, S., Jr., Ayres, S. M., and Buehler, M. E.: Effect of pulmonary blood flow upon lung mechanics. J. Clin. Invest., *46:*1625–1642, 1967.

3734. Giuntini, C., Maseri, A., and Bianchi, R.: Pulmonary vascular distensibility and lung compliance as modified by dextran infusion and subsequent atropine injection in normal subjects. J. Clin. Invest., *45:*1770–1790, 1966.

3735. Tammeling, G. J., Nieveen, J., and Sluiter, H. J.: Studies on anomalous collateral systemic-pulmonary circulation. Circulation, *35:*457–470, 1967.

3736. Plum, F., and Brown, H. W.: Hypoxic-hypercapnic interaction in subjects with bilateral cerebral dysfunction. J. Appl. Physiol., *18:*1135–1145, 1963.

3737. Hunziker, A., Frick, P., Regli, F., and Rossier, P. H.: Chronic alveolar hypoventilation of central origin due to thrombosis of the posterior inferior cerebellar artery (Wallenberg's syndrome). Deutsch Med. Wschr., *89:*676–680, 1964.

3738. Sobol, B. J., and Weinheimer, B.: Assessment of ventilatory abnormality in the asymptomatic subject: an exercise in futility. Thorax, *21:*445–449, 1966.

3739. Weiss, W.: Validation of a screening procedure for chronic nonspecific respiratory disease. Arch. Environ. Health, *16:*844–852, 1968.

3740. Sluis-Cremer, G. K., and Sichel, H. S.: Ventilatory function in males in a Witwatersrand town. Amer. Rev. Resp. Dis, *98:*229–239, 1968.

3741. Dempsey, J. A., Redden, W., Rankin, J., and Balke, B.: Alveolar–arterial gas exchange during muscular work in obesity. J. Appl. Physiol., *21:*1807–1814, 1966.

3742. Barrera, F., Reidenberg, M. M., and Winters, W. L.: Pulmonary function in the obese patient. Amer. J. Med. Sci., *254:*785–796, 1967.

3743. Sharp, J. T., Henry, J. P., Sweany, S. K., Meadows, W. R., and Pietras, R. J.: Inertance and its gas and tissue components in normal and obese men. J. Clin. Invest., *43:*503–510, 1964.

3744. Sharp, J. T., Henry, J. P., Sweany, S. K., Meadows, W. R., and Pietras, R. J.: The total work of breathing in obese men. J. Clin. Invest, *43:*728–739, 1964.

3745. Sharp, J. T., Henry, J. P., Sweany, S. K., Meadows, W. R., and Pietras, R. J.: Effects of mass loading the respiratory system in man. J. Appl. Physiol., *19:*959–966, 1964.

3746. Couture, J., Picken, J., Trop, D., Ruff, F., Lousada, N., Housley, E., and Bates, D. V.: Airway closure in normal, obese, and anesthetized supine subjects. Fed. Proc., *29:*269(Abs.), 1970.

3747. Barrera, F., Reidenberg, M. M., Winters, W. L., and Hungspreugs, S.: Ventilation perfusion relationships in the obese patient. J. Appl. Physiol., *26:*420–426, 1969.

3748. Milic-Emili, J., and Tyler, J. M.: Relation between work output of the respiratory muscles and end-tidal CO_2 tension. J. Appl. Physiol., *18:*497–504, 1963.

3749. Cherniack, R. M.: Work of breathing and the ventilatory response to CO_2. In: *Handbook of Physiology,* Volume 2, Section 3: Respiration. Washington, D.C., American Physiological Society, p. 1469.

3750. Brendenberg, C. E., James, P. M., Collins, J., Anderson, R. W., Martin, A. M., Jr., and Hardaway, R. M.: Respiratory failure in shock. Ann. Surg., *169:*392–403, 1969.

3751. Collins, J. A.: The causes of progressive pulmonary insufficiency in surgical patients. J. Surg. Res., *9:*685–704, 1969.

3752. Stern, L., Ramos, A. D., Outerbridge, E. W., and Beaudry, P. H.: Negative pressure artificial respiration: use in treatment of respiratory failure of the newborn. Canad. Med. Assoc. J., *102:*595–601, 1970.

3753. *Uses and Dangers of Oxygen Therapy.* Scottish Health Services Council. Her Majesty's Stationery Office, 13A Castle Street, Edinburgh, 1969.

3754. Flenley, D. C.: Respiratory failure. Scot. Med. J., *15:*61–72, 1970.

3755. Bedon, G. A., Block, A. J., and Ball, W. C., Jr.: The "28%" venturi mask in obstructive airway disease. Arch. Intern. Med., *125:*106–113, 1970.

3756. Schaffner, F., Felig, P., and Trachtenberg, E.: Structure of

rat lung after protracted oxygen breathing. Arch. Path., *83*:99–107, 1967.
3757. Kistler, G. S., Caldwell, P. R. B., and Weibel, E. R.: Development of fine structural damage to alveolar and capillary lining cells in oxygen-poisoned rats. J. Cell. Biol., *32*:605–628, 1967.
3758. Caldwell, P. R. B., Lee, W. L., Jr., Schildkraut, H. S., and Archibald, E. R.: Changes in lung volume, diffusing capacity, and blood gases in men breathing oxygen. J. Appl. Physiol., *21*:1477–1483, 1966.
3759. Fisher, A. B., Hyde, R. W., Puy, R. J. M., Clark, J. M., and Lambertsen, C. J.: Effect of oxygen at 2 atmospheres on pulmonary mechanics of normal man. J. Appl. Physiol., *24*:529–536, 1968.
3760. Catterall, M., Kazantzis, G., and Hodges, M.: The performance of nasal catheters and a face mask in oxygen therapy. Lancet, *1*:415–417, 1967.
3761. McLelland, R. M. A.: Complications of tracheostomy. Brit. Med. J., *2*:567–569, 1965.
3762. Luft, U. C., and Finkelstein, S.: Hypoxia: a clinical-physiological approach. Aerospace Med., *39*:105–110, 1968.
3763. *Leading Article: Endotracheal intubation or tracheostomy?* Lancet, *1*:258–259, 1967.
3764. Brewis, R. A. L.: Oxygen toxicity during artificial ventilation. Thorax, *24*:656–666, 1969.
3765. Nunn, J. F.: Influence of age and other factors on hypoxaemia in the postoperative period. Lancet, *2*:466–468, 1965.
3766. Adams, E. B., Holloway, R., Thambiran, A. K., and Desai, S. D.: Usefulness of intermittent positive-pressure respiration in the treatment of tetanus. Lancet, *2*:1176–1180, 1966.
3767. Downes, J. J., Kemp, R. A., and Lambertsen, C. J.: The magnitude and duration of respiratory depression due to Fentanyl and Mepiridine in man. J. Pharmacol. Exp. Ther., *158*:416–419, 1967.
3768. Shepard, F. M., Johnston, R. B., Jr., Klatte, E. G., Burko, H., and Stahlman, M.: Residual pulmonary findings in clinical hyaline membrane disease. New Engl. J. Med., *279*:1063–1071, 1968.
3769. Lewis, S.: A follow-up study of the respiratory distress syndrome. Proc. Roy. Soc. Med., *61*:771–773, 1968.
3770. Colgan, F. J., and Whang, T. B.: Anesthesia and atelectasis. Anesthesiology, *29*:917–922, 1968.
3771. Cross, C. E., Packer, B. S., Altman, M., Gee, J. B. L., Murdaugh, H. V., and Robin, E. D.: Determination of total body exchangeable O_2 stores. J. Clin. Invest., *47*:2402–2410, 1968.
3772. Ambiavagar, M., Robinson, J. S., Morrison, I. M., and Jones, E. S.: Intermittent positive pressure ventilation in the treatment of severe crushing injuries of the chest. Thorax, *21*:359–366, 1966.
3773. Finley, T. N.: Anesthesia and atelectasis. Anesthesiology, *29*:863–864, 1968.
3774. Moore, F. D., Lyons, J. H., Pierce, E. C., Morgan, A. P., Drinker, P. A., MacArthur, J. D., and Dammin, G. J.: *Post-Traumatic Pulmonary Insufficiency*. Philadelphia, W. B. Saunders Co., 1969, p. 234.
3775. Berlyne, G. M., Lee, H. A., Ralston, A. J., and Woolcock, J. A.: Pulmonary complications of peritoneal dialysis. Lancet, *2*:75–78, 1966.
3776. Nahas, R. A., Melrose, D. G., Sykes, M. K., and Robinson, B.: Post-perfusion lung syndrome. Lancet, *2*:251–254, 254–256, 1965.
3777. Gibson, D. G.: Hemodynamic factors in the development of acute pulmonary oedema in renal failure. Lancet, *2*:1217–1220, 1966.
3778. Slapak, M., Lee, H. M., and Hume, D. M.: Transplant lung—a new syndrome. Brit. Med. J., *1*:80–83, 1968.
3779. Rotheram, E. B., Safar, P., and Robin, E. D.: CNS Disorder during mechanical ventilation in chronic pulmonary disease. J.A.M.A., *189*:993–996, 1964.
3780. Harris, R. S., and Lawson, T. V.: The relative mechanical effectiveness and efficiency of successive voluntary coughs in healthy young adults. Clin. Sci., *34*:569–577, 1968.
3781. Bethune, D. W., and Collis, J. M.: An evaluation of oxygen therapy equipment. Thorax, *22*:221–225, 1967.
3782. Noble, M. I. M., Trenchard, D., and Guz, A.: The value of diuretics in respiratory failure. Lancet, *2*:257–260, 1966.
3783. Sukumalchantra, Y., Dinakara, P., and Williams, M. H., Jr.: Prognosis of patients with chronic obstructive pulmonary disease after hospitalization for acute ventilatory failure: a three year follow up study. Amer. Rev. Resp. Dis., *93*:215–222, 1966.
3784. Jessen, O., Kristensen, H. S., and Rasmussen, K.: Tracheostomy and artificial ventilation in chronic lung disease. Lancet, *2*:9–12, 1967.
3785. Edwards, G., and Leszczynski, S. O.: A double-blind trial of five respiratory stimulants in patients with acute ventilatory failure. Lancet, *2*:226–229, 1967.
3786. Tisi, G. M., Twigg, H. L., and Moser, K. M.: Collapse of left lung induced by artificial airway. Lancet, *1*:791–793, 1968.
3787. Therapy of acute respiratory failure: A statement by the committee on therapy of the American Thoracic Society. Amer. Rev. Resp. Dis., *93*:475–480, 1966.
3788. Bendixen, H. H., Egbert, L. D., Hedley-White, J., Laver, M. B., and Pontoppidan, H.: *Respiratory Care*. St. Louis, C. V. Mosby Co., 1965, p. 252.
3789. Addington, W. W., Kettel, L. J., and Cugell, D. W.: Alkalosis due to mechanical hyperventilation in patients with chronic hypercapnia. Amer. Rev. Resp. Dis., *93*:736–741, 1966.
3790. Addis, G. J.: Bicarbonate buffering in acute exacerbation of chronic respiratory failure. Thorax, *20*:337–340, 1965.
3791. Campbell, E. J. M.: The J. Burns Amberson Lecture. The management of acute respiratory failure in chronic bronchitis and emphysema. Amer. Rev. Resp. Dis., *96*:626–639, 1967.
3792. Campbell, E. J. M., and Gebbie, T.: Masks and tent for providing controlled oxygen concentrations. Lancet, *1*:468–469, 1966.
3793. Cherniack, R. M., and Young, G.: An evaluation of ethamivan as a respiratory stimulant in barbiturate intoxication, and alveolar hypoventilation in emphysema and obesity. Ann. Intern. Med., *60*:631–640, 1964.
3794. Clarke, D. B.: Tracheostomy in a thoracic surgical unit. Thorax, *20*:87–92, 1965.
3795. Auchincloss, J. H., Gilbert, R., and Mullison, E.: A new self inflating tracheostomy cuff of silicone rubber for use in patients requiring mechanical aid to ventilation. Amer. Rev. Resp. Dis., *97*:706–709, 1968.
3796. Reid, D. H. S., Tunstall, M. E., and Mitchell, R. G.: A controlled trial of artificial respiration in the respiratory distress syndrome of the newborn. Lancet, *1*:532–533, 1967.
3797. Bowden, D. H., Adamson, I. Y. R., and Wyatt, J. P.: Reaction of lung cells to high concentrations of oxygen. Arch. Path., *86*:671–675, 1968.
3798. Palmer, K. N. V., and Diament, M. L.: Postoperative changes in gas tensions of arterial blood and in ventilatory function. Lancet, *2*:180–182, 1966.
3799. Mithoefer, J. C., Mead, G., Hughes, J. M. B., Iliff, L. D., and Campbell, E. J. M.: A method of distinguishing death due to cardiac arrest from asphyxia. Lancet, *2*:654–656, 1967.
3800. Whitehouse, A. C., and Petty, T. L.: Recovery in Landry Guillain Barré syndrome after prolonged respiratory support. Lancet, *1*:1029–1030, 1969.
3801. Grillo, H. C.: The management of tracheal stenosis following assisted respiration. J. Thorac. Cardiov. Surg., *57*:52–71, 1969.
3802. Cullen, J. H., and Kaemmerlen, J. T.: Acute ventilatory failure in chronic obstructive lung disease. Amer. Rev. Resp. Dis., *98*:998–1002, 1968.
3803. Reynolds, E. O. R., Roberton, N. R. C., and Wigglesworth, J. S.: Hyaline membrane disease, respiratory distress and surfactant deficiency. Pediatrics, *42*:758–768, 1968.
3804. Shook, C. D., MacMillan, B. G., and Altemeier, W. A.: Pulmonary complications of the burn patient. Arch. Surg., *97*:215–224, 1968.
3805. Palamarchuk, U. P.: Atelectasis of the lungs in the burned. Vestn. Rentgen. Radiol., *43*:3–9, 1968.

3806. Border, J. R., Tibbetts, J. C., and Schenk, W. G., Jr.: Hypoxic hyperventilation and acute respiratory failure in the severely stressed patient: massive pulmonary arteriovenous shunts? Surgery, *64:*710–719, 1968.

3807. Avery, M. E.: *The Lung and Its Disorders in the Newborn Infant.* 2nd Ed. Philadelphia, W. B. Saunders Co., 1968.

3808. Usher, R., McLean, F., and Maughan, G. B.: Respiratory distress syndrome in infants delivered by cesarian section. Amer. J. Obstet. Gynec., *88:*806–815, 1964.

3809. Strang, L. B., Anderson, G. S., and Platt, J. W.: Neonatal death and elective cesarean section. Lancet, *1:*954–956, 1957.

3810. Rudolph, A. M., and Yuan, S.: Response of the pulmonary vasculature to hypoxemia and H+ ion concentration changes. J. Clin. Invest., *45:*399–411, 1966.

3811. Chu, J., Clements, J. A., Cotton, E. K., Klaus, M. H., Sweet, A. Y., and Tooley, W. H.: Neonatal pulmonary ischaemia. Pediatrics, (Supplement) *40:*709–782, 1967.

3812. Lieberman, J.: Clinical syndromes associated with deficient lung fibrinolytic activity. New Engl. J. Med., *260:*619–626, 1959.

3813. Clements, J. A.: Surface phenomena in relation to pulmonary function. Physiologist, *5:*11–28, 1962.

3814. Karlberg, P., Cook, C. D., O'Brien, D., Cherry, R. B., and Smith, C. A.: Studies of respiratory physiology in the newborn infant: observations during and after respiratory distress. Acta Paediat., *43:*397–411, 1954.

3815. Stahlman, M.: Management of respiratory failure in the newborn infant. (Discussion.) Pediat. Res., *2:*400, 1968.

3816. Delivoria-Papadopoulos, M., and Swyer, P. R.: Assisted ventilation in terminal hyaline membrane disease. Arch. Dis. Child., *39:*481–484, 1964.

3817. Stahlman, M. T., Young, W. C., Gray, J., and Shepard, F. M.: The management of respiratory failure in the idiopathic respiratory distress syndrome of prematurity. Ann. N.Y. Acad. Sci., *121:*930–941, 1965.

3818. Silverman, W. A., Sinclair, J. C., Gaudy, G. M., Finster, M., Bauman, W. A., and Agate, F. J.: A controlled trial of management of respiratory distress syndrome in a body-enclosing respirator. Pediatrics, *39:*740–748, 1967.

3819. Bell, A. G.: A vacuum jacket. Bein Bhreagh Recorder, vol. 4, 1910. (Quoted in reference 3752.)

3820. Gross, N. J., and Hamilton, J. D.: Correlation between the physical signs of hypercapnia and the mixed venous P_{CO_2}. Brit. Med. J., *2:*1096–1097, 1963.

3821. Guz, A., Noble, M. I. M., Trenchard, D., Cochrane, H. L., and Makey, A. R.: Studies on the vagus nerves in man: their role in respiratory and circulatory control. Clin. Sci., *27:*293–304, 1964.

3822. Guz, A., Noble, M. I. M., Widdicombe, J. G., Trenchard, D., Mushin, W. W., and Makey, A. R.: The role of vagal and glossopharyngeal afferent nerves in respiratory sensation, control of breathing, and arterial pressure regulation in conscious man. Clin. Sci., *30:*161–170, 1966.

3823. Campbell, E. J. M., Freedman, S., Clark, T. J. H., Robson, J. G., and Norman, J.: The effect of muscular paralysis induced by tubocurarine on the duration and sensation of breath-holding. Clin. Sci., *32:*425–432, 1967.

3824. Eisele, J., Trenchard, D., Burki, N., and Guz, A.: The effect of chest wall block on respiratory sensation and control in man. Clin. Sci., *35:*23–33, 1968.

3825. Nunn, J. F.: Applied Respiratory Physiology with Special Reference to Anesthesia. London, Buttenwatts, 1969.

3826. Gilson, Albert J., and Smoak, William M.: Pulmonary Investigation with Radionuclides. Springfield, Illinois, Charles C Thomas, 1970, p. 371.

3827. Anthonisen, N. R., Bass, H., and Heckscher, T.: ^{133}Xe studies of patients after pneumonectomy. Scand. J. Resp. Dis., *49:*81–91, 1968.

3828. Astrand, P-O., and Rodahl, K.: Textbook of Work Physiology. Toronto, McGraw-Hill, 1970, p. 669.

3829. Breathing: Hering-Breuer Centenary Symposium. Ciba Foundation Symposium. Edited by Ruth Porter. London, J & A Churchill, 1970, p. 402.

3830. Bates, D. V., Bell, G., Burnham, C., Hazucha, M., Mantha, J., Pengelly, L. D., and Silverman, F.: Problems in studies of human exposure to air pollutants. Canad. Med. Assoc. J., *103:*833–837, 1970.

3831. Mosher, J. C., Macbeth, W. G., Leonard, M. J., Mullins, T. P., and Brunelle, M. F.: The distribution of contaminants in the Los Angeles Basin resulting from atmospheric reactions and transport. J. Air Pollution Control Assoc., *20:*35–42, 1970.

3832. Wang, N-S., and Thurlbeck, W. M.: Scanning electron microscopy of the lung. Human Path., *1:*227–231, 1970.

3833. Macklem, P. T.: Airway obstruction and collateral ventilation. Physiol. Rev. *In Press.*

3834. Naimark, A., DuGard, A., and Rangno, R. E.: Regional pulmonary blood flow and gas exchange in hemorrhagic shock. J. Appl. Physiol., *25:*301–309, 1968.

Index of First Authors of Cited Literature

C

G

I

J

K

L

M

Q

R

S

T

U

V

W

Y

Z

Subject Index

See the first page of each chapter for main headings of subjects, and see specific measurement for values in separate disease entities.